www.harcourt-international.com

Bringing you products from all Harcourt Health Sciences companies including Baillière Tindall, Churchill Livingstone, Mosby and W.B. Saunders

- ▶ **Browse** for latest information on new books, journals and electronic products

- ▶ **Search** for information on over 20 000 published titles with full product information including tables of contents and sample chapters

- ▶ **Keep up to date** with our extensive publishing programme in your field by registering with eAlert or requesting postal updates

- ▶ **Secure online ordering** with prompt delivery, as well as full contact details to order by phone, fax or post

- ▶ **News** of special features and promotions

If you are based in the following countries, please visit the country-specific site to receive full details of product availability and local ordering information

USA: www.harcourthealth.com

Canada: www.harcourtcanada.com

Australia: www.harcourt.com.au

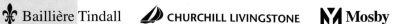 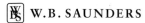
Baillière Tindall   CHURCHILL LIVINGSTONE   Mosby   W.B. SAUNDERS

Children's Orthopaedics and Fractures

Second Edition

Commissioning Editor: Deborah Russell
Project Development Manager: Paul Fam
Project Manager: Hilary Hewitt

Children's Orthopaedics and Fractures

Second Edition

Edited by

Michael KD Benson MBBS, FRCS

Consultant Orthopaedic Surgeon, Nuffield Orthopaedic Centre, Oxford, UK

John A Fixsen MChir, FRCS

Honorary Consultant Orthopaedic Surgeon, Great Ormond Street Hospital for Sick Children, Great Ormond Street, London, UK

Malcolm F Macnicol BSc(Hons), MCh, FRCS, FRCP, FRCSEd(Orth), Dip. Sports Med.

Consultant Orthopaedic Surgeon, Royal Hospital for Sick Children and Princess Margaret Rose Orthopaedic Hospital, Edinburgh, UK

Klaus Parsch MD

Professor, Department of Orthopaedic Surgery, Pediatric Centre, Olgahospital, Stuttgart, Germany

Reference

WE168
BEN

H0305044

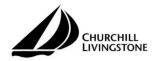

CHURCHILL LIVINGSTONE

London • Edinburgh • New York • Philadelphia • St Louis • Sydney • Toronto 2002

CHURCHILL LIVINGSTONE
An imprint of Harcourt Publishers Limited

First edition published 1994
Second edition published 2002

ISBN 0 443 06459 8

British Library Cataloguing in Publication Data
A catalogue record for this book is available from the British Library

Library of Congress Cataloging in Publication Data
A catalog record for this book is available from the Library of Congress

Note
Medical knowledge is constantly changing. As new information becomes available, changes in treatment, procedures, equipment and the use of drugs become necessary. The editors, authors, contributors and the publishers have taken care to ensure that the information given in this text is accurate and up to date. However, readers are strongly advised to confirm that the information, especially with regard to drug usage, complies with the latest legislation and standards of practice.

Existing UK nomenclature is changing to the system of Recommended International Nonproprietary Names (rINNs). Until the UK names are no longer in use, these more familiar names are used in this book in preference to rINNs, details of which may be obtained from the British National Formulary.

Typeset by Phoenix Photosetting, Chatham, Kent
Printed in China

Contents

Contributors   ix
Preface   xv
Foreword   xiii
E. E. Bleck

SECTION I: Overview

1. General principles   3
   G. C. Bennet

2. Growth and its normal variants   11
   G. C. Bennet

3. The disabled child in society   29
   G. M. Cochrane

4. Regional analgesia and pain relief in children   41
   E. Doyle

5. Paediatric imaging   51
   D. Wilson and G. Allen

SECTION II: Generalised disorders

6. Bone, cartilage and fibrous tissue disorders   67
   W. G. Cole

7. Metabolic and endocrine disorders of the skeleton   93
   R. Smith

8. Blood disorders and AIDS   109
   C. A. Ludlam and J. Jellis

9. Infections of bones and joints   119
   K. Parsch and S. Nade

10. Skeletal tuberculosis   147
    S. M. Tuli

11. Children's orthopaedics in the tropics   161
    Abdul-Hamid Abdul-Kadir and S. Ibrahim

12. Juvenile idiopathic arthritis   177
    M. Swann

13. Bone tumours   191
    D. H. Gray and J. W. van der Eijken

SECTION III: Neuromuscular disorders

14. Neurology overview   215
    J. Wilson

15. Hereditary and developmental neuromuscular disorders   223
    E. E. Bleck

16. Neural tube defects, spina bifida and spinal dysraphism   241
    M. B. Menelaus and H. Kerr Graham

17. Poliomyelitis   261
    E. K. W. Ho and J. C. Y. Leong

18. Orthopaedic management of cerebral palsy   273
    J. E. Robb and R. Brunner

19. Arthogryposis multiplex congenita   293
    J. A. Fixsen

SECTION IV: Regional disorders

20. The upper limb
    20.1 Developmental anomalies of the hand   301
         P. Burge
    20.2 The shoulder   316
         J. A. Fixsen

21. Obstetrical brachial plexus injuries
    21.1 Management of the injury   321
         A. Gilbert
    21.2 Late sequelae   327
         R. Birch

22. Classification and management of lower limb reduction anomalies   335
    J. A. Fixsen

23. The limping child   347
    G. Hansson and F. S. Jacobsen

24. Developmental dysplasia of the hip   359
    M. K. D. Benson and M. F. Macnicol

25. Legg-Calvé-Perthes' disease   383
    A. Catterall

26. Slipped capital femoral epiphysis   397
    M. F. Macnicol and M. K. D. Benson

27. The knee   409
    M. F. Macnicol and A. M. Jackson

28. Leg length discrepancy   427
    A. M. Jackson, M. F. Macnicol and M. Saleh

29. The foot and ankle
    29.1 General   449
         J. A. Fixsen, A. Catterall and S. S. Coleman
    29.2 Early assessment and management of
         the club foot   464
         A. Catterall
    29.3 Club foot: later problems and relapse   478
         J. A. Fixsen
    29.4 Pes cavus   483
         S. S. Coleman and J. A. Fixsen
    29.5 Congenital vertical talus (congenital
         convex pes valgus)   487
         S. S. Coleman and J. A. Fixsen

30. Congenital disorders of the cervical spine   491
    R. N. Hensinger

31. Thoraco-lumbar spine
    31.1 Back pain in children   505
         M. A. Edgar
    31.2 Spinal deformities   512
         R. A. Dickson
    31.3 Spondylolisthesis   547
         R. A. Dickson

SECTION V: Fractures

32. Principles of fracture care   557
    M. F. Macnicol

33. Fracture epidemiology   575
    L. A. Landin

34. Polytrauma in children   579
    M. J. Bell

35. Management of growth plate injuries   587
    B. K. Foster and E. W. Johnstone

36. Birth injuries and non-accidental injuries   599
    P. J. Witherow

37. Fractures of the shoulder, upper limb and hand   609
    J. de Pablos and A. Tejero

38. Fractures of the pelvis, femoral neck,
    lower limb and foot
    38.1 Fractures of the pelvis   633
         P. Engelhardt
    38.2 Femoral neck fractures   635
         P. Engelhardt
    38.3 Femoral shaft fractures   640
         K. Parsch
    38.4 Fractures of the knee and tibia   646
         C. Hasler
    38.5 Fractures of the foot   654
         P. Engelhardt

39. Spinal fractures
    39.1 Traumatic disorders of the cervical spine   657
         R. N. Hensinger
    39.2 Fractures of the thoracic and lumbar spine 669
         R. N. Hensinger and C. L. Craig

SECTION VI: Appendix

Growth charts   694

Index   697

List of Contributors

Abdul-Hamid Abdul-Kadir MBBS(Singapore), FRCSE, MChOrth (Liverpool)
Consultant Orthopaedic Surgeon
Pantai Medical Centre
Kuala Lumpur
Malaysia

Gina M. Allen BM, DCH, MRCGP, MRCP, FRCR
Consultant Radiologist
West Wales General Hospital
Camarthen
UK

Michael J. Bell FRCS
Consultant Orthopaedic Surgeon
Department of Paediatric Orthopaedic Surgery
Sheffield Children's Hospital
Sheffield
UK

George C. Bennet BSc, MB, ChB, FRCS
Consultant Orthopaedic Surgeon
The Royal Hospital for Sick Children
Glasgow
UK

Michael K. D. Benson MBBS, FRCS
Consultant Orthopaedic Surgeon
Nuffield Orthopaedic Centre
Oxford
UK

Rolfe Birch MChir, FRCS
Consultant Orthopaedic Surgeon
Peripheral Nerve Injury Unit
Royal National Orthopaedic Hospital
Brockley Hill
Stanmore
Middlesex
UK

Eugene E. Bleck MD
Professor Emeritus, Orthopaedic Surgery
Stanford University
California
USA

Reinald Brunner MD
Head of Neuro-orthopaedic Unit
Department of Paediatric Orthopaedics
Neuro-orthopaedic Unit
Children's University Hospital
Basle
Switzerland

Peter Burge FRCS
Consultant Hand Surgeon
The Nuffield Orthopaedic Centre
Headington
Oxford
UK

Anthony Catterall MChir, FRCS
Consultant Orthopaedic Surgeon
Royal National Orthopaedic Hospital
Brockley Hill
Stanmore
Middlesex
UK

George M. Cochrane MA, MB, BChir, FRCP, FRCPE, DPhysMed
Retired Physician with special interests in severely disabled people and rehabilitation
Previously Mary Marlborough Lodge
Nuffield Orthopaedic Centre
Oxford
UK

William G. Cole MBBS, MSc, PhD, FRACS, FRCSC
Professor of Surgery, and Head, Division of Orthopaedics
The Hospital for Sick Children
Toronto
Ontario
Canada

Sherman S. Coleman MD
Senior Consultant Services
Department of Orthopedics
University of Utah Health Services Center
Salt Lake City
Utah
USA

Clifford Craig MD
Clinical Associate Professor
Orthopedic Surgery Section
Mott Children's Hospital
University of Michigan
Ann Arbor
Michigan
USA

Robert A. Dickson MA, ChM, FRCS, DSc
Professor and Head
Department of Orthopaedic Surgery
University of Leeds;
Consultant Orthopaedic Surgeon
St James's University Hospital
Leeds
UK

Edward Doyle MD, FRCA
Consultant Paediatric Anaesthetist
Royal Hospital for Sick Children
Edinburgh
UK

Mike A. Edgar MA, MChir, FRCS
Consultant Orthopaedic/Spinal Surgeon
The Middlesex Hospital
London
UK

Jan W. van der Eijken PhD
Professor
Onze Lieve Urouwe Gasthuis; and Academisch Medisch Centrum
Amsterdam
The Netherlands

Peter Engelhardt MD
Professor
Head of Orthopaedic Department
St Joseph Krankenhaus
Berlin
Germany

John A. Fixsen MChir, FRCS
Honorary Consultant Orthopaedic Surgeon
Great Ormond Street Hospital for Sick Children
Great Ormond Street
London
UK

Bruce K. Foster MBBS, MD(Adel), FRACS
Clinical Associate Professor
University of Adelaide;
Staff Orthopaedic Surgeon
Department of Orthopaedic Surgery
Women & Children's Hospital
North Adelaide
Australia

Alain Gilbert MD
Associate Professor of Orthopaedic Surgery
Clinique Jouvenet
Paris
France

H. Kerr Graham MD, FRCS(Ed), FRACS
Professor of Orthopaedic Surgery
Department of Orthopaedics
Royal Children's Hospital
Parkville
Australia

D. Harley Gray MB, ChM, MMedSc, FRACS
Formerly, Professor of Orthopaedic Surgery
Department of Orthopaedic Surgery
Middlemoore Hospital
Auckland
New Zealand

Göran Hansson MD, PhD
Associate Professor
Department of Orthopaedics
Central Hospital
Halmstad
Sweden

Carol-Claudius Hasler MD
Head of Traumatology
University Children's Hospital
Basel
Switzerland

Robert N. Hensinger MD
Professor and Section Head, Orthopedic Surgery
Section of Orthopedic Surgery
University Hospital
Ann Arbor
Michigan
USA

Eric K W Ho FRCS, FRACS
Formerly Senior Lecturer
Department of Orthopaedic Surgery
The University of Hong Kong
Queen Mary Hospital; and
Formerly Medical Director & Consultant Orthopaedic Surgeon
Duchess of Kent Children's Hospital
Hong Kong

Sharif Ibrahim MBChB(Cairo), FRCS(Glasg), MS Orth(UKM)
Associate Professor and Paediatric Orthopaedic Surgeon
Department of Orthopaedics and Traumatology
National University Hospital
Kuala Lumpur
Malaysia

Andrew M. Jackson FRCS
Consultant Surgeon
Harley Street
London
UK

F. Stig Jacobson MD
Paediatric Orthopaedic Surgeon
Marshfield Clinic
Marshfield
Wisconsin
USA

John E. Jellis OBE, FRCS, FRCSE
Professor of Orthopaedic Surgery
Zambian–Italian Orthopaedic Hospital
Lusaka
Zambia

Edward W. Johnstone PhD
Senior Research Officer
Department of Orthopaedic Surgery
Women's & Children's Hospital
North Adelaide
Australia

Lennart A. Landin MD, PhD, SOE
Consultant Orthopaedic Surgeon
Department of Orthopaedics
Helsingborg Hospital
Helsingborg
Sweden

John C. Y. Leong OBE, FRCS, FRCS(Edin), FRACS, JP
Professor & Head
Department of Orthopaedic Surgery and
Chief of Services
Department of Orthopaedics and Traumatology
The University of Hong Kong
Queen Mary Hospital; and
Consultant Orthopaedic Surgeon
Duchess of Kent Children's Hospital
Hong Kong

Christopher A. Ludlam PhD, FRCPEd
Consultant Haematologist
Department of Haematology
Edinburgh Royal Infirmary
Edinburgh
UK

Malcolm F. Macnicol BSc(Hons), MCh, FRCS, FRCP,
FRCSEd(Orth), Dip. Sports Med.
Consultant Orthopaedic Surgeon
Royal Hospital for Sick Children and
Princess Margaret Rose Orthopaedic Hospital
Edinburgh
UK

Malcolm B. Menelaus MD, FRCS (deceased)
Formerly, Senior Orthopaedic Surgeon
Department of Orthopaedics
Royal Children's Hospital
Parkville
Victoria
Australia

Sydney Nade DSc, MD, MB BS, BSc(Med), FRCS, FRACS,
MRCP(UK), FAOrthA
Clinical Professor
Department of Surgery
Westmead Hospital
The University of Sydney
Sydney
Australia

Julio de Pablos MD, PhD
Consultant in Orthopedics
Orthopedic Department
Hospital of Navarra
Pamplona
Spain

Klaus Parsch MD
Professor
Department of Orthopaedic Surgery
Pediatric Centre
Olgahospital
Stuttgart
Germany

James E. Robb BSc (Hons), MB, ChB, FRCS
Consultant Orthopaedic Surgeon
Princess Margaret Rose Orthopaedic Hospital and
Royal Hospital for Sick Children
Edinburgh
UK

Mike Saleh MB, ChB, MSc(Bio-Eng), FRCS, FRCSEd
Professor
Northern General Hospital
Sheffield
UK

Roger Smith MD, PhD, FRCP
Consultant Physician
Nuffield Orthopaedic Centre
Headington
Oxford
UK

Malcolm Swann MBBS, FRCS
Consultant Orthopaedic Surgeon
Wexham Park Hospital
Slough
UK

A. Tejero MD
Consultant in Orthopedics
Orthopedic Department
Hospital of Navarra
Pamplona
Spain

S. M. Tuli MB, BS, MS, PhD, FAMS
Senior Consultant Orthopaedics & Spinal Diseases
Vidyasagar Institute of Mental Health & Neurosciences
New Delhi
India

Andrew J. Unwin BSc FRCS(Orth)
Consultant Orthopaedic Surgeon
Windsor Orthopaedic Clinic
Phoenix House
Nightingale Walk
Windsor
UK

David J. Wilson MBBS, BSc, FRCP, FRCR
Consultant Radiologist
Nuffield Orthopaedic Centre
Headington
Oxford
UK

John Wilson PhD, FRCP, FRCPCH
Consultant Paediatric Neurologist (Retired)
Great Ormond Street Children's Hospital
London
UK

Peter J. Witherow MB, ChB, FRCS
Formerly Consultant Orthopaedic Surgeon
Bristol Royal Hospital for Sick Children
Bristol
UK

Foreword

Once again the European editors have reached across the Atlantic to the Pacific shore of the United States to graciously invite me to write a foreword to the second edition. They have succeeded in collaring authoritative (but not authoritarian) paediatric orthopaedic surgeons to share with us their knowledge, the current status of diagnosis and treatment, and perspectives. The number of new authors in this second edition has increased from 37 in the first to 51 representing 15 nations befitting the global extent of orthopaedic surgery and the explosion of interest in paediatric orthopaedics. Globalisation is nothing new to us in medicine. We all have the same bones, muscles, nerves, blood vessels and organs underneath our varied coloured skins. And, we all share the same genetic and acquired diseases and injuries although conditioned by geography, culture and racial traits.

Seven years ago when the first edition was launched, electronic prophets might have expected confirmation of their predictions that by 2001 books would be outmoded by the World Wide Web. Although the http://www and CD-ROMs greatly facilitate access to the voluminous medical literature in titles and abstracts, the resultant retrieval can be disjointed. In contrast, a book synthesises the topic in one accessible and portable space. With a book in hand you can read it anywhere – on the sand of the beach or desert, in the mountains and forests, on the seas and rivers, and in your own garden under a tree. You can turn the pages back to re-read and reflect. A book never gives you a message that you have performed 'an illegal operation', that 'access is denied', nor will it electronically crash in the midst of a read. You don't have to make a backup copy or delete messages and advertising. A book is ecological. You don't have to use reams of new paper to print the text to read, file and save.

As with the first edition, this new edition is directed toward a readership of registrars and residents (but seasoned orthopaedic surgeons and general medical practitioners will find it informative too). The contents of the chapters are not exhaustive, but are more than enough to give the physician a firm working knowledge of the state of the art. The texts can serve as springboards to leap into the Internet and get more details from the search engines of the medical literature databases. I am reminded of the preface of *The Compleat Pediatrician*, by the late Wilbur Davidson, M.D., Dean of the Duke University School of Medicine. 'Most books are like the old-fashioned hoop skirt. They cover the subject without touching it. This book is more like a G-string. It barely touches the subject while covering it – in other words, the bare facts.' Enjoy!

EEB
2001

Preface

In the preface to the first edition we recorded our debt to the children we treat. It is a singular privilege to care for the disabled child but privilege carries responsibility. We need a thorough understanding of normal child development and when a child deviates from this. We must try to understand how children grow so that we harness their growth to minimise and not exacerbate deformity. Children are not just 'small adults': diseases in childhood are often very different from those in adult life and we must recognise how they differ and plan accordingly. We must understand the natural history of disease and how our treatment may modify it, both in the short-term and in the long-term throughout adult life. When we win the confidence and co-operation of a young child it facilitates treatment which may extend over many years.

In this second edition Klaus Parsch has strengthened the editorial team. We have expanded substantially the sections on trauma to include more detailed descriptions of individual injuries and their management. We have already drawn contributors from around the world to describe the musculoskeletal disorders which affect children both in the developing and the developed world. Our original contributors have updated their chapters but it is a pleasure to recognise several new contributors. It is with great sadness that we record the death of Malcolm Menelaus. When the first edition of this book was discussed Malcolm was most supportive and encouraging: we honour his memory.

Within this book are included sections on assessing the stages of childhood development, common disorders of the skeletal, haemopoietic and neuromuscular systems and those inherited and acquired conditions to which the immature musculoskeletal system is vulnerable. We are grateful to neurological, anaesthetic and paediatric colleagues for their unique contributions.

We recognise that no text book can be completely comprehensive. We have attempted, however, to be concise and relevant so that the book will be of particular value to those surgeons in training for whom examinations loom. The text should continue to be a straightforward reference for those in established practice since it discusses areas of diagnostic and management difficulty.

The selected references at the end of each chapter should stimulate further reading. The principles of common surgical procedures are described but this is not an operative manual: we believe that paediatric surgical skills should be learned by daily experience under supervision, coupled with frequent reference to surgical atlases.

It is a real pleasure to record our thanks to our contributors; without their enthusiasm, expertise and time this volume would not have been produced. They share with us the aim of improving care for the child with musculoskeletal disability throughout the world.

To you the reader we wish every success both in your years of training and in the years of practice beyond.

MKDB, JAF, MFM and KP
Oxford, London, Edinburgh and Stuttgart

Section I
Overview

Chapter 1

General principles

G. C. Bennet

INTRODUCTION

As medicine has become more 'scientific', less attention has been paid to those more traditional aspects of the art that might be collectively termed the 'bedside manner'. Medical students, and indeed more senior trainees, are not taught to talk to patients, but rather are expected to 'pick it up as they go along'. This seems very strange because adequate communication, usually in the setting of the consultation, is the very bedrock of our specialty. If the subject is considered at all, undue stress is usually laid on the taking of a history. It is as if the highest, and indeed sometimes the only, peak is diagnosis. In this scenario, the doctor sits back taking notes and emitting the occasional encouraging, albeit carefully modulated, grunt whilst the patient tells their story. In due course the diagnosis is pronounced. The story seems to stop here. When therapeutic efforts were of limited efficacy, this was indeed the case. Even when effective treatment became available, but still in the days when the doctor instructed and the patient obeyed, this was acceptable. Not so now. There is a shift away from the authoritarian figure of the doctor and he is but one source of advice competing for acceptance, on equal terms, with grandmothers, friends, women's magazines and quacks. He has to convince. If we wish the patient to comply with our advice, we should be able to convey to them what is wrong, what should be done, and why. The factors that may influence the chances of success or failure in this undertaking are the subject of this chapter.

THE DOCTOR

Nowadays, medical competence is taken for granted. Something more is expected. The patients first and foremost expect the doctor to listen to their story, to understand their problems, and then to communicate their conclusions and recommendations in terms they can understand. Korsch et al (1968) found a much higher percentage of satisfactory consultations in which the doctor was perceived to be friendly (as opposed to businesslike). A smile, an introduction, and a word or two to the child give the right impression. There is something to be said for the old adage that haemorrhoids are a useful disease for a doctor to have, as they give him the proper demeanour of concern and slight anxiety.

It is not just what is said that counts. If you are dressed in jeans and a T-shirt, it makes no difference at all to the standard of medicine you practise, but it may not meet with the patient's expectations of a medical man, so that the proportion of satisfactory consultations goes down. In paediatric practice, the wearing of white coats is an issue that is best left to the individual surgeon. There are arguments both for and against. Against is the fact that children are said to be alarmed by the sight of them, but it is probably the behaviour of those inside them that is alarming, rather than the coats themselves. Nevertheless, there is something to be said for not wearing them, as an informal atmosphere is something to be encouraged in a paediatric setting.

THE CLINIC

Children and adults do not mix terribly well in the hospital outpatient department; they are better segregated. Indeed, the facilities required for paediatric consultations are in some respects different from those required for adults. Planning should start with consideration of the facilities outside the hospital building. Parking should be available close to the clinic entrance; parents cannot be expected to walk a long way with a handicapped child and perhaps other children in tow. There should be a supply of buggies and wheelchairs and staff should be on hand to give help where necessary and before it is requested.

The atmosphere of the hospital should be cheerful, bright and welcoming. Good signposting is vital. One way that patients and their parents are kept subjugated is to keep them lost. Whilst they are vainly looking around trying to orientate themselves, staff sweep past with an air of superiority. The parents' irritation and feeling of unease is transmitted to the child and the surroundings are perceived as unwelcoming. Make it fun! Footsteps marked on the floor are far better than arrows on the wall. Even these, however, can be made more interesting (Fig. 1.1). In the waiting area there should be child-sized furniture but, as the parents' comfort must also be taken into account, it is inadvisable to make it all this size. Try to keep the parents comfortable, with a supply of magazines and the prospect of a coffee. Perhaps as important as anything, get someone to keep the children entertained within their sphere of vision. Playleaders or suitably trained volunteers are invaluable in this respect. The provision of an abundance of safe toys is essential. When children are brought to hospital, some parents seem to think that they then automatically become the responsiblity of the staff. Supervision is therefore desirable. There will be lots of noise and mess, but this must be accepted.

Nowadays, there is no place for block booking or hopeless

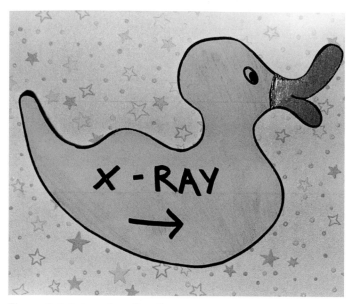

Figure 1.1 Interesting directions.

overbooking of clinics. Quite apart from the fact that it is no longer acceptable and represents bad medicine, it boils down to a matter of self-preservation. Waiting makes both children and parents irritable. If a child has just received a smack in the waiting room and is then ushered in, still in tears, to see the doctor, the start of the consultation will be a little tricky. The parents and children are unlikely to be very well disposed to the doctor at that stage; the usual light-hearted introductory approach is not well received, and jokes are liable to fall a little flat. Once the tears stop, they are usually replaced by sullen rebellion, and there is likely to be little co-operation during the rest of the meeting.

There is a rather strange list of other requirements that aid the successful running of a children's orthopaedic clinic. All hospitals no doubt carry a supply of nappies for the youngsters that attend, but perhaps not all keep spare trousers and underpants for those, often not long out of nappies, who find the whole experience too frightening or too exciting. Perhaps we need them only because our patients wait too long. Spare shoes are another necessity: many parents do not seem to anticipate the removal of plaster casts, so that something to put on little Johnny's feet may be required. A sweet jar that can be produced after an unpleasant experience such as blood letting is a good way of soothing hurt arms and feelings. The odd little trinket hidden away for those children who are called to the hospital on their birthday will do wonders for the reputation of the place. Little badges or certificates for children who are subjected to X-rays or other procedures raise the spirits and keep everyone a little happier than might otherwise have been the case.

THE CONSULTATION

Children are different, and this must be recognised. One cannot transpose adult methods to children, as they will not

work predictably and will lead to more dissatisfied customers than is necessary. Nothing will be said in the clinic, but views will be made known to the world at large. Unfortunately, those who undertake only occasional children's clinics may fail to realise that they could get better results and more patient satisfaction if they changed their techniques from those they use in adults. One clinic a week is just not enough for such a change to be made subconsciously. In the paediatric setting the doctor must not only satisfy the patient, but also the parents and whoever else is behind a complaint. Children have their own ideas of what to expect from the doctor; these will not change, so we have to adapt our behaviour patterns to fit in with their expectations. Do not be too rigid or too embarrassed to enter into the spirit of things.

The parents' expectations too will differ, and must be satisfied. Your behaviour should be tailored to what you consider these expectations to be. It is obvious that the approach, for example, to a handicapped child being seen for the first time will be more sober than that when seeing an old friend who has been known to you for years, when a bit of leg pulling and jollity is in order. The expectations of parents can sometimes be better estimated by trying to assess the thinking behind the consultation, and who is behind a complaint. This may be clarified by noting who is present. In this country, the norm is for the mother to accompany the child. If this is not the case, or someone else appears in the consulting room, think again. Their presence may suggest that they are the one making the complaint, and that a change in the method of conducting the interview is indicated.

Perhaps the most common deviation from the norm is that the father is present. Usually he appears with a first-born baby. Then, he will be in the background, carrying the large bag of equipment (all brand new) that seems to accompany first-born children wherever they go. His presence under these circumstances is of no special significance. Similarly, he may be present if there is a large gap between the last-born child and the present. By that time, usually an older parent, he sits in the background looking faintly embarrassed but nevertheless rather pleased with himself.

Our obstetric colleagues have produced a new subgroup who have become parents by the use of such techniques as *in vitro* fertilisation. My impression is that such parents are similar to, but have rather more exaggerated characteristics than, those of the first-born group, and tend to be rather intense about it all.

Of more significance is when both parents are there under other circumstances. Almost invariably, both are present when they are seeking a second opinion. By that stage they will probably have fallen out with their previous surgeon and may well be looking for support in their criticisms of him or her. Be guarded and do not disparage their efforts; they may well be seeing your failures! Where serious disease is suspected and bad news expected, both parents may be present in anticipation of the need for mutual support.

When only the father accompanies the child, it may signify nothing more than that the mother is home minding other siblings or working. On the other hand, it may point to paternal ambition for the child, usually in the field of sporting endeavours. Most often the patient is an adolescent girl. Then, dad sits in the background, often looking rather disapproving and saying little, whilst the girl tells her story. Commonly, she will be found to be suffering from an overuse syndrome.

Grandmothers are often there to make sure that the true state of affairs (i.e. their view) is put forward. This is done in their role as the fount of all knowledge on the subject of child rearing in the family. Sometimes they are right and certainly they are always worth listening to. Teachers also may be invoked as the reason for the child having been brought to clinic. When the parents state that the teacher said it 'ought to be seen to', they are invoking a higher authority whom they feel you will be more likely to believe.

Physiotherapists most commonly accompany children with cerebral palsy or other chronic handicaps. They may be there to stop you doing something (usually surgical) or to impress upon you the desirability of a particular line of treatment (usually non-surgical) but, more often than not, they are there because they are unsure what to do next and are looking for advice. This is most useful and is much better than an exchange of letters, which is impersonal and leaves much unsaid. Mother, physiotherapist and surgeon can have a sensible discussion and plan future management.

Lastly, there is the vexed question of medical parents! Expect anything from neuroticism to embarrassed neglect. You will find nothing but surprises. Be thankful that they tend not to beat a path to your door until you have been in practice for a while so that, by that stage, you will have had a chance to work out all these things for yourself.

These observations gradually become second nature and are made subconsciously. That you were making them may become apparent only when you realise that an assessment was wrong. Perhaps a child that you felt sure was an only child proves to have siblings. Then, the rest of the consultation can be spent trying to work out where you went wrong. The importance of these signposts is brought into relief only when you cannot use them, for example when an immigrant or foreign family is seen. There is no doubt then that the consultation seems to suffer as a result.

The starting point of most consultations is a letter of referral. Do not be surprised, however, if the presenting complaint mentioned there does not seem to be the main concern of the mother. At the initial medical contact, it is not uncommon for the parents to put forward a complaint that they think will be acceptable to the doctor and that will attract his attention – for example a limp. Once the object of their ruse has been gained, they feel free to broach the hidden agenda.

Parents want to be heard rather than spoken to. You must let them have their say; if you do not, they will be resentful. Being a good listener is a characteristic much appreciated by the general public. If you interrupt the parents' story too soon by trying to elicit the salient points of the history, this may cause irritation because they feel that the course of the consultation is being dictated by the doctor. If the consultation does not then proceed in the way they envisaged, they will become sullenly anxious and uncommunicative.

First, ask why they came, why now and what worries them most; you may be surprised at some of the answers. In an interesting and illuminating study by Korsch et al (1968), the expectations that the parents had of the consultation – for example that X-rays or injections would be performed or the child would be admitted to hospital – were not even mentioned in 65% of cases. Even more startling was that in only 24% of cases was the parents' main worry mentioned to the doctor.

Aim the questions at the mother unless the child is an adolescent, in which case they should be asked directly. Talk directly to handicapped children, to avoid the 'does he take sugar?' syndrome. If the child is incapable of answering, the parent will step in and provide the responses. Be ready for disagreements, usually between adolescent girls and their parents, about how long the problem has been present, how it affects them, and so on. Whatever the frustrations, let them tell their story. If not given the chance, they will feel that you have not understood their concerns and, as a result they will be disinclined to take, or indeed even to listen to, advice.

The functional effect of the symptoms upon the child should be elicited. What effect does the complaint have on schooling? Are there problems in keeping up with other children? Are there any problems with friends, with a lack of them, or at home?

Whatever the age group, a birth and developmental history should be taken: the course of the pregnancy, the method and type of delivery, the birth weight and birth order should all be ascertained. Check the motor milestones. The age of sitting and walking should suffice in most cases. With first-born children, the age of walking is often given as impossibly early. After the first, parents learn to be in no rush to get their children mobile and, indeed, to appreciate that there are definite advantages in keeping them as immobile as possible for as long as possible. Any deviation from the norm in any of the above should indicate the need for further inquiry and investigation, and perhaps referral.

EXAMINATION

All the time that you are talking to the parents, the child will be looking at you and making up their mind as to whether or not you pose a threat. If the conclusion is that you do not, then the consultation should go smoothly. The more obviously you and the parents seem to get along well, the more likely it is that the child's decision will be in your favour.

Children sometimes associate getting undressed with staying in hospital. Get them undressed a bit at a time. Always ask for their permission to look at, for example, their legs. Once this is granted, there is seldom any trouble. Do not take off more than is necessary to examine a particular part at any one time. Taking off the shoes and socks is probably the least threatening, so start there. Proceed as seems best to fit the situation. This is not to say the whole child should not be examined, but rather that the approach should be a little different than that followed in adult practice. Children should not be undressed before the doctor even puts in an appearance. It just has to be accepted that the consultation will take a little longer. In older children, do not forget their modesty. Always offer them the opportunity to undress in private and not under the gaze of their parents.

If a child is young and a bit uncertain, they are best examined on the mother's knee; continued co-operation may depend upon maintaining contact with the mother. Such an examination technique avoids the lachrymocutaneous reflex described by Rang (1982) – when the skin touches the couch, the tears begin to flow. Do not try to lie a child down until the end of the examination, as many children seem to feel threatened in this position. A cuddle from the mother at the top may keep the child happy long enough for the doctor to do what is necessary at the other end. Leave any potentially painful or embarrassing procedures until the end.

In babies, the general examination should include a rough appraisal of the child's motor development (Fig. 1.2). The

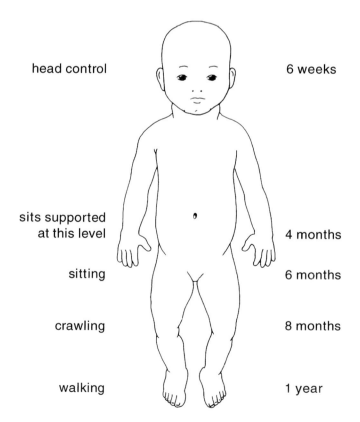

head control — 6 weeks

sits supported at this level — 4 months

sitting — 6 months

crawling — 8 months

walking — 1 year

Figure 1.2 Motor development. This develops in a craniocaudal direction. If you remember a few basic milestones, you can easily estimate the developmental stage reached between them.

examination should look at the whole baby to exclude any skin lesions, such as haemangiomata or hairy patches suggestive of spinal dysraphism. Plagiocephaly, bat ears, scoliosis and torticollis will be routinely sought. No young child should be allowed to leave the clinic without the hips being tested. All this is in addition to the more detailed examination of the part complained of. In the older child, the examination varies widely, depending upon the nature of the presenting complaint, so that it is a little difficult to generalise. Nevertheless, in most cases it will start with the child walking. This gives a general idea of the gait in addition to, for example, the presence of any limp or torsional abnormality. Whilst the child is undressing, look at the pattern of wear on their shoes. If the patient is old enough, have them hop, first on one foot and then on the other. Perform a Gower's sign (Fig. 1.3). Check the Trendelenburg test if indicated. Take a look at the feet. Are the arches flattened or too high? Is there forefoot/hindfoot malalignment? Are the toes in their normal positions? If a back disorder is suspected, ask the child to bend over, and check for scoliosis and assess back movements.

Only then should the child mount the throne of the examination couch. Look at the leg lengths and the shape and comparative size of the lower limbs. Exclude any generalised pathology by examining for organomegaly, lymphadenopathy, swellings or rashes. A complete examination, even if negative, shows thoroughness and concern, and will reinforce the fact that you have taken the complaints seriously.

Do not forget that a large proportion of parents will be dissatisfied if X-rays or blood tests are not taken, as they will otherwise feel that their complaint has been dismissed as trivial. Under these circumstances it may be worthwhile undertaking these measures, for therapeutic reasons. If the parents have unrealistic expectations, however, there is little one can do to satisfy them.

At the end of the consultation, the aim is to know the location of the pathology, to have a rough idea what the problem is and to have in one's mind what confirmatory tests, if any, should be done. If a diagnosis has not been reached, but radiographs indicate no serious pathology, then explain this to the parents. They want a diagnosis, but do understand that not all aches and pains in children can be described diagnostically. Explain that there is no serious underlying problem and offer to see them again at some time, with the proviso that, should the symptoms get worse before then, then you will be happy to see them sooner. If you really are unsure, be honest and say that you do not know what the problem is, but would like to do a few tests to make a diagnosis or to exclude any of the more serious complaints. Failure to make any diagnostic statement leads to dissatisfaction.

If a diagnosis is reached, it is important that it is explained properly. As has been stressed throughout, satisfied patients are more likely to comply with the advice subsequently given. Explanations should be tailored to the perceived ability of the parents to understand. Such explanations are

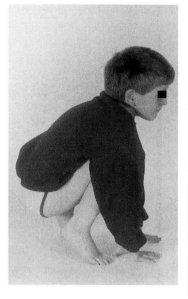

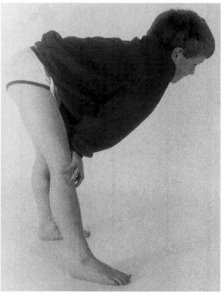

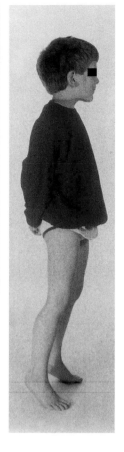

A

B

C

Figure 1.3 Gower's sign. The child with muscular dystrophy can only get up by first getting into the quadriped position and then extending his hips by 'walking' up his thighs with his hands.

often helped by the use of handouts or, particularly, drawings, which can often make a point far more tellingly (Fig. 1.4). They can also be taken away and used to explain to grandmother. Parents will remember only one or two points – usually the last – so try to limit the number of messages. If, at the end of the consultation, the parents do not seem to be too certain about specific points, offer to let them come back for further discussions. If they are immigrants with a

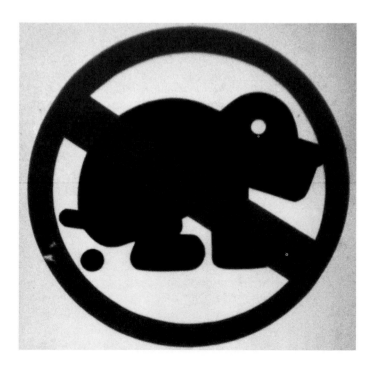

PLEASE DO NOT LET

YOUR DOG FOUL

THE CAR PARK

Figure 1.4 Drawings speak louder than words.

poor grasp of English, ask them to return with a relative who can translate, or ask them to wait whilst an interpreter is found.

It is the parents', rather than the doctor's, perception of the seriousness of the illness that dictates whether they will comply with the doctor's advice. Furthermore, their compliance depends upon whether or not they feel that the doctor has understood their problems and their related concerns; nowhere in life will people act on the advice of someone they feel does not have a clear understanding of their problem. Patients come with expectations; these must be satisfied before the physician can be successful in management. If expectations are not met, it is likely that there will be parental dissatisfaction. Ideally, if they cannot be met, they should at least be acknowledged. Avoid medical jargon; this will widen the gap. Be specific, and let the family know what you are going to do. This should be spelt out in detail. For example, mention that a bone scan involves an injection, otherwise they will be unable to prepare the child, and will feel let down by you.

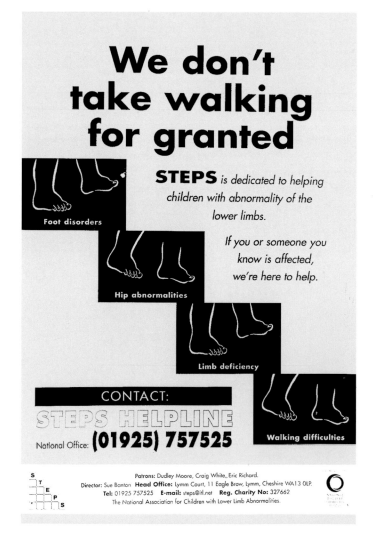

Figure 1.5 Example of an advertisement for a helpline and support group.

Whilst there is an understandable desire to know the diagnosis, the desire to know *why* something has developed should not be underestimated. Reassure the parents that they are not at fault. If this is not done, they may well blame themselves. Mother may feel that part of her role is to keep her children healthy. Try to make her feel that she is doing well, and that the illness in no way reflects badly upon her or her competence as a mother. This will do wonders for her self-esteem and lead to a better relationship between you. Parents need support at such worrying times, not criticism or condescension. If the news is more serious, they may appreciate a chat with their family practitioner. Suggest that you write to or telephone him or her. Help may also be sought from various voluntary bodies such as those for cerebral palsy or spina bifida. Counselling officers with these societies are invaluable and can offer all sorts of additional practical advice and help. They can assess the parents and child and arrange for them to meet someone with similar problems that have been successfully overcome (Fig. 1.5).

PREADMISSION POLICY

In the UK, about 6% of all children are admitted to hospital each year. By the age of 5 years, about one in four will have been admitted on at least one occasion: of these, about one in seven will have been admitted to an adult ward. Although, at the time, the child may be apparently resigned to the situation, they are likely to have angry feelings and there may be a cycle of protest, despair and detachment. Psychological upsets are a common sequel. After discharge from hospital, the child may be unusually difficult with the parents, as if testing them to see if he or she is still loved or likely to be sent away again. Feeding and sleeping difficulties are common.

How can a preadmission programme help? We must first realise that the requirements differ with the age of the child. Obviously, the programme should take this into account. Up to the age of 5 years, the greatest fear of being in hospital relates to separation whereas, in the slightly older child between the ages of 5 and 7 years, the fear is not only of separation but also of the operation. In the 7–10-years age group, worries about the anaesthetic begin to appear, and after the age of 10 years anaesthetic fears predominate (Jenner et al 1952). However, as well as dealing with the child's fears, preadmission programmes should also take into account the feelings of the mother.

If you are not in a specialist children's hospital with such a facility available, arrange for the child to go up to the ward so that they can be shown round by a suitable person – it matters not whether it is the sister or ward clerk – so that they can see how things work. If possible, let them speak to another child who has undergone a similar procedure. They will learn much more of the practicalities of the undertaking than you will be able to tell them. The mother too will appreciate the opportunity to talk with another mother in the same situation.

The easiest of the fears to put at rest is that of separation. Having the mother (or the father) resident is a choice that should be readily available to all parents. Unrestricted visiting, which is the minimum alternative that should be offered, is very much a second best. From the point of view of the staff it is useful to have the mother stay for, although her enthusiasm may at times need restraining, there is no doubt that she is the best person to handle the child and can be of immeasurable help. She must, however, be kept informed about what is happening.

Nevertheless, there are certain problems associated with living in. Particularly when an illness is a serious one, it is very easy for the child and resident mother to become isolated from the rest of the family. Just when the family needs to be together to support each other, they are apart. Encourage the parents to get out a bit by themselves and, if the mother is resident, for her to get out and about a little each day to try to retain her sanity. This is something that they are often loathe to do. Point out that they will give their child much more help and comfort if they themselves are fit. Easy access for the siblings should also be offered.

The hospital stay is made less frightening if the child and mother know a little about what to expect. The best thing of all is to have someone that they can identify with. There is evidence that watching a film of a child having a procedure done painlessly has positive benefits and reduces the anxiety levels when the child comes in (Melamed 1977). The greater the perceived similarity, the greater the effect of the film; in other words, the more closely the child can identify with the star of the film, the more beneficial will be the result. Encouraging the child to play with stethoscopes, masks and caps seems to allay their fears further. Details such as the extent of a plaster can easily be demonstrated to the parents either by their meeting a similarly treated child or, if this is not possible, by showing them photographs (Fig. 1.6).

An informal and relaxed ward atmosphere can do nothing but good. Whilst there is often a great deal of tension simmering under the surface, try to minimise the effects of

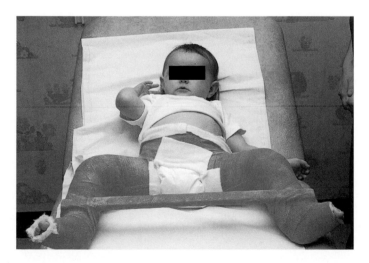

Figure 1.6 A hip spica explained.

this by striving for a friendly atmosphere in which the routines are mainly for the sake of the patients rather than the staff. It is useful to give a booklet to the parents before they come in, so that they can describe to the children what the ward routine is, what to bring in, whom they will meet there and what day-to-day activities to expect. Encourage them to bring in some items from home to make the place a little more cheerful.

BAD NEWS AND HANDICAP

Imparting bad news should be done by the most senior member of the medical team. Both the parents should be present, along with other members of the close family. All the senior medical staff likely to be involved in the care of the child, such as oncologists and haematologists, should all be there to outline an accurate plan of treatment and answer any questions.

It is useful to start by finding out what the parents know. This gives a starting point. Be open and honest. Stress the positive as well as the negative aspects of the situation. It is, for example, much easier nowadays to tell parents that their child has an osteosarcoma than it was some years ago, when there was little hope for survival. When the interview is over, the parents may wish to be left alone or to continue to talk to someone such as the nurse looking after their child. Make sure that there is a contact point and an offer that they can come again to talk at any time they like. Always make another definite appointment so that the plan can be gone over again once the news has had a chance to sink in and they are better able to take part in the discussion about the future.

The news of serious disease changes family life for good. This is also the case when a child has a chronic handicap. The parents grieve for the child that has been affected. They go through the same stages as if the child had died, namely shock, anger, denial and, it is to be hoped, eventually acceptance. Whilst all move through these stages at varying speeds, not everyone reaches the last. Help from colleagues in the psychology department may be necessary. Unless the stage of acceptance is reached, the parents' energies cannot be channelled into useful help for the child – and, indeed, for the rest of the family, as they too are handicapped by the presence of a chronic illness.

Various events bring home a disability to the parents, even after the initial diagnosis. A handicapped baby in a pram looks no different from any other baby. With age, the gap becomes wider and worry increases, for example when the 'record of needs' is compiled and the decision made as to whether the child will go to a normal school. If they are accepted at such a school, then the worry is what the reaction of the other children, parents and teachers will be. In the early stages of school much help comes from other children who do not have adult prejudices and who treat a handicapped child with natural acceptance. At some stage, all this changes, and children may be unbelievably cruel and hurtful. Teachers in schools vary. Some will make every

3

effort to help; often this reflects their experience of other children with handicaps. In these circumstances, necessary equipment will be in place and attitudes adjusted. Failing such enlightenment, there may be problems; fire regulations or flights of stairs are often invoked as a deterrent to accepting the child. If the child is accepted at a school, the attitude – positive or negative – of one teacher may well be transmitted to other children, who will then change their treatment of the handicapped child to fall into line with that shown by the adult role model.

REFERENCES

Jenner L, Blom G, Walford S 1952 Emotional implications of tonsillectomy and adenoidectomy in children. In: Eissler R S (ed) The psychoanalytical study of the child. International Universities Press, New York

Korsh B M, Gozzi E K, Francis V 1968 Doctor–patient interaction and patient satisfaction. Pediatrics 42: 855–869

Melamed B 1977 Psychological preparation for hospitalisation. In: Rachman S (ed) Contributions to medical psychology, vol 1. Pergamon Press, Oxford

Rang M 1982 The Easter Seal guide to children's orthopaedics. Easter Seal Society, Ontario

Chapter 2

Growth and its variants

G. C. Bennet

INTRODUCTION

Many children seen in orthopaedic clinics have nothing wrong with them. Rather, they deviate in some respect from someone's idea of how a child should be at a particular age. That someone may have a very limited knowledge of child development. In our own department, over half the children referred from family practitioners were within normal limits (Roberts & Conner 1987). Similarly, Craxford et al (1984) found that 49% of their referrals were for flat feet or intoeing, both of which can be regarded as normal variants.

These figures merely serve to emphasise that there is great ignorance of what represents normality. If one cannot appreciate what is normal, then one is unlikely to distinguish reliably the abnormal. What constitutes normality does of course change with age, and what would be normal at one age would not be accepted at another.

The vital difference between adults and children is that children grow. Consequently, in children, static problems are practically unknown. Whilst there may be a non-progressive lesion, this does not mean that it is unchanging, so that more frequent and close observation of a child is required than would be the case for an adult; only then can one appreciate whether something is getting better or worse. This is, however, one of the fascinations of children's orthopaedic surgery. In many cases, the natural history of a condition is still incompletely known, so that simple clinical examination over a prolonged period produces very useful, and in some cases original, data.

The fact that growth is taking place means it may be harnessed to aid recovery. This is particularly so in the management of fractures. In spite of its occasional unpredictability, growth can still be of great assistance compared with the problems met in dealing with unchanging adult tissues.

GROWTH

As a child gets older, it gets bigger. This we take for granted. When expressed graphically, size increase tells us little about how the child is growing, how fast and where (see growth charts in the Appendix). The rate of growth, for example, is neither equal throughout the body, nor does it take place at a uniform rate during childhood.

BODY PROPORTIONS

In proportion to the trunk, the infant's legs and arms are comparatively short. As growth occurs, the limbs enlarge more than the trunk, so that this disproportion is gradually corrected until the adult form is reached.

At 1 year of age, the sitting height is 63% of total body height. This reduces to 60% at 2 years and, at maturity, is 52% in males and 53% in females. From birth to maturity, the sitting height increases by 67%, whereas the legs increase by 145%.

The child's spine changes shape as it grows. When the child gains head control, a cervical lordosis develops, usually by the age of 3 months, and as sitting balance develops, so does a lumbar lordosis. Before this, the spine is in a long, smooth C curve, without the two areas of lordosis that we associate with the adult back.

GROWTH VELOCITY

Much more information can be obtained from growth velocity rather than from simple growth charts (see Appendix). As can be seen, the rate of growth at birth is very fast but slows down to a much slower rate around the age of 5 years. The rate then remains fairly constant until the adolescent growth spurt is entered. This occurs between 10 and 12 years for girls and 12 and 14 years for boys. Before that, the rate of growth is the same for girls and boys. As girls enter the growth spurt earlier, for a time they become bigger than boys. As the growth spurt is longer and more dramatic in males, they gradually catch up with girls around the age of 14 or 15 years, and then overtake them. Allowing for great individual variation, girls on average stop growing by 15 years, whereas boys may go on growing until the age of 18 years.

There is also great variation between individuals as to when they enter the growth spurt and at what age maximum growth velocity occurs. Anderson et al (1963) pointed out the inherent inaccuracy of using chronological age as a basis of growth prediction. Estimates of future growth based on this parameter are very inaccurate, because of the variability of the time of the growth spurt. It follows that children with the same chronological age may have a very different number of years of growth remaining to them. In younger children who obviously have not entered the growth spurt, however, the chronological age is more accurate than in older children.

The alternative to chronological age is to estimate the skeletal age. This is done using standards for various age groups (Greulich & Pyle 1950): by comparing a radiograph of the left hand and wrist with these standards, an estimate

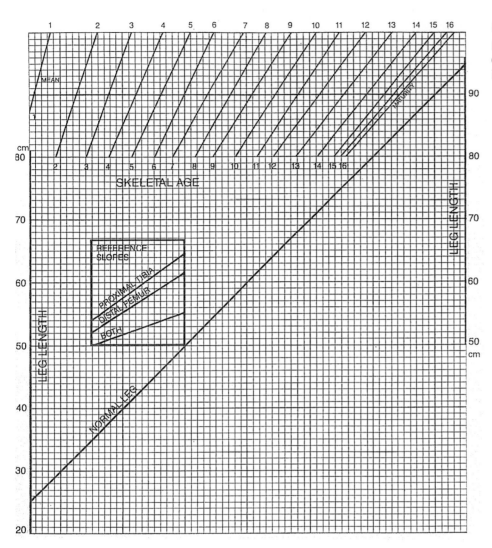

Figure 2.1 The Moseley chart for predicting growth and terminal discrepancy in cases of limb length inequality.

of the skeletal age can be made. The method is very subjective, so that inaccuracies are inevitable. In an attempt to overcome these, Tanner et al (1975) produced an alternative method. This attributes numerical values to the maturity of anatomical landmarks in the hand and wrist. In each of the ages between 8 and 18, the standard deviation for skeletal age is about 1 year, so it is within normal limits for a child to be either advanced or retarded by as much as 2 years compared with the chronological age. The prediction of growth remaining and the likely discrepancy at maturity in the case of limb length inequality can be calculated using the Moseley chart (Fig. 2.1). By plotting the length of both the long and the short legs, and the bone age, increasingly accurate predictions of terminal discrepancy can be obtained after 18 months.

MECHANISM OF GROWTH

Bone can only grow by adding tissue to its outer surface. Growth in length occurs by deposition of new bone at the ends, where it is laid down on a pre-existing cartilaginous scaffold – enchondral ossification. Growth in circumference

is mediated by the periosteum, which lays bone down directly on the surface of the cortex – membranous ossification.

Growth plate

The primary function of the growth plate or physis is to contribute to the longitudinal growth of a bone. Some growth plates, for example the tibial tubercle and the lesser trochanter, have tendons inserted into them and do not add to longitudinal growth. They are known then as apophyses.

Anatomy and function

A typical physis has three areas:

1. Cartilage: this is further subdivided into several distinct regions.
2. Bone.
3. Fibrous tissue, which surrounds the periphery of the plate and forms the perichondrial ring of Lacroix.

The cartilaginous zone is where growth takes place and is the most important part of the physis. This has been studied by Brighton (1983) and the following account is based largely on his work. He described the following functional regions:

a. Germinal or reserve zone (Fig. 2.2). This lies adjacent to the bony epiphysis. It contains few cells, but much matrix. The cells are known to contain glycogen and to synthesise protein. In the matrix, the collagen fibres are distributed randomly. The partial pressure of oxygen (pO_2) is low, so that the blood vessels that pass through the region obviously do not supply it. Chondrocytes do not seem to proliferate here. Its function is not entirely clear, but it is possibly one of storage. Alternatively, it may be that, in view of the collagen and protein synthesis that takes place there, the function is to make matrix (Moseley 1996).

b. The proliferative zone. Here, flattened chondrocytes are arranged with their longitudinal axes at right angles to the long axis of the bone. The chondrocytes in this area are the true germinal cells of the growth plate and, with few exceptions, are the only ones that divide. It follows, therefore, that longitudinal growth can be calculated by multiplying the rate of cell production by the maximum size that the cells reach at the bottom of the hypertrophic zone. The number of cells in each cell column is relatively constant so that, as they are added at the top of this zone, they are removed at the bottom. In the main, these occur at the same rate, otherwise the plate would widen or narrow. Because of its rich blood supply, the pO_2 is greater here than at any other part of the physis. The abundant blood supply is necessary for the continued vitality of the germinal cells. Anything that results in a change in the blood supply will later be reflected in a change in the growth of the plate.

c. Hypertrophic zone. As the cells move down from the proliferative to the hypertrophic zone, the flattened chondrocytes expand and enlarge, becoming spherical in the process. By the time they have reached the bottom of this zone, they are five times the size they were when they entered it. Near the middle of the zone the cytoplasm loses all glycogen-staining ability and the cells then appear nonviable. By the bottom of the zone, the lacunae are empty and the chondrocytes dead. The upper one-third of the zone is metabolically active (as indicated by a high pO_2) and aerobic metabolism occurs. Glycogen is stored in the mitochondria in the form of adenosine triphosphate (ATP). The pO_2 decreases by the middle of the zone, so that anaerobic metabolism then takes place. This consumes glycogen. Somewhere in the top half of the zone, the mitochondria switch from forming ATP to accumulating calcium. As we have already seen, by the middle of the zone all the glycogen has disappeared and, as there is no other source of energy, calcium is released as its uptake and retention are energy dependent. The presence of calcium in the matrix makes it less easy for nutrients to permeate into the cells, so that anaerobic glycolysis becomes even more important.

d. Metaphysis. This begins just distal to the last transverse septum and ends where the wide metaphysis meets the

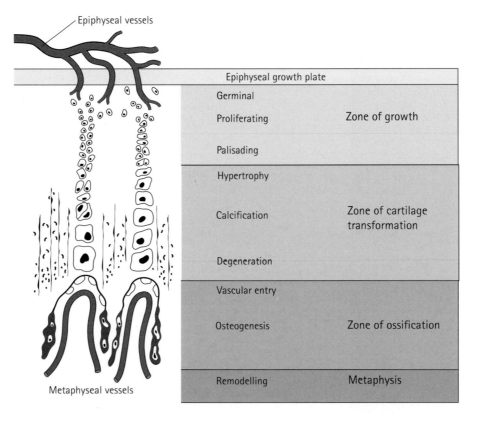

Figure 2.2 The epiphyseal growth plate.

narrower diaphysis. It is a region of vascular stasis. The capillaries invade the hypertrophic zone and osteoblasts, which presumably originate from the vascular endothelium, follow. These lay down bone – the primary spongiosum. Subsequent remodelling, or *funellisation*, occurs on the periosteal surface as well as within the metaphysis. Only if it occurs is the diameter of the metaphysis reduced to that of the diaphysis; when it fails, the bone is an abnormal shape (Fig. 2.3).

e. Fibrocartilage peripheral structure. Around the growth plate is a well-defined group of cells – the ossification groove – and a band of tissue – the perichondrial ring. These are subdivisions of the same structure, but have different functions. The ossification groove contributes to lateral growth of the plate by adding chondrocytes around the periphery. The perichondrial ring is a fibrous band continuous at one end with the periosteum of the metaphysis and at the other with the fibroblasts and collagen fibres of the ossification groove. Its function is to provide mechanical support.

f. Blood supply. There are two main groups of vessels supplying the physis. The first originates on the epiphyseal side and passes through the resting zone to enter the germinal layer of the proliferative zone. The second group comes from the bony side of the physis and supplies the area of the plate where ossification occurs. These vessels arise

from the metaphyseal vessels and from the terminal branches of the nutrient artery of the shaft. They have a role in removing degenerate cartilage and in the formation of bone.

Control of growth plate

The function of the growth plate is influenced by many factors, both specific and non-specific. For example, it is well known that diet has an effect on height. Undernutrition will lead to stunting. More specifically, hormones exert a powerful influence on the growth plates. Which hormones are being secreted at the time dictates the relative growth of different parts of the body and thus its proportions at various stages of development.

By such general control, adult body proportions are reached. If, for any reason, growth stops prematurely, the limbs are proportionately too short for the body. Conversely, if growth continues for too long, the reverse will apply.

Growth hormone secreted by the anterior pituitary has a major effect on enchondral bone formation. If it is deficient, all cartilage proliferation is arrested and the cartilage columns are replaced by bone. Excessive secretion before closure of the plate results in widening of the proliferative zone of the physeal plate and gigantism.

Thyroid hormone influences enchondral bone formation. A deficiency results in a delay in the appearance of ossific nuclei, whereas excessive secretion results in an advanced bone age. Steroids also affect the growth plate and are certainly implicated in its closure. Excessive androgens or oestrogens can cause premature closure. They cannot be the only factors, however, as different growth plates close at different times. The concentration of growth hormone does not change during the time of plate closure, so it is unlikely that its absolute value has any great effect. It is more likely that it is the relative proportions of growth to steroid hormones that in some way cause closure. In addition to these general factors, more localized ones such as muscle tension can affect growth plate function. In paralysis, for example, the shape and texture of a bone may alter because of differential muscle pull. Coxa valga, for example, is commonly found in association with decreased power of the hip abductors.

As mentioned above, growth plates close at different times. During the time they are functioning, they also grow at different rates. For example, 65% of all leg growth takes place at the knee, with 39% occurring in the distal femur and 26% in the proximal tibia. The proximal femur accounts for only 15% of the length of the limb and the distal tibia 20%. To put this another way, the femur contributes 54% of the total length of the limb and the tibia 46%. In the femur, the distal end gives approximately 70% of the ultimate length of the bone and, in the tibia, the proximal end gives 60%. This can be quantified by using the data of Anderson et al (1963). Menelaus (1966) calculated that the distal end of the femur grew 0.95 cm per year and the proximal tibia 0.64 cm per year. If it is assumed that girls stop growing at a chronological age of 14 years, and boys at 16 years then it is possible

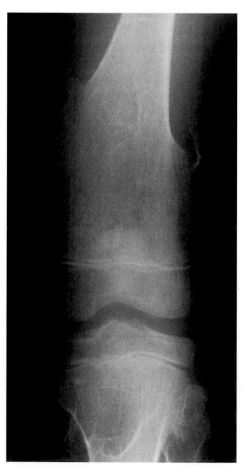

Figure 2.3
Failure of remodelling in diaphyseal aclasis.

to calculate any anticipated leg length difference. The method presumes a constant rate of growth in the upper tibia and lower femur; in spite of this, it seems to be almost as accurate in its predictions as those based on skeletal age. Further details of limb length calculations in growth can be found in Chapter 28.

Growing pains

These are considered here not because they are known to have any connection with growth but because they occur in growing children. Initially, they were considered to be caused by rheumatic disease. The symptom complex is very common, but just how common is not quite clear. Oster & Neilson (1972) found an incidence of 13% in boys and 18% in girls. Peterson (1977) estimated that it affected somewhere between 4% and 25% of all children. Naish & Apley (1951), using strict diagnostic criteria, found an overall incidence of 4.2% (4% in boys and 4.7% in girls).

Affected children complain of pain, usually in the evening or at night, and not specifically related to joints. It is of a severity to interrupt normal activities, for example sleep. The same authors felt that such children could be divided into two groups: those with night pain and those with diurnal pain. Nocturnal pains were always worse in the lower limbs, whereas diurnal pain could affect either the upper or the lower. The classic history is of a child who, after a fairly active day, goes to bed and wakes up screaming with pain in the thighs, calves or behind the knee. The pain responds to parental rubbing, and after anything from a few minutes to half an hour it disappears and the child goes back to sleep. The next morning he is absolutely fine. There is no history of a limp, and no abnormal physical findings. The cause is not known.

The peak incidence of growing pains is between the ages of 4 and 8 years, and yet this is a time that the growth velocity is slowing. Affected children have the same growth curves as other children, and there is no relationship apparent between growth velocity or weight. Children that are affected often also have headaches and abdominal pain. Naish & Apley (1951) found this association to be almost invariable, and also found that these children tended to come from pain-prone families. They concluded that the condition was likely to be an emotional disturbance. After about the age of 11 years in girls and 13 years in boys, its incidence decreases.

In view of the fact that growing pains are such a vague disturbance, treatment is of necessity given on an empirical basis. Once serious diseases have been excluded, then usually reassurance is all that is needed. The natural history is that the condition tends to decline and disappears after 18–24 months. Baxter & Dulberg (1988) felt that it may be a problem of muscle fatigue. On this basis, they tried stretching the quadriceps and hamstrings in one group, whereas another group with similar symptoms were treated with only explanation and reassurance. The average number of episodes occurring over a period of 18 months was

recorded, and found to be much reduced in the treated group compared with the control group.

THE DEVELOPMENT OF GAIT

When children start walking independently at around the age of 1 year, they do so in a fairly standard manner, with a gait pattern that differs significantly from that of an adult. In a surprisingly short time, however, their gait matures so that, by the age of 3 years, it is very similar to that of an adult. An early study of gait was done by Statham & Murray (1971), using interrupted light photography. They found that, as the child's walking improved, so it walked faster, but that this increased velocity did not correlate with the increasing height of the child. Although the gait cycle became more reproducible as walking ability improved there were, at each age, certain characteristics that distinguished the immature from the mature gait. Some of these are due to neurological immaturity, whereas others are related to stature.

As we have already seen, the average child sits at around 6 months and crawls at 9 months. It will walk with support at 12 months, without at 15, and be able to run at 18 months. On first starting to walk, the child has a gait that is rather jerky, unsteady and wide based. The arms are held abducted and initially extended at the elbows. The manner of initial ground contact is variable: it may be heel–toe, whole foot or toe–heel. Certainly in the early stages it is not reproducible. Whereas adults make the heel strike with the knee extended and proceed to flexion, in early stance phase, children tend to strike the floor with the knee flexed then extend the knee with the onset of weight bearing. This increase in stance-phase knee flexion is not caused by lack of quadriceps function, because electromyographic studies have shown prolonged activity in this phase compared with that found in adults. More probably, it is related to the comparative weakness of the plantar flexors (Sutherland et al 1980). Children at this age spend less time in single limb stance and have wider step length (Fig. 2.4). With maturation, the base diminishes, the movements become smoother, a reciprocal swing of the upper limb begins, and step length and walking velocity increase.

Sutherland et al (1980) found that heel strike, knee flexion and reciprocal arm swing in addition to an adult pattern of joint angles, were acquired at an early age and certainly before the development of mature cadence, step length and walking velocity. Heel strike and reciprocal arm swing were found consistently 22 weeks after starting to walk. Both were established by 18 months. Compared with 1-year-olds, children in the 2-year-old group showed increased velocity and step length, and diminished cadence. The time spent in single limb stance was increased. Heel strike was more common and the ankle was dorsiflexed when heel strike took place, as opposed to the foot dragging. Most adult patterns were established by the age of 3 years, but changes in velocity and cadence continued up to the age of 7. Sutherland et al (1988) showed that the characteristics of a

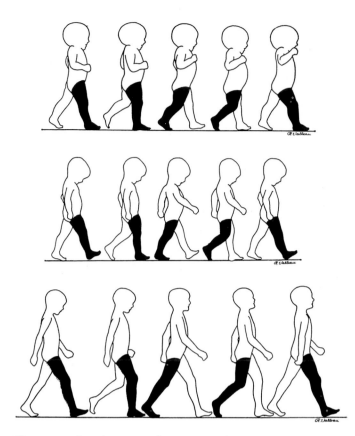

Figure 2.4 Development of a mature gait. *Top*: 1-year-old. Note the flexed elbows and lack of arm swing. The foot is plantar flexed at contact. *Middle*: 3-year-old. Arm swing is now present, as is heel strike. *Bottom*: 6-year-old. There is now an adult-type gait.

7-year-old were very similar to those of an adult. They found five significant determinants of mature gait:

1. Duration of single limb stance;
2. Walking velocity;
3. Cadence;
4. Step length;
5. Relation of pelvic span to step width.

The appearance of adult values for these parameters was the best indicator of mature gait.

On first starting to walk, many children do so on tiptoe. This is normally a fairly transient phase and they soon get down on to their heels and establish a more mature gait as described above. In a small proportion, toe walking persists. Then the concern is whether the children can simply be classified as idiopathic toe walkers or whether they have some more serious underlying condition such as cerebral palsy or Duchenne muscular dystrophy.

Hicks et al (1988) found that, in idiopathic toe walking, the main disability was increased plantar flexion at the ankles. Such children had either toe strike or flat foot at contact. Children with cerebral palsy had normal dorsiflexion at initial contact, but struck with a flat foot because the limb approached the floor with the knee bent. Even a

child with mild cerebral palsy has some hamstring tightness. Clinically, an idiopathic toe walker has a contracted heel cord and no hamstring tightness, whereas the child with cerebral palsy has the opposite. Kalen et al (1986) studied children with idiopathic toe walking and cerebral palsy. Using electromyography, they did not find any pattern that was characteristic of idiopathic toe walking. This therefore remains a clinical diagnosis.

FEET

Parents pay an enormous amount of attention to their children's feet. Many see it as one of their duties as parents that their children end up with 'good' feet. They themselves may have been treated with insoles or special shoes. They may expect the same for their children.

The focus of such attention is often the longitudinal arch. In a baby, the arch is barely perceptible as it is obscured by a fat pad. This may persist for several years. When a child first starts to walk, its broad-based gait and knock knees throw its weight onto the medial borders of the feet. A position of eversion and forefoot abduction is adopted. Once muscular control of the foot is gained (as a consequence of neurological maturation as well as lessening of ligamentous laxity with age), it usually adopts a more typically adult position. This tendency is reinforced by the resolution of genu valgum. In a normal weight-bearing child, the line of the calf and foot should be continuous (Bleck & Berzins 1974).

Up to about 5° of valgus is acceptable. This usually occurs in a hypermobile valgus foot in which loading causes the calcaneum to rotate under the talus. The anterior end of the talus then loses some of its support. It falls into a more vertical position, giving the appearance of a flat arch when the child is standing, but a normal-looking foot when it is not. Morley (1957) studied the development of the longitudinal arch from sole prints. Among children aged 2 years, she found that 97% had a flat footprint, compared with 4% at the age of 10 years. She found no difference between those who wore shoes and those who did not. Harris & Beath (1947), in their classic study in the Canadian army, found that 22% of their population had flattened longitudinal arches, most of them the result of simple depression; 2% were found to have a flattened arch secondary to peroneal spastic flat foot, and 6% had a short tendo-Achilles, associated with a hypermobile flat foot.

Staheli (1987) studied the development of the arch in children and adults. Using footprints, he measured the width of the heel and the width of the foot at the midpoint of the arch; this he termed the arch index. The arch index was therefore greater than unity when the measurement across the arch was greater than that at the heel. He used the average of both feet. For each age group, the arch index and the two standard deviations on either side were plotted. For practical purposes, there was no difference between the sexes but there was marked individual variation. The extent of this may be illustrated by the fact that, in infancy, normal values ranged from 0.7 to 1.35. This means that a child with an arch 1.3 times broader than the heel can still be considered normal. After mid-childhood, the arch index ranges from 0.3 to 1 and this is maintained through adult life. Staheli concluded that there was no evidence that flexible flat foot produced any disability. Indeed, he quoted Giladi et al (1985) as having shown that stress fractures are less common in army recruits with lower arches. It goes without saying that, if a child's measurements fall within the normal range, there is no need to modify shoes or provide any other sort of treatment. Most flat feet therefore represent biological variability.

FLAT FEET

This subject is still poorly understood. There is no doubt at all that children with apparent flat feet are still grossly overtreated. Many parents put their children into one sort of shoe or another with the express aim of trying to ensure that an 'adequate' arch develops. Why a rather flat longitudinal arch should come to be regarded as a 'bad thing' is not known. Obviously, one should decide at the outset whether this is merely a normal temporary phenomenon of childhood or, alternatively, that it represents something altogether more serious that may cause problems in adult life. If it is the former, then no treatment is required, but if the latter, preventive steps should be taken.

Children with this supposed disorder often present because of some comment that has been made by a well-wishing relative or shoe-shop assistant. Often, some pronation of the foot is mirrored in what the parents consider abnormal wear to the shoe. In more obese children, there may be pain associated with 'flat feet' from foot strain, particularly in the presence of marked genu valgum.

Examination allows division into further categories. In 'mild' flat foot, the longitudinal arch is depressed but still visible. In the 'moderate' category, the arch is not visible on standing, whereas in 'severe' cases, the arch is absent and the medial border of the foot is convex, with the head of the talus palpable on the plantar surface of the foot. When non-weight-bearing, such feet look normal (Fig. 2.5).

If the hind foot is held in inversion and dorsiflexion attempted, shortening of the tendo-Achilles may be found. Tachdjian (1990) attempted to delineate where the sag is taking place according to whether or not the arch is restored when the child stands on tip-toe, or on dorsiflexion of the big toe. Barry & Scranton (1983) suggested radiographic assessment, specifically a standing dorsoplantar view, in which the normal talo-calcaneal angle should be 15–35°, and a standing lateral view in which the talo-calcaneal angle is normally in the same range. Oblique views should be taken to exclude tarsal coalition.

Deformities from a plantar flexed talus are the most common and are the result of persistent laxity. The diagnosis of such flexible 'flat feet' is one of exclusion. Conditions to

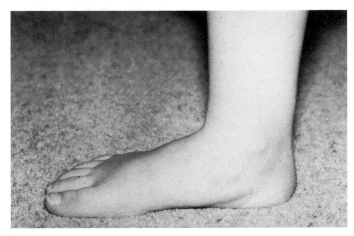

A

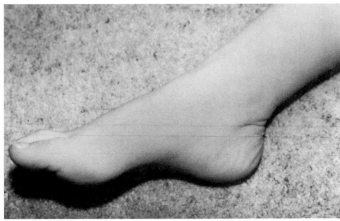

B

Figure 2.5 A flexible foot, rather than a flat foot. The arch disappears on weight bearing (**A**), but reappears when weight is removed (**B**).

be excluded include juvenile chronic arthritis and tarsal coalition, both of which are considered later. Only a small proportion of flexible 'flat feet' will persist into adult life, and only rarely will they become symptomatic.

Treatment

If a flexible foot falls within the normal range, there is obviously no need to treat it. Whilst most people would agree with that, there the agreement ends. Many forms of management have been used. Thomas heels, scaphoid cookies and heel cups are perhaps the most popular. To be effective, treatment must alter the natural history of a condition. As we have seen above, the natural history is towards resolution with age, so that any trials must compare the effect of a treated group with those who are not receiving such treatment, as they too will undoubtedly improve. Trials that merely show improvement whilst a specific treatment is being undertaken are worthless.

Wenger et al (1989) looked at a group of children, all of whom had a talo-calcaneal angle of more than 35°. These children were treated with Helfet heelcups, inserts, or corrective shoes. They found that any improvement in foot shape over the 3-year period of the trial was independent of the method of treatment used, and none had any effect on the development of the longitudinal arch. Their conclusion was that corrective shoes or inserts were of no value for typical flat feet. Staheli (1990) concurs with this opinion, concluding that it is a benign problem, unaffected by treatment.

If the apparent flattening of the foot is caused by a tight tendo-Achilles, the results from lengthening the tendon are good (Hall & Salter 1967). In the absence of such a finding, or evidence of other pathological processes, it is doubtful if any of the several operations described for this simple condition (Tachdjian 1990) is ever indicated.

SHOES

Shoes have been around for a long time – at least 10 000 years. Sandals were the most common footwear in classical times. Stewart (1972) noted atrophy on the little toe of Greek and Roman statuary and suggested that this might have been caused by its being rubbed by a sandal strap. Heels made their appearance in the 12th century. King Edward II of England was the first to introduce sizing for shoes, and did so for tax reasons. Their length was determined by barley corns, these being units of measurement of $1/3$ inch (0.85 cm). This is still the basis of shoe sizes today. Children's shoe sizes start at 3 inches (1.6 cm) and adults at 7 inches (17.78 cm).

Although almost invariably used in Western society, footwear is not absolutely necessary. Many people do without. Basically, shoes afford protection from rough surfaces and keep the feet warm. Sim-Fook & Hodgson (1958) compared the feet of groups who did and did not wear shoes. The latter lived on boats. They were found to have hypertrophy of the skin of the sole of the foot and the toenails. Most had well-developed arches. There was a tendency for the forefoot to spread between the hallux and the second toe, and it was interesting that good prehensile strength of the hallux was maintained. The conclusion was that mobility and flexibility were inversely related to the wearing of shoes. Those that wore shoes had an increased risk of developing deformities (Table 2.1).

Twenty-one percent of surveyed parents admitted buying

Table 2.1 Deformities of the feet in the shod and the unshod

	Shod (%)	Unshod (%)
Hallux valgus	33	1.9
Hallux rigidus	17	10.3
Varus 5th toe	14.4	3.7
Hammer toe	11	4.7
Flat feet	10.1	7.5

From Sim-Fook & Hodgson (1958) © The Journal of Bone and Joint Surgery.

shoes on the recommendation of their medical adviser (Staheli & Griffin 1980). Their major concern was the fit. For this reason, they replaced the shoes at 3-monthly intervals because, in 91% of cases, the children were felt to have outgrown them. Children's shoes, therefore, do not need to be expensive and long lasting. Wenger et al (1983) studied this aspect of the subject. Traditionally, children's feet are said to need a half-size bigger every 2 months up to the age of 6 years. Wenger's group found that, from 12 to 18 months, all children required at least a half-size change every 3 months, with 50% requiring a full-size change; they recommended, therefore, that children this age should be measured every 2 months. From 18 to 30 months, the average growth was half a size every 3 months; they therefore recommended that children of this age should be examined every 3 months. From the age of 21 months to 4 years, children's feet increased in length by less than half a size every 3 months and therefore remeasurement every 4 months would be adequate. Finally, between the ages of 4 and 6 years, the foot grew only one-quarter of a size every 3 months and therefore examining children of this age every 6 months was sufficient. After this age, growth of the foot reduced significantly.

It goes without saying that the shape of children's shoes should be the same as that of children's feet. Unfortunately, this is not always so. Most children have straight feet (Bleck 1971), yet many children's shoes are shaped to fit a varus forefoot. Obviously, if the shoe and the foot are different shapes, pressure and pain are the likely consequences.

There are many opinions as to what constitutes a 'good' shoe, but it should be remembered that they are based on prejudice rather than on fact. There is little evidence that expensive 'good' shoes are superior in any way to a cheap pair of trainers. Parents, however – even those who are not well off – often feel obliged to spend more than they can afford on buying what they consider to be an adequate pair of shoes for their child.

ANGULAR DEFORMITIES

Just like flat feet, angular deformities at the knee have received an inordinate amount of attention, quite out of proportion to their importance. Previously, they were considered a manifestation of more serious disease such as rickets. More recently, most have been recognised as part of normal development. Salenius & Vankka (1975) studied 979 children who were in hospital for reasons other than lower limb problems. All had radiographs taken of their knees and legs. The radiographic appearances correlated well with the clinical appearances. The angle between tibia and femur was measured on each radiograph and for each age a mean angle was established (Fig. 2.6). There was no sex difference.

The tibio-femoral angle was in marked varus in newborns and in children younger than 1 year old. After this, the legs started to straighten, and during the second and third years of life the angle changed to valgus. Between 3 and 7 years,

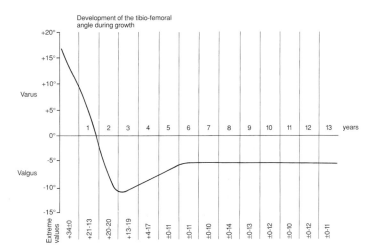

Figure 2.6 The relationship of the tibio-femoral angle with age. (From Salenius & Vankka 1975.)

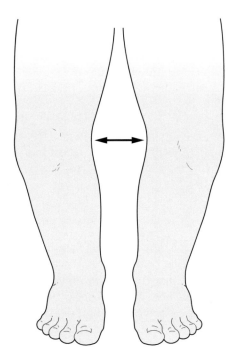

Figure 2.7 The intercondylar distance in genu varum. For accurate measurement, the medial malleoli should just touch.

valgus decreased to the normal adult value. Even if an angular deformity persists, it is not known what relationship this has with the later development of osteoarthritis of the knee (Staheli 1990).

GENU VARUM

As can be seen from Fig. 2.6, varus angulation is normal in infants, but should resolve by the age of 18–24 months. The cosmetic effect of a varus deformity in this age group is often exaggerated by the coexistence of medial tibial torsion. Often, the normal falls of the toddler stage are blamed on the existence of this combined deformity.

Clinical evaluation should include a dietary and family history; the chances of resolution are much less when there is a family history of deformity. The child's height and weight should be recorded, as these are reduced in rickets. With the child standing, the feet should be placed together, pointing forwards, and the intercondylar distance measured (Fig. 2.7). Note the location of any angulation. The torsional profile (see below) should be checked during walking. Salenius & Vankka's (1975) chart (Fig. 2.6) is the key to management. If the child deviates by more than 2 standard deviations from the mean, or if the deformity is asymmetrical, an underlying cause should be excluded. In the vast majority of cases it is not necessary to obtain a radiograph. If, however, there is a suspicion of rickets, X-rays will show the classical changes of widening of the physeal plate, loss of definition, and cupping of the metaphysis. Bone biochemistry confirms the diagnosis. Blount's disease is the other condition to be excluded. This is common in Scandinavians, Blacks and West Indians. It appears to be part of a continuum with physiological genu varum and, initially, it is impossible to tell the difference between the two.

In physiological genu varum, there is simple medial angulation of the upper one-third of the tibia and the lower end of the femur. There may also be thickening of the medial cortex of the tibia. The epiphyseal plate is normal and the deformity is usually symmetrical. In tibia vara or Blount's disease, the proximal tibial metaphysis is fragmented medially. The proximal shaft remains almost straight, but there is sharp angulation of the medial cortex. The lateral half of the cortex of the tibia remains straight, whereas the medial side angulates sharply. In physiological genu varum, both sides angulate gently.

Traditionally, the tibio-femoral angle has been measured to assess the amount of deformity. Levine & Drennan (1982) felt, however, that this reflected only the deformity at the knee of the involved extremity, and they suggested instead the use of the metaphyseal-diaphyseal angle, which more accurately depicts the angulation of the proximal part of the tibia where, as we have seen, the most severe deformity in tibia vara is located. They studied 58 extremities with a metaphyseal-diaphyseal angle of less than 11°. Only three of these children subsequently developed tibia vara at follow-up. Of 30 that had an angle greater than 11°, 29 subsequently developed the condition.

Treatment

The use of splints to treat angular deformities has long been practised. Takatori & Iwaya (1984) demonstrated an effect from splintage, and felt that some of their patients might otherwise have developed significant tibia vara. There is no doubt, however, that in the vast majority of these deformities no treatment is required.

The aim of management is to rule out serious causes of angulation. The parents should then be assured that the 'deformity' is normal and will correct with growth. It is worthwhile warning that some children will later develop knock knees. The familial type, however, is less likely to correct and, if severe, a very small proportion may require surgical correction. Some surgeons feel that, if pronounced angular deformity is present after the age of 10 years, surgical treatment is the only option, because spontaneous correction will not occur. Vankka & Salenius (1982), however, showed that, even at this late age, it often does. If Blount's disease is diagnosed in the younger patient, bracing may lead to improvement. Corrective osteotomy may still be required on one or more occasions, particularly in the older child (McDade 1977).

GENU VALGUM

This condition, also, is now appreciated to be usually physiological. From observation, most knock knees tend to correct spontaneously (Salenius & Vankka 1975). Howorth (1971) found a racial difference, in that knock knees were seldom found in the Japanese, whereas bow legs were common. Similar findings have been described in Eskimos. Between the ages of 2 and 6 years, up to 15° of valgus is commonly found. This is usually, but not always, symmetrical. If the deformity is marked, the child walks with the knees rubbing together and the feet pronated. Affected children seldom run well, always looking rather awkward. Pain in the calf and anterior thigh is common. If there is a severe deformity, patellar subluxation may develop.

Clinically the deformity is best recorded by asking the child to stand with the knees together and the feet pointing forwards. The intermalleolar distance is then measured (Fig. 2.8). Morley (1957) studied this measurement in 1000 children of various ages. She found that it increased up to the age of 3½ years and then declined. Between the ages of 3 and

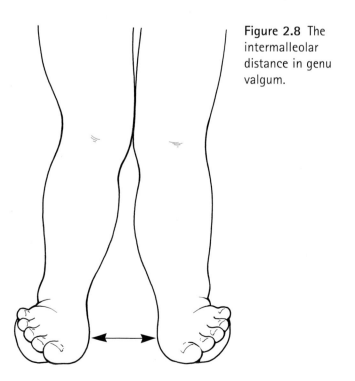

Figure 2.8 The intermalleolar distance in genu valgum.

3½ years, 52% of children had between 2.5 and 5 cm between the malleoli, and 22% had more than 5 cm. The mean weight of children with knock knees was greater than those without. Morley felt that, in children younger than 7 years, genu valgum could be safely ignored unless severe or asymmetrical, in agreement with Salenius & Vankka (1975).

In the past, even physiological valgus has been treated quite actively. The methods ranged from splintage to horse-riding, depending on the social status of the patient. If it is present between the ages of 2 and 6 years, 95% of cases will correct and no treatment is required. During this time, however, particularly if the child is obese, symptoms of foot strain may develop and can be lessened by shoe wedges.

Even when genu valgum is asymmetrical and pathological, the natural history is towards resolution. The child depicted in Fig. 2.9 sustained a proximal metaphyseal fracture of the right tibia and, as a consequence, developed a unilateral valgus deformity (Fig. 2.9A). One year later, it was lessening (Fig. 2.9B), and by 2 years the valgus was symmetrical (Fig. 2.9C).

Tachdjian (1990) recommended a knee–ankle–foot orthosis with knock-knee pads and thigh and calf cuffs. He admitted, however, that there is no documentary evidence that this corrects the deformity. If the condition persists into adolescence, the pressure to intervene becomes greater. Affected children seldom run well. They may well have patello-femoral problems. Should correction be undertaken? The worry is that malalignment may lead to premature degenerative changes, the hypothesis being that shear stresses caused by the angular deformity cause cartilage breakdown. This is questionable. Dietz & Merchant (1990) found no evidence to suggest that this occurs. They studied a group of adults who had sustained limb fractures up to 30 years previously. All had healed in varying degrees of varus or valgus deformity. At follow-up, no relationship was found between the amount of deformity, its direction, and the presence of osteoarthritic changes.

In the past stapling of the growth plate has been used to correct the deformity, but because the amount of correction obtained may be unpredictable, it is now less widely used. There are various recommendations for osteotomy. Griffin (1986) felt that surgery should at least be considered if the deformity is more than 15–20°. The angulation should be corrected at the site of the deformity, and in most cases this will be at the distal femur.

Steel et al (1971) stressed the complications of proximal tibial osteotomy. These operations have to be done rather more distally in children than in adults, to avoid damage to the physis. At this level, the risk of vascular complications is greater, because it is here that the anterior tibial artery penetrates the interosseous membrane. In 46 operations (25 for valgus and 21 for varus), nine children developed complications, including loss of sensation on the dorsum of the foot, pain and impaired circulation. Although most of these complications resolved by moving the divided bone back to its original position, some were left with permanent sequelae.

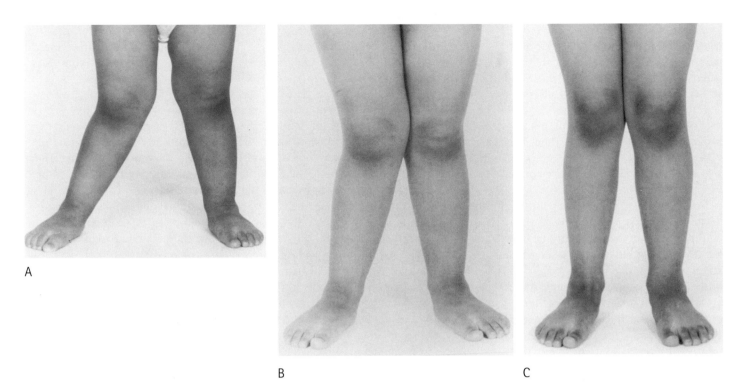

Figure 2.9 Natural resolution of unilateral valgus deformity. **A** Initial deformity, resulting from proximal metaphyseal fracture of the right tibia. **B** Improvement 1 year later. **C** Symmetry regained after 2 years.

TORSION

Torsion is the twisting of a long bone on its longitudinal axis. For practical purposes, it is only of importance in the lower limbs. In itself, it is of little importance, but it assumes greater significance because it is so common; indeed, it is the most common problem in childhood that is seen by orthopaedic surgeons. The children present because of the effect torsion has on the gait. Scrutton (1968) found that 18% of an unselected group of children walked with an in-toed gait. Hutter & Scott (1949) found that 30% of 2–3-year-old children intoed, usually as a result of internal tibial torsion; the prevalence was 8–10% in the 5–7-year age group, and 8–9% in adolescents. The range of normal is wide.

A torsional deformity is said to be present if it is more than 2 standard deviations from the mean. Some abnormalities are flexible and secondary to the intrauterine position (e.g. metatarsus varus or tibial torsion), whereas others are hereditary. They occur in otherwise normal children. Most resolve spontaneously and do not lead to long-term disability, but a small proportion persist and in such cases treatment may be required.

Aetiology

Heredity

Femoral torsion can certainly be familial and may be a dominant trait, although the exact mode of inheritance is unclear. In contrast, tibial torsion is more likely to be acquired. If applied continuously and for long enough, abnormal pressure can alter the shape of a bone. *In utero*, the hips are flexed and laterally rotated, resulting in more lateral than medial rotation. The legs and feet are medially rotated. Spontaneous resolution usually occurs. Habitual sleeping or sitting positions may, however, interfere with this process of natural resolution, i.e. some positions may cause the fetal limb rotation to persist or, indeed, to become more severe, rather than resolve. However, children may also adopt the positions that are associated with persistent torsion, such as the 'W' position, because they are comfortable.

The effect of external pressure on bones has been well described. Katz et al (1990) found that the rate and direction of the growth of a physis could be modified by stress. Appleton (1934) showed that, by dividing certain muscles and thus altering the stress, the shape of a bone could be altered. The deformity produced is predictable.

Clinically, we know that abductor weakness at the hip leads to a valgus deformity. Wilkinson (1962) produced femoral anteversion in rabbits by keeping the hip internally rotated; lateral rotation produced retroversion. Moreland (1980) felt that such rotations occurred across the epiphyseal plate, and that there was none in the metaphyseal or diaphyseal regions. There is, of course a limit to the alteration in shape that can occur in a bone. The basic shape is genetically determined, as indicated by the fact that a bone grown in tissue culture will still grow into a recognizable shape, in spite of the fact that it is free from external forces other than gravity.

Evaluation

In spite of the availability of imaging techniques such as computed tomography, clinical examination still provides the basis for management of these conditions. Its purpose is to localise the deformity and assess its magnitude.

The most useful tool in this respect is the *torsional profile* described by Staheli et al (1985). It allows localisation of any torsional deformity of the foot, leg, or thigh, so that a distinction may be made between a simple deformity affecting one bone, and a more complex one affecting more than one segment.

Staheli et al (1985) considered that children falling within 2 standard deviations of the mean for rotational variation could be considered as having torsional *problems* and to be within the normal range, whereas those falling outside 2 standard deviations were considered to have torsional *deformities*. They performed a study of 1000 normal limbs in a group ranging in age from less than 1 year to 70 years. They divided them up into 22 groups. Those aged between 1 and 14 years were considered at yearly intervals. The foot-progression angle, hip rotation, thigh-foot angle and the angle of the trans-malleolar axis were measured. Medial rotation of the hip was found to be significantly different between males and females, but otherwise there was no sex difference.

Foot-progression angle

The foot-progression angle (Fig. 2.10) is the angle that the feet make with the line of progression. Most children younger than 4 years have a few degrees of in-toeing, and most adults toe-out a little. The mean value is +10°, with a range of −3° to +20°.

The other parts of the torsional profile must, of course, be taken into account. If there is medial femoral torsion, for example, the gait angle or foot-progression angle may be either negative or positive. The latter occurs if there is compensatory external tibial torsion. The foot-progression angle is most variable in infancy. Adult values are achieved in early childhood.

Hip rotation

There appears to be a fairly close relationship between the range of hip rotation (Fig. 2.11) measured clinically and anteversion measured radiographically (Staheli et al 1985). Hip rotation is best measured with the child in the prone position. The knees are flexed to 90°, and the thighs rotated until resistance is felt. External rotation of the hip to 90° is common in infancy but, steadily reduces up to the age of 3 years. After that, internal rotation is slightly more than external (Engel & Staheli 1974). Total rotatory excursion of the hip is 120° up to the age of 2 years, and then decreases to 95–110° in later childhood. Medial rotation ranges from 15–60° in girls and from 15–65° in boys, whereas lateral rotation measures 25–65° in both sexes.

A torsional abnormality is said to be present if lateral rotation is less than 20°. It is classified as *mild* if medial rotation is 70–80° and lateral is between 10° and 20°, *moderate* if the internal rotation is 80–90° and lateral less than 10°, and *severe* if medial rotation is more than 90° and no external rotation is possible.

Thigh-foot angle

With the child in the same position as for measurement of hip rotation (prone with the knees flexed to 90°), for measurement of thigh-foot-angle (Fig. 2.12) light pressure is applied to the sole of the foot to bring the ankle up to neutral. The angle made by a line along the foot with a line along the thigh (this can be judged by looking down from above) is known as the thigh-foot angle. This is taken to be a measure of tibial torsion. A positive value denotes external rotation and a negative figure indicates internal torsion. The mean is around +10°. In this position, the sole

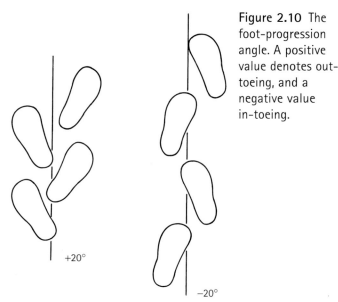

Figure 2.10 The foot-progression angle. A positive value denotes out-toeing, and a negative value in-toeing.

+20°

−20°

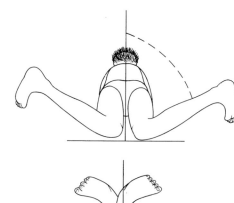
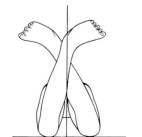

Figure 2.11 Hip rotation measured prone (top is internal rotation and bottom external).

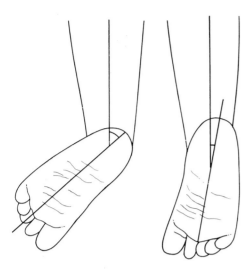

Figure 2.12 The thigh-foot angle.

of the foot can also be inspected to exclude metatarsus adductus.

The transmalleolar axis also gives a measure of tibial torsion. The values correspond roughly to the thigh-foot angle, but under certain conditions may differ. This axis can be measured with the child prone. A line joining the tips of the medial and lateral malleoli is drawn across the heel. A second line is then drawn perpendicular to this, and the angle between this line and the angle of the thigh is equivalent to the transmalleolar axis. Alternatively, it can be estimated with the child sitting over the edge of a couch or table with the thigh perpendicular to the edge. The tips of the lateral and medial malleoli are palpated. A goniometer is then pressed next to the edge of the couch and its arm swivelled until it is parallel to the line joining the tips of the malleoli. The transmalleolar axis can then be read off the goniometer.

Luchini & Stevens (1983) studied the accuracy of the torsional profile. They asked eight examiners to study seven patients twice each. The average age of the patients was 21.1 months (range 14–30 months). The ranges of error in these examinations were collated. The investigators concluded that, to be of significance, the foot-progression angle should change by at least 7°; less than this may merely be attributable to inter-observer error. Similarly, the thigh-foot angle would have to change by 25°.

TIBIAL TORSION

Tibial torsion is defined as the twist in the tibia as measured by the angle formed by the coronal planes constructed through the longitudinal axes of the proximal and distal tibial articular surfaces (Bleck & Minaire 1983). The proximal line bisects the articular surface of the tibia and the distal axis bisects the malleolus and the lateral aspect of the distal tibial articular surface.

Natural history

The natural history of tibial torsion has been intensively studied. Staheli & Engel (1972) found that there is a gradual change from internal to external torsion with age. Hermosh et al (1971) found that this change averaged 1.3° per year, although the rate of change was not uniform.

Internal torsion appears to be due to intrauterine position. Katz et al (1990) studied 104 infants with a birth weight of less than 1500 g and a gestational age of between 24 and 36 weeks. Torsion was measured by the thigh-foot angle. Medial tibial torsion was deemed to be present if this measured −5° or less.

Using this criterion, medial tibial torsion was found in 1.9% of the study population. Metatarsus adductus was present in 1.4%. Only one of the children found with internal tibial torsion had a gestational age of less than 30 weeks. In 92% of preterm children with a gestational age of 31–36 weeks, there was an average of 15° of medial torsion. In those with a gestational age less than 31 weeks, however, the average thigh-foot angle was 25°. This study would appear to support the view that postural deformities tend to occur in the later weeks of pregnancy, and that internal tibial torsion is not found in the younger age group. This can be explained on the basis of Wilkinson's observations (1985). In the later weeks of pregnancy, the feet are in plantar flexion and internally rotated, such that there is a medial torsional force on the tibia. Before this, the ankles are dorsiflexed and everted.

At birth, the medial malleolus is usually found to be behind the lateral malleolus. When the child starts to walk the tips are level and later, when walking is fully established, the medial is in front of the lateral. Merrill et al (1976) felt that torsion was part of normal infant development. They found that, at birth, there was a mean of 4° external torsion (range −5° to +25°). At 6 months the mean was 6° (range 0–12°), at 12 months it was 10° (range 6–25°) and at 24 months, 11°. No sex or racial differences were found. Negative values were much more common in younger children. From another approach, Hutter & Scott (1949) found, that in the second year of life, 30% of children walked with an in-toed gait. Between the ages of 5 and 7 years, 10% of boys and 8.5% of girls were found to have internal tibial torsion. There seems to be little spontaneous correction after the age of 8 years. There is some racial difference, in that internal tibial torsion is common in the Japanese community who habitually sit on the floor with their feet tucked under them.

The difference between the sexes is not marked, although the reaction to the deformity may be. Five percent of women have internal tibial torsion that, in 2%, is severe enough to give problems with walking; 3% of males are said to have torsion and in around 1% it is severe enough to give rise to psychological problems.

Bleck & Minaire (1983) drew attention to the presence of a group who had an in-toeing gait but no internal tibial torsion. They ascribed this to medial deviation of the talar neck. Merrill et al (1976) were of the same opinion. In a dissection of an affected stillborn, they found medial deviation of the talar neck such that the foot was internally rotated with respect to the transmalleolar axis and that in-toeing was possible, even when the transmalleolar axis was neutral or, indeed, externally rotated. Bleck & Minaire (1983) pointed out that at the 25 mm stage, medial deviation of the talar neck is 20°. This increases to between 20° and 40° at birth. In most, the axial deviation of the foot that this produces resolves spontaneously. Lateral torsion is usually acquired, most commonly as a compensatory mechanism for internal femoral torsion.

Long-term effects

Turner & Smillie (1981) studied 1200 consecutive patients in a knee clinic. All had their tibial torsion measured, as did 137 controls with no known knee pathology. Only those (836) who fell into known diagnostic categories were considered further. In the control group, the average lateral torsion was 19° (±4.8°). Among the patients, 84% fell in the normal range between 15° and 25° with only 12% below and 4% above. There were three groups outside that range. Those with unstable patello-femoral joints had, on average, more than 24.5° external torsion. More than 50% were above the normal range. Among those with Osgood–Schlatter's disease, 47% were also above the normal range. In the presence of panarticular disease, 64% were below the normal range, but when the disease was unicompartmental most had normal values. Turner & Smillie concluded that internal tibial torsion increases the risk of the later development of osteoarthritis.

Treatment

In the vast majority of children, medial tibial torsion will resolve spontaneously. Such children have long been treated (quite unnecessarily) with various devices such as Denis Browne splints. These merely force the foot into abduction and cause genu valgum. Indeed, it might be that the early correction associated with the use of a Denis Browne splint is due to rotation taking place through the ankle joint. There is really no evidence that non-operative treatment alters the outcome. Shoes are ineffective, and night splinting is of unproven value. As pointed out above, the tibia normally rotates laterally with time. External rotation, therefore, may get worse rather than better. Griffin (1986) claimed that it may lead to biomechanical problems by increasing stresses on the feet, reducing the ability to run. This remains unproven.

Various suggestions as to the indications for surgery have been put forward. These include a family history, lack of spontaneous correction, torsion exceeding 40°, or torsion in a child older than 8 years of age with a thigh-foot angle more than 3 standard deviations beyond the mean (medial torsion more than 15° or lateral torsion more than 30°). In all these groups, supramalleolar osteotomy has been advocated, but is not universally accepted. High tibial osteotomy is never indicated, because it is associated with a significant complication rate.

FEMORAL TORSION

Femoral torsion may be defined as the inclination of the axis of the femoral neck with reference to the transcondylar plane of the femur. Because of the intrauterine position, there may be as much as 60° anteversion during fetal development. At birth, it measures around 40°, and it gradually declines to an adult value of around 10°. Values for females are about 5° greater.

Measurement

Clinical

The basic premise of clinical assessment is that the range of rotation of the hip can be correlated with the amount of anteversion of the femur, increased medial rotation indicating increased anteversion. This is considered below. Anteversion can also be measured by palpating the midpoint of the greater trochanter, then rotating the limb until that point is at its most lateral position. The degree of rotation of the femoral condylar plane is noted, and this is the angle of anteversion. It is, of course, somewhat inaccurate.

Ultrasound

Phillips et al (1985) felt that the most commonly used radiographic methods had the drawback of excessive radiographic exposure. They found that ultrasound was a reasonable alternative and was accurate up to around 40°, after which it became increasingly inaccurate. However, other methods (Dunn 1952) have similar problems and have to be adjusted at higher levels. Using ultrasound, Moulton & Upadhyay (1982) found the average anteversion value was around 8° in adults and tended to be symmetrical. Anteversion was markedly increased on the affected side when in-toeing had been present in childhood. They suggested that the ultrasound technique could be used to screen patients, and that other methods could then be used in the presence of high values.

Radiographic

These methods are all similar, and share the same essential features in that the neck-shaft angle is measured on an anteroposterior film. A frame is then used to position the hips for the lateral view, in about 90° of flexion and 10–30° of abduction. Graphs provide a calculation of the true from the apparent angle obtained (Dunn 1952, Fabry et al 1973). The values obtained have been very useful in establishing the natural history of the condition. Fabry et al (1973) found the average to be 32° at the age of 1 year and 16° at the age of 16 years. Interestingly, in their study they found that, when internal rotation exceeded external rotation, abnormal torsion was present. There was no change in anteversion after the age of 8 years.

Computed tomography scanning

This is now the method of choice. The values obtained by this method correlate well with those measured by either bipolar radiography or ultrasound. The method obviously exposes the child to a significant amount of radiation, but allows a direct and accurate measurement to be made. Indeed, where there is limitation of movement at the hip, it may be the only practicable way of obtaining a measurement. However, it should not be used routinely, but only for those in whom surgical correction is being considered.

Clinical diagnosis

In children aged between 3 and 12 years, abnormal femoral anteversion is the most common cause of in-toeing. It is usually bilateral and symmetrical, and affects twice as many females as males. On looking at the legs it will be obvious that, when the child stands with the feet together, the patellae point inwards (Fig. 2.13). The torsion may be diagnosed by examination of the range of rotation of the hips. Increased internal rotation and decreased external is the rule. Paradoxically, anteversion is at its maximum at birth and gradually decreases with time. The in-toeing associated with femoral torsion, however, is not seen until the age of 3 years. This is because, although anteversion is at its maximum at an early age, it is not clinically evident, as it is masked by the fixed external rotation normally found in infants. This is a consequence of capsular and soft-tissue contractures. Standing provides the stimulus to rotate the hips internally.

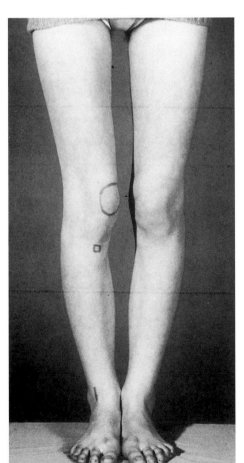

Figure 2.13
Internal femoral and compensatory external tibial torsion. The patella, the tibial tubercle, and the midpoint between the malleoli are all marked on the skin.

McSweeney (1971) found that 13.6% of normal children in-toed, two-thirds because of internal femoral torsion. They tend to be brought to medical attention for cosmetic reasons in girls and because of supposed loss of athletic activity in boys. Tachdjian (1990) has pointed out that, while the hip is extended, no external rotation may be possible, but once flexed, lateral rotation to 45° may be possible. Soft-tissue tension plays a role. Gelberman et al (1987) studied the changes in rotation of the hip in different positions in a number of children. Two groups were studied: those with more internal than external rotation in flexion, and *vice versa*. The first group had a mean anteversion angle of 49°, compared with one of 32° in the latter group. In the control group, there was approximately equal internal and external rotation in flexion and extension. The investigators felt that rotation in extension did not correlate well with measured anteversion. In those patients with more than 70° of internal rotation in extension, the amount of anteversion ranged from 22° to 66°. These findings suggest that there are reasons for limitation of rotation other than anteversion. Of those children with excessive internal rotation in extension, one-third did not have increased anteversion or acetabular malrotation to account for the toe-in gait. In these children, the gait abnormality may be caused by a tight anterior capsule and soft tissues: the capsule is tight in extension and relaxed in flexion. The increase in the range of rotation in flexion supports this view. An abnormal amount of anteversion can be inferred clinically only when there is more internal than external rotation of the hips in both extension and flexion.

Natural history

Although the clinical syndrome of in-toeing usually improves spontaneously, this often occurs without any concomitant change in the amount of anteversion. Such improvement is probably due to stretching of the capsule and soft tissues around the hip, although in some cases it may be explained by the development of compensatory external tibial torsion. McSweeney (1971) found that, of those who ceased to toe-in, only one-third had normal femoral anteversion angles, whereas one-third of those who had no spontaneous improvement had normal angles of anteversion. He suggested that this might be explained by some alteration in the inclination of the acetabulum. All are agreed that the deformity is relatively common and tends to resolve before adolescence. Hosby et al (1987) performed femoral osteotomies in cats, producing internal or external rotation of 25°; the other femur was used as a control. Anteversion was measured radiographically before the operation and 58 weeks after the operation. As the bone grew, the amount of rotation gradually reduced and tended to return to that of the control side.

What of the long-term effect on function? Staheli (1990) has shown that there is no relationship between anteversion and athletic performance. Hubbard et al (1988) studied its association with the later development of osteoarthritis. This has, of course, been one of the reasons put forward in favour of correcting the deformity in childhood. They used two groups – those with osteoarthritis, and a control group with normal hips; no difference was found. They concluded that anteversion does not lead to the later development of osteoarthritis. They also questioned the validity of other studies that purport to show the opposite, mainly because they had used the opposite 'normal' hip as a control.

Treatment

The only treatment usually required is observation and reassurance. In the vast majority of cases, the deformity corrects by the age of 7 or 8 years. There is no need for radiography during this time. It is unlikely that posture has any effect on the long-term outcome, and the sitting position of these children is more likely to be the effect, rather than the cause; altering the way the child sits has little effect. Non-operative methods of treatment are no better than doing nothing. Thus Fabry et al (1973) showed that twister cables and Denis Browne splints were ineffectual, and Knittle & Staheli (1976) showed the same with shoe wedges.

The only method that is proven to be effective is femoral osteotomy. The indications are variable. Fabry et al (1973) felt that a child aged more than 8 years with a measured anteversion of more than 50°, medial rotation of more than 85° and lateral of less than 10° might require osteotomy. Kling & Hensinger (1983) suggested osteotomy for children in whom there was significant functional or cosmetic disability in the presence of proven anteversion in excess of 40°. External tibial torsion of more than 35° is a relative contraindication.

Tachdjian (1990) recommends that the child should be seen for at least 2 years before operation, to see if any spontaneous improvement is taking place. The function or appearance should be such that the parents or child demand that something be done. A collapsing gait secondary to inward rotation of the knees or persisting groin pain are relative indications for the operation.

The aim of the procedure is to provide equal internal and external rotation. Whilst this is usually achieved, the operation is not without problems. Fonseca & Bassett (1988) studied 14 patients who had undergone derotation osteotomies. In two, a progressive valgus deformity developed postoperatively. Staheli et al (1980) examined the results of 146 osteotomies, all but 16 performed at the subtrochanteric level. There were significant complications in 15%, two had loss of fixation and needed replating, there were errors in the amount of rotation in three, one developed a heel ulcer, one an infection, and three femurs fractured. At follow-up, all these patients walked with the foot in external rotation and most had symmetric hip rotation. Anteversion measured within normal limits. The operation is thus effective, but not without complications. Sveningsen et al (1990) performed subtrochanteric osteotomy for anteversion in 52 patients. In 17, the outcome was some retroversion, and there was little tendency for this to correct spontaneously if it exceeded 10°. Gait was then likely to be impaired and to be cosmetically unacceptable. Leg length inequality may also result from unilateral derotation procedures if the neck-shaft angle is allowed to alter or from overgrowth.

REFERENCES

Anderson M, Green W, Mesner M 1963 Growth predictions of growth of the lower extremities. Journal of Bone and Joint Surgery 45A: 1–14

Appleton A B 1934 Positional deformities and bone growth: an experimental study. Lancet 1: 451–454

Barry R, Scranton R 1983 Flat feet in children. Clinical Orthopaedics and Related Research 181: 68–75

Baxter A, Dulberg C 1988 'Growing pains' in childhood. Journal of Pediatric Orthopaedics 8: 402–406

Bleck E E 1971 The shoeing of children; sham or sciences? Developmental Medicine and Child Neurology 13: 188–191

Bleck E, Berzins U 1974 Conservative management of pes valgus with plantar flexed talus, flexible. Clinical Orthopaedics and Related Research 122: 85–94

Bleck E, Minaire P 1983 Persistent medial deviation of the neck of the talus: a common cause of intoeing in children. Journal of Pediatric Orthopaedics 3: 149–159

Brighton C 1983 The femoral capital growth plate. In: Katz J, Siffert R (eds) Management of hip disorders in children. J Lippincott, Philadelphia

Craxford A, Minns R J, Park C 1984 Plantar pressures and gait parameters; a study of foot shape and limb rotation in children. Journal of Pediatric Orthopaedics 4: 477–481

Dietz F R, Merchant J C 1990 Indications for osteotomy of the tibia in children. Journal of Pediatric Orthopaedics 10: 486–490

Dunn D M 1952 Anteversion of the neck of the femur. Journal of Bone and Joint Surgery 34B: 181–186

Engel G M, Staheli L T 1974 The natural history of torsion and other factors influencing gait in childhood. Clinical Orthopaedics and Related Research 99: 12–17

Fabry G, McEwan G, Shands A 1973 Torsion of the femur; a follow up study in normal and abnormal conditions. Journal of Bone and Joint Surgery 55A: 1726–1738

Fonseca A, Bassett G 1988 Valgus deformity following derotation osteotomies to correct medial femoral torsion. Journal of Pediatric Orthopaedics 8: 295–299

Gelberman R, Cohen M, Desai S, Griffin P, Saloman P, O'Brien T 1987 Femoral anteversion. Journal of Bone and Joint Surgery 69B: 75–79

Giladi M, Milgram C, Stein M et al 1985 The low arch: a protective factor in stress fractures. Orthopedic Review 14: 81–84

Greulich W W, Pyle S I 1950 Radiographic atlas of skeletal development of the hand and wrist. Oxford University Press, Oxford

Griffin P 1986 Tibial torsion. In: Lovell W, Winter R B (eds) Pediatric orthopedics. J B Lippincott, Philadelphia

Hall J, Salter R B 1967 Congenital short tendo Achilles. Journal of Bone and Joint Surgery 49B: 695–697

Harris R I, Beath T 1947 Army foot survey: an investigation of foot ailments in Canadian soldiers. National Research Council of Canada, Ottawa

Hermosh O K, Lior G, Weismann S 1971 Tibial torsion in children. Clinical Orthopaedics and Related Research 79: 25–31

Hicks R, Durinick N, Gage J 1988 Differentiation of idiopathic toe walking and cerebral palsy. Journal of Pediatric Orthopaedics 8: 160–163

Hosby O S, Sudmann B, Gjerdet N R, Hitland S, Sudmann E 1987 Spontaneous correction of femoral torsion in diaphyseal osteotomies studied in kittens. Acta Orthopaedica Scandinavica 58: 113–118

Howorth B 1971 Knock knees. Clinical Orthopaedics and Related Research 77: 233–246

Hubbard D D, Staheli L, Chew D, Musca V S 1988 Medial femoral torsion and osteoarthritis. Journal of Pediatric Orthopaedics 8: 540–542

Hutter C, Scott W 1949 Tibial torsion. Journal of Bone and Joint Surgery 31A: 511–518

Kalen V, Alder N, Bleck E 1986 Electromyography of idiopathic toe walking. Journal of Pediatric Orthopaedics 6: 31–33

Katz K, Naor N, Merlob P, Weilunsky E 1990 Rotational deformities of the tibia and foot in preterm infants. Journal of Pediatric Orthopaedics 10: 483–485

Kling T F, Hensinger R N 1983 Angular and torsional deformities of the limbs in children. Clinical Orthopaedics and Related Research 186: 136–142

Knittle G, Staheli L 1976 The effectiveness of shoe modifications for intoeing. Orthopedic Clinics of North America 7: 1019–1025

Levine A, Drennan J 1982 Physiological bowing and tibia vara. Journal of Bone and Joint Surgery 64A: 1158–1163

Luchini M, Stevens D B 1983 Validity of the torsional profile. Journal of Pediatric Orthopaedics 3: 41–44

McDade W 1977 Bow legs and knock kness. Pediatric Clinics of North America 24: 825–839

McSweeney A 1971 A study of femoral torsion in children. Journal of Bone and Joint Surgery 53B: 90–95

Menelaus M B 1966 Correction of leg length discrepancy by epiphyseal arrest. Journal of Bone and Joint Surgery 48B: 336–339

Merrill A, Ritter G, De Rose P, Babcock J 1976 Tibial torsion. Clinical Orthopaedics and Related Research 120: 159–163

Moreland M 1980 Morphological effects of torsion applied to growing bones. Journal of Bone and Joint Surgery 62B: 230–237

Morley J 1957 Knock knees in children. British Medical Journal 2: 976–977

Moseley C 1996 Growth. In: Morrissy R, Weinstein S (eds) Lovell and Winter's pediatric orthopaedics. J B Lippincott, Philadelphia

Moulton A, Upadhyay S 1982 A direct method of measuring femoral anteversion using ultrasound. Journal of Bone and Joint Surgery 62B: 230–237

Naish J M, Apley J 1951 Growing pains – a clinical study of nonarthritic limb pains in children. Archives of Disease in Childhood 26: 134–140

Oster J, Neilson A 1972 Growing pains. Acta Paediatrica Scandinavica 61: 329–334

Peterson H 1977 Leg aches. Pediatric Clinics of North America 24: 731–736

Phillips H, Green W, Guilford B et al 1985 Measurements of femoral torsion: comparison of standard roentgenographic techniques with ultrasound. Journal of Pediatric Orthopaedics 5: 546–549

Roberts A P, Conner A N 1987 Referrals to a children's orthopaedic clinic. Health Bulletin 45: 174–178

Salenius P, Vankka E 1975 The development of the tibiofemoral angle in children. Journal of Bone and Joint Surgery 57A: 259–261

Scrutton R 1968 The gait of fifty normal children. Physiotherapy 54: 363–368

Sim-Fook L, Hodgson A R 1958 A comparison of foot forms among the non shoe and shoe wearing Chinese populations. Journal of Bone and Joint Surgery 40A: 1058–1062

Staheli L 1987 The longitudinal arches. Journal of Bone and Joint Surgery 69A: 426–428

Staheli L 1990 Lower positional deformity in infants and children: a review. Journal of Pediatric Orthopaedics 10: 559–563

Staheli L, Engel G 1972 Tibial torsion. Clinical Orthopaedics and Related Research 86: 183–186

Staheli L, Griffin L 1980 Corrective shoes for children. A survey of current practice. Pediatrics 65: 13–17

Staheli L, Clawson D K, Hubbard D P 1980 Medial femoral torsion: experience with operative treatment. Clinical Orthopaedics and Related Research 146: 222–225

Staheli L, Corbett C, Wyss C, King H 1985 Lower extremity rotational problems in children. Journal of Bone and Joint Surgery 67A: 39–47

Statham L, Murray M P 1971 Early walking patterns of children. Clinical Orthopaedics and Related Research 79: 8–24

Steel H H, Sandrou R, Sullivan P 1971 Complications of tibial osteotomy in children for genu valgum or varus. Journal of Bone and Joint Surgery 53A: 1629–1635

Stewart S 1972 Footgear – its history, uses and abuses. Clinical Orthopaedics and Related Research 88: 119–130

Sutherland D, Olshen R, Cooper L, Woo S 1980 The development of mature gait. Journal of Bone and Joint Surgery 62A: 336–353

Sutherland D, Olshen R, Biden E, Wyatt M 1988 The development of mature walking. McKeith Press, Oxford

Sveningsen S, Terjessen T, Apalset K, Anda S 1990 Osteotomy for femoral anteversion. Acta Orthopaedica Scandinavica 61: 360–363

Tachdjian M O 1990 Pediatric orthopedics. W B Saunders, Philadelphia

Takatori Y, Iwaya T 1984 Orthotic management of severe genu varum and tibia vara. Journal of Pediatric Orthopaedics 4: 633–635

Tanner J M, Whitehouse R M, Marshall W, Healey M, Goldstein H 1975 Assessment of skeletal maturity and prediction of adult height (TW2 method). Academic Press, London

Turner M S, Smillie I S 1981 The effect of tibial torsion on the pathology of the knee. Journal of Bone and Joint Surgery 63B: 396–398

Vankka E, Salenius P 1982 Spontaneous correction of severe tibiofemoral deformity in growing children. Acta Orthopaedica Scandinavica 53: 567–570

Wenger D, Mauldin D, Morgan D, Sobol M, Pennebaker M, Thaler R 1983 Foot growth rate in children after the age of six. Foot and Ankle 3: 207–210

Wenger D, Mauldin D, Speck G, Morgan D, Leiber R 1989 Corrective shoes and inserts as treatment for flexible flat feet in infants and children. Journal of Bone and Joint Surgery 71A: 800–810

Wilkinson J A 1962 Femoral anteversion in the rabbit. Journal of Bone and Joint Surgery 44B: 386–397

Wilkinson J A 1985 Congenital displacement of the hip joint. Springer Verlag, Berlin

Chapter 3

The disabled child in society

G. M. Cochrane

INTRODUCTION

The Office of Population Censuses and Surveys (1989) reports of disability (Bone & Meltser 1989) showed that 3% of Britain's 11.3 million children younger than 16 years of age have disabilities. The prevalence rates at all levels of severity were greater for boys than for girls: 56 per 1000 compared with 37 per 1000. The large majority of disabled children live at home; only 1.5% – a tiny proportion of the 34 000 most severely disabled – live in communal establishments.

The causes, nature and severities of chronically disabling diseases change. Progress in housing, sanitation, nutrition and preventive and curative medicine have brought immeasurable gains; more will come as the incidence of inherited disorders, for which at present there is no cure, will be reduced as a result of the identification of specific gene defects. Formerly, most profoundly disabled children with severe brain damage, metabolic disorders and malformation syndromes died early in childhood. Currently, through intensive medical and surgical treatment, the median survival of the most severely disabled children with cerebral palsy is 30 years. Children with Down's syndrome have a long life expectancy because chest infections are cleared promptly and heart disease is usually treated surgically. The prognosis for children with cystic fibrosis, the most common lethal genetic disease in the white population, has steadily improved to a median survival of more than 20 years, thanks to dietary supplements of pancreatin, vitamins and adequate calorie intake, twice daily chest physiotherapy and prompt control of pulmonary infections.

Changes in the behaviour of society bring new disasters to children: conspicuously, major trauma caused by high-speed transport, abuse of fire arms, armed conflicts and local total war. Economic collapse in eastern Europe has caused the reappearance of 'poverty diseases' in children (malnutrition, diphtheria, tuberculosis and poliomyelitis) and in their families (human immunodeficiency virus infection, drug and alcohol misuse) and an increase in the rate of suicide (United Nations Children's Fund 1999). Several of these catastrophes occur to children in Western societies; in addition, inequalities in wealth inevitably bring inequalities in health, social environment, education and opportunities.

The birth rate has decreased more than child survival has increased, with a net decrease in the number of children. Women are having children at an older age. In England and Wales in 1997, 63% of births to married women in social classes I and II were to women aged 30 years and older; in social classes IV and V the corresponding number was 41% of births (Office of National Statistics 1987, 1997). The number of women older than 30 years who seek financial help for their disabled child has increased over the past 18 years, from 38% to 57% (Social Policy Research Unit 1999). There is an underclass of children, many of them born to younger mothers, who are unwanted, growing up in poverty, retarded in communication, untrained in social behaviour, frequently absent from school, and exposed to violence, abuse and exploitation.

The immense contributions of orthopaedic surgery to disabled children are essential elements of a disparate whole, each component of which must mesh with the others in the child's development – the parents, members of the Health and Social Services, teachers from nursery to leaving school, and voluntary agencies. Without a co-ordinator, usually a paediatrician, the services of these various groups are fragmented and there is piecemeal understanding of the child and family.

THE FAMILY FIRST

The parents' joy at a new birth is turned to anguish when they learn that their child is in any part deficient, deformed or abnormal in function. Emotional reactions vary in kind and intensity and cascade. Initial shock may be followed by disbelief, denial, anger, guilt, shame, isolation, and sometimes extreme reactions of rejection or overprotection, before final acceptance and adjustment. Most parents prefer to be informed together, as soon as possible, and with the baby present. They need explanation, confidence in touching, handling and feeding their baby. They need advice on the chances of future offspring being affected, the programme of remedial and surgical treatment, and the decisions that they may be asked to reach. Their physical and emotional strain, feelings of inadequacy, conflicts of responsibilities and limited time for themselves may break up the home. Disruption of family life inevitably affects other children, who may feel neglected, disadvantaged and resentful. Among parents of children severely disabled by spina bifida, the rates of separation and divorce are 10 times higher than the national average, and three times greater if the child died (Kew 1975). In a survey of 25 families of children with Duchenne muscular dystrophy, more than 50% had serious marital problems, and 25% were divorced (Buchanan et al 1979).

Success of treatment and education is measured by the

accomplishments of the child, the behaviour of the parents and siblings, and the wholeness of the family.

ASSESSMENT OF DEVELOPMENT

Continuing throughout the early years, at least until the child starts school, the health visitor and family doctor maintain surveillance, alert to any developmental delay. The stepping stones of normal development must be known, so that deviations are recognised and access is given to all available services. In nearly every Health District there is a child development assessment centre directed by a paediatrician and attended by many specialists. The disabled child should be referred to the centre when a few months old, and the health visitor may accompany the family to ensure optimal liaison. Every member of the multidisciplinary team contributes in compiling an accurate profile of the child and family. Duplication is avoided by combined medical and functional assessments. Thorough examination and appropriate further investigation establish the diagnosis in full. The child's posture, reactions, head control, tone, movements of the trunk and limbs, and fine manipulations are recorded. Appraisals are made of vision and hearing, speech and language, and social behaviour at play. The assessment report is shared with the parents; they are partners in the programme, which must take account of their values, priorities and limitations. The conclusion is a summary of the major functional difficulties, the need for the advice of other specialists, and plans for continuing management, periodic reviews and support for the family.

MULTIDISCIPLINARY TRAINING

Treatment begins early. It is based upon the sequences of normal development and involves the parents intimately. Therapists explain the child's next physical and mental needs.

The *physiotherapist* has particular responsibility for assessing sitting, standing, balancing, walking, climbing and transferring between two surfaces. He/she advises about the need for simple orthoses, walking aids and wheelchairs. Asymmetric deformities should be prevented; such deformities arise through intrinsic forces of muscle imbalance and spasticity, and the extrinsic force of gravity. The position of the head can influence posture by initiating the asymmetric tonic neck reflex. This causes unequal muscle tone on the two sides of the body. Through physiotherapy, the child learns sequences of movements, control of posture, the gross motor skills of sitting, standing and walking, and fine manipulative skills. The child and parents are given weekly learning goals and a chart that describes the skill to be developed through practice.

The *occupational therapist* advises on everyday activities of feeding, drinking, micturition and defecation, clothing and dressing, washing and bathing, play and learning, and recommends seating for good posture, controlled movements and two-handed activities. Appropriate adaptations

of the home, such as the installation of rails, are recommended.

The *speech and language therapist* uses tests of comprehension and articulation of language, and of expression in words and writing. The levels of the child's attainment are compared with normal development. The therapist assesses and treats children who have speech, language and hearing difficulties. To be most effective, the programme of language stimulation should start early. A child copies actions and speech sounds. The desire to communicate must be encouraged. Vocabulary is taught as the child recognises objects and pictures of them. The child is assisted to play imaginatively, to express by words and gestures, and to discriminate, sequence and remember.

The *educational psychologist* uses three sets of evidence in assessing the child's mental abilities and levels of attainment:

- the combined report of the paediatrician and therapists
- observations at home, at school and at play of the child's concentration span, distractibility and perseverance for selected tasks and interactions with others of the same age
- the results of a battery of tests of intelligence, reasoning, visuomotor and visuoperceptual skills, memory and abilities with words.

The early assessments of difficulties and needs are essential, but premature conclusions about a child's potential must be avoided: they may prove to be inaccurate and may adversely affect the judgement and expectations of those concerned with the child.

Cerebral palsy, spina bifida with hydrocephalus, and Duchenne muscular dystrophy are three frequently occurring examples of chronic disabling diseases. They require the mutual understanding and collaboration of orthopaedic surgeons and many other professionals in the health, education and social services.

CEREBRAL PALSY

The orthopaedic management of cerebral palsy is described in Chapter 18. Here the problems and major goals of management are described. The fixed, non-progressive brain lesion occurs before, at or soon after birth, interfering with the developing central nervous system. The causes may include hypoxia in the third trimester or at birth, trauma with subdural haemorrhage, toxicity due to Rhesus incompatibility, maternal uraemia, diabetes mellitus, drugs, rubella, toxoplasmosis and cytomegalovirus.

TREATMENT

The purpose of treatment is to achieve, within the limits of his or her motor and associated disorders, the child's maximal independence in daily living activities, communication and mobility. Each professional makes a particular contribution; team work is essential. Even children severely affected can gain some independence in self-care, which pleases them and lessens the burden on the carers. Seizures require the use of anticonvulsants for their control. In spastic syndromes, the long-term use of spasmolytics, such as baclofen, dantrolene or diazepam is *not* recommended.

Remedial treatment

The disabilities of those with *hemiplegia* are relatively mild, and the child usually achieves independence. The child is urged to be mindful of his hemiplegic limbs and to make symmetric movements. Ahead of his achievements, the physiotherapists and parents induce him to move from lying to sitting, to protract the affected shoulder, to crawl, to stand and, rotating the affected side of the pelvis forwards, to balance, transfer weight and walk. Two-handed activities are promoted in drinking, feeding and playing, practising dressing, pushing a toy wheelbarrow, swimming and riding a cycle or a pony. Extensor thrust causing plantar flexion of the foot can be controlled by a moulded polypropylene ankle-foot orthosis. Fixed deformities may be prevented by positioning, passive stretching and corrective bracing. When the child is older, shortening of the leg by more than 1.25 cm may be treated by raising the sole of the shoe. Elongation of the tendo-Achilles should be undertaken if contracture develops, but should seldom be performed in children younger than 7 years.

In *spastic paraplegia*, *diplegia* and *quadriplegia* unwanted postures may be controlled by lying the child prone, carrying with the hips astride, sitting symmetrically in a seat with a tray (Fig. 3.1), and by inhibiting the primitive reflexes that persist and impede motor development. Flexing the trunk, hips and knees inhibits a strong extensor thrust; pulling the child forwards by one arm from lying supine induces a propping reaction in the other arm, with abduction at the shoulder, extension at the elbow, supination and extension at the wrists and of the fingers. Exercises over rolls and a large ball may assist hip extension, trunk balance and rotation. In standing, flexion at the knees may be prevented by knee braces. A standing frame with the feet plantigrade helps to lessen extensor posturing (Fig. 3.2).

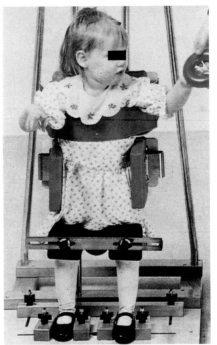

Figure 3.2 Rifton adjustable standing frame.

Orthopaedic management is sought early, before persisting adduction, internal rotation and flexion of the hips lead to contracture and progressive subluxation. Despite conservative measures, secondary deformities may occur. Conspicuous among these is the 'windswept' position of the legs, from persistence of the asymmetric tonic neck reflex: the adducting hip becomes dislocated, the pelvis tilts up on the same side and scoliosis progresses, convex on the abducting side. The treatments are surgical, followed by an individually shaped supporting seat (Fig. 3.3).

Difficulties in feeding

Feeding is impeded by persistence of primitive rooting, bite and gag reflexes, hypersensitivity of the lips and palate, tongue thrust, weak lip closure, and lack of head control. In the process of teaching the child to feed independently, the speech therapist guides the parents and carers in controlling

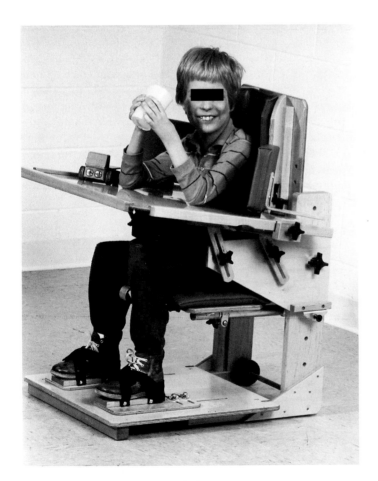

Figure 3.1 Rifton adjustable chair.

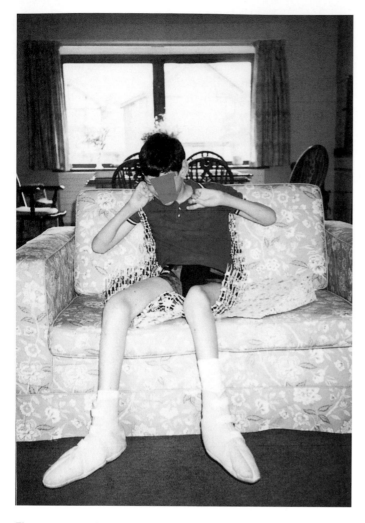

Figure 3.3 An individually shaped supporting seat.

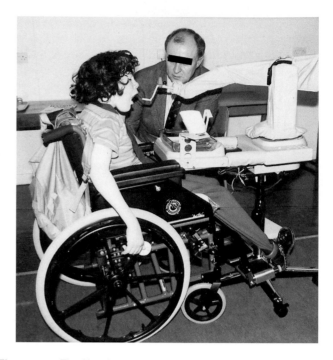

Figure 3.4 The Handy 1 robotic aid to eating.

COMMUNICATION

Speech therapy

Speech demands co-ordination of ventilation, control of the larynx for varying the pitch, volume and modulation of sounds, and control of movements of the lips, tongue and palate to form words. Poor control of exhalation causes speech to be interrupted: the sounds fade or only one or two words come with each breath. Training is given in posture when sitting, controlled breathing, coughing, and phonation. Children with athetosis may have severe dysarthria and depend upon those who know them to interpret their needs. Involuntary movements and speech are worse under stress.

Alternative methods of communication

A child who is unable to speak uses alternative means such as gestures, signs or tailor-made communication boards. From a simple picture-board, the child can progress to Blissymbols (pictographs representing objects, ideographs to convey ideas, and signs for words which recur frequently). These are displayed on a board, conveniently arranged and colour coded, and indicated by finger, fist or head pointer, or on a computer screen (Fig. 3.5). The Rebus and Makaton systems use simple pictographs that are easier for children with both communication and learning difficulties (Fig. 3.6).

The range of portable electronic communication aids is expanding rapidly (Thursfield 1995). Speech output is in the form of synthesised or digitised speech. The former refers to the electronic reproduction of speech, and the latter to real speech that has been stored by the device to be played back as required. Speech output can be used by a non-speaking person to communicate by telephone. A very wide range of

the trunk and head. Techniques are taught that desensitise the lips, tongue and palate, and overcome tongue thrust, first in sucking and then by assisted feeding and promoting chewing.

The Handy 1 robotic aid to eating enables a child with cerebral palsy and severely impaired arm function, but with control of head movements, to select food from the plate and eat it (Fig. 3.4). The device is controlled by a single switch positioned conveniently. The robotic arm scoops up food from the glass dish and presents it to the child at a preprogrammed position; the child can then take the food from the spoon. A drinking cup is also available.

Treatment of dribbling

Dribbling interferes with play, school work, social activities, feeding and speaking. A child hates their clothes to be sodden. Training is aimed at the ability to hold the head up with the lips closed, and to swallow. The ducts of the submandibular salivary glands that secrete a substantial proportion of saliva are directed forwards; surgical re-routing of the ducts towards the back of the mouth lessens drooling (Burton et al 1991).

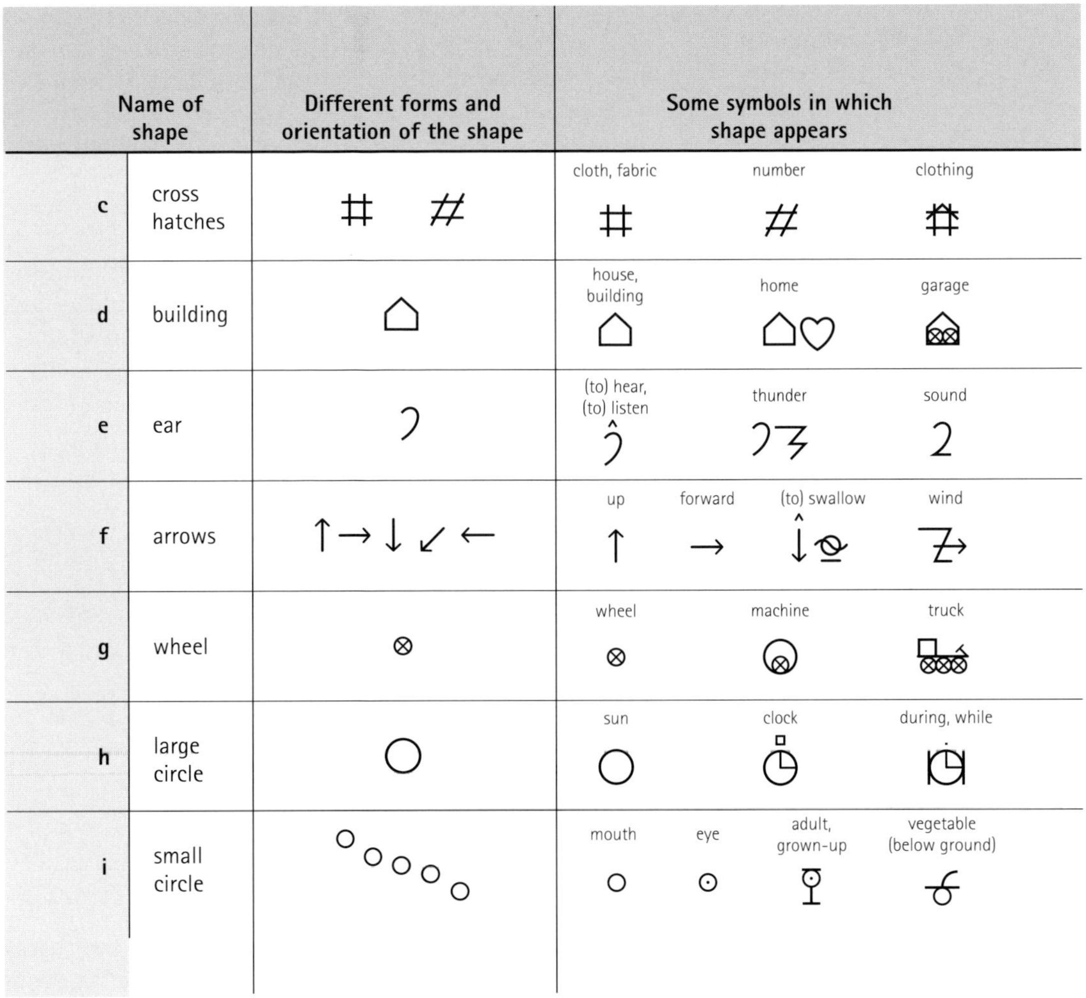

Figure 3.5 Blissymbols.

	Name of shape	Different forms and orientation of the shape	Some symbols in which shape appears		
c	cross hatches	＃ ⧣	cloth, fabric ＃	number ⧣	clothing ⊞
d	building	⌂	house, building ⌂	home ⌂♡	garage ⌂
e	ear	⌒	(to) hear, (to) listen	thunder	sound 2
f	arrows	↑ → ↓ ↙ ←	up ↑	forward →	(to) swallow / wind
g	wheel	⊗	wheel ⊗	machine ⊙	truck
h	large circle	○	sun ○	clock	during, while
i	small circle	○○○○○○	mouth ○	eye ⊙	adult, grown-up / vegetable (below ground)

WHEELCHAIRS

For some children, wheelchairs are their only means of mobility, giving independence at home, at school and with their friends. In Britain, wheelchairs are obtained in four ways:

- free of charge on permanent loan from the District Wheelchair Services of the National Health Service (NHS)
- by 'partnership option': the user is assessed by the Wheelchair Service and may choose to accept a voucher, equal to the cost of a wheelchair that would have been offered on loan. This voucher may be used to contribute towards the cost of a preferred, and usually more expensive, wheelchair. The user pays the extra cost, but the wheelchair remains the property of the NHS
- on temporary loan from the British Red Cross
- by private purchase, using a voucher from the Wheelchair Services towards part of the cost: the user owns the chair and is responsible for its maintenance.

switches is available to enable even the most severely disabled people to use a communication aid (Fig. 3.7).

The range of wheelchairs, cushions, individual seating, accessories and adaptations is wide, and personal choice is extended in design, quality, performance, low weight, manoeuvrability and comfort.

A wheelchair with accessories appropriate to the child's needs is best selected by a rehabilitation engineer and occupational therapist in the Wheelchair Service. Decisions are better for having impartial advisors who have experience of severely disabled children and are experienced in wheelchairs, special seating, controls and adaptations.

A child disabled by cerebral palsy may sit in a wheelchair most of the day. It must be easy for the carer to lift the child in and out. Cushions, restraining straps, supportive pads and individually shaped body support may be needed for comfort, function and the avoidance of pressure sores. Forces supporting the child must be well distributed to avoid tissue deformation and ischaemia. Different types of pressure-distributing cushions are available with the wheelchair (Cochrane 1998). For comfort, relief of pressure, postural support, hygiene and ventilation, the choice is made by trial.

When a child has extensor spasms and the pelvis shifts

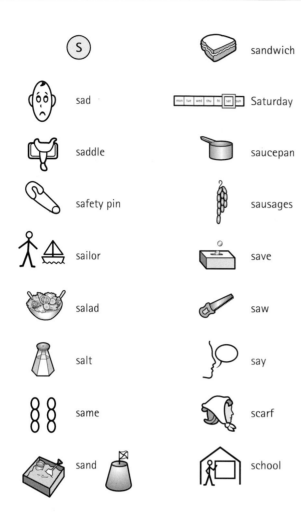

(S)	sandwich
sad	Saturday
saddle	saucepan
safety pin	sausages
sailor	save
salad	saw
salt	say
same	scarf
sand	school

Figure 3.6 Rebus symbols.

forwards towards the front of the seat, the seat may be wedged higher at the front and the pelvis restrained by a strap that pulls down and back towards the junction of the seat and backrest. Abduction at the hips decreases the tendency to subluxation at the hips, widens the sitting base, improves pelvic stability and encourages lumbar lordosis

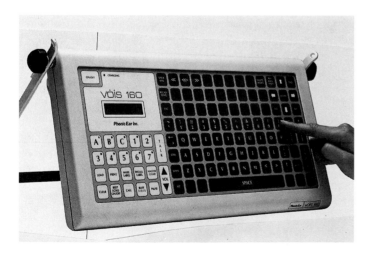

Figure 3.7 VOIS 160 communication aid.

(Fig. 3.8). A pommel shaped to the medial sides of the thighs applies abduction forces, or straps lined with sheepskin can hold the legs apart. Windswept legs – one hip adducted and internally rotated and the other abducted and externally rotated – can be controlled by applying forces appropriately (Fig. 3.9).

Control of the trunk in sitting

Postural support may be achieved by straps passing around the waist and thorax and over the shoulders and attached to a high backrest by lateral pelvic and thoracic supports (Fig. 3.10). Alternatively, an individually shaped

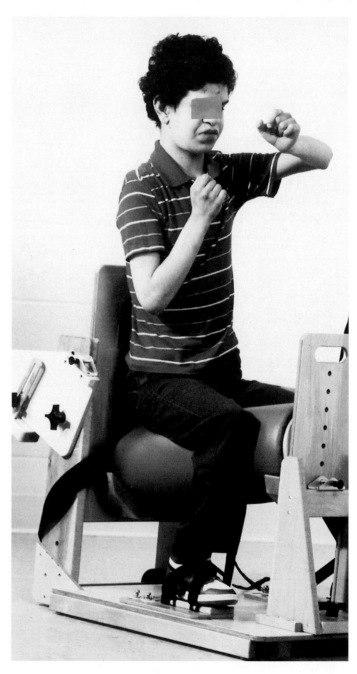

Figure 3.8 Bolster chair, inhibiting extension spasms and encouraging abduction at the hips.

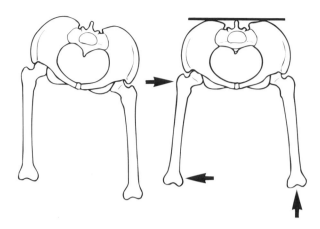

Figure 3.9 Application of forces to control windswept hips.

seat may be fashioned by thermoplastic moulding (Fig. 3.11) or from a sheet of repeating units that can be locked or unlocked to allow readjustment for growth or change in shape (Fig. 3.12). The seat is mounted on an aluminium tubular frame and upholstered with quilted, flame-retardant Terrylene cloth and foam. Commonly, children with

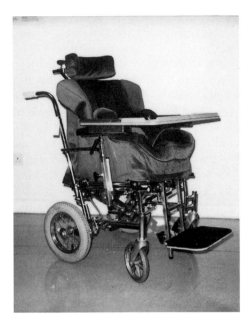

Figure 3.11 Upholstered thermoplastic moulded seat.

cerebral palsy need two different seats, one in the alert position for education, feeding and hand function, and the other with less support, to stimulate voluntary postural control.

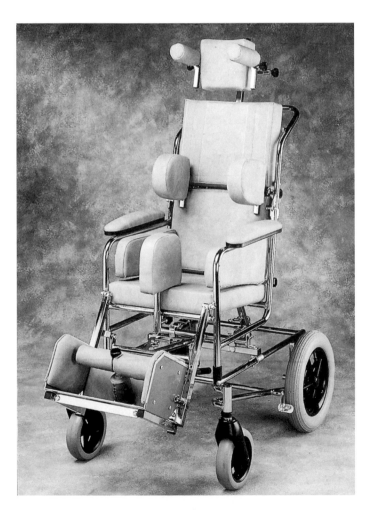

Figure 3.10 Wheelchair with high backrest and adjustable supports.

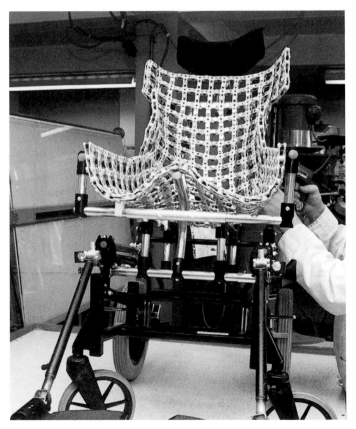

Figure 3.12 A seat shaped from a sheet of repeated units.

AN EDUCATION PROGRAMME FOR MOTOR-IMPAIRED CHILDREN

Education programmes have been inspired by 'conductive education', pioneered at the Peto Institute in Budapest, which encourages motor development and, at the same time, the whole range of learning experiences enjoyed by other pre-school and school-age children.

As soon as the child is identified as having a special need, a pre-school teacher-counsellor and a physiotherapist collaborate in a programme at the child's home, with fortnightly visits, giving the parents the necessary skills to handle their child. The child and mother are invited to attend opportunity play groups for social experience and to gain support and confidence through meeting other adults and children. Through this early intervention in the education programme and the provision of a continuing physical component, the children gain independence and extend their opportunities at school.

SPINA BIFIDA WITH MYELOMENINGOCELE

Spina bifida cystica is the most common of all central nervous system malformations. The defect may occur anywhere along the length of the neural tube, most commonly in the lumbar, lower thoracic and sacral regions. Hydrocephalus occurs frequently, from block of the fourth ventricle, aqueduct stenosis or the Arnold–Chiari malformation in which the cerebellar tonsils protrude through the foramen magnum and the upper cervical spinal cord is thickened. Hydrocephalus may be present at birth or may increase after closure of the defect.

Progressive hydrocephalus requires a shunt operation. The ventriculo-peritoneal shunt has replaced the ventriculo-atrial shunt, being safer and requiring fewer revisions. Subsequently, ventricular size is monitored by ultrasonography and computed tomography. If the valve fails, the symptoms of increased intracranial pressure develop; the signs are neck stiffness, papilloedema, optic atrophy, palsy of cranial nerve VI, bulbar weakness, spasticity and ataxia. The valve and shunt may need to be removed and replaced. The surgical management of the child's spine and limbs is discussed in Chapter 16.

INTELLECTUAL DEVELOPMENT

In general, the intellect of children with spina bifida is shifted towards the lower normal range, and is lower in those with shunts and especially if the ventricles are very large or abnormally small. Verbal ability and the use of complex language structures often exceed understanding and practical skills. Attention and concentration are diminished and numeracy is usually below average. Visual perception and actions based on perception are most affected. The 'cocktail party syndrome' describes the bright social chatter that may mask intellectual limitation.

PARALYSIS AND SENSORY LOSS

When the lumbo-sacral nerve roots are involved, as is usual, varying degrees of paralysis occur below the involved level. The paralysis usually affects the sphincters of the bladder and rectum, and the resulting urinary disorder can, eventually, lead to severely damaged kidneys.

Vulnerability of anaesthetic tissue

The risk is ever present that pressure and friction over a prominent scar or kyphus may cause ischaemia, necrosis and ulceration, which heal very slowly. Always, there must be vigilance and diligent care. Anaesthetic skin is liable to damage from undetected and unrelieved high pressure, shear, friction, humidity, local increase in temperature, and contamination. To minimise such damage, the child's back support may be shaped to receive the kyphus, or a protective dome may be made.

Besides the back, the tissues most at risk are those over the sacrum, ischial tuberosities, perineum, greater trochanters, backs of the thighs and malleoli, and where there is pressure because of deformities, orthoses and tight shoes. The danger to buttocks and thighs is greater in sitting than in lying, because the axial loading is restricted to a smaller surface area. The rules of care must be observed throughout life:

- protection of anaesthetic skin
- control of incontinence
- changes of position at night and three times in every hour by day, using effective and sustained push-ups on the wheelchair arm rests
- a seat cushion that distributes the load as evenly as possible over the greatest surface area
- avoidance of coins and keys in pockets, and of tight trousers with prominent seams
- care in transferring between two surfaces
- daily inspection of all anaesthetic skin; the first suggestion of tissue ischaemia must be recognised and all pressure relieved until healing is complete.

MOBILITY

Children with hydrocephalus may have upper motor neurone signs and ataxia above the level of the spinal lesion. Balance in sitting depends upon the level of the neural defect. Different chairs are needed for feeding, play and travelling. For many, the Chailey chariot (Fig. 3.13) is a good start, followed by a self-propelling wheelchair, and a buggy wheelchair suitable for the parents to push for short distances outside the home.

ORTHOSES

Complete paralysis below the midthoracic segments does not prevent standing and walking if the child is supplied with the correct orthoses. Success in walking encourages young

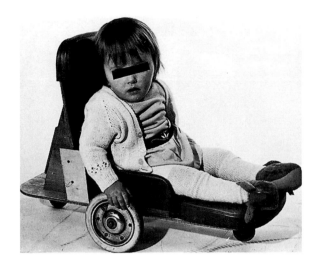

Figure 3.13 Chailey chariot.

people to continue to use the orthoses through adolescence into adult years. Their values are in standing upright, physical exercise, stimulation of circulation and osteogenesis in the lower part of the body, drainage of the bladder, further development of the shoulder girdle and upper limbs, and feelings of achievement and wellbeing.

Children younger than 4 years who have thoracic or upper lumbar neural defects may stand and walk using a swivel walker (Fig. 3.14). After 4 years of age, a child with a thoracic defect will walk with a hip guidance orthosis (HGO), and those with an upper lumbar defect will walk with either an HGO or a reciprocating gait orthosis (RGO) The HGO 'Para Walker' (Fig. 3.15), and the RGO (Fig. 3.16) differ. The hip joints on the HGO are free between flexion and extension stops, whereas on the RGO cables link the two sides, so that extension on one side causes flexion on the other. On the HGO the child's shoes fit into metal plates with rocker soles; the foot section of the RGO is a plastic ankle-foot orthosis and fits inside the shoe. The RGO is designed to be worn under the clothes; the HGO was originally worn outside the clothes. Largely for cosmetic reasons, older children may prefer the RGO (Health Equipment Information 1989).

The methods of walking in the two orthoses are different. To walk in the HGO, the arms are used to move the trunk forwards, the weight being taken on the leg which is in front. By pushing downwards and backwards with the opposite arm and hand on the rollator or crutch, the child leans towards the supporting leg and gravity causes the other leg to swing forwards and to take a step, assisted by contraction of the latissimus dorsi twisting the pelvis forwards on that side. The cycle is repeated for the other side, to advance the leg that has been left behind. In walking with the RGO, the forward motion is achieved by pushing down with both arms and hands, pulling the pelvis forwards and elevating it on one side. The walking action is assisted by the cable linking the two legs.

If, at 4 years of age, a child has sufficient strength in latissimus dorsi to sit unsupported with the arms raised above

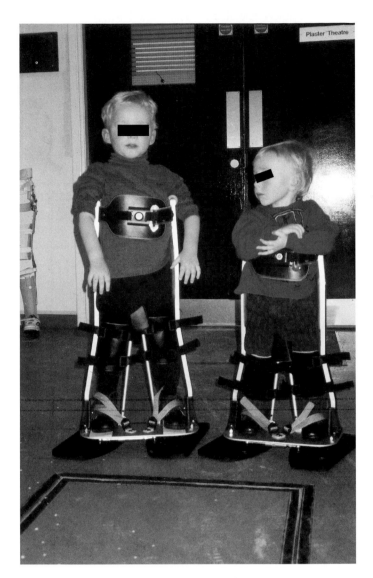

Figure 3.14 Swivel walkers.

the head and has normal power in both triceps, the child will succeed in walking reciprocally. Until they are older than 8 years, children will require someone to put them in the orthosis and help them to stand. Older children, who are strong in their upper limbs, will use elbow crutches for support.

Children with lower lumbar and incomplete lesions need less bracing and depend on crutches. For speed, many prefer to swing both legs forwards together, moving the elbow crutches together; they accelerate by swinging their legs in front of the crutches.

URINARY INCONTINENCE

A neuropathic bladder does not drain adequately, and the urine is likely to become infected. Recurrent urinary infections lead to trabeculation of the bladder, diverticula, bladder calculi, uretero-vesical incompetence, and ureteric reflux. Impaired renal function may follow.

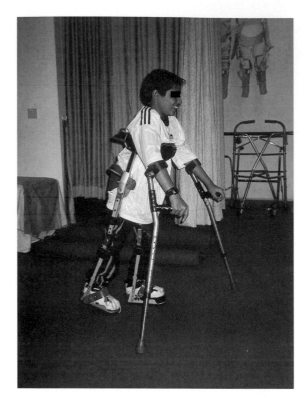

Figure 3.15 The 'Para Walker' hip guidance orthosis (HGO).

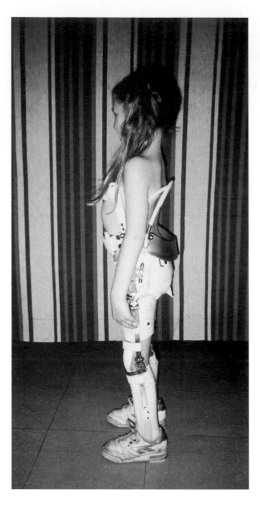

Figure 3.16 The reciprocating gait orthosis (RGO).

The urine should be cultured every 3 months, or earlier if the urine is offensive. Every 6 months, the serum urea and creatinine should be measured, and every 3 years, isotope scanning should be undertaken to demonstrate the size, shape and function of the kidneys. Ultrasonography will demonstrate bladder and renal size.

Urinary infection should be treated if there is illness, fever, the concentration of pathogens exceeds 100 000/ml or there is known to be ureteric reflux. Prophylactic treatment should be prescribed for ureteric reflux or recurrent urinary tract infections. A high fluid intake should be encouraged.

Reflex emptying of the bladder may be achieved in infants by stimulating the skin over the lumbo-sacral area, lower abdomen or inner sides of the thighs. The bladder may be emptied by manual expression if there is no ureteric reflux. When boys are 3 years old, urinary incontinence can be managed by a pubic pressure urinal; at about 10 years old, management is possible with a small disposable urinary condom rolled over an adhesive strip applied spirally to the penis. Clean intermittent catheterisation is the preferred method of managing urinary incontinence in girls, and self-catheterisation is encouraged from the age of 6 years (Lapides et al 1972).

FAECAL INCONTINENCE

Faecal incontinence is due to deficient sensation in the lower bowel, diminished reflex peristaltic activity, and a paralysed anal sphincter. Bowel training is slow, but can usually be achieved. When the child wants to be clean, regular periods of twice-daily bowel training for 10 minutes begin, with the child lying on their side. One bisacodyl suppository may be inserted 20 minutes before. The child learns to push down and the mother assists by manual evacuation, and later by perianal pressure.

EDUCATION

Attendance at a preschool play group should be followed by primary education at 5 years in an ordinary school whenever possible. Besides the child's physical disabilities, intelligence may be lower than normal. The child needs accommodation suitable for a wheelchair and management of incontinence, a personal carer, access to therapists for physical treatment and training in personal care, and teachers with special experience. When learning is delayed, individual teaching is possible in remedial classes.

The decision as to whether a mainstream secondary school may be attended is based on the child's intellectual level, difficulties in learning, the availability of therapists, proximity of the school to the home, and the wishes of the parents. Education is directed towards social skills, self confidence and future career.

DUCHENNE MUSCULAR DYSTROPHY

This sex-linked recessive disorder typically presents in boys aged 3–7 years as proximal muscle weakness that causes a waddling gait, toe walking, lordosis, frequent falls and difficulties in standing up and climbing stairs. The pelvic girdle is affected first, then the shoulder girdle. Creatine kinase concentrations are markedly increased, even before symptoms develop. Progression of the disease is steady, and most boys are confined to a wheelchair by the age of 12. Flexion contractures and scoliosis ultimately occur, and most boys die by the age of 20 years. About 50% of boys have lower intelligence than non-affected siblings. As yet, no cure is available, but successful gene therapy can be expected in the first decade of the 21st century.

TREATMENT

Much can be done to improve the boy's quality of life by stimulating activity, avoiding excess gain in weight, preventing contractures, and preserving ventilatory function. Active exercises do not have a deleterious effect, and swimming is recommended because buoyancy makes movements easier. Passive movements may retard contractures when performed twice daily every day, stretching the shortening flexor muscles of the limbs. Such exercises may be complemented by daily intermittent compression splinting using a Flowtron for about 1 hour, and by ankle-foot orthoses worn at night, holding the feet in the neutral position. Compliance is good when orthoses are individually made, light, and with smooth surfaces to slide on the sheets. Standing with support and the feet plantigrade will delay scoliosis and contractures at the hips, knees and ankles. Once contractures have developed, passive stretching is ineffectual and causes pain. As soon as there is equinus deformity, percutaneous Achilles tenotomy will enable the child to stand plantigrade and, wearing knee-ankle-foot orthoses, to continue walking.

When a boy is too weak to walk, he can continue to stand in a frame or stand-up wheelchair (Fig. 3.17), if flexion contractures do not prevent this.

Fractures
Because of osteoporosis and falls, fractures of the long bones occur not infrequently. They heal normally, and should be treated with minimal splintage and early resumption of usual activities.

Scoliosis
If a boy with scoliosis is able to stand, the lumbar lordosis is exaggerated, but in sitting the boy slumps into kyphosis. In the majority, there is progressive paralytic scoliosis, with one arm dedicated to propping. In a small proportion of affected individuals, hyperlordosis persists, with increasing stiffness throughout the spine from fibrosis of the paraspinal muscles. Asymmetric loading on the ischia causes discomfort.

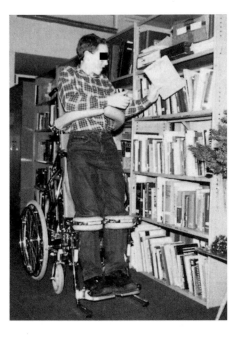

Figure 3.17
Stand-up wheelchair.

Compression of the sciatic nerve results in tingling and altered sensation in the lower leg and foot. Pulmonary ventilation diminishes as the intercostal muscles and diaphragm weaken, and is made worse by progressive thoracic deformity.

The surgical correction of scoliosis by Luque's segmental stabilisation has proved successful and is often undertaken early rather than late for curve progression.

Progressive cardiomyopathy is inevitable, with interstitial fibrosis beginning in the posterobasal part and becoming more diffuse in the left ventricle. The electrocardiogram shows sinus tachycardia, tall R waves in lead V1, a shortened P–R interval, depressed Q waves in leads V5–6, right bundle branch block, altered T waves, and left axis deviation. Echocardiography demonstrates impaired left ventricular function, with a dilated left ventricle, thinned myocardium and, occasionally, mitral valve prolapse.

Sinus tachycardia, artrial and ventricular fibrillation, and cardiac arrest may occur during surgery. Succinylcholine should be avoided, as it has been implicated in rhabdomyolysis causing myoglobinuria. During the early postoperative days, intensive paediatric care must be given because of the hazards of weak ventilatory muscles and retained bronchial secretions, gastric dilatation, myoglobinuria and hyperkalaemia.

Impaired respiratory function
The vital capacity is a prognostic index and closely reflects the degree of respiratory disability. It deteriorates after the age of 11 years. The higher the peak value in excess of 1.2 litres, the better the prognosis. The diaphragm is not selectively involved, and only late in the disease is there a significant decrease in vital capacity when the position is changed from sitting to lying. Coughing becomes ineffective because of low lung volume, diminished lung compliance, and

reduced dynamic airway compression. Six factors contribute to respiratory failure:

- intercostal and diaphragmatic muscle weakness
- scoliosis and mechanical abnormalities of the thorax
- widespread microatelectasis, with reduced lung compliance
- weak cough, with retained secretions and repeated infections
- ventilation-perfusion imbalance
- recurrent nocturnal hypoxaemia.

Arterial puncture is very difficult in these boys, and earlobe or finger oximetry detects important abnormalities in oxygen saturation.

In advanced Duchenne muscular dystrophy, the boys are at risk of hypoxaemia during rapid eye movement sleep. The symptoms of ventilatory failure, which worsens at night, are restless sleep with frequent arousals, followed by morning confusion and headaches.

Assisted ventilation by intermittent positive pressure ventilation can normalise blood gases, lessen recurrent arousals, relieve symptoms, and benefit the boy and his carers (Heckmatt et al 1990). Most boys die from impaired pulmonary function, and when assisted ventilation prolongs life, the proportion of deaths due to cardiomyopathy increases.

DISABLED SCHOOL LEAVERS

Before and during the school years of the disabled child, the Health and Education services have been the key agencies, and the paediatrician has been the co-ordinator. After the young adult leaves school, the local authority Social Services Department assumes a major role, but money for day care, short-term residential care, incontinence laundry services and practical support diminishes. A fragile family may break down.

In Britain about 11 000 disabled adolescents leave special schools, and more than this number leave ordinary schools, each year. They have poorer chances than able-bodied school leavers of being employed, of receiving training and of further education. Only 31% of disabled people of working age are in employment (Office of Population Censuses and Surveys 1989), and at times of high unemployment, they suffer disproportionately (McRae 1987). To prevent the physical and psychological deterioration that accompanies unemployment, it is essential to think ahead. Continuing discussion is necessary between the young person, parents, school careers advisor, the Career Advisory Service and the paediatrician; early in the final year at school, they should hold a school leavers' conference. Here, the nature of the disabling disease, the prognosis and any complications are made plain and the adolescent's skills, speed and dexterity of movements, personal independence and need for equipment at work are defined. The young person's aptitude and preferences, intellect and educational achievements are established, as are the integrity of the home and the reliability of parental backing.

It is absolutely clear that young disabled people who are trained are much more readily accepted by the labour market (Pugh & Walker 1981). Higher education or a place in a technical college with a promise of training within a firm gives a much better prospect. If work is not practicable the school leaver becomes eligible for State Benefits. The Social Services Department is not alone in having a continuing obligation to the disabled person and family.

REFERENCES

Bone M, Meltser H 1989 The prevalence of disability among children. OPCS surveys of disability among children in Great Britain. Report 3. HMSO, London

Buchanan D C, Larbarera C J, Roelofs R, Olson W 1979 Reactions of families to children with Duchenne muscular dystrophy. General Hospital Psychiatry 1: 262–269

Burton M J, Leighton S E J, Lund W S 1991 Long-term results of submandibular duct transposition for drooling. Journal of Laryngology and Otology 105: 101–103

Cochrane G M 1998 Wheelchairs; powered wheelchairs and scooters; and wheelchair accessories. Disability Information Trust, Oxford

Health Equipment Information 1989 A comparative evaluation of the Hip Guidance Orthosis (HGO) and the Reciprocating Gait Orthosis (RGO). HMSO, London

Heckmatt J Z, Loh L, Dubowitz V 1990 Night-time nasal ventilation in neuromuscular disease. Lancet 335: 579–582

Kew S 1975 Handicap and family crisis. Pitman Medical, London

Lapides J, Diokno A C, Silber S J, Lowe B S 1972 Clean intermittent self-catheterization in the treatment of urinary tract disease. Journal of Urology 107: 458–461

McRae S 1987 Young and jobless – the social and personal consequences of long-term youth unemployment. Policy Studies Institute, London

Office of National Statistics 1987 Birth statistics for England and Wales. HMSO, London

Office of National Statistics 1987 and 1997 Birth statistics for England and Wales. HMSO, London

Office of Population Censuses and Surveys 1989 OPCS surveys of disability in Great Britain – Report 4. Disabled adults: services, transport and employment. HMSO, London

Pugh G, Walker A 1981 Employment experiences in handicapped school-leavers. International Journal of Rehabilitation Research 4: 231

Thursfield C 1995 Communication and Access to Computer Technology. Disability Information Trust, Oxford.

United Nations Children's Fund (Unicef) 1999 After the fall: the human impact of ten years of transition. Unicef Research Centre, Florence

Chapter 4

Regional analgesia and pain relief in children

E. Doyle

ANAESTHESIA

The majority of children undergoing orthopaedic surgery are healthy, with no intercurrent disease to complicate anaesthesia. A minority have significant cardiac, respiratory or neuromuscular disease. The use of local anaesthetic techniques alone without general anaesthesia is much less common in children than in adult orthopaedic patients, and is usually most suitable for those whose intercurrent disease makes general anaesthesia potentially dangerous. The combination of a light general anaesthetic and a local anaesthetic technique is very common. This reduces the requirement for anaesthetic agents and opioids during surgery and allows children a rapid pain-free recovery from anaesthesia. For most children and their families, particularly those who undergo multiple procedures, the main problems associated with anaesthesia are preoperative anxiety or fear and poorly treated postoperative pain. Attention to these areas and to the delivery of anaesthesia itself is essential for the wellbeing of paediatric orthopaedic patients.

A combination of psychological and pharmacological methods is used to alleviate anxiety and fear. The opportunity to visit the hospital, ward and reception area of the operating theatres before admission is often helpful in familiarising the patient and their parents with what will happen during their hospital stay. This provides an opportunity for children to watch an explanatory video of the admission and anaesthetic procedures, and to be given an unhurried explanation, appropriate to their age, of what their admission to hospital will entail. Many paediatric hospitals now have dedicated play specialists who will spend time with children in order to discover any anxieties or misconceptions. They provide reassurance, explanation of what will happen, and distraction during the induction of anaesthesia. In most paediatric hospitals, parents now accompany children to the anaesthetic room and remain until the child is anaesthetised. This helps to ensure a calm and co-operative patient. Should a child remain anxious despite preoperative preparation, pharmacological sedation or premedication shortly before the induction of anaesthesia is helpful. The use of benzodiazepines for this purpose usually produces amnesia for the events immediately preceding surgery, and may be particularly helpful in children who are to undergo a series of procedures.

Because much orthopaedic surgery is peripheral in nature and amenable to local anaesthetic analgesic techniques, the use of neuromuscular blockade, intermittent positive pressure ventilation and large doses of opioids is uncommon. These factors mean that there is no need for endotracheal intubation in many elective cases, and the airway may be maintained during anaesthesia by means of a laryngeal mask airway (Fig. 4.1). This is a soft, flexible form of airway, which sits in the pharynx and allows the patient to breathe through it, unlike an endotracheal tube, which is passed through the larynx and vocal cords to lie in the trachea. Furthermore, unlike endotracheal intubation, the laryngeal mask airway does not require a deep level of anaesthesia or neuromuscular blockade. The use of a laryngeal mask airway also avoids some of the complications that may be caused by endotracheal intubation, in particular, laryngeal irritation, which may cause postoperative laryngeal spasm, hypoxia and croup. The avoidance of these complications is particularly important in patients undergoing surgery on a day-case basis.

In those infants who undergo correction of congenital lesions in the first 6 months of life, drug elimination is very variable, owing to diminished clearances and prolonged half-lives. The volume of distribution of opioids and local anaesthetics is greater than in older children, and there are reduced plasma concentrations of proteins (especially α-1-acid glycoprotein), with consequent high concentration levels of free drugs. Clinically, there is an increased sensitivity to the depressant effects of anaesthetic agents and opioids in the first 6 months of life; the metabolism and elimination of local anaesthetic agents are also not fully developed. These factors necessitate reduced doses, longer intervals between doses, or reduced infusion rates for anaesthetic and analgesic drugs in this age group.

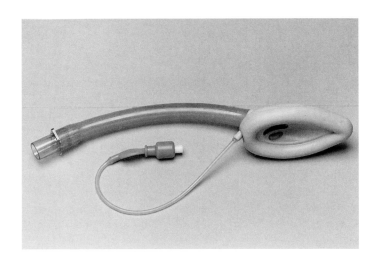

Figure 4.1 Laryngeal mask airway.

There is an incidence of corrected and uncorrected congenital heart disease in the paediatric orthopaedic population and the pathophysiological effects of this may require modification of the anaesthetic technique. Respiratory function may be impaired, particularly in patients undergoing correction of severe scoliosis. Preoperative physiotherapy may help, but often there is little that can be done. In view of the decline in respiratory function that is seen after major surgery, some patients will require postoperative ventilation of the lungs in an intensive care unit until respiratory function improves sufficiently to allow extubation. A variety of conditions that require orthopaedic surgery are associated with neuromuscular diseases that increase sensitivity to opioids and neuromuscular relaxants, and increase the risk of postoperative respiratory depression. These include the muscular dystrophies, dystrophia myotonica and arthrogryposis. Other conditions that may complicate anaesthesia are osteogenesis imperfecta, juvenile idiopathic arthritis and cervical spine anomalies such as Klippel–Feil syndrome, which may make airway management and endotracheal intubation difficult.

In patients undergoing anaesthesia for emergency surgery after trauma, there is a significant risk of pulmonary aspiration of gastric contents. Whenever possible, this surgery should be delayed until the following day, to allow gastric emptying to resume. Immediate surgery should be undertaken only if delay will compromise the outcome. Whenever possible and feasible, children at risk of aspiration of gastric contents should undergo a rapid-sequence induction of anaesthesia to synchronise the onset of muscle relaxation and endotracheal intubation, in order to minimise the chance of pulmonary aspiration of gastric contents.

During surgery in the exsanguinated limb there is a steady decrease in pH and oxygen tension and an increase in lactate and carbon dioxide tension within the limb. After deflation of the tourniquet, release of the products of anaerobic metabolism into the circulation can cause a transient, mixed respiratory and metabolic acidosis. Acid metabolites are buffered by bicarbonate with the production of carbon dioxide, and there may be a temporary increase in arterial and end-tidal carbon dioxide tensions in the region of 0.5–1.5 kPa. These effects are greater if two limbs rather than one are involved, if legs rather than arms are affected, and if there has been a prolonged period of exsanguination. Tourniquets reduce the effective body surface area available to dissipate heat, and may occasionally cause an increase in body temperature. Other than these, adverse effects of tourniquets are very rare. Recommendations for safe tourniquet use usually emphasise a duration of use less than 90 minutes and an increase in pulmonary ventilation just before and just after release, in order to enhance the elimination of excess carbon dioxide.

For many paediatric orthopaedic patients, the provision of adequate venous access for the intraoperative and postoperative period may be a major challenge. In well-nourished infants, especially those who will be put into a hip spica or bilateral leg plasters, there are limited options for venous access. In the event of failed cannulation in the upper limbs, the external jugular or scalp veins may be used. Unfortunately, these may not be available for long in the postoperative period and, if reliable postoperative venous access is necessary, central venous access via the internal jugular veins may be required. This technique requires dedicated equipment and some expertise, and has a small but definite incidence of complications such as pneumothorax and puncture of the carotid artery. Well-designed paediatric equipment is available for central venous cannulation, and this should be available for immediate use if required. For patients in whom the groins are accessible, the femoral veins are usually easy to cannulate and offer a route for central venous access, with fewer potential complications.

In an emergency, intraosseous access may be used in place of intravenous access. This involves siting a short wide-bore cannula through the cortex into the medulla of a long bone. The most common site for this is the anterior surface of the tibia, 1 cm below the tuberosity to avoid the growth plate. This allows immediate fluid resuscitation and drug administration until adequate venous access is secured at a more leisurely pace. Unlike venous access, and particularly central venous cannulation, intraosseous access requires no special expertise and may be performed by any doctor if necessary. It is widely used in paediatric accident and emergency departments.

POSTOPERATIVE ANALGESIA

The provision of postoperative analgesia for children undergoing orthopaedic surgery is very rewarding. The peripheral nature of much orthopaedic surgery and the absence of a prolonged postoperative ileus allow a multimodal approach to be used. Dense intraoperative analgesia provided by a local anaesthetic technique means that a light anaesthetic is possible. This reduces the requirement for anaesthetic agents and opioids during surgery, and allows children to experience a rapid, pain-free recovery from anaesthesia, with little or no postoperative vomiting. These children are then able to resume oral intake rapidly and, provided adequate oral analgesia is both prescribed and administered before the local anaesthetic block has regressed, the postoperative course is usually smooth. In general, it is preferable to prescribe oral analgesic drugs on a regular as opposed to an 'as required' basis over 24 hours for children who will certainly experience pain once an intraoperative local anaesthetic block becomes ineffective. This ensures timely administration of analgesia and avoids unnecessary delays in the administration of adequate analgesia. If parents have to ask for medication, and the nurses to verify that the child is in pain, before analgesia is given, the beneficial effect is suboptimal.

Barriers to the provision of adequate postoperative analgesia include a persistent belief that children do not feel pain to the same extent as adults, an exaggerated perception of the incidence and magnitude of the side effects of analgesic drugs, a lack of adequate facilities and equipment, and difficulties in the assessment of pain in children. The prescription of analgesic drugs is usually delegated to the most inexperienced medical staff, and this often produces poor prescribing in terms of the dosages and the frequency of administration of analgesic drugs. Children often receive smaller doses of analgesics than adults on a dose-to-weight basis, and at longer intervals. When doses are prescribed on an 'as required' basis, they are often administered in the smallest dose and at the longest intervals prescribed. It is therefore possible to improve the provision of postoperative analgesia to children in an institution if senior medical, nursing and pharmacy staff agree on simple and practical procedures for adequate dosages and administration of analgesic drugs. These procedures must then be followed by junior members of staff, confident to prescribe and administer adequate analgesia within a framework supported by their seniors and their employer.

Pain in children can be treated by physical, psychological and pharmacological methods. Simple measures such as ensuring warmth, swaddling and early feeding may all be useful. The presence of parents, reassurance and distraction are also important. Older children should be given a simple explanation of what is to happen and an assurance that any pain experienced will be treated. The main groups of drugs used for analgesia after surgery or trauma are the same as in adults: local anaesthetics, opioids, and non-steroidal anti-inflammatory drugs (NSAIDs), including paracetamol.

Mild pain of brief duration can be adequately treated with a single analgesic agent, but it is usually impossible to provide adequate analgesia with one type of analgesic after major surgery or trauma. Under these circumstances, analgesia has traditionally been provided by the systemic administration of opioids. It is difficult to provide complete analgesia with opioids alone without a significant risk of side effects, including respiratory depression, nausea and over-sedation. Multimodal or combined analgesic regimens are superior. It is often desirable to use two or more analgesic drugs, such as a local anaesthetic block plus an opioid, or a combination of opioid, a local anaesthetic technique and an NSAID. These combinations tend to have synergistic effects and can be used to provide analgesia equivalent or superior to that obtained with opioids alone, but with a reduction in dose and in the incidence of side effects.

Table 4.1 summarises a scheme of approach to the use of surgical and postoperative analgesia.

Table 4.1. Scheme of approach to surgical and post-operative analgesia

Severe pain

Epidural infusion of local anaesthetic solution and opioid started in theatre and continued after operation

or

Single-injection local anaesthetic technique given in theatre to last into the postoperative period followed postoperatively by a combination of *intravenous* opioids, NSAIDs and paracetamol

or

Intravenous opioids given in theatre followed postoperatively by a combination of intravenous opioids, NSAIDs and paracetamol. Whenever possible, opioids, NSAIDs and paracetamol should be used together if there are no contraindications.

Intravenous opioids
Intravenous morphine sulphate infusion or patient-controlled analgesia
NSAIDs
Diclofenac or Ibuprofen

Moderate pain

Single-injection local anaesthetic technique given in theatre to last into the postoperative period followed postoperatively by a combination of *oral* opioids, NSAIDs and paracetamol.
Intravenous opioids given in theatre followed postoperatively by a combination of *oral* opioids, NSAIDs and paracetamol.
This combination of *oral* opioids, NSAIDs and paracetamol should be used after major surgery when intravenous opioids are no longer required.

Oral opioids
Morphine sulphate or dihydrocodeine
NSAIDs
Diclofenac or ibuprofen

Mild pain

Paracetamol
Can be given with opioids and NSAIDs

PAIN ASSESSMENT

The effective provision of analgesia requires valid assessments of pain to be made at frequent intervals. These assessments should be able to determine the presence of pain, to estimate its severity, and to determine the effectiveness of analgesic intervention. Several tools for pain assessment have been validated for use in children of different ages, and may be used clinically to guide the provision of analgesia, or in research studies to quantify pain. These tools include the visual analogue scale (Berde et al 1991), a simple four-point self-report scale (Maunuksela et al 1987), an objective pain score based on observations of behaviour (Hanallah et al 1987), and features of facial expression (Grunau & Craig 1987). In order to ensure the delivery of effective postoperative analgesia, nursing staff should perform regular formal assessments of pain and act upon unsatisfactory scores in a fashion similar to the monitoring of other postoperative physiological variables such as heart rate, blood pressure, urine output and temperature.

LOCAL ANAESTHETIC TECHNIQUES

Various local anaesthetic techniques combined with general anaesthesia now play a major part in the provision of good analgesia for children. Dense analgesia will last into the postoperative period and results in a reduced requirement for anaesthetic agents and opioids, with rapid recovery and a reduction in the incidence and severity of opioid-induced side effects. Local anaesthetic techniques include infiltration of the surgical field, single-nerve blockade, plexus blockade, and central neuraxial blockade (epidural and spinal analgesia). Local anaesthetics produce a lack of sensation, which may distress children if it has not been explained beforehand, and may present the potential risk of injuries from incorrect positioning of a limb, plaster casts, or compartment syndromes.

TOPICAL CUTANEOUS ANAESTHESIA

The use of topical cutaneous anaesthesia before venepuncture should now be an essential part of anaesthesia for elective surgery, and adequate time should be included in the preoperative period to enable it to be instituted between the time of the child's admission to hospital and the induction of anaesthesia. This is particularly important for children who will undergo a series of surgical procedures. Late admission before surgery may prevent preoperative preparation and result in unnecessary pain and distress being experienced by the child and parents. This may make future admissions stressful for the patient, parents, nurses and medical staff.

EMLA cream is an effective topical anaesthetic agent with a very low incidence of side effects. It should be applied 2 hours before venepuncture, to ensure efficacy. More recently, a preparation of amethocaine has been marketed that has a reduced onset time of 40 minutes and a longer duration of action than EMLA cream. One of these preparations should be used in every child undergoing venepuncture for the induction of anaesthesia or blood sampling.

INFILTRATION ANALGESIA

Infiltration techniques are widely used in most areas of paediatric surgery, particularly those limited to the body surface. Local infiltration under direct vision is a technique that can be carried out simply, without the identification of landmarks or a knowledge of the anatomy of nerves; it is relatively free from complications. However, analgesia is limited to the skin and superficial tissues, and for anything other than superficial procedures it is insufficient as the sole analgesic technique.

PERIPHERAL NERVE BLOCKS (Table 4.2)

Brachial plexus blockade

Upper limb blockade is usually carried out by the axillary route, as this is free of the risks of pneumothorax, phrenic nerve block and recurrent laryngeal nerve block, which are associated with the supraclavicular and parascalene techniques. The axillary approach to the brachial plexus is of particular value in hand and forearm procedures. More proximal brachial plexus blocks will provide analgesia of the shoulder and may include areas innervated by the cervical plexus. Analgesia of the ulnar nerve distribution may, however, be less predictable. In a series of 142 brachial plexus blocks combined with intravenous sedation, carried out on 109 children (mean age 14.4 years) undergoing surgery on the upper limb, 134 were performed by the axillary route. There was a high success rate, with only three children requiring supplementation of the block by the surgeon, and six requiring general anaesthesia (Wedel et al 1991). Unsupplemented brachial plexus block is tolerated by few children, and is most useful as an adjunct to general anaesthesia to provide perioperative analgesia. In addition, it has been used to provide sympathetic blockade and enhance postoperative blood flow to the arm or hand (Audenaert et al 1991). The technique is usually contraindicated if there is a risk of a postoperative compartment syndrome.

Table 4.2 Peripheral nerve blocks	
Block	**Area affected**
Brachial plexus	Upper limb
Bier's block	Upper limb
Femoral and sciatic	Unilateral lower limb
Fascia iliaca compartment	Unilateral lower limb
Three-in-one	Unilateral lower limb
Metatarsal	Forefoot

Bier's block

Intravenous regional anaesthesia (or Bier's block) is an effective anaesthetic technique in older children. The limb is exsanguinated and a tourniquet inflated to 50 mmHg above systolic blood pressure. Prilocaine 7 mg/kg is the local anaesthetic of choice for this technique, and is injected via an intravenous cannula placed distal to the operative site. The tourniquet should be left inflated for a minimum of 20 minutes, even if the surgical procedure is of shorter duration than this. The main limitation to this technique is the patient's tolerance of the tourniquet, which restricts its use to procedures of 30–60 minutes' duration.

Lower limb blocks

Lower limb blocks are of particular value in paediatric practice. Two of the most common indications are fractured shaft of femur and surgery below the knee. Femoral nerve blockade is used for the former, whereas both sciatic and femoral nerve blockade are usually required for adequate analgesia after surgery below the knee.

Femoral nerve block

This may be performed as a single injection technique (with or without a nerve stimulator) below the inguinal ligament lateral to the femoral artery. This technique has the benefit of simplicity. The use of continuous femoral nerve blockade by means of an indwelling catheter has been described as an analgesic technique for fractures of the femur that avoids the use of opioids in patients with head injuries (Tobias 1994).

Sciatic nerve block

Blockade of the sciatic nerve will provide anaesthesia of the anterolateral leg and the foot. If it is used in combination with a saphenous or femoral nerve block, anaesthesia of the leg below the knee is obtained. There are three principal approaches to the proximal sciatic nerve: posterior, anterior and lateral. The posterior approach is the most commonly used. In this technique, the patient is supine with the thigh and knee flexed to 90°. The sciatic nerve lies midway between a line drawn between the greater trochanter and the ischial tuberosity. As the leg is flexed, the nerve tends to be fixed in a groove against the pelvis as it emerges from the greater sciatic foramen. Use of a nerve stimulator elicits dorsiflexion of the foot and allows safe identification of the nerve. A short-bevelled stimulating needle is introduced and is advanced while a stimulus of 1 mA/s is produced. Once dorsiflexion is obtained, the needle should be localised to the nerve by reducing the stimulating current to approximately 0.5 mA. If the sciatic nerve is blocked at the buttock, the back of the thigh will be anaesthetised, because of the proximity of the posterior cutaneous nerve of the thigh.

Fascia iliaca compartment block

The fascia iliaca compartment block has been described as an alternative to femoral nerve block and 'three-in-one' block for the provision of unilateral analgesia in the legs. The technique has been shown to have a significantly greater success rate (95%) than the three-in-one block (20%) in children (Dalens et al 1989). The fascia iliaca compartment block does not require the use of a nerve stimulator or the production of paraesthesia, and is performed away from blood vessels and nerves, so that the chances of inadvertent nerve injury or intravascular injection of local anaesthetic are remote.

Digital nerve block

This is a simple and effective technique for procedures limited to single digits. In the hand, 0.5–1 ml of 0.25% or 0.5% bupivacaine is injected on either side of the base of the digit, keeping the needle at right angles to the plane of the hand. This allows both palmar and dorsal branches to be blocked. A similar technique is used for blockade of the toes, although metatarsal block may be more effective. For this, the needle is introduced on the dorsal surface of the foot and directed towards the sole, passing the side of the metatarsal neck in the space to be blocked. Before the sole is punctured, the needle is aspirated and local anaesthetic is deposited as the needle is slowly withdrawn. The process is repeated on the other side of the metatarsal. Similar volumes of local anaesthetic are used. Adrenaline should not be used, because of the risk of vasoconstriction leading to ischaemic damage.

CENTRAL NEURAXIAL BLOCKADE

Epidural analgesia

This increasingly popular technique allows effective analgesia to be achieved in children both during and after operation. The introduction of small-gauge epidural needles and fine epidural catheters has made epidural analgesia feasible in the smallest of children. Single injection, intermittent, and infusion epidural analgesia have become popular, often permitting light anaesthesia, minimal use of opioids and early extubation. Physiological differences between adults and children – namely a reduced sympathetic tone and reduced blood volume in the splanchnic circulation and lower limbs in children – result in remarkable cardiovascular stability in infants undergoing high central neuraxial blockade that, in adults, would cause hypotension because of sympathetic blockade.

Approaches to the epidural space in children have been described at thoracic, lumbar, sacral and caudal levels. These techniques are demanding and there is a significant failure rate, particularly in smaller children. In infants aged up to 6–12 months it is usually possible to cannulate the epidural space via the caudal hiatus, and this avoids the potential complications of higher approaches.

The main concern must be to keep the total dose of local anaesthetic low in order to minimise the possibility of systemic toxicity. In general, an opioid is required in addition to local anaesthetic after major surgery. It acts synergistically with the local anaesthetic to improve analgesia and reduce the requirement for local anaesthetics, and will also treat discomfort not blocked by the epidural and provide a mild degree of sedation.

Side effects

The use of epidural analgesia requires close nursing supervision of the child. Potential side effects of epidural analgesia include urinary retention, leg weakness, and intravenous or subarachnoid injection. Hypotension is rarely a problem, especially in children younger than 8 years, but the lack of sensation may cause problems if not anticipated. Pressure sores may occur in analgesic skin unless patients are repositioned regularly, and after trauma the technique is generally contraindicated because of the possibility of a compartment syndrome. Wilson & Lloyd-Thomas (1993) reported an 11% incidence of urinary retention among patients receiving epidural infusions of 0.125% bupivacaine and diamorphine. This often requires urinary catheterisation, which has a low but definite incidence of complications.

Caudal epidural analgesia

The technique of epidural analgesia using a single injection of local anaesthetic to the epidural space via the caudal approach combines the advantages of a simple technique with a high success rate and is one of the most commonly used local anaesthetic techniques in paediatric anaesthesia. The technique has a wide range of indications, including lower limb and pelvic orthopaedic surgery. Reports on several large studies describe the high success rate and low incidence of complications associated with the technique. Injection is made through the sacral hiatus (Figs. 4.2 and 4.3), which is formed by a deficiency in the neural arch of the 5th sacral vertebra and is covered by a ligamentous membrane known as the sacrococcygeal membrane. The landmarks for this hiatus are the sacral cornua superiorly and the coccyx inferiorly. Under aseptic conditions, a needle is advanced through the sacrococcygeal membrane until a 'pop' or loss of resistance is felt. After a negative aspiration

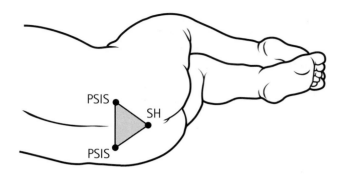

Figure 4.3 Child positioned for caudal epidural injection. The sacral hiatus (SH) lies at the apex of an equilateral triangle formed by the posterior superior iliac spines (PSIS) and the coccyx. (Adapted from McKenzie et al 1997.)

test, the selected dose of local anaesthetic solution is injected slowly.

Side effects

Failure of this technique is usually due to failure to deposit the local anaesthetic in the correct space; the primary determinant of this is the experience of the anaesthetist. The 'failed caudal' may also be due to an inappropriate indication, with the use of an inadequate volume to block the required nerve roots. In older children, there may be failure of the technique because of the development of fibrous septa within the epidural space, which can result in unilateral or limited blocks despite appropriate volumes being injected. Weakness of the legs is common and may be found in more than 30% of young patients given 0.5% bupivacaine (Dalens et al 1986). The incidence of motor block is reduced when more dilute solutions of local anaesthetic are used; however, in many cases there is no requirement for a child to be able to walk in the first few postoperative hours after operation.

Spinal (subarachnoid) anaesthesia

Subarachnoid anaesthesia may be used in high-risk patients, including those with congenital abnormalities or muscular and neuromuscular disease, as these conditions increase operative and anaesthetic risk.

OPIOIDS

The most commonly used opioid is morphine; more experience has been gained with this than with any of the other opioids. In addition to producing analgesia, opioids cause a similar spectrum of side effects. They have the disadvantage of a relatively narrow therapeutic range and marked variability in response between patients because of differing pharmacokinetics and pharmacodynamics. This is particularly marked in children younger than 6 months, as drug elimination is very variable owing to diminished clearance and a prolonged half-life. There is also an increased sensitivity to the depressant effects of these drugs. Nevertheless,

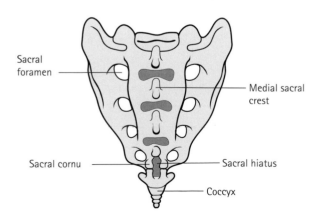

Figure 4.2 Posterior view of the sacrum 1997. (Adapted from McKenzie et al 1997.)

it is still possible to provide excellent analgesia with safety in these infants if sensible dosage regimens and appropriate monitoring procedures are used. There are, of course, older children who can be expected to be particularly susceptible to the depressant effects of opioids because of specific conditions or sensitivities. These include those with severe respiratory disease, upper airway obstruction, and renal or hepatic impairment. The concurrent administration of other centrally acting sedative drugs, such as benzodiazepines, with opioids puts any patient at considerable risk of over-sedation and respiratory depression. These classes of drugs should rarely be administered concurrently.

The analgesic effect of opioids depends upon the brain concentration of active compounds, which in turn is related to plasma concentrations. Intermittent intramuscular administration is unlikely to produce steady plasma concentrations and may result in widely fluctuating concentrations of opioids. This tends to produce periods of analgesia and excessive sedation alternating with periods of inadequate pain relief. Furthermore, intramuscular injections may cause such distress to children that they are not requested. These factors may lead to long periods of inadequate pain relief when intermittent intramuscular injections are used.

The intermittent administration of intravenous bolus doses of an opioid on an 'as required' basis has the potential to provide extremely good analgesia, with a high degree of safety. If pain is assessed conscientiously and analgesia given when required, then excellent relief is achieved. However, because this is a relatively labour-intensive method of administering opioids, intermittent intravenous bolus dose administration is rarely used. Despite this, it is a very useful and safe method of giving analgesia to children and is particularly applicable in the emergency department for the treatment of pain caused by trauma.

Opioids by infusion

The technique of continuous intravenous infusion of an opioid solution has become popular because of its efficacy, simplicity and wide range of indications. Continuous infusion will maintain a steady blood concentration of opioids once equilibration is reached, and makes repeated injections unnecessary. A loading dose is required to avoid the prolonged period of four to five half-lives required to reach a steady state. Dosages of morphine in the range 10–40 μg/kg per hour are adequate in most patients, and infusions are usually started in the middle of this range for children older than 6 months, and at 5–10 μg/kg per hour for the younger child. The effective use of intravenous infusions requires close nursing supervision so that the infusion rate is adequate and is titrated against changing requirements during mobilisation and physiotherapy.

An alternative method of delivering a continuous infusion of an opioid is to use the subcutaneous route of administration. This technique has been shown to be effective in adults and children. It is subject to the same potential dangers as the intravenous route.

Patient-controlled analgesia

Patient-controlled analgesia is an analgesic technique whereby the patient is able to self-administer bolus doses of opioid with a degree of flexibility within a prescription that sets the bolus dose administered, the obligatory delay between boluses (lockout interval) and the presence or absence of a background infusion. Most machines comprise an infusion pump with software allowing the use of a trigger device to deliver bolus doses with or without a variable background infusion.

When used appropriately, patient-controlled analgesia has the potential to provide good analgesia that is flexible enough to respond to the changing needs of patients with time. It takes account of events such as physiotherapy and mobilisation by the prophylactic administration of a bolus. The technique also adjusts for the great variability between patients in terms of the perception of pain and their pharmacokinetic and pharmacodynamic behaviour. Patients who perceive that their pain requires treatment are able to self-administer within the prescription limits without reference to medical or nursing staff.

Selection of patients suitable for patient-controlled analgesia depends on a number of features, including the age of the child, the developmental stage, and intelligence. The absolute requirements are the ability to understand the concepts of demand analgesia and a lockout interval, and to be physically able to operate the trigger of the patient-controlled analgesia machine. Sensible use of a patient-controlled analgesia machine requires preoperative tuition of the child and parent(s) and postoperative reinforcement of this tuition, particularly the concept of a lockout interval. With adequate explanation and postoperative supervision, many children aged 8 years and more can use patient-controlled analgesia appropriately.

A variation on patient-controlled analgesia that has been used successfully in children is nurse-controlled analgesia. With this technique, a modest infusion of morphine (10–20 μg/kg per hour) is supplemented by boluses of 10–20 μg/kg given at the discretion of the nurse caring for the child, subject to a lockout interval. This offers the advantages of avoiding a generous, fixed infusion rate that may be excessive in some children, while offering a basal level of analgesia that can be supplemented as required and titrated to the needs of the child. It also has the advantage of requiring an obligatory assessment of the patient by the nurse before any opioid boluses are administered. When used appropriately, nurse-controlled analgesia is a very effective and safe form of postoperative analgesia, which combines some of the better features of both fixed infusions and patient-controlled analgesia (PCA).

The use of morphine sulphate in these various techniques is summarised in Table 4.3.

Table 4.3 Suggested dilutions and dosages for the use of morphine sulphate

Technique	Dilution	Dose
Bolus dose (intramuscular or intravenous)		100–200 µg/kg
Intravenous infusion	1 mg/kg in 50 ml 0.9% saline (20 µg/kg per ml)	10–40 µg/kg per hour (0.5–2 ml/hour); 5–20 µg/kg per hour if younger than 6 months
Subcutaneous infusion	1 mg/kg in 20 ml 0.9% saline (50 µg/kg per ml)	10–40 µg/kg per hour (0.2–0.8 ml/hour)
Patient-controlled analgesia	1 mg/kg in 50 ml 0.9% saline (20 µg/kg per ml)	Bolus dose 20 µg/kg (1 ml); lockout interval 5 minutes
Nurse-controlled analgesia	1 mg/kg in 50 ml saline 0.9% saline (20 µg/kg per ml)	Infusion 10 µg/kg per hour (0.5 ml/hour); bolus dose 20–40 µg/kg (1–2 ml); lockout 20 minutes
Oral dose		300 µg/kg 4-hourly

Monitoring

The potential problems that may occur with opioid infusions or patient-controlled analgesia can be divided into those resulting from errors by medical and nursing staff, from misuse by the patient or others, and from faults in the equipment. These necessitate the implementation of some form of monitoring procedure that will detect potential problems at an early stage and provide warnings that can be acted upon to prevent the situation from deteriorating. The features of interest are a measure of respiratory depression or hypoventilation, an assessment of the level of sedation or consciousness, the opioid consumption, and machine performance. The intermittent recording of the rate of ventilation has been shown to be a late and insensitive monitor of hypoventilation, and this cannot be relied upon to give early warning of this problem. The use of pulse oximetry while breathing air is a more sensitive monitor of hypoventilation (Hutton & Clutton-Brock 1993) and, in the absence of other causes of hypoxia such as impaired gas exchange, mild hypoxia (arterial oxygen saturation (SaO_2) <94%) indicates mild hypoventilation.

Somnolence caused by opioids tends to occur at an early stage and is a valuable early warning of excessive opioid administration. When used in conjunction with pulse oximetry, this helps to discriminate between the possible causes of hypoxia. To be used properly, the measure of sedation should be as objective as possible, to avoid bias between observers and with time. This should ensure that different observers looking at the same patient will give the same sedation score, and that important changes in the status of

the patient are reflected by changes in the score. Those components of the Glasgow Coma Scale that relate to eye opening fulfil these requirements. With experience, paediatric nurses can discriminate between a child who is naturally asleep and one who is receiving excessive opioid. A child who is asleep has a good colour and peripheral perfusion, and breathes in an easy unobstructed manner with an SaO_2 greater than 94% while breathing air. A child becoming over-sedated has a less good colour, and may breathe with the mouth hanging open and be partially obstructed; an SaO_2 of less than 94% is usually present.

Regular checks of the performance of the infusion pump or patient-controlled analgesia machine are necessary, to ensure that appropriate doses of opioid are being administered and that the machine has not failed or over-delivered.

NON-STEROIDAL ANTI-INFLAMMATORY DRUGS (NSAIDS)

There are several groups of NSAIDs that exert an analgesic effect by means of an anti-inflammatory action – specifically the inhibition of the enzyme, cyclo-oxygenase – to reduce the synthesis of the inflammatory mediators, prostaglandins, thromboxane and prostacyclin. Their efficacy has been well described in minor surgery when used in combination with local anaesthetic techniques when they prolong the effective duration of regional blocks (Gadiyar et al 1995). In combination with opioids after major orthopaedic surgery they exert a useful opioid-sparing effect – of the order of a 30% reduced requirement (Teiria & Meretoja 1994). The main limitation of NSAIDs is their relative lack of potency, with a ceiling effect on the analgesia provided, which makes the drugs inadequate for use in single-analgesic techniques after intermediate and major surgery.

Adverse effects of NSAIDs include peptic ulceration, impaired platelet function, bronchospasm and renal impairment. Prostaglandins inhibit gastric acid secretion and stimulate the production of mucus. Blood flow to the gastric mucosa is reduced by inhibitors of prostaglandin synthesis and this may play a part in the spectrum of gastric effects that NSAIDs produce, including erosions, petechiae and

Table 4.4 Non-steroidal analgesic drugs

Drug	Dosing regimen
Diclofenac sodium	0.5–1 mg/kg 8-hourly oral or rectal Maximum 3 mg/kg per day Maximum adult dose 150 mg/day
Ibuprofen	5 mg/kg 6-hourly oral Maximum 20 mg/kg per day Maximum adult dose 400 mg 6-hourly
Paracetamol	15 mg/kg 4-hourly oral 20 mg/kg 6-hourly rectal Maximum 90 mg/kg per either route Maximum adult dose 4 g/day

ulcers. In paediatric practice, the potential side effects of these drugs, including peptic ulceration, impaired platelet function, bronchospasm and renal impairment, have rarely been major problems. Most anaesthetists and surgeons are prepared to use these drugs for a variety of orthopaedic procedures, provided there are no contraindications.

Commonly used and effective NSAIDs include diclofenac sodium, ibuprofen and paracetamol. Typical dosing regimens are described in Table 4.4. Paracetamol in a dose of 15 mg/kg 6-hourly is a useful analgesic in many forms of minor surgery or non-specific pain. Its antipyretic effect is of great value and will not prevent the recognition of postoperative infective complications. It is effective and safe in neonates. The drug has a wide therapeutic ratio and few contraindications. It does not cause gastritis or renal impairment, and may be given rectally, although this affords a lower bioavailability than the oral route and doses in the region of 20–30 mg/kg are required.

REFERENCES

Audenaert S M, Vickers H, Burgess R C 1991 Axillary block for vascular insufficiency after repair of radial club hands in an infant. Anesthesiology 74: 368–370

Berde C B, Lehn B M, Yee J D, Sethna N F, Russo D 1991 Patient-controlled analgesia in children: a randomised prospective comparison with intramuscular administration of morphine for postoperative analgesia. Journal of Pediatrics 118: 460–466

Dalens B, Tanguy A, Haberer J 1986 Lumbar epidural anesthesia for operative and postoperative pain relief in infants and young children. Anesthesia and Analgesia 65: 1069–1073

Dalens B, Vanneuville G, Tanguy A 1989 Comparison of the fascia iliaca compartment block with the 3-in-1 block in children. Anesthesia and Analgesia 69: 705–713

Gadiyar V, Gallacher T M, Crean P M, Taylor R H 1995 The effect of a combination of rectal diclofenac and caudal bupivacaine on postoperative analgesia in children. Anaesthesia 50: 820–822

Grunau R V E, Craig K D 1987 Pain expression in neonates: facial action and cry. Pain 28: 395–410

Hanallah R S, Broadman L M, Belman A B, Abramowitz M D, Epstein B S 1987 Comparison of caudal and ilioinguinal nerve blocks for control of post-orchidopexy pain in pediatric ambulatory surgery. Anesthesiology 66: 832–834

Hutton P, Clutton-Brock T 1993 The benefits and pitfalls of pulse oximetry. British Medical Journal 307: 457–458

Maunuksela E, Olkkola K T, Korpela R 1987 Measurement of pain in children with self-reporting and behavioural assessment. Clinical Pharmacology and Therapeutics 42: 137–141

McKenzie I M, Gaukroger P B, Ragg P G, Kester Brown J C 1997 Manual of Acute Pain Management in Children. Churchill Livingstone, London

Teiria H, Meretoja O A 1994 PCA in paediatric orthopaedic patients: influence of a NSAID on morphine requirement. Paediatric Anaesthesia 4: 87–91

Tobias J D 1994 Continuous femoral nerve block to provide analgesia following femur fracture in a paediatric ICU population. Anaesthesia and Intensive Care 22: 616–618

Wedel D J, Krohn J S, Hall J A 1991 Brachial plexus anesthesia in pediatric patients. Mayo Clinic Proceedings 66: 583–588

Wilson P T J, Lloyd-Thomas A R 1993 An audit of extradural infusion analgesia in children using bupivacaine and diamorphine. Anaesthesia 48: 718–723

Chapter 5

Paediatric imaging

D. Wilson and G. Allen

GENERAL PRINCIPLES

Children pose particular problems for imaging, partly because it is vital to limit the dose of radiation. The younger the child, the more radiosensitive the bone marrow and the greater the potential harm. Children also have to be persuaded to co-operate if adequate imaging is to be obtained, and specific radiographic skills are essential.

When plain X-rays are undertaken, a fast screen/film system with short exposure times and good collimation can reduce the radiation dose. The gonads should be adequately protected, unless examination of the central or lower pelvis is essential (Fig. 5.1). Protection for the thyroid and breast tissue should be provided where necessary, as they are particularly radiosensitive. Ultrasound and magnetic resonance imaging (MRI) should be considered as alternatives to X-ray, although sedation or anaesthesia may be needed for MRI, making it less practical in children.

The environment in which imaging is performed should be 'child friendly', with pictures and soft toys. Parents should be made welcome, but care should be taken to protect them if necessary – for example when a mother is pregnant

and her child is undergoing an X-ray examination. Fluoroscopy and computed tomography should be performed only for specific indications in which the potential benefit outweighs the risk.

The referring clinician should be aware of the risks of ionising radiation, and should be prepared to discuss the issues involved with the child's parents or guardian. On occasion it may be necessary to refer to a radiologist for additional advice.

In the UK, Europe, and many other countries, a doctor with sufficient training and experience to understand the risks, radiation-limiting techniques and alternative non-ionising methods must clinically direct any examination involving ionising radiation. Statutes and directives have been and continue to be published to indicate that the specialised training necessary to meet these requirements takes several years; in practice, this means that a qualified radiologist is essential. The individual clinically directing the exposure has a personal responsibility to the patient and should not accept referrals that contravene principles of safety. In general, the referring doctor should request an examination for a specified clinical indication and expect advice when alternative techniques may be indicated.

Table 5.1 illustrates the dose of radiation and the risks of harm incurred with a single radiograph of the chest, pelvis or skull.

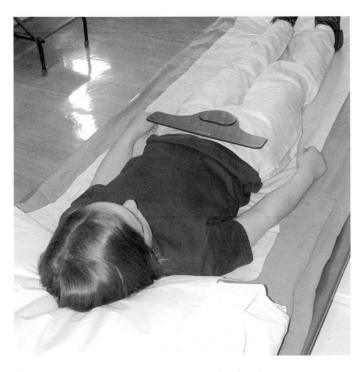

Figure 5.1 A child with gonad protection in place.

Table 5.1 Dose of common X-rays, and associated risks			
Examination	Age group	Effective dose (mSv)	Risk of harm (detriment)
AP/PA chest	1–<12 months	0.011	1 in 71 000
	1–<5 years	0.010	1 in 78 000
	5–<10 years	0.009	1 in 84 000
	10–<16 years	0.008	1 in 92 000
AP hip	1–<12 months	0.024	1 in 32 000
	1–<5 years	0.032	1 in 24 000
	5–<10 years	0.021	1 in 37 000
	10–<16 years	0.087	1 in 89 000
AP skull	1–<12 months	0.009	1 in 890 000
	1–<5 years	0.011	1 in 730 000
	5–<10 years	0.012	1 in 660 000
	10–<16 years	0.015	1 in 530 000

mSv, millisievest – unit of dose equivalent; 1/Sv = 1/J/kg.
AP, anteroposterior view; PA, posteroanterior view.
(Courtesy of Dr A. Woodward; calculated from Kyriou et al 1996.)

To give some idea of these risks, 0.25 msV of radiation is equivalent to:

- smoking 10 cigarettes
- 15 minutes of rock climbing
- travelling 4000 miles by air
- travelling 600 miles by road
- 1:100 000 risk of fatality.

NORMAL DEVELOPMENTAL ANATOMY AND NORMAL VARIANTS

One of the most challenging aspects of interpreting a child's X-ray is recognising normal developmental anatomy and normal variants (Fig. 5.2).

It is impossible for even the dedicated paediatric musculoskeletal radiologist to memorise all the epiphyseal centres and the age at which they appear – or, indeed, the many variants that occur in bone. Help is at hand in the excellent bench books (Keats 1996, Keats & Smith 1988, Kohler & Zimmer 1993). For the assessment of age in an overdeveloped or underdeveloped child, the left hand radiograph (Fig. 5.3) has also been well documented by Greulich & Pyle (1959) and Tanner et al (1983). The former uses standard images of male and female children for direct comparison, indicating the time of appearance of the ossification centre in the epiphysis of each bone of the digits and carpus, with the timing of their fusion. The latter volume describes a more complex and arguably more accurate method: each bone of the carpus and digits is individually scored. This is a

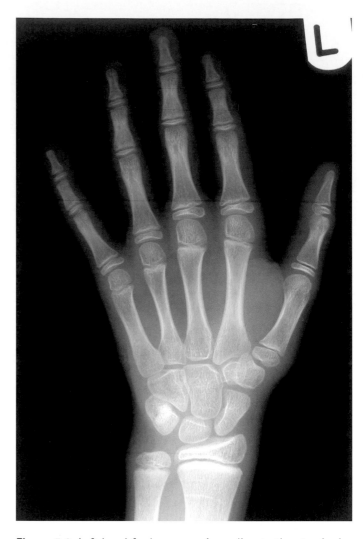

Figure 5.3 Left hand for bone age. According to the standards set by Greulich & Pyle (1959), this is the hand of a child aged 11 years 6 months (standard deviation 10.5 months).

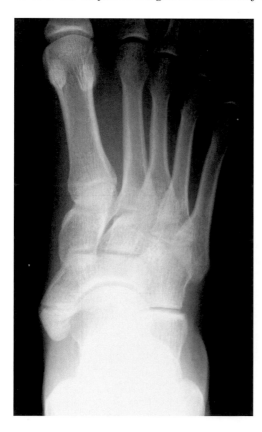

Figure 5.2 Os tibiale externum, an accessory ossification centre of the navicular, which is a normal variant.

time-consuming process, but it may be worthwhile when management choices are dependent critically upon the precise bone age. When either method is used, we recommend that the standard deviation of normal is recorded.

The elbow poses a particular challenge to the clinician because of its ossification centres. A good aide-memoire for these is 'CRITOL':

C	Capitellum	2 months–2 years
R	Radial head (bipartite)	3–6 years
I	Internal (medial) epicondyle	4–7 years
T	Trochlea (two centres)	
	Lateral condyle	1–2 years
	Medial (bipartite)	8–10 years
O	Olecranon (bipartite)	8–10 years
L	Lateral epicondyle	10–13 years

Fusion of the epiphyses starts with the radial head and ends with the lateral epicondyle, the others fusing at approximately the same age.

TECHNIQUES AVAILABLE

PLAIN FILMS

Plain radiographs remain the workhorse of imaging. They are mandatory in cases where trauma is suspected, and when there is implanted metal in a joint or bone. With more than 100 years of accumulated experience in interpreting plain radiographs, radiologists and clinicians are more familiar at interpreting abnormalities than they are with more modern imaging techniques. Plain radiographs, however, have significant limitations. They use radiation and give only very limited information about muscles, ligaments, tendons and soft tissues. Furthermore, plain radiographs may appear normal in cases of significant bony abnormality; for example in early osteonecrosis, osteomyelitis or subtle fractures.

A number of techniques may reduce the dose of radiation. The newest film screen combinations using rare-earth screens should always be used in paediatric practice; indeed, they should probably be used in all forms of radiological imaging, whatever the age of the patient. When thicker or wider areas of the body such as the chest or abdomen are being examined, scattering artefact may degrade the quality of the image. A Bucky or grid placed between the film and the patient reduces the scatter, but increases the dose of radiation required to achieve the same exposure. In general, Bucky techniques are not required in the peripheral skeleton and probably should be avoided in smaller children. More modern plain X-ray systems allow for computed radiography. Here, a phosphor plate replaces the film and a separate piece of apparatus reads the image from this plate directly into a computer archive. The films may be viewed on a monitor or printed on laser film. These systems have much wider latitude to faulty exposure. Over- and under-exposures are less likely to obscure or over-penetrate the image; as a result, fewer repeated exposures are required, and the radiation load to the patient is reduced. These images have the advantage that they may be viewed on different window levels to allow for a more penetrated examination of bone, or a softer view of the muscles and subcutaneous tissues.

Recently developed direct digital capture systems allow the image to be transferred instantly to the computer archive for viewing in storage, in the same way as computed radiography. These latest systems have advantages similar to those of computed radiography and also considerably decrease the time it takes to perform an examination.

ULTRASOUND

Musculoskeletal ultrasound has improved considerably over the past few years. Better equipment with high frequency probes, plus an increased understanding of the relevant anatomy and pathology have lead to its widespread use in orthopaedic, rheumatological and other musculoskeletal practice. It is an easy technique that does not use ionising radiation. The principal disadvantage of the technique is that it is very observer dependent, and there is a considerable learning curve.

Children generally tolerate ultrasound examination very well. It is advantageous if the contact jelly is warmed, either in hot water or on a nearby radiator; if you do not use a purpose-built warmer, always test the temperature before use. A careful explanation, including a demonstration on the examiner's limb, usually proves effective in calming anxiety. Ultrasound is the examination of choice in the assessment of developmental dysplasia of the hip, irritable hip, tendon disease and soft tissue lumps. It is also useful in guiding biopsies and aspirations.

COMPUTED TOMOGRAPHY

Most hospitals are being re-equipped with helical computed tomography (CT) machines. These are less precisely described as 'spiral CT machines', and differ from conventional CT in their speed of examination and the ability to produce much better quality reconstructions in orthogonal planes. Their principal disadvantage is that it is very tempting to use CT over extensive areas and thus significantly increase the dose of radiation; care must therefore be taken in planning and judging the area of interest.

CT remains the main workhorse in the district general hospital for cross-sectional imaging. However, its use in children should be limited, because of the dose of radiation involved.

CT is the best technique for examining the pathology of bone in detail and for studying complex fractures. It is extremely useful for detecting the nidus in osteoid osteoma, as this may not be visible on MRI. For this condition, MRI is useful to detect an area of bone oedema and CT is then a second-line test to confirm its nature by using very thin sections at the site of MRI abnormality. CT is now rarely used in the assessment of bone and soft tissue tumours, having been replaced by MRI, but CT is of particular value in bony coalitions and abnormalities of the skeleton. These include complex spinal malformations and hindfoot coalitions.

MAGNETIC RESONANCE IMAGING

MRI is of particular value in children, because it does not use ionising radiation. Children vary considerably in their tolerance of the technique, particularly when using a solenoid (conventional bore-type) magnet: claustrophobia can be a distinct problem. Open MRI systems reduce this risk and also have the advantage that the child's parents can sit nearby, but if the field strength (Tesla) of the magnet is low, this can lead to long examination times. More recently, high-field open systems have achieved good quality images in less time, while preserving the advantage of the open architecture.

Radiographers experienced in examining children can normally perform good quality studies on any child able to understand the explanation of the study. In general, children younger than 4 years are very difficult to examine without sedation or anaesthesia. If a small infant is in a plaster cast, it may be practical to perform the examination despite lack of co-operation. It is always wise to attempt MRI without sedating the patient when there is even an outside chance of achieving a diagnostic study. If sedation or anaesthesia are necessary for children in an MRI unit, it should be performed by an experienced paediatric anaesthetist with full monitoring equipment. MRI-safe monitoring and anaesthetic devices are available, but they are very expensive and are usually installed only in systems with a particular requirement for anaesthesia. An MRI room is a difficult environment in which to observe the response to sedation, and monitoring is complex.

MRI is the investigation of choice in patients suspected to have an internal disruption of a joint, bone infection, bone tumour, soft tissue tumour, spinal anomaly, or congenital malformation.

NUCLEAR MEDICINE

Nuclear medicine is now used less often, since ultrasound and MRI have become more widely applicable. The radiation burden of the technique is significant, and most of the examinations require intravenous injections. The scans can, however, be easily repeated if a child moves. A disadvantage of nuclear medicine is that it is expensive, because of the cost of radiopharmaceuticals; in many institutions, it costs as much as, if not more than, MRI.

Bone scintigraphy is still particularly useful for assessing metastases – both for the detection of lesions and to assess their extent. It can detect or exclude osteomyelitis, especially the multifocal form, but MRI now rivals this technique and is the preferred imaging method. Indium chloride labelled white cell studies and gallium citrate scintigraphy may be used, with or without emission computed tomography, in obscure cases of osteomyelitis. In children, the interpretation of bone scintigrams may be confused by high activity at the growth plates, which may obscure significant disease such as tumours and infections.

OTHER IMAGING

Angiography is important in the treatment of complex venous malformations, when embolisation is indicated. This is an area of special expertise only available in specialist centres. Luckily, MRI can be used diagnostically in assessing the extent of congenital vascular lesions before a decision as to the need for such intervention is made.

Dual energy X-ray absorptiometry scans quantitate bone density in osteoporosis and osteogenesis imperfecta. They can also be used to monitor the treatment of osteoporosis. However, they require sedation in the very young, because of the length of time needed for data acquisition.

APPLICATIONS

ANTENATAL DIAGNOSIS

One of the most significant contributions imaging can make is in the antenatal diagnosis of skeletal disorders. The routine use of ultrasound in pregnancy at 20 weeks gestation helps both clinician and parent-to-be to plan ahead for the newborn if fetal anomalies are detected and the pregnancy is allowed to continue.

Ultrasound may detect serious abnormalities such as arthrogryposis, neural tube defects and limb reduction defects, but it is also useful in the diagnosis of subtle problems such as clubfoot and polydactyly. In hereditary disorders, ultrasound guides amniocentesis for DNA analysis and other tests.

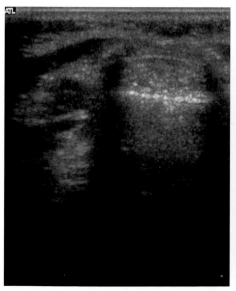 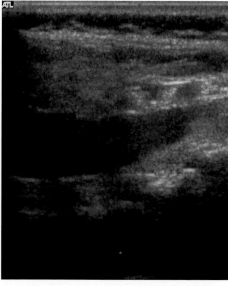

Figure 5.4 Ultrasound images of an infant with a tethered cord. The canal should only contain the cauda equina on the axial view (**A**), and the tip of the conus can be seen too low down on the longitudinal image (**B**).

A
B

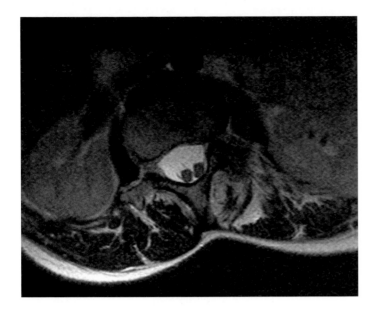

Figure 5.5 MRI of diastematomyelia.

SPINAL ANOMALIES

Ultrasound is the screening technique of choice in infants suspected of spine anomalies.

In the newborn with a sacral dimple or hair tuft, the spinal canal can be visualised with ultrasound. This allows the diagnosis of an occult spina bifida or a tethered spinal cord (Fig. 5.4).

In the newborn with other skeletal abnormalities, an ultrasound of the cord is an accepted screening test to exclude associated spinal anomalies. Spinal cord tethering, myelomeningocele, syringomyelia, and diastematomyelia can be diagnosed. The only alternative technique would be MRI (Figs 5.5–5.8); however, infants are difficult to examine, and the images provided by even the best MRI systems in anaesthetised infants lack the resolution of good quality ultrasound.

DEVELOPMENTAL DYSPLASIA OF THE HIP

There is a window of opportunity to treat children with hip dysplasia. Splintage for instability and dysplasia is most effective in the first 6–8 weeks of life. Ultrasound examination is proven to enhance the accuracy of clinical assessment and is now established as routine practice in many centres. Frank dislocation is usually detected clinically; ultrasound is principally of use in showing milder forms of acetabular dysplasia that might lead to late subluxation or even dislocation (Figs 5.9 and 5.10). In the newborn, the hips are commonly subluxable, but within 4 weeks most stabilise. It is wise to delay the initial examination for 3–4 weeks to reduce the number of positive examinations but keeping within the treatment window of 6–8 weeks.

A variety of methods are used for the examination of infants' hips by ultrasound. Each has its advocates, but all

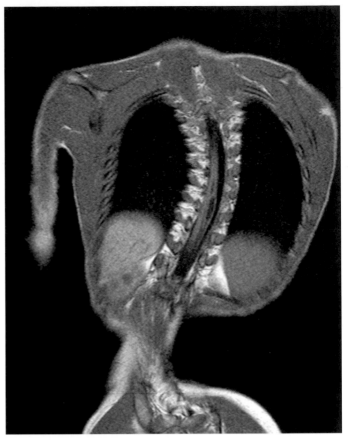

A

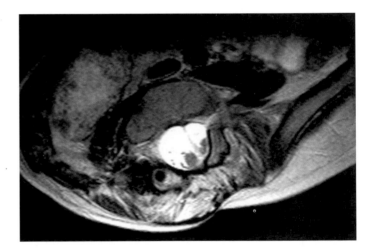

B

Figure 5.6 MRI of tethered cord. **A** Coronal. **B** Axial.

that have been reported are similar in their efficacy. Rather than argue the merits of a particular technique, it is more useful to advise that a standard technique is used by each hospital, so that there is a method of quantifiable measurement of acetabular depth, which can be reproduced. It is recommended that dynamic studies be used as an adjunct. For all methods, a precise coronal or axial plane should be recorded. The choice of method will depend on the

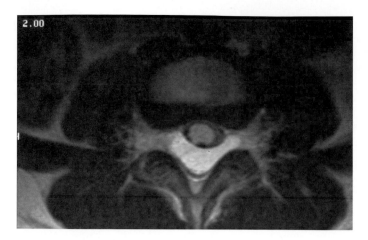

Figure 5.7 MRI of lipoma of the cord.

institution, but those described by Graf (1982), Morin (1999) and Harke & Grisson (1999) are all effective. It is important to arrange regular audit and clinical outcome review, as this allows the maintenance of high standards and enhances the continued training of sonographers.

Radiographs are of limited value in infants younger than 3 months; thereafter they are the preferred method of judging hip morphology.

IRRITABLE HIP

Investigation and management of this common condition concentrates upon excluding those conditions that require urgent treatment – in particular, septic arthritis. Ultrasound

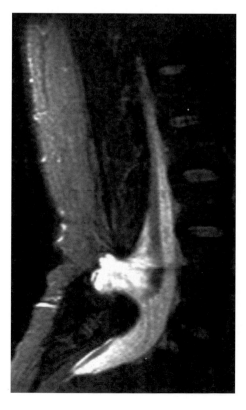

Figure 5.8 MRI of myelomeningocele.

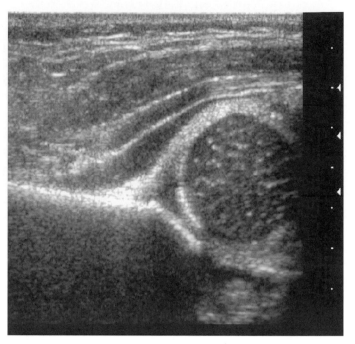

Figure 5.9 Ultrasound image of a shallow (dysplastic) hip.

is a sensitive and powerful method of detecting hip joint effusion: less than 1 ml of excess fluid can be detected by careful technique. The hip is examined with the patient supine. The anterior part of the hip capsule is relatively slack. An oblique ultrasound plane along the axis of the femoral neck provides an image that will demonstrate fluid as a dark (echo-free) collection. Comparison is made with the opposite side, and a difference of 2 mm or more in depth of the synovial space indicates an effusion (Fig. 5.11). Unfortunately, the characteristics of the fluid or synovial

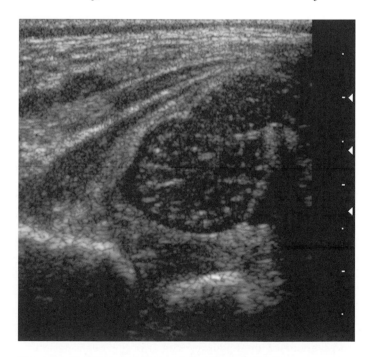

Figure 5.10 Ultrasound image of a dislocated hip.

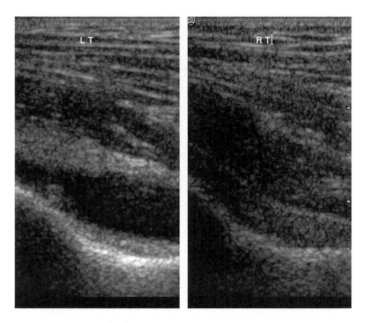

Figure 5.11 Ultrasound image of an irritable hip, showing an effusion on one side as a result of transient synovitis.

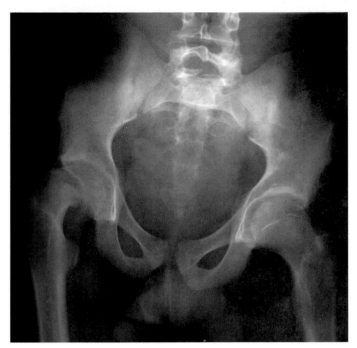

Figure 5.12 Plain film of a child with a slipped upper femoral epiphysis.

hypertrophy do not differentiate a clear effusion from blood or pus; indeed, some septic joints in children occur without any clinical or serological markers, and they may produce only a small effusion.

We, with others, feel that emergency ultrasound-guided aspiration has great merit. Any tamponade is relieved and the patient rapidly becomes pain free. Sepsis may be excluded by Gram stain and culture. If the initial Gram stain is negative, it is safe to discharge the patients, provided immediate recall is possible if the cultures subsequently grow organisms. This approach reduces the duration of symptoms for all, and saves many overnight admissions. The techniques involved are easy to learn and have proved to be safe. If a local anaesthetic skin cream is applied 90 minutes before the patient undergoes imaging by ultrasound, the hip aspiration is less traumatic than a blood test. However, for this system to be effective, a procedure must be in place for the rapid receipt and feedback of the microbiology results.

SLIPPED UPPER FEMORAL EPIPHYSIS

Ultrasound may also detect a slipped upper femoral epiphysis (SUFE) or fragmentation of the epiphysis in Perthes' disease. Unexplained and persistent joint effusions should be investigated further, to exclude osteomyelitis, Perthes' disease and other subarticular pathology. A plain film can be helpful, but the most useful test is MRI, as most abnormalities are ruled out by a normal study.

Children older than 8 years who present with hip pain should always be suspected of suffering from SUFE (Fig. 5.12). A frog or lateral view of both hips is mandatory in all cases. It may be argued that the conventional anteroposterior view may be omitted, as 14% of anteroposterior films may be normal in the presence of a SUFE; some authors, however, claim that the frog lateral view can provoke the slip. Remember that 75% of children with SUFE show a joint effusion on ultrasound and may be confused with those suffering from transient synovitis. The inclusion of a plain film with an appropriate projection should remove the risk of oversight in this age group.

If there is doubt about minor degrees of slip, especially on the 'normal' side when SUFE is apparent in one hip, MRI using an oblique plane of imaging is very useful. It could be argued that all patients with a unilateral SUFE should undergo MRI, because in some studies the incidence of bilateral slipping has been reported as 60%.

LIMB LENGTHENING

Operations to correct leg length discrepancies or fracture deformity should be monitored by a combination of ultrasound and plain films (Fig. 5.13). The gap at the osteotomy will contain callus that is forming; too slow a distraction may allow premature bridging, whereas too fast a distraction can cause haemorrhagic cysts to form in the gap, preventing healing. Weekly or fortnightly review with the combination of a radiograph that includes a measurement marker plus ultrasound measurement of the width of the gap allows these problems to be overcome. If the gap is filling too fast, more speedy distraction is indicated. If there is delayed filling on ultrasound, with or without cysts, it is wise to slow down. Cysts that do not resolve rapidly may be aspirated, using ultrasound guidance.

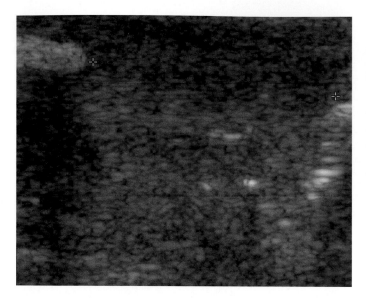

Figure 5.13 Ultrasound image of the gap during a leg lengthening procedure; there are no cysts.

SCOLIOSIS

Children present with scoliosis because of deformity, pain or a rib hump. Imaging is useful in assessing the degree of scoliosis, underlying congenital bony abnormalities, and underlying neurological tissue abnormalities.

Imaging is particularly important before surgery. Defects of neural tissues including tethering, myelomeningocele and diastematomyelia are especially dangerous if they are undiagnosed before the corrective surgery. The routine follow-up for patients with spinal deformity is a concern, because of the substantial radiation dose to organs and tissues that are sensitive in young people.

The initial diagnosis to include the assessment of the degree of curvature and bony abnormalities should be made on anteroposterior and lateral plain films of the entire spine, taken with the child in a standing position. The angle of curvature (scoliosis or kyphosis) may be measured from these films. A line should be drawn along the endplate of the vertebral body, at the point at which the curve reverses, effectively measuring the maximum angle within each element of the curve (Cobb's angle) (see Ch.31). Curvature is described by the direction of the convexity. Marks made on the film should be in erasable crayon, to avoid obscuring details that may be clinically important at a later stage.

There should be a description of hemivertebrae, fused vertebrae, butterfly vertebrae and other segmentation anomalies.

In cases of simple scoliosis without congenital vertebral anomalies, further imaging for the neurological structures is not normally indicated until such time as surgery is considered or planned. If there are significant bony abnormalities, it would be reasonable to perform an MRI series early in the conduct of the case (Fig. 5.14). Most surgeons

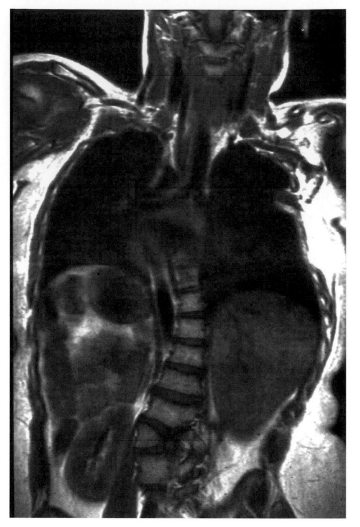

Figure 5.14 MRI of scoliosis with a butterfly vertebra.

would now consider MRI to be a requirement before elective surgery for scoliosis. The sequences used should include images of the foramen magnum for Chiari and other hindbrain abnormalities. Sagittal images are required to assess spinal cord tethering and lipoma of the cord. Coronal images are particularly useful, to look for vertebral anomalies and to assess the adjacent organs. Renal abnormalities are commonly associated with spinal deformity. A series of axial images should be taken throughout the spinal cord, as diastematomyelia and syringomyelia may be very difficult to identify on the sagittal and coronal images alone. The MRI protocol for scoliosis imaging is a lengthy procedure, but exclusion of any of these images leads to the risk of missing a significant abnormality:

- sagittal FSE T2 (thoraco-lumbar)
- coronal CSE T1 (thoraco-lumbar)
- axials through the apex of the curve (FSE T2 or GE T2)
- axial FSE T2 from conus to filum terminale
- sagittal FSE T2 (cervical spine).

(FSE, fast spin echo; CSE, conventional spin echo; GE, gradient echo. T1, T2, weighted images.)

The assessment of curvature may include plain-film bending views. Reactive and secondary curves will be obliterated by motion, but the primary structural curve will remain. Follow-up studies may be usefully achieved by using photographic methods of assessing the shape of the back – for example, the ISIS scanner marketed by Oxford Metrics, or Moiré Fringe techniques (Fig. 5.15). These methods have the advantage of not using ionising radiation and being recorded in a repeatable and electronic form. They also, probably, afford a better assessment of the physical deformity of the patient, giving a measure of the degree of rib hump in addition to the abnormalities of curvature in the spine. They are particularly useful for serial assessments after conservative or surgical treatment.

After operations, plain films are mandatory to assess the placement and integrity of instrumentation. When there is doubt over the positioning, especially of pedicle screws, CT is the best means of assessing their location; metal artefact reduction software is improving and it is usually possible to define the position of the implants with considerable accuracy. However, if there is a question of impingement on nerve roots or spinal cord, CT may not be sufficient to make this diagnosis and an attempt should be made to use MRI. Fast spin echo techniques with the minimum of additional radiofrequency pulses (pre-saturation, fat saturation, etc.) produce the least artefact. Low-field systems have the advantage over high-field systems in that they produce fewer artefacts with metal implants. If MRI fails, it may be necessary to resort to conventional myelography, with or without CT. These are difficult examinations and need to be performed by radiologists with expertise in myelography; as the technique is nowadays used very rarely, such individuals are proving more difficult to find.

OSTEOMYELITIS

Isotope scintigraphy detects multifocal areas of infection. Children are restless, but after one injection of isotope they can be repeatedly examined as necessary. Whole-body MRI may be the technique of the future, as (unlike scintigraphy) it locates precisely the anatomical sites of multifocal infection.

Ultrasound identifies early infection, as it demonstrates subperiosteal abscesses before they can be revealed by X-ray. It is useful in the extremities, but for spinal infection MRI is mandatory, not only to look at the skeleton, but also for the possibility of epidural and disc involvement. Plain films may strongly suggest infection – for example the well-defined metaphyseal lesion of a Brodie's abscess – and therefore the initial investigations for possible infection should be ultrasound and plain X-ray.

The organism that has caused the infection may give a characteristic appearance on imaging, but specimens should always be obtained after adequate imaging, to guide the appropriate antibiotic therapy (Fig. 5.16).

JUVENILE IDIOPATHIC ARTHRITIS

The plain radiograph has long been used to look for erosive changes in the skeleton; magnetic resonance imaging and ultrasound have now been shown to detect erosions and other soft tissue abnormalities earlier in the disease process, enabling earlier and perhaps more effective treatment. MRI is the most sensitive imaging in patients with

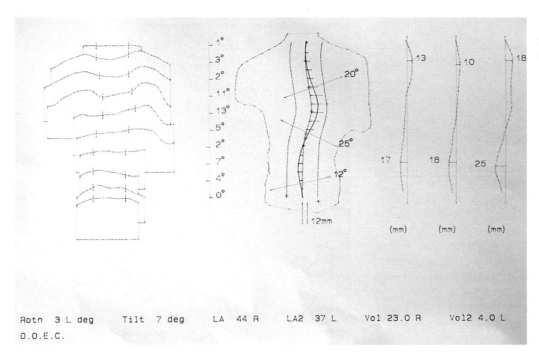

Figure 5.15 Printout of an 'ISIS' study of a child with scoliosis and a rib hump.

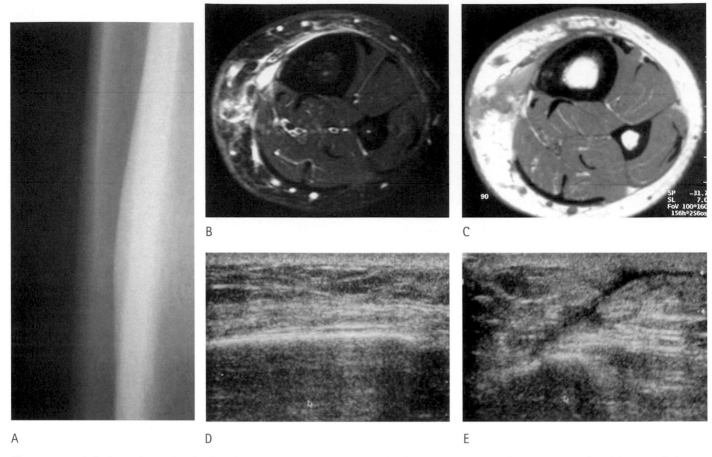

A   D   E

Figure 5.16 A Periosteal reaction in the tibia, caused by osteomyelitis. **B, C** MRI shows the soft tissue extension. Ultrasound shows the periosteal reaction (**D**) and the sinus track through the muscle (**E**).

juvenile idiopathic arthritis, but ultrasound is a good screening test. Ultrasound is easier than MRI to use in children, and it is also more sensitive than the plain X-ray, as it detects the synovitis. The benefit of contrast agents for ultrasound is still being investigated. The use of gadolinium-enhanced MRI is accepted practice in looking for synovitis (Fig. 5.17).

TUMOURS – SOFT TISSUE AND BONE

In any child who presents with bone pain, malignancy must be excluded. A plain film will show most lesions, but if it appears normal and doubt remains as to the diagnosis, an MRI study should be performed.

For soft tissue lesions, ultrasound is the best initial screening test. It may give a definite diagnosis, such as a popliteal cyst or ganglion, but it will also detect those lesions that require further imaging when the diagnosis is in doubt. In general, echogenic or mixed-echo pattern lesions require further investigation by MRI and, probably, biopsy.

All lesions should be investigated by a staged approach, with assessment of local and distant spread only after a definitive diagnosis of malignancy is made. MRI should be

performed to assess the extent of local involvement of bone or soft tissue before a biopsy is performed, and any biopsy

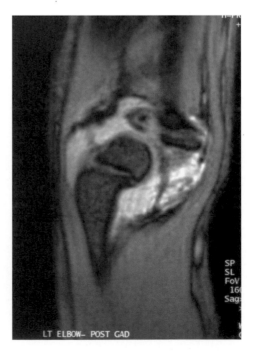

Figure 5.17 Gadolinium-enhanced MRI arthrogram of the elbow of a child with juvenile rheumatoid arthritis and profound synovitis.

should be undertaken by a route that may be excised at operation if the lesion is found to be malignant. Preliminary discussion with the involved tumour surgeon is mandatory. Biopsies of soft tissue and bone lesions with soft tissue extension (e.g. sarcomas) may be performed with ultrasound guidance. MRI angiography can also be used to assess the vascularity and vascular involvement of a lesion, allowing the surgeon to plan excision of the lesion or to assess the need for embolisation of the area before operation (Fig. 5.18).

FRACTURES

Exclusion of fractures is the most common reason for imaging a child's skeleton. Radiographic examination is routine after trauma or suspected trauma. The necessity for good quality images cannot be overemphasised. When an X-ray is not clinically indicated and the parents are expectant, the risks and benefits of radiation should be discussed. When an X-ray examination is normal but a fracture is strongly suspected, other imaging techniques should be considered.

CT is the workhorse in casualty departments. Details not easily seen on plain films will be revealed, and this is invaluable in cases of complex fracture, before surgical reconstruction. This is especially true for injuries to the

pelvis and face. However, the dose of radiation delivered to the patient is high, and it is tempting to use modern helical CT systems to excess. Another disadvantage has been that, even with very thin slices, there is a risk with CT that fractures in the plane of the section may be obscured by volume-averaging artefact. The use of coronal and sagittal reformatting to reduce such errors of interpretation is now accepted practice. Three-dimensional surface reconstruction may aid in surgical planning (Fig. 5.19). Radiologists will insist on seeing plain films before undertaking CT, and the examination will be easier and safer if these films are available in the CT room. The use of lead shielding to the radiosensitive areas of the patient should also be considered, as these areas are nearer to the radiation beam in a child.

Ultrasound can help in trauma. It may show subperiosteal haematoma at the fracture site, a break in the cortex, or periosteal reaction in fractures a few days old. Around the elbow, it may show a posterior effusion, often difficult to see on radiographs, especially as a true lateral radiograph may be impossible in a painful elbow. The presence of an effusion supports the diagnosis of a fracture. In addition, the technique may show synovitis, suggesting infection or arthropathy. It could be argued that ultrasound should be a first-line test in the very young infant, but the current availability of machines and, more

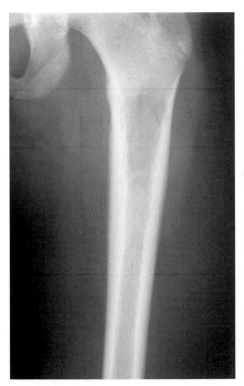 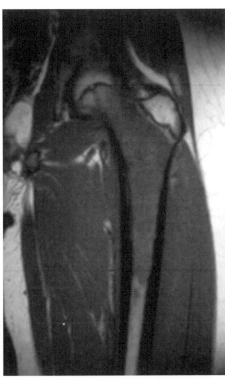 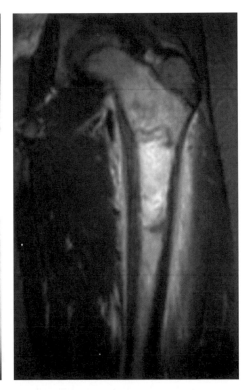

A   B   C

Figure 5.18 A Plain film of a destructive lesion in the femur. **B, C** MRI shows a more extensive lesion. The diagnosis on biopsy was Ewing's Sarcoma.

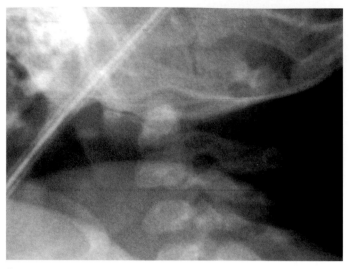

A

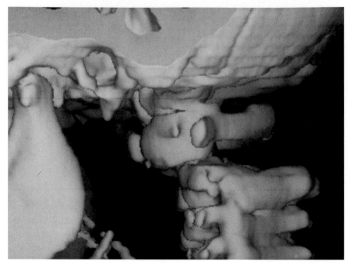

B

Figure 5.19 Images in a child who suffered C1/2 subluxation in a road traffic accident. **A** plain film. **B** CT three-dimensional surface reconstruction.

importantly, practitioners with expertise, limits its application.

MRI also can be used as an adjunct to plain films. This may show subtle fractures invisible on plain films. If there is doubt about the extent of an epiphyseal lesion, MRI may help the surgeon to decide whether to operate – for example, if Salter Harris IV fracture fragments involve the articular surface, reduction and fixation are indicated, but if the fracture stops in the epiphysis it is stable. MRI can also determine the displacement of a fracture fragment. It is a tomographic technique and may reveal detail inside bone that is not seen on plain films. Haematoma and soft tissue injury are readily apparent, therefore, although MRI is not currently used routinely in trauma, this may change in the future.

NON-ACCIDENTAL INJURY

A skeletal survey for non-accidental injury should be performed only if there is clinical evidence of abuse. Signs that raise this suspicion include retinal haemorrhage, a torn frenulum, and skin lesions. Non-accidental injuries may also be suspected after detecting unusual fracture patterns – for example, fractures not corresponding to the history of injury, fractures of differing ages, metaphyseal fractures, anterior and posterior rib fractures or long bone fractures in the infant younger than 1 year (see Ch. 36). It is important that all the administrative procedures and film labelling associated with these radiographs are exemplary, because they may be used in future legal proceedings. In addition, parent, nurse, doctor or social worker must accompany the child during the procedure.

Routine X-ray views should include:

- skull: anteroposterior and lateral views (plus Towne's view, if there is an occipital fracture)
- thoracic and lumbar spine: lateral
- chest: anteroposterior supine view
- both arms: anteroposterior view
- both hands (if clinically suspicious): oblique view
- abdomen and pelvis: supine
- both legs: anteroposterior view
- both feet (if clinically suspicious): anteroposterior view.

Coned-down views, centred on the joints, are required to see metaphyseal fractures; the 'babygram' is not acceptable, as it centres over the body so that the extremities are blurred. If a fracture is suspected or demonstrated, lateral views of the affected limb must be obtained.

Other imaging that may be useful includes isotope bone scintigraphy, which may show occult fractures and confirm the presence of metaphyseal fractures. Bone scans can help to resolve the issue of ambiguous fractures on plain X-rays and are positive within 7 hours of injury. If they are negative but clinical suspicion is high, they should be repeated 3 days later. Repeat X-rays after examination of doubtful significance may show callus at 10 days.

Ultrasound may show periosteal elevation at sites of suspected fracture. It can also be used to look for intracranial haemorrhage, or to detect small amounts of fluid in the abdomen if abdominal injuries are suspected. CT may be useful in detecting intracranial haemorrhage and significant abdominal trauma, whereas MRI can be used to judge the age of subdural collections of blood. MRI also affords the best means of examining the brain stem and posterior fossa and of detecting subtle structural or ischaemic changes, for all of which CT is poor. Whole-body MRI may become important in detecting fractures, but this approach is not yet established.

Table 5.2 A guide to the assessment of fracture age on plain X-ray

Feature	Likely age of fracture
Resolution of soft tissue swelling	4–10 days
Fracture without periosteal reaction	< 7 days
Slight periosteal reaction	4–7 days
Peak periosteal reaction	10–14 days
Blurring of fracture line	2–3 weeks (earliest 10 days)
Well-defined florid callus	>3–6 weeks (earliest 2 weeks)
Bony union/remodelling	3 months – 1 year (earliest 1 month)

Table 5.2 gives a guide to the age of a fracture from its appearances on plain films.

CONCLUSION

Imaging has a crucial role in the management of paediatric musculoskeletal disorders. A proper understanding of the risks of radiation, the variants that may simulate disease, and the strengths and weaknesses of each technique is essential to clinical practice. The more recently developed methods provide a powerful range of investigations that have significantly changed the management of disease in children. The field is evolving rapidly, and further innovation and improvement is inevitable.

REFERENCES AND FURTHER READING

Adam R, Hendry G M A, Moss 1986 Arthrosonography of the irritable hip in childhood: a review of 1 years experience. British Journal of Radiology 59: 205–208

Alexander J E, Seibert J J, Glasier C M et al 1989 High resolution hip ultrasound in the limping child. Journal of Clinical Ultrasound 17: 19–24

Beek F J A, Boemers T M L, Witkamp T D 1995 Spine evaluation in children with anorectal malformations. Paediatric Radiology 25: S28–S32

Berman L, Klenerman L 1986 Ultrasound screening for hip abnormalities: preliminary findings in 1001 neonates. British Medical Journal 293: 719–722

Berman L, Fink A M, Wilson D J, McNally E 1995 Technical note: identifying and aspirating hip effusions. British Journal of Radiology 68: 306–310

Boles C A, el-Khoury G Y 1997 Slipped capital femoral epiphysis. Radiographics 17: 809–823

Burgan H E, Furness M E, Foster B K 1999 Prenatal ultrasound diagnosis of clubfoot. Journal of Pediatric Orthopaedics 19: 11–13

Castelein R M, Sauter A J M, de Vlieger M, van Linge B 1992 Natural history of ultrasound hip abnormalities in clinically normal newborns. Journal of Pediatric Orthopaedics 12: 423–427

Castriota-Scanderbeg A, Orsi E 1993 Slipped capital femoral epiphysis: ultrasonographic findings. Skeletal Radiology 22: 191–193

Cook J V, Shah K, Pablot S, Kyriou J, Pettett A, Fitzgerald M 1999 Guidelines on best practice in the Xray imaging of children

Cowell H R 1966 The significance of early diagnosis and treatment of slipping of the capital femoral epiphyses Clinical Orthopaedics and Related Research 48: 89–94

Del-Beccaro M A, Champoux A N, Bockers T, Mendelman P M 1992 Septic arthritis versus transient synovitis of the hip: the value of screening laboratory tests. Annals of Emergency Medicine 21: 1418–1422

Derbyshire N D, Simpson A H 1992 A role for ultrasound in limb lengthening. British Journal of Radiology 775: 576–580

Eggl H, Drekonja T, Kaiser B, Dorn U 1999 Ultrasonography in the diagnosis of transient synovitis of the hip and Legg-Calve-Perthes' disease. Journal of Pediatric Orthopaedics B8: 177–180

Fink A M, Berman L, Edwards D, Jacodson S K 1995 The irritable hip: immediate ultrasound guided aspiration and prevention of hospital admission. Archives of Disease in Childhood 72: 110–113

Greulich W W, Pyle S I 1959 Radiographic atlas of skeletal development of the hand and wrist. Stanford University Press, Oxford

Graf R 1982 What possbilities does sonography of infantile hips offer? Wien Med Wochenschr 132: 499–506

Gupta P, Lenke L G, Bridwell K H 1998 Incidence of neural axis abnormalities in infantile and juvenile patients with spinal deformity. Is a magnetic resonance image screening necessary? Spine 23: 206–210

Gylys-Morin V M 1998 M R imaging of pediatric musculoskeletal inflammatory and infectious diseases. MRI Clinics of North America 6: 537–559

Hadi H A, Wade A 1993 Prenatal diagnosis of unilateral proximal femoral focal deficiency in diabetic pregnancy: a case report. American Journal of Perinatology 10: 285–287

Harcke H T, Grissom L E 1999 Pediatric hip sonography. Diagnosis and differential diagnosis. Radiology Clinics of North America 37: 787–796

Jaramillo D, Treves S T, Kasser J R, Harper M, Sundel R, Laor T 1995 Osteomyelitis and septic arthritis in children: appropriate use of imaging to guide treatment. American Journal of Roentgenology 165: 399–403

Kaiser S, Jorulf H, Hirsch G 1998 Clinical value of imaging techniques in childhood osteomyelitis. Acta Radiologica 39: 523–531

Kallio P E, LeQuesne G W, Paterson D C, Foster B K, Jones J R 1991 Ultrasonography in slipped capital femoral epiphysis. Journal of Bone and Joint Surgery 73B: 884–889

Keats T E 1996 Atlas of normal roentgen variants that may simulate disease. Mosby, St Louis

Keats T E, Smith T A 1988 An atlas of normal developmental roentgen anatomy. Mosby, St Louis

Kleinman P K 1998 Diagnostic imaging of child abuse, 2nd edn. Mosby, St Louis

Kohler A, Zimmer E A 1993 Borderlands of the normal and early pathologic in skeletal roentgenology. Grune and Stratton

Korsvik H E, Keller M S 1992 Sonography of occult dysraphism in neonates and infants with MR correlation. Radiographics 12: 297–306

Kyriou J C, Fitzgerald M, Pettett A, Cook J V, Pablot R M 1996 Comparison of doses and techniques between specialist and non-specialist centres in the diagnostic x-ray imaging of children. British Journal of Radiology 69: 437–450

Lang P, Johnston J O, Arenal-Romero F, Gooding C A 1998 Advances in MR imaging of pediatric musculoskeletal neoplasms. MRI Clinics of North America 6: 579–604

Larcos G, Antico P J, Cormick W, Gruenewald S M, Farlow D C 1994 How useful is ultrasonography in suspected acute osteomyelitis? Journal of Ultrasound in Medicine 13: 707–709

Marks D S, Clegg J, Al-Chalabi A N 1994 Routine ultrasound screening neonatal hip instability. Can it abolish late-presenting congenital dislocation of the hip? Journal of Bone and Joint Surgery 76: 534–538

Morin C, Zouaoui S, Delvalle-Fayada A, Delforge PM, Leclet H 1999 Ultrasound assessment of the acetabulum in the infant hip. Act Orthop Belg 3: 261–265

Nath A K, Arunchala U 1992 Use of ultrasound in osteomyelitis. British Journal of Radiology 65: 649–652

Novick G S 1988 Sonography in pediatric hip disorders. Radiology Clinics of North America 26: 29–53

Ostreich A E, Young L W, Young Poussaint T 1998 Scoliosis circa 2000: radiologic imaging perspective 1. Diagnosis and pretreatment evaluation. Skeletal Radiology 27: 591–605

Pagnotta G, Maffulli N, Aureli S, Maggi E, Mariani M, Yip K M H 1996 Antenatal sonographic diagnosis of clubfoot: a six-year experience. Journal of Foot and Ankle Surgery 35: 67–71

Petrikovsky B M 1999 Fetal disorders: diagnosis and management. Wiley-Liss

Ranner G, Ebner F, Fotter R, Linhart W, Justich E 1989 Magnetic resonance imaging in children with acute hip pain. Pediatric Radiology 20: 67–71

Rao P, Carty H 1999 Non-accidental injury: review of the radiology. Clinical Radiology 54: 11–24

Rockwood C A, Wilkins K E, Beaty J H (eds) 1996 Fractures in children. Lippincott Williams and Wilkins, Philadelphia

Saifuddin A, Burnett S J, Mitchell R 1998 Pictorial review: ultrasonography of primary bone tumours. Clinical Radiology 53: 239–246

Sundaram M, McDonald D Engel E, Rotman M, Siegfried E 1996 Chronic recurrent multifocal osteomyeltis: an evolving clinical and radiological spectrum. Skeletal Radiology 25: 333–336

Tanner J M, Whitehouse R H, Cameron N, Marshall W A, Healey M J R, Goldstein H 1983 Assessment of skeletal maturity and prediction of adult height (TW2 method), 2nd edn. Academic Press, London

Terjesen T 1993 Ultrasonography in the primary evaluation of patients with Perthes' disease. Journal of Pediatric Orthopaedics 13: 437–443

Terjesen T, Benum P, Rossvoll I, Svenningsen S, Floystad Isem A E, Nordbo T 1991 Leg-length discrepancy measured by ultrasonography. Acta Orthopaedica Scandinavica 62: 121–124

Thornton A, Gyll C 1999 Childrens fractures. WB Saunders, Philadelphia

Treadwell M C, Stanitski C L, King M 1999 Prenatal sonographic diagnosis of clubfoot: implications for patient counseling. Journal of Pediatric Orthopaedics 19: 8–10

Umans H, Liebling M S, Moy L, Haramati N, Macy N J, Pritzker H A 1998 Slipped capital femoral epiphysis: aphyseal lesion diagnosed by MRI, with radiographic and CT correlation. Skeletal Radiology 27: 139–144

Wakefield R J, McGonagle D, Green M J et al 1997 A comparison of high resolution sonography with MRI and conventional radiography for the detection of erosions in early rheumatoid arthritis. Arthritis and Rheumatism 40: S511

Wakefield R J, Gibbon V W V, O'Connor P 1998 High resolution ultrasound. A superior method to radiography for detecting cortical bone erosions in rheumatoid arthritis. British Journal of Rheumatology 7: S197

Weisz I, Jefferson R J, Turner-Smith A R, Houghton G R, Harris J D 1988 ISIS scannning: a useful assessment technique in the management of scoliosis. Spine 13: 405–408

Wilson D J, Green D J, MacClarnon J C 1984 Arthrosonography of the painful hip. Clinical Radiology 35: 17–19

Wirth T, LeQuesne G W, Paterson D C 1992 Ultrasonography in Legg–Calve–Perthes' disease. Pediatric Radiology 22: 498–504

Young J W R, Kostrubiak I S, Resnik C S, Paley D 1990 Sonographic evaluation of bone production at the distraction site in Ilizarov limb-lengthening procedures. American Journal of Roentgenology 154: 125–128

Section II
Generalised disorders

Chapter 6

Bone, cartilage and fibrous tissue disorders

W. G. Cole

INTRODUCTION

The disorders to be considered in this chapter are mostly inherited conditions of the musculoskeletal system. There are many hundreds of them, but only the major ones will be considered because the purpose of this chapter is to provide an approach to diagnosis and treatment, rather than to provide an encyclopaedic account of every known inherited disorder of bone, cartilage and fibrous tissue.

GENERAL PRINCIPLES

AETIOLOGY

The connective tissues contain a wide range of cell types and extracellular matrix components. It is to be expected that mutations of each of the matrix proteins and of the enzymes involved in their synthesis, modification and degradation will produce diseases with major skeletal involvement. Various examples will illustrate this point. First, mutations of type I collagen, the major collagen of bone, ligaments, tendons, dentin and sclera, produce osteogenesis imperfecta and one form of the Ehlers–Danlos syndrome. Secondly, mutations of type II collagen, the main collagen of cartilage and intervertebral discs, produce a range of dysplasias with major anomalies of the growth plates, epiphyses, articular surfaces and intervertebral discs.

The composition of the connective tissues alters during development, ageing and repair. During skeletal development of the limbs, there is a complex series of tightly regulated events that produces mesenchymal and cartilage models of the skeleton. Primary and secondary ossification centres subsequently develop, with definition of the growth plates and articular cartilages. Some of the genes that regulate the embryological events have been identified. They include genes that encode growth factors, growth factor receptors and transcription factors that switch other genes on and off. For example, a family of genes, the Hox genes, encode transcription factors that regulate segmental development of the axial and peripheral skeleton. Many of the embryological skeletal events are reproduced during fracture healing, and remodelling of the skeleton and articular surfaces occurs throughout adulthood.

The pathogenesis of the skeletal dysplasias characterised to date can be attributed to a deficiency of a normal component of the tissue, to the addition of mutant components that do not function normally, to the accumulation of normal metabolic intermediates, or to abnormal regulation of development. The tissue distribution of the changes conforms to the normal tissue expression patterns of the relevant genes.

It is to be expected that the genetic causes of an increasing number of the dysplasias will be determined, with consequent improvements in the diagnosis, classification, prediction of prognosis, counselling, and treatment. There are two general approaches to defining the genetic defects. The first approach involves linkage studies, in which co-inheritance of genetic markers and the clinical phenotype are sought in large families. Such studies can be undertaken quickly, because of the ready availability of genetic markers. Linkage analysis was used to identify the fibrillin-1 gene, *FBN1*, as the Marfan syndrome gene and the fibroblast growth factor receptor 3 gene, *FGFR3*, as the achondroplasia gene. The second approach is to produce a short-list of likely candidate genes in which the known distribution of the gene product matches the distribution of the phenotypic features of the disease. The candidate genes are then studied in detail. The candidate gene approach has been successfully used to characterise type I collagen mutations in osteogenesis imperfecta and type II collagen mutations in some of the cartilage dysplasias, such as spondyloepiphyseal dysplasia.

Within a short period, the DNA sequence of the human genome will be complete. It is to be expected that all genes involved in normal development, remodelling and repair of the skeleton will be identified. A major challenge will be to identify the genes responsible for each of the many hundreds of skeletal dysplasias. The Online Mendelian Inheritance of Man world wide web site – www3.ncbi.nlm.nih.gov/Omim/ – provides descriptions of each skeletal dysplasia, in addition to the latest details concerning the relevant disease genes.

CLINICAL DIAGNOSIS

A child may first be suspected of having an inherited disorder of the skeleton because of obstetric and birth abnormalities, abnormal growth, specific musculoskeletal complaints, family history or radiographic findings. A detailed history is required, and should include information about the family history, pregnancy, birth, growth, development, and the presenting complaints.

A careful clinical examination is also required. If there have been progressive changes in the appearance of the child, then families should be asked to provide photographs at various ages for review. It is also useful to examine other affected members of the family in order to assess the variability of the disease and the likely prognosis.

Most children with inherited disorders of the skeleton are either abnormally short or tall, and their bodies are often disproportionate. The limbs may be short relative to the spine, as in short-limbed forms of dwarfism, or long relative to the spine, as in short-trunk forms of dwarfism. The limb segments may also be disproportionate, with more shortening in one segment than in another. For example, children with achondroplasia have more proximal or rhizomelic shortening, whereas those with mesomelic dysplasias have more shortening of the forearms and shins, and those with acromelic dysplasias have more involvement of the hands and feet. Many children also have anomalies of the head and face.

The height and weight of the child should be recorded on growth charts. Previous measurements and birth measurements are also plotted. Arm span and upper to lower segment ratios are recorded, particularly in patients with marfanoid features. Normally, the upper segment measured from the crown to the pubis is equal to the lower segment measured from the pubis to the heel.

The alignment of the limbs and spine, ranges of movement and stability of joints, limb length discrepancies and gait anomalies are also recorded.

In many instances, a provisional clinical diagnosis can be rapidly made from the general appearance of the child. This diagnostic process involves pattern matching, in which the clinician compares the general appearance of the child with the features of other children that have previously been seen with known diseases. Syndrome atlases and computer-based diagnostic systems are commonly used to supplement the clinician's memory.

RADIOGRAPHIC DIAGNOSIS

Some disorders, such as achondroplasia, produce characteristic clinical appearances that are unlikely to be confused with other disorders. However, despite confidence in a clinical diagnosis, it is wise to confirm it with radiographs. Furthermore, in many instances a firm clinical diagnosis cannot be made, in which case the definitive diagnosis will rely on the radiographic appearances of the skeleton.

A skeletal survey, using standard plain radiographs, is essential and should include the skull, spine, pelvis, and all bones of one arm and one leg. Computed tomography or magnetic resonance imaging may be needed for the investigation of specific lesions such as anomalies of the spinal canal with cord compression. Other imaging methods such as isotope bone scans and ultrasonography are rarely needed for diagnosis.

As the skeletal features of many bone dysplasias change with growth, it is essential that previous radiographs, including birth X-rays, are obtained and kept. All available X-rays are displayed in chronological order. A quick scan of them will reveal which bones are most affected, and these can be examined in detail before re-examining the whole skeleton.

The radiographic pathology is assessed in a manner similar to that applied to a pathology specimen, taking note of the size, shape and texture of the bone, and the details of localised anomalies. Abnormalities will usually be more marked in one region of the bone, although not necessarily confined to it. The abnormal features are systematically identified and categorised. For example, a dysplasia that has its major effects on epiphyseal development is classified as an epiphyseal dysplasia, such as multiple epiphyseal dysplasia. If there is also major spinal involvement, it is classified as a spondyloepiphyseal dysplasia. If the changes are mostly in the metaphyses, the disorder is classified as a metaphyseal dysplasia, such as metaphyseal chondrodysplasia. Similarly, changes that are greatest in the diaphysis are classified as diaphyseal dysplasia.

The distribution of changes between the proximal, middle and distal segments of the limb is also noted, as is that in the skull and spine. If a child has metaphyseal dysplasia and frontal bone anomalies, the disorder is descriptively named craniometaphyseal dysplasia. Some limb disorders preferentially affect one segment more than another. If the radius, ulna, tibia and fibula are mainly affected, the disorder is classified as a mesomelic dysplasia.

Various classifications of inherited disorders of the skeleton are available, but all are complex. The most widely used is the International Nomenclature of Constitutional Diseases of Bone, which is revised periodically (McKusick 1990).

BIOCHEMICAL AND PATHOLOGICAL DIAGNOSIS

Routine biochemical diagnosis is available for only a few of the bone dysplasias. Urinary screening tests and enzyme assays are used in children with suspected storage disorders, such as the mucopolysaccharidoses.

Characteristic histopathological changes are present in many skeletal dysplasias, but they are infrequently used for diagnosis. However, specimens should always be obtained for biochemical and histological examination, whenever a child is having an operation on affected tissues.

GENERAL MANAGEMENT

Although there are many inherited disorders of the skeleton, each one is rare and as a result most children should be reviewed by staff who are experienced in the field. Many children's hospitals have multidisciplinary bone dysplasia clinics that involve an orthopaedic surgeon, medical geneticist, social worker and associated specialists as required. Children should be referred for assessment once an inherited abnormality of the skeleton is suspected.

An accurate diagnosis is essential in order to be able to provide families with appropriate information. It is needed for the prediction of mature height, associated anomalies, prognosis, treatment and genetic counselling. A diagnosis should not be made if there is any uncertainty about it; it is preferable to follow the child's progress until the diagnosis becomes obvious when other features appear. Syndrome atlases and computer systems with clinical and radiographic illustrations stored on a laser disc can also be used as aids in diagnosing an unknown syndrome.

The child's height and weight are recorded at each clinic visit. Specific areas, which will vary with the different disorders, are also reviewed. For example, regular ophthalmological examinations are required in children with spondyloepiphyseal dysplasia, Marfan's syndrome, homocystinuria, Stickler syndrome and Ehlers–Danlos syndrome. Infants with achondroplasia need regular assessment by ear, nose and throat specialists. Regular cardiovascular assessments are also required in patients with Marfan's syndrome.

Apart from some of the metabolic disorders, considered in the next chapter, no specific treatment is available for any of the inherited disorders of the skeleton. Treatment is, therefore, symptomatic. Initially, the focus is on providing appropriate verbal and written information for the parents about their child's disorder and the risk of recurrence in future pregnancies. This information must be reinforced by regular visits to a bone dysplasia clinic. Medical social workers and various self-help organisations such as the Little People's Associations and Brittle Bone Societies can also provide valuable support.

Specific assistance will often need to be given when the child starts kindergarten and primary school, in the transition from secondary to tertiary education, and when entering the workforce. Obtaining a driving licence is a challenge that also requires expert assistance. Additional information is often sought by affected individuals when marriage and children are contemplated.

GENETIC COUNSELLING

Genetic counselling is requested by most families, but should only be undertaken by those experienced in the specialty. It involves a discussion of the clinical disorder, the risk of recurrence in an individual with an inherited disease with the parents of an affected child, and consideration of the burden of the disorder. An unequivocal diagnosis is clearly essential before such discussions commence.

Intrauterine diagnosis by biochemical means is available for a few bone dysplasias, such as the mucopolysaccharidoses and osteogenesis imperfecta. Many bone dysplasias are diagnosed *in utero* by ultrasonography. The lengths and shapes of individual long bones can be determined with remarkable accuracy, as can anomalies of vertebral development and deformities of the spine and limbs. Fractures can be detected, and osteoporosis is likely if there is a poor echogenic signal from the skeleton.

ORTHOPAEDIC MANAGEMENT

Many children need minimal, if any, orthopaedic treatment, whereas others have major orthopaedic anomalies that almost defy treatment. In general, orthopaedic management is directed towards preventing and correcting deformities, stabilising lax and dislocated joints, supporting fragile bones, and correcting limb length discrepancies. The treatment is usually more complex than for similar problems in otherwise normal children. It is undertaken with paramedical staff who assist the children to be independent in their activities of daily living.

Some deformities, such as talipes equinovarus, are present at birth, but many of them develop later. Deformities such as tibia vara and valga may progress rapidly when the mechanical axis of the limb is disturbed to such an extent that abnormal growth from asymmetrical loading of the growth plates is added to the pre-existing growth disturbance. Such deformities should be corrected before they deteriorate rapidly; they may need to be corrected several times during growth.

Malalignment of the limb is corrected surgically because orthoses, particularly in dwarfed children, are tolerated poorly and are largely ineffective. The correction of limb alignment often requires osteotomies at multiple levels. The deformities are usually complex, with both angulatory and rotational anomalies, and the adjoining joints may be unstable or stiff. Careful preoperative planning is required, and both limbs are corrected at the same operation or within a short time of each other. Plaster fixation cannot be relied upon in children with short limbs, so that internal fixation or external unilateral or ring fixation are preferable. Hemiphyseal stapling can be used near the end of growth to correct some angular deformities.

Spinal deformities often develop at an early age, and are severe and rigid. Orthoses are of limited value in children of short stature, because they markedly restrict mobility and are ineffective in children with soft bone and lax tissues. Localised spinal fusions or non-fusion rodding may be needed before the vertebrae are big enough for definitive internal fixation and arthrodesis. Atlanto-axial instability is common in dysplasias with major spinal involvement; atlanto-axial fusion may be required for gross instability and to relieve cervical myelopathy. Decompression of the lumbar spinal canal and its nerve root canals is frequently required in adults with achondroplasia and cauda equina syndrome.

Premature osteoarthritis is a common outcome of many bone dysplasias. Replacement arthroplasties may be required, and can be expected to improve function greatly.

SPECIFIC BONE DISORDERS

This section will be confined to osteogenesis imperfecta; metabolic and endocrine disorders affecting bone are presented in Chapter 7.

OSTEOGENESIS IMPERFECTA

Osteogenesis imperfecta (OI) is one of the most common and best known of the skeletal dysplasias. It is a form of genetically determined osteoporosis for which orthopaedic treatment is frequently required.

Aetiology

The birth incidence is approximately 1:20 000. About 80% of cases of OI are caused by mutations of the type I collagen genes. Type I collagen is the principal collagen of bone, ligament, dentin and sclera, which are the tissues most affected in OI. The majority of cases result from autosomal dominant mutations that are either inherited from a parent or develop spontaneously as a new mutation. A number of affected children may occur in families with apparently normal parents, as a result of autosomal recessive inheritance or gonadal mosaicism. Autosomal recessive inheritance, in which an abnormal allele is inherited from both parents, has a recurrence risk of 25% with each pregnancy. In contrast, gonadal mosaicism, in which one parent carries an autosomal dominant mutation in the sperm or ova, has an unpredictable risk of recurrence. Overall, the recurrence risk of apparently normal parents having a second child with osteogenesis imperfecta is about 7%.

The autosomal dominant mutations of the genes for type I collagen produce two general categories of protein defects. In the first group, the mutations inactivate one copy or allele of the gene and result in a 50% reduction in the amount of normal type I collagen in bone. These patients usually have a mild form of the disease (type I OI). The bone is osteoporotic, with osteoid seams that are about half the normal thickness. Lamellar bone is found in the trabecula of the metaphysis, and lamellar bone and Haversian systems are present in the diaphysis. In the second group, the tissues contain a reduced amount of normal collagen, in addition to type I collagen molecules that contain one or two mutant collagen chains. The patients are usually severely affected, and may have a perinatal lethal disease. The bone morphology is grossly abnormal, with defects of bone modelling and lack of normal cortical bone formation. The bone is of a woven type, with minimal amounts of osteoid and without lamellar bone and Haversian systems.

In general, the severity of the clinical disease is greater in those with mutant collagen in the tissues than it is in those with only a reduced amount of normal type I collagen.

Clinical and radiographic features

Osteogenesis imperfecta is a heterogeneous disorder that has been classified into four broad categories as indicated in Table 6.1. The main clinical and radiographic features in the absence of treatment, and the inheritance patterns, are outlined below.

Type I OI (blue sclerae and autosomal dominant inheritance)

This is the most common and mildest clinical form. It is the classical type, with blue sclerae, bone fragility, minimal deformities, premature deafness and autosomal dominant inheritance. The birth weights and lengths are normal, but one or more bones may be fractured. A family history of OI will prompt careful assessment of the scleral colour, as it is the most consistent feature of OI in large families. Although most neonates have light blue sclerae, those with type I OI have dark blue sclerae with a grey tinge.

The osteoporotic skeleton is well formed and modelling of the metaphyses is also normal. The skull usually contains wormian bones. Fractures commonly occur for the first time when the child starts to walk. The blue sclerae may then be observed for the first time in children with sporadic new mutations. The severity of osteoporosis and the frequency of fractures may differ considerably between affected members of large pedigrees.

The types of fractures that occur in type I OI are similar to those seen in normal children, except that they occur more easily. The fractures heal well, although occasionally a rapidly growing hypertrophic callus, resembling a sarcoma, will develop. Fractures are less common after puberty, but may increase later in life as the effects of age- and sex-related osteoporosis are superimposed upon the effects of the underlying OI.

Dentinogenesis imperfecta also occurs in some patients with type I OI, and premature deafness is common.

Type II OI (lethal perinatal form)

This is the most severe type of OI and is usually fatal within hours of birth, but some babies survive for several months. The babies are dwarfed and have grey-blue sclerae and short, bowed limbs. The skull is soft and the face is small.

Table 6.1 Classification of osteogenesis imperfecta

Type	Features	Inheritance
I (dominant, blue sclerae)	IA: Bone fragility, blue sclerae and normal teeth. IB: Same as IA but with dentinogenesis imperfecta	Autosomal dominant
II (lethal perinatal)	Severe porosis with multiple fractures and malformed skeleton	Autosomal dominant
III (progressive deforming)	Multiple fractures at birth with progressive deformities, normal sclerae and dentinogenesis imperfecta	Autosomal recessive
IV (dominant, white sclerae)	IVA: Bone fragility, white sclerae and normal teeth. IVB: Similar to IVA but with dentinogenesis imperfecta	Autosomal dominant

Radiographs show severe osteoporosis, with multiple fractures. The long bones are frequently short and crumpled, and the calvarium contains minimal bone. Most cases are the result of new autosomal dominant mutations of the type I collagen genes.

Type III OI (progressively deforming type)

Babies with type III OI have severe bone fragility, with multiple fractures at birth. In contrast to babies with type II OI, the chest is usually well formed, with few or no fractures of the ribs. The inheritance is autosomal recessive or autosomal dominant.

The birth weight and length of these babies are nearly normal. The sclerae are pale blue, and fade over the following years to become white. The limbs are bowed and the calvarium is large relative to the small triangular face (Fig. 6.1). The long bones progressively bow with growth, and multiple fractures are common. The shafts of the long bones may be wide at birth, but narrow later. The epiphyses appear large in proportion to the narrow shafts, and the growth plates may fracture into many pieces, which round up to form islands of endochondral ossification. These islands produce a 'popcorn' appearance on radiographs (Fig. 6.2), but eventually they disappear, leaving an enlarged lucent epiphysis.

Progressive bowing, multiple fractures and disruption of the growth plates account for the very short skeleton. Progressive flattening of the vertebral bodies and kyphoscoliosis are common. The chest becomes barrel shaped, with a pectus carinatum. As the lumbar spine shortens, the wide rib cage overlaps the narrow pelvis. The iliac wings flare outwards as the hip joints migrate towards each other. Severe shortening of the trunk and limbs results in very short stature and reduced sitting height. Most children with type III OI eventually cease to walk.

Dentinogenesis imperfecta is frequent.

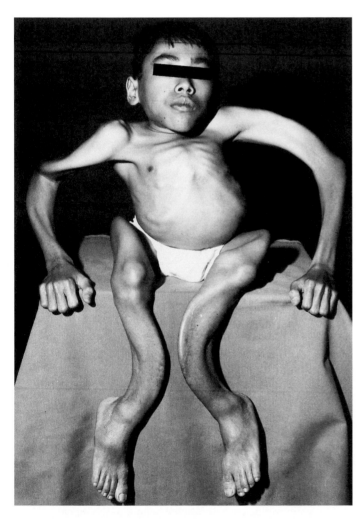

Figure 6.1 Osteogenesis imperfecta type III. This child presented with multiple deformities and minimal previous treatment.

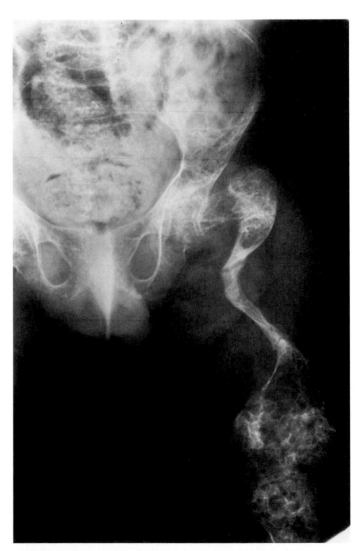

Figure 6.2 Osteogenesis imperfecta type III. Radiograph showing 'popcorn' femur and tibia, with shepherd's crook femoral deformity and multiple fractures. (Courtesy of Dr R. Smith.)

Type IV OI (white sclerae with autosomal dominant inheritance)

This is a form of OI in which there is autosomal dominant inheritance, white sclerae, a moderate number of fractures and variable severity of bone deformity. It resembles type I OI, except that the sclerae are normal in colour. Dentinogenesis imperfecta is common.

Investigations

In most instances, the diagnosis of OI can be made from the clinical appearance of the individual, the family history and plain radiographs. Diagnostic difficulty is frequent in patients with sporadic forms of type IV OI because such individuals may have normal sclerae and teeth and no bone malformations. In infancy, this form of OI is frequently misdiagnosed as 'child abuse' (see Chapter 36). Careful assessment of the radiographs may reveal osteoporosis, slender bones with fine cortices, and wormian bones. Dental assessment may also demonstrate subclinical evidence of dentinogenesis imperfecta.

The diagnosis of type IV OI should be suspected in a school-aged child who has repeated fractures and none of the usual clinical features of OI. In this situation, measurement of the bone mineral density is helpful in determining whether osteopenia is present; normal bone density standards for children are available, and help to exclude the condition. Type I collagen analyses provide the definitive evidence of OI.

Management

General care

As with other bone dysplasias, families should be referred to an orthopaedic surgeon and geneticist who specialise in this field, once the diagnosis is suspected.

Specific treatment

There is currently no specific treatment that will correct the underlying type I collagen mutations. Specific treatment, using somatic gene therapy, is likely to be difficult to achieve, as each family with OI has their own particular mutation. In addition, major improvements in somatic gene therapy methods will be needed before the technique can be considered seriously. However, non-specific bisphosphonate treatment of severe and moderately severe types of OI appears to be successful in relieving bone pain, improving strength, reducing the number of fractures, and improving the density of the bones; the effects appear to be greatest when it is commenced within a few months of birth. Current evidence indicates that the natural history of type III and IV OI is significantly improved after bisphosphonate treatment, which reduces bone resorption: histological studies of iliac crest biopsies show that it significantly increases the thickness and density of the iliac crest. Further trials are in progress to determine the effectiveness of bisphosphonates in the mild type I form of OI.

Treatment of fractures and deformities

Severely affected babies usually have multiple fractures, in varying stages of healing, at birth. Unstable fractures require simple splintage to reduce pain and to aid in nursing. Analgesics may also be required. The pain usually decreases after several weeks as the fractures heal. These babies are difficult to nurse, and parents need assistance in learning to care for their child. Home visits and regular clinic assessments are essential in the first few months of life. Bisphosphonate treatment may be commenced in the neonatal period.

Thermoplastic splints for upper and lower limbs are provided for home treatment of fractures. The splints are easy to apply and provide good first-aid support for the fractured limb. Radiographs may be obtained, but in many instances it is appropriate to rely on the clinical diagnosis of a fracture. The methods of treating fractures in OI are the same as in normal children, except that the period of immobilisation is kept to a minimum. Home gallows traction kits are useful in the treatment of femoral shaft fractures in young children with OI. Standing and walking with lower limb plasters are encouraged in previously mobile children.

The role of external and internal splintage of the skeleton requires evaluation in children receiving bisphosphonate treatment. External supports such as inflatable suits or polypropylene orthoses can be used to support the limb; they are most effective after deformities have been corrected by osteotomies or osteoclasis. As an alternative, the support can be provided internally, using intramedullary rods (Fig. 6.3). Fragmentation and rodding was popularised by Sofield et al (1952). It dramatically reduces the number of fractures in the involved bone, but has the disadvantage that, with growth,

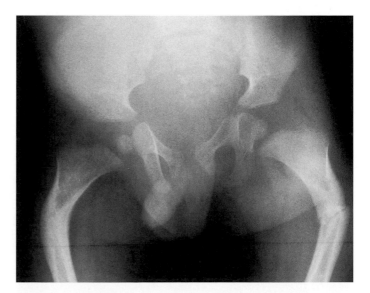

Figure 6.3 Osteogenesis imperfecta type IV. Radiograph showing subtrochanteric deformities and a pathological fracture of the femur. This child is able to walk, but correction of the femoral deformities and insertion of intramedullary rods were required to prevent recurrent fractures.

the bone bows beyond the rod and re-fractures. Stress-shielding from the rod also leads to further thinning of the diaphysis. These rods may need to be changed several times during growth. To avoid these problems, the telescoping rod was developed; however, this must be inserted correctly otherwise there is a high technical failure rate, and the bone needs to be sufficiently strong to provide an anchor for the ends of the rod or it will not extend. Multiple osteotomies are frequently required to correct deformities and are best made as closing wedge osteotomies with minimal periosteal stripping.

In adolescents and adults with OI it is usually appropriate to use the internal fixation systems that are commonly used in the management of trauma. Modern intramedullary rods with cross-bolt fixation can provide excellent internal splintage of long bones. The cross bolts are removed once the fracture is healed, but the rod is best left in place.

Scoliosis and kyphoscoliosis are common in untreated, severe forms of OI. In some, arthrodesis with spinal instrumentation is appropriate. In many children with severe OI, however, the vertebral bodies flatten within the first few years of life and scoliosis develops rapidly. Orthotic or plaster management is not practical in most, because the chest wall deforms without any change in spinal shape. The small and severely osteoporotic vertebrae are also unsuitable for most forms of internal fixation. However, the prevalence of spinal deformities requires evaluation in children receiving bisphosphonates. Restoration of vertebral height may follow bisphosphonate treatment.

Mobility

All parents are keen for their child with OI to walk. Bisphosponates appear to improve significantly the walking ability of children with severe forms of OI. In the absence of bisphosphonates, community walking is rarely achieved in children with type III OI and is not achieved in some patients with severe type I or IV OI. The children who are unable to walk have severe osteoporosis, severe deformities, and muscle weakness. In such children, it is important to set achievable goals in therapy. If the child shows no signs of wishing to walk, it is unlikely that the correction of deformities with external or internal splintage will transform the child into an effective walker. Under these circumstances, it is more desirable to focus on other methods of achieving mobility; children as young as 2 years can use electric mobility devices. Provision of such devices gives the child more independence and stimulates motivation. The provision of an electric mobility device at an early age does not prevent later attempts to stand and walk.

SPECIFIC CARTILAGE DISORDERS

ACHONDROPLASIA

Achondroplasia is the most common and best known form of dwarfism. The clinical and radiographic appearances are remarkably constant.

Aetiology

Achondroplasia is an autosomal dominant disorder and about 80–90% of cases result from new mutations of the *FGFR3* gene. Histological assessment of growth plates has shown relatively normal architecture, except that the cartilage columns are short and lack the usual linear array of cells.

Clinical features

At birth

The most obvious features at birth are the abnormal facies and disproportionate shortness. The skull is large, with a prominent forehead, biparietal bossing and flattening of the occiput. The nasal bridge is depressed, with midface hypoplasia and prominence of the lower jaw.

Achondroplasia is a rhizomelic, short-limbed form of dwarfism. The limbs are relatively short compared with the trunk and the proximal segments of the limbs are relatively short compared with the middle and distal segments. The finger tips usually reach to the iliac crests or greater trochanters. The amount of skin, subcutaneous fat and muscle appears excessive. The hands are short, and the stubby fingers produce a 'trident' appearance when extended.

The limbs are well aligned at birth. The elbows have fixed flexion deformities of about 30°, whereas most other joints are lax.

During childhood

The disproportionate short stature becomes more obvious during childhood (Figs 6.4 and 6.5). Gross motor development is delayed by about 6 months because of hypotonia

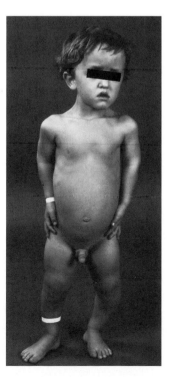

Figure 6.4 Achondroplasia. Note the frontal bossing, flat nasal bridge, long torso relative to the short limbs. This child has rhizomelic shortening of the limbs; he developed progressive bowing of the left tibia.

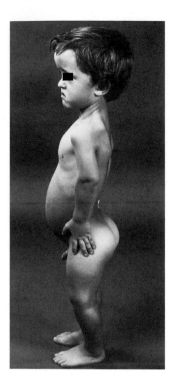

Figure 6.5 Achondroplasia. Side view of patient shown in Fig. 6.4. Note the prominent calvarium, midface hypoplasia, excessive lumbar lordosis, and rhizomelic shortening of the limbs.

and joint laxity. Delay beyond this time may be due to stenosis of the foramen magnum, with compression of the medulla oblongata and cervical spinal cord.

Rapid calvarial development occurs during the first 12–18 months of life. True hydrocephalus can develop, although shunting of cerebrospinal fluid is rarely required. Recurrent middle ear infections are common in the preschool and early school age child. They are due to facial hypoplasia with constriction and hypoplasia of the Eustachean tubes. Deafness is a frequent sequel unless treated early. Dental crowding may also result from hypoplasia of the jaw.

The children are slow to develop head control, because the skull is relatively large and the spinal muscles are hypotonic. The large head, muscle hypotonia and ligament laxity also contribute to the rounded thoraco-lumbar kyphosis that develops when the child first starts to sit. The kyphosis is postural in most children. Once the child starts to walk, the kyphosis changes to a marked lumbar lordosis, and the abdomen and buttocks become prominent. A few children develop an angular thoraco-lumbar kyphosis as a result of wedging of the vertebral bodies at this level. Progressive thoraco-lumbar kyphosis is likely to follow.

The knee is hypermobile because of ligament laxity. Mediolateral stability is present when the knee is hyperextended. The walking child usually has mild genu varum and internal tibial torsion. These deformities give little trouble in early childhood, but later may cause aching over the lateral side of the knee as a result of stretching of the lateral collateral ligament. In addition, the overlong fibula may abut against the calcaneum and prevent valgus of the subtalar joint.

The restricted elbow joint motion usually persists. Fixed flexion deformities of the hips are also common in later childhood, but are rarely troublesome.

During adolescence and adulthood

The average adult height is 131 cm for men and 124 cm for women with achondroplasia. The principal musculoskeletal problem arising in the mid to late teens and early adulthood is neurological deterioration resulting from spinal stenosis. The spinal canal is much smaller than normal, but several additional factors add to the stenosis; these include excessive lumbar lordosis secondary to an angular thoraco-lumbar kyphosis, and osteophytes and herniation of degenerative intervertebral discs.

The earliest clinical indication of stenosis is decreased exercise tolerance. Aches and paraesthesiae in the limbs may be incorrectly attributed to osteoarthritis of peripheral joints. However, osteoarthritis of peripheral joints is infrequent, and such symptoms are usually due to spinal stenosis. In the early stages, these symptoms are relieved by flexion of the spine and hips, or by sitting. Later, progressive neurological impairment occurs, with persistent backache and overt neurological signs caused by compression of the cauda equina. An abrupt deterioration in neurological status may follow an injury.

Radiographic features

The radiographic features of achondroplasia are present at birth and are diagnostic. Radiographs of the skull, lumbar spine and pelvis are the minimum required to make a diagnosis. The calvarium is large, with prominence of the frontal, parietal and occipital bones. The base of the skull and foramen magnum are hypoplastic and 'occipitalisation' of the atlas is frequent. The characteristic feature of the achondroplastic spine is the progressive narrowing of the interpedicular distances from the thoracic to the sacral spine, in contrast to the normal widening of the interpedicular distances. The pedicles and the anteroposterior diameters of the vertebral bodies are also short, and posterior scalloping of the vertebrae is usual (Fig. 6.6).

A rounded thoraco-lumbar kyphosis is common in infancy, but lumbar lordosis develops after walking commences. The sacrum becomes more horizontal as a result of increasing angulation at the lumbo-sacral junction. In contrast to these normal changes with growth, a few infants develop wedging of the 12th thoracic and 1st lumbar vertebral bodies. It is commonly associated with a progressive gibbus and, later, cauda equina compression.

The pelvis also has a characteristic shape. The ilia are wide, the greater sciatic notches are deep, and the superior margins of the acetabulum are horizontal. The femoral necks are short, but the neck-shaft angles are usually normal. The shafts of the femora and other long bones are broad, with flared metaphyses.

An oval-shaped lucency is common at birth in the proximal humeri and femora, but disappears over several years. In infancy, the distal femoral growth plate also has a

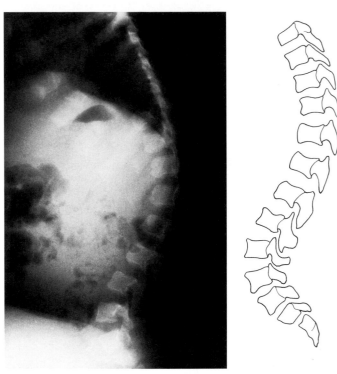

Figure 6.6 Achondroplasia. Lateral radiograph of the spine of a 1-year-old child, showing short pedicles and posterior scalloping of the vertebral bodies.

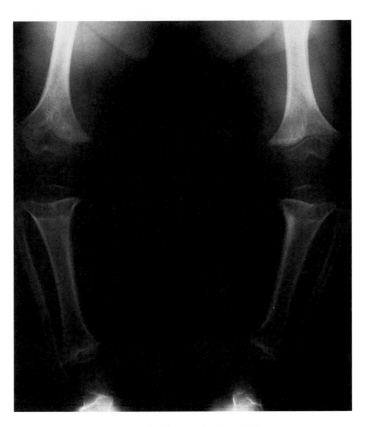

Figure 6.7 Achondroplasia. Same child as in Fig. 6.6. Radiograph of legs, showing the short broad bones with inverted-V shaped distal femoral growth plates.

characteristic inverted-V shape, with a correspondingly shaped ossific centre of the distal femoral epiphysis (Fig. 6.7). The growth plate becomes more horizontal with growth. The fibula is longer than the tibia, and may be associated with tibia vara. The distal fibula may also abut against the calcaneum.

Progressive deformity of the radial head and posterior bowing of the radius is frequent, and results in posterior subluxation and dislocation of the radial head in later childhood.

Management

A clinical and radiographic diagnosis of achondroplasia can usually be confidently made at birth. The features are characteristic and there is little clinical and radiographic variability. Achondroplasia needs to be distinguished from other dwarfing conditions evident at this time, including diastrophic dysplasia, lethal short-limbed dwarfing syndromes, and spondyloepiphyseal dysplasia congenita; in the past, many of these conditions were misdiagnosed as achondroplasia.

In school age children, achondroplasia can resemble hypochondroplasia. This latter dysplasia shares many of the features of achondroplasia, but is less severe. Achondroplasia and hypochondroplasia are both caused by mutations of the *FGFR3* gene.

Treatment is symptomatic. Initial treatment focuses on providing parents with verbal and written information about

achondroplasia. Additional information and continuing support is also available from the Little People's or related Associations.

Infants and young children are reviewed regularly in order to provide general support and to follow the child's development and growth. The height and weight can be plotted on normal growth charts and on normal achondroplastic growth charts. The particular medical problems that may require investigation and treatment are recurrent middle ear infections, possible hydrocephalus, possible cervical cord compression, thoraco-lumbar kyphosis, and tibia vara.

It may be necessary to insert grommets into the middle ears to provide drainage. Computed tomograms and magnetic resonance imaging of the brain and cervical cord are undertaken in infants with possible hydocephalus or spinal cord compression; a general anaesthetic is usually required for these investigations. A cerebrospinal fluid shunt may occasionally be needed to correct hydrocephalus, and occasionally a posterior fossa decompression is needed to release the contents of the posterior fossa and the upper cervical spinal canal.

Infants with wedging of the bodies of the vertebrae at the thoraco-lumbar junction need orthotic treatment in an attempt to prevent progressive kyphosis. Anterior release and grafting may be required in the few children with progressive wedging of the vertebral bodies and an increasing gibbus. Orthoses are unnecessary and expensive for 'normal' achondroplastic infants who have a rounded thoraco-lumbar kyphosis without anterior wedging of the vertebral bodies.

The treatment of spinal stenosis in early adulthood is difficult. Neurological investigation has been aided considerably by magnetic resonance imaging of the cauda equina and spinal cord. Lumbar myelography is often difficult and dangerous because of the narrow spinal canal and partial or complete blockage of the subarachnoid space. Cisternal puncture is also difficult, because of the overhanging occiput and basilar impression. Posterior decompression of the stenotic spinal canal and nerve root canals is usually required to relieve spinal stenosis. The surgery is difficult because of the thick bone and the cramped space, and the results are unpredictable.

Progressive unilateral or bilateral tibia vara and internal tibial torsion may develop in early childhood and require correction. Careful preoperative planning is required to ensure full correction of each component of the deformity. Standing radiographs and photographs are essential because the knee is lax. Both legs are draped and sterile tourniquets are used, so that the alignment of both limbs can be observed. The tibial osteotomy is undertaken below the proximal growth plate. A piece of the distal one-third of the fibula is excised to enable the deformities to be corrected. The varus and internal torsion deformities are corrected and the tibial osteotomy is held with Kirschner wires. Care is taken to ensure that recurvatum does not occur, and the ends of the wires are buried. Radiographs are taken of the whole limb. A hip spica is applied, because the legs are too short for long leg plasters to be effective. The spica is removed 3 weeks later when the osteotomies are stable, and long-leg plaster casts are applied for a further 3 weeks. The wires are removed several weeks after removal of the casts. Correction of tibia vara is usually long lasting.

Lengthening of the femora, tibiae and humeri as a means of increasing height and arm length can be undertaken, but its place in the management of achondroplasia remains controversial.

PSEUDOACHONDROPLASIA

This dysplasia is distinct from achondroplasia. It is also known as the pseudoachondroplastic form of spondyloepiphyseal dysplasia, in order to highlight the widespread changes in the skeleton.

Aetiology

Pseudoachondroplasia is an autosomal dominant trait. The cartilages are disorganised and the chondrocytes contain intracellular inclusions. Mutations of the cartilage oligomeric matrix protein gene, *COMP*, have been identified in patients with this condition.

Clinical features

The child appears normal at birth. By the 2nd to 3rd year, growth retardation, waddling gait and angular deformities of the legs are observed (Figs 6.8 and 6.9). This is a short-limb form of dwarfism, with body proportions resembling those of achondroplasia. However, the head and face are normal. The lumbar lordosis is exaggerated, and scoliosis may develop.

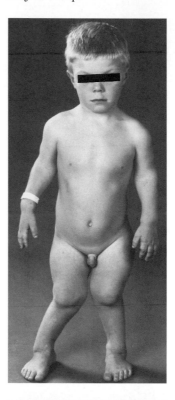

Figure 6.8
Pseudoachondroplasia. Note the short stature, normal facies and severe deformities of lower limbs.

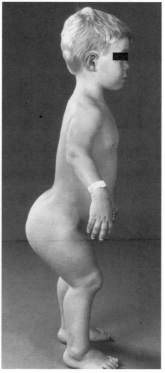

Figure 6.9
Pseudoachondroplasia. Side view of patient shown in Fig. 6.8. Note the normal skull and face, the short limbs, and flexion contractures of elbows, hips and knees. The spine is flat.

Ligament laxity and progressive lower limb deformities are common in young children. Typically, the lower limbs have a 'windswept' appearance, with genu valgum and an adducted hip on one side and genu varum and an abducted hip on the other. Occasionally, symmetric bow legs or knock knees develop.

The windswept deformities are progressive. The adducted hip subluxates and is associated with pelvic obliquity and scoliosis. The valgus knee also subluxates. The adducted hip drives the femoral condyles anteromedially, whereas the tibial plateau translates posterolaterally and rotates externally. In late childhood, the patella is chronically dislocated and there is minimal contact between the tibial and femoral condyles. At this stage, the patient may have great difficulty standing and mobility is severely restricted. The ankles may also subluxate. Premature osteoarthritis is usual.

The adult height is between 82 and 130 cm.

Radiographic features

The long bones are short, broad and misshapen, and the metaphyses are cupped and flared. The epiphyses are delayed in their appearance, and are small and irregular (Fig. 6.10). The pubis and ischium are hypoplastic, and the acetabular roof is horizontal. The vertebral bodies are irregular and biconvex, with central projections (Fig. 6.11). Odontoid hypoplasia is frequent, but atlanto-axial instability is uncommon (Fig. 6.12). The ribs are spatulate.

Management

Pseudoachondroplasia may be confused with achondroplasia. However, babies with pseudoachondroplasia are

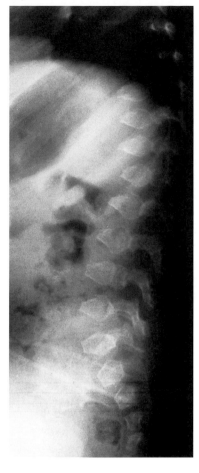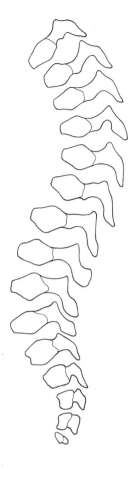

Figure 6.11 Pseudoachondroplasia. Lateral radiograph of the spine in the same patient as in Fig. 6.10, showing biconvex vertebral bodies with central projections.

normal at birth. Later, when some of the disproportionate features of achondroplasia develop, the pseudoachondroplastic child is noted to have a normal head and face, and there are major differences in the radiographic features of the spine and peripheral skeleton compared with those of an achondroplasic child.

The major orthopaedic problems during childhood involve the alignment of the lower limbs. Progressive deformity usually merits surgical correction. Multiple osteotomies may be required to restore the weight-bearing line and the plane of the various joints. However, epiphyseal development is grossly delayed, so that the shape of the joints is impossible to determine from standard radiographs. Magnetic resonance imaging, ultrasonography or arthrograms can be used to determine the plane and shape of the cartilaginous epiphyses. In addition, it is necessary to assess with care the laxity of the knee joints, and to determine the alignment with the knee fully extended and when weight bearing. Rotatory malalignment is also noted. Weight-bearing radiographs and photographs are essential for record keeping and for surgical planning.

Corrective lower limb surgery is undertaken with both legs

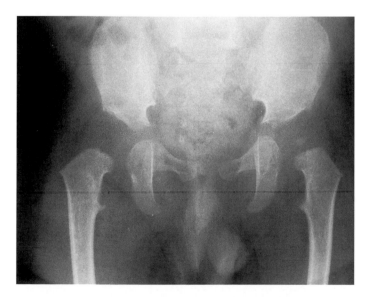

Figure 6.10 Pseudoachondroplasia. Radiograph of the pelvis in a child aged 2 years. Note the delayed ossification of the femoral epiphyses, the abnormal contour of the acetabulum, and the abnormal ossification of the pubis and ischium.

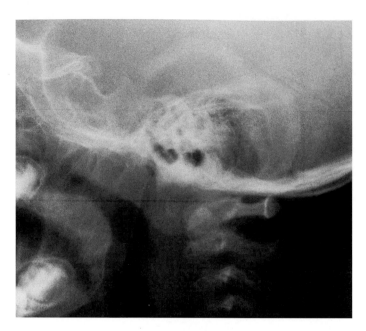

Figure 6.12 Pseudoachondroplasia. Lateral radiograph of the cervical spine in the same patient as in Figs 6.10 and 6.11, showing odontoid hypoplasia.

and the pelvis prepared and draped. Multiple osteotomies are often required, and it is best to commence proximally. Three-dimensional corrections are required at most sites. The proximal femoral osteotomies are fixed with a blade-plate or screw plate, but distal osteotomies are fixed with crossed Kirschner wires and the limb is further supported in a hip spica. The second side is corrected 3 weeks later, when the osteotomies are stable on the first side. In older children, monolateral or circular frames can be used to maintain alignment of the limbs. Lengthening the limbs in pseudo-achondroplasia may increase the likelihood of premature osteoarthritis. Many of the older children are obese, and it is desirable to reduce their weight before corrective surgery is undertaken.

Despite the enthusiasm for corrective surgery that exists in some centres, recurrence of deformities is common. None-theless, if no procedures are undertaken in young children, many will not be able to walk later in childhood. Total joint arthroplasty, particularly of the hip, may be required in the young adult.

Atlanto-axial instability is not as common as in other forms of spondyloepiphyseal dysplasia. Scoliosis of moderate degree is usually seen in patients with pelvic obliquity. Treatment is directed towards restoring pelvic symmetry. Arthrodesis and instrumentation of the spine are rarely required.

Mobility becomes an increasing problem for older children and adolescents with pseudoachondroplasia. Pain, stiff-ness and instability of joints, short limbs and obesity contribute to their inability to keep up with their peers. A mobility device such as a wheelchair or skateboard is often required for school excursions and other group activities,

and walking is usually possible within the schoolroom, home and workplace.

EPIPHYSEAL DYSPLASIAS

Many skeletal dysplasias affect the epiphyses. However, the two main groups to be considered here are multiple epiphy-seal dysplasia, which has minimal spinal involvement, and the spondyloepiphyseal dysplasias.

MULTIPLE EPIPHYSEAL DYSPLASIA

Aetiology

Multiple epiphyseal dysplasia is an autosomal dominant disorder with wide variability in its expression. Families tend to have either the mild Ribbing type or the more severe Fairbank type of dysplasia. The radiographic and patholog-ical features suggest that the patients have an anomaly of the matrix of the hyaline cartilage of the growth plates, epiphyses and articular cartilages. Mutations have been identified in the cartilage oligomeric matrix protein and type IX collagen genes.

Clinical features

Multiple epiphyseal dysplasia is not evident at birth. It first becomes apparent because of joint pain and stiffness in childhood. The hips, knees and ankles are usually involved. The hands and fingers are often short, and the fingers may lack full movement.

Some children have progressive physical difficulties during childhood. They may not be able to keep up with their peers, and attempts to do so increase their pain and limp, and accentuate nocturnal limb pain. Hand fatigue is also common during writing. Growth is slower than normal, although dwarfism is rare. Adult heights range from 145 to 170 cm. The facies is usually normal.

Radiographic features

Radiographs of the pelvis, spine, knees, ankles and wrists are required to make the diagnosis. The epiphyseal changes are usually most evident in the proximal femora (Fig. 6.13), where the ossific nuclei are small and irregular or frag-mented. The features resemble Perthes' disease, but they lack the progressive changes seen in that condition. Any child believed to have bilateral Perthes' disease should be consid-ered to have an epiphyseal dysplasia until proven otherwise, particularly when the radiographic changes are symmetrical.

The severity of the epiphyseal dysplasia varies between families. In some families, the ossific nucleus of the femoral head is fragmented, with multiple centres of ossification, and the femoral neck is short and broad. The fragmented areas coalesce to produce a flattened and often incongruous femoral head. Premature osteoarthritis is common in adoles-cence and early adult life. In other families, the ossific nucleus of the femoral head is small and irregular, but well contained within a relatively normal acetabulum. A

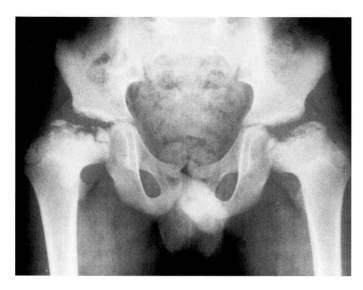

Figure 6.13 Multiple epiphyseal dysplasia. Radiograph of the pelvis of a child aged 6 years, showing abnormal ossification of the femoral heads and short, broad femoral necks. He developed incongruous hips, with premature osteoarthritis.

congruous hip usually results: it also is prone to premature osteoarthritis, but usually several decades later than those with a fragmented epiphysis.

The epiphyses of other bones are often less affected, but ossification is delayed and the ossific nuclei are small and misshapen.

The spine is minimally affected. There may be a minor amount of platyspondyly, and the vertebral bodies may be slightly ovoid. If there is more marked spinal involvement, the patient is likely to have spondyloepiphyseal dysplasia.

Management

The diagnosis is currently based on the clinical and radiographic features of the patient and family. DNA diagnoses are available in specialised centres. Treatment is symptomatic. Mild short stature is usual, but is rarely a clinical problem.

Severe hip pain and limp are treated by rest and crutches. Paracetamol taken before going to bed is useful in children with increasing nocturnal limb pain. At other times, the children are encouraged to participate in activities within their limits of comfort. Pain in the hand when writing is eased by using pens with a wide grip.

It is uncertain whether 'containment' procedures, such as the Salter osteotomy or femoral osteotomy, alter the prognosis of the hips. Premature osteoarthritis of the hip is difficult to treat, because the patients are often young and the disease is bilateral. Femoral osteotomy may be used to delay the need for total hip arthroplasty.

SPONDYLOEPIPHYSEAL DYSPLASIAS

Spondyloepiphyseal dysplasia is the term used to describe a diverse range of conditions involving delayed and abnormal ossification of epiphyses and the spine. Some of the condi-

tions have known causes and are classified separately. For example, several patterns of spondyloepiphyseal dysplasia are features of congenital hypothyroidism and the mucopolysaccharidoses. These conditions will not be considered here.

Spondyloepiphyseal dysplasia varies in its severity. It includes achondrogenesis, which is lethal, spondyloepiphyseal dysplasia congenita, which produces severe dwarfism, and spondyloepiphyseal dysplasia tarda, which produces mild short stature and premature osteoarthritis. The Stickler syndrome (hereditary arthro-ophthalmopathy) and Kniest dysplasia are also included in this family of dysplasias. The features of spondyloepiphyseal dysplasia congenita and tarda and of the Stickler syndrome will be described.

SPONDYLOEPIPHYSEAL DYSPLASIA CONGENITA

Aetiology

Spondyloepiphyseal dysplasia congenita is an autosomal dominant disorder in most families. Mutations involving the type II collagen gene have been characterised in some families. This collagen gene was considered to be the likely candidate gene, as it is expressed in growth plate and articular cartilage, intervertebral disc and vitreous humor.

Clinical features

At birth
Fetal growth is delayed, and short-trunk dwarfism is evident at birth. The face is flat, with malar hypoplasia and wide-set eyes. Club feet and a cleft palate may be present.

During childhood
Hypotonia is usual and motor development is delayed, although most children walk by 2 years of age. Excessive delay in walking may be due to cervical myelopathy with atlanto-axial instability and odontoid hypoplasia.

After weight bearing commences, the lumbar lordosis worsens, causing further shortening of the trunk (Fig. 6.14). A waddling gait is usual and is due to coxa vara. The coxa vara is progressive and is often associated with a triangular metaphyseal fragment. The hips are also flexed and externally rotated. A moderate degree of bow leg and internal tibial torsion are common.

Children with spondyloepiphyseal dysplasia congenita are prone to develop cervical myelopathy at any age, because of atlanto-axial instability. Progressive kyphoscoliosis may also develop in early childhood.

During adolescence and adulthood
Shortness of stature is severe, with an adult height of between 84 and 120 cm. Retinal detachments, with or without myopia, are common (they occur in up to 50% of children) and preventable.

Decreasing endurance and increasing limb pain are common and may be due to premature osteoarthritis or cervical myelopathy.

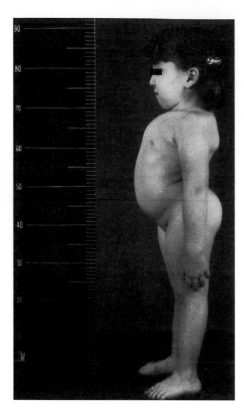

Figure 6.14 Spondyloepiphyseal dysplasia congenita. Clinical appearance in a child aged 3 years, showing short stature, short trunk and relatively long limbs. This girl has excessive lumbar lordosis and prominence of the sternum.

Radiographic features

Radiographic abnormalities are present at birth. The ossification centres of the pubis, lower femur and proximal tibia are severely retarded and the vertebrae are ovoid and flattened.

Ossification of the femoral head is absent throughout most of childhood (Fig. 6.15). Progressive coxa vara is accompanied by a high greater trochanter, short femoral neck, and a triangular metaphyseal fragment. The development of other epiphyses is also delayed. Premature osteoarthritis in the hips and knees is common.

The spinal anomalies worsen with growth. The lumbar lordosis becomes severe and is associated with decreased vertical height of the posterior margins of the vertebral bodies and elongation of the pedicles (Fig. 6.16). A thoracic kyphoscoliosis may also develop. The odontoid is hypoplastic and is often associated with atlanto-axial instability.

The feet and hands are relatively normal at all ages.

Management

The clinical and radiographic features of spondyloepiphyseal dysplasia congenita are usually characteristic. When there is any doubt, mucopolysaccharidosis screening tests are required, and the results of neonatal screening tests for hypothyroidism should be checked and may need to be repeated.

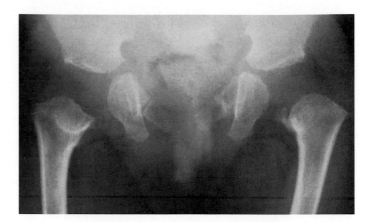

Figure 6.15 Spondyloepiphyseal dysplasia congenita. Radiograph of the pelvis from the same 3-year-old child shown in Fig. 6.14. Note the absence of ossification in the femoral heads, the short broad femoral necks and the triangular metaphyseal fragment of the left proximal femur. The child developed progressive coxa vara that was treated by a Pauwel's Y-shaped intertrochanteric osteotomy of the femur.

As with other forms of dwarfism, the initial treatment focuses on providing families with appropriate information about the disorder. A full radiographic skeletal survey is required for diagnostic purposes and for comparison with later radiographs.

Regular review is required to check for atlanto-axial instability and cervical myelopathy. If cervical myelopathy is suspected, flexion and extension radiographs of the cervical spine and magnetic resonance imaging of the spinal cord and brain stem are indicated. Atlanto-axial fusion may be required to restore stability.

Coxa vara is usually progressive, and may be associated with a triangular metaphyseal fragment, as seen in infantile coxa vara. Coxa vara can be corrected by a Pauwel's Y-shaped intertrochanteric osteotomy that corrects the plane of the growth plate and provides support for the triangular metaphyseal fragment. Progressive tibia vara and internal tibial torsion infrequently require correction by osteotomy. Progressive tibia valga may occasionally occur and requires correction by osteotomy or hemiepiphyseal stapling. Osteoarthritis of multiple joints is common in adulthood and total joint arthroplasties, particularly of the hips, may be required.

Regular ophthalmological examinations are recommended during childhood, as a means of prevention of retinal detachments.

SPONDYLOEPIPHYSEAL DYSPLASIA TARDA

Aetiology

Spondyloepiphyseal dysplasia tarda is an X-linked disorder caused by mutations of the *SEDL* gene. This gene produces a protein that is involved in the transport of proteins from the chondrocyte.

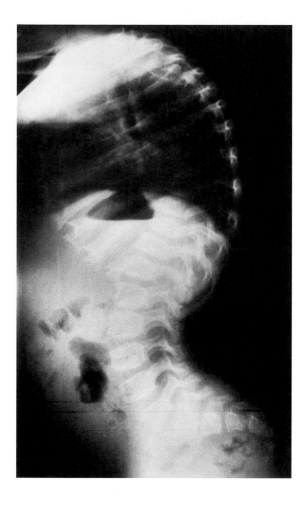

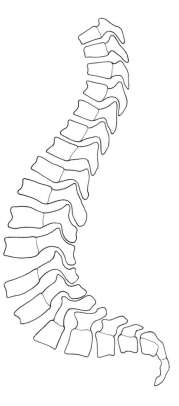

Figure 6.16 Spondyloepiphyseal dysplasia congenita. Radiograph of the spine from the same 3-year-old child shown in Figs 6.14 and 6.15. Note the excessive lumbar lordosis and thoracic kyphosis, the decreased height of the posterior margins of the vertebral bodies, and the elongation of the pedicles.

Clinical features

The clinical manifestations appear in late childhood. The patients have a short trunk and the adult height ranges from 125 to 157 cm. The chest is broad, and there is moderate pectus carinatum. Spine and joint pains are common. Premature osteoarthritis, particularly of the hips and shoulders, develops in the second and third decades of life.

Radiographic features

There is generalised platyspondyly, with central humps of bone on the upper and lower plates of the lumbar vertebrae. The ring epiphyses are poorly developed. There may also be a thoracic kyphosis or mild scoliosis.

The pelvis is small and the femoral necks are short and broad. The hip joints may also be misshapen, and premature osteoarthritis is common.

Management

The clinical and radiographic features are usually sufficient to allow a diagnosis of spondyloepiphyseal dysplasia tarda. The extensive involvement of the spine distinguishes this condition from multiple epiphyseal dysplasia, and the widespread changes within the spine distinguish it from Scheuermann's disease.

The major orthopaedic abnormalities are short stature and premature osteoarthritis. Total joint replacements may be required to relieve progressive osteoathritis.

STICKLER SYNDROME (HEREDITARY ARTHRO-OPTHALMOPATHY)

Aetiology

Stickler syndrome is transmitted as a dominant trait with highly variable expression. In some families, the phenotype has been linked to the type II and XI collagen genes.

Clinical features

Children have a marfanoid habitus, with hypotonia and joint hypermobility. The facies is flat, with midface and mandibular hypoplasia, a depressed nasal bridge and epicanthal folds. Other cranio-facial features include cleft palate, deafness and ocular anomalies. Progressive myopia, beginning in childhood, is common and may give rise to retinal detachments in young adulthood. The joints are large, and progressive joint degeneration occurs in the second and third decades of life.

Radiographic features

In childhood, there is a mild epiphyseal dysplasia of the proximal femora and distal tibiae. The tubular bones have long narrow shafts and wide metaphyses. The vertebral bodies show mild flattening and anterior wedging.

Management

The treatment required will vary according to the phenotypic features. A cleft palate may need repair. The joints wear prematurely, and arthroscopic lavage may be required in adolescence, to lesser symptoms. Some patients show symptomatic improvement with anti-inflammatory agents. However, arthroplasties are the only means of treating a severely arthritic joint in adult life.

MUCOPOLYSACCHARIDOSES

Aetiology

The mucopolysaccharidoses represent a class of storage disorder in which intermediate metabolites from the partial degradation of proteoglycans are stored in various tissues, including the bone marrow and connective tissues. They are caused by autosomal recessive and X-linked recessive genetic deficiencies of various enzymes involved in the degradation of proteoglycans and glycosaminoglycans. The clinical and chemical anomalies are summarized in Table 6.2.

Clinical and radiographic features

The mucopolysaccharidoses are heterogeneous, with various types and subtypes attributable to different enzyme deficiencies in the cascade of enzymatic steps in the degradation of the glycosaminoglycan components of proteoglycans. The major clinical features are mental retardation, dwarfism, corneal clouding and dysostosis.

The typical progressive features of the mucopolysaccharidoses are well shown by Hurler's syndrome. The babies appear normal up to about 6–8 months of age; they subsequently become large babies with rhinorrhoea, stiff joints and thoraco-lumbar kyphosis. Over the following year, the accumulation of metabolic intermediates in the tissues produces increasing coarseness of the face, stiffness of joints, hepatosplenomegaly, corneal clouding, severe growth retardation, and developmental delay. These changes progress, with death between 6 and 10 years of age.

Table 6.2 Main features of the mucopolysaccharidoses

Classification	Enzyme deficiency	Excreted glycosaminoglycan	Main organs affected	Appearance	Mental state
IH Hurler	α-L-Iduronidase	Dermatan sulphate Heparan sulphate	CNS, skeleton, viscera	Hurler ('gargoylism')	Rapid deterioration
IS Scheie	α-L-Iduronidase	Dermatan sulphate Heparan sulphate	Skeleton, viscera	Coarse features	Normal
IH/S Hurler/Scheie	α-L-Iduronidase	Dermatan sulphate Heparan sulphate	Intermediate phenotype	Coarse features	Variable
II Hunter	Iduronate sulphate sulphatase	Dermatan sulphate Heparan sulphate	CNS, skeleton, viscera	Like Hurler	Variable deterioration
III A Sanfilippo–III D	Four distinct biochemical types. Identical phenotype	Heparan sulphate	CNS	Not characteristic	Severe mental deterioration
IV Morquio	Galactosamine 6-sulphatase	Keratan sulphate	Skeleton. Severe deformities. Flat, beaked vertebrae. Thoraco-lumbar gibbus. Odontoid hypoplasia	Not diagnostic	Normal
VI Maroteaux–Lamy	N-Acetylgalactosamine 4-sulphatase	Dermatan sulphate	Skeleton	Like Hurler	Variable
VII–	β-Giucuronidase	Dermatan sulphate Heparan sulphate	CNS, skeleton, viscera	Like Hurler	Variable

Note that all these disorders are inherited as autosomal recessive disorders, with the exception of mucopolysaccharidosis (MPS) II (Hunter), in which the enzyme deficiency is inherited as an X-linked recessive.
There are common skeletal abnormalities in this group of disorders (referred to as dysostosis multiplex); these are seen typically in Hurler's syndrome (MPS I). Specific features occur in MPS IV (Morquio syndrome).
In MPS I there is a large skull, with a J (shoe)-shaped pituitrary fossa: in the spine, persistence of infantile biconcave vertebrae gives way to a thoraco-lumbar kyphosis: in the thorax, the ribs are paddle shaped; in the hands, the phalanges are pointed distally ('bullet shaped'), and the metacarpals proximally.
In MPS IV, excessive joint mobility combines with typical skeletal deformity. The spine initially resembles MPS I. Later, platyspondyly with an anterior projecting central tongue is typical. The odontoid is small or absent. There is gross deformity of the chest, shortening of the spine, and genu valgum. The small bones of the hand are well modelled.

The radiographic features in Hurler's syndrome are often referred to as 'dysostosis multiplex'. The principal changes are enlargement of the calvarium, with lack of the normal digital markings. The long bones have expanded diaphyses as a result of the storage of metabolic intermediates in the bone marrow. The hands show characteristic features, with proximal pointing of the metacarpals; the metacarpals and phalanges are wider than normal. There is generalised platyspondyly, with anterior beaking of the vertebral bodies and a thoraco-lumbar gibbus with wedging of the apical vertebra.

Orthopaedic surgeons may be referred children with the milder forms, such as Morquio, Scheie, Hunter (Fig. 6.17) or Maroteaux–Lamy syndromes. The orthopaedic problems are likely to consist of progressive kyphoscoliosis, flexion deformities of joints, foot deformities, and altanto-axial instability.

Management

The key to management is to have a biochemical diagnosis, so that the likely progress of the disease can be predicted. There is little point in undertaking orthopaedic procedures in a child with rapid general deterioration. However, progressive deformities may need to be corrected in a child with slow progression and a good life expectancy. For example, soft-tissue releases of flexion contractures and correction of foot and spinal deformities may need to be undertaken. Enzyme replacement therapy is effective in some patients. It is to be hoped that somatic gene therapy in the future will provide a lasting supply of the deficient enzyme.

METAPHYSEAL CHONDRODYSPLASIAS

This group of dysplasias is characterised by defective endochondral ossification. In metaphyseal chondrodysplasia, the metaphyses and growth plates are abnormal, whereas in spondylometaphyseal dysplasia the spine is also abnormal. The spondylometaphyseal dysplasias are extremely rare, and will not be described.

Metaphyseal chondrodysplasia is heterogeneous, with a typical mild-to-moderate Schmid type, a very rare severe Jansen type, a cartilage-hair form also referred to as the McKusick type, a Shwachman–Bodian type associated with pancreatic insufficiency and cyclical neutropenia, and the Davis type associated with thymolymphopenia. The features of the Schmid type are outlined below.

SCHMID TYPE OF METAPHYSEAL CHONDRODYSPLASIA

Aetiology

This is inherited as an autosomal dominant trait with variable expression. Histologically, there is disorganised growth and ossification of the growth plate. Mutations of the type X collagen gene, *COL10A1*, which is specifically produced by hypertrophic chondrocytes, have been identified in patients with the Schmid form of metaphyseal chondrodysplasia.

Clinical features

Affected children appear normal at birth. Short stature, bow legs, a waddling gait and increased lumbar lordosis are noted at about 2 years of age. The facies is normal. Exercise-related and nocturnal leg pain is common.

The adult height is between 130 and 160 cm. Premature osteoarthritis is unusual.

Radiographic features

The abnormalities are noted principally at the ends of the fastest-growing bones. All long bones are short and curved; the growth plates are wide and the metaphyses are irregular and wide (Fig. 6.18). The appearances are like those of rickets, particularly X-linked hypophosphataemic rickets, except that the bones are normally mineralised and have a normal texture in metaphyseal chondrodysplasia. The epiphyses are normal. There is bilateral coxa vara, with short and broad femoral necks.

Management

The clinical and radiographic features of metaphyseal chondrodysplasia are very similar to those of X-linked hypophosphataemic rickets. They can be distinguished by the osteopenia, and by the abnormal serum calcium, inorganic phosphate and alkaline phosphatase concentrations in those with rickets.

Osteotomies may be required to correct tibia vara, should the bow legs be progressive (Figs 6.18 and 6.19). The osteotomies are planned and undertaken in the same manner as described for achondroplasia. If femoral osteotomies are also required, each limb is corrected in turn. Monolateral or ring fixators can be used to provide three-dimensional control of multiple osteotomies in older children.

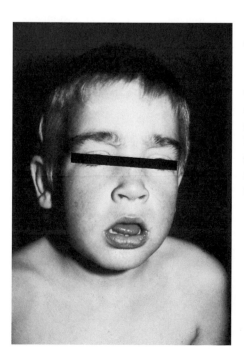

Figure 6.17 A 9-year-old with Hunter's syndrome. Note the coarse features – thick eyebrows and lips, and wide nostrils. Unlike Hurler's syndrome, there is no corneal clouding.

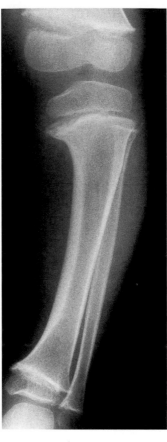

Figure 6.18 Metaphyseal chondrodysplasia. Radiograph of the tibia of a 3-year-old child, showing tibia vara and widening and irregularity of the growth plates.

EXOSTOSIS SYNDROMES

Exostoses in childhood are usually osteochondromata rather than true exostoses. They develop from the margins of the growth plates and protrude from the surface of the metaphysis. Rarely, they develop from epiphyses, giving rise to dysplasia epiphysealis hemimelica.

Solitary osteochondromas are common and sporadic; they will not be considered further. Multiple osteochondromata typically occur in diaphyseal aclasis, but they also occur as part of other syndromes. The features and management of diaphyseal aclasis and dysplasia epiphysealis hemimelica are described below.

DIAPHYSEAL ACLASIS (HEREDITARY MULTIPLE EXOSTOSES)

Aetiology
Diaphyseal aclasis is an autosomal dominant trait. About 30% of cases are new mutations, involving the *EXT1* and *EXT2* genes.

The growth plates of the osteochondromata grow in a manner similar to the normal growth plates. They close at similar times, so that the lesions do not enlarge in adult life unless malignant transformation occurs.

Clinical features
Osteochondromata first become apparent in infancy and increase in both number and size with growth. They stop growing when the growth plates close, unless there is malignant transformation, which occurs in less than 2% of cases. The common sites for osteochondromata are the ends of the long bones, pelvis, shoulder girdle and fingers; the spine and skull are rarely affected. They may be unsightly and give rise to pressure effects on tendons and neurovascular structures. Joint stiffness is common and some children may complain of aching.

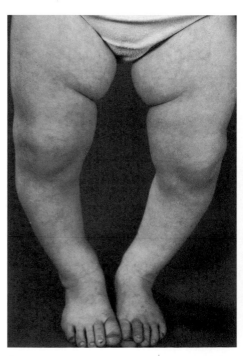

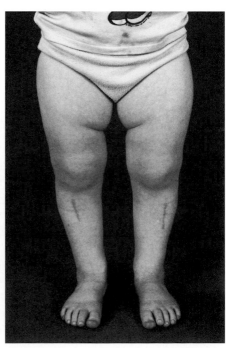

Figure 6.19 A Metaphyseal chondrodysplasia. Clinical appearance of same child as in Fig. 6.18, at 4 years of age. Note the bilateral bowing and internal tibial torsion. B Clinical appearance of the same child after correction of the bow legs and internal tibial torsion by tibial osteotomies at 4 years of age.

A   B

Osteochondromata can also produce major skeletal distortions because of pressure and growth effects. At the deep surface of the scapula, they produce winging of the scapula; at the distal radius and ulna they may produce a Madelung deformity; at the distal tibia or fibula they may distort the ankle mortice, producing a deformed and unstable ankle; and at the femoral neck they may subluxate the hip. Osteochondromata of the phalanges may produce angular deformities of the fingers and joint stiffness.

The average final height of affected individuals is 169 cm for males and 159 cm for females.

Radiographic features

The trabecular and cortical bone of the osteochondromata are continuous with the equivalent components of the metaphysis (Fig. 6.20). The attachment to the metaphysis may be broad, referred to as sessile, or narrow, referred to as pedunculated. The metaphysis is poorly modelled. Computed tomography is a useful means of defining the circumferential extent of osteochondromata, particularly around the distal femur and proximal tibia. The lumps may be felt to be discrete, whereas the scan may show them to be continuous, rather like a mountain range with a common base and a series of peaks. Each osteochondroma is much larger than the radiographic appearance because of its radiolucent cartilage cap.

The bone of the osteochondromata has a well-ordered trabecular pattern that is continuous with the underlying metaphyseal bone. Some lesions may have a smooth external surface, whereas others are more lobulated, with a cauliflower appearance. The appearance of bone destruction

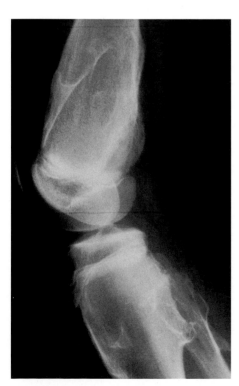

Figure 6.20
Diaphyseal aclasis. Radiograph of the knee in an adolescent of 13 years, showing sessile and pedunculated osteochondromata.

or patchy calcification after maturity is likely to indicate malignant transformation.

Madelung's deformity frequently develops as a result of disproportionate shortening of the ulna with bowing of the radius. The growth of the distal radius and ulna is often grossly abnormal. Shortening and bowing of the distal fibula and widening of the ankle mortice are also common.

Management

The diagnosis is usually obvious. Osteochondromata occur in other syndromes such as the Langer–Giedon form of acrodysplasia, which is also called trichorhinophalangeal dysplasia, type II. However, such children have a characteristic facies, with a bulbous pear-shaped nose, sparse hair and cone-shaped phalangeal epiphyses.

The clinical diagnosis may also be confused with multiple enchondromatosis, which gives metaphyseal lumps. Madelung's deformity is also a feature of dyschondrosteosis, but children with that condition lack the widespread osteochondromata that are characteristic of diaphyseal aclasis.

Excision of selected osteochondromata may be required because of pain, dysfunction or deformity. If the base of the lesion abuts the growth plate, it is wise to delay removal until the growth plate has grown away from it, otherwise cautious removal of the lesion is likely to lead to recurrence, or complete removal of it may lead to a partial growth plate arrest. A surgical approach is selected that provides direct access to the base of the lesion rather than to the cap. The cap is often large and obstructs access to the base. Vital structures may also be closely applied to the base of the lesion. For example, the femoral or popliteal artery may wind around the base of osteochondromata of the distal femur. In such situations, the surgical approach should not only provide direct access to the base of the lesion, but should also allow the vessels to be isolated above and below the lesion, so they can be retracted from the base before excision.

It is essential that the cartilage cap, with its growth plate, is completely removed, or the lesion may recur. This is easily achieved with small osteochondromata, but considerable care is required when removing large, cauliflower lesions. After removal of the lesion, the metaphysis should have the normal concave shape of a well-modelled metaphysis.

Removal of sessile lesions from the distal femur and proximal tibia is often difficult because the lesions are circumferential. Computed tomography will confirm the clinical extent. Under these circumstances, specific lesions that are causing symptoms may be removed, but recurrence is common.

Madelung's deformity is difficult to treat. Removal of exostoses, epiphyseolysis and realignment osteotomy of the radius, and lengthening of the ulna have been recommended, but the results are unpredictable.

Osteochondromata of the distal tibia or fibula may widen the ankle mortice. Regular radiographs of the ankles are advisable and if this complication appears likely, the osteochondromata should be excised. It is difficult to restore the ankle mortice to normal once the inferior tibio-fibular joint has been separated.

All excised osteochondromata should be sent for pathological examination, although malignant transformation is rare in childhood. In adults, it is wise to regard any lesion that starts to enlarge or to become painful as being a chondrosarcoma. The radiograph may show some new areas of calcification and bone destruction. Such lesions, even without radiographic evidence of a sarcomatous degeneration, should be removed immediately. The clinical behaviour of the lesion is the best indication of whether it is malignant. Biopsy is not helpful in the early stages, and if a suspicious lesion is left alone it may become very large and difficult, or even impossible, to remove later. In general, malignant transformation is more likely in proximal and flat bone lesions.

DYSPLASIA EPIPHYSEALIS HEMIMELICA

This disorder is also known as Trevor's (1950) disease or osteochondroma of the epiphyses.

Aetiology
The aetiology of this condition is unknown, because most cases are sporadic. The lesions are similar to those of external osteochondromata, except that they develop from the epiphysis and protrude into the joint.

Clinical and radiographic features
Affected children present with pain, swelling and deformity; the wrist, ankle and foot are the most frequent sites of complaint. A lump is palpable on the epiphysis, and is often associated with angular deformity of the joint. Radiographs reveal multiple sites of ossification over one-half of the epiphysis, at the ends of the long bones of one or more segments of a limb or of the tarsal bones (Fig. 6.21). The multiple centres of ossification gradually coalesce and, by the end of growth, the trabecular pattern is continuous with that of the underlying epiphysis. The end result is enlargement of one side of the epiphysis of one or more long bones or of the tarsal bones.

Management
The diagnosis is usually obvious from the clinical and radiographic appearances. Chondrodysplasia punctata also produces stippling of epiphyses. However, in chondrodysplasia punctata, the stippling has usually disappeared by the time the child is aged 2 years, whereas dysplasia epiphysealis hemimelica becomes apparent at or after this age.

Growth of the epiphyseal osteochondroma frequently leads to angular deformities of the knee or to distortion of the ankle mortise. In both situations, paring down of the osteochondroma may be indicated. This can be undertaken using curved scalpel blades. It is best done when the centres of ossification are deep in the lesion, otherwise more superficial ossific centres are exposed as the lesion is pared. In later childhood, it is preferable to leave epiphyseal osteochondroma of the

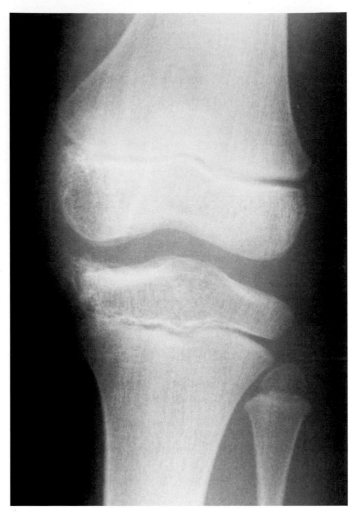

Figure 6.21 Dysplasia epiphysealis hemimelica. Radiograph of the knee in a child of 7 years of age, showing abnormal ossification of the medial margin of the proximal tibial epiphysis. A similar lesion of the distal femur was shaved off when the child was 3 years of age.

distal tibia and femur alone and to correct limb alignment by osteotomy. However, subluxation of the hip or ankle at any age requires excision of the intra-articular lesions.

ENCHONDROMATOSIS

Enchondromatosis, also called Ollier's disease, is a skeletal dysplasia that may involve one or more bones. When it is associated with haemangiomata, it is called Maffucci's syndrome. There are also more rare variants in which enchondromata are associated with osteochondromata.

Aetiology
The aetiology is unknown, because most cases are sporadic.

Clinical and radiographic features
There are two main presentations. The first is with multiple lumps on the fingers or toes. The second is with deformity

and limb length discrepancy (Fig. 6.22). Pathological fractures can also occur.

The radiographs show multiple metaphyseal lesions. Lesions in the metacarpals or phalanges usually have the typical features of benign enchondromata. They expand the bone and the enlarging surface is covered by a thin layer of subperiosteal new bone. The lesion may contain some speckled calcification, characteristic of a cartilage lesion. The number and size of the lesions in the digits often increase during childhood, but they stop growing after skeletal maturity.

The masses of hyaline cartilage in the metaphyses of long bones give rise to long metaphyseal lucencies in the radiographs. The lesions are usually present bilaterally, but the severity of involvement is asymmetric (Fig. 6.23). The more severely affected limb, commonly the leg, is short and bowed and the metaphyses are enlarged. Mild shortening of one leg may be evident at birth, without evidence of enchondromata.

The lesions stop growing at puberty and remodelling occurs, with replacement of the cartilaginous masses by bone, although some cartilage islands usually remain. Malignant degeneration occurs rarely.

The diagnosis is usually obvious from the clinical and radiographic features. It should be distinguished from diaphyseal aclasis, metaphyseal chondrodysplasia and fibrous dysplasia.

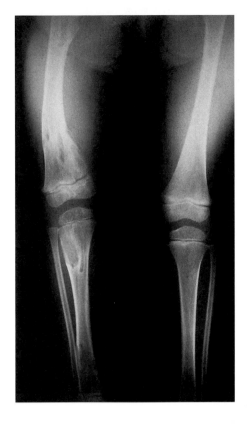

Figure 6.23 Ollier's disease. Radiograph of legs of same girl as shown in Fig. 6.22. Note the normal long bones of the left leg. The right femur and tibia are short and the distal femur is bowed. The metaphyses of the right leg are abnormal because of the persistence of cartilage columns.

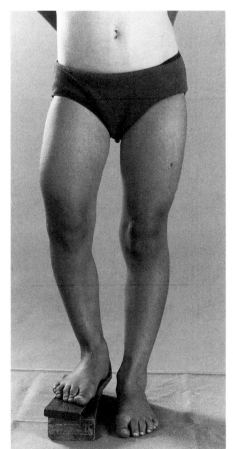

Figure 6.22 Ollier's disease. Clinical appearance in a girl aged 4 years, showing shortening of the right leg, with bowing and internal torsion of the femur.

Management

Surgical treatment of finger lumps may be required to improve finger function and to correct deformities. Selected lesions of the phalanges and metacarpals are treated by curettage, with care to avoid damage to the growth plate if the lesion adjoins it. Asymmetric lesions rarely need bone grafting, because the normal bone acts as a stable buttress and the subperiosteal bone can be invaginated into the defect. An osteotomy may be undertaken at the same time if asymmetric growth of the bone produces a significant angular deformity. For symmetric lesions, a corticocancellous bone graft may be needed to maintain alignment and length of the bone after subperiosteal excision of the lesion.

No attempt is made to excise enchondromata from the long bones of the leg, as the masses of cartilage are continuous with the growth plates. However, severe and progressive angular deformities often need to be corrected in early childhood, by osteotomy; for example, varus of the distal femur is corrected by metaphyseal osteotomy. Both limbs are prepared and draped free and a sterile tourniquet is applied high on the affected thigh. An osteotomy is made perpendicular to the bone and the deformity is overcorrected. The osteotomy is fixed with two crossed Kirschner wires, and the limb is immobilized in a well-moulded hip spica.

The osteotomy through the abnormal metaphysis heals in the normal time; however, the deformities in the lower limb recur, and the leg length discrepancy worsens progressively. Correction of the angular and rotary deformities and the leg length discrepancy are undertaken together in later childhood. Monolateral or ring fixator methods of limb lengthening and deformity correction provide the three-dimensional control required to achieve correction in Ollier's disease. Multiple osteotomies may be required in the tibia and femur to achieve the correct alignment.

Malignant transformation in Ollier's disease is rare. It is, however, common in Maffucci's syndrome. Reactivation of growth of any lesion in adult life should be considered to be the result of sarcomatous transformation.

SPECIFIC FIBROUS DISORDERS

MARFAN'S SYNDROME

This is a relatively common and well-known connective tissue disease.

Aetiology

Marfan's syndrome is an autosomal dominant disorder with variable expression. About 15% of patients have new mutations. The abnormal fibrillin-1 gene, *FBN1*, encodes a microfibrillar protein that is found in the various tissues affected by Marfan syndrome.

Clinical and radiographic features

Patients with Marfan's syndrome are tall, with disproportionately long slim limbs, arachnodactyly and a decreased upper to lower segment ratio. Pectus carinatum or excavatum are common. The face is long and narrow, with a high arched palate. Ocular problems are common and include lens subluxation (usually upwards), myopia and retinal detachment. Mitral valve prolapse and aneurysms of various types are also common.

There are three patterns of spinal deformity: thoraco-lumbar kyphosis, 'flat back' and scoliosis. Thoraco-lumbar kyphosis is noted in late infancy. It is flexible and is caused by hypotonia and ligament laxity. It usually improves as muscle power increases. The flat back consists of flattened lumbar and thoracic spines. Scoliosis is common, and may commence in infancy (Fig. 6.24). The curves are usually progressive, and more than half are double structural curves.

Congenital hip dislocation and dysplasia may occur, as may protrusio acetabuli. The foot is long and narrow with an abnormally long big toe, and rolls into planovalgus (Fig. 6.25). Hallux valgus is common.

The diagnosis of Marfan's syndrome is a clinical one at present. It is straightforward in the typical case, but many children lack some of the usual features and either have another syndrome or are classified as having a marfanoid habitus.

There are many syndromes with a marfanoid habitus. Homocystinuria, which is very similar to Marfan's syndrome, is an autosomal recessive disease that can be diagnosed by urine analysis. It is important to distinguish it from Marfan's syndrome, because patients with homocystinuria are prone to major thromboses during or after surgery unless precautions are taken. Patients with congenital contractural arachnodactyly (Beal's syndrome) have the marfanoid habitus and contractures of the knees, elbows and hands at birth. The face

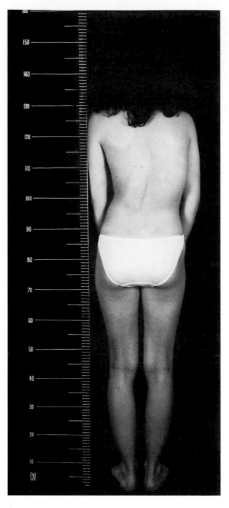

Figure 6.24 Marfan syndrome. Note the right thoracic scoliosis.

is oval, with micrognathia, and the pinnae are crumpled and flattened. The feet are often held in calcaneus with hindfoot valgus and forefoot adductus and supination; the contractures tend to improve with growth. Patients with Stickler's syndrome (hereditary arthro-ophthalmopathy), Klinefelter's syndrome, diaphyseal dysplasia and frontometaphyseal dysplasia may all show some marfanoid features.

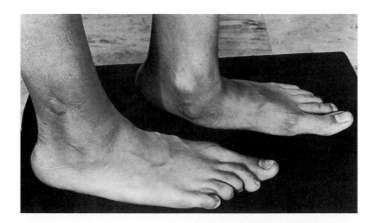

Figure 6.25 Marfan syndrome. Severe planovalgus feet that were treated with inlay triple fusions because of persistent pain.

Management

Orthopaedic care is best provided in conjunction with a paediatrician or geneticist, because of the general and life-threatening complications that may occur. Ankle-foot orthoses may be required in infancy to provide a stable base for the child during stance. Progressive scoliosis may require fusion and instrumentation in late childhood or adolescence. Non-fusion Harrington rods may be used in early childhood if the scoliosis is severe and progressive. Progressive genu valgum may occur in late childhood and can be corrected by hemiepiphyseal stapling. Pes planoabductovalgus foot deformities may produce pain or excessive shoe wear. An inlay triple fusion improves the shape, stability and comfort of the foot. To ensure a solid arthrodesis, it is usually also necessary to inlay bone graft along the medial joints of the foot and to use staples or heavy Kirschner wire fixation.

Cardiovascular assessment, including ultrasonography of the heart valves and aorta, is required before undertaking any major orthopaedic surgery in older children and teenagers. Aortic replacement, with or without aortic valve replacement, is frequently required and is best undertaken early, because vascular complications are the usual cause of premature death. It is usually wise to keep the blood pressure below 'normal'.

EHLERS–DANLOS SYNDROME

The Ehlers–Danlos syndrome (EDS) is a heterogeneous disease producing laxity in soft connective tissues (Fig. 6.26).

Aetiology

There are many types of Ehlers–Danlos syndrome, listed in Table 6.3. They are genetically determined and involve autosomal dominant, autosomal recessive and X-linked

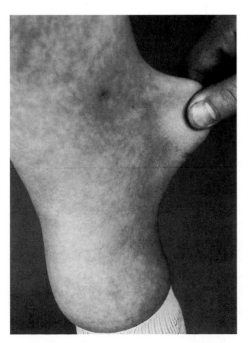

Figure 6.26 Ehlers–Danlos syndrome. Child with type I EDS, showing marked laxity of the skin of the thigh.

inheritance patterns. Abnormalities of various connective tissue macromolecules have been identified in most forms of the syndrome. In the types of EDS that involve collagen abnormalities, the connective tissue laxity and fragility appear to be due to the presence of mutant and poorly cross-linked collagen in the tissues.

Clinical features

There are at least 10 main types of Ehlers–Danlos syndrome. Their features and aetiology, when known, are outlined below.

Type I EDS (gravis or classic type)

Type I EDS is an autosomal dominant disease caused by mutations of type V collagen. This type of collagen is involved in regulating the size and shape of the thick, type I collagen-containing fibrils of dermis, tendon, ligaments, bone and blood vessels. The principal features include soft, velvety, hyperextensible and fragile skin that is prone to forming paper-thin scars, easy bruising, hypermobility of joints, flat feet and valvular incompetence. There are also a wide diversity of visceral complaints.

Type II EDS (mitis or mild type)

Type II EDS is also an autosomal dominant disease caused by mutations of type V collagen. The clinical features are similar to those of EDS-I, but are much milder.

Type III EDS (benign hypermobility syndrome)

The aetiology of type III EDS is unknown, but this type also is inherited as an autosomal dominant disease. Joint hypermobility is severe and dislocations are common. The skin is soft, but otherwise normal.

Type IV EDS (ecchymotic type)

Type IV EDS is caused by mutations, usually autosomal dominant, of type III collagen, which is the major collagen in vessels and viscera. The skin is thin, and bruising is common. The finger joints are hypermobile, but otherwise there are few skeletal anomalies. Most of the abnormalities involve the vessels and viscera. Premature death may result from vascular ruptures.

Type V EDS (X-linked type)

Type V EDS has an appearance similar to that of EDS-II. The molecular defect remains uncertain.

Type VI EDS (ocular-scoliotic type)

Type VI EDS is an autosomal recessive disease caused by a deficiency of the enzyme lysyl hydroxylase, which is an important collagen-modifying enzyme. The skin is soft and is prone to scarring and bruising. Ocular fragility, keratoconus and progressive scoliosis are common.

Type VII EDS (arthrochalasis multiplex congenita)

This is characterised by marked joint hypermobility and multiple dislocations at birth. The skin is soft, but not exces-

Table 6.3 Classification of the Ehlers-Danlos syndrome

Type	Features	Inheritance
I (gravis or classic type)	Lax, fragile skin and lax joints	Autosomal dominant
II (mitis or mild type)	Mild type I features	Autosomal dominant
III (benign hypermobility syndrome)	Severe hypermobility with multiple dislocations	Autosomal dominant
IV (ecchymotic type)	Vascular fragility; mild distal joint hypermobility and thin skin	Autosomal dominant and recessive forms
V (X-linked type)	Type II features	X-linked
VI (ocular-scoliotic type)	Skin laxity and fragility, ocular fragility and scoliosis	Autosomal recessive
VII (arthrochalasis multiplex congenita)	Multiple joint dislocations with mild skin laxity	Autosomal dominant and recessive forms
VII (periodontitis type)	Skin and joint laxity with periodontitis	Autosomal dominant
IX (occipital horn syndrome)	Cutis laxa	X-linked
X	Skin laxity and fragility and easy bruising	Autosomal recessive

sively lax. It includes autosomal dominant forms with deletions involving the amino-terminal proteinase cleavage sites of the pro-α1(I) and pro-α2(I) chains of type I procollagen. There is a more rare autosomal recessive form in which there is a deficiency of the amino-proteinase enzyme. These mutations prevent the removal of the amino-terminal propeptide that normally occurs in the processing of procollagen to collagen. The persistent attachment of the propeptide interferes with fibril formation and collagen function.

Type VIII EDS (periodontitis type)
Type VIII EDS is an autosomal dominant trait of unknown cause. In addition to the usual features of skin and joint laxity, affected patients have periodontitis.

Type IX EDS (occipital horn syndrome or X-linked cutis laxa)
Type IX EDS is an X-linked recessive disease involving copper metabolism. Lysyl oxidase activity, which is important for collagen cross-linking, may be reduced as a result of abnormal copper metabolism, as it is a copper-dependent enzyme. This form of EDS has been reclassified as X-linked cutis laxa.

Type X EDS (fibronectin abnormality)
Type X EDS is an autosomal recessive form caused by defects in fibronectin, which is a widespread glycoprotein of the connective tissues. The skin is moderately hyperextensible and is prone to scarring and bruising. Platelet function is abnormal.

Management
It is important first to decide whether a patient has the Ehlers–Danlos syndrome and then to determine which type. It may be difficult to be sure whether a patient has the disease, in which case the diagnosis should not be made. Difficulty is often encountered in children who have hypermobile joints or hypermobility, particularly in selected joints such as the shoulders and knees.

The general aspects of management include referral to a genetics clinic for diagnosis and assessment for ocular, cardiovascular and visceral involvement. Correct typing of the EDS also assists in genetic counselling.

Skin fragility is a major problem in many young children because they fall so frequently. A protective head orthosis may be temporarily required to protect the skin of the forehead, which can otherwise become extensively scarred from simple falls.

The orthopaedic problems associated with EDS include congenital dislocation of the hips, congenital laxity of multiple joints, flat feet and scoliosis. Congenital dislocations of the hips are difficult to treat because the hip joint capsule remains lax and voluminous, despite prolonged use of harnesses and other abduction devices (Fig. 6.27). The hips may dislocate easily for many months. If the hips remain unstable, it may prove necessary to splint the joints

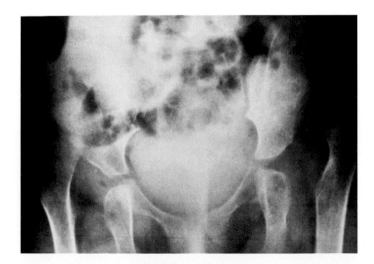

Figure 6.27 Ehlers–Danlos syndrome. Radiograph of the pelvis of a child with type VII EDS The dislocations were very unstable. Stability was achieved by open reductions and innominate osteotomies.

for several months in a hip spica, or to carry out an open reduction and capsular reefing. Femoral or acetabular osteotomy is required to ensure that a stable reduction is achieved and maintained. Soft tissue procedures alone are rarely adequate, owing to the torsional abnormality.

Laxity of multiple joints can produce pain, frequent injuries and impaired function. Limited motion orthoses are often helpful in protecting a joint. For example, pain in the elbow, as a result of hyperextension, is a common complaint in many sporting activities. An orthosis with an extension stop will often allow a child to continue comfortably with sports. Knee orthoses may also be required. Patellar instability is common, and is best managed conservatively because soft tissue procedures usually fail.

Severe planovalgus deformity is common and is a source of discomfort and of excessive shoe wear. In young children, ankle-foot orthoses prevent excessive valgus. Although the laxity does diminish with growth, a soft or plastic foot orthosis will usually be needed. In some adolescents a triple arthrodesis of the foot, commonly of the inlay type, will be required. It is undertaken in the same manner as in Marfan's syndrome.

Scoliosis is also a common problem. The deformity is often quite flexible. Arthrodesis with spinal instrumentation may be required in later childhood or adolescence.

Patients with EDS are prone to excessive bleeding during and after surgery, and wound dehiscence and spreading of healed wounds are common. Meticulous haemostasis should be obtained. Subcuticular dermal sutures need to be carefully inserted, as the dermis is often thin. The wound should be supported for several months, with adhesive plastic strips or wound dressings.

FIBROUS DYSPLASIA

Aetiology

In fibrous dysplasia, the bone and bone marrow are replaced with fibrous connective tissue containing some fragments of bone. There are two forms of this disease: a monostotic form and a polyostotic form. In the latter form, skin pigmentation may be present, and some children have endocrine anomalies producing the McCune–Albright syndrome. Mutations of protein have been identified in the two forms of the disease.

Clinical features

The monostotic form is more common than the polyostotic disease. It may produce pain, fracture or swelling, usually in teenagers, and may occasionally be an incidental finding on an X-ray taken for some other purpose. The most common sites are the proximal femur and tibia. The lesion may progress during growth, but usually ceases to grow after puberty.

The polyostotic form produces symptoms in the first decade of life. Although many bones may be affected, the condition is often worse in one leg, producing deformity, fractures and severe shortening. Cranio-facial involvement

is common. The McCune–Albright syndrome occurs in girls and causes precocious sexual development, premature closure of epiphyses, and short stature. The skin lesions consist of multiple, well-demarcated melanotic patches that stop at the midline and have irregular margins.

Radiographic features

The typical appearance is of a lytic area in the medullary cavity of a long bone, producing a 'ground glass' appearance. As the lesion expands it erodes and scallops the cortex, but is covered by the remaining cortex or by subperiosteal new bone. Additional bone may form on the concave side of the lesion – an appearance that is common in the tibia, where it produces a sabre type of appearance. Progressive coxa vara is common, and in polyostotic forms the proximal femur may produce the characteristic 'shepherd's crook' deformity (Fig. 6.28).

Management

Many monostotic lesions have a typical radiographic appearance and biopsy is not required to confirm the diagnosis. Similarly, polyostotic fibrous dysplasia also produces a typical clinical and radiographic appearance and biopsy is not required for diagnosis. Bisphosphonate treatment improves the bone density and strength in some children.

Fractures are usually treated by standard methods, but the lesion usually persists. Repeated fracture of a deformed bone, such as the proximal femur, requires correction of the deformity and internal fixation, preferably with an intramedullary rod. Bisphosphonate treatment may minimise the deformities, improve implant fixation and reduce the likelihood of recurrent deformities.

Malignant transformation has been reported, but is rare.

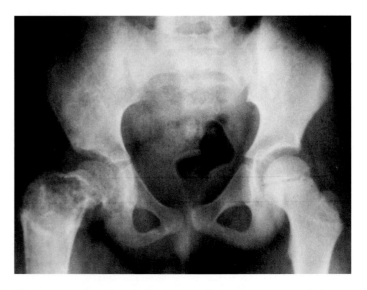

Figure 6.28 Polyostotic fibrous dysplasia. Radiograph of the pelvis, showing the abnormal bone of the proximal right femur and pelvis. Progressive coxa vara was treated with a Pauwel's Y-shaped intertrochanteric osteotomy of the femur.

SUMMARY

The variety of disorders of bone, cartilage and fibrous tissue is wide, and most are genetically determined. It is essential to make the correct diagnosis, so that families can be given appropriate information regarding the future, associated anomalies, and the risks of recurrence in future pregnancies. Orthopaedic anomalies are frequent, often severe, and progressive. Treatment needs to be carefully planned. It should take into account the specific requirements of children with short limbs and trunks, and those with lax and fragile or stiff tissues.

REFERENCES AND FURTHER READING

Briggs M D, Mortier G R, Cole W G et al 1998 Diverse mutations in the gene for cartilage oligomeric matrix protein in the pseudoachondroplasia – multiple epiphyseal dysplasia disease spectrum. American Journal of Human Genetics 62: 311–319

Chan D, Cole W G, Rogers J G, Bateman J F 1995 Type X collagen multimer assembly in vitro is prevented by a Gly618 to Val mutation in the alpha 1(X) NC1 domain resulting in Schmid metaphyseal chondrodysplasia. Journal of Biological Chemistry 270: 45558–45562

Cole W G 1997 The molecular pathology of osteogenesis imperfecta. Clinical Orthopaedics 343: 235–248

Cole W G 1997 Abnormal skeletal growth in Kniest dysplasia caused by type II collagen mutations. Clinical Orthopaedics 341: 162–169

Cordes S, Dickens D R, Cole W G 1991 Correction of coxa vara in childhood. The use of Pauwel's Y-shaped osteotomy. Journal of Bone and Joint Surgery 73B: 3–6

Dreyer S D, Zhou G, Baldini A et al 1998 Mutations in LMX1B cause abnormal skeletal patterning and renal dysplasia in nail patella syndrome. Nature Genetics 19: 47–50

Giunta C, Superti-Furga A, Spranger S, Cole W G, Steinmann B 1999 Ehlers–Danlos syndrome type VII: clinical features and molecular defects. Journal of Bone and Joint Surgery 81A: 225–238

Glorieux F H, Bishop N J, Plotkin H, Chabot G, Lanoue G, Travers R 1998 Cyclic administration of pamidronate in children with severe osteogenesis imperfecta. New England Journal of Medicine 339: 947–952

Hecht J T, Deere M, Putnam E et al 1998 Characterization of cartilage oligomeric matrix protein (COMP) in human normal and pseudoachondroplasia musculoskeletal tissues. Matrix Biology 17: 269–278

Jones K L 1988 Smith's recognizable patterns of human malformation. W B Saunders, Philadelphia

McGrory J, Weksberg R, Thorner P, Cole W G 1996 Abnormal extracellular matrix in Ehlers–Danlos syndrome type IV due to the substitution of glycine 934 by glutamic acid in the triple helical domain of type III collagen. Clinical Genetics 50: 442–445

McKusick V A 1990 Mendelian inheritance in man. Catalogs of autosomal dominant, autosomal recessive, and X-linked phenotypes. The Johns Hopkins University Press, Baltimore

Michalickova K, Susic M, Willing M C, Wenstrup R J, Cole W G 1998 Mutations of the alpha2(V) chain of type V collagen impair matrix assembly and produce Ehlers–Danlos syndrome type I. Human Molecular Genetics 7: 249–255

Mundlos S, Otto F, Mundlos C et al 1997 Mutations involving the transcription factor CBFA1 cause cleidocranial dysplasia. Cell 89: 773–779

Schipani E, Langman C B, Parfitt A M et al 1996 Constitutively activated receptors for parathyroid hormone and parathyroid hormone-related peptide in Jansen's metaphyseal chondrodysplasia. New England Journal of Medicine 335: 708–714

Sillence D O, Senn A, Danks D M 1979 Genetic heterogeneity in osteogenesis imperfecta. Journal of Medical Genetics 16: 101–116

Smith R, Francis M J O, Houghton G R 1983 The brittle bone syndrome. Osteogenesis imperfecta. Butterworths, London

Sofield H A, Page M A, Mead N C 1952 Multiple osteotomies and metal-rod fixation for osteogenesis imperfecta. Journal of Bone and Joint Surgery 34A: 500–502

Susic S, McGrory J, Ahier J, Cole W G 1997 Multiple epiphyseal dysplasia and pseudoachondroplasia due to novel mutations in the calmodulin-like repeats of cartilage oligomeric matrix protein. Clinical Genetics 51: 219–224

Treble N J, Jensen F O, Bankier A, Rogers J G, Cole W G 1990 Development of the hip in multiple epiphyseal dysplasia. Natural history and susceptibility to premature osteoarthritis. Journal of Bone and Joint Surgery 72B: 1061–1064

Trevor D 1950 Tarso-epiphyseal aclasis. Journal of Bone and Joint Surgery 32B: 204–213

Wenstrup R J, Langland G T, Willing M C, D'Souza V N, Cole W G 1996 A splice-junction mutation in the region of COL5A1 that codes for the carboxyl propeptide of pro alpha 1(V) chains results in the gravis form of the Ehlers–Danlos syndrome (type I). Human Molecular Genetics 5: 1733–1736

Chapter 7

Metabolic and endocrine disorders of the skeleton

R. Smith

INTRODUCTION

This chapter deals with the metabolic and endocrine disorders that affect the skeleton, the results of excess and deficiency of vitamins, and the toxic effects of metals on bone. It also concerns itself with inherited conditions, such as osteopetrosis, that result from abnormal bone cell biology; with polyostotic fibrous dysplasia, in which endocrine disturbances may also occur; and with ossification in the soft tissues, particularly when this is inherited. Osteogenesis imperfecta – an important metabolic disorder that has become a subject of its own – and the skeletal dysplasias are dealt with in Chapter 6.

Within the past two decades, the scope of metabolic bone disease has widened. There is an increasing recognition of the importance of the organic matrix of bone, particularly collagen. There is also greater understanding of how hormones affect the skeleton and of the many factors produced from bone cells and the non-collagenous matrix that contribute to the function of the skeleton. This does not mean that classic metabolic bone diseases such as rickets are of diminished importance, but it emphasises that the term 'metabolic bone disease' covers a wider range of skeletal disorders than previously envisaged (Smith 1996).

PHYSIOLOGY

An outline of the physiology of bone, presented here, is necessary to an understanding of the cause, diagnosis and management of metabolic bone disorders; the subject is reviewed extensively by Bilezikian et al (1996). The important components of the skeleton are cells, organic matrix and mineral. There are two widespread misconceptions about the skeleton: first that it is inert, and second that it is composed entirely of chalk. Both conclusions are superficially logical, the first because of the mechanical properties of the skeleton and its persistence after death, the second from the fact that the skeleton contains 99% of the body's calcium. However, neither is correct.

BONE CELLS

Bone cells comprise the osteoblasts, the osteocytes and the osteoclasts. Osteoblasts, which come from preosteoblasts of the mesenchymal stromal system, become transformed to osteocytes that occupy lacunae in mineralised bone. In contrast, osteoclasts are derived from the haemopoietic system.

Osteoblasts have many functions and may be regarded as the most important bone cells (Fig. 7.1). They produce all the components of the organic matrix including collagen, and important non-collagen proteins such as osteocalcin, and control the mineralisation of this matrix. They influence the activity of other bone cells, particularly the osteoclasts, by the use of short-acting messengers (cytokines), only some of which have been identified. Osteoblasts respond to a number of systemic hormones (such as parathyroid hormone, oestrogens and growth hormone) by virtue of their surface receptors.

The functions of the osteocytes are not so well defined. They appear to be responsible for the integrity of bone and communicate with each other via their extensions in the canaliculi, modulating the response of the skeleton to mechanical stimuli.

Whereas osteoblasts are synthetic cells, osteoclasts are concerned particularly with bone resorption. Contrary to previous belief, osteoclasts do not have receptors to hormones such as parathormone and dihydroxycholecalciferol $(1,25(OH)_2D)$, and appear to be largely controlled by the osteoblasts. However, they do respond directly to calcitonin, which temporarily suppresses their activity. The osteoclast has polarity, and resorption begins when the cell seals off an area on the bone surface adjacent to its ruffled border. The

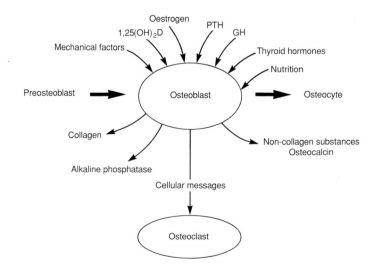

Figure 7.1 The central position of the osteoblast. Fine arrows indicate factors that influence the osteoblast, and some functions of the osteoblast. Broad arrows indicate the origin of the osteoblast and osteocyte.

production of lysosomal enzymes and a very acid environment via a proton pump utilising the enzyme carbonic anhydrase II leads to the digestion of bone.

BONE MATRIX

The major component of the organic bone matrix is collagen, interspersed with a complex mixture of non-collagen proteins and proteoglycans. Defects in the synthesis of collagen lead to the inherited disorders of connective tissue, notably osteogenesis imperfecta (see Ch. 6). Abnormal breakdown of the complex proteoglycan (mucopolysaccharide) molecules produces a large variety of disorders known as the mucopolysaccharidoses. The enzyme defects responsible produce a variety of skeletal defects.

The skeleton contains more than 50% of the body's collagen, which is essential for its strength and for correct mineralisation. Many collagens exist, each with different functions and different polypeptide α-chains controlled by their own specific genes, localised to different chromosomes. In normal adult bone, the only collagen is type I, a heteropolymer with two α-1 chains and one α-2 chain, each represented as $(Gly\ X\ Y)_{338}$. An absolutely accurate triple helix with glycine in every third position in the α-chains is essential for the structural integrity of collagen. The chains are formed as precursors within the osteoblast and fibroblast and then exported as triple helical procollagens. These are converted to collagen and self-assemble in the form of fibrils and fibres that overlap by 25% of their length and subsequently cross-link. This cross-linking provides both the strength of collagen and an organised matrix with hole zones upon which early mineralisation occurs.

MINERALISATION

Mineralisation appears to be an active phenomenon controlled by osteoblasts or components derived from them (matrix vesicles), both of which contain alkaline phosphatase. This enzyme acts also as a pyrophosphatase, and it has been proposed that the local removal of pyrophosphate, itself an inhibitor of mineralisation, initiates mineralisation at selected sites. The importance of alkaline phosphatase is well demonstrated by the defective mineralisation in hypophosphatasia. Mineralisation normally occurs in the region of matrix vesicles found in most, if not all, mineralising tissues, particularly bone and cartilage. It also occurs, apparently without vesicles, on the organised matrix of bone collagen.

MINERAL HOMEOSTASIS

Little is known of matrix homeostasis; in contrast, there are many factors known to affect the absorption and excretion of calcium and its intracellular and extracellular concentrations. Phosphorus remains a neglected but important ion – for instance, in inherited hypophosphataemia. Calcium is essential for life, regulating neuromuscular transmission,

reproduction, endocrine function, blood clotting and many widespread processes. It circulates in the plasma at a concentration of 2.25–2.60 mmol/l in protein-bound (46%), ionised (47%) and complexed forms. Its concentration is maintained by a sensitive balance between intestinal absorption, renal reabsorption and bone resorption, controlled by the classic calciotropic hormones parathyroid hormone, vitamin D (as its $1,25(OH)_2$ derivative) and calcitonin, by the relatively newly discovered parathyroid-related protein (PTHrP), and by a host of locally acting factors in addition to hormones with other important functions, such as growth hormone and oestrogens. The actions of these are illustrated in Fig. 7.2; their clinical effects are listed in Table 7.1.

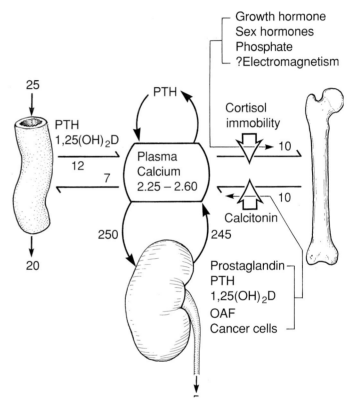

Figure 7.2 Calcium homeostasis. The figures represent the daily exchange in adults (in mmol), and the concentration in the plasma (in mmol/l). To convert values to mg, multiply by 40. PTH, parathyroid hormone; OAF, osteoclast activating factor(s).

Parathyroid hormone

Parathyroid hormone (PTH) is synthesised as a precursor (preproPTH), in the manner of proteins packaged for export. It is secreted in response to hypocalcaemia, and is produced in excess in primary hyperparathyroidism. PTH increases plasma calcium by stimulating intestinal absorption (via its effect on the synthesis of $1,25(OH)_2D$), by increasing renal reabsorption of calcium, and by increasing osteoclastic bone resorption (via the osteoblasts). Its effects on receptor cells are mediated through two separate systems that involve adenyl cyclase and inositol triphosphate. Recent work has

Table 7.1 The main clinical actions of hormones on the skeleton

	Excess	Deficiency
Parathyroid hormone	Increased bone resorption Osteitis fibrosa cystica Also osteosclerosis and osteoporosis	Skeletal changes in pseudohypoparathyroidism
Vitamin D (via 1,25(OH)$_2$D)	Increased metaphyseal density	Defective mineralisation
Thyroxine	Osteoporosis (resorption increased more than formation)	Delayed bone age: fragmented epiphyses
Cortisol	Osteoporosis: short stature	None
Sex hormones	Early epiphyseal closure	Osteoporosis
Pituitary	Acromegaly and gigantism (before growth ceases)	Pituitary dwarfism Osteoporosis associated with hypogonadism

Note that neither deficiency nor excess of calcitonin produces any clinical effect on the skeleton.

demonstrated important calcium sensing receptors in the parathyroid and other tissues (Brown et al 1996); mutations in the genes for these receptors can cause inherited alterations in plasma calcium.

Vitamin D

Vitamin D produces its effects via its active metabolite, 1,25(OH)$_2$D. The main physiological source of vitamin D is the skin, where cholecalciferol (vitamin D$_3$) is synthesised from its precursor, 7-dehydrocholesterol, under the influence of ultraviolet light. Vitamin D also comes from the diet, mainly in the form of ergocalciferol (vitamin D$_2$). Both vitamins D$_2$ and D$_3$ (collectively referred to as vitamin D), undergo hepatic conversion to 25(OH)D and subsequent renal conversion to 1,25(OH)$_2$D, the active vitamin D metabolite. As 25(OH)D is the major circulating vitamin D metabolite, it provides an accurate measure of vitamin D status. It is reduced in nutritional rickets, in Asian immigrants, and in geriatric patients.

The effects of 1,25(OH)$_2$D are mediated through its widely distributed receptor. The gene for this receptor has been cloned, and mutations within it cause very rare forms of type II vitamin-D-dependent rickets (see below). The main effects of vitamin D on mineral metabolism are to increase intestinal calcium absorption and osteoclastic bone resorption. However, the effects of vitamin D (via 1,25(OH)$_2$D) are not limited to mineral metabolism, as 1,25(OH)$_2$D is known to have important effects on growth, on differentiation of cells, and on immunological processes.

Calcitonin

Calcitonin directly suppresses the osteoclast, thereby reducing bone resorption. It is secreted in response to hypercalcaemia, but its physiological role is undefined. It has been proposed that it prevents bone resorption in times of physiological stress, such as growth and pregnancy.

Parathyroid–hormone–related peptide

Recent investigations of hypercalcaemia in non-metastatic solid tumours have identified a hormone with considerable amino-terminal homology with PTH, now known as PTHrP. It has actions very similar to those of PTH and appears to use the same receptor mechanisms. Apart from its secretion by some tumours, there is evidence that it is a naturally occurring fetal hormone that may control calcium flux across the placenta. It is also important in early development of bone and cartilage. Activating mutations in the PTHrP receptor can cause the very rare Jansen metaphyseal dysplasia.

CLINICAL ASPECTS OF METABOLIC BONE DISEASE IN CHILDREN

Metabolic and endocrine bone disease in children differs from that in adults in the relative frequency of its causes, its relationship to growth, and the physiological variations in its biochemistry. The importance of growth is emphasised in Chapter 2. Accurate and consecutive measurements of height against percentile charts for a normal population will detect abnormality and the effects of treatment such as thyroxine in hypothyroidism or phosphate in inherited hypophosphataemia. Short stature is the most frequent abnormality of height. Dwarfism is proportional in some genetic conditions, and in coeliac disease, hypopituitarism or malnutrition. Disproportionate short stature is most commonly caused by a skeletal dysplasia, which may lead to relative shortness of the limbs, as in achondroplasia, or relative shortness of the spine, as in spondyloepiphyseal dysplasia.

The normal biochemical reference ranges differ with age. Thus plasma phosphate concentration in children is about twice the adult normal level and declines rapidly after puberty. Both alkaline phosphatase and urinary total hydroxyproline are related to growth velocity and increase temporarily during the adolescent growth phase. The interpretation of new bone markers based on collagen-derived fragments is difficult in children. The radiographic changes, which will be described in the appropriate sections, occur mainly at the growing regions of the bones. The clinical and biochemical features of the main disorders discussed in this chapter are summarised in Table 7.2.

Table 7.2 Metabolic and endocrine disorders of the skeleton: main features

	Clinical	Biochemical	Comments
Rickets	Many causes Most frequent in northern UK Nutritional rickets	Ca ↓ P ↓ Phosphatase ↑	For variations see Table 7.3
Osteoporosis (see Table 7.4)	Uncommon in childhood	Normal unless immobilised	
Hyperparathyroidism	Some have osteitis fibrosa cystica	Ca ↑ P ↓ Phosphatase ↑	Phosphatase sometimes increased if bone disease present
Hypoparathyroidism	Features of hypocalcaemia	Ca ↓ P ↑ Phosphatase N	Those with PHP have short metacarpals, mental simplicity, etc. (see text)
Hypothyroidism	Lack of development Dull, slow, cold	Low T4, high TSH	Skeletal features resemble mucopolysaccharidoses
Hypophosphatasia	Severe: lethal Juvenile: with cranial synostosis Adult: with long bone fractures	Low alkaline phosphatase Phosphoethanolamine in urine	Different forms
Osteopetrosis	Fracture, blindness, etc	In some acid phosphatase ↑	Several different types
Idiopathic hypercalcaemia	Mental simplicity, aortic stenosis	Plasma Ca ↑	Associated with elfin face syndrome

N, Normal; PHP, pseudohypoparathyroidism; T4, thyroxine; TSH, thyroid-stimulating hormone; phosphatase, total alkaline phosphatase.

RICKETS

Rickets (and osteomalacia in the adolescent and adult) is, with rare exception, caused by a deficiency of vitamin D or a disturbance in its metabolism. The bone matrix fails to mineralise and, histologically, there is an excess of osteoid. The causes, some of which are very rare, can be understood in relation to vitamin D metabolism (Fig. 7.3, Table 7.3). The features of nutritional rickets will be described, and the specific differences in other forms outlined.

Table 7.3 The causes of rickets

	Biochemistry		Comments
	Plasma	Urine	
Vitamin D deficiency (nutritional rickets)	Ca ↓ P ↓ Phosphatase ↑	Ca↓	Asian immigrants
Malabsorption	Ca ↓ P ↓ Phosphatase ↑	Ca↓	Main cause coeliac disease
Inherited hypophosphataemia	Ca N P ↓ Phosphatase ↑	Ca N	X-linked inheritance
Fanconi syndrome	Ca ↓ P ↓ Phosphatase ↑	Ca↓ N Aminoaciduria	Many causes Often systemic acidosis Generalized aminoaciduria
Renal glomerular failure	Ca ↓ P ↑ Phosphatase↑	Ca↓	Biochemistry of uraemia
Vitamin-D-dependent rickets (pseudovitamin D deficiency)	Ca ↓ P ↓ Phosphatase ↑	Ca↓	Two forms, both recessive: Type I $1,25(OH)_2D$ ↓ Type II $1,25(OH)_2D$ ↑
Tumour rickets	Ca N P ↓ Phosphatase ↑		Associated with haemangiomatous tumours $1,25(OH)_2D$ ↓

N, Normal.

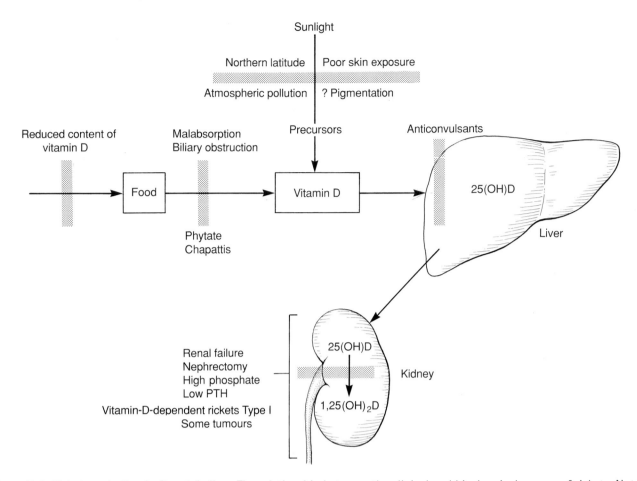

Figure 7.3 Rickets and vitamin D metabolism. The relationship between the clinical and biochemical causes of rickets. Note that chapattis may also increase the requirement for vitamin D by accelerating its breakdown.

VITAMIN-D-DEFICIENCY RICKETS

This occurs in underprivileged populations throughout the world, particularly in the Northern hemisphere. In the UK, it is most common in the Asian immigrant population of northern cities. Affected children lack the exposure to ultraviolet light necessary for the dermal synthesis of vitamin D, and receive a diet poor in vitamin D in which the components (high fibre and high cereal) contribute to the excessive breakdown of vitamin D (Smith 1990).

Clinical features

The child with nutritional rickets has delayed growth, bony deformity, proximal myopathy, and tenderness and pain in the bones. Classic changes (Fig. 7.4) are enlarged epiphyses in the long bones, enlarged costochondral junctions ('rickety rosary'), bossing of the vault of the skull, and deformities of the long bones that depend upon the age at which rickets occurs. Bow legs are common, and knock knees and asymmetric deformity can also occur. Proximal myopathy is a striking feature of rickets (and also of osteomalacia); its cause is unknown, but it can produce delay in standing and walking and, at a later age, difficulty in rising from a low chair or climbing stairs. Hypocalcaemia may produce tetany, carpopedal spasm and, occasionally, stridor.

Radiographic features

In rickets there is failure of the orderly replacement of mineralised cartilage with bone. Radiographs show a widening of the growth plate, with a ragged, cupped and widened metaphysis. Additional radiographic changes are due to secondary hyperparathyroidism with bone resorption induced by hypocalcaemia. This can occur in relation to the periosteum at the end of the long bones, the phalanges, the medial ends of the clavicles, and elsewhere. Finally, in the adolescent, Looser's zones are diagnostic of osteomalacia. These are ribbon-like areas of failure of mineralisation that typically occur symmetrically on the medial borders of the long bones, the pubic rami, and the borders of the scapulae and the ribs.

Biochemistry

Plasma calcium concentration is low or normal, phosphate low, and alkaline phosphatase increased. The typical findings vary with the stage of rickets and its cause (see Table 7.3). Secondary hyperparathyroidism will tend to correct hypocalcaemia, but increase hypophosphataemia. The increase in plasma alkaline phosphatase is related to the degree of osteoblastic activity (despite the fact that mineralisation is defective, osteoblastic activity is increased). In

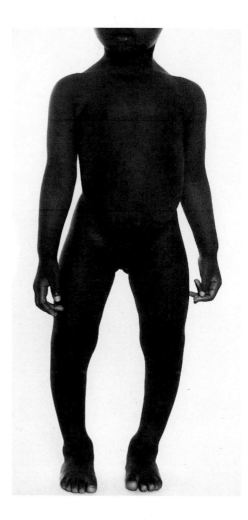

Figure 7.4
Nutritional rickets. The thickened epiphyses at wrist and ankle and the genu varum are evident.

vitamin D deficiency, the plasma 25(OH)D concentration is low. The urine calcium excretion is also very low. Aminoaciduria (which is reversible) may occur in vitamin D deficiency, as in the inherited renal tubular syndromes.

Histology

It is rarely essential to examine bone histologically in order to diagnose rickets, but bone will show an excess of unmineralised bone matrix (osteoid), with increased thickness and coverage of the mineralised surfaces.

Prevention and treatment

Nutritional rickets is prevented by exposing the skin to summer sunlight. Where this is not possible or unacceptable, physiological amounts of oral vitamin D (up to 25 µg or 1000 U) daily are effective. Successful preventive programmes have been used in Asian rickets.

Differential diagnosis

In its classic form, nutritional rickets is unlikely to be misdiagnosed. Rare causes may present difficulties.

OTHER FORMS OF RICKETS

These are outlined in Table 7.3, and will be summarised here.

Rickets due to malabsorption

This will have the added features of the underlying disease – such as coeliac disease.

Rickets due to renal disease

The term 'renal rickets' is an over-simplification. Rickets occurs in renal tubular disorders and renal glomerular failure. The causes, clinical features, management and treatment are different.

Renal tubular rickets

Inherited hypophosphataemia (vitamin-D-resistant rickets) is inherited as an X-linked dominant and, excluding Asians, is probably the most frequent cause of rickets in orthopaedic practice in the UK (Thakker & O'Riordan 1988, Glorieux 1996). The incidence is about 1 in 20 000 births, and the mutant gene has been localised to the X chromosome. Boys carrying the mutant gene may be more severely affected than girls, who have an additional normal X chromosome. Particular features are short stature, lower limb deformity (Fig. 7.5), absence of proximal myopathy, and persistent hypophosphataemia. In later years there is a widespread enthesiopathy, sometimes with ligamentous calcification leading to paraplegia. The exact cause of the renal loss of phosphate is not known, but the mutant protein is similar to an endopeptidase and may control phosphate metabolism. The main differential diagnosis is from other forms of rickets and from metaphyseal dysplasias (especially the Schmid type). Treatment combines oral phosphate (up to 2 g daily in divided doses) and 1-α-hydroxycholecalciferol (up to 1 µg daily). Corrective surgery requires considerable planning, because the deformities are complex. Surgery should only be undertaken when adequate, sustained medication has failed to prevent deformity (Fig. 7.6).

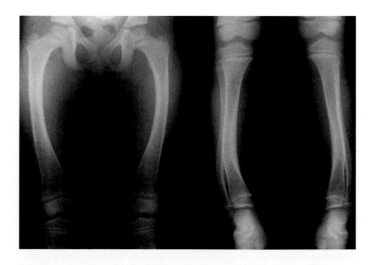

Figure 7.5 Vitamin-D-resistant rickets. Bowing of the femora and tibiae with metaphyseal flaring, especially at the distal femora.

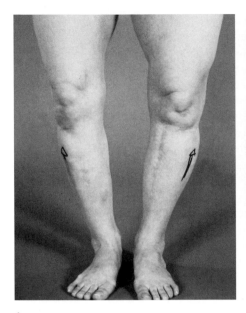
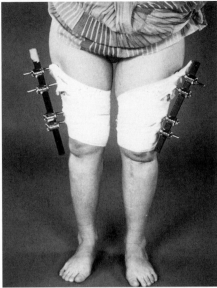

A   B

Figure 7.6 A Hypophosphataemic rickets in a 15-year-old. The tibiae have been straightened by osteotomy, but anterolateral femoral bowing leaves residual deformity. **B** Following femoral osteotomy, stabilised by external fixation.

Rickets and the Fanconi syndrome

The term 'Fanconi syndrome' refers to multiple renal tubular abnormalities, with generalised aminoaciduria. In children the most frequent cause is cystinosis, or cystine storage disease (Gahl et al 1989). In this condition, inherited as a recessive trait, cystine crystals progressively accumulate in the tissues. This leads to multiple renal tubular defects, with rapid dehydration as a result of failure of reabsorption of water, severe acidosis, hypophosphataemia and a form of renal tubular rickets. Cystinosis can be rapidly confirmed by the finding of cystine crystals in the eyes; this is often associated with photophobia (Fig. 7.7).

The underlying biochemical cause of cystine storage is unknown, although defects in the transport of cystine out of the cell have been demonstrated. The renal aspects of the disorder can be dealt with by renal transplantation. The rickets is alleviated by correction of the severe acidosis with oral bicarbonate and by giving 1-α-hydroxycholecalciferol.

Renal glomerular rickets (renal glomerular osteodystrophy)

When renal failure predominantly involves the glomeruli (as in chronic renal failure, for instance secondary to undiagnosed renal obstruction) the sequence of events differs from that in tubular disease (Fig. 7.8). Hyperphosphataemia leads to hypocalcaemia, secondary hyperparathyroidism and bone resorption. This is superimposed on failure of bone mineralisation and rickets as a result of a lack of $1,25(OH)_2D$, and produces a rapidly deforming bone disease that particularly affects the growing ends of the long bones, giving a 'rotting stump' appearance (Fig. 7.9). Other skeletal changes include osteosclerosis (producing the 'rugger-jersey' spine), osteoporosis, osteonecrosis, and deposits of amyloid in the bone.

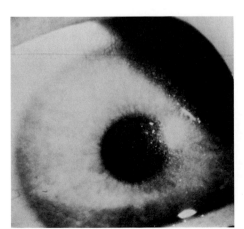

Figure 7.7 Cystine crystals in the eye in a child with cystinosis. (Reproduced with permission from Smith 1979.)

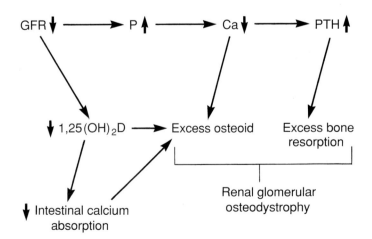

Figure 7.8 The biochemistry of renal glomerular osteodystrophy. GFR, glomerular filtration rate. P, Ca, PTH and $1,25(OH)_2D$ refer to circulating concentrations.

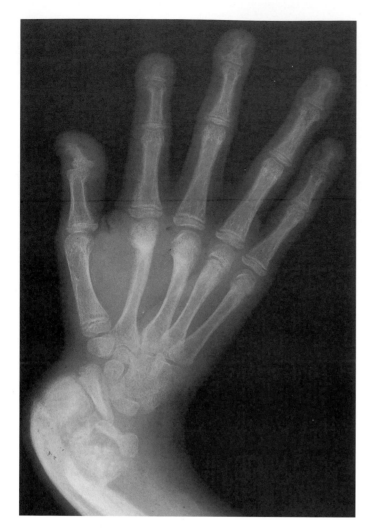

Figure 7.9 Renal glomerular osteodystrophy. To show excessive bone resorption and gross deformity in a child with chronic renal failure.

In addition, severe renal glomerular failure delays growth and bone age.

Diagnosis is based upon the association of severe rickets and deformity with renal glomerular failure. Medical treatment of renal glomerular osteodystrophy is based on replacing the deficiency of 1,25(OH)$_2$D and, where necessary, reducing plasma phosphate.

Prolonged dialysis may produce problems of its own, such as aluminium bone disease. Successful renal transplantation is clearly the most effective treatment.

Vitamin-D-dependent rickets

This is a very rare form of severe rickets that occurs without vitamin D deficiency. Two types exist, both inherited as recessive traits. In the first (type I), the 1-α-hydroxylase enzyme is defective; in the second (type II), there is apparent end-organ resistance to 1,25(OH)$_2$D. This resistance appears to be caused by single base mutations in the gene for the vitamin D (1,25(OH)$_2$D) receptor, affecting either the DNA or steroid binding sites. Interestingly, this form of rickets, also known as 1,25-vitamin-D-resistant rickets, has additional features of abnormal teeth and alopecia. Treatment is difficult, but there is a good response to prolonged intravenous calcium, and spontaneous improvement occurs with age.

Although some causes of rickets are very rare, they emphasise the close relationship between the clinical features and the known biochemistry of vitamin D (Fig. 7.3).

Finally, rickets may also occur in osteopetrosis, neurofibromatosis and fibrous dysplasia, for reasons that are obscure.

Oncogenic rickets

Certain tumours, such as non-ossifying fibromas, fibrosing haemangiomata and haemangioperiocytomas, are associated with rickets, which is cured by their removal. It is likely (although the mechanism is not proved) that the tumour interferes with the hydroxylation of 25(OH)D.

OSTEOPOROSIS

In osteoporosis there is a reduction in the amount of bone per given volume, without a change in its composition Marcus et al 1996); microarchitectural failure leads to fragility predisposing to fracture. The increasing use of dual X-ray absorptiometry has led to another definition of osteoporosis, namely a bone mass, measured as BMD or BMC, which is 2.5 SD or more below the mean peak bone mass. This is useful in adults, but normal ranges for children have not been widely established. Osteoporosis is, however, uncommon in children. Known causes of osteoporosis, such as Cushing's syndrome, have their own features in addition to the bone disease that they produce. Visual impairment is associated with osteoporosis in the rare, recessively inherited, osteoporosis pseudoglioma syndrome (Gong et al 1996). Rarely, osteoporosis occurs without an identifiable cause, sometimes associated with pre-adolescent growth (Smith 1995).

IDIOPATHIC JUVENILE OSTEOPOROSIS

The underlying change in this condition appears to be temporary formation of abnormal osteoporotic bone at the growing ends of the long bones and in the vertebrae, associated with a reduction in osteoblastic activity. Fractures occur in the metaphyses and shafts of the long bones and in the vertebrae, and growth velocity decreases. Backache, a kyphosis and characteristic pain around the lower ends of the tibia on weight bearing develop. The child walks slowly and with difficulty. Radiographically, the compression fractures may simulate Looser's zones; widespread wedging of the vertebrae may produce a fish-like spine with extensive biconcave vertebral collapse (Fig. 7.10). Routine plasma haematology and biochemistry are normal. Because pain in the bones with fracture is uncommon in children, the differential diagnosis is important (Table 7.4). It is particularly important to exclude leukaemia by bone marrow examina-

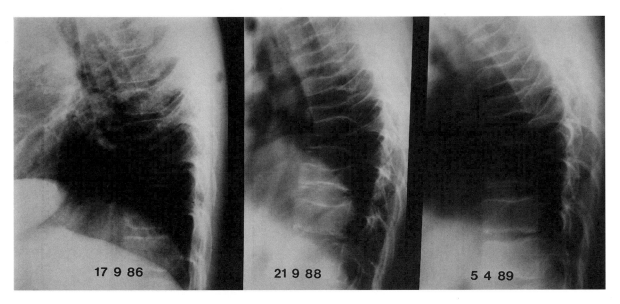

Figure 7.10 Radiological appearance of the spine in a 14-year-old boy with idiopathic juvenile osteoporosis. There is progressive vertebral collapse, with spontaneous improvement.

Table 7.4 Differential diagnosis of idiopathic juvenile osteoporosis
Other causes of juvenile osteoporosis
Cushing's syndrome
Homocystinuria
Turner's syndrome
Osteogenesis imperfecta (type I)
Osteoporosis pseudoglioma syndrome
Other diseases
Rickets
Acute leukaemia

tion, which can be done at the same time as bone biopsy. In a significant proportion of affected individuals, the bone disorder begins to improve with the onset of puberty, so that the vertebrae may resume an almost normal shape (sometime leaving a shadow of the osteoporotic bone within them). In others, the bones continue to be fragile and to fracture, so that it is important to be as certain as possible that mild forms of osteogenesis imperfecta (types I and IV) have been excluded (see Ch. 6), although this can be difficult if a family history is absent.

Provided the diagnosis of idiopathic juvenile osteoporosis is correct, treatment is for symptoms only. Some reports suggest a lack of 1,25(OH)$_2$D and an improvement when this is administered. More recently bisphosphonates, particularly those with an amino substitution, have been used (Brumsen et al 1997).

PARATHYROID DISORDERS

Primary hyperparathyroidism and its associated bone disease is uncommon in childhood, but secondary hyper-parathyroidism may be associated with the hypocalcaemia of rickets. The skeleton also alters in pseudohypoparathyroidism (PHP).

HYPERPARATHYROIDISM

Skeletal changes are the same as in the adult, with excessive osteoclastic activity, fibrosis, and the formation of cyst-like areas within the bones combining to produce osteitis fibrosa cystica. Bone resorption occurs at the growing ends of the long bones and subperiosteally, especially on the medial border of the phalanges. In those children with bone disease, the diagnosis of primary hyperparathyroidism is confirmed by the characteristic biochemistry: an increase in the plasma calcium, reduced plasma phosphate and increased alkaline phosphatase. Treatment is surgical removal of the primary tumour. The differential diagnosis is from other causes of hypercalcaemia in childhood (Table 7.5).

HYPOPARATHYROIDISM

Secretion of parathyroid hormone may be defective, or the hormone itself may be ineffective. Hypoparathyroidism may present in the neonatal period as a transient or persistent

Table 7.5 Causes of hypercalcaemia in childhood
Hyperparathyroidism
Vitamin D overdose
Idiopathic hypercalcaemia
Neoplastic disease
Immobilisation
Hypophosphatasia

disorder. It may be associated with maternal hyperparathyroidism, magnesium deficiency, or as part of the Di George syndrome. In childhood, hypoparathyroidism may be an autoimmune disorder or the result of thyroidectomy.

The skeletal abnormalities are restricted to PHP, in which there is end-organ resistance to the action of parathyroid hormone as a result of a loss of function mutation in a component of the G protein signalling system. The circulating PTH concentration is high, yet there is hypocalcaemia and hyperphosphataemia. The typical phenotypic changes of PHP are delayed growth, mental retardation, cataracts and subcutaneous ossification, together with characteristic skeletal changes that mainly affect the hands and feet, with short 4th and 5th metacarpals or metatarsals. This last feature can be demonstrated by asking the patient to clench their fist and noting that the knuckles are not in line.

PHP may be familial, and the expression of the dominant gene is variable. Patients within such families may have the PHP phenotype without any biochemical changes. The diagnosis of PHP is important since lifelong treatment with 1-α-hydroxycholecalciferol and calcium may be necessary to prevent complications.

HYPOTHYROIDISM AND OTHER HORMONAL DISORDERS

The skeleton is affected by altered secretion of other systemic hormones, with the most striking effects occuring in hypothyroidism. This is rarely recognised at birth, but by the time the child is about 6 months of age defective thyroid function leads to the clinical features of cretinism. The child becomes sluggish and sleepy, with noisy ventilation and a large tongue. Nasal obstruction and a large abdomen gradually became apparent. The temperature is subnormal, the skin is dry and cold, and there is difficulty in feeding. Importantly, there is marked delay in growth and skeletal age.

The diagnosis is made biochemically: circulating TSH is high, thyroxine is low, and the plasma cholesterol is increased. Radiographs show delayed bone age and stippling of the upper femoral epiphyses, which ossify late. The first lumbar vertebra may be hypoplastic, with anterior beaking. The diagnosis of cretinism in an infant is not difficult, but should be differentiated from multiple epiphyseal dysplasia, spondyloepiphyseal dysplasia, or one of the mucopolysaccharidoses.

Prolonged thyrotoxicosis causes bone disease in the adult, but it does not occur in childhood. The growing skeleton may also be affected by an excess of corticosteroids – most often administered therapeutically and less frequently in Cushing's syndrome – and by hypogonadism, hypopituitarism, or hyperpituitarism.

The effects of these and other hormone disturbances on the skeleton have been summarised in Table 7.1.

HYPOPHOSPHATASIA

Hypophosphatasia is a rare condition associated with a reduction in the tissue non-specific plasma alkaline phosphatase (TNSALP) (Whyte 1996). The incidence is about one in 100 000 live births. The inheritance of the severe form is recessive, and in some cases there is consanguinity. For reasons that are not fully understood, there is wide phenotypic variation, from a lethal perinatal disease to a virtually asymptomatic condition in childhood. Numerous missense mutations have now been described in the *TNSALP* gene in hypophosphatasia.

The main effect of the absence or reduction of alkaline phosphatase is to produce a disorder of mineralisation that histologically resembles rickets, with excessively thick osteoid seams. This is associated with an increase in the urinary excretion of phosphoethanolamine and an increase in plasma pyrophosphate.

PERINATAL LETHAL HYPOPHOSPHATASIA

This recessive condition is one of the causes of perinatal lethal short-limbed dwarfism, which includes type II osteogenesis imperfecta, thanatophoric dwarfism and achondrogenesis. The differential diagnosis (Table 7.6) depends on the radiological appearances. The skeleton shows grossly defective mineralisation, with large Y-shaped defects in the long bones as a result of patchy failure to mineralise (Fig. 7.11). The cranial bones are ossified only in their central portion. Prenatal diagnosis is possible by ultrasound and radiography, by measurement of alkaline phosphatase in amniotic fluid cells, and by genetic linkage studies.

INFANTILE HYPOPHOSPHATASIA

This condition occurs before the age of 6 months and is characterised by poor feeding, inadequate weight gain, and the development of rachitic-type deformities. Hypercalcaemia,

Table 7.6 Differential diagnosis of lethal hypophosphatasia

Condition	Features
Osteogenesis imperfecta (type II)	Multiple fractures, new mutation
Achondrogenesis	Absent ossification vertebral bodies and sacrum
Thanatophoric dwarfism	Short ribs, H-shaped vertebrae, short curved femora
Asphyxiating thoracic dystrophy	Small thorax, very short horizontal ribs
Chondroectodermal dysplasia	Very short limbs, polydactyly, hypoplastic nails

Note that the diagnosis in these conditions depends on accurate interpretation of whole-body radiographs.

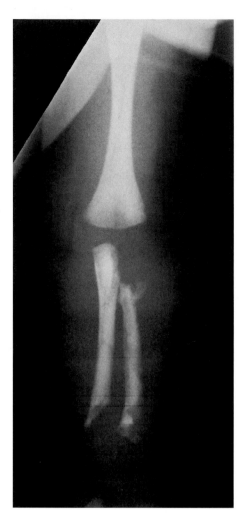

Figure 7.11 Lethal perinatal hypophosphatasia. There are large mineralisation defects in the metaphyses of the long bones.

and hypercalciuria with nephrocalcinosis and renal failure are also features. The sclerae may be blue. Premature fusion of the cranial sutures may produce papilloedema and proptosis; radiographs show irregular translucencies within the metaphyses.

CHILDHOOD HYPOPHOSPHATASIA

This is characterised by early loss of deciduous teeth (before 5 years of age), the incisors being shed first. Where the teeth, but not the skeleton, are affected the term 'odontohypophosphatasia' may be used.

There is short stature, delayed walking and a waddling gait, with rachitic deformities. Cranial synostosis may lead to proptosis and brain damage if cranial osteotomy/cranioplasty is not undertaken. As in intantile hypophosphatasia, radiographs may show tongues of radiotranslucency extending from the growth plate into the metaphyses.

ADULT HYPOPHOSPHATASIA

In the mild form of the disease, the adult develops pathological fractures across the shafts of the long bones. Chondrocalcinosis (possibly related to an excess of pyrophosphate) may occur. Such adults may represent the

heterozygous form of the alkaline phosphatase gene mutation.

MANAGEMENT

Treatment depends on the severity of the disease. In the infantile form, hypercalcaemia may be reduced by dietary restriction of calcium and glucocorticoid therapy. The transfusion of alkaline-phosphatase-enriched plasma from patients with Paget's disease has proved unsuccessful. Long bone fractures are probably best treated with intramedullary rods. For the severe infantile form, transplantation of bone marrow-derived stromal cells may be possible in the future.

THE OSTEOPETROSES (AND OSTEOSCLEROSES)

In a number of conditions, there is excessive formation of mineralised bone. In many (see Ch. 6) the cause is unknown, but as they are both familial and present in childhood, they probably have a metabolic cause. In marble bone disease (Albers–Schönberg disease), the cellular changes are partly understood.

MARBLE BONE DISEASE (OSTEOPETROSIS; ALBERS–SCHÖNBERG DISEASE)

Marble bone disease has a variable phenotype, with a severe, recessive infantile form and a dominantly inherited mild adult form (Key & Ries 1996), which has recently been further subdivided according to biochemistry and radiology. Rickets is occasionally associated with the disorder. Most advances in understanding and treatment have been made in the severe form. In this type, at least, there are variable defects in the osteoclasts: for instance, some may lack their ruffled border, whereas others have a defect in their carbonic anhydrase II enzyme. The causes of infantile recessive osteopetrosis are multiple, which helps to explain why some infants are cured by bone marrow transplantation containing compatible normal osteoclasts, whereas others are not.

Severe infantile osteopetrosis
The failure of resorption of calcified cartilage and bone leads to excessive amounts of bone because formation probably continues unabated. This produces two main effects: one is a lack of bone marrow with a progressive pancytopenia; the other is cranial nerve compression, with deafness, blindness and eventual death. Diagnosis is based on these clinical features, together with various deformities, including those of the face and skull and typical radiographic appearances. A number of radiographic changes are described: the two most important are an increase in bone density affecting the skull and long bones, and a lack of bone remodelling.

Mild osteopetrosis
The mild form of osteopetrosis is dominantly inherited and does not have the severe complications of the infantile form.

It may be asymptomatic and diagnosed only by radiographs. Characteristically, there is a variation between dense unmodelled bones and less dense bone with normal modelling. This leads to striation (osteopathia striata), which is transverse in the long bones and circumferential in the pelvis, and to the appearance of a 'bone within a bone' in the vertebrae and the small bones of the hands and feet (Fig. 7.12). The complications of mild osteopetrosis include an increased tendency to fracture, which affects the long bones and also the phalanges (the fractures are typically transverse, as are most pathological fractures), anaemia (especially at time of increased physiological requirements), and a tendency to develop mandibular osteomyelitis. Deafness, loss of vision, psychomotor delay, osteoarthritis and carpal tunnel syndrome have all been recorded. In some patients, there is an isolated increase in plasma acid phosphatase.

MANAGEMENT

This differs according to the severity of the disease. Bone marrow transplantation is a complex and dangerous procedure that should be reserved for life-threatening disease in infancy. Successful grafting of allogeneic bone marrow has produced excellent improvement in a few patients, but not all respond.

Other forms of treatment have included restriction of dietary calcium, high-dose calcitriol to encourage bone resorption, and high-dose glucocorticoids for malignant osteopetrosis with pancytopenia. Deterioration of vision and other signs of cranial nerve compression may benefit from surgery. In the rare form of osteopetrosis that is caused by carbonic anhydrase II deficiency, there is no evidence that correction of the systemic acidosis decreases bone density.

ECTOPIC MINERALISATION

Mineral may be deposited outside the skeleton, with or without the formation of ectopic bone matrix. Ectopic calcification (without bone formation) can be due to biochemical abnormalities, such as vascular calcification in hyperparathyroidism, basal ganglia calcification in hypoparathyroidism, and tumoral calcinosis in inherited hyperphosphataemia. Alternatively, it may occur with normal biochemistry in damaged tissues – for instance, in the dystrophic calcification in systemic sclerosis. In contrast, all the components of bone may be laid down in the soft tissues. This often occurs after spinal injury, after some forms of surgery, and in the ligaments of adults with inherited hypophosphataemia. Progressive ossification in muscles occurs in the rare inherited condition of myositis (or fibrodysplasia) ossificans progressiva. Despite its extreme rarity (fewer than 1 per million), this is an important disease to recognise.

FIBRODYSPLASIA (MYOSITIS) OSSIFICANS PROGRESSIVA

Ossification in the skeletal muscles progresses from infancy, leading to fixation of major joints and gross disability combined with typical skeletal abnormalities, particularly

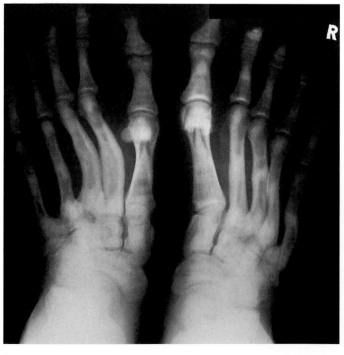

A

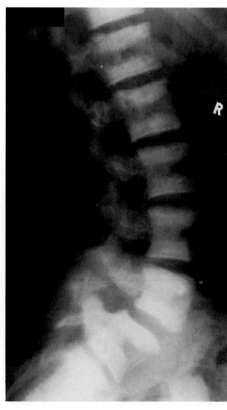

B

Figure 7.12 The skeleton in dominantly inherited mild osteopetrosis demonstrates variable bone density. **A** AP view of the feet, which shows evidence of previous fractures. **B** Lateral view of the lower thoracic and lumbar spine.

monophalangic big toes and fusion of the cervical spine (Smith 1998). The disease is most often regarded as the result of a dominant mutation, although good family studies are limited. Recent research suggests that the mutation leads to overexpression of one or more of the bone morphogenetic proteins (Shafritz et al 1996).

Ossification usually begins in the paraspinal muscles, and at least 50% of patients have had episodes of myositis by the age of 3 years. Typically, there is swelling, redness, and pain in the affected muscle, which feels very hard. At this acute stage, various diagnoses are considered, particularly infection and soft-tissue sarcoma. Biopsy shows oedematous muscle with many inflammatory cells and fragmented myofibrils. Later, true bone forms, associated with cartilage, and this subsequently mineralises. Clinically, the swelling subsides but is replaced by palpable masses of solid bone that fix the larger joints. The paraspinal muscles are involved early and the major muscles around the hip late, but all major striated muscles can become involved. Small muscles such as those of the hands and feet, smooth muscle, and cardiac muscle escape ossification. At birth and in infancy, the big toes show abnormal centres of ossification and are short and deviated laterally, so that a diagnosis of congenital hallux valgus may be made. Attempted surgical correction leads to ossification, and subsequent fusion of the epiphyses leads to a short and rigid big toe (Fig. 7.13).

In the cervical spine the vertebral bodies are small in comparison with the pedicles and spinous processes. There is progressive fusion of all these elements. At this stage, erroneous diagnoses such as Still's disease and the Klippel–Feil syndrome may be made.

Because episodes of myositis are quite unpredictable, it is difficult to give a prognosis. However, myositis is less frequent with increasing age, although it may follow injury at any time. There is no evidence that any current form of treatment influences the progress of the condition. Surgical removal of ectopic bone is followed by rapid recurrence and increasing disability. Corticosteroids have been used in an attempt to reduce the frequency and effects of myositis, and bisphosphonates to slow down mineralisation; neither produces a predictable result.

VITAMINS AND MINERALS

VITAMIN C DEFICIENCY

Scurvy occurs typically between the age of 6 and 9 months in infants fed exclusively on vitamin-C-deficient food. Vitamin C, ascorbic acid, is necessary for the hydroxylation of proline to hydroxyproline, a vital post-translational step in the synthesis of collagen. In its absence, the under-hydroxylated collagen is not correctly exported from the cell.

The onset of scurvy may be precipitated by an acute infection. Perifollicular petechial haemorrhage in the skin may be the earliest sign, and peridontal haemorrhage also occurs. The scorbutic infant is irritable, anorexic, and fails to gain weight. The main skeletal problems are subperiosteal haemorrhage, with characteristic epiphyseal and metaphyseal changes. The limbs are tender and painful and the infant adopts a frog position. The subperiosteal lesions produce painful swellings along the shafts of the long bones, radiological changes being most marked where growth is rapid – at the knees, the wrists and the costochondral junctions. There is a loss of bone density, with a thin cortex and a ground-glass appearance of the cancellous bone. The outline of the epiphyses is accentuated to give a ringed appearance, and there is a dense line with spurs at the ends of the metaphyses. Subperiosteal haemorrhages become radiologically more obvious after treatment is commenced. The changes in the metaphyses resemble those of non-accidental injury (see Ch. 33). Treatment is with vitamin C.

VITAMIN A EXCESS

Retinoic acid and its derivatives have profound effects on osteoblastic function. Two main skeletal abnormalities result from an excess of vitamin A: cortical hyperostosis, and ectopic ossification of the ligaments. In children, prolonged overdose with vitamin A causes pain and tenderness in the long bones and localised swelling. The cortical density of the long bones is increased, but the bones are abnormally fragile and liable to fracture. In adults, the prolonged use of retinoic acid derivatives for skin disease such as psoriasis and ichthyosis can lead to calcification of the ligaments, especially around the spine, with new bone formation, stiffness and reduced mobility.

VITAMIN D TOXICITY

This may occur from therapeutic overdosage in inherited hypophosphataemia. In addition to the features of hypercalcaemia (nocturia, polyuria, thirst, constipation, anorexia and vomiting), nephrocalcinosis and renal failure can develop. As in idiopathic hypercalcaemia (below), there are deposits of dense bone at the metaphyses of the long bones, and increased density of the spine, ribs and pelvis.

IDIOPATHIC HYPERCALCAEMIA

The condition known as idiopathic hypercalaemia of infancy (the elfin face syndrome; the Williams' syndrome) has been attributed to an excess of vitamin D, although doubt exists as to its true cause. Mild and severe types are described. In the severe type, symptomatic hypercalcaemia is associated with supravalvular aortic stenosis, a characteristic face with low-set ears, and mental impairment. Further study of this disorder suggests an abnormal regulation of 25(OH)D, concentrations of which may be increased when the patient is hypercalcaemic. Radiographs of the long bones show increased metaphyseal density. Recent work has localised a mutation to the elastin gene (Langman 1996).

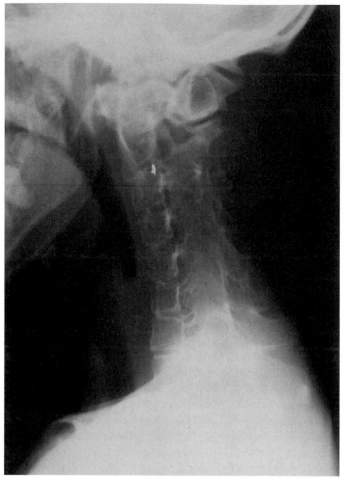

A

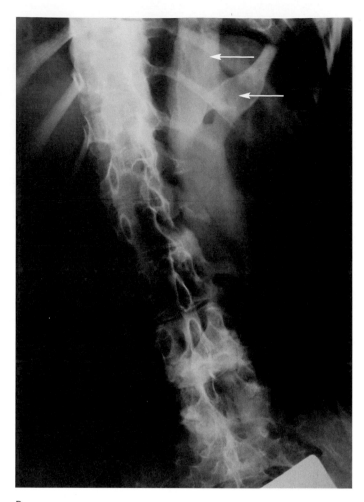

B

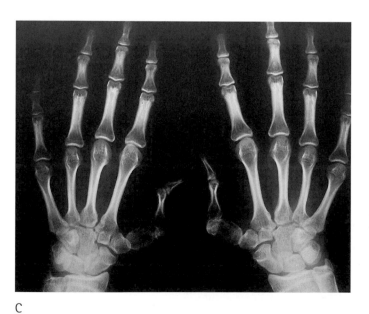

C

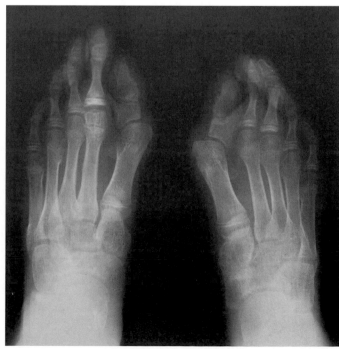

D

Figure 7.13 Fibrodysplasia ossificans progressiva. **A** Neck: abnormal vertebrae with fusion. **B** Ectopic ossification: radiograph with bars of ectopic bone (arrows). **C** Hands: short abnormal thumbs. **D** Toes: the typical appearance of shortened (valgus) big toes.

LEAD POISONING

Increased radiographic density of the metaphyses in children may be produced by an excess of lead, phosphorus, mercury or bismuth (Nordin 1984). The extent of environmental lead poisoning is not clear, but established causes include the ingestion of lead-containing paint or of water stored in lead pipes, and exposure to exhaust fumes. Lead has effects upon the gastrointestinal, neuromuscular and haematological systems, causing constipation, myopathy, and anaemia, with characteristic punctuate basophilia. Radiographs may demonstrate deposits in the gastrointestinal tract and widening of the sutures of the skull as a result of increased intracranial pressure. However, the most characteristic feature is the lead line – a dense metaphyseal band of varying thickness seen after about 1 month of chronic lead poisoning. Repeated lead lines may form with variations in lead exposure and during the treatment of lead poisoning with chelating agents.

FLUOROSIS

The skeletal effects of fluoride are most often seen in adults treated for osteoporosis with sodium fluoride. The fluoride ion stimulates the osteoblasts to produce new bone, although this is woven rather than lamellar and, unless additional calcium is given, is poorly mineralised. Fluoride is not given therapeutically to increase bone density in children, except possibly for osteogenesis imperfecta, but low concentrations are recommended to prevent dental caries.

Fluoride poisoning is uncommon in Western societies, but may be produced by inhalation of fluoride vapour in the cryolith industry, by the ingestion of vegetables contaminated with fluorine-containing dust, and from a high concentration in the drinking water. Endemic fluorosis is well described in India.

The changes in the teeth affect the permanent dentition, mainly the incisors, and are seen only if the high fluoride intake begins before the age of 8 years. The teeth are arranged irregularly and the enamel is translucent with patchy opaque areas. The bones are dense but more fragile than normal, the cortex is thick and the metaphyses are widened, with an irregular edge. The skull is thick and dense, as are the vertebral bodies. Calcium is deposited in the spinal ligaments and at the insertions of tendons into the long bones. The skeletal signs of fluorosis increase with age, and the calcification in the spine can lead to spinal and nerve root compression.

ALUMINIUM EXCESS

An excess of aluminium leads to a form of osteodystrophy in patients maintained on haemodialysis. The aluminium, derived from the dialysis fluid itself or from tap water, accumulates in the skeleton, where it is deposited at the calcification front. Histologically, there is a failure of normal osteoblast function and of mineralisation, producing an aplastic bone disease that is resistant to treatment with vitamin D. Aluminium osteodystrophy, 'dialysis bone disease', also causes bone pain and fracture. Another feature of the skeleton of patients maintained on prolonged dialysis is the deposition of amyloid.

COPPER DEFICIENCY

Copper is essential for the function of many enzymes, particularly amino acid oxidases, and for the hydroxylation of proline and lysine residues. The main skeletal effect of copper deficiency probably arises from its effect on collagen synthesis. Acquired deficiency of copper occurs in premature or low-birthweight babies maintained on parenteral nutrition, although it may occur as a transient phenomenon in otherwise normal infants or in protein-energy malnutrition. The effects of copper deficiency on the skeleton are similar to those of scurvy; in the differential diagnosis, non-accidental injury and the brittle bone syndrome should be excluded.

Menkes' syndrome is an inherited disorder of copper metabolism that is closely related to the occipital horn syndrome (now called Ehlers–Danlos syndrome IX). In both, the inheritance is X-linked. In Menkes' syndrome, the face and hair (steely hair) are abnormal. Progressive cerebral degeneration, hypopigmentation, arterial rupture and thrombosis, and bone changes occur. In the skeleton, there is osteoporosis, and widening of the flared metaphyses with spiky protrusion. Rib fractures and Wormian bones occur. Again, non-accidental injury and osteogenesis imperfecta must be excluded.

The occipital horn syndrome is so named because of the palpable protrusions of bone from the occiput. Other features include inguinal herniae, skin and joint laxity, and widespread arterial tortuosity.

POLYOSTOTIC FIBROUS DYSPLASIA

Fibrous dysplasia is a relatively common disorder of bone. Typically, isolated lesions are found in the long bones, ribs or skull. They may be first discovered incidentally, or as a result of a pathological fracture, for instance in the femoral neck. The rarer polyostotic form may be associated with ipsilateral pigmentation and endocrine abnormalities – particularly sexual precocity in girls (McCune Albright syndrome). Cushing's syndrome, thyrotoxicosis and hypertension are also described.

The skeletal lesions are often unilateral and widespread. Cranio-facial fibrous dysplasia causes severe deformity, which can sometimes be corrected surgically, whereas advanced fibrous dysplasia involving the proximal femur leads to 'shepherd's crook' deformities, which may be bilateral. Rarely, polyostotic fibrous dysplasia is associated with hypophosphataemic osteomalacia. It is now known (Weinstein 1996) that the cause of fibrous dysplasia (both monostotic and polyostotic) is an activating mutation in the G protein involved in cell signalling. The severity of the condition depends on the proportion of cells affected (mosaicism). The skeletal lesions may respond to an amino-bisphosphonate (Weinstein 1997).

SUMMARY

The number of metabolic and endocrine disorders known to affect the skeleton is increasing now that disorders previously thought of as skeletal oddities are found to have a metabolic basis. With the definition of new syndromes and the increased understanding of rarities, the management of metabolic bone disease in children is more than ever a team effort, and should involve a physician and geneticist in addition to the orthopaedic surgeon.

REFERENCES

Bilezikian J P, Raisz L G, Rodan G A (eds) 1996 Principles of bone biology. Academic Press, San Diego

Brown E M, Harris H W, Vassilev P M, Hebert S C 1996 The biology of the extracellular Ca^{2+}-sensing receptor. In: Bilezikian J, Raisz L G, Rodan G A (eds) Principles of bone biology. Academic Press, San Diego, pp 243–262

Brumsen C, Hamdy N A T, Papapoulos S E 1997 Long-term effects of bisphosphonates on the growing skeleton. Medicine 76: 266–283

Gahl W A, Renlund M, Thoene J G 1989 Lyososomal transport disorders. In: Scriver C R, Beaudet A L, Sly W S, Valle D (eds) The metabolic basis of inherited disease, 6th edn. McGraw Hill, New York, pp 2619–2647

Glorieux F H 1996 Hypophosphatemia: vitamin D resistant rickets. In: Favus M J (ed) Primer on the metabolic bone diseases and disorders of mineral metabolism, 3rd edn. Lippincott-Raven, Philadelphia, pp 316–319

Gong Y, Vikkula M, Boon L et al 1996 Osteoporosis-pseudoglioma syndrome, a disorder affecting skeletal strength and vision is assigned to chromosome region 11q12–13 American Journal of Human Genetics 59: 146–151

Key L L, Ries W L 1996 Osteopetrosis. In: Bilezikian J, Raisz L G, Rodan G A (eds) Principles of bone biology. Academic Press, San Diego, pp 941–950

Langman C B 1996 Hypercalcemic syndromes in infants and children. In: Favus M J (ed) Primer on the metabolic bone diseases and disorders of mineral metabolism, 3rd edn. Lippincott-Raven, Philadelphia pp 209–212

Marcus R, Feldman D, Kelsey J 1996 Osteoporosis, Ist edn. Academic Press, San Diego

Nordin B E C 1984 Metabolic bone and stone disease, 2nd edn. Churchill Livingstone, Edinburgh

Shafritz A B, Shore E M, Gannon F H et al 1996 Overexpression of an osteogenic morphogen in fibrodysplasia ossificans progressiva. New England Journal of Medicine 335: 555–561

Smith R 1979 Biochemical disorders of the skeleton. Butterworths, London

Smith R 1990 Asian rickets and osteomalacia. Quarterly Journal of Medicine 76: 899–901

Smith R 1995 Idiopathic juvenile osteoporosis; experience of twenty-one patients. British Journal of Rheumatology 34: 68–77

Smith R 1996 Disorders of the skeleton. In: Weatherall D J, Ledingham J G G, Warrell D A (eds). Oxford textbook of Medicine, 3rd edn. Oxford University Press, Oxford, pp 3053–3097

Smith R 1998 Fibrodysplasia (myositis) ossificans progressiva. Clinical lessons from a rare disease. Clinical Orthopaedics and Related Research 346: 7–14

Thakker R V, O'Riordan J L H 1988 Inherited forms of rickets and osteomalacia. Ballière's Clinical Endocrinology and Metabolism 2: 157–191

Weinstein L S 1996 Other skeletal diseases resulting from G protein defects – fibrous dysplasia and McCune Albright syndrome. In: Bilezikian J, Raisz L G, Rodan G A (eds) Principles of bone biology. Academic Press, San Diego, pp 877–887

Weinstein R S 1997 Long-term aminobisphosphonate treatment of fibrous dysplasia: spectacular increase in bone density. Journal of Bone and Mineral Research 12: 1314–1315

Whyte M P 1996 Hypophosphatasia: nature's window on alkaline phosphatase function in man. In: Bilezikian J, Raisz L G, Rodan G A (eds) Principles of bone biology. Academic Press, San Diego, pp 951–968

Chapter 8

Blood disorders and AIDS

C. A. Ludlam and J. Jellis

INTRODUCTION

Disorders of either the haemostatic system or the bone marrow may lead to impaired musculoskeletal development. Haemostatic diatheses are of two main types:

1. Those affecting the plasma coagulation factors (e.g. haemophilia), leading predominantly to joint and muscle haemorrhage.
2. Disorders of platelets and von Willebrand factor, in which the bleeding is usually from mucosal surfaces (e.g. epistaxis, gastrointestinal haemorrhage and menorrhagia).

Permanent damage may follow joint and muscle bleeds, particularly if these are recurrent at the same site or if treatment is delayed (Duthie 1997, Madhok 1997). In contrast, musculoskeletal changes are rare in individuals with platelet disorders and von Willebrand disease.

In congenital disorders of haemopoiesis, hypertrophy of the bone marrow occurs; it is particularly marked in the thalassaemias, but to a lesser extent it accompanies haemoglobinopathies such as sickle-cell disease. Increased erythropoiesis leads to hypertrophy and deformity of the surrounding bone, and in sickle-cell disease bone infarction occurs. Acute lymphatic leukaemia in childhood infiltrates the marrow, but it is uncommon for this to lead to orthopaedic complications. However, back pain from vertebral involvement, a swollen joint, or a limp should alert the orthopaedic surgeon to this possibility, particularly if the child is systemically ill. Occasionally, localised malignant deposits of other tumours cause osteolytic lesions that may cause pathological fracture.

HAEMOPHILIA

Congenital deficiencies of the plasma coagulation factors VIII and IX result in haemophilia A and B respectively. As genes for both these proteins are on the X chromosome, the diseases are inherited as sex-linked disorders; consequently, in the majority of instances, only males are clinically affected. Haemophilia A and B are clinically indistinguishable (Rizza 1997). Approximately one-third of cases arise 'sporadically', without a family history. A variety of gene defects, including point mutations or deletions, result in the synthesis of a coagulant protein with decreased activity. As the same genetic defect is present in all individuals within a family, the affected individuals have haemophilia with the same degree of severity.

The propensity to haemorrhage depends upon the level of coagulant protein in the plasma (Table 8.1). Individuals with severe haemophilia with less than 2% factor VIII activity usually have frequent, apparently spontaneous joint bleeds, whereas those with levels of 2–10% have moderate disease and bleed significantly following minor trauma; those with more than 10% factor VIII/IX only haemorrhage excessively after trauma or surgery.

Factor VIII is synthesised principally in the liver. In the plasma it is bound to the carrier protein von Willebrand factor. Its plasma half-life is approximately 12 hours. The basal concentration can be increased in response to a variety of stimuli, such as stress and exercise. Haemophilia B is caused by a deficiency of factor IX. This protein is also synthesised in the liver, but has a longer half-life of approximately 18 hours.

In children with severe haemophilia, bleeding is uncommon until the age of approximately 6 months, when excessive bruising may be seen as the baby becomes more active. These infants may initially be assumed to be victims of non-accidental injury or child abuse (see Ch. 36) and it is important that, in all instances in which this diagnosis is suspected, appropriate tests of the haemostatic system are performed at an early stage of investigation. An earlier diagnosis may be made if the baby is circumcised, as prolonged haemorrhage will almost inevitably occur. Diagnosis can be made at birth by measuring the factor VIII concentration, and it is appropriate to do so if the mother is known to have a high probability of being a carrier.

Haemarthrosis results in a distressed infant who is resistant to all attempts at comforting. An arm or leg is held rigidly and the elbow or knee may be swollen. As children become older, they realise a bleed is starting as they experience a characteristic discomfort that precedes joint swelling. If treatment is not given at this early stage, stiffness and severe pain ensue and the joint becomes markedly warm and swollen. It is held in partial flexion by

Table 8.1 Classification of severity of haemophilia	
Factor VIII/IX level	Clinical manifestation
Severe (<2%)	Frequent, 'spontaneous' bleeds
Moderate (2–10%)	Bleeds following minor trauma
Mild (>10%)	Only bleed after surgery or trauma

For surgery in all patients it is necessary to increase the factor VIII/IX level to greater than 50% of normal.

surrounding muscle spasm and any attempt at movement greatly exacerbates the pain. After relatively few haemarthroses, joint changes become established. The synovium hypertrophies and forms a pannus over the articular cartilage; its increased vascularity and size predispose to further haemorrhage. Cartilage is eroded both by the hypertrophied synovium and by leucocyte enzymes liberated from blood within the joint cavity (Fig. 8.1). During resolution of an acute haemarthrosis, iron accumulates in synovial macrophages, which become laden with haemosiderin. Subchondral haemorrhage and bleeds into the matrix further weaken the bone. Hyperaemia of the joint ensues, causing bone overgrowth. Osteoporosis and disuse atrophy of the surrounding muscles develop, and joint instability and deformity progress (Arnold & Hilgartner 1977).

Recurrent haemarthroses result in fibrosis in the joint capsule and surrounding muscles. This, with the bony changes, leads to permanent loss of joint movement. Fixed flexion deformities of the knee and hip result in apparent shortening of the leg and the resultant compensatory pelvic tilt may induce later spinal symptoms. Thus haemophilic arthropathy of the lower limbs may produce compensatory

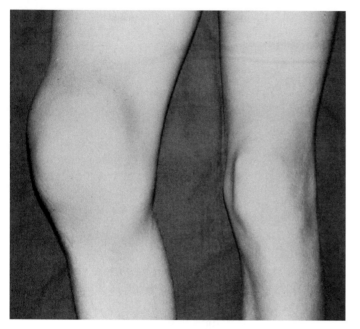

A

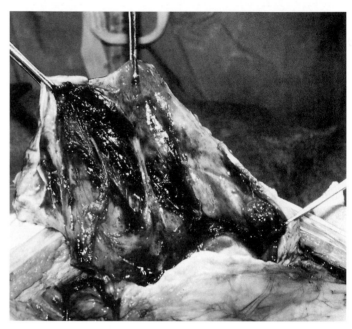

B

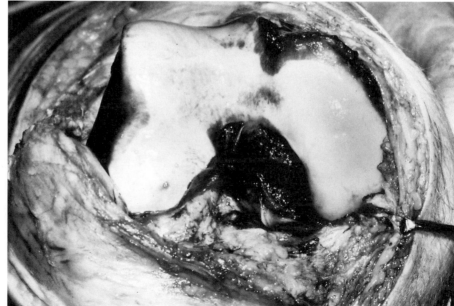

C

Figure 8.1 The severe synovitis provoked by repeated haemarthroses leads to erosion of the cartilage.

skeletal deformities remote from the sites of haemarthroses.

The incidence and sites of haemarthroses vary with age. Bleeding frequency is greater in children than in adults, probably because of greater physical activity and joint laxity early in life. An individual joint particularly prone to recurrent haemarthroses is termed a 'target' joint; it is imperative that effective therapeutic measures are initiated to prevent a rapid decline in its function.

The knee is the most common site of haemarthrosis (Fig. 8.2). Ridging of the tibial condyles and posterior subluxation may prevent full extension. Wasting of the quadriceps group, particularly vastus medialis, becomes obvious. If knee bleeds are not treated early and promptly in childhood, by mid-adult life ankylosis of the knee in partial flexion is frequently observed. It is important in the long term to minimise the development of fixed flexion deformity by prompt treatment of bleeds, splinting, and physiotherapy if necessary. Once fixed flexion is greater than 20°, walking becomes extremely difficult and the joint quickly flexes further. This, along with osteoarthritis of the hips and ankles, inevitably causes severe physical disability.

The elbow is the next most commonly affected joint, particularly on the non-dominant side (Högh et al 1987). Recurrent bleeds lead to loss of flexion and extension, and supination is particularly impaired as a result of enlarge-ment of the radial head. Typical features of ulnar neuritis may develop if the nerve is trapped as it passes behind the medial epicondyle.

Acute bleeds into the hip joint cause pain and spasm of the surrounding muscles, limiting all movement. Such bleeds must be distinguished from an ilio-psoas haematoma or acute appendicitis. Relatively few acute episodes of haemarthroses may initiate chronic progressive degenerative arthropathy, possibly because the femoral head readily undergoes ischaemic necrosis. It is therefore particularly important to treat promptly and aggressively all acute bleeds into the hip joint.

As in other joints, acute haemarthrosis in the shoulder leads to loss of articular cartilage and 'squaring' of the proximal humeral epiphysis (Petterson et al 1980). Marked loss of abduction and rotation can be compensated for by movement of the scapula, provided that the gleno-humeral joint adopts a position of function.

Recurrent ankle bleeds are a characteristic problem in young children. These result in ankle and subtalar arthropathy. The talus has a particularly vulnerable blood supply, which can become impeded by the pressure of a haemarthrosis. This leads to avascular necrosis and collapse of the talar dome (Macnicol & Ludlam 1999). Early changes in joint pathology may be discernible by MRI before any

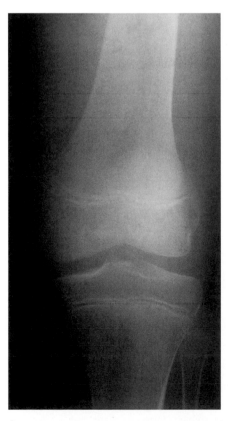
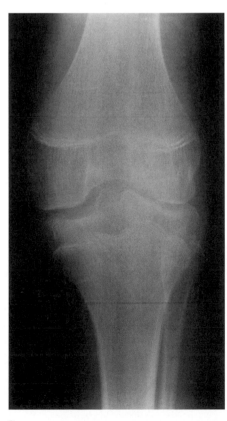
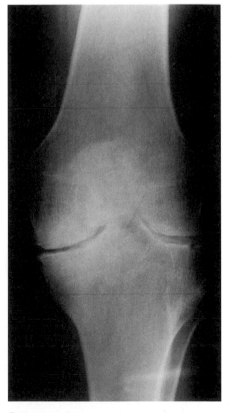

A   B   C

Figure 8.2 Progressive changes of left knee haemophilic arthropathy in a young person aged 11 years (A), 14 years (B) and 17 years (C).

changes become visible on plain X-ray (Fig. 8.3). In later life, loss of ankle joint movement is rarely a handicap, but the pain of the chronic arthropathy can be very disabling. Equinus should be controlled by splintage, and an arthrodesis is occasionally indicated.

Muscle haematomas are less common than haemarthroses, but are potentially very serious and require early vigorous treatment with factor VIII or IX concentrate. Haemorrhage dissects between the muscle planes, producing ischaemia, which may lead to necrosis and subsequent fibrosis. If the muscle is contained within an inflexible, tough sheath, such as the gastrocnemius and soleus, and haemorrhage continues unabated, compartment pressure increases to the point when the arterial supply is occluded, leading to further muscle ischaemia and subsequent necrosis. The resultant fibrosis causes shortening and, in the case of the calf muscle, equinus deformity. In the forearm, a similar process will lead to contracture of the flexor muscles – Volkmann's ischaemic contracture.

A bleed into the ilio-psoas muscle may present with pain in the lower abdomen, groin, thigh or knee. The hip is flexed in an attempt to relieve the tension in the muscle. Entrapment of the femoral nerve, by pressure from the enlarged haematoma as it passes under the inguinal ligament, causes paraesthesiae over the thigh and inner calf and gross weakness of the quadriceps. The ipsilateral knee jerk may be depressed.

Pseudotumours are rarely seen nowadays, because patients receive early and effective treatment with factor VIII or IX concentrate. Previously, these tumours arose particularly in the thigh and pelvis as a result of inadequately treated haematomas into which chronic oozing continued unabated. The haematoma, surrounded by a fibrous capsule, gradually expands and then may erode adjacent structures, including bone, causing pathological fractures. Infection may supervene and the ensuing septicaemia can be fatal. Treatment with long-term factor VIII/IX replacement therapy and antibiotics prevents the progression of these cysts and their later surgical excision may be indicated in some instances.

Haemorrhage may also occur at other sites. Excessive bleeding during dental extraction and all such procedures must be prevented by appropriate haemostatic cover. Haemorrhage may occur into the central nervous system, and if not promptly treated is often fatal. Haematuria was previously a common symptom, but is now rarely seen. Bleeding is believed to arise from the renal parenchyma, but can be from bladder lesions. When peptic ulcers were more common, upper gastrointestinal bleeding was a major source of morbidity and mortality. With the use of H_2-antagonists and the decline in the prevalence of ulcers, this is now much less of a problem. However, increasing numbers of patients are developing hepatic cirrhosis as a result of hepatitis C-induced progressive liver disease, and the prevalence of

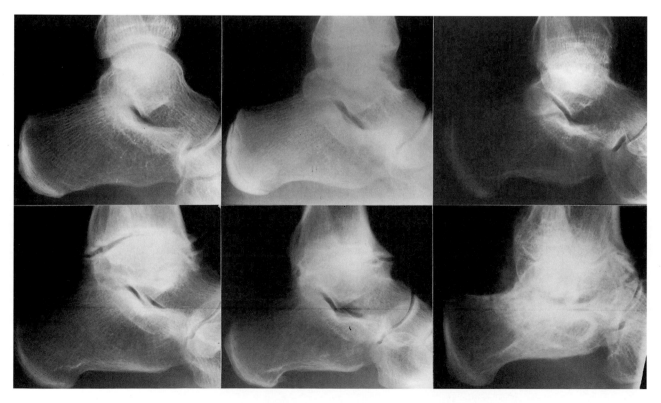

Figure 8.3 The stages of talar body collapse in late adolescence are shown from top left to bottom right. Once the contour of the dome has flattened and anterior ankle joint impingement is present, the joint is irreversibly stiffened.

associated oesophageal varices is increasing. Haemorrhage from these is liable to be catastrophic. At the distal bowel, fresh bleeding from haemorrhoids and fissures is commonly reported by haemophiliacs and should be treated by operation if persistent.

MANAGEMENT OF HAEMOPHILIA

Prophylactic factor VIII/IX therapy

For children with severe haemophilia, optimal therapy is to give injections of factor VIII/IX concentrate to prevent bleeds. This prophylactic treatment prevents most haemorrhages and allows the child to lead a nearly normal life, without the worry and disruption that bleeds cause. Furthermore, by preventing most haemarthroses, this strategy enables the child to grow into adulthood with the prospect of normal joints and a life unaffected by severe arthritis. As the half-life of factor VIII is only 12 hours, injections need to be given on alternate days, whereas factor IX, because of its longer half-life of 18 hours, need be given only twice weekly (Berntorp 1996).

If a haemophiliac patient who is not receiving regular prophylaxis suffers recurrent bleeds into a single joint – often termed a 'target' joint – a short period of prophylaxis for several weeks or months, along with physiotherapy, reduces the propensity to bleed. Prophylaxis breaks the vicious circle of bleeds and subsequent muscle atrophy, which otherwise leads to further joint deformity and recurrent haemarthroses.

Treatment of acute haemorrhage

Early treatment of acute haemarthroses with intravenous factor VIII/IX concentrate delays the onset of chronic, crippling haemophilic arthropathy. The child should be taught to report when he considers a bleed has started and his parents should ensure he receives treatment quickly. With children younger than about 3 years, parents usually find it difficult to give intravenous therapy. Once a child reaches school age, it is often possible for the parents to give treatment at home (Fig. 8.4). This is the best arrangement, because there is less delay than when the child is brought to hospital.

The amount of factor VIII required to be infused depends upon the size of the child and the severity of the bleed. Spontaneous haemarthroses require less treatment than those after trauma. If there is delay before treatment is given, larger doses for a more prolonged period may be necessary. If a small spontaneous haemarthrosis is treated promptly, a single infusion of concentrate is sufficient to stop bleeding and allow restitution of normal joint function. If the haemorrhage is more severe, injections may need to be given twice daily for several days. Provided there is no doubt about the diagnosis of a haemarthrosis, aspiration of the joint is not advisable unless an HIV-positive haemophiliac patient has a fever, with an 'atypical' joint swelling suggestive of septic arthritis.

If the haemarthrosis is other than minor, the joint should

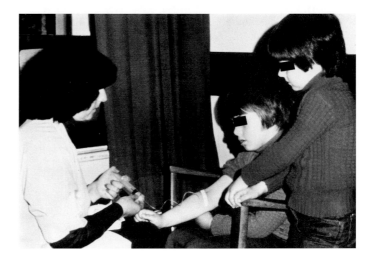

Figure 8.4 Home therapy with factor VIII/IX should eventually prove possible.

be rested. With a severe haemarthrosis, this can be aided by means of a lightweight polypropylene splint (Fig. 8.5). The application of icepacks is found helpful by some patients.

Minor bleeds treated early in children usually do not require rest or subsequent physiotherapy. However, if a child has a major haemarthrosis, gentle physiotherapy should be initiated once the bleeding has stopped. It may be necessary to continue factor VIII/IX therapy at a low dose for several weeks, in order to prevent further bleeding during the phases of mobilisation and more intense physiotherapy.

In patients with mild haemophilia, it may be appropriate to offer treatment with desmopressin. This vasopressin analogue increases factor VIII concentrations three- to fourfold above the basal level after intravenous infusion. It is therefore sometimes useful for patients with relatively minor bleeds or to cover surgical procedures, such as dental extraction or lymph node biopsy. The advantage of using

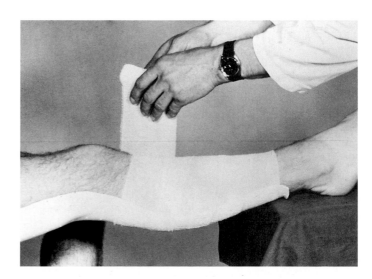

Figure 8.5 Polypropylene splintage of the knee affected by a bleed.

desmopressin, as opposed to factor VIII concentrate, is that it avoids exposing the patient to a pooled plasma product and the potentially serious adverse effects described below and summarised in Table 8.2.

Table 8.2 Major complications of haemophilia treatment
Antifactor VIII antibodies
Virus transmission
Human immunodeficiency virus
Hepatitis viruses B, C and D
Parvovirus
HIV infection and AIDS
Hepatitis, cirrhosis, liver failure and hepatocellular carcinoma

Complications of factor VIII/IX concentrates

The tragedy of human immunodeficiency virus (HIV) transmission by factor VIII/IX concentrate is well known. Other viruses, however, have also been transmitted by pooled blood products. All patients should be vaccinated to prevent infection with hepatitis A and B viruses. At present there is no vaccine against the hepatitis C virus, which appears to cause the majority of cases of chronic hepatitis. It is now believed that many individuals infected with this virus will develop chronic active hepatitis and about 25–30% will develop cirrhosis with its attendant complications – oesophageal varices, liver failure, and hepatocellular carcinoma (Lee 1996).

Before 1985, HIV transmission by factor VIII/IX concentrates was common, particularly in individuals with haemophilia A. In the UK, approximately 60% of all patients with severe haemophilia A and 6% of those with haemophilia B became infected. The risk of HIV transmission is now minimal because high-risk donors are asked not to give blood. In addition, each individual unit is screened for HIV antibodies, and finally the product is treated during manufacture either by solvent/detergent or by heating to inactivate viruses. With the current virucidal processes, introduced in the mid 1980s, the risk of transmission of hepatitis C virus (HCV) is now remote. Provided a child has only received virally inactivated concentrates, he should not become infected with HIV or HCV. These infections are therefore not found in children younger than 10 years. However, if a child has received an inadequately virally inactivated concentrate, or a fresh blood product such as cryoprecipitate, then there is a chance of HIV or HCV infection. Recombinant factors VIII and IX are free from the risk of HIV and HCV.

The transfusion of factor VIII concentrate leads to the development of antibodies to factor VIII in 10–30% of patients with severe haemophilia. When this occurs, the infused factor VIII is rapidly neutralised and does not readily stop haemorrhage. It is therefore much more difficult to give clinically effective therapy. The antibody titre can be quantified and, if it is low, it is often possible to stop bleeding by transfusing large doses of factor VIII concentrate. If the antibody titre is high, alternative therapy with other blood products (activated factor IX concentrates, porcine factor VIII or recombinant factor VIIa) may be effective. In haemophilia B, antibodies to factor IX are rare.

Surgery in haemophiliac patients

Provided a patient does not have an anti-factor VIII/IX inhibitor, surgery can be safely undertaken (Houghton & Duthie 1978). Immediately before operation, concentrate is infused to bring the level to 100% and repeated infusions are given postoperatively. Initially, it is necessary to keep the factor VIII level about 50%, but this can be gradually reduced during the second and third weeks after surgery. After major orthopaedic surgery, gentle mobilisation can begin the day after operation, but treatment with factor VIII/IX should continue for approximately 2–3 weeks.

Synovectomy is useful in young haemophiliac patients with a target joint, when there is significant synovitis. The principal aim is to reduce the frequency of bleeding, but this is often achieved at the expense of some reduction in the range of joint movement.

If malalignment of the knee joint causes recurrent bleeds or painful arthritis, a proximal tibial osteotomy is occasionally indicated. Such a procedure may improve gait and reduce pain and the frequency of haemarthoses. In the adult, total joint replacement and arthrodesis are indicated when arthropathic pain and stiffening are severe.

Haemophilia centres

Within the UK, all haemophiliac individuals are registered at haemophilia centres, which offer comprehensive care from haematologists, orthopaedic and dental surgeons, specialist physiotherapists, nurses and social workers. In addition to treating the acute and chronic haemorrhagic problems, the haemophilia team is able to offer parental support, and advise nurseries, schools and prospective employers. Genetic counselling of potential carriers is important, particularly now that molecular genetic techniques are available for antenatal diagnosis.

THALASSAEMIAS

In the thalassaemias, overactivity of the marrow as a result of ineffective erythropoiesis and haemolysis results in widening of the medullary cavity and thinning of cortical bone. The skull radiograph shows widening of the diploic space, giving the typical 'hair-on-end' appearance. Overgrowth of the maxillary and temporal bones reduces the volume of the sinuses. The thickened cranium and prominent cheek bones, depressed nasal bridge and overgrowth of the maxillae produce a distinctive appearance. Cortical thinning may predispose to pathological fractures of long bones.

Management consists of regular red cell transfusions, to ensure that the haemoglobin concentration remains relatively normal. This reduces erythropoietic activity and prevents the characteristic skeletal deformities. Furthermore, because these children have nearly normal haemoglobin values, their growth approaches that of their peers, in marked contrast to the stunted appearance seen in those given only occasional transfusions. To reduce the risk of iron overload, such patients require regular iron chelation therapy with desferrioxamine.

HAEMOGLOBINOPATHIES

In many countries of sub-Saharan Africa, up to 25% of the population carry the sickle-cell gene. From unions of these individuals, children are born with sickle-cell disease (HbSS) and comprise about 1% of the indigenous paediatric population. Affected children have chronic haemolytic anaemia, with haemoglobin concentrations between 5 and 8 g/dl. They may suffer episodes of acute haemolysis – sickle-cell crises – in which they become jaundiced and the haemoglobin concentration decreases further. In West Africa, haemoglobin C disease (HbSC) and thalassaemia complicate the situation, but the effects are generally milder than the homozygous HbSS state. The child with sickle-cell disease has between 75% and 100% of the abnormal haemoglobin which, in heterozygous (HbAS) individuals, comprises less than 50% of their total haemoglobin. Sickling tests may be positive in both homozygous and heterozygous individuals, but the homozygous state can be distinguished by haemoglobin electrophoresis; furthermore, heterozygous children do not suffer the clinical manifestations of sickle-cell disease.

Children with sickle-cell disease are usually small for their age, and thin (Fig. 8.6). Frontal and parietal bossing of the skull is typical, and the fingers are short (Fig. 8.7). Clinical anaemia and intermittent jaundice are usually obvious. The abdomen is typically protuberant with hepatosplenomegaly.

Children with sickle-cell disease are prone to bacterial infections, the clinical effects being very similar to those with advanced HIV infection. They are prone to bone and joint infections, and commonly have otitis media. Acute, subacute and chronic osteomyelitis, septic arthritis, aseptic bone infarction and Perthes' disease are the usual presentations to the orthopaedic surgeon and it may be difficult to differentiate between them. During a sickling (haemolytic) crisis, the child will have fever, tachypnoea, bone pains and tenderness, joint pains and, possibly, abdominal pain and peritonism. An attack of malaria gives a similar picture and may, indeed, precipitate a crisis. Bone pain and tenderness, or joint pain and effusion, may be either aseptic as a result of infarction, or septic from septicaemia. Where facilities exist, blood cultures and cultures of synovial fluid or from needle aspirates from painful bones should be obtained before antibiotic treatment is commenced. If a joint is found to contain pus, arthrotomy and lavage are indicated. Similarly, any subperiosteal collections of pus should be drained. Every precaution should be taken, however, to ensure that anaesthesia will be safe; repeated aspirations may be necessary if doubt exists.

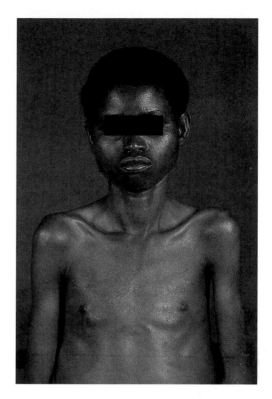

Figure 8.6 Patient with sickle-cell disease, showing slight jaundice and frontal bossing of the skull.

Hypoxia and acidosis cause the abnormal haemoglobin of sickle-cell disease to form liquid crystals that distort the erythrocytes, rendering them fragile and encouraging clumping. Haemolysis, blockage of small vessels and infarction are the result. Preoperative determination of haemoglobin concentrations and the further investigation of anaemic patients is essential to avoid disasters of rapid circulatory collapse and death, which may occur within a few hours of surgery. Before surgery, the haemoglobin concentration should be increased to as near to 8 g/dl as possible. Malaria prophylaxis and folic acid are routinely given. In an emergency situation, or immediately before major surgery, exchange transfusion or the transfusion of

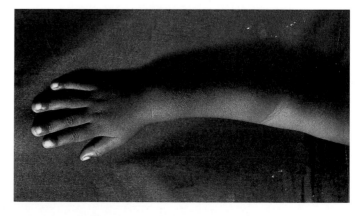

Figure 8.7 The short stubby fingers of a patient with sickle-cell disease. There is also osteomyelitis of the radius.

packed cells should be considered. During induction and maintenance of anaesthesia, hypoxia and dehydration must be avoided. After operation, oxygen should be given for at least 24 hours and the arterial pO_2 monitored by pulse oximetry. Drugs that diminish respiratory drive (such as a narcotic analgesic) should be given with great caution or avoided. Regional analgesia should be used, if practicable.

The use of tourniquets in patients with sickle-cell disease remains controversial. A bloodless field may shorten surgery, make it safer and minimise blood loss; these are all important factors, especially if no blood is available for transfusion. Conversely, theoretically, any blood that remains in the limb distal to a tourniquet will sickle and the hypoxia and acidosis that are present in a limb when the tourniquet is deflated could have deleterious effects. We have carefully monitored systemic pO_2, using pulse oximetry, and have not seen any marked decrease in its value after tourniquet deflation in such patients. If the limb is thoroughly exsanguinated, using an Esmarch bandage before tourniquet inflation, very little blood remains in the limb. The benefits afforded by the use of a tourniquet should be balanced against the dangers, and a decision made for each operation.

Osteomyelitis in children with sickle-cell disease tends to have a subacute onset and is often polyostotic. It affects the upper limbs (Fig. 8.7) almost as commonly as the legs, and both the diaphyses (Fig. 8.8) and the metaphyses. The common infecting organisms are *Staphylococcus aureus* and *Salmonella* spp.; antimicrobial treatment that will cover both possibilities should be used pending culture results. A

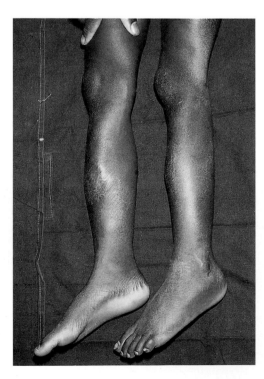

Figure 8.8 Sickle-cell osteomyelitis. Note that most of the swelling is diaphyseal.

combination of ampicillin and cloxacillin or chloramphenicol is given intravenously in high dosage and the limb immobilised and elevated while the child is prepared for surgery. In general, the bone infection is more diffuse and surgery to remove large sequestra less often needed than in the staphylococcal osteomyelitis commonly seen in children without sickle-cell disease. Conversely, involucrum formation is often poor and the weakened bone should be protected by traction or casting. During the periods of often prolonged bed rest, it is essential to keep painful joints from stiffening in flexion.

The orthopaedic manifestations of sickle-cell disease are crippling and often life-threatening, but some patients with sickle-cell disease do survive into adulthood. Early diagnosis and effective treatment are needed to obtain consistently successful outcomes. Ankylosis of the hip, for example, may necessitate total hip arthroplasty, which can be successfully undertaken – despite a reported higher complications rate – with great benefit to the patient, provided all the precautions described are observed, and suitably small prostheses can be obtained.

ACQUIRED IMMUNE DEFICIENCY SYNDROME

Children can be infected by HIV either by maternal transmission or after the infusion of infected blood or blood products (Neilson & Bryson 2000). Children who were infected by transfusions in the early 1980s are now entering their teenage years. With the current rigorous screening of blood donors, HIV antibody testing of each donation and the safe manufacture of factor VIII/IX concentrates, the risk of HIV transmission today is remote. However, the infection is commonly transmitted heterosexually and women so infected are liable to infect children with HIV by prenatal or neonatal transmission of the virus. Such women are often unaware of their infection and therefore the child is not perceived as being at risk.

HIV primarily infects CD4 lymphocytes (T helper cells) and leads to a steady decline in their number. The CD4 cells have a pivotal role in the control of the immune system and their loss inevitably impairs immune mechanisms. After infection of an individual cell by the RNA virus, a DNA copy is made by the enzyme, reverse transcriptase; this copy is then incorporated, as a provirus, into the nuclear DNA, where it is immortalised. If the cell undergoes mitosis, each daughter cell will contain HIV in its nucleus. Expression of the proviral DNA leads to the assembly of many virus particles, which are shed to infect other cells: in addition to T cells and B lymphocytes, glial cells within the central nervous system and epithelial cells within the gut can also become infected. Infected monocytes and macrophages harbour the virus in sanctuary sites, where it evades some antiviral drugs.

The clinical manifestations of HIV depend upon the route of infection (Lindegren et al 2000). Children infected at or before birth initially appear healthy, but later fail to gain weight and thrive. Recurrent bacterial infection is a prominent feature initially, but later there are classical opportunistic infections, such as pneumocystis pneumonia. The common opportunistic infections vary according to the particular organisms most prevalent in the environment: whereas in Western Europe and USA, *Pneumocystis pneumoniae* is the most common infective agent, in sub-Saharan Africa, tuberculosis and cryptococcal infection are much more common. As the immune system involutes, high-grade non-Hodgkin lymphomas occur; they are peculiarly resistant to chemotherapy. The lymphomas appear not infrequently at extranodal sites – for example, the central nervous system. Kaposi's sarcoma, a manifestation of sexually transmitted HIV, is not observed in those infected by transfusion.

The classification of HIV disease is different in children than adults, and is summarised in Table 8.3. Various

classifications are necessary because the clinical manifestations are so diverse.

Management of HIV is less well defined for infected children than for adults. Any child with HIV infection, or whose mother is known to have HIV infection, should be regularly reviewed. Many infants at birth have passively acquired maternal anti-HIV antibody and therefore all children of infected mothers should be investigated. HIV infection can be established by culturing the virus, identifying it by polymerase chain reaction, or by detecting the presence of antibody after the child has reached 18 months of age. Even if these investigations remain negative, it is still possible that a child may be infected, and all at-risk children must have long-term follow-up.

Infections should be treated promptly. If bacterial infections recur despite prophylactic antibiotics, regular infusions of intravenous immunoglobulin may be of benefit. When the CD4 count decreases to less than about 200×10^6/litre it is reasonable to consider prophylaxis against the prevailing opportunistic infection, for example, co-trimoxazole for pneumocystis pneumonia, or triple therapy against tuberculosis. Antiviral therapy should be given (usually as a combination of anti-HIV agents) and the parents should be asked to bring their child for medical attention immediately they become unwell.

Children with HIV infection will require the same spectrum of surgical procedures as non-infected children. Some HIV-infected individuals are thrombocytopenic. This must be corrected by either platelet infusion or intravenous immunoglobulin before surgery.

The prospects for HIV-infected children are progressively improving as greater experience is gained in the management of the clinical difficulties experienced. Anti-viral drugs and the prompt treatment of infections, fortunately, seem to improve the prognosis for this unfortunate group of children.

Table 8.3 Classification of HIV disease in children

P–0 Indeterminate infection
P–1 Asymptomatic infection
P–2 Symptomatic infection
  A: Non-specific findings
  B: Progressive neurological disease
  C: Lymphoid interstitial pneumonitis
  D: Secondary infectious diseases
    (e.g. pneumocystis carinii pneumonia)
    Toxoplasmosis
    Recurrent bacterial infections
  E: Cancers
    Lymphomas
    Kaposi's sarcoma

REFERENCES

Arnold W D, Hilgartner M W 1977 Hemophilic arthropathy. Current concepts of pathogenesis and management. Journal of Bone and Joint Surgery 59A: 287–305

Berntorp E 1996 The treatment of haemophilia, including prophylaxis, constant infusion and DDAVP. Baillière's Clinical Haematology 9: 259–271

Duthie R B 1997 Musculoskeletal problems and their management. In: Rizza C R, Lowe GDO (eds) Haemophilia and other inherited bleeding disorders. WB Saunders, London, pp 227–274

Högh J, Ludlam C A, Macnicol M F 1987 Hemophilic arthropathy of the upper limb. Clinical Orthopaedics and Related Research 218: 225–231

Houghton G R, Duthie R B 1978 Orthopaedic problems in haemophilia. Clinical Orthopaedics and Related Research 138: 197–216

Lee C A 1996 Transfusion-transmitted disease. Baillière's Clinical Haematology 9: 369–394

Lindegren M L, Steinberg S, Byers R H 2000 Epidemiology of HIV/AID in children. Pediatric Clinics of North America 47: 79–108

Macnicol M F, Ludlam C A 1999 Does avascular necrosis cause collapse of the talus in haemophilia? Haemophilia 5: 139–142

Madhok R 1997 Musculoskeletal bleeding in hemophilia. In: Forbes CD, Madhok R, Aledort L (eds) Haemophilia. Arnold, pp 115–122

Neilsen K, Bryson Y J 2000 Diagnosis of HIV infection in children. Pediatric Clinics of North American 47: 39–63

Petterson H, Ahlberg A, Nilsson I M 1980 A radiologic classification of hemophilic arthropathy. Clinical Orthopaedics and Related Research 149: 153–159

Rizza C R 1997 Clinical features and diagnosis of haemophilia, Christmas disease and von WIllebrand's disease. In: Rizza C R, Lowe GDO (eds) Haemophilia and other inherited bleeding disorders. WB Saunders, London, pp 87–113

Chapter 9

Infections of bones and joints

K. Parsch and S. Nade

'Infection must be considered as a struggle between two organisms . . . the parasite and its host. This brings about adaptations on both sides.'

Elie Metchnikoff 1891

INTRODUCTION

A parasite is an organism that resides on or within another living organism in order to find the environment and nutrients it requires for growth and reproduction. Most successful parasites do no harm to their host and live in a balance that ensures the survival of both. *Infection* is the process whereby a parasite enters into a damaging relationship with the host. If the parasite injures the host to a sufficient degree, the manifestations result in disease. The combination of the presence of microorganisms, inflammation and tissue destruction constitutes *clinical infection.*

Once infection is established, the outcome of the contest between the host and parasite determines the effects of the infection. The possibilities are:

1. Microorganisms are repelled and eradicated, with restitution of host tissues to their normal state.
2. The microorganisms cause such tissue damage that the host is unable to survive.
3. Most commonly, the host eradicates the invading microorganism, but tissue destruction, inflammation and subsequent repair leave a scar at the site of invasion.

With clinical resolution of the disease, organisms may remain dormant in the tissues. It is the effect of the tissue response that determines the functional recovery of the host – that is, the *clinical outcome.*

In order to achieve infection there must be:

1. Entrance of the parasite into the host.
2. Establishment and multiplication of the parasite within the host.

AETIOLOGY AND BIOLOGICAL CAUSE

In order to *produce disease*, parasites must be able to invade host tissues, multiply and spread, and produce toxic substances. The ability to produce disease is known as *pathogenicity*, and the comparative pathogenicity of different organisms is expressed as *virulence*. Very small numbers of virulent organisms are able to produce disease, whereas larger numbers of less virulent organisms are required. The *invasiveness* of microorganisms is not clearly related to their toxic properties, but enzymes produced by them may allow both spread by tissue dissolution and protection from host phagocytes.

Infection starts with the pathogen colonising its portal of entry: colonisation depends upon the size of the inoculum and attachment to the site of entry. The infection can continue only if the pathogen multiplies. The host tissue must be able to support the growth of the microorganism and the pathogen must be able to overcome the host defence mechanisms. The pathogen may form products that aid its multiplication in the host; these may be either secretions, or breakdown products of the cell. Such substances may act against natural host bactericides by inhibiting phagocytosis or phagocyte migration, or by destroying phagocytes.

Portals of entry

There are several ways in which organisms gain access to bones and joints:

1. *Haematogenous* spread from primary site of colonisation (skin, mouth, gut) if the barriers to spread have been breached.
2. *Direct access* by puncture of the skin and deeper tissues after *injury.*
3. *Direct access* at the time of elective *surgery*, or after surgery for open injury.
4. *Local spread* from infected adjacent tissues (for example from a subcutaneous abscess into the adjacent bone or joint).

The tissues that harbour the infection

An infective process depends, not only upon the nature of the pathogen, its initial inoculum size and its portal of entry to the involved tissues, but also upon the nature of the tissue itself. Those tissues regularly in contact with the external environment, such as skin, mucous membrane, and cornea resist invasion by microorganisms, and a breach of the tissue surface is needed for an infection to occur. Deeper tissues, such as bone, joint and muscle do not appear to have the same natural barriers to infection.

Factors known to alter host defence mechanisms

Host resistance may be reduced, both to organisms of known pathogenicity and to organisms not normally pathogenic. Host defences may be altered by:

1. Reduction of normal commensal flora.
2. Disrupted anatomical barriers and secretions.
3. Changes in inflammatory responses.
4. Abnormal immune responses.

The increasing number and use of drugs that specifically interfere with cell function (antimetabolites, corticosteroids, cytotoxics and antibiotics) must alert the clinician to bone and joint infections presenting in a cryptic fashion, unlike the presentation in classical descriptions of disease.

PATHOLOGY OF BONE INFECTION

Bacteria lodge adjacent to the physis, probably in relation to terminal metaphyseal vessels. The acute inflammation results in vascular engorgement, oedema, polymorphonuclear cellular responses, and tissue death secondary to ischaemia from either venous or arterial obstruction. The growing bacterial colonies provoke acute suppurative inflammation and liquefactive necrosis of medullary tissues. Trabeculae of cancellous bone become fragmented, lose their vascular relationships and die. They lie in the pus as small sequestra.

The inflammatory process extends from the marrow and contained trabecular bone to the adjacent cortex (Fig. 9.1). This spread within the cortex probably initially follows the natural pathways of Haversian and Volkmann canals. Both osteoclastic and non-oesteoclastic bone resorption occur. Periosteal tissues may be lifted, thereby disrupting the periosteal blood supply entering the cortex. Further spread through periosteum and soft tissues may lead to spontaneous discharge of pus to the exterior. The lifting of periosteum from bone ruptures the intra-to-extramedullary vascular connections, thereby increasing the volume of bone made ischaemic. The displaced periosteum is stimulated to produce bone, which may be seen, on radiographic examination, initially (about 7–10 days after the onset of infection) as fine layers, and later perhaps as a thick involucrum.

In the absence of treatment, some of the physeal and metaphyseal bone dies and this dead bone, seeded as it is with bacteria, may act as a permanent reservoir for recurrent infection. The spontaneous or surgical drainage of pus is followed by repair, in favourable cases, through apposition of new bone. The cortex may become thickened by the newly formed bone of the repair process. Where the blood supply is inadequate, necrotic bone persists, as osteoclastic resorption can only take place under conditions of cell viability. Small abscesses are eventually replaced by cellular or fatty bone marrow, whereas large abscesses may be transformed into cystic cavities. The presence of residual abscesses or sequestra predisposes to recurrent or chronic osteomyelitis.

The usual clinical course

Trueta (1959), in his attempt to correlate the clinical features with his hypothesis of the underlying pathology of bone infection, described three clinical stages:

Stage I he described as a 'boil' in bone. This produces pain that is quite severe, constant and described as 'deep' or 'in the bone' and is often not localised to the focus of infection. It is more useful to ask the child to point to the site of pain. Tenderness, usually accurately localised, is constant in position and intensity, and is exquisite. At this stage there is no redness, no swelling, no heat and no fluctuation.

Stage II occurs when there is pus in the medulla and the subperiosteal space. The symptoms and signs are more marked, and systemic symptoms such as malaise, fever, other aches and pains, and headache develop.

Stage III is characterised by pus in the soft tissues. Galen's signs of acute inflammation, calor, dolor, rubor, tumor, and functio laesa, are now present.

These days, presentation may be rather different. Initially, the child may complain that a limb hurts. Some trauma

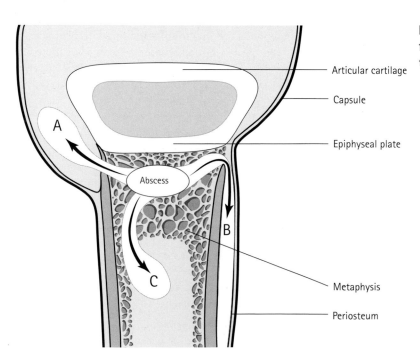

Figure 9.1 The spread of pus from a metaphyseal focus into the joint (A), the subperiostal tissue (B), and the medullary canal (C).

Articular cartilage

Capsule

Epiphyseal plate

Abscess

Metaphysis

Periosteum

might have occurred. Very soon the pain becomes so severe that the child finds it hard to bear.

Pathology of haematogenous osteomyelitis in infants

The basic process in the infant is similar to that in the child. Because of the presence of transphyseal vessels, the infection may spread across the physis and epiphysis into the joint. Whereas in childhood the infection does not usually involve the germinal cells of the physis and hence does not interfere directly with growth, these cells in the infant may be inhibited or die; growth aberrations and deformity can then occur. The amount of growth disturbance that follows is related to:

1. The volume of physis destroyed.
2. The location of such destruction (e.g. germinal or hypertrophic layers, central or peripheral).
3. The invasion and destruction of the epiphysis and its cartilage canal systems.

Epiphyseal growth, which controls the 'sphericity' of the bone ends and the shape of the articulating surfaces, may also be jeopardised, as the epiphysis has its own separate mechanism for endochondral growth.

Osteomyelitis in infancy is also characterised by extensive involucrum formation, often involving the entire length of the diaphysis. Despite gross early radiological changes, subsequent growth and remodelling eventually leave little evidence of diaphyseal cortical involvement.

Pathology of subacute and chronic osteomyelitis

The balance between microbe and host is such that the destructive and repair processes do not take place as rapidly as in acute infection. The fundamental problem is the persistence of organisms as a result of sequestration, unrecognised antibiotic resistance, or compromised host defences. The result is a bone abscess, most often in the metaphysis of long bones. The proximal tibia, distal femur, proximal or distal humerus or distal radius are frequently affected. The calcaneum and metarsals are also common locations.

The clinical appearance is usually of a mild, sometimes intermittent limb pain, present for days or weeks, with loss of function and local tenderness, but little or no systemic signs. Sometimes the chronic form of osteomyelitis may change into an acute form with more dramatic clinical signs of infection and the formation of a *bone abscess*. The causative organisms are sometimes elusive, especially if antibiotics have been used.

Pathology of acute septic arthritis

Septic arthritis may destroy synovial joints, because erosion of articular cartilage is usually irreversible and progressive. As a result of the success of modern treatment and subsequent lack of post-mortem material, there are very few reports about the pathogenesis and sequential development of the disease in man, but a strong association has been observed between pus and cartilage destruction in septic arthritis.

An intra-articular infective dose of bacteria produces oedema, hyperaemia and acute inflammation of the synovium. Polymorphonuclear neutrophils, often in clumps, can be seen within synovial vessels, outside those vessels in the synovium, and within the joint lumen. Synovial fluid dynamics are altered, leading to an effusion. If treatment is commenced early and is successful, resolution of the inflammatory process may take place. If the disease process is not controlled, there may be complete loss of articular cartilage, leading eventually to fibrous ankylosis of the joint. Although modern antimicrobial agents are efficient, they do not remove pus sufficiently, or do not do so rapidly enough, to avoid permanent damage to the cartilage. The majority of paediatric orthopaedic surgeons therefore agree that it is important to remove purulent fluid from a joint as soon as its presence is suspected.

In infants in particular, but sometimes also in children, intracapsular inflammation, with synovial proliferation and an exudate or transudate of fluid, may distend the joint capsule, causing laxity, subluxation or dislocation. Pus contained in the joint, by virtue of the thick anatomical barriers around it, increases intra-articular pressure and favours destruction of the articular cartilage. Later, when cartilage has been destroyed, there may be focal or patchy bone loss in the subchondral region. Osteopenia resulting from disuse and hyperaemia appear quickly.

The infection of a joint by blood-borne spread has been outlined. Bacteria may also gain entry by direct penetrating injury, by diagnostic or therapeutic puncture, as a complication of venepuncture, or arthrotomy. The virulence of the infecting organism and the resistance of the host determine whether suppuration ensues. Infancy, trauma or prior arthropathy appear to reduce the resistance to spread of infection. *In any acute and painful joint disease, infection must be suspected.*

Why are bones infected?

In haematogenous infection of bone, the bacterial replication and tissue destruction take place remote from the site that is primarily involved. Why haematogenous infections select bone, and even certain bones more than others, remains an enigma.

Trueta (1959) first drew attention to the fact that acute osteomyelitis in infants, children and adults has different clinical features. He postulated that the reason for this might be the *different vascular anatomy in these three age groups*. In the infant, many epiphyses have not begun to ossify and are entirely cartilaginous. Some vessels may cross the physis directly, linking metaphysis and epiphysis, and thereby providing a direct path from the nutrient artery to the joint. Furthermore, epiphyseal vessels are end-arterial. The adult has no physis, so that vessels link one subchondral articular region to the other.

Why are joints infected?

Articular cartilage has few blood vessels, and it is improbable that haematogenous spread of bacteria leads to their

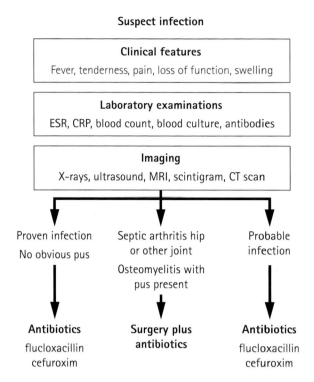

Suspect infection

| **Clinical features** |
| Fever, tenderness, pain, loss of function, swelling |

| **Laboratory examinations** |
| ESR, CRP, blood count, blood culture, antibodies |

| **Imaging** |
| X-rays, ultrasound, MRI, scintigram, CT scan |

Proven infection
No obvious pus

Septic arthritis hip
or other joint
Osteomyelitis with
pus present

Probable
infection

Antibiotics
flucloxacillin
cefuroxim

**Surgery plus
antibiotics**

Antibiotics
flucloxacillin
cefuroxim

Figure 9.6 Algorithm for the management of skeletal infection.

aseptic technique, and to avoid needle passage through potentially septic sites in skin or soft tissues.

The traditional indication for aspiration of suspected septic joints has been modified by modern imaging methods. If the clinical picture, laboratory findings of a high CRP and sedimentation rate, together with ultrasound documentation suggest a septic joint, it seems sensible and kind to aspirate this under general anaesthesia followed by arthroscopy or arthrotomy to wash out the infected joint. In doubtful cases, aspirations may help clarify whether further procedures are necessary.

Aspiration in acute osteomyelitis must also be seen in the light of new imaging methods. If MRI has identified an active bone marrow infection with a subperiostal abscess, it is more sensible to drain this immediately than wait two days for the bacteriological result of the aspirate.

In doubtful cases, or in the absence of modern imaging, aspirating the painful bone helps. If pus is present, this is an indication for operative surgery. A needle aspirate should not be delayed for fear of spreading infection to bone. If pus is not present, the risk of introducing infection to 'tender' bone that is not necessarily infected must be considered. If correct aseptic technique is used, the procedure need not carry a high risk of iatrogenic infection.

Bone should not be repeatedly traumatised, nor any attempt made to use the aspirating needle as a trephine to enter the medullary cavity.

Antibiotics
The treatment of infections of the musculoskeletal system often requires both surgical removal of infected tissues and antimicrobial chemotherapy. Antibiotic management requires consideration of:

- the choice of drugs to be administered
- the dose to be used
- the route of administration
- the duration of treatment.

As newer antibiotics become available, their performance must be compared with established drugs. Changes to treatment protocols must be based upon a clear appraisal of what is expected from the drug.

The choice of antibiotics
The chosen antibiotic must be effective against the bacteria causing the infection. Before an organism has been identified, or while antibiotic sensitivity of known organisms is being determined, the selection of antibiotic is 'provisional', based on a 'best guess'. Once identification and sensitivity are known, the 'definitive' or 'specific' treatment can be used.

The choice of antibiotics is determined by:

1. The organism(s) to be eradicated.
2. Patient allergy to particular drugs.
3. Associated diseases.
4. Characteristics of the antibiotic (toxicity, activity and specificity, expense and potential hypersensitivity).

The dose of antibiotics
In infants and children, the dose relates to body weight. The efficiency of elimination of an antibiotic should be considered when the frequency of administration is being decided. The concentration of antibiotic in the blood should be greatest soon after administration of a dose and still therapeutic just before a subsequent dose. The aim of treatment is to maintain effective serum (and tissue) concentrations. The popular teaching is that a concentration of the antibiotic that is approximately four times the minimum inhibitory concentration (MIC) should be achieved in patients with normal defences; in patients with abnormal defences, or infections at anatomical sites where there may be locally impaired defence mechanisms or poor penetration of antibiotic, the prescriber should achieve drug concentrations that are at least eight times the MIC.

If antibiotics are administered intravenously, the physician can be assured of serum concentrations in the therapeutic range, given correct dosage. If they are given orally, absorption from the gut must also be taken into consideration.

If manufacturers' instructions are followed with regard to dosage schedules and timing of administration, regular monitoring of serum concentrations is not usually necessary. However, when using toxic antibiotics, such as aminoglycosides, it is important to measure serum concentrations and renal function frequently, and to adjust the drug dose accordingly. Table 9.1 lists the average doses for various

Table 9.1 Average doses of antibiotics used for musculoskeletal infections in children older than 4 weeks*

Drug	Dose
Penicillin G	60–120 mg/kg (4)
Cloxacillin	50–100 mg/kg (4)
Flucloxacillin	50–100 mg/kg (4)
Cefuroxim	50–100 mg/kg (4)
Cefotaxime	50–100 mg/kg (3)
Gentamicin	7.5 mg/kg (3)
Vancomicin	30–50 mg/kg (3)
Clindamycin	8–16 mg/kg (4)
Fusidic acid	20–40 mg/kg (3)
Erythromycin	30–40 mg/kg (3)

*These drugs are given in divided doses (number per day in parentheses).

antibiotics when used to treat musculoskeletal infections in children.

The route of administration

Possible routes of administration are intravenous, intramuscular, oral, rectal, and local in the infected area by irrigation or slow release. In acute infections, when the patient is unwell, nauseated or dehydrated, oral treatment is not advised. The most effective route is *intravenous*. Entry to the blood stream is ensured, and the exact dose calculated can be given. Because of antibiotic protein binding and excretion patterns, it is preferable to give a bolus of antibiotic at regular intervals (4–6 hours), rather than a continuous low concentration infusion. If peak and trough serum concentrations are monitored, the correct dose can be calculated.

Oral preparations are available for most classes of antimicrobials (except aminoglycosides). The major problems with oral use are the breakdown of the drug by gastric secretions or poor absorption across the gastrointestinal mucosa. With the ability to measure blood concentrations of antibiotic drugs and a knowledge of their MIC, oral administration can be used once the acute phase of the disease has passed.

The criteria for a change to oral administration are:

1. Satisfactory clinical response to initial parenteral therapy.
2. Isolation of a bacterial pathogen that is susceptible to orally administered drugs.
3. Patient tolerance of an oral agent.
4. Adequate serum bactericidal activity with oral therapy.
5. Compliance by the patient.

Subacute and chronic infections may respond to oral treatment from the outset. However, if surgical intervention is indicated (abscess drainage, implantation of PMMA + gentamicin beads), the intravenous route should be used initially.

In chronic osteomyelitis, irrigation with antibiotic solutions can achieve high local concentrations. Antibiotic-impregnated methacrylate cement as a stent or as wire-threaded beads placed into the septic bone cavity is used in severe cases of acute or chronic osteomyelitis.

Duration of therapy

There are very few studies which compare the duration of therapy in musculoskeletal infections. The spectre of chronic osteomyelitis from the pre-antibiotic era still looms large, and many clinicians believe that prolonged treatment should be used for all bone and joint infections. What needs to be determined is the minimum period of treatment necessary to prevent chronicity and relapse of infection. This should be balanced against the cost, exposure to toxicity, and duration of parenteral treatment. If surgical drainage of an acute osteomyelitis or chronic abscess has been performed, antibiotic treatment duration can be shortened to 2–3 weeks.

It seems best to follow the clinical progress in addition to CRP and ESR values. A minimum of 2 weeks parenteral antibiotic treatment is recommended by most authors; after that, there is a divergence of opinion. It is not clear how long parenteral treatment should be continued, or for how long oral antibiotics should be given. Anderson et al (1980) suggested that antibiotics should be continued intravenously for 6 weeks, and recommended a similar length of oral treatment.

We prefer to follow the clinical course and monitor the CRP. In septic arthritis, normalisation might take as few as 7 days. The following oral medication will normally be given for another 2 weeks, with another check on CRP and ESR at that stage.

Whether the child needs to remain in hospital is debatable and is more a matter of domestic circumstance than medical need. After surgical intervention and for the safety of intravenous antibiotic treatment, the acute phase is better taken care of with the patient in hospital. Increasingly, it is possible to give intravenous medication at home thereafter.

WHAT IS THE PLACE OF SURGERY?

In septic arthritis and osteomyelitis, the major problem is deciding whether surgical intervention is necessary. In many centres, surgery is advised only if previous aspiration has demonstrated pus in the location. The authors prefer to identify the focus by clinical examination and imaging using radiography, ultrasound, bone scan or MRI.

The *indications* for surgery are:

1. Suspected septic arthritis confirmed by ultrasound (see Fig. 9.5) and possibly aspiration.
2. The presence of an abscess, as judged clinically, by ultrasound or MRI (see Fig. 9.2).
3. Osteomyelitis in a child who is severely ill despite adequate nourishment and hydration.
4. Inadequate clinical response with increasing local tenderness and swelling and failure to see a decrease in temperature within 12–24 hours of the commencement of treatment.

Contraindications to surgery include dehydration, a bleeding disorder (unless haemostasis can be assured) and parental refusal. Surgical treatment of osteomyelitis is largely empirical, based on concepts that have gained wide acceptance, often without scientific documentation. The suggestion of Mollan & Piggot (1975) that all children with osteomyelitis should undergo operation cannot be supported. In contrast, acute septic arthritis is an absolute indication for surgery.

When an operation is indicated, it should be performed as follows:

1. In septic arthritis, by the shortest and most direct approach to the joint. In septic arthritis of the knee joint (Fig. 9.7), arthroscopy is useful (Skyhar & Mubarak 1987, Stanitski et al 1989).

2. In acute osteomyelitis, the incision should be centred on the point of maximum tenderness, to allow release of pus in the soft tissues and beneath the periosteum.
3. Excision of obvious necrotic tissue, ensuring that specimens are taken for histology and culture.
4. Thorough saline irrigation of the infected area.
5. In osteomyelitis with a large osteolytic zone, with implantation of PMMA beads impregnated with gentamicin.
6. Wound closure over a suction drain.

The limb should (initially) be immobilised in such a way that the wound can be inspected. Should pus subsequently accumulate in the soft tissues, a secondary intervention should not be delayed.

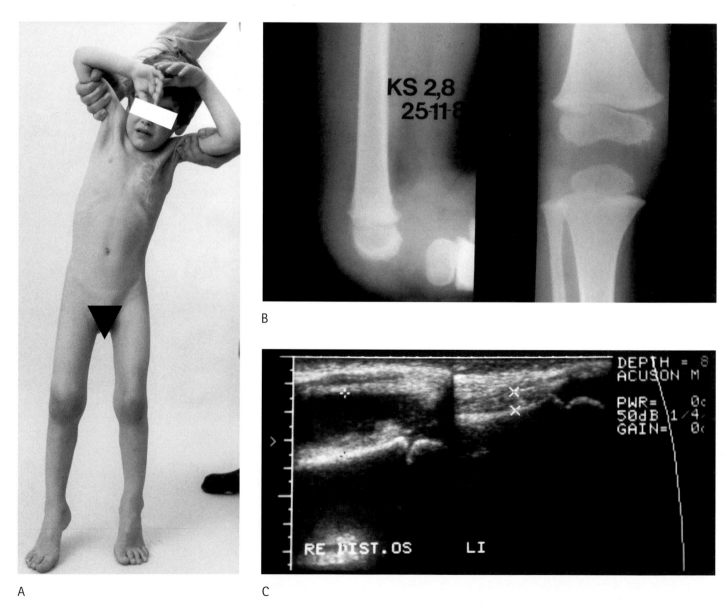

A   C

Figure 9.7 Septic arthritis of the right knee in a boy 2 years and 8 months old. **A** Clinical appearance of the right knee, with swelling and inability to bear weight. **B** An X-ray of the right knee shows no visible changes. **C** Ultrasound picture of right knee, showing 1.5 cm effusion (+). Left side shows normal joint fluid (××).

ACUTE HAEMATOGENOUS OSTEOMYELITIS

Acute haematogenous osteomyelitis is an acute illness characterised by fever, bone tenderness and reduced function after the establishment of a bacterial colony in bone. Pain and inflammation develop quickly and progress rapidly.

INCIDENCE

Osteomyelitis severe enough to require hospital admission is predominantly a disease of children, affecting boys more often than girls. The incidence appears to be greater in countries at lower latitudes, and multifocal disease is more frequently seen there. Seasonal variations, with a peak in autumn and spring, suggest an environmental effect. Although there is an association with lower socioeconomic status, acute osteomyelitis occurs also in children who are perfectly healthy and who live in a good environment.

LABORATORY SIGNS

Increased C-reactive protein is the most sensitive parameter in laboratory investigation. Quantitative measurements are mandatory. Initial values greater than 8 mg/dl may increase rapidly, to as much as 30 mg/dl.

The sedimentation rate may similarly increase quickly to values as high as 100 mm in the first hour.

For differential diagnosis, a complete cell count is mandatory in cases of suspected acute haematogenous osteomyelitis. The white blood cell count may be increased to 15 000 or more, but these values are of little reliability.

IMAGING

Plain radiography is of very little value in the early stage of acute osteomyelitis. Bony rarefaction may be visible after a few days. Soft-tissue swelling with subperiostal spread of the bone infection is more obvious. At a later stage (10–14 days after the onset), lytic lesions and periosteal new bone formation become visible (see Fig. 9.3).

Technetium bone scans become positive 2–3 days after onset of the disease. They are mainly of use in unusual sites such as the sacrum or the spine.

Ultrasonography shows changes only after the metaphyseal abscess has perforated the cortex and lifted the periosteum.

Magnetic resonance imaging (if available) has become the imaging tool of choice. There is a clear identification of the bone infection, even in the earliest phase. It should be performed as an emergency in any case of suspected acute osteomyelitis. STIR sequences allow visualisation of the bone marrow changes. With gadolinium contrast, differentiation may be possible between acute infection and tumour infiltration.

DIAGNOSIS

The diagnosis of acute haematogenous osteomyelitis in the early phase relies on five features:

1. Clinical examination with severe pain and inability to move or to bear weight.
2. Increased C-reactive protein and ESR.
3. Negative plain radiography, but with possible soft-tissue swelling.
4. Ultrasound imaging identifying epi- or subperiosteal abscess.
5. MRI images in STIR sequences with additional gadolinum contrast demonstrating infection in bone marrow and possible invasion into periosteum and adjacent tissue.

TREATMENT

The principles of treatment are as follows:

1. The appropriate antibiotic will achieve cure in the very early phase, before pus has formed.
2. Systemic antibiotics cannot sterilise avascular tissues and pus; therefore, these should be surgically removed.
3. Systemic antibiotics can then prevent the further formation of pus; primary suture of the skin is safe after surgery.
4. Bone is damaged by ischaemia; therefore surgery, if performed, should not put the already ischaemic bone at further risk. Pus removal aims to restore the disrupted continuity of the periosteum and cortex (see Fig. 9.3) and allows intramedullary blood flow.
5. Antibiotic treatment should be started immediately after surgery, or should be continued if already given before surgery.

The principal areas of debate over the management of patients with acute haematogenous osteomyelitis concern:

- which antibiotic to choose
- the value of early operative intervention
- the duration of treatment
- immobilisation.

Immobilisation had been advised for many years, but has been abandoned by most centres, especially since the introduction of continuous passive motion by Salter et al (1981). Especially after surgery, early mobilisation without weight bearing is encouraged.

Antibiotics: which should be used?

It is not always possible to identify the infecting organism, or to determine its antibiotic sensitivity; organisms are grown from clinically diagnosed cases of haematogenous osteomyelitis in only 50–66% of patients. The majority of infections are caused by *Staph. aureus* and β-haemolytic *Streptococcus*.

Bactericidal anti-staphylococcal and anti-streptoccal

antibiotics should be administered parenterally in adequate doses. The critical problem, however, is whether all cases should be treated as if they were attributable to *Staph. aureus*, with the administration of one antibiotic alone, or treated with a combination of antibiotics, to cover more organisms.

Cefuroxim (100 mg/kg) has been an effective drug for more than 10 years, with very rare exceptions to its sensitivity. The antibiotic is applied parenterally for at least 2 weeks.

Oral therapy is introduced when the child is clinically well, has no fever, and the local signs have decreased. Flucloxacillin or cephaclor is administered between meals, because of the effect of gastric contents on drug absorption. The dose to be given by mouth is controlled initially on a body weight basis (50–100 mg/kg per day, in divided doses), but is adjusted according to peak and trough serum values to provide a concentration in excess of the MIC for the causative organism, or to 20 µg/ml (trough) if no organism is grown.

For streptococcal osteomyelitis, benzyl penicillin should be given intravenously ($0.25–1.0 \times 10^6$ units, every 6 hours) for as long as the intravenous route is necessary. When intravenous is replaced by oral administration, phenoxymethyl penicillin is given in a dose of 100 mg/kg per day every 6 hours. If the child is intolerant of penicillin, a cephalosporin such as cephrazine or cephalexin can be given in a dose of 100 mg/kg per day, either intravenously or orally.

When investigation of a suspected infection indicates a probable infection, the selection of antibiotics may be based on the *age* of the child:

- neonates: gentamicin + flucloxacillin
- age 6 weeks – 2 years: flucloxacillin + ampicillin
- age over 3 years: flucloxacillin.

Surgery

In established acute abscess detected either by radiography or in an earlier phase by MRI, surgical decompression is mandatory. This gives quick relief from pain and offers the chance of rapid recovery. After decompression, a swab is taken for bacteriology and a specimen for the pathologist. Antibiotic parenteral treatment with a second generation cephalosporin is started immediately after the swab has been taken.

Surgical cleansing of bone marrow and periosteum of pus and debris is followed by thorough rinsing of the infected zone. Gentamicin-impregnated PMMA beads aligned in a chain to fill the gap can be implanted (see Fig. 9.2). The wound is closed with a drain left in place. The PMMA chain is removed after a fortnight, which provides the opportunity of a 'second look' operation and another curettage.

Some centres prefer the use of an irrigation suction system for several days. However, there can be compliance problems, especially in small children.

Immobilisation of the involved limb is for as short a time as possible; as soon as the patient is able to move it without pain, he or she may do so. Weight bearing is permitted only after 4–6 weeks, when laboratory signs have returned to normal.

In very aggressive infections with virulent organisms, occasionally a second, or even a third, operation is necessary. As soon as there are signs of the infection spreading, one should not hesitate to look again. This offers a better chance for a complete recovery than a 'wait and see' strategy.

Sequelae are more frequent in the infant group. With an aggressive surgical approach to any patient with an acute abscess, sequelae can be reduced, even in severe disease. Major disturbances are seen if surgery is delayed.

OUTCOME

Death rarely occurs in acute haematogenous osteomyelitis today. When it does, it is from overwhelming septicaemia with involvement of multiple organs. The risk of *chronic osteomyelitis* remains a major reason for seeking to improve early management in acute haematogenous osteomyelitis. If the child presents early enough and the principles of treatment are followed meticulously, chronic osteomyelitis should become a disease of the past.

Another complication is *aberration of growth*. Whether the function of the growth plate is retarded or accelerated depends on the effect of the metaphyseal infection upon the germinal cells at the epiphyseal edge of the growth plate. It is often stated that overgrowth of the affected bone is a normal sequel of acute osteomyelitis; however, in one series of patients who had osteomyelitis in infancy, there was some shortening of the affected limb in every case reviewed at adolescence. Unequal growth has clinical significance only if it is considerable, affects only a portion of the growth plate, producing an angulatory deformity (Fig. 9.8), or affects one of a pair of bones (in the forearm or leg). Anatomical deformity of the contour of a bone does not necessarily produce significant clinical, functional or cosmetic deformity.

Involvement of an *adjacent joint* leads to suppurative arthritis. This is seen more frequently in infants, in whom the growth plate is anatomically different from that of children because of the presence of transphyseal vessels.

Local extension into *adjacent soft tissues* may occur in untreated cases, with spontaneous discharge of pus through the skin. The process of resorption of bone, either in the acute phase, or more often in the chronic phase, may lead to pathological fracture.

Weakness of bone may be the result either of bone loss or of osteoporosis; pathological fracture may result if the bone is not protected by external support. Provided that the infection is controlled, such fractures usually unite when treated by conventional non-operative methods.

A very difficult sequel to treat is *diaphyseal loss*. This may

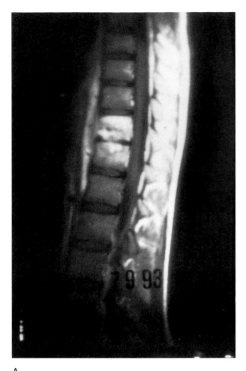
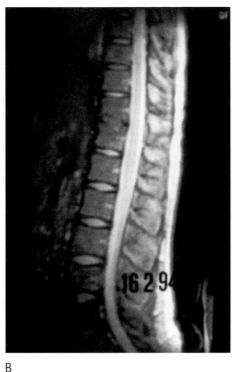

Figure 9.8 Spondylitis and discitis in a 13-year-old girl with acute back pain, fever and inability to walk. **A** T1 weighted MRI shows spondylodiscitis at T10/11 and adjacent spondylitis. **B** Five months later, after 6 weeks of antibiotic treatment and bed rest T2-weighted MRI shows residual signals at T10/11. The child is symptom free.

A   B

involve a long segment of bone. It usually implies that the ability of the surrounding periosteum to produce reparative involucrum has been lost and that spontaneous restoration of bone, even when infection is eradicated, cannot occur. A bone graft or bone transfer must be used to replace the missing bone (Daoud & Saighi-Bouaouinna 1989). There is some suggestion that such diaphyseal loss as a consequence of chronic osteomyelitis is much more frequent in those children in whom multiple drill-holes have been made along the diaphysis in an early stage of treatment of acute osteomyelitis, or who have undergone overenthusiastic sequestrectomy at an inappropriate time.

SUBACUTE OSTEOMYELITIS

FREQUENCY

The estimated incidence of subacute osteomyelitis is 0.4–0.9 per 100 000 per year, and the majority of patients are younger than 20 years. In a service area of approximately 2 million people, we see about 15 cases of subacute osteomyelitis per year. Males are more commonly affected. Several bones and joints can be affected (multifocal subacute osteomyeltis). Recurrence is seen in special forms such as Garré's chronic and hypersclerotic osteomyeltis (Garré 1893, Mollan et al 1984).

HEREDITY

There is no direct hereditary link between infections of bones and joints and particular families, although people with HbS-sickle-cell disease are more likely to have osteomyelitis caused by *Salmonella* spp.

CLINICAL PICTURE

Subacute osteomyelitis presents as a mild, sometimes intermittent local limb pain of a few days or weeks duration, with mild systemic signs. A characteristic of subacute presentation is a long history (usually more than 14 days) of symptoms dominated by pain. Fever is slight or absent, and constitutional symptoms are rare. Loss of function is obvious in most cases, but may be dramatic in spinal infection.

Unlike the acute osteoarticular infections, the diagnosis of subacute infection depends greatly on imaging techniques, particularly radiology.

IMAGING

The majority of cases of subacute osteomyelitis are metaphyseal abscesses, but 25–33% present with a cortical diaphyseal lesion. Epiphyseal abscesses are rare.

Radiological signs are normally established at the time of presentation and include absorption, sclerotic margination and sequestration. This has led to a classification based on the radiological appearances (Gledhill 1973, Roberts et al 1982) (Table 9.2, Fig. 9.9). Ross & Cole (1985) preferred to use two other radiological categories: aggressive lesions and metaphyseal or epiphyseal abscesses. Most lesions occur in the metaphysis of the tibia and femur, but the tarsal bones, particularly the os calcis, may be affected (Table 9.3).

Nuclear imaging is a valuable investigation in an early subacute presentation in which the radiological changes are obscure or poorly developed, particularly in the pelvis, but once the radiological changes are established, there is no

being the more frequent, the more deceptive in presentation, and the more devastating, merits special attention.

The neonate and infant

In septic arthritis of the hip in the infant, delay in diagnosis is common. The major features are those of a septicaemia. The very young child with fever and a serious illness may not manifest classic local signs of arthritis. The infective process in a joint, particularly the hip joint, is frequently not obvious, and subtle changes in posture are important. When infection in an infant is suspected, great care must be taken in clinical examination: all bones should be palpated, and all joints moved. The traditional clinical signs of inflammation, such as swelling and reddish colour, may be lacking.

In any infant with a septicaemia, involvement of the hip joint must be suspected. This is manifest by one or more of the following:

• abnormal posture of the leg
• pain on palpation of the hip or passive movement
• lack of active movement of the leg
• a palpable bulge over the buttock or in the perineum
• asymmetric buttock creases.

Among these, *Pseudoparalysis* (the limitation of spontaneous movement of the affected limb) may be obvious, and is the most common sign of bone and joint infection in the neonate (see Fig. 9.12). In contrast, in a small child the amount of soft-tissue swelling around the buttock creases may be dramatic, and this may give rise to confusion in diagnosis.

In septic arthritis of a shoulder joint, abnormal posture of

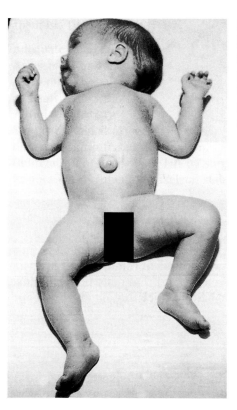

Figure 9.12
External rotation and flexion with pseudoparalysis of the left hip, resulting from septic arthritis.

the arm, painful reactions to passive movement, and pseudoparalysis should foster suspicion. Arthritis in the knee or elbow joint is more obvious: these joints have less muscle and soft tissue to cover them.

The main differential diagnosis is perinatal injury with epiphyseolysis, for example, in the hip, shoulder, or knee joint.

The older child

In contrast to the infant, the older child with septic arthritis usually presents with an acute illness. *Severe pain* uniformly about the involved joint, muscle spasm and reluctance to move the joint or even the whole limb are important criteria. Fever and tachycardia are common, together with evidence of joint effusion (see Fig. 9.7).

LABORATORY SIGNS

Measurements of CRP and ESR are the key instruments for diagnosing septic arthritis. CRP concentrations greater than 0.8 mg/dl indicate an acute infection. If there is uncertainty, the test should be repeated. In some patients, rapid changes are seen, with the concentrations increasing from 3 mg/dl to 15 mg/dl within 12 hours. In the case of the ESR also, if in doubt, repeat the tests. The white cell count is less reliable, but should nevertheless also be monitored.

IMAGING

Plain radiographs may demonstrate capsular swelling and joint distension. Late radiographic changes due to infection are seen with a delay of some days, with metaphyseal involvement adjacent to the joint, or joint destruction with or without dislocation.

Ultrasound is most reliable to visualise joint effusion. Septic arthritis of the hip, the shoulder or any other joint can be assessed, although differentiation between blood, purulent or simply excessive joint fluid is not possible. For this reason, information collected from the clinical appearance, laboratory analysis and ultrasound must be considered together. Even in neonates, capsular swelling and fluid inside the hip joint can clearly be identified. This is particularly important, as ultrasound is positive immediately after the onset of infection, and days before plain radiography shows any changes (see Fig. 9.5).

MRI images and CAT scans are similarly useful to visualise a joint effusion. In practical terms, ultrasound is preferred, as it can be undertaken without anaesthesia.

DIFFERENTIAL DIAGNOSIS

In acute septic arthritis, diagnosis in the crucial period is clinical. Conditions that may produce some difficulty in differential diagnosis (Kocher et al 1999) are:

1. *Acute osteomyelitis*, which may present a picture very similar to that of acute septic arthritis, with a sympathetic joint effusion adjacent to the involved

metaphysis. The two conditions may occur together, particularly in the hip or the shoulder joint. In acute osteomyelitis, gentle clinical examination usually allows some joint movement, which is always very painful.

2. *Juvenile idiopathic arthritis*, in which the initial manifestation may be monoarticular. There is considerable swelling and joint effusion, but little pain.
3. *Irritable hip or Perthes' disease*, which may present with hip or knee joint discomfort, and restriction of movement by muscle spasm. Ultrasound and radiology, together with negative laboratory signs, will reveal the true cause.
4. *Post-traumatic joint effusion*, in which a definite history of trauma is not always available, particularly in the child with an 'irritable' hip.
5. *Cellulitis*, which usually shows more local skin redness and oedema than septic arthritis, and a wider area of local tenderness. Lymphadenopathy usually accompanies cellulitis and the swelling is not circumferential.
6. *Acute rheumatic fever*, in which the symptoms tend to flit from joint to joint. This can also occur during the septicaemia of acute septic arthritis.
7. *Haemophilia*, which may present a diagnostic problem as the first presentation of a coagulation disorder.
8. *Henoch–Schonlein purpura*, which may present with single or multiple arthralgia before the cutaneous manifestations appear.

TREATMENT

There are two essentials for effective treatment of septic arthritis: first, the joint must be adequately cleaned, and second, antibiotics must be given to diminish the systemic effects of sepsis. If unstable, a septic joint must be rested in a stable position. If there is metaphyseal infection, pus and debris should be evacuated at the same operation.

Aspiration, irrigation or arthrotomy?
Treatment should sterilise the joint, evacuate bacterial products and debris, relieve pain and prevent deformity. Patients with septic arthritis require surgical drainage of the affected joint (see Fig. 9.13).

Most authors believe that early arthrotomy is less likely to produce an adverse long-term result than late arthrotomy after repeated arthrocentesis. Paterson (1970) advised against repeated joint aspiration and antibiotic joint irrigation as treatment. His reasons were:

1. Broad-spectrum antibiotics are irritant to cartilage.
2. The tension within the joint recurs.
3. The procedure is painful.
4. The results are uncertain.
5. Pus is often thick and cannot be aspirated, even when under tension.

The view of George Lloyd-Roberts (1972) that "the misguided conservatism of the needle should yield to the conservatism of the knife" is short, simple and sensible.

For the hip joint, there is no disagreement. Drainage can be posterior, medial or anterior, but the most reasonable is the anterior approach, making a wide hole in the capsule by a partial excision that can be used as a biopsy; a swab is taken for culture of causative germs. Adequate irrigation is followed by primary skin closure.

For the knee joint, arthrotomy can provide very thorough debridement. It may need to be repeated on two or three occasions. Some make a case for *arthroscopic lavage* under vision (Stanitski et al 1989, Shaw & Kasser 1990). This may achieve joint cleansing for the expert arthroscopist, but the less experienced should consider arthrotomy for all joints. Open arthrotomy is helpful in checking, and possibly debriding, a metaphyseal septic abscess.

After adequate debridement of the joint at arthrotomy, closure of the skin with a *suction drainage* left inside for 2–3 days is perfectly adequate. Some surgeons use a suction–irrigation system for a few days. Comparative randomised studies of the techniques have not been reported, but our own experience has been of problems of compliance with the suction–irrigation system, especially in the small infant.

Postoperative management
In the neonate, after surgical drainage, splintage of the hip should be in modest abduction and flexion, to prevent dislocation (Fig. 9.5) Appropriate antibiotics are administered systemically.

The causative germs
Staph. aureus and *Strep. pyogenes* are the most common causative organisms of acute septic arthritis in infants and children, but many other organisms have been isolated from septic joints. In 1966, Nelson & Koontz drew attention to the increasing importance of *Haemophilus influenzae* in the infant; however, during the past 12 years, not a single case was found in our community. This is probably due to routine immunization against *Haemophilus influenzae* in infancy and has been commented on in recent literature (Howard et al 1999). It is important to bear such changes in mind when choosing antibiotics before the results of bacterial culture and antibiotic sensitivity are known. Other causative organisms reported include *Strep. pneumoniae*, *E. coli*, *Proteus* spp., *Salmonella* spp., *Serratia marcescens*, *Clostridium welchii*, *Neisseria* spp., *Staph. albus*, *Aerobacter* spp., *Bacteroides* spp., and *Paracolon bacillus*.

However, organisms are not grown from the aspirates or biopsies in all cases: about 30% are sterile. Several reasons have been proposed for the inability to obtain bacteriological proof of infection:

1. Prior use of antibiotics.
2. Inadequate anaerobic cultures.
3. The standard of microbiological laboratories.
4. The changing prevalence of the organisms involved (e.g. *H. influenzae*) and their cultural characteristics.
5. Failure to obtain blood for culture or to perform adequate aspiration or arthrocentesis.

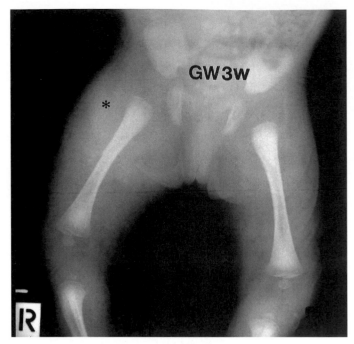

A

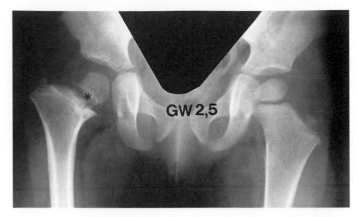

B

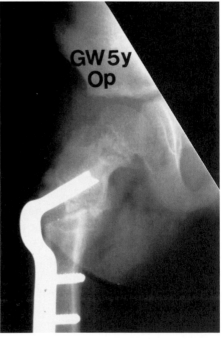

C

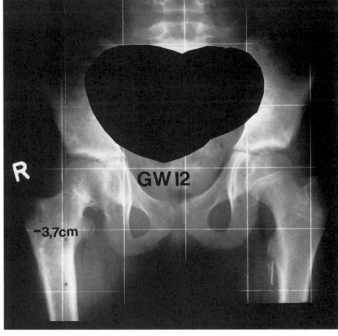

D

Figure 9.13 Follow-up over 12 years of septic arthritis and proximal femoral metaphyseal osteomyelitis. **A** Septic arthritis of the right hip in an infant aged 3 weeks, showing characteristic soft-tissue swelling. Therapy consisted of repeated aspirations and antibiotic treatment. **B** Coxa vara and metaphyseal gap (*) as sequelae of metaphyseal osteomyelitis in the same child aged 2 years and 5 months. **C** At 5 years of age, after valgus osteotomy the metaphyseal gap has closed, and the neck shaft angle is satisfactory. **D** At 12 years of age, premature closure of the proximal femoral physis has caused a leg length discrepancy of 3.7 cm.

Unusual organisms are more likely to appear when there has been penetration of the joint by a foreign body, the retention of a foreign body within a joint, systemic disease altering the immunological status of the patient, or treatment with corticosteroids.

The choice of antibiotics

Among cases in which a clinical diagnosis is made, an aetiological agent is found in only about 60%. In the infant younger than 6 months, the most likely organisms are staphylococci or streptococci; in children between 6 months and 2 years they are staphylococci or *H. influenzae*, where immunization is not routinely undertaken, and in those older than 2 years, a similar spectrum is found, staphylococci and streptococci being seen most frequently.

The provisional or 'best-guess' antibiotics should be based upon age (and smear findings):

1. *In the neonate*, flucloxacillin (75 mg/kg per day in four to six divided doses) and gentamicin (5–7.5 mg/kg per day in three divided doses).
2. *In the age group 6 months to 2 years*, flucloxacillin (100 mg/kg per day in four to six divided doses) or a cephalosporin such as cefuroxim (50–100 mg/kg) or cephotoxime is given as the initial treatment.
3. *For children older than 2 years*, flucloxacillin (100 mg/kg per day in four to six divided doses) or cefuroxim (100 mg/kg) is recommended, preferably by intravenous therapy.

Obviously, when organisms have been cultured and their antibiotic sensitivity is known, the definitive bacteriocidal antibiotic should be used in effective dosage.

The duration of antibiotic treatment

The duration of antibiotic therapy in acute septic arthritis remains empirical. Studies such as those performed by Blockey & Watson (1970) regarding the duration of antibiotic therapy in acute haematogenous osteomyelitis have not been performed on patients with septic arthritis. An empirical period of antibiotic treatment lasting 6 weeks is more than adequate, as long as adequate blood concentrations have been maintained.

If CRP concentrations and ESR values decrease rapidly and the clinical picture shows a return to normality with no symptoms of pain, a shorter course of antibiotic treatment suffices.

Immobilisation of a joint is unnecessary, unless the hip is unstable. We then use spica cast in the human position (see Fig. 9.5) or an abduction splint for a limited period of time.

OUTCOME

Unfortunately, there is no clear statement of the outcome after septic arthritis. It is generally accepted that progno-

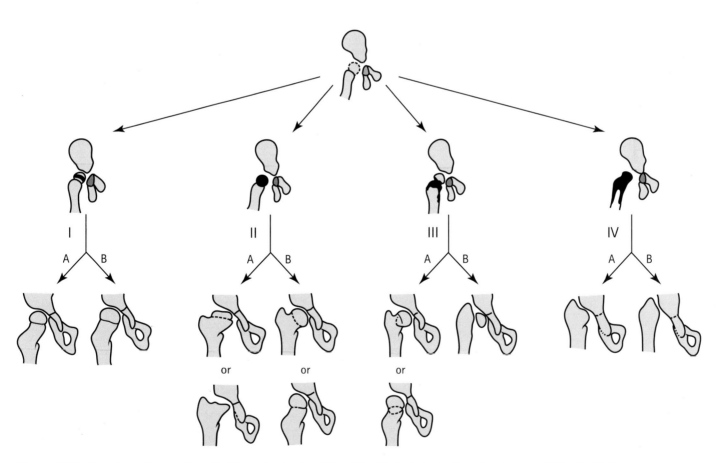

Figure 9.14 Sequelae after septic arthritis and osteomyelitis of the hip in infants. Type I – A: normal hip; B: slight coxa magna, minimal shortening. Type II – A: coxa brevis; B: coxa vara/valga. Type III – A: coxa vara and brevis, head in joint. B: pseudarthrosis with residual head in joint; Type IV – A: complete loss of femoral head with dislocation; B: loss of head and high-riding metaphyseal stump. (Reproduced with permission from Choi et al 1990 © Journal of Bone and Joint Surgery.)

sis after hip infection in neonates is poor (Bergdahl et al 1985), but for the other joints the introduction of antibiotics has improved the prognosis. Factors predicting outcome in the individual have not been defined. Complications may occur, in particular, in children younger than 1 year or who have had symptoms for three or more days before diagnosis and treatment were established.

The *potential sequelae* of hip sepsis (Choi et al 1990; Fig. 9.14) are:

I.   Recovery: A, with no deformity; or B, with mild coxa magna (see Fig. 9.5).
II. Coxa brevis with deformed head causing: A, progressive coxa vara; or B, coxa valga as a result of premature physeal closure.
III. Slipping of femoral epiphysis: A, with coxa vara or coxa valga; and B, with pseudarthrosis. The femoral head remains in the acetabulum.
IV. Destruction of femoral head and neck: A, with small medial remnant of head; or B, with complete loss of head and neck and no articulation of hip.

Late reconstructions of coxa vara by valgus osteotomy can be advantageous. (see Fig. 9.13).

The *risk of recurrence of acute osteomyelitis* decreases rapidly as time passes after the acute illness. If the overall recurrence rate is 20%, a child who has had no recurrence by 6 months has less than a 10% chance of further infection, and if no recurrence has occurred by 1 year, less than a 5% risk of further problems remains. The risk of recurrence seems to be lower in children who have their abscess drained surgically. Such figures are of value in counselling the patient and parents.

REFERENCES AND FURTHER READING

Alderson M, Nade S M L 1987 The natural history of acute septic arthritis in an avian model. Journal of Orthopaedic Research 5: 261–273

Anderson J R, Orr J D, MacLean D A 1980 Acute haematogenous osteitis. Archives of Diseases in Childhood 55: 953–957

Bergdahl S, Ekengren K, Eriksson M 1985 Neonatal hematogenous osteomyelitis: risk factors for long-term sequelae. Journal of Pediatric Orthopaedics 5: 564–568

Bjorksten B, Gustavson K H, Erikson B, Lindholm A, Nordstrom S 1978 Chronic recurrent multifocal osteomyelitis and pustulosis palmoplantaris. Journal of Pediatrics 93: 227–231

Blockey N J, Watson J T 1970 Acute osteomyelitis in children. Journal of Bone and Joint Surgery 52B: 77–87

Choi I H, Pizzutillo P D, Bowen J R, Dragann R, Malhis T 1990 Sequelae and reconstruction after septic arthritis of the hip in infants. Journal of Bone and Joint Surgery 72A: 1150–1165

Cole W G 1990 The management of chronic osteomyelitis. Clinical Orthopaedics and Related Research 264: 84–89

Couture A, Baud C, Ferran J L, Veyrac C 1988 Echographie de la hanche chez l'enfant. Axone, Montpellier, pp 145–160

Daoud A, Saighi-Bouaouinna A 1989 Treatment of sequestra, pseudarthroses and defects in the long bones of children who have chronic haematogenous osteomyelitis. Journal of Bone and Joint Surgery 71A: 1448–1468

Deeley D M, Schweitzer M E 1997 MR imaging of bone marrow disorders. Radiologic Clinics of North America 35: 193–212

Erdman W A, Tamburro F, Jayson H T, Weatherall P T, Ferry K B, Peshock R M 1991 Osteomyelitis: characteristics and pitfalls with MR imaging. Radiology 180: 533–539

Fletcher B D, Scoles P V, Nelson A D 1984 Osteomyelitis in children: detection by magnetic resonance. Radiology 150: 57–60

Gamble J G, Rinsky L A 1986 Chronic recurrent multifocal osteomyelitis: a distinct clinical entity. Journal of Pediatric Orthopaedics 6: 579–584

Garré C 1893 Über besondere Formen und Folgezustände der akiuten infektiösen Osteomyelitis. Beiträge der Klinischen Chirurgie 10: 257–265

Gideon A, Holthusen W, Masel L F, Vischer D 1972 Subacute and chronic 'symmetrical' osteomyelitis. Annales de Radiologie (Paris) 15: 329–342

Gillespie W J, Nade S M L 1987 Musculoskeletal infections. Blackwell, Melbourne

Gledhill R B 1973 Subacute osteomyelitis in children. Clinical Orthopaedics and Related Research 96: 57–69

Gold R H, Hawkins R A, Katz R D 1991 Bacterial osteomyelitis: findings on plain radiography, CT, MR and scintigraphy. American Journal of Roentgenology 157: 365–370

Hallel T H, Salvati E A 1978 Septic arthritis of the hip in infancy. Clinical Orthopaedics and Related Research 132: 115–128

Hamdy R C, Lawton L, Carey T, Wiley J, Marton D 1996 Subacute hematogenous osteomyelitis: are biopsy and surgery always indicated? Journal of Pediatric Orthopaedics 16: 220–223

Howard A W, Viskontas D, Sabbagh C 1999 Reduction in osteomyelitis and septic arthritis related to *Haemophilus influenzae* type B vaccination. Journal of Pediatric Orthopaedics 19: 705–709

Kallio P, Ryöppy S, Jappinen S, Siponmaa A K, Jääskeläinen J, Kunnamo I 1985 Ultrasonography in hip disease in children. Acta Orthopaedica Scandinavica 56: 367–374

Knudsen D J M, Hoffman E B 1990 Neonatal osteomyelitis. Journal of Bone and Joint Surgery 72B: 846–851

Kocher M S, Zurakowski D, Kasser J R 1999 Differentiation between septic arthritis and transient synovitis of the hip in children: an evidence-based clinical prediction algorithm. Journal of Bone and Joint Surgery 81A: 1662–1670

Lindenbaum S, Alexander H 1984 Infections simulating bone tumors. Clinical Orthopaedics and Related Research 184: 193–203

Lisbona R, Rosenthal L 1977 Radionuclide imaging of septic joints and their differentiation from periarticular osteomyelitis and cellulitis in pediatrics. Clinical Nuclear Medicine 2: 337–343

Lloyd-Roberts G C 1972 Orthopaedics in infancy and childhood. Butterworth, London

Majd M, Frankel R 1976 Radionuclide imaging in skeletal inflammatory and ischemic disease in children. American Journal of Roentgenology 126: 832–841

Mandelll G A 1996 Imaging in the diagnosis of musculoskeletal infections in children. Current Problems in Pediatrics 26: 218–237

Mazur J M, Ross G, Cummings R J, Hahn G A, McClusky W P 1995 Usefulness of magnetic resonance imaging for the diagnosis of acute muskuloskeletal infections in children. Journal of Pediatric Orthopaedics 15: 144–147

Mollan R A B, Piggot J 1975 Acute osteomyelitis in children. Journal of Bone and Joint Surgery 59B: 2–7

Mollan R A B, Craig B F, Biggart J D 1984 Chronic sclerosing osteomyelitis. Journal of Bone and Joint Surgery 66B: 583–585

Nade S 1983 Acute haematogenous osteomyelitis in infancy and childhood. Journal of Bone and Joint Surgery 55B: 109–119

Nelson J D, Koontz W C 1966 Septic arthritis in infants and children: a review of 117 cases. Pediatrics 38: 966–971

Parsch K, Savvidis E 1997 Die Koxitis beim Neugeborenen und Säugling Orthopäde 26: 838–847

Paterson D C, 1970 Acute suppurative arthritis in infancy and childhood. Journal of Bone and Joint Surgery 52B: 474–482

Peltola H, Vahvanen V, Aalto K 1984 Fever, C-reactive protein, and erythrocyte sedimentation rate in monitoring recovery from septic arthritis. Journal of Pediatric Orthopaedics 4: 170–174

Roberts J M, Drummond D S, Breed A L, Chesney J 1982 Subacute haematogenous osteomyelitis in children. A retrospective study. Journal of Pediatric Orthopaedics 2: 249–254

Ropes M W, Bauer W 1953 Synovial fluid changes in joint disease. Harvard University Press, Massachusetts

Ross E R S, Cole W G 1985 Treatment of subacute osteomyelitis in childhood. Journal of Bone and Joint Surgery 67B: 443–448

Salter R B, Bell R S, Keeley F W 1981 The protective effect of continuous passive motion on living articular cartilage in acute septic arthritis. Clinical Orthopaedics and Related Research 159: 223–247

Shaw B A, Kasser J R 1990 Acute septic arthritis in infancy and childhood. Clinical Orthopaedics and Related Research 257: 212–225

Skyhar M J, Mubarak S J 1987 Arthroscopic treatment of septic arthritis of the knees in children. Journal of Pediatric Orthopaedics 5: 647–651

Smith T 1874 On the acute arthritis of infants. St Bartholomew's Hospital Reports 10: 189–204

Stanitski C L, Harvell J C, Fu F H 1989 Arthroscopy in acute septic knees. Clinical Orthopaedics and Related Research 241: 209–212

Tang J S H, Gold R H, Bassett L W, Seeger L L 1988 Musculoskeletal infection of the extremities: evaluation with MR imaging. Radiology 166: 205–209

Thomson A 1906 Observations on the circumscribed abscess of bone (Brodie's abscess). Edinburgh Medical Journal 19: 297–309

Trueta J 1959 The three types of acute haematogenous osteomyelitis. A clinical and vascular study. Journal of Bone and Joint Surgery 41B: 671–677

Unger E, Moldofsky P, Gatenby R, Hartz W, Broder G 1988 Diagnosis of osteomyelitis by MR imaging. American Journal of Roentgenolgy 150: 605–610

Wegener W A, Alavi A 1991 Diagnostic imaging of muskuloskeletal infection. Roentgenography; gallium, indium labeled white blood cell, gammaglobulin, bone scintigraphy; and MRI. Orthopedic Clinics of North America 22: 401–418

Wenger D R, Davids J R, Ring D 1994 Discitis and
.   osteomyelitis. In: S L, Weinstein (ed) The pediatric spine: principles and practice. Raven Press, New York, pp 813–835

Wilson D J, Green D J, McClarnon J C 1984 Arthrosonography of the painful hip. Clinical Radiology 35: 17–19

Wingstrand H, Egund N, Lindgreen L, Sahlstrand T 1987 Sonography in the septic arthritis of the hip in the child. Journal of Pediatric Orthopaedics 7: 206–209

Zieger M, Dörr U, Schulz R 1987 Ultrasonography of hip joint effusions. Skeletal Radiology 16: 607–611

Chapter 10

Skeletal tuberculosis

S. M. Tuli

OSTEOARTICULAR TUBERCULOSIS

EPIDEMIOLOGY AND PREVALENCE

Tuberculous bacilli have lived in symbiosis with mankind since time immemorial. At present there are nearly 30 million people suffering from tuberculosis worldwide, and of these 1–3% have involvement of the skeletal system.

Tuberculosis will exist for as long as there are pockets of malnutrition, poor sanitation and overcrowding. Exanthematous fevers, repeated pregnancies and immunodeficiency also predispose towards the disease. The source of infection is a person with sputum positive for pulmonary tuberculosis. One cough can produce 3000 droplet nuclei, which can stay in the air for a long time, especially in indoor conditions with poor ventilation. Three factors determine a child's risk of getting the infection: the concentration of droplet nuclei in the air, the duration of his breathing the air, and his immunity status.

Regional distribution

Vertebral tuberculosis is the most common form of skeletal tuberculosis, accounting for 50% of all cases in reported series (Martini 1988, Tuli 1991). The major areas of predilection are, in order of frequency, the spine, hip, knee, foot, elbow, hand, shoulder, bursal sheaths and other sites.

PROPHYLAXIS AGAINST TUBERCULOSIS

Selective immunisation of groups at special risk is strongly recommended. The protection afforded by bacillus Calmette-Guérin (BCG) in the control of tuberculosis is estimated to be in the region of 80%. In developing countries, it is customary to vaccinate children at 1–3 months of age. About 1 in 10 000 vaccinated children in European countries may develop BCG osteitis; more rarely, a child may develop a generalised BCG infection. Fortunately, these patients respond favourably to modern anti-tubercular drugs. Chemoprophylaxis (using isoniazid with ethambutol) in addition to vaccination is appropriate for infants and children in contact with an infected mother or attendants.

PATHOLOGY AND PATHOGENESIS

An osteoarticular tubercular lesion results from haematogenous dissemination from a primarily infected focus that may be active or quiescent, apparent or latent, and in the lungs, lymph glands or other viscera. The infection reaches the skeleton through vascular channels – generally the arteries – as a result of bacteraemia or, rarely, in the axial skeleton, through Batson's plexus of veins. Simultaneous involvement of the paradiscal parts of contiguous vertebrae in a typical spinal tuberculous lesion lends support to the concept that the bacilli are blood-borne; 20% of patients at routine investigation reveal tuberculous involvement of the viscera, lymph nodes, or parts of the skeletal system, suggesting spread of infection through the arterial blood supply. Development of clinical tuberculosis of the skeletal system is a reflection of a weakened immune status of the patient.

IMMUNOPATHOGENESIS OF TUBERCULOSIS AS A RESULT OF HUMAN IMMUNODEFICIENCY VIRUS INFECTION

The helper subset of T lymphocytes is central to cell-mediated immunity against tuberculous infection. These cells carry the CD4 antigen on their surface (CD4$^+$ lymphocytes). The human immunodeficiency virus HIV enters and infects CD4$^+$ lymphocytes, kills these cells, and progressively leads to a decline in the immunity of the host.

Experimental tuberculosis

Hodgson et al (1969) tried to produce spinal tuberculosis in animals by a variety of methods. The only technique that was successful was injection of bacilli into the kidney, prostate and other abdominal and pelvic organs. This observation suggests that infection may spread directly from visceral foci to the vertebral column through the paravertebral veins.

Chronic osseous lesions were induced consistently in 8–10-week-old unvaccinated guinea pigs (Tuli et al 1974) by the insertion of Gelfoam impregnated with *Mycobacterium tuberculosis* into the metaphyseal region through a drill hole in the distal part of the femur. Localised tissue necrosis and prolonged contact between the bacilli and the damaged bone tissue markedly increased the likelihood of osteomyelitis.

Osteoarticular disease

Tubercular bacilli reach the joint space via the blood stream through subsynovial vessels, or indirectly from epiphyseal lesions that erode into the joint space. Destruction of the articular cartilage begins peripherally, and the weight-bearing surfaces are preserved for a few months, providing the potential for good functional recovery with effective treatment.

The future course of the tubercle

Before the availability of anti-tubercular drugs, the 5-year follow-up mortality of patients with osteoarticular tuberculosis was about 30%. Modern anti-tubercular agents have greatly changed the outlook. Depending upon the sensitivity pattern, the host resistance, and the stage of the lesion at the inception of treatment, the tuberculous lesion may behave as follows:

1. It may resolve completely.
2. The disease may heal with residual deformity and loss of function.
3. The lesion may be completely walled off and the caseous tissue may calcify.
4. A low-grade, chronic, fibromatous, granulating and caseating lesion may persist.
5. The infection may spread locally by contiguity and systemically by the blood stream.

THE ORGANISM

Before pasteurisation, the bovine type of bacillus was responsible for a great deal of osteoarticular tuberculosis; now, most skeletal tuberculosis is caused by bacilli of the human type. Because skeletal tuberculosis is a paucibacillary disease, positive cultures for acid-fast bacilli in osteoarticular tuberculous lesions are obtained in fewer than 50% of patients.

The best microbiological specimens appear to be those obtained from centrifuged material from an abscess, curettings from the walls of a cold abscess, or curettings from the lining of sinus tracts as close to the base (source) as possible.

Sensitivity of the organism

There are only a few reports regarding the culture and sensitivity of tubercle bacilli isolated from osteoarticular lesions. Resistance to various drugs is as follows: 7–10% for streptomycin; 4–10% for para-amino salicylic acid; 8–20% for isoniazid; 5–15% for thioacetazone; 2–9% for ethambutol; and about 2% for rifampicin. The development of resistant strains is minimised by multi-drug therapy.

Disease caused by atypical mycobacteria

The term 'atypical mycobacteria' refers to mycobacteria other than *M. tuberculosis* and *M. bovis*. Rarely, these organisms may be responsible for infective lesions in the skeletal system. Synovial sheath infections are more common with atypical mycobacteria than infection of osseous tissues. With atypical mycobacterial infections, human-to-human transmission is uncommon. Often a history of trauma such as a puncture wound, steroid injections, surgery or exposure to contaminated marine life is found. Many patients may have concomitant diabetes or immunodeficiency.

DIAGNOSIS AND INVESTIGATIONS

Skeletal tuberculosis mostly occurs during the first three decades of life. The characteristics are insidious onset, mono-articular or single bone involvement and the constitutional symptoms of low-grade fever, lassitude (especially in the afternoon), anorexia, loss of weight, night sweats, tachycardia and anaemia. Local symptoms and signs are pain, night cries, painful limitation of movements, muscle wasting and regional lymph-node enlargement. In the acute stage, protective muscle spasm is severe. During sleep, the muscle spasm relaxes and permits movement between the inflamed surfaces, resulting in pain and the typical night cries.

Diagnosis

In developing counties in general, the diagnosis of tuberculosis of bones and joints can be made reliably on clinical and radiological examination. However, in affluent countries tuberculosis has been reduced to the status of a rare disease, and the present generation of doctors is unfamiliar with the skeletal manifestations of the disease. In such situations, and whenever there is doubt, positive proof of the disease must be obtained by semi-invasive or invasive investigations. Skeletal tuberculosis must be included in the differential diagnosis of chronic or subacute mono-articular arthritis, chronic abscess, a draining sinus, or chronic osteomyelitis.

Radiography and imaging

Localised osteoporosis is the first radiological sign of active disease. The articular margins and bony cortices become hazy, and there may be areas of trabecular or bony destruction and osteolysis. The synovial fluid, thickened synovium, capsule and pericapsular tissues produce soft-tissue swelling, and the joint space narrows. As the destructive process advances, bone architecture collapses and joints deform or displace (see Fig. 10.4). The epiphyseal growth plate may be destroyed, producing irregular growth, angulation, or premature fusion. With healing of the disease process there is remineralisation, reappearance of bony trabeculae, and sharpening of cortical and articular margins.

In the centre of a tuberculous cavity, there may be a sequestrum of cancellous bone or calcification of the caseous tissue, which gives the appearance of an irregular, feathery nidus in a cavity.

If secondary infection supervenes, subperiosteal new bone formation can be seen along the involved bones. The subperiosteal reaction occurs much earlier in pyogenic osteomyelitis. Plaques of irregular (dystrophic) calcification in the wall of a chronic abscess or sinus are almost diagnostic of long-standing tuberculous infection.

Computed axial tomography (CAT) and magnetic resonance imaging (MRI) demonstrate the localisation and extent of bone and soft-tissue lesions, and improve diagnosis of the disease at a very early stage (3–6 weeks).

MRI and bone scintigraphy in the earliest stages reveal 'inflammation' and not 'infection' – just as radioisotope scintigraphy may show a hot area during the active stage of the disease. However it is neither specific, nor does it differentiate between the osseous and soft-tissue pathology (Fig. 10.5). The feathery tubercular sequestra and dystrophic calcification are discernible on CAT scans, but cannot be seen by MRI.

Blood

A relative lymphocytosis, low haemoglobin, and increased erythrocyte sedimentation rate (ESR) are often found in the active stage of disease. A raised ESR, however, is not necessarily proof of activity of the infection. Its repeated estimation at 3–6-month intervals gives a valuable index of the activity of the disease.

Mantoux test

As a rule, a positive result on Mantoux testing is present in a patient infected with tuberculosis for more than one month. A negative test, in general, excludes the disease. Rarely, the tuberculin test may be negative, although active tuberculosis is present, such as in immune deficiency states.

Biopsy

Whenever there is doubt (particularly in the early stages), it is mandatory to prove the diagnosis of tuberculosis by biopsy of the diseased tissue (granulations, synovium, bone or lymph nodes, or the margins of tuberculous ulcers or sinuses). Microscopic examination of an aspiration, core biopsy, needle biopsy or open biopsy will reveal typical tubercles in untreated cases. The presence of epithelioid cells surrounded by lymphocytes, even without central necrosis or peripheral foreign-body giant cells, is adequate histological evidence of tuberculous pathology in a patient who is suspected to be suffering from the disease. At the time of open biopsy of a joint or bone, the orthopaedic surgeon should perform therapeutic synovectomy or curettage.

The infections of bone and joint that present as granulomatous lesions are, in order of frequency: tuberculosis, mycotic infection, brucellosis, sarcoidosis and tuberculoid leprosy.

Guinea pig inoculation

The tuberculous pus, joint aspirate, or diseased material obtained at biopsy is injected intraperitoneally into a guinea pig. Examination in positive cases discloses tubercles on the peritoneum 5–8 weeks later. Although no longer considered a cost-effective test, this is perhaps the most reliable proof of tuberculous pathology.

Smear and culture

The material prepared for guinea pig inoculation may also be submitted for smear and culture examination for acid-fast bacilli.

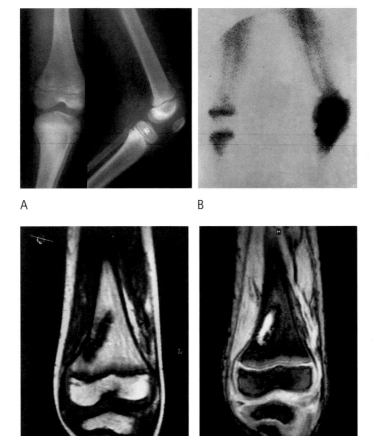

A   B

C   D

Figure 10.5 **A** Anteroposterior and lateral radiographs of the distal end of the femur, showing a lytic lesion in the metaphysis. **B** An isotope bone scan reveals a hot area in the distal part of the thigh and knee, attributable to localised hyperaemia associated with active disease. MRI T1-weighted (**C**) and T2-weighted (**D**) images show that the extent of the disease is greater than suggested radiologically. Histology confirmed the diagnosis of tuberculosis and the disease responded to multidrug treatment.

MANAGEMENT OF OSTEOARTICULAR TUBERCULOSIS

General principles

Modern drugs (see Table 10.2) promote the healing of sinuses, ulcers and abscesses previously resistant to extensive surgery. They also eliminate the danger of postoperative miliary and meningeal disease caused by dissemination of the tuberculous infection.

Death as a result of uncontrolled disease, meningitis, miliary tuberculosis, amyloidosis, paralysis and crippling is now rare. If a patient is diagnosed early and treated vigorously, healing can be accomplished without residual joint ankylosis.

SYMPTOMS

The usual c
anorexia, ni
in temperatu
may develc
Vertebral mt
clinically. N
monitoring a
in the diagr
invariably ir

Pain refer
cholecystitis
tuberculosis
with neural

THE VERTEE

In the majo
characterisec
endplates an
see also Figs
all spinal les
intact for a l

1. The anter
   (Fig. 10.6
2. The poste
   spinous p
3. The centr
   concentri

Rarely, the t
ital or atlant

Abscesses a
Abscesses or
travel along
paraspinal r
gles and the
lumbar spine
the lumbar
inguinal liga

Figure 10.6
central; 3, an
Spondylodisc
involvement

the his
epithel
unrecc
lymph
disapp
advan

Multi
Six n
patien
destru
contin
active
despite
reserv
quinol
in con
85%
regime

1. Lev
   at v
2. BC(
   giv
3. On
   inje
   per
   1 n

SURG

No su
tuberc
adequ
arthrit
arthrit
  Sur
condit
ment,
a mini
any m

Exten
Fusio
cated
lar c
debric
juxta-
despit
of the
tuberc
synov
debric
lesion
opera
infect
Repet

Table 10.4 Main indications for various operations in vertebral tuberculosis
Decompression (± fusion) for neurological complications that fail to respond to 3–6 weeks of conservative treatment or are too advanced.
Debridement (± fusion) for failure of response after 3–6 months of non-operative treatment
Doubtful diagnosis
Fusion for mechanical instability after healing
Debridement ± decompression ± fusion in recurrence of disease or neural complication
Prevention of severe kyphosis by debridement anteriorly + posterior fusion by panvertebral operation in young children with extensive dorsal lesions

Laminectomy has no place in the treatment of tuberculosis of the spine except for extradural granuloma/tuberculoma presenting as 'spinal tumour syndrome', or for a case of old healed disease (without much deformity) presenting with 'vertebral canal stenosis', or refractory posterior spinal disease.

- patients with spinal caries develop neurological complications during conservative treatment
- patients with neurological complications become worse (flaccid paralysis, severe flexor spasm, sphincter disturbance)
- patients suffer a recurrence of neurological complication
- patients with prevertebral cervical abscess develop neurological signs or difficulty in swallowing and breathing.

Because of the efficacy of modern anti-tubercular drugs, the absolute indications for surgical decompression have been reduced to nearly 5% of uncomplicated cases, and to about 60% of those with neurological deficit. An approach to the management of children with vertebral tuberculosis and neural complications is presented in the flow chart (Fig. 10.8).

Radiological healing of vertebral tuberculosis without operation

In patients with early disease in whom the intervertebral spaces are preserved, long-term follow-up reveals that the radiological appearance of the disc space remains intact. At 5 years following the start of disease, patients with classical paradiscal or metaphyseal tubercular spondylitis show the following radiographic appearances: 19% have fibrous, 12% have fibro-osseous, and 69% have osseous replacement of the intervertebral space. Complete destruction of the disc usually results in bony ankylosis.

NEUROLOGICAL COMPLICATIONS

The overall incidence of neurological complications has been reported to be between 10% and 30% in various studies. Disease below the level of the first lumbar vertebra rarely causes paraplegia (Fig. 10.9), which is commonest in

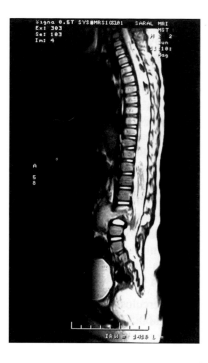

Figure 10.9 MRI of a 2-year-old child who was still walking, despite a destructive lesion of the 3rd lumbar vertebral body, with significant perivertebral and predural abscess formation. Note the arachnoiditis-like changes in the posterior part of cerebrospinal space of the dorsal spine.

tuberculous disease of the lower thoracic region. Tetraplegia from cervical involvement is less common. The youngest child to have been reported as having tuberculous paraplegia was 1 year old (Tuli 1991).

Tuberculous paraplegia has been classified into two main groups (Griffiths et al 1956):

1. *Early onset paraplegia* occurs within the first 2 years of the disease. The underlying pathology includes inflammatory oedema, granulation tissue, caseating abscess or the (rare) ischaemic cord lesion.
2. *Late onset paraplegia* develops more than 2 years after the vertebral infection. Neurological complications may result from recrudescence of the disease or mechanical pressure on the cord. Compression results from tuberculous caseous tissue, tubercular debris, sequestra from vertebral body and disc, internal gibbus, stenosis of the vertebral canal or severe deformity.

A more rational classification is paraplegia associated with 'active disease' or with 'healed disease'. In most early-onset paraplegia associated with active disease, inflammation causes compression and the prognosis for recovery is favourable. The basic pathology in most cases of late onset paraplegia associated with healed disease is mechanical. Surgical removal of mechanical compression is mandatory, but the prognosis is less favourable. The usual pathology responsible for neurological complications is shown in order of frequency in Table 10.5.

Myelography and imaging

When there is little difficulty in determining the level of cord compression from clinical, neurological and radiological examination, myelography is considered unnecessary. However, in cases of paraplegia without radiological

Table 10.5 Usual causes of neurological complications in tuberculosis of the spine

Inflammatory

1.	Inflammatory oedema	Recovers with rest and drug therapy
2.	Tuberculous granulation tissue	Mostly recovers with rest and drug therapy
3.	Tuberculous abscess	Recovers with conservative therapy; rarely requires evacuation and decompression
4.	Tuberculous caseous tissue	May subside with conservative therapy; sometimes requires evacuation and decompression

Mechanical

5.	Tubercular debris	Solid debris requires operative removal and decompression
6.	Sequestra from vertebral body and disc	Require operative removal and decompression
7.	Constriction of cord due to stenosis of vertebral canal	Requires operative decompression
8.	Localised pressure due to angulation (internal gibbus) along anterior wall of vertebral canal	Requires operative decompression

Intrinsic

9.	Prolonged stretching of the cord over a severe deformity	(i) Stretched cord may be more vulnerable to other causes; then decompression, release of cord, and anterior transposition may lead to recovery
		(ii) Rarely, stretching leads to interstitial gliosis, syrinx formation or atrophy of cord (difficult to prove/disprove), does not recover, probably seen as myelomalacia on MRI
10.	Infective thrombosis/endarteritis of spinal vessels	Difficult to prove/disprove; does not recover, probably seen as myelomalacia on MRI
11.	Pathological dislocation of spine	Rare complication, usually results from rough manipulation by masseur or panvertebral lesion or indiscriminate laminectomy for crisis spine; irreparable severance of cord
12.	Tuberculous meningomyelitis	Difficult to prove/disprove; myelitis seen on MRI does not recover completely
13.	Syringomyelic changes	Seen on MRI; poor recovery

Spinal tumour syndrome

14.	Diffuse extradural granuloma or tuberculoma or peridural fibrosis	Present as spinal tumour syndrome; surgical approach is by laminectomy

As a rule more than one cause may be acting in the same case. MRI, whenever available, can demonstrate atrophy of cord, myelomalacia, syringomyelia, infarction and arachnoiditis in cases that fail to recover despite adequate surgical decompression.

evidence of the disease, as in 'spinal tumour syndrome', or in cases with multiple vertebral lesions, myelography is helpful in determining the level of obstruction. Another situation in which myelography is indicated arises when a patient has not recovered after surgical decompression. A myelographic block indicates inadequate mechanical decompression and warrants a second decompression. If a block is not present, failure to recover may be due to intrinsic damage to the cord. Myelography is now being replaced by MRI scanning: T2-weighted images give a myelographic effect, although a block to the flow of contrast medium obviously cannot be portrayed.

Prognosis for recovery of cord function

Recovery depends on many factors (Table 10.6). However, treatment should never be withheld, as there are many patients with advanced disease who partially recover after a satisfactory mechanical decompression.

Treatment of Pott's paraplegia

The prevention of paraplegia in tuberculous disease of the spine is of paramount importance. In the usual paradiscal

lesion the anterior cord is compressed. Decompression is achieved through an anterior or an anterolateral approach. Laminectomy is contraindicated, as it provides inadequate decompression and renders the vertebral column unstable. The role of costotransversectomy is extremely limited; it

Table 10.6 Clinical factors influencing prognosis in cord involvement

Cord involvement	Better prognosis	Relatively poor prognosis
Degree	Partial	Complete
Duration	Shorter	Longer (>12 months)
Type	'Early onset'	'Late onset'
Speed of onset	Slow	Rapid
Age	Younger	Older
General condition	Good	Poor
Vertebral disease	Active	Healed
Kyphotic deformity	<60°	>60°
MRI	Healthy cord	Myelomalacia ± syringomyelia
Operative findings	Wet lesion	Dry lesion

first trimester. In a large general hospital in Malaysia, among an annual average of 20 new cases of syphilis, eight to 10 infants present with congenital syphilis. Antenatal check-ups in most tropical countries routinely include screening for syphilis.

The infant presents with pseudoparalysis and swollen joints in the first 4 months of life. Hepatosplenomegaly, anaemia, desquamating skin lesions on the hands and soles of the feet, and systemic illness develop. The primary skeletal involvement is a bilaterally symmetric polyostotic condition, with moth-eaten rarefaction of the diaphysis and erosive or exuberant callus in the metaphysis. Dactylitis of the hands and feet is also seen. Pathological fractures occur in the destructive lesions. The presentation is very similar to the battered baby syndrome (Rasool & Govender 1989).

Treatment of congenital syphilis in hospitals includes immobilisation of fractures and antibiotic therapy with procaine penicillin 10 000 U/kg per day for 10 days.

FUNGAL INFECTION OF BONE

Fungal infections of bone are rare in South-East Asian countries, but are encountered in India, Egypt and Africa. The mycotic infection is acquired by inhalation or inoculation through the skin. Actinomycosis (caused by *Actinomyces israelii*) and maduramycosis are the two common fungal infections of bone. The infection spreads locally, blood-borne only in actinomycosis, and occasionally in the lymphatics in maduramycosis.

Maduramycosis is caused by *Nocardia madurae*, a saprophyte in soil and plants. The infection, which affects the hands and feet, is seen periodically in India, Sudan, Somalia, Ethiopia, West Africa and Central and South American countries. Treatment is with dapsone (diamino-diphenylsulphone) 100 mg twice daily for 2 years.

MUSCULOSKELETAL TUMOURS

In developing countries, about 40% of the population is younger than 15 years of age. The impact of malignant cancers is lessened by the high mortality from serious infections, parasitic diseases, and malnutrition. Childhood cancers account for fewer than 10% of all malignancies in tropical countries. Accurate data are not available, as there has only recently been a move to establish cancer registries in most countries in the region.

Among the common childhood tumours are Burkitt's tumour, neuroblastoma, retinoblastoma and nephroblastoma. Leukaemia is recognised as the most common tumour (35%) in children younger than 15 years. Other tumours affecting the musculoskeletal system involve the central nervous system (17%), sympathetic nervous system (10%), soft-tissues (10%) and bone (4%).

Spinal tumours in children are rare, and form less than 1% of all childhood cancers; 60% present before the age of 6 years, and malignant neuroblastomas make up 75% of them.

After the age of 6 years, the common spinal tumour is aneurysmal bone cyst.

Malignant tumours such as osteosarcoma, chondrosarcoma and Ewing's sarcoma are encountered periodically, along with benign bone tumours such as osteochondroma and osteoma (see Ch. 13).

OSTEOSARCOMA

Osteosarcoma ranks as the most common malignant bone tumour in children and adolescents; the distal femur accounts for 30% of cases. The incidence per million of the population in Nigeria, Uganda and Fiji ranges from 37 to 128. The incidence per million of population in the 0–14-years age group is 27 in India, 36 in the Philippines, 30 in Hong Kong, 48 for Singapore Chinese and 31 for Singapore Malays. In an epidemiological study carried out in Malaysia, the incidence per 100 000 population per year was 0.11 for ethnic Malays, 0.23 for Chinese and 0.23 for Indians. These figures are comparable to the incidence in Sweden of 0.28 per 100 000.

Children with osteosarcoma frequently present late, after traditional treatment with massage, herbal fomentation and spiritual exhortations. The tumours by then assume considerable dimensions and sometimes ulcerate and fungate. On occasion, patients come to hospital in a very serious condition, only to refuse the offer of what may be no more than palliative surgery, aimed at reducing their persistent discomfort and pain and improving the quality of their remaining life (Fig. 11.11).

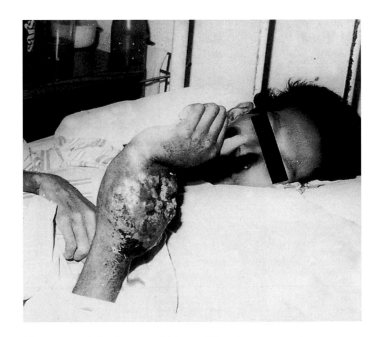

Figure 11.11 A 13-year-old boy with osteosarcoma in an unusual site. He was admitted three times before this photograph was taken, refusing amputation each time. On the occasion of this photograph, there were metastases in his axillary nodes and the lungs.

EWING'S SARCOMA

Ewing's sarcoma is a malignant, small, round-cell tumour of bone arising from medullary reticulo-endothelial supportive tissue. It affects flat bones, such as the scapula, in addition to the long bones. It is rare in black Africans and black African-Americans, Chinese and Japanese. In tropical countries, the range of incidence for children younger than 14 years is 7–36 per million. Classically described as arising from the diaphysis of long bones, the tumour may also develop at the metaphysis. Children present with a febrile illness similar to acute osteomyelitis. Tissue biopsy is important to establish the diagnosis.

SOFT-TISSUE TUMOURS

The cumulative incidence of soft-tissue sarcomas in tropical countries is in the range of 34–130 per million, with an upper-scale incidence in Nigeria, Uganda and Zimbabwe. The main soft-tissue tumour encountered is rhabdomyosarcoma. The embryonic variety affects the small muscles of the hand (Fig. 11.12), foot and the inner ear. The prognosis is extremely poor.

MISCELLANEOUS CONDITIONS

POST-INJECTION FIBROSIS OF MUSCLES

Post-injection fibrosis of muscles is an iatrogenic, intramuscular complication of repeated injections administered during infancy or childhood, and is periodically seen in tropical countries. In contracture of the extensor mechanism of the knee, children present with knee stiffness or genu recurvatum, and a variable degree of anterior tibial subluxation. The history in some cases suggests that the disability was present at birth, but most often the limitation of movement is noticed at 2 or 3 years of age, often following an illness during which injections have been given (Gunn 1969). The injection would have been given repeatedly into the thigh, usually between the ages of 6 months and 2 years, for diseases such as tuberculosis, poliomyelitis, enteritis, tetanus or protracted febrile illnesses. The condition must be distinguished from habitual dislocation of the patella and congenital conditions causing limitation of knee flexion. Knee stiffness varies from gross limitation to less than 30°. The child with contracture of the extensor mechanism compensates by lateral displacement of the patella to achieve flexion, with resultant instability of the knee (Bose & Chong 1976).

The muscles affected are commonly the vasti lateralis and intermedius and, less often, the rectus femoris and the iliotibial band. The fibrotic change is maximal at about the mid-thigh or just distal, but rarely proximal, to it. Surgical release and excision of the fibrotic area followed by intensive physical therapy will achieve up to 90° of flexion, sometimes after repeated operations. Postoperative extensor lag, however, may remain for some time (Sengupta 1985).

Other muscles involved in post-injection fibrosis are the deltoid, which leads to abduction–internal rotation contracture of the shoulder, and the gluteal muscles, producing atrophic buttocks and abduction contracture of the hip and, sometimes, pelvic tilt. These are also treated by excision of fibrotic muscle segments, followed by stretching and intensive physical therapy.

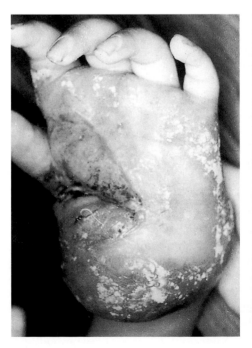
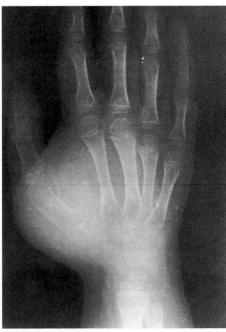

Fig. 11.12 Embryonic rhabdomyosarcoma in the left hand of a 6-year-old girl. The parents refused amputation at the time of initial diagnosis. **A** Appearance of the hand 1 year later after topical herbal application, 2 weeks before the child succumbed to massive, widespread systemic metastases. **B** X-ray of the hand.

A

B

PERTHES' DISEASE

There is a significant geographical variation in the incidence of Perthes' disease, influenced by socioeconomic factors. It is frequent in dark-skinned people, aborigines, American Indians and Polynesians. An epidemiological study in South India found an incidence of 4.4 per 100 000 children in Udupi, on the west coast – 10 times more than that in Vellore on the east but lower than in southern England (6.6 per 100 000 children). This regional study in India concluded that Perthes' disease occurred more commonly in the south-west coastal plains of the Indian subcontinent, more in the rural than in the urban settings, and in children of an older age group (Joseph et al 1988).

Studies in the UK have found the condition to be more common in the lower socioeconomic classes and in children born to manual labourers. This finding, however, does not explain the low incidence of Perthes' disease in many countries in the tropics with low socioeconomic status, and implies that other genetic and environmental factors are involved (see Ch. 25).

IDIOPATHIC SCOLIOSIS

Infantile and juvenile scoliosis in most tropical countries is less common than in developed countries. A study in Johannesburg reported an incidence of 2.5% in white populations and 0.03% in Bantus. The incidence of scoliosis in schoolchildren in Jerusalem, with curves of more than 10%, was 1.5% in a group of 10 000 children aged 10–16-years. The reported prevalence in developed countries ranges between 1.6% and 4.6% in children of susceptible age.

A Singapore study using the forward-bending test and a standing radiograph of the spine, and taking a curve of more than 5° as positive, showed the prevalence of scoliosis to range from 0.1% for boys in the 6–7-year age group to 3.2% for girls in the 16–17-year age group. The survey also determined the ethnic distribution of idiopathic scoliosis in Singapore, and reported 3.5% for Chinese, 1.7% for ethnic Malays and 1.7% for girls in the 16–17-year age group (Daruwalla et al 1985).

Children usually report late for treatment (Fig. 11.13), possibly because parents do not detect the spinal curvatures early. This may be related, to some extent, to cultural requirements for children, particularly girls, to be fully covered at all times, at home and even during games and sports activities.

JUVENILE IDIOPATHIC ARTHRITIS

There appears to be wide variation in the incidence and severity of polyarticular arthritis, particularly rheumatoid arthritis, in tropical countries, but there are no community-based studies available. Data collected in the Mayo Clinic provided an incidence of 13.9 cases per 100 000 per year (Towner et al 1983). A hospital-based study in Kuala Lumpur, Malaysia, revealed an incidence of 7.2 per 10 000

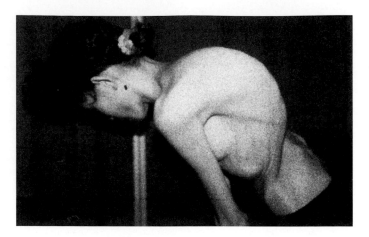

Figure 11.13 Idiopathic right thoracic scoliosis in a 15-year-old girl. No medical consultation or treatment had been sought.

paediatric admission under 13 years of age; the mean age at presentation was 7.03 years and ranged from 1 to 14 years (Cheah 1996). In India, the prevalence of juvenile idiopathic arthritis was one-sixth that of adult rheumatoid arthritis and the median age of onset was 8.8 years (Agarwall & Misra 1994). There appears to be a preponderance of males afflicted in India, Thailand and Malaysia, but in the West, girls are more affected.

Juvenile idiopathic arthritis is the most frequent major connective tissue disease in children (see Ch. 12). It is one of the more common chronic illnesses of childhood and a major cause of functional disability and eye disease – chronic anterior uveitis – leading to blindness (Cheah 1996). The disease in tropical Africa is more benign than in temperate zones; in South-East Asian countries, the disease tends to be intermediate in severity.

HAEMOPHILIC PSEUDOTUMOUR

Haemophilic pseudotumours are rare, and occur in 1% of patients with severe factor VIII or IX deficiency (see Ch. 8). These swellings are enlarging, encapsulated pseudotumours produced by recurrent bleeding, and may be purely within the fascial envelope of muscle or in the subperiosteal region, immediately adjacent to the bone, causing bony erosion by interference with the periosteal blood supply. They may also develop within the bone itself, destroying its architecture. The tumours often occur in the ilium and femur in adults, but in children the lesion is more common in the small bones of the hands and feet (Ibrahim et al 1994) (Fig. 11.14).

Early cases of haemophilic pseudotumour can be treated by compression, immobilisation and factor replacement therapy, but needle aspiration or evacuation of the haematoma should be avoided, as these may lead to wound breakdown, chronic fistula or secondary infection. There is a risk of sarcomatous change and, in children, growth-plate damage. When necessary, excision or amputation should be carried out, with meticulous attention to surgical technique and haemostasis. The factor VIII concentration must be

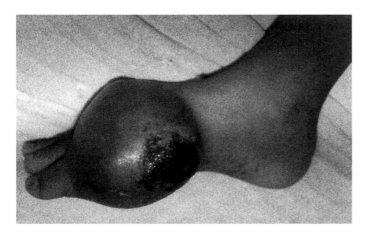

Figure 11.14 Haemophilic pseudotumour of the foot in a 10-year-old boy, caused by poor control of haemophilia.

maintained at 100% or more during surgery, and 50–60% until wound healing is complete.

SNAKE BITES

Snakes are cosmopolitan in distribution, other than in the Arctic and Antarctic regions. They thrive best in damp and humid areas of the world, such as the tropics. The types of snakes seen in the tropics are reticulated pythons, cobras and the krait in South-East Asia, India and Africa.

Most snakes are poisonous and the venom, which is a complex mixture of enzymatic proteins and different toxins, is classified as either haemotoxic or neurotoxic; it may cause severe illness and sudden death. Symptoms generally include swelling, discolouration and severe pain at the site of the bite. Skin necrosis may occur eventually (Fig. 11.15). Victims may feel weak and dizzy, perspire heavily and experience nausea and vomiting – all being symptoms of shock. Early administration of anti-venom may help to neutralise the venom.

A 5-year study in Kelantan, a state on the north-east coast of the Malaysian peninsula, recorded the admission to a general hospital of 83 children between the ages of 6 months and 12 years, with bites mainly from elapids, fewer from vipers, and none from sea-snakes. Anti-venom was administered only when indicated, as there was also a high possibility of adverse reactions to the serum. The study recorded two deaths from snake venom (Tan et al 1990).

In a study carried out in one district in West Bengal, India, there were 31 deaths among a total of 307 victims of snake bites (Hati et al 1992). More than 65% of the victims had received treatment from *ozahs* (traditional healers).

ORTHOPAEDIC TRAUMA

The WHO predicts that by the year 2020, trauma will be the first or second leading cause of years of life lost in both developed and developing countries. On the basis of current

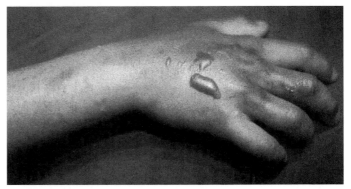

A

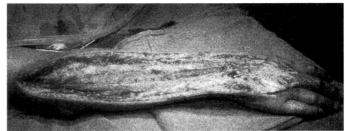

B

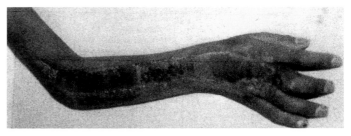

C

Figure 11.15 A The dorsal aspect of the forearm of a 10-year-old boy who was bitten by a snake, showing bite marks at the middle finger, bullous eruptions and ascending thrombophlebitis. Necrosis of the extensor compartment followed a few days later (**B**), requiring extensive debridement and split-skin grafting (**C**).

population projection there are about 190 million disabled children in the world. Three-quarters of disabled children lived in developing countries in 1975, but by the year 2000 this proportion is expected to be four-fifths.

More children are injured in the home and its environs than on the road. The common supracondylar fracture results from children falling at home or on the playing field. In the tropics, children also fall from fruit trees – particularly the rambutan tree, which bears a fleshy fruit with a hairy skin, and which is too slender to take even the weight of a child. Fractures in patients from the rural areas are often treated by traditional bone-setters and healers, with massage and herbal pastes, both of which increase the swelling and sometimes cause local skin reactions (see Fig. 11.5). When these patients finally reach hospital with deformities and complications the salvage treatment is difficult and prolonged, and the final functional result at best is just acceptable.

Face and hand injuries occur during festive seasons, when children play with firecrackers or home-made explosive devices.

NON-ACCIDENTAL INJURIES

Non-accidental injury to children as a result of child abuse (the battered baby syndrome) is a social malady and often poorly recognised in the casualty department. The abused children present, understandably, with severe physical and emotional distress, and are withdrawn and sullen. There were 776 cases of child abuse admitted to the General Hospital, Kuala Lumpur, during the period 1985–1991. Physical abuse accounted for 55.5% of the cases in children younger than 5 years. Orthopaedic injuries included multiple fractures, intracranial injuries and cuts and bruises, in addition to burns and scalds inflicted with lit cigarette ends, hot irons, and boiling water. Among the 41 deaths (5.3%) in this series, the most common cause was intracranial haemorrhage. Usually the suspected perpetrators were the natural parents, acting together or individually (Krishnan et al 1994).

Adults are imprisoned if found guilty by the legal process. The abused children are returned to their parents after counselling, or to the care of relatives or professionals.

ROAD TRAFFIC ACCIDENTS

The incidence of fatalities from road traffic accidents in most tropical countries varies between 0.12 and 0.81 per 10 000 population. The major vehicle involved in road traffic accidents in Malaysia, Thailand and the Philippines is the motorcycle. In 1998, 49% of all road traffic accidents in Malaysia involved motorcycles, and 46% (or 3291) of deaths were accounted for by motorcycle riders or pillion riders, compared with 26.4% accidents involving motorcars and 23.4% (or 799) deaths of drivers or passengers in cars. The number of children younger than 15 years who died as a result of road traffic accidents in Malaysia in 1988 was 373, representing 15% of the total number of fatalities. The figure decreased slightly to 233 in 1998. Children are also fatally injured as pedestrians on the road: in 1998, 167 children younger than 15 years died, among a total of 668 pedestrian deaths. Those who survive road traffic accidents sustain the entire range of fractures and severe soft tissue injuries.

Morbidity and mortality from road traffic accidents are a matter of serious concern in most developing countries, because of the great increase in the number of vehicles, with inadequate development of thoroughfares, careless and speeding drivers, and poor enforcement of existing laws. Safety belt restraints are mandatory for the driver and the front-seat passenger in cars, but there are no specific regulations for children and infants. It is common to see children travelling in the front seats, and infants with no harness, being held by adults. Public transport is also unsafe and poorly controlled.

Light motorcycles in tropical countries provide a cheap and convenient form of transport for the riders to move quickly through crowded roads and tracks. Although the legal age for obtaining a motorcycle licence is 17 years, children younger than that are known to ride motorcycles – a practice that often ends in severe fractures and head injury, and sometimes with loss of life. Children and infants are often sandwiched between parents, on a motorcycle, although the law forbids more than two riders on such vehicles. Safety helmets are mandatory, but quality control of the helmets is poor, and riders often wear them incompletely fastened. Persons wearing turbans or *Haji* caps are excused from the obligation to wear safety helmets, and heat and humidity also discourage riders from wearing heavy protective gear.

WORKPLACE ACCIDENTS

The International Labour Organisation (ILO) Convention 138 (1973) on the subject of child labour stipulated that the minimum age for employment was 15 years. These laws are often flouted, as the socioeconomic status of families requires children to supplement their income and in many situations children are the sole breadwinners. Working children are exposed to biological, chemical, physical and psychosocial hazards.

The ILO estimates the number of working children between 5–14 years of age, world-wide, to be 120 million, the majority of them in developing countries: 61% in Asia, 32% in Africa and 7% in Latin America. Rapid mechanisation in urban and agricultural industries has been responsible for many injuries, not only amongst children in family industries and workshops. In India, where 50% of the labour force are women, some 20% of the working children in the 10–14-year age group are girls (Srivastava, personal communication 1988). Long hours of work and exhaustion contribute to accidents in the workplace, and the injuries mainly involve upper limbs, particularly the hand (see Fig. 11.1). Children employed in construction and heavy industries suffer a variety of musculoskeletal injuries, including fractures and spinal injuries. Fishing at sea or in rivers using explosives also produces serious physical injuries (Fig. 11.16) or drowning.

LANDMINE INJURIES

Landmines or booby traps are primarily designed to maim and mutilate rather than cause instant death and for this reason are described as weapons that kill in slow motion. It is estimated that there are 100 000 000 mines strewn across 64 war-torn countries, including Angola, Ethiopia, Iraq, Kuwait, Laos, Mozambique, Myanmar, Somalia, Sudan, Vietnam, Uganda, Sri Lanka, Cambodia, and the former Yugoslavia. Landmines affect the lives and livelihoods of more than 26 000 innocent people every year, with one casualty occurring every 20 minutes. In Angola, about 1.5%

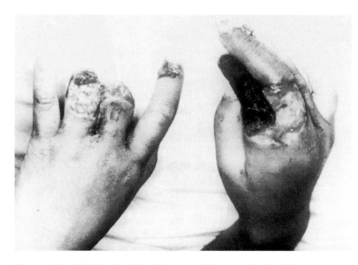

Figure 11.16 Hands of a 14-year-old boy who had been fishing using explosives.

of the population has been injured by mines and unexploded devices. One Angolan in 334 is an amputee. In Cambodia, one person in every 236 has lost a leg, hand or eye (Global Health Watch 1997). During the conflict in Somalia, two-thirds of mine-injured persons were combatant soldiers; after the cessation of fighting, however, 90% of casualties were among civilians, and 75% of these were between the ages of 5 and 15 years (Grant 1997).

Children are more likely to detonate mines and sustain injuries, for a number of reasons. Young children do not understand the signs that mark known minefields. They tend to 'explore' areas beyond cleared tracks and paths, and set off mines while playing in the fields. Because they are small and the body is closer to the landmines, children sustain more serious bodily harm (Fig. 11.17). It is estimated that 85% of child victims of landmines never reach a hospital.

Some landmines are designed to look like toys: during the Afghan conflict, brightly coloured land mines shaped like

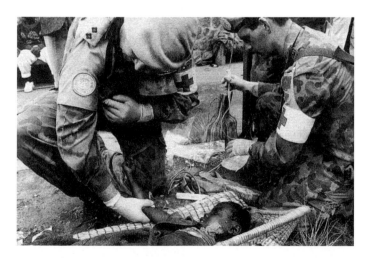

Figure 11.17 UN medical soldiers attend to a child wounded by a landmine, outside the Central Hospital in Kigali, Rwanda. (Source/Photographer: UNICEF/94–0454/Betty Press).

butterflies were strewn from the air, the ulterior motive probably being to injure children specifically, and indirectly create emotional and psychological stress in the adult population (Fig. 11.18). Although there are world-wide aid organisations seeking to rehabilitate child victims of landmines, a more concerted international commitment is needed to ban the use of these mines.

AMPUTATIONS IN CHILDREN

Amputation in children, for whatever reason, is an unfortunate and heart-breaking event. However, amputations for non-fatal diseases, besides those caused by landmines, are required with alarming frequency in many developing countries. In a study of amputations carried out in the General Hospital, Kuala Lumpur, among children and young adults younger than 18 years, tumour and trauma contributed to 15% of all major lower limb amputations (Abdul-Hamid & Han, 1988). A report from Tanzania analysing 49 amputations in children younger than 18 years gave the following breakdown: complications after medical treatment for osteomyelitis 12, burns 9, bone tumours 8, hyena and snake bite gangrene 7, and idiopathic tropical lower-limb gangrene 4. Of the nine amputations for burns, four were in toddlers injured by open cooking fires at floor

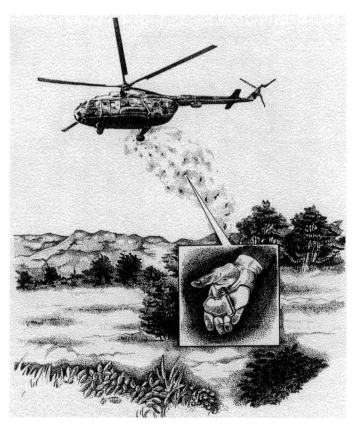

Figure 11.18 The 'butterfly' anti-personnel mine, brightly coloured and dropped from aeroplanes, becomes activated on landing on the ground. Kicking or stepping on it causes the mine to explode.

level in huts. The amputations following osteomyelitis were in children in whom aggressive sequestrectomy had been carried out in the acute stage of the infection, leading to extensive bone loss (Loro et al 1994).

ACKNOWLEDGEMENTS

The authors record with gratitude the assistance rendered by Professor S Sengupta (Department of Orthopaedics, University of Malaya), Dr K S Sivananthan (Fatimah Hospital, Ipoh, Perak, Malaysia), Dr M Subramaniam (Consultant Plastic Surgeon, Ipoh, Malaysia), and Dr V K Pillay (Singapore), who have provided clinical material for inclusion in this chapter. We also thank Mr Alias Omar (Orthopaedic Department) and the staff of the Medical Illustrations Department of the Faculty of Medicine, University Kebangsaan Malaysia, for their assistance in preparing the illustrations.

REFERENCES AND FURTHER READING

Abdul-Hamid Abdul-Kadir 1986 Correction of claw fingers in leprosy by the Brand four-tailed tendon graft operation. The Medical Journal of Malaysia 41: 264–268

Abdul-Hamid Abdul-Kadir, Myint Han 1988 Major lower limb amputations. Medical Journal of Malaysia 43: 218–223

Adeyemo A A, Akindele J A, Omokhodion S I 1993 Klebsiella septicaemia, osteomyelitis and septic arthritis in neonates in Ibadan, Nigeria. Annals of Tropical Paediatrics 13: 285–289

Agarwall A, Misra R 1994 Juvenile chronic arthritis in India: is it different from that seen in Western countries? Rheumatology International 14: 53–56

Belsey M A 1993 Child abuse: measuring a global problem. World Health Statistics 46: 69

Bose K, Chong K C 1976 The clinical manifestation and pathomechanics of contracture of the extensor mechanisms of the knee joint. Journal of Bone and Joint Surgery 58B: 478–484

Bovil E G, Silva J F, Subramaniam N 1975 An epidemiological study of osteogenic sarcoma in Malaysia. Clinical Orthopaedics and Related Research 113: 119–127

Brand P W 1958 Paralytic claw hand. Journal of Bone and Joint Surgery 40B: 618–625

Chacha P B 1970 Muscle abscesses in children. Clinical Orthopaedics and Related Research 70: 174–180

Cheah Y K 1996 Juvenile chronic arthritis – University Hospital experience 1980–1994 Masters Thesis in Paediatrics, University of Malaya

Daruwalla J S, Balasubramaniam P, Chay S O, Rajan U, Lee H P 1985 Idiopathic scoliosis: prevalence and ethnic distribution in Singapore school children. Journal of Bone and Joint Surgery 67B: 182–184

Global Health Watch 1997 Landmines: a global health crisis. In: (eds) The landmine epidemic. IPPNW Global Health Watch Report No. 2

Gomez V R 1996 Clubfeet in congenital annular constricting bands. Clinical Orthopaedics and Related Research 323: 155–162

Govender S, Chotai P R 1990 Salmonella osteitis and septic arthritis. Journal of Bone and Joint Surgery 72B: 504–506

Grant J P 1997 War, children and the responsibility of the international community. In: Levy B S, Sidel V W, (eds) War and public health. Oxford University Press (in cooperation with the American Public Health Association), New York, pp 12–24

Gunn D R 1964 Contracture of the quadriceps muscle. Journal of Bone and Joint Surgery 46B: 492–497

Gunn D R 1969 Orthopaedic surgery in South and East Asia. University of Malaya Press, Singapore

Halder D, Quah B S, Malik A S, Choo K E 1996 Neonatal septic arthritis. South-East Asian Journal of Tropical Medicine and Public Health 27: 600–605

Hati A K, Mandal M, De M K 1992 Epidemiology of snake bite in the district of Burdwan, West Bengal. Journal of the Indian Medical Association 90: 145–147

Hodgson A R, Skinsnes O K, Leong J C Y 1967 Pathogenesis of Pott's paraplegia. Journal of Bone and Joint Surgery 49A: 1147–1156

Huckstep R L 1979 Poliomyelitis: a guide for developing countries. ELBS/Churchill Livingstone, Edinburgh

Ibrahim S, Noor M A, Dhillon M 1994 Haemophilic pseudotumour of the foot – a case report. Journal of Orthopaedic Surgery 2: 71–74

Ismail H I, Lal M 1993 Poliomyelitis in Malaysia – two confirmed cases after 6 years without polio. Annals of Tropical Paediatrics 13: 339–343

Joseph B, Chacko V, Rao B S, Hall A J 1988 The epidemiology of Perthes' disease in South India. International Journal of Epidemiology 17: 603–607

Krishnan R, Rivara F, Arokiasamy J 1994 Child abuse in injuries in Malaysia (monograph), pp 73–85

Lavy C B D, Lavy V R 1995 Salmonella septic arthritis in Zambian children. Tropical Doctor 1995: 163–166

Loro A, Franceschi F, Lago A D 1994 The reasons for amputation in children (0–18 years) in a developing country. Tropical Doctor 24: 99–102

Meleney F L 1933 A differential diagnosis between certain types of infectious gangrene of the skin. Surgery, Gynecology and Obstetrics 56: 847–867

Mok P M, Reilly B J, Ash J M 1982 Osteomyelitis in the neonate. Radiology 145: 677–682

Molyneux E M, French G 1982 Salmonella joint infection in Malawian children. Journal of Infection 4: 131–138

Omene J A, Odita J C, Okolo A A 1984 Neonatal osteomyelitis in Nigerian infants. Paediatric Radiology 14: 318–322

Parkin D M, Stiller C A, Terracini B, Young J L (eds) 1988 International incidence of childhood cancer. IARC Scientific Publication WHO, Geneva

Pillay V K, Hesketh K T 1965 Intra-uterine amputations and annular limb defects in Singapore. Journal of Bone and Joint Surgery 47B: 514–519

Rasool M N, Govender S 1989 The skeletal manifestations of congenital syphilis. Journal of Bone and Joint Surgery 71B: 752–755

Razak M, Nasiruddin J 1998 An epidemiological study of septic arthritis in Kuala Lumpur Hospital. The Medical Journal of Malaysia 53 (Suppl): 86–94

Royal Malaysian Police 1998 Statistics on road crashes. Royal Malaysian Police, Kuala Lumpur

Saez-Llorens X, Velarde J, Canton C 1994 Paediatric osteomyelitis in Panama. Clinical Infectious Diseases 19: 323–324

Sengupta S 1981 Congenital annular defects. Malaysian Journal of Surgery 6: 11–17

Sengupta S 1985a Musculoskeletal lesions in yaws. Clinical Orthopaedics and Related Research 192: 193–198

Sengupta S 1985b Pathogenesis of infantile quadriceps fibrosis and its correction by proximal release. Journal of Pediatric Orthopaedics 5: 187–191

Shanmugasundaram T K 1983 Bone and joint tuberculosis. Kothandaram, Madras

Shanmugasundaram T K 1985 Current concepts in bone and joint tuberculosis. Kumudam, Madras

Sivananthan K S 1975 Congenital constriction bands and intra-uterine amputations. MChOrth Thesis, University of Liverpool

Soosai A P, Cheah I G S, Lim N L, Lim A, Ibrahim S B 1995 Group B beta-haemolytic streptococcus – a rare cause of neonatal necrotising fasciitis. Malaysian Journal of Child Health 1: 66–69

Stover E, Cobey J C, Fine J 1997 The public health effects of land mines: long-term consequences for civilians. In: Levy S B, Sidel V W (eds) War and public health. Oxford University Press (in cooperation with American Public Health Association), New York, pp 137–146

Tan K K, Choo K E, Ariffin W A 1990 Snake bite in Kelantanese children: a five-year experience. Toxicon 28: 225–230

Torpin R, Knoblich RR 1969 Foetal malformations of amniotic origin. Journal of Medical Associations of Georgia 58: 126–127

Towner S R, Michet C J Jr, O'Fallon W M, Nelson AM 1983 The epidemiology of juvenile rheumatoid arthritis in Rochester, Minnesota. Arthritis and Rheumatology 26: 1208–1213

Tuli S M 1975 Tuberculosis of the spine. Amerind, New Dehi/New York

World Health Statistics 1988 WHO, Geneva

World Health Report 1998 Life in the 21st century: a vision for all. WHO, Geneva

Chapter 12   JUVENILE IDIOPATHIC ARTHRITIS

M. Swann

INTRODUCTION

Because of its relative rarity, juvenile chronic arthritis continues to cause confusion regarding its nature and patterns (Fig. 12.1). Some surgeons still refer to it as Still's disease (a generic title for all varieties of the condition), whereas others believe it is a form of rheumatoid arthritis in children. In fact, George Frederick Still (1896) described a subgroup of the condition with systemic features.

Juvenile chronic arthritis is a heterogeneous group of diseases of unknown cause. However, it is generally considered that these disease are autoimmune in origin, with well-documented associations with genetic markers. There are no specific tests to pinpoint the diagnosis, but there is evidence of inflammation reflected in the increased erythrocyte sedimentation rate and C-reactive protein concentration.

In the USA, the term 'juvenile rheumatoid arthritis' is preferred. In Europe, the term 'juvenile chronic arthritis' has been accepted until recently. However, this has now given way to the term 'juvenile idiopathic arthritis' (Ansell 1998). The orthopaedic surgeon's perspective would have been best served by naming this group of diseases 'juvenile idiopathic chronic arthritis'. The following criteria are required for the diagnosis (Wood 1982): there must be a persistent arthritis of one or more joints lasting 3 months or longer in a patient younger than 16 years at disease onset, and other known and identifiable causes of persistent arthritis must be excluded. The 'other causes' are so important to the surgeon handling these patients that they are listed here:

1. Septic arthritis and post-infective arthropathies.
2. Non-rheumatological conditions such as Perthes' disease and osteochondritis dissecans.
3. Arthropathies associated with specific, non-rheumatological disease, including haematological disorders, villonodular synovitis, haemangiomata, immunological abnormalities and neoplastic diseases.
4. Distinct conditions affecting the musculoskeletal system, including systemic lupus erythematosus, polymyositis and dermatomyositis.
5. Acute rheumatic fever.

Epidemiological studies in Great Britain suggest that about one child in 5000 younger than 16 years will suffer an episode of swelling in one or more joints and meet the criteria for juvenile idiopathic arthritis. The long-term prognosis is favourable: about 75% of the children will undergo remission or heal without serious joint damage. The persistence of active disease greatly influences the prognosis.

CLASSIFICATION

The simple classification to be described has been expanded by the 1999 task force of the International League Against Rheumatism to include seven different types of disease. However, this is unnecessarily confusing and unhelpful for the orthopaedic surgeon, who would be wise to adopt a more practical approach, whereby juvenile idiopathic arthritis may be broadly classified into three subgroups according to the mode of onset. This is important, because of their differing complications and varying prognosis (Ansell & Swann 1983). The presentation may be as a systemic illness followed by a persistent arthritis, as a polyarthritis at onset with five or more joints affected within the first 3 months of the illness, or as pauci-articular arthritis with fewer than five joints involved. The last is the most common, accounting for approximately 50% of cases. The features of these subgroups vary as follows.

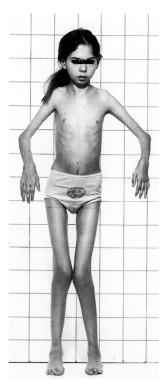

Figure 12.1 This 12-year-old patient developed seronegative polyarthritis at 2 years of age. She has had multiple joints affected, some of which remain swollen (such as the fingers), whereas others have developed contractures. Note the underdeveloped jaw, rigid cervical spine, contractures and deformities of the arm joints. There are adduction and flexion contractures of the hips associated with femoral neck anteversion. The patellae are squinting and there is a secondary lumbar lordosis. Genu valgum has developed together with secondary external tibial torsion. The feet are rigid and in varus.

SYSTEMIC ILLNESS

This represents the subgroup described by Still. The systemic illness affects boys and girls equally, with the most common age of onset between the first and fourth birthdays. It is characterised by fever, a rash, lymphadenopathy, often hepatosplenomegaly, and sometimes pericarditis, together with severe constitutional symptoms. Although, initially, arthralgia and myalgia may predominate, about 50% of the patients will develop a severe arthritis. The course may be protracted, with systemic features persisting for several years and progressive joint problems. These children are at particular risk of developing serious intercurrent infections, and it is in this group that the potentially fatal complication of amyloidosis occurs.

POLYARTHRITIS

This group can be subdivided into those patients who carry the immunoglobulin M rheumatoid factor and those who do not. The seropositive group accounts for about 10% of all chronic childhood arthritis and particularly affects girls older than 10 years. These patients display many of the features of adult rheumatoid arthritis.

As the age at disease onset in these patients approaches skeletal maturity, surgical management is similar to that in the adult.

Seronegative polyarthritis also predominantly affects girls, but may occur in infancy or at any time during childhood. There is less tendency to joint destruction but, from the surgical point of view, the overriding problems are the severe stiffness and contractures that occur in these children.

PAUCI-ARTICULAR DISEASE

The pauci-articular group may be further subdivided according to age of onset and sex. Thus very young girls, and only occasionally boys, may present with a single swollen joint such as the knee or ankle and commonly display localised growth anomalies (Fig. 12.2). These children usually carry antinuclear antibodies and they often develop chronic iridocyclitis, which requires slit-lamp examination for its recognition. These patients must all be seen by an ophthalmic surgeon for routine examination, as severe untreated forms of the condition can lead to blindness (Kanski 1990).

The remaining members of this group are boys of 9 years and upwards who present with an arthropathy in the lower limb and carry the HLA B27 antigen. This may be the first manifestation of juvenile spondylitis, because sacro-iliitis and spinal problems do not arise until the late teens or early 20s.

SURGICAL MANAGEMENT

The surgical management of children with juvenile idiopathic arthritis outlined in this chapter relates to those younger than 16 years at the time of operation, and embraces the particular problems posed by inflammatory

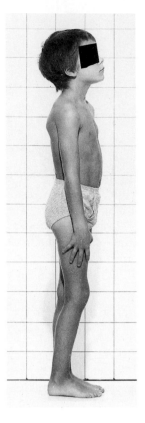

Figure 12.2 This 6-year-old boy with pauci-arthritis presented with a swollen knee. This can be the first joint involved in many conditions. The orthopaedic surgeon must never assume this to be 'IDK' (internal derangement of the knee).

arthritis in the growing skeleton. We are less concerned with the treatment of secondary degenerative change in the burnt-out disease of the mature skeleton (Haley & Charnley 1975, Arden 1978).

Approximately 10% of more than 5000 patients who have been under the care of our paediatric rheumatology unit have required single or multiple surgical procedures. If those who have undergone invasive procedures, such as injections under general anaesthetic are included, the number so treated increases to about 25% of the total. It is interesting to note that, whereas 10% of all the patients with juvenile idiopathic arthritis are seropositive, in our surgical series, 50% of the cases are seropositive. It is important, therefore, to appreciate the great difference in management of patients who are seropositive and those who are not. Patients with seropositive arthritis show a clinical picture akin to the adult with rheumatoid arthritis, but it tends to be very much more aggressive and destructive in a short time. A chronic effusion leads to destruction and instability of the joints. In contrast, in seronegative disease after the initial effusion has passed, many patients develop a tight joint contracture, with limited movement and the rapid development of intra-articular adhesions. Their joints are thus destroyed, deformed and stiff, but not unstable. The cervical spine illustrates the contrasts: in seropositive disease, there is instability, particularly at the atlanto-axial level, whereas in seronegative disease the posterior elements of the spine tend to fuse spontaneously, leading to rigidity and often almost total lack of neck movement (Fig. 12.3). Both pathological processes may lead to difficulties, particularly during general anaesthesia.

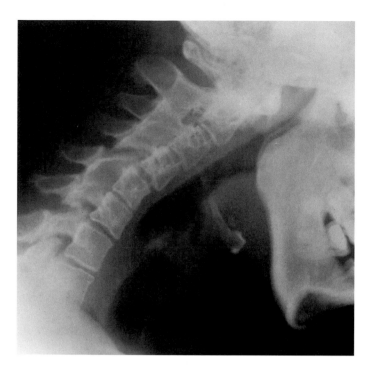

Figure 12.3 This 17-year-old developed pauci-arthritis, spreading to polyarthritis, at the age of 6 years. Fusion of the posterior elements of the cervical spine is seen, and the danger of the condition evident.

WHY SURGERY?

"Juvenile chronic arthritis is a rheumatological disorder and the mainstay of management is medical control by the paediatric rheumatologist" (Woo et al 1990). All patients undergo a full assessment and investigation and are then directed to a regimen of medication, splintage and physiotherapy. The cause of the condition is not known and complete cure is not available. Conservative measures can ameliorate the local and systemic effects of the disease, but complete control is often not possible; surgical intervention can be indicated when there is failure to control the disease or when early diagnosis has been missed. Conservative treatment usually fails either because facilities were not available or because the patient failed to take medication or comply with the exercise regimens.

THE PATHOLOGICAL PROCESS

The surgeon will be asked to deal with a combination of pain, stiffness and deformity. It is of paramount importance to identify the specific cause of the problem before planning treatment. For instance, a patient can lose movement in a knee because the patella has become adherent to the underlying femoral condyle; it would be fruitless and unkind to attempt to force unobtainable movement by physiotherapy when a simple surgical release of the patella might solve the problem. Some patients develop a fixed contracture of the hip and walk with a very awkward lumbar lordosis. To some extent this gait and posture must be accepted, because it is

associated with increased and persistent anteversion of the femoral neck. The patient only feels comfortable and stable by flexing the pelvis over the hip and, in such patients, trying to gain full extension by physiotherapy will be unrewarding, as will soft-tissue release of the anterior structures.

Inflammatory synovial proliferation spreads as a pannus over the articular surface that it destroys. Direct attack upon bone may occur at the articular margins through vascular foramina. A marked effusion during the early phase, together with synovial thickening, causes an increase in pressure and palpable swelling. This leads to tamponade and, in the case of the capital femoral epiphysis, avascular necrosis may develop. Fibrosis and contracture of the periarticular tissues follow, and the synovial membrane later undergoes similar changes. The tendency for contractures to develop is greater in seronegative patients; seropositive patients tend to suffer a proliferative synovitis similar to that in their adult counterparts. The final fate of the articular surface depends upon the activity of the disease. If this abates, some degree of repair by fibrocartilage produces a serviceable surface. If the disease fails to remit or cannot be controlled, fibrous or bony ankylosis may develop.

In the later stages, when bone destruction has occurred, the synovial membrane and periarticular tissues contain products of bone and cartilage destruction, and also organised fibrin. The presence of these elements contributes to the capsular and periarticular fibrosis. Direct involvement of tendon sheaths by adhesions and contractures is not uncommon.

These patients suffer not only a generalised retardation of growth, but also local growth defects. Hypertrophy, irregular growth or premature fusion of an epiphysis can occur and interfere with the normal pattern of development, causing deformities. Examples of this are anteversion of the femoral neck, hypertrophy of the lesser trochanter, exaggerated bowing of the femur, and overgrowth of the medial side of the lower femoral epiphysis. Asymmetric growth defects in the foot are very common (Fig. 12.4) (Ansell & Swann 1996). Rotational deformity of the leg below the knee is frequently seen, and is an example of a problem induced by a number of the factors described. Anteversion of the femoral neck causes a compensatory external rotation of the leg below the knee; painful joints in the feet cause the patient to walk with the feet turned out, imposing torsion on the tibia. A contracture of the ilio-tibial band may also cause torsion and the line of pull of the quadriceps is translated laterally, inhibiting its power and control of the knee (Fig. 12.5). All these problems must be appreciated if surgical planning is to be rational.

Frequently, these children are unable to walk because of the pain caused by polyarthritis or because of their constitutional illness. This contributes to the failure of joints, particularly the hip, to develop properly. Osteoporosis and muscle weakness add to the problem.

A spectrum of available treatment is designed to tackle the problems at various stages of this pathological process.

Infection

These children carry a high risk of postoperative infection. They commonly suffer from intercurrent infections, particularly in systemic disease, and the problem is compounded by long operations, poor healing and steroid medication. These patients must have an adequate course of per- and postoperative antibiotics and adequate blood replacement.

SURGICAL PROCEDURES

Because of the complex problems surrounding the care of these patients, it is recommended that those who are to undergo operation should do so preferably in a paediatric or adolescent ward, under the overall care of a paediatric rheumatologist. The rigorous supervised programme of medication, physiotherapy and splintage must continue in the postoperative period to ensure success.

It has been emphasised that it is of the utmost importance to identify the actual cause of a deformity or loss of movement before embarking on surgery to overcome the problem. Thus soft-tissue problems may be overcome by the application of plaster of Paris, traction, intra-articular steroids or soft-tissue operation and, occasionally, synovectomy. When deformity in the bone or joint has occurred, an osteotomy may be indicated. Sometimes, epiphyseal stapling to correct an angular deformity is necessary. In the severely destroyed joint, under exceptional circumstances, joint replacement may have to be considered. Ideally, the patient is seen early in the course of the disease, because timely intervention such as a simple soft-tissue release may obviate the need for more radical operations.

Examination under anaesthetic

Examination under anaesthetic is recommended in many cases in which apprehension may preclude proper assessment. Manipulation under anaesthetic probably should never be performed, as there is a significant risk of damage or fracture to the articular surfaces or the porotic bone. Likewise, serial plaster correction, if indicated, must always be undertaken without anaesthetic; it is only reasonable for minor degrees of deformity, probably not exceeding 10–15° at the knee. If forced, the three-point pressure holds the patella firmly against the underlying condyle, where it may cause damage or adhesions. In general, flexion contractures greater than 15° should be treated surgically.

Traction, splints, insoles, callipers and moulded supports all have a part to play where a deformity can be corrected and needs to be held. However, it must be emphasised that these methods cannot be used to overcome an established deformity.

Intra-articular and intrathecal corticosteroids

These agents afford a useful method of controlling disease activity and reducing swelling in a persistently active joint (Earley et al 1988). They are particularly helpful in pauci-articular disease and in the larger joints such as the hip, knee, ankle and subtalar joints, together with the wrist, elbow and shoulder. Intra-articular injections are given under anaesthetic in the younger child and the drug of choice is triamcinalone hexacetonide (10 mg per injection for those younger than 10 years and 20 mg for those older than 10 years); the dose should be modified depending on the size of the target joint and the number of joints that are injected at any one session. Consultation with the paediatric rheumatologist should be made with regard to the dose, in particular as it relates to other medication that the patient may be receiving. Early studies have shown few complications and encouraging results, but it is recommended that injections are given no less than 6 months apart, with a total of three injections for any one joint. Similarly, intrathecal injections of hydrocortisone into the flexor sheaths of the hand have produced excellent results; this is an area where surgical intervention and attempts at synovectomy may lead to intractable stiffness, and injections are an excellent alternative.

OPEN SURGICAL PROCEDURES

The procedures to be described are used by orthopaedic surgeons who treat many conditions in routine orthopaedic practice. In indicating their special place in the surgery of juvenile idiopathic arthritis, we will make main reference to the hip and knee joints, as these are by far the most common sites requiring attention. They illustrate the principles that are applicable to other joints.

SYNOVECTOMY

Opinions vary as to the place of synovectomy in rheumatoid arthritis, and even more so in juvenile idiopathic arthritis. The child who perhaps would benefit most from synovectomy often has multiple joint involvement and is systemically ill, thus precluding operation. It has already been mentioned that there are some sites at which synovectomy is contraindicated, such as the flexor tendon sheath of the hand, although it may occasionally be necessary to clear a synovitis of the dorsal sheaths and occasionally an isolated metacarpo-phalangeal joint in a patient with seropositive disease (Harrison 1978). An absolute indication for synovectomy is when a single joint, such as a knee, is the site of persistent activity in pauci-arthritis, leading to continuous effusion, synovial swelling and overgrowth (Rydholm et al 1986) (Fig. 12.6). The authors feel that synovectomy should be a therapeutic, rather than a prophylactic, operation – particularly as the activity in an individual joint is variable and unpredictable and the disease often burns itself out without the need for operation; thus no controls are available. Finally, it has already been indicated that these operations are very painful, and it may be difficult to secure the co-operation of the child for the essential postoperative regimen of early movement. The continuous passive motion machine may help in gaining early mobility.

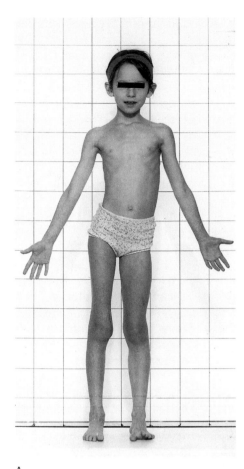

A

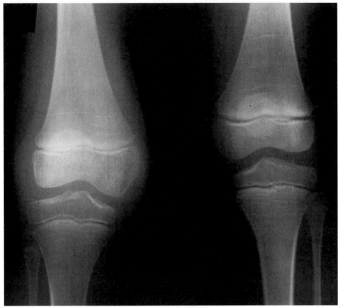

B

Figure 12.6 **A** This 10-year-old girl developed pauci-arthritis of the right knee at the age of 5 years. There is wasting of the leg, with overgrowth in length and a compensatory scoliosis. A synovectomy has now been performed and she has subsequently developed minor problems in a wrist and an ankle. **B** X-rays of the same patient, comparing the right knee with the left, normal knee.

SOFT-TISSUE-RELEASE PROCEDURES

The authors lay great store by these relatively simple procedures, which serve to correct a contracture, increase the total range of movement, and decompress a joint. The last of these may account for the immediate and dramatic relief of the severe pain experienced by some patients.

If the contracture is overcome and the pain relieved, the patient will move the joint readily, so overcoming stiffness and promoting joint nutrition. Secondary benefits include an overall increase in mobility and improved joint position. This may help to re-establish walking and overcome muscle wasting, weakness and secondary osteoporosis. Benefit will also be felt by other unaffected joints. The operation has been used extensively at the hip and knee, although it can be applied to other joints, using the same principles. At the hip, an open approach is made through the groin and the adductor longus and gracilis muscles are divided (Swann & Ansell 1986). The finger is then passed across the surface of the adductor brevis to seek the psoas tendon at its attachment to the lesser trochanter. A psoas tenotomy is performed. More radical soft-tissue release of the hip appears to add little, and more extensive procedures are very painful, limiting the patient's postoperative mobilisation. Immediately after soft-tissue release, the patient undergoes intensive physiotherapy, with traction in abduction and prone lying when possible. As soon as the wound has healed, hydrotherapy can be started.

The principles for surgery at the knee are exactly the same (Clarke et al 1988), although the operation itself is more difficult. Knee flexion contracture is usually associated with backward subluxation of the tibia on the femur. Preliminary imaging should confirm that, as it becomes possible to straighten the joint, good articular surfaces are available for weight bearing. In the absence of this confirmation, it is probably better to straighten the knee by supracondylar osteotomy. The operation of soft-tissue release of the knee is made by posteromedial and posterolateral incisions with the patient prone. It is thus possible to sling the neurovascular bundle out of the way by retracting it backwards, and with the knee in its flexed position, it is possible to pass under the heads of the gastrocnemius muscle to incise the capsule. It is important that the capsular soft-tissue release is carried around towards the front of the joint, to include that part of the retinaculum which is preventing extension. Post-operatively, the leg is immobilised for 48 hours in a plaster cylinder, which is then bivalved and active movements commenced, including weight bearing, using the posterior half of the plaster as a support during walking and as a night splint (Fig. 12.7). If the original contracture is severe,

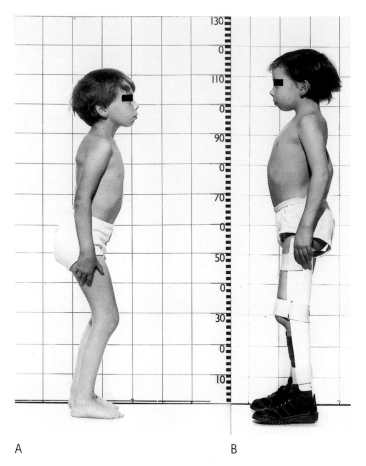

A   B

Figure 12.7 A This 12-year-old boy developed pauci-arthritis, spreading to polyarthritis, at the age of 5 years. Despite a full regimen of conservative treatment, he had residual flexion contractures of both hips and both knees. **B** After soft-tissue-release operations of both hip joints and both knee joints. Splints are worn when the patient is walking and at night during the postoperative phase.

straightening must be staged, to prevent problems with the popliteal nerves and vessels.

These soft-tissue release operations are essentially extra-articular. However, intra-articular adhesions may need to be divided, and occasionally the anterior cruciate ligament in the knee has to be released to correct the subluxation of the tibia. Adhesions may form in the suprapatellar pouch and, in particular, between the overgrown and distorted patella and the femoral condyle. It is possible in some cases to introduce an arthroscope into the joint, but not if adhesions have formed, because these preclude the distension of the joint with fluid. Arthroscopy may be used diagnostically if there is a distensible joint; it is particularly important when a secondary problem exists: juvenile idiopathic arthritis does not preclude a patient suffering from a loose body or osteo-chondritis dissecans.

The success of soft-tissue surgery depends on many factors, not least the overall disease activity and its activity in the particular joint. In the majority of patients, there is an immediate and significant improvement in terms of pain relief, movement and loss of deformity. More than 50% of our patients have shown a significant radiological improvement in the hip with evidence to suggest that healing by fibrocartilage can occur (Fig. 12.8). In those patients who continue to suffer from active disease within the operated joint, there is nevertheless a temporary improvement in function and an overall improvement in position, so that later surgical procedures such as total replacement can be undertaken in a more favourable anatomical setting.

OSTEOTOMY

There appear to be many instances when a corrective osteotomy might prove helpful in the correction of a deformity. However, two issues mitigate against the success of this procedure: first, the patients are often so porotic that it is impossible to fix the bone with metal plates, screws or other devices, and second, the alternative method of immobilisation

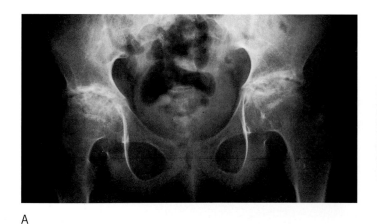

A

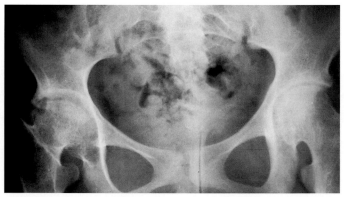

B

Figure 12.8 A This 13-year-old developed polyarthritic-onset arthritis at the age of 3 years. X-rays show erosive changes and narrowing of the joint space. **B** Two years after soft-tissue-release operations, there has been 'healing', particularly of the left hip. Note, in addition, the premature arrest of the capital epiphysis and overgrowth of the lesser trochanter.

in plaster sometimes leads to devastating and intractable stiffness. There are exceptions, however, when this method can be used, and in particular at the knee. Some patients demonstrate severe combined flexion and valgus deformity of the knee in a joint that may be quite badly damaged. In these patients a supracondylar osteotomy is indicated, using an osteotomy-osteoclasis technique through a small medial approach. A plaster cylinder is then applied and walking encouraged from the first day after operation. Cancellous bone in this area and the compression thus obtained encourage rapid union, so that the cylinder can usually be removed after 4 weeks and movement encouraged to overcome the problem of stiffness. Occasionally, there is sufficient bone stock for an osteotomy to be performed at the hip when the joint is beginning to sublux and where adequate internal fixation can be anticipated. A preoperative requisite is that the joint can be centred, and this must be checked under the image intensifier. Some cases of subluxation are due to coxa magna and cannot be contained.

STAPLING

This method still has some supporters for correction of valgus deformities at the knee or overgrowth of the limb (Rydholm et al 1987). Nevertheless, it has not found favour with the authors, as the timing for correction is totally unpredictable in these children with stunted growth. The porotic bone offers a poor grip for the staples, and a further operation is required to remove them.

JOINT REPLACEMENT

The hip

Total hip replacement is not to be undertaken lightly. However, in 9% of patients with juvenile idiopathic arthritis,

the hip is involved within 1 year of disease onset; its development is impaired by loss of the stresses of normal weight bearing and later by the destructive arthritis. The disease affects many joints, but involvement of the hips is the single most important cause of loss of mobility. Consequent social and educational isolation, with increasing dependence upon relatives, hospital and residential institutions, often affects the child at the most important stage of adolescent development. Our practice has been to replace both components of the hip joint, using a cementing technique. The joints are usually totally destroyed and the remnants of the femoral head often have to be removed piecemeal with bone nibblers. This type of advanced disease has precluded methods such as resurfacing the joints, which have been described by other workers (Mogensen 1982). We have reported the use of uncemented hips (Kumar & Swann 1998) in 16 patients with juvenile idiopathic arthritis. These patients were, however, of an older average age (24.9 years), with largely burnt-out disease and adequate bone stock. The average follow-up of only 4.5 years has given encouraging results, but the longer-term outcome is awaited.

There are many technical problems encountered in joint replacement. The surgeon must be prepared for considerable bleeding. He may also find a very anteverted neck and a femoral shaft greater in its sagittal than its coronal diameter. A range of small prostheses, including ultra-small cups, must be available, and a full preoperative assessment of the type of joint required must be made (Fig. 12.9). In the past, we have mainly used the Howse or mini-Howse prostheses, because these have come in sizes sufficiently small in both the socket and the stem. Other smaller sizes are now available 'off the shelf' from a number of manufacturers; however, some of our patients have required custom-made prostheses for their small skeletons.

These are time-consuming procedures because of the

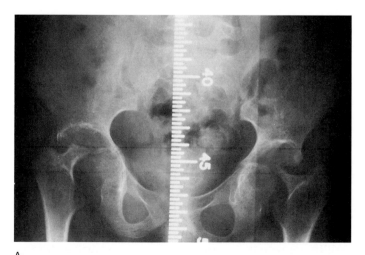 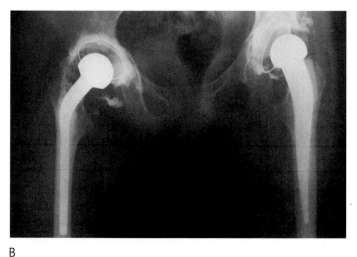

A   B

Figure 12.9 A This 15-year-old patient developed systemic-onset arthritis at the age of 1 year. The acetabulum is severely eroded, and the femoral head is a fibrous nubbin. **B** Custom, made prostheses were necessary. As a result of the total hip replacement, the patient walked for the first time in 4 years.

bleeding and the fragility of the bone. Our long-term studies show that they carry a greater risk of infection and prosthetic loosening. A review of 96 hip replacements with a follow-up of 6–18 years (average follow-up 10 years) revealed that 30% failed and the appearance of lucent lines and hip migration, even in the asymptomatic patients, suggested that this rate would increase with time (Witt et al 1991). Twenty-four patients (34 hips) had revision operations (Witt & Swann 1999). They were followed up for an average of 4.3 years, during which time only three of the revised components had failed. However, concern remains about the future of these hips in patients who are still so young at the time of their first revision arthroplasty. Of 42 children reviewed in 1986 after total hip replacement (Ruddlesdin et al 1986), four had died of amyloid disease and four remained with a pseudarthrosis after a late onset infection requiring removal of the prosthesis. Nevertheless, those who reach late teenage or early adult life are clearly physically transformed in their ability to integrate with the community, particularly in terms of work, leisure and social contacts. We continue to be highly selective when considering joint replacement, reserving it for those who are in great pain and who are becoming wheelchair-bound. It is hoped that the new generation of hip replacement prostheses and a better understanding of bone biology will produce longer-lasting results.

The knee

Similar considerations as those for the hip apply to replacement of the knee (Rydholm 1986). Until recently, no small prosthetic knees were available, other than the Attenborough, which came in three sizes. It was therefore possible to fit a prosthesis 75% of the adult size into even the smallest of candidates. Since 1989, the press-fit condylar knee has been used in 55 knee arthroplasty procedures in which a considerable number of size 1 components have proved satisfactory for the smaller skeletons. This series of patients is under review, with an average follow-up of 5.7 years (unpublished work 1999). Fortunately, none of the components has been revised to date. Compared with the outcome of total knee replacement in other conditions, the overall results of the clinical and functional score appear disappointing using the Knee Society clinical rating system; however, this is largely a reflection of the overall pathology, including involvement of many other joints. Nevertheless, careful selection, aimed particularly at the need to relieve intractable pain, has brought a satisfactory outcome in individual patients. With a similar selection of patients as was made in the case of hips, the results of this operation have been worthwhile in terms of pain relief and mobility.

Other joints

The case can be made occasionally for relieving a severe problem of the shoulder, elbow, or wrist by arthroplasty. These joints individually, or together, and often bilaterally, can become extremely painful and stiff. Functionally,

youngsters with such problems may be severely handicapped, in particular with respect to feeding and toilet. Arthroplasty is quite feasible in those approaching skeletal maturity with adequate bone stock. This has proved beneficial in a few patients, but experience and follow-up are limited to date.

The Benjamin double osteotomy of the shoulder has produced dramatic pain relief in some patients, and, although superseded by arthroplasty, might still be considered if the latter is not appropriate.

SURGERY OF THE FOOT

The ankle and tarsus are involved in 40% of patients with juvenile idiopathic arthritis. All the joints in this region are liable to be affected, although the disease pattern may be specific. Thus seronegative arthritis has a predilection for the tarsus, whereas seropositive disease more commonly affects the forefoot (Ansell & Swann 1996).

Problems with the foot arise as a result of the direct involvement of its joints or as a result of fixed deformity at the knee, rotation of the leg, or within the foot itself, where failure of function in one element stresses another. For example, stiffness or fusion in the subtalar and midtarsal complex may stress and produce pain in the ankle. Identification of joint disease within the foot may be apparent from clinical and radiological appraisal, but the source of pain must be clearly identified, as it does not necessarily arise from the joints most obviously affected radiologically.

In common with other non-rheumatic diseases of the foot, deformity *per se* does not necessarily present a problem if it is combined with mobility. Fixed deformity, however, is constant in producing symptoms at the points of pressure and at other sites within the foot that become stressed. The aim of the clinician should be to anticipate and prevent the onset of deformity and make every effort to keep the foot plantigrade and mobile.

From a practical point of view, the chief problems experienced are toe deformities of various kinds, including clawing and hallux valgus, metatarsalgia with painful plantar callosities, midtarsal pain and pain and deformity in the hindfoot. The last of these may be caused by ankle or subtalar joint involvement, or both. There may be differential rates of growth because of epiphyseal involvement and, not infrequently, the feet may differ in size.

The forefoot and toes

In seronegative disease, the interphalangeal joints bear the brunt of the problem (see Fig. 12.4) and respond by inequality of growth, dislocation and occasional effusion. It is difficult to prevent these deformities occurring, because splintage is not a practical solution. It is therefore easier to deal with these problems as they arise. Trimming of bone irregularity or excision arthroplasty can afford rapid relief of symptoms.

In seropositive disease, we see a pattern similar to that in adult rheumatoid disease. Involvement of the metatarso-phalangeal joints leads to their destruction and dorsal phalangeal dislocation. At the same time, the toes tend to claw at the interphalangeal joints. The metatarsal heads are driven plantarwards, and painful callosities appear on the sole of the foot. The foot widens and the gait loses its normal spring, so that the patient tends to plod with the feet turned out. The big toe does not claw like the others, but responds by developing a valgus deformity.

The spectrum of the condition will vary from early passively correctable clawing to total destruction of the metatarso-phalangeal joint with dislocation and fixed clawing. Patients with early clawing and only minimal radiological changes can be treated conservatively by physiotherapy, metatarsal insoles and, sometimes, simple tenotomy of the flexor tendons. Single or multiple oblique osteotomies of the metatarsal necks have afforded relief in patients in whom simpler methods failed and joint destruction was not marked.

When dislocation of the metatarso-phalangeal joints is complete and articular destruction advanced, forefoot excision arthroplasty is indicated. Hallux valgus can be treated by first metatarsal osteotomy or excision arthroplasty. Mayo's excision of the first metatarsal head is often appropriate.

The hindfoot

This excludes the ankle, but includes all the joints of the tarsus and, in particular, the triple complex of subtalar, talo-navicular and calcaneo-cuboid joints. These joints are frequently affected by other influences or by the primary disease. It is often difficult to define the site of joint pain. An intra-articular injection of local anaesthetic may help define the source. No set pattern of deformity occurs, but varus, valgus, pronation or supination can occur. Painful collapse of the foot into valgus is most common, but spasm of the peroneal muscles may equally produce this deformity (Fig. 12.10). A steroid injection into the sinus tarsi may be helpful. The hindfoot and forefoot usually diverge in the same direction, and a careful assessment of any supination or pronation must be made, because this implies that the patient is walking on the outer or inner side of the foot. This is more important to deal with than pure valgus, which may be compatible with a plantigrade and symptomless foot. In the early stages, if passive correction is obtainable, the planti-grade position should be held by a below-knee plaster applied under anaesthetic. If primary joint inflammation of the hindfoot is confirmed, an intra-articular steroid injection may be used. Four weeks in plaster is usually sufficient. Any sign of relapse can be controlled by a below-knee iron and T-strap. Surgery is rarely required but, occasionally, a selective midtarsal arthrodesis may be indicated, particularly if the talo-navicular joint is painful. A number of patients have undergone a full triple arthrodesis and, in some patients, a Dwyer's os calcis osteotomy has been helpful.

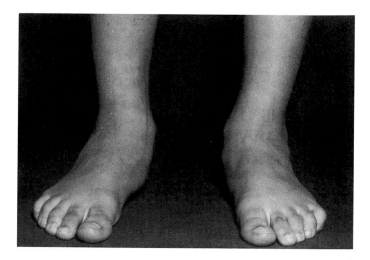

Figure 12.10 This 11-year-old patient developed peroneal spastic flat foot. However, his erythrocyte sedimentation rate was increased, and he was HLA B27 antigen positive. Spondyloarthropathy may present at about this age and more commonly affects the knee, but both hip and ankle may be involved. Spinal manifestations do not appear until about 20 years of age.

The ankle

Disease may directly affect the joint; occasionally, the talus may undergo avascular necrosis secondary to disease in the sinus tarsi. Stress on the ankle is increased when tarsal mobility is lost. The ankle can be treated like the tarsal joints by a period of immobilisation in a below-knee walking plaster, with a steroid injection if it is the site of disease activity. The surgical choice lies between arthrodesis and arthroplasty; several patients have had successful arthrodesis, but arthroplasty has not been performed to date.

Soft tissue of the foot

The synovial sheaths of tendons in the feet and toes are frequently affected by juvenile idiopathic arthritis – in particular, the flexor sheath of the toes and that of the tibialis posterior as it courses round the inner side of the ankle. The tendo-Achilles and the plantar fascia are also occasional sites at which pain and swelling demand treatment. In all these sites, a local injection of steroid with anaesthetic has often been useful in controlling symptoms. Rarely, surgical decompression or synovectomy is indicated.

FRACTURES

Patients with juvenile idiopathic arthritis are protected from sports injuries because of their inability to participate. Nevertheless, they are more vulnerable to pathological fractures because of the stiffness of their joints and porosity of their bones. Immobility rapidly leads to joint stiffness, so that it is important to keep splintage light and of short duration. Ideally, internal fixation might seem suitable, but

1

Chapter 13

Bone tumours

D. H. Gray and J. W. van der Eijken

INTRODUCTION

Dysplasias and tumours of bone have always commanded the interest of orthopaedic surgeons, because of the biological questions they pose and the challenging clinical management problems they present. As this book is related to childhood, some of the conditions to be described will present as a result of abnormalities in development or maturation of the physis. The opportunity may be taken to use tumour behaviour to study both normal growth and the influence of tumours upon this process. The solutions to be offered will need to take into account the prospect of continued growth in the same or contralateral limb and the influence that any treatment proposed may have on limb length. One must also consider aspects of durability, because many of these patients have a long life expectancy, with considerable functional demands. It is also necessary to balance the iatrogenic consequences (e.g. infections, pseudarthrosis, problems with prostheses) with the life expectancy of the patient.

The propensity for local recurrence in many paediatric benign lesions and the highly aggressive nature of the common malignancies indicate that an understanding of the biology of tumours is critical in developing appropriate treatment programmes. In particular, knowledge of the nature of the host–tumour interaction and the behaviour of the tissues at this interface is essential if the incidence of local recurrence, which has plagued the management of both benign and malignant lesions, is to be reduced.

This chapter is not presented as a catalogue of the common paediatric musculoskeletal tumours and dysplasias. It is proposed to emphasise the biological reaction, at a local level, between the tumour and the host, and to highlight the need to manage lesions by their behaviour pattern rather than by tissue type alone.

It is opportune to point out that it is the duty of the orthopaedic surgeon, in dealing with these patients and their families, to manage the individual and his/her family, not merely the lesion. The need for a caring attitude, patience in explanation, and the requirement for frankness without raising unnecessary fears and anguish is a challenging and time-consuming task. Both surgery and radiotherapy may be mutilating and disfiguring, and modern chemotherapy regimens are prolonged and stressful to the patient and the family. Limb salvage surgery requires a considerable degree of surgical skill, so that only those surgeons possessing appropriate attitudes, aptitudes and experience should become involved.

As will become apparent, the management of bone tumours in children involves surgeons, radiologists and pathologists in the staging process. The skills of one complement the other in this important activity, and no clinician can master more than a small facet of the problem. Similarly, treatment involves surgeons, oncologists, radiotherapists, counsellors and, sometimes, engineers and prosthetists. A willingness to consult at each stage of the decision-making process and an ability to work in a team are essential attributes for each player.

DEFINITIONS

TUMOUR

For the purposes of this discussion, a tumour is defined as an abnormal mass of tissue, the growth of which exceeds and is unco-ordinated with that of normal tissues and persists in the same excessive manner after cessation of the stimuli that evoke the change (Walter & Israel 1987). Benign tumours proliferate slowly; they are well differentiated and do not metastasise. Malignant tumours are characterised by the ability to invade locally and, more particularly, to metastasise.

An underlying theme of this chapter is that the surgeon should think of bone tumours as occupying a continuous spectrum of disease from those characterised by benign, indolent behaviour through to those exhibiting uncontrollable aggression. It is not always helpful to attempt to classify lesions as being discontinuous in their behaviour – that is, as being either strictly benign or malignant.

DYSTROPHY AND DYSPLASIA

A dystrophy may be defined as a disorder, usually congenital, of the structure or function of an organ or tissue as a result of its perverted nutrition. This can include agenesis, hypertrophy, hyperplasia and metaplasia. The word 'dysplasia' is often used in musculoskeletal pathology as an alternative term when a disorder is believed to be developmental. The term usually implies that the exact nature of the lesions under consideration is not known.

METAPLASIA

Metaplasia is the replacement of one differentiated tissue by another differentiated tissue. In the true sense of the term, it is seldom seen in musculoskeletal pathology.

INCIDENCE

Fewer than 1 in 600 children will develop a malignancy before the age of 15 years. Tumours of bone account for 5% of these malignancies, and tumours of soft tissue for an additional 8%. The prevalence of benign lesions is clearly much greater, but, as many are asymptomatic, the true frequency will never be known. The most common benign lesions are osteochondromas, various forms of non-ossifying fibroma, osteoid osteoma and fibrous dysplasia. The approximate incidence of primary malignant bone tumours is 5 per million under 15 years of age (Altman & Schwartz 1978).

AETIOLOGY

This is largely unknown. Prenatal radiation may be a factor and, clearly, osteosarcoma can develop after therapeutic radiation (Kim et al 1978). This almost invariably follows exposure of 30 Gy or more, with a long interval between exposure and sarcomatous change. The effect of ingestion of bone-seeking nuclides is well known.

The peak incidence of malignant bone tumours occurs during the second decade of life, which corresponds to the period of greatest bone growth. Children with osteogenic sarcoma tend to be taller than average; bone sarcomas occur much more commonly in large dogs than in smaller breeds: clearly growth is related to oncogenesis. It is interesting to note that many of the recently described growth factors are derived from proto-oncogenes. The following conditions may be precancerous in bone:

1. Radiation.
2. Chronic infection.
3. Cartilage lesions, e.g. enchondromata and osteochondromata.
4. Dysplasias, e.g. fibrous dysplasia, melorheostosis.
5. Bone infarction.
6. Paget's disease.

HEREDITARY FACTORS

Diaphyseal aclasis, or multiple osteochondromatosis, is a classic autosomal dominantly inherited musculoskeletal tumour. Gardner's syndrome is a variant of multiple polyposis coli (autosomal dominant) with skull tumours that include osteomas, fibromas and jaw cysts. Osteosarcoma has a greater incidence in those children with inherited bilateral retinoblastoma, but, in general, musculoskeletal tumours are not associated with chromosomal abnormalities or single gene defects as heritable factors, although some tumours such as Ewing's sarcoma show identifiable characteristic chromosomal abnormalities (Aurias et al 1983).

PATHOLOGY

In general, tumours grow by expansion and their increase in size is, commonly, irregular. An understanding of the nature of events occurring at the interface between the tumour and the host is fundamental to a rational approach to treatment (Enneking 1983, 1986).

Any lesion consists of four zones:

1. Tumour.
2. Capsule.
3. Reactive zone.
4. Normal host tissue.

TUMOUR

The tumour zone consists of the tumour cells and their associated stroma, e.g. chondrocytes and a matrix of cartilage in an enchondroma.

CAPSULE

In general, the tumour expands along the path of least resistance and the fibrous connective tissue at the margin formed by compression of the host tissue constitutes a capsule that is only a few cells thick. As the tumour commonly extends along perivascular spaces, the host tissue containing the vessels may form septae, which invaginate into the tumour mass. More formal resistance is offered by dense fascia, tendon sheaths and capsules, and the septal walls that form the compartments for limbs. In these situations the abutting capsule will be smooth. When the tumour arises in bone, a capsule is formed from elements of the bone marrow, the endosteum and the periosteum. The structure of trabecular bone may mean that this capsule follows a very convoluted path.

THE REACTIVE ZONE

The host response outside the capsule includes:

1. Proliferation of fibrous connective tissue.
2. Formation of new vessels.
3. Infiltration with inflammatory cells.

The *connective tissue response* may include the formation of bone, cartilage or fibrous tissue, and the nature of this reaction is more likely to reflect the rapidity of growth of the tumour and its site, rather than its histological type. A slow-growing tumour will allow time for the host to form mature tissue, whereas an invasive, rapidly growing tumour may expand and infiltrate so quickly that the host response is overwhelmed.

The *vascular component* includes new vessels formed from those already present where their structure and form approach normality. In addition, particularly in more aggressive lesions, a more haphazard thin-walled vasculature develops; this system may communicate with the abnormal vessels present within the tumour mass. The vascular pattern varies, depending upon the aggressive qualities of the tumour and its type.

The third component of the host reaction is the *inflammatory response*, which contains non-specific chronic inflammatory cells and, in some cases, a more specific component of B and T lymphocytes that are believed to represent an immunological defence process (Enneking 1983). This response is variable in its magnitude and, in general, the inflammatory component may be absent or very thick, depending upon the nature and behaviour of the lesion.

PATTERNS OF HOST–TUMOUR INTERACTION

The hallmark of the benign lesion is encapsulation; that of the malignant lesion is locally aggressive behaviour, and its ultimate characteristic is metastatic spread. Each tumour should be considered as a parasite on its host: the outcome depends upon the qualities of that individual tumour and the ability of that individual host to respond. The experienced surgeon will recognise that the interaction in any one individual case will be a part of a virtually continuous spectrum of behaviour. Within this spectrum, certain patterns at the host–tumour margin, as determined by imaging techniques or histological appearances, can provide a guide to the behaviour of the lesion, and enable the development of an appropriate investigative programme and, eventually, a treatment plan. The classification of tumour behaviour may be summarised thus (after Enneking 1986):

- Benign
  - latent
  - active
  - aggressive
- Malignant
  - low grade
  - high grade

BENIGN LATENT LESIONS

These lesions are slow growing and well encapsulated, with a tendency to heal with skeletal maturity. There is very little reactive zone, with minimal inflammatory response and no tumour vessel formation. In the soft tissues, the cleavage plane between the capsule and the host is well defined and smooth in contour. The host has time to respond and such lesions are characterised by good reactive bone formation at the margin. The cleavage plane is between the thin reactive zone and normal tissue in bone. A typical example is the mature simple bone cyst, or fibrous dysplasia (see Figs 13.4 and 13.5).

BENIGN ACTIVE LESIONS

These tumours are more aggressive; they tend not to heal and, although there is good capsule formation, it is irregular, with more invasion of the capsule by tumour. The reactive zone is thicker than that in benign latent tumours, and the inflammatory and vascular responses are more active. The obvious plane of cleavage at surgery is within the reactive zone, so that enucleation may leave some of this layer in the tumour bed. Tumour excision should be complete in soft tissue. In bone, the host response in the reactive zone is mature trabecular bone formation, but the more uneven aggressive nature of the boundary zone between host and tumour makes excision more hazardous. Aneurysmal bone cysts are typical examples of these lesions (see Fig. 13.3).

BENIGN AGGRESSIVE LESIONS

The edge of a benign aggressive lesion is irregular, and nodule formation is common. The reactive zone is much more prominent than that in latent or active lesions, with increased vascular response. Tumour nodules may penetrate into the reactive zone along tracks created by blood vessels; the tumour mass is continuous, however, and a simple shell-out procedure may well leave tumour tissue behind. Examples of these lesions include giant-cell tumours and chondroblastomas (see Fig. 13.9).

MALIGNANT LOW-GRADE LESIONS

These tumours metastasise late, but they are characterised by penetration of the tumour into the reactive zone. *Nodules are present in this location that are no longer continuous with the main tumour mass.* In these lesions, the reactive zone is more prolific, with invagination into normal tissues, particularly along vascular and other preformed channels. Clearly a shell-out procedure through the reactive zone will inevitably leave tumour cells able to give rise to an 'apparent' local recurrence. The parosteal sarcoma typifies this lesion.

MALIGNANT HIGH-GRADE LESIONS

These tumours have an aggressive local behaviour and a high propensity for early recurrence and metastasis. Capsular formation is poor, because the capsule may be destroyed by the tumour or the host may have little time to form one. Tumour now actively invades the reactive zone and the vascular and inflammatory components are prominent. *In particular, tumour masses discontinuous from the primary focus are seen in the apparently normal adjacent tissue.* In benign lesions, bone resorption is carried out by osteoclasts, but in high-grade lesions the tumour cells appear to be able to resorb bone directly. Tumour may be seen in the vessels adjacent to the lesion. In general, the more aggressive the tumour, the more it invades by infiltration and destruction rather than by expansion and compression. The more rapid the growth, the less time the host has to respond. An example of such lesions is the osteosarcoma (see Fig. 13.14).

CORRELATION BETWEEN PLAIN RADIOGRAPHIC APPEARANCE AND RATE OF GROWTH

A system commonly referred to as the Lodwick system (Lodwick et al 1980) has been devised for correlating the radiographic appearance of bone tumours with their rate of growth. It is based upon the concept that geographic, moth-eaten or permeated patterns of destruction are fundamentally different from each other and can usefully be applied to help determine the behaviour pattern of the process under investigation. However, combinations of appearances may be seen. With *geographic* destruction, the observer can detect a relatively well-defined area of bone destruction, although the content of the lesion will obviously vary. Such lesions that are static or slow growing are circumscribed, confined within the bone, and, in cancellous bone, are surrounded by a sclerotic rim. In the cortex, their expansion occurs with the formation of a new periosteal shell of bone. With an increase in rate of growth, these responses become less organised and obvious. Lodwick described three grades of geographic destruction, IA, IB and IC, corresponding to benign, active and aggressive disease, respectively (see Figs 13.3–13.5, 13.9, 13.10 and 13.13).

In the case of *moth-eaten* destruction, there is an apparently random array of focal areas of destruction of varying size in a bone (see Fig. 13.16). The cortex is destroyed. The involved area may still be moderately circumscribed. In a *permeative* lesion, the extent is ill defined and there are small areas of bone destruction of a uniform size visible in the cortex and cancellous bone, but the general form of the bone is preserved (see Figs 13.14 and 13.16). These two patterns correspond to Lodwick grade II if they have a geographic boundary (Fig. 13.16), and grade III if the changes are diffuse (Figs 13.14 and 13.15).

Table 13.1 sets out some helpful criteria of malignancy. Size refers to tumour volume with respect to that of the host bone, and reaction refers to the degree of sclerotic margin in cancellous bone or periosteal new bone formation in the cortex. This is merely a guide and not a set of absolute criteria.

Table 13.1 Characteristics of benign and malignant lesions

	Benign	Malignant
Size	Small	Large
Host reaction	Present	Absent
Cortical destruction	Minimal	Present
Soft-tissue mass	Absent	Present

(After H J Mankin, personal communication.)

CORRELATION BETWEEN OTHER INVESTIGATIVE MODALITIES AND TUMOUR BEHAVIOUR

Bone scanning

This investigation has great value both in determining the activity of the primary lesion and in excluding osseous metastases. In general, the more aggressive the primary lesion, the greater is the increase in isotope uptake. Furthermore, uptake beyond the radiographic extent of the lesion correlates with invasive behaviour.

Angiography

The more aggressive the tumour, the greater is the new vessel formation and the more atypical its appearance, particularly for limb salvage. This method is now rarely used to help decision-making as the quality of magnetic resonance imaging (MRI) has improved and gives ample information in most cases. However, it is sometimes helpful to clarify the location of vessels in connection with the tumour. Sometimes it is useful for embolising very vascular tumours.

Computed tomography

This investigation helps greatly in determining the anatomical margin and extent of the lesions. Latent lesions show a clear margin with a good capsule, and this becomes more indistinct with evidence of host bone destruction with increasing aggressivity. The modality helps particularly with determining the extent of a soft-tissue mass. Computed tomography (CT) of the chest is the most reliable technique for determining the presence of pulmonary metastases.

Magnetic resonance imaging

The role of MRI in the detection and staging of musculoskeletal bone tumours continues to evolve. The modality is far superior to CT for detecting the intramedullary spread of malignant tumours and tumour extension into the soft tissues. It is particularly helpful for imaging in the sagittal and coronal planes.

None of these investigations is reliable in determining the tissue type of a tumour, and for this information biopsy is essential.

STAGING OF MUSCULOSKELETAL TUMOURS

Staging is determined by:

1. Compartmental containment.
2. Tumour grade.

COMPARTMENTS

For the staging of a tumour by compartmental containment, the limbs are divided into sets of compartments (Table 13.2). The outer boundary consists of the envelope of deep fascia that encases the principal limb segments. From this sheet, septa pass to the bone. Benign latent and benign active lesions are confined within compartments, but aggressive lesions, because of their ability to penetrate capsules, are able to escape from compartments, be they bone, fascia or muscle. Malignant tumours clearly have the capacity to cross compartmental boundaries (Enneking 1986).

GRADE OF TUMOURS (HISTOLOGICAL)

In the past, Broders' system of four histological grades of tumours has been used, but the modern approach is to grade sarcomas as high and low grade. Benign tumours are graded

Table 13.2 Surgical sites as determined by compartments

Intracompartmental	Extracompartmental areas
Intraosseus	Extension from any compartment, e.g. from bone into adjacent soft tissue
Paraosseus	
Intra-articular	
Superficial to the deep fascia	
Intrafascial compartments	Extrafascial spaces and planes
Ray of hand or foot	Midfoot and hindfoot
Posterior calf	Popliteal space
Anterolateral leg	Femoral triangle
Anterolateral thigh	Intrapelvic
Medial thigh	Midhand
Posterior thigh	Antecubital fossa
Buttocks	Axilla
Volar forearm	Periclavicular
Dorsal forearm	Paraspinal
Anterior arm	Head and neck
Posterior arm	
Pericapsular	

(After Enneking 1986.)

Table 13.3 Staging systems by grade and compartment

Benign		
Latent	Intracompartmental	
Active		
Aggressive	May be extracompartmental	
Malignant		
	Intracompartmental	Extracompartmental
Low grade	IA	IB
High grade	IIA	IIB
Metastasis, any grade	IIIA	IIIB

(After Enneking 1986.)

and the presence of any local or regional metastases should be sought. Osseous metastases are less common in children than in adults; however, a careful examination for lymphadenopathy, splenomegaly and abdominal masses is essential. High-quality radiographs of the lesion should then be obtained.

MANAGEMENT

Tables 13.4 and 13.5 outline the decision-making tree for management of benign and malignant lesions from this point. In all but the most innocuous lesions, a standard haematological and biochemical evaluation should be performed as a routine. It is important to note that, if a tumour is believed to be benign, aggressive or malignant, the full local staging procedures should be carried out before biopsy; CT of the lungs and other distant staging manoeuvres can be delayed.

BIOPSY

Considerable thought needs to be given to the methodology of biopsy. The authors favour the use of a Yamshidi needle biopsy and only ocasionally perform open biopsy. *Before undertaking the procedure, the surgeon must discuss with the radiologist and pathologist* the optimal site for the procedure; in general, this should be at the edge of the lesion, encompassing both normal and abnormal tissue. An adequate quantity of tissue (four or five cylinders) must be removed. For an intraosseous tumour, a drill hole is made under fluoroscopic control, after which the Yamshidi needle can be introduced. If an open biopsy is necessary, the limb can be exsanguinated by elevation and a tourniquet applied, but an Esmarch bandage must not be used.

The approach should take into account any likely second-stage surgical procedures. The incision must always be longitudinal to the limb, and as few tissue planes as possible should be opened to reach the lesion. One should open the compartment that is already contaminated by tumour or, if there is no soft-tissue extension of the tumour, that compartment through which the resection will take place.

as G0. Low-grade malignant (G1) tumours have few mitotic bodies, little cellular atypia, no necrosis, are well differentiated and have a mature matrix. They tend not to invade vessels, and they metastasise late. In contrast, high-grade lesions (G2) have many mitoses and much atypia with poor differentiation, and the cells are pleomorphic. Any matrix is immature and atypical, necrosis is present, and vascular invasion is common.

In the assessment of the final grade of a tumour, the radiographic and isotopic appearances should be correlated with the histological evaluation before classification is carried out. As has been emphasised above, tumours form a virtually continuous spectrum of behaviour and it is helpful to attempt to locate a lesion within that spectrum, rather than struggle to make it fit exactly into one of the categories outlined above.

The staging system based on grade and site is outlined in Table 13.3.

STAGING PROCEDURES

Patients may present with pain, a mass or a pathological fracture. Sometimes lesions are found incidentally on radiographs taken for other purposes.

The surgeon should proceed to take a specific history related to the lesion, noting previous episodes of infection or trauma, and the duration and growth of any noted mass. The presence of previous tumours, radiation and the family history should be noted. The physical examination should include a definition of the characteristics of the local lesion

Table 13.4 Management of benign lesions

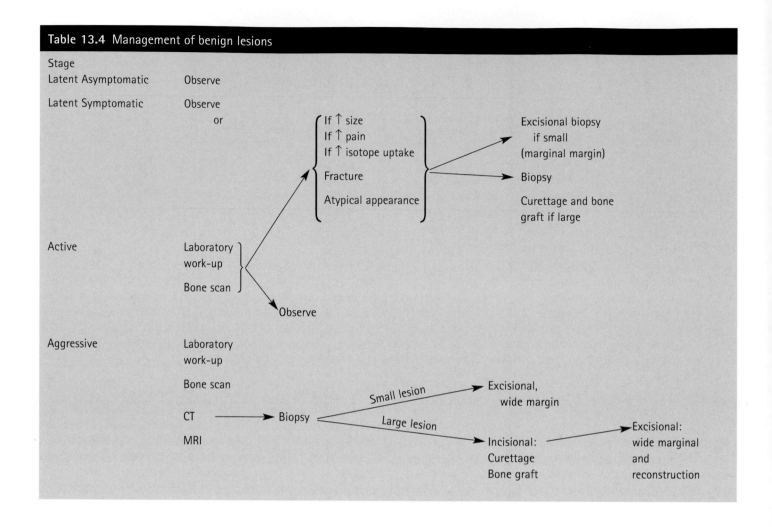

Stage		
Latent Asymptomatic	Observe	
Latent Symptomatic	Observe or	

If ↑ size
If ↑ pain
If ↑ isotope uptake
Fracture
Atypical appearance

→ Excisional biopsy if small (marginal margin)

→ Biopsy

Curettage and bone graft if large

Active   Laboratory work-up   Bone scan

Observe

Aggressive   Laboratory work-up

Bone scan

CT → Biopsy

MRI

Small lesion → Excisional, wide margin

Large lesion → Incisional: Curettage Bone graft → Excisional: wide marginal and reconstruction

Table 13.5 Management of malignant lesions

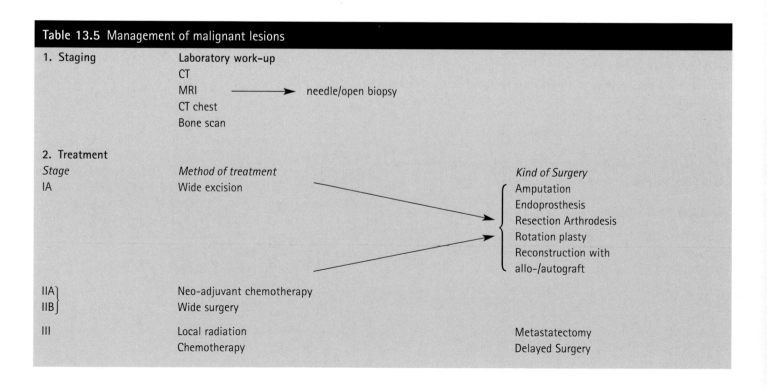

1. Staging   Laboratory work-up
CT
MRI → needle/open biopsy
CT chest
Bone scan

2. Treatment

Stage	Method of treatment		Kind of Surgery
IA	Wide excision		Amputation Endoprosthesis Resection Arthrodesis Rotation plasty Reconstruction with allo-/autograft
IIA IIB	Neo-adjuvant chemotherapy Wide surgery		
III	Local radiation Chemotherapy		Metastatectomy Delayed Surgery

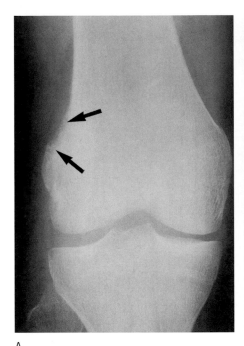
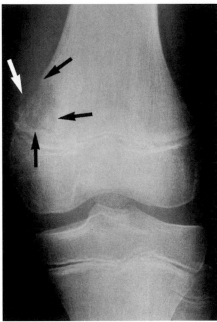

A   B

Figure 13.1 A This destructive lesion of the metaphyseal cortex of the lateral aspect of the lower right femur was a typical osteosarcoma histologically. **B** Radiograph of the lower end of the femur of a 12-year-old male presenting with staphylococcal subacute osteomyelitis. Note the similar appearances of these two lesions.

Careful haemostasis should be achieved to minimise the spread of tumour cells. If a drain is necessary, it must be brought out in line with and close to the incision. Some surgeons perform a biopsy without tourniquet, in an effort to force good haemostasis and reduce the size of any tumour cell bolus produced at the time of tourniquet release.

An open biopsy is undertaken when the pathologist cannot reach a diagnosis after needle biopsy.

On every occasion, tissue must be sent for both histology and culture, because infection can mimic almost any tumour radiologically (Fig. 13.1). It is helpful to ask for a smear or a frozen section to be made of the fresh tissue, to demonstrate that tumour has actually been sampled. Unless evaluation is performed by very experienced pathologists, it is advisable to defer definitive surgery, particularly amputation, until the result of the paraffin sections is available. There is no evidence that needle or incisional biopsy influences longterm outcome (Mankin et al 1996, Skrzynski et al 1996).

SURGICAL MARGINS

Table 13.6 shows the classification of surgical margins that can be expected after biopsy or therapeutic manoeuvres. Note that an amputation is still classified by the extent to which the compartment containing the tumour is removed by the ablation. It is important to note that virtually all limb salvage manoeuvres will incorporate a wide-margins excision together with adjuvant therapy, some of which may be administered before the definitive surgical procedure. When a benign aggressive lesion is being dealt with, the risk of recurrence can be reduced by cryotherapy (liquid nitrogen), the application of phenol, or the use of cement to fill a bone cavity, which may result in thermal sterilisation of this margin.

OVERVIEW OF TUMOURS

A summary of the characteristics of benign and malignant tumours is given in Tables 13.7 and 13.8; flow diagrams for their management were shown in Tables 13.4 and 13.5. Figure 13.2 presents a schematic diagram of the common lesions, examples of which will be considered in more detail in the remainder of this chapter.

Table 13.6 **Surgical margins**		
Margin type	Plane	Microscopy
Intracapsular	Within lesion	Some residual tumour
Marginal	In reactive zone	Leaves tumour in aggressive benign and malignant lesions
Wide[†]	In normal tissue outside reactive zone	May leave tumour in high-grade malignant tumours
Radical	Extracompartmental	Leaves only normal tissues ± metastases

[†]Ideally, a wide margin should include a cuff of normal tissue at least 1 cm thick.
(After Enneking 1986.)

Table 13.7 Characteristics of benign tumours

	Latent	Active	Aggressive
Symptoms	Absent/minor	Mild	Pain/mass
Growth	Slow, self-limiting, ceases with maturity	Steady, not self-limiting	Rapid, aggressive
Bone deformity	Nil	Deformed, expanded	Some deformity, more destruction
Radiology	Demarcated, cortical type reactive bone Lodwick IA	Thin, reactive ring of bone, may be irregular Lodwick IB	Poor or absent reactive bone, permeative border Lodwick IC
CT	Clear margin	Expanded thin margin	Indistinct margin
Compartment	Contained	Contained	May be extracompartmental
Bone scan	No change	Increased uptake at lesion	Increased uptake beyond lesion
Histology	Benign Litte reactive zone	Benign Osteoclastic bone resorption ↑ reactive zone	Benign More invasion, capsule broached Marked reactive zone
Cleavage plane	Between capsule and normal tissue Regular smooth plane	Irregular margin, capsule nodular Cleavage in reactive zone	Irregular margin, tumour left in irregular cleavage plane in reactive zone
Preferred treatment	Observation Injection Intralesional curettage	Marginal resection or curettage Bone grafting	Wide-margin excision if possible, or lesser ± adjuvant, e.g. cryosurgery, phenol

Table 13.8 Characteristics of malignant tumours

	Low grade	High grade
Symptoms	Indolent, minor, late symptoms	Rapid growth, symptoms pain, fracture
Bone destruction	Variable margin destruction rather than expansion	Poor or absent margins Loss of cortex Soft-tissue mass
CT	Irregular margin Some invasion Intracompartmental = IA Extracompartmental = IB	Wide invasion of adjacent bone, soft tissue Intracompartmental = IIA Extracompartmental = IIB
Bone scan	Increased uptake at lesion	Increased uptake beyond radiographic extent of lesion
Histology	Malignant, scant mitoses, moderate cell/matrix ratio, little pleomorphism Separate discrete tumour in reactive zone	Malignant, mitoses bizarre forms, high cell/matrix ratio, anaplasia, necrosis, pleomorphism Tumour in adjacent normal tissues
Metastases	Late, scant	Early, widespread
Treatment	IA wide margin resection IB wide margin if possible, may need amputation Radical resection not easily achieved Adjuvant therapy of little benefit All stage I suitable for limb salvage	IIA, wide excision neoadjuvant chemotherapy IIB, wide margin + adjuvant or radical +adjuvant Limb salvage or through-femur amputation for lesions at knee

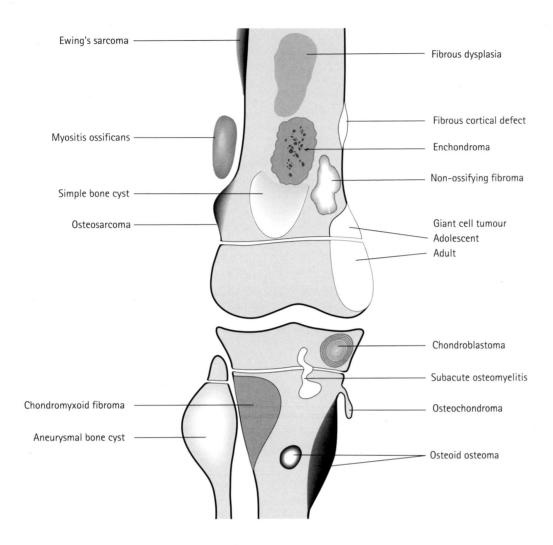

Figure 13.2 Common sites and configurations of bone lesions.

DYSPLASIAS OF BONE

SOLITARY BONE CYSTS

Definition
A solitary bone cyst is a benign, fluid-filled unicameral defect. It is common, and has a predilection for fracture and recurrence. It is a dysplasia rather than a tumour (Fig. 13.3).

Clinical features
Most commonly, the lesions occur in the upper metaphyseal region of the humerus or femur. They occur in the first and second decades of life. The male:female ratio is 3:1. Cysts have been subclassified as:

1. Active, where there is less than 1 cm of cancellous bone between the lesion and the growth plate.
2. Latent, where there is more than 1 cm of normal bone between the margin and the growth plate.

The cause is unknown. The symptoms may include pain or aching, but in 70% of cases (Mulder et al 1993), the child presents with a pathological fracture after minor to moderate trauma.

Behaviour
Radiologically, cysts fall into the latent or active category. There is destruction of cancellous bone, with a failure of remodelling of the metaphyseal area, so that the bone appears dilated. Simple cysts usually do not expand the bone beyond the width of the adjacent growth plate. The cyst fluid is clear in the unfractured situation and the lining is a simple fibrous one, with some areas of granulation tissue. Ridges in the cyst wall may give the radiographic appearance of septa.

Differential diagnosis
The differential diagnosis usually includes aneurysmal bone cyst, in which the lesion is often eccentric and expansile, and fibrous dysplasia, in which there is a ground-glass appearance of the cyst content.

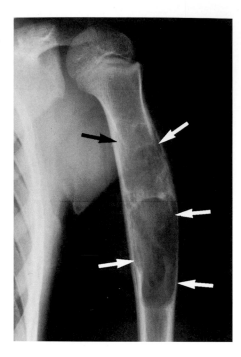

Figure 13.3 Left humerus of an 8-year-old boy, demonstrating a large simple bone cyst that recurred after bone grafting. This is a latent lesion in the old classification system because there is more than 1 cm of intact metaphyseal bone between the adjacent growth plate and the cyst. In the system used here, it is a benign active defect, Lodwick IB.

Treatment

The natural history of the lesion is that it almost invariably ceases to be a problem with achievement of skeletal maturity. The surgeon therefore needs to plan with this time-course in mind.

Patients who present with a fracture should have appropriate immobilisation to allow the fracture to heal. There is no impediment to fracture healing in this disorder: some 15% of lesions will subsequently heal.

Management of symptomatic lesions can be by observation or more definitive. The latter approach consists of placing a wide-bore needle in the lesion: if clear fluid is obtained, the lesion must be a simple bone cyst; if no fluid is obtained, the surgeon may proceed to biopsy to make a definite diagnosis.

In the event of the nature of the lesion being confirmed, the surgeon can proceed to:

1. Observation.
2. Injection of the cyst with methyl prednisolone.
3. Curettage and bone grafting.

For the second of these, a two-needle technique, in which one needle allows drainage of fluid and the other needle is used to inject the steroid, is favoured by most. It is advisable first to inject X-ray contrast fluid in order to ensure there is only one cavity. If there are more cavities, each is needled separately. If the cyst does not involute, these injections may be repeated several times before an open procedure is considered. Some authors prefer injection with bone marrow (Lokiec & Weintroub 1998).

Between 50 and 67% of patients will respond either to steroid injection or to curettage and bone grafting. The former procedure results in much less morbidity. Recurrence

is definitely more common in the young, and this factor is probably more important than the size of the lesion or its proximity to the growth plate. Fractures at the upper end of the humerus seldom lead to great disability and, in general, there is little indication for more radical procedures for lesions in the upper humerus, where the consequences of fracture are not great.

If there are recurrent problems with fracture at the upper end of the femur where it may be difficult to hold position, then more aggressive manoeuvres may be required. The initial treatment should consist of injection, possibly followed by curettage and grafting for recurrence. Resection of the lesion with a marginal margin, while almost invariably curative, is seldom indicated because of the known natural history.

The author's preferred option is aspiration and injection in the young, with grafting for recurrent fracture. Treatment should be less aggressive with the approach of maturity (Campanacci et al 1986).

NON-OSSIFYING FIBROMA AND FIBROUS CORTICAL DEFECT

Definition

These are geographic fibrous defects in the metaphyseal parts of long bones. A fibrous cortical defect represents a small asymptomatic disturbance of ossification in the cortex; the name non-ossifying fibroma can be applied to the larger lesions involving cancellous bone (Fig. 13.4).

Clinical features

These lesions exhibit no predilection for either sex and are found in about 30% of the population. Fracture occurs

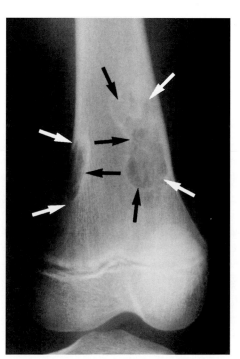

Figure 13.4 Radiograph of the lower end of the femur of an 11-year-old boy, demonstrating the classic image of a fibrous cortical defect on the left and a larger non-ossifying fibroma involving the cancellous bone on the right. These are benign latent lesions, Lodwick IA.

rarely. Most are asymptomatic and found incidentally on X-ray examination.

Behaviour

The character of these lesions is benign and latent, with a geographic sclerotic margin. Unlike the lesions of fibrous dysplasia, they do not have a ground-glass appearance. Histologically, there is a fibrous stroma interspersed with some giant cells and foam cells. There is no new bone formation unless there has been a previous fracture. The lesions may wax and wane in size and seldom cause a problem in the mature skeleton.

Treatment

Although curettage and bone grafting are curative, most lesions should be managed by observation. Operation is indicated only for impending fracture. If there is no doubt about the diagnosis, biopsy is not required, and if there has been no change in the radiographic appearance over 6–12 months, the patient need be seen only if symptoms develop in the future.

FIBROUS DYSPLASIA (see Ch. 6)

Definition

This is a benign, relatively common fibro-osseous, monostotic or polyostotic, sharply defined pathological abnormality of bone; it is of unknown aetiology. The bone is characteristically replaced by fibrous tissue containing small islands of osseous tissue (Fig. 13.5).

Clinical features

Sites of predilection include the ribs, femur and tibia. The bone is usually expanded, with thinning of the cortex. It is

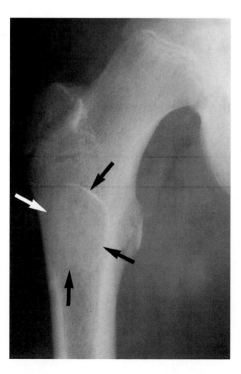

Figure 13.5
Radiograph of a 12-year-old male, showing a classic area of fibrous dysplasia in the metaphyseal region. There is a well-defined geographic boundary with a ground-glass appearance in the lesion. This is a benign latent lesion, Lodwick IA.

replaced by a homogeneous mass that appears on X-ray as of ground-glass appearance. Polyostotic cases are encountered in Albright's syndrome, with precocious puberty and pigmentation. If the facial bones are involved, there may be considerable deformity. Significant problems can occur with deformation of weight-bearing bones. Coxa vara is a particularly troublesome complication, sometimes culminating in a 'shepherd's crook' deformity of the proximal femur.

Behaviour

These lesions classically fall into the benign active category; they may present with fracture. Fibrous dysplasia, like Paget's disease, may involve the entire length of a bone, and is characterised particularly by internal scalloping; external scalloping is seen in neurofibromatosis. Histologically, the lesion consists of a cellular fibrous mass containing islands of woven bone in the form of an 'alphabet soup'. The osseous fragments do not show osteoblastic rimming. Malignant transformation is rare. Most lesions mature in the adult skeleton.

Differential diagnosis

This may include simple bone cyst and non-ossifying fibroma; histologically, the lesion may be confused with fibrosarcoma or osteosarcoma. When there are focal collections of giant cells, giant-cell tumour may also be misdiagnosed in the mature skeleton.

Treatment

Management for small lesions may be expectant; for others, curettage and bone grafting may help prevent fracture. Grafting of femoral neck lesions with cortical bone (fibula) may control deformity. The authors' preferred treatment is observation for small lesions, and curettage and bone grafting with or without internal fixation for those with symptoms (aching or repetitive fracture, particularly in those not approaching maturity) (Stephanson et al 1987).

CARTILAGE-FORMING LESIONS OF BONE

OSTEOCHONDROMA

Definition

An osteochondroma is a cartilage-capped bony projection most often located at the metaphysis in the juxta-epiphyseal area of the long tubular bones. It can involve any bone that develops from cartilage.

Clinical features

These are the most common tumours of bone; they may be solitary or multiple, and in the latter case they are often hereditary. Lesions are most common at the lower end of femur, the upper end of tibia and the upper end of humerus. In the hereditary multiple form, there may be significant skeletal deformity (Fig. 13.6).

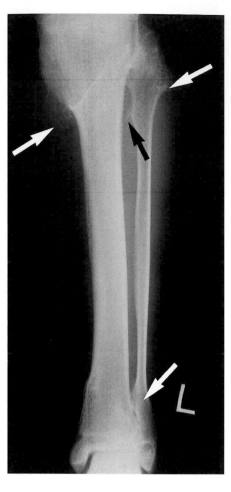

Figure 13.6 Multiple familial osteochondromatosis in a 17-year-old youth, demonstrating distortion of both tibia and fibula.

Behaviour

The tumours may be pedunculated or sessile, and there is usually little difficulty in establishing a diagnosis radiographically. The lesions consist of a bony base with a cartilage cap, and probably arise as a defect in the biology of the perichondrial ring at the physis. The risk of malignancy is low, probably of the order of 1%. The propensity for malignant change per lesion is probably the same in the isolated and multiple forms; in the latter, the risk per patient is cumulative. There is no indication to excise these tumours because of a potential malignant change. When malignant transformation occurs, it does so most often in axial lesions involving the spine, shoulder or pelvis.

Differential diagnosis

The radiographic appearance is characteristic. However, in certain projections the stalk of an osteochondroma may be seen end-on and be confused with a fibrous cortical defect. Inspection of an appropriately directed oblique film will demonstrate the presence or absence of the osteochondroma with its stalk and cap. In adults who present with a large dense tumour, there is always the possibility of a chondrosarcoma.

Treatment

Individual lesions may need excision if they impair the function of adjacent muscles, tendons and joints; occasionally,

impingement upon nerves or arteries may dictate the need for surgical intervention. It is often useful to carry out a preoperative CT scan. Lesions that increase rapidly in size, develop a large, speckled cartilaginous cap or become 'hot' on bone scan, particularly in the mature patient, should be regarded with suspicion: growth of the cartilage cap should cease with maturity. In the patient with multiple osteochondromas, it may be advisable to perform a bone scan at the cessation of growth; if malignant degeneration of one of the osteochondromas is subsequently suspected, a new bone scan may then be compared with that taken at the cessation of growth.

ENCHONDROMA

Definition

Enchondroma is a benign lesion characterised by cartilage formation within a bone; the stroma in the mature individual may become patchily calcified. The disorder may well be a dysplasia, rather than a true benign neoplasm. The cartilage cells are probably derived from the growth plate.

Clinical features

Many lesions are found incidentally in the pelvis or upper femur. Some may give rise to minor symptoms of aching. In the periphery, particularly in the hand, multiple phalanges and metacarpals may be involved, with considerable deformity (Fig. 13.7). There is a rare form of multiple enchondromatosis that affects many of the long bones in any one individual and is known as Ollier's disease (Fig. 13.8). The problem in this disorder is its potential for malignant change and the considerable deformities of angulation and shortening that arise.

Maffucci's syndrome is characterised by enchondromatosis that is predominantly unilateral, and haemangioma

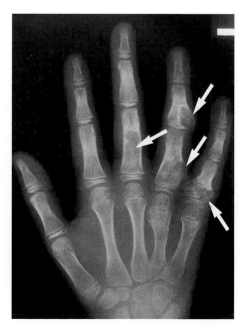

Figure 13.7 Multiple enchondromas of the fingers in an 11-year-old boy.

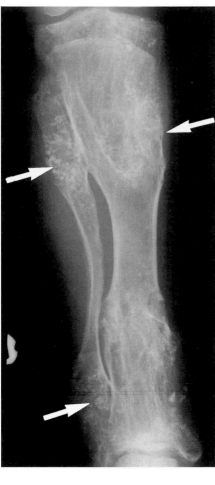

Figure 13.8 Radiograph of the lower limb of a patient (aged 16 years) with multiple enchondromas. He succumbed to chondrosarcoma of the shoulder when aged 40 years. Multiple punctate areas of calcification are typical of chondroid lesions.

formation. Malignancy in the form of chondrosarcoma is a common complication (occurring in 30–50% of affected individuals), although extraskeletal sarcomas and carcinomas also occur (Schwartz et al 1987).

Behaviour

Lesions in the pelvis and large limb bones present as a geographical area of bone destruction with an indistinct margin. They commonly contain an area of spotty calcification. Lesions in the small bones of the hand are more aggressive, with expansion and destruction of the cortex, but there is usually a clearly defined margin. The radiographic appearance of isolated metaphyseal and pelvic lesions is so classical that biopsy is seldom required.

Differential diagnosis

This includes bone infarct, fibrous dysplasia and non-ossifying fibroma.

Treatment

Malignant transformation in enchondromas is more common with defects in the limb girdles and proximal limb bones. There is, however, no indication for aggressive management of lesions found incidentally. In this circumstance, the authors' policy is to carry out a CT examination and bone scan at cessation of growth, as reference data for

measuring any change should symptoms develop. Malignant transformation, characterised by the development of pain, an increase in mass, an increase in radioisotope uptake and expansion on X-ray examination with loss of the margin, is seen in an older age group.

Multiple enchondromas in the hands may give rise to significant cosmetic and functional losses. The authors favour curettage and bone grafting as indicated. Malignant transformation is not a problem with these distally placed lesions.

PERIOSTEAL CHONDROMA

This is a true, benign tumour of cartilage, formed under the periosteum, which can have active or aggressive characteristics. The lesion presents as an erosion of the cortex, with elevation of the periosteum. The cartilage content is seldom calcified. The lesion may occur in any bone, but has a predilection for the shaft of the humerus. Recurrence is common and a wide-margin excision with appropriate reconstruction is advised.

CHONDROBLASTOMA

Definition

This is a rare, benign tumour of cartilaginous origin, with a predilection for the epiphyses (Fig. 13.9).

Clinical features

The common sites are the proximal end of the humerus and the knee. Chondroblastoma is most frequently seen in teenagers and has a significant preponderance in males. Patients may present with aching discomfort or joint symptoms (Springfield et al 1985).

Behaviour

Radiographically, chondroblastoma is a benign active lesion (although it can show aggressive characteristics as shown in Fig. 13.9) that is characteristically in the epiphysis, but may

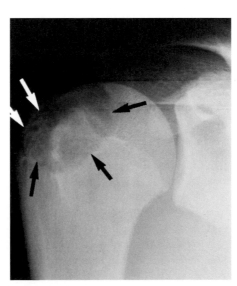

Figure 13.9 Chondroblastoma of the upper end of the right humerus in a 16-year-old youth, demonstrating transgression of the epiphyseal scar and destruction of the cortex of the greater tuberosity. This is a benign aggressive disease, Lodwick IC.

cross the growth plate to involve the metaphysis. There is usually a thin sclerotic rim, and tomography reveals a fine speckled calcification. Histologically, there are aggregations of chondroblast-like cells that secrete an immature matrix. Between the aggregations there is a fibrous stroma, which may contain areas of haemorrhage and giant cells.

Differential diagnosis

Chondroblastoma is the only tumour or dysplasia that commonly affects the epiphysis in the immature skeleton. Transgression of the growth plate, however, is not uncommon. The principal differential diagnosis is with subacute osteomyelitis, in which disorder there is usually increased sclerosis at the margin, no speckled calcification within the lesion, and a path of destruction that has a burrowing characteristic.

Treatment

The proximity of the lesion to growth plates and joint surfaces in the younger individual makes treatment difficult. As the lesion is moderately aggressive, those approaching skeletal maturity should have a wide-margin excision carried out together with bone grafting. In younger patients, it is reasonable to stage the lesion and, after establishing the diagnosis by biopsy, to adopt a policy of observation. Should the progress of bone destruction be slow, it is wise to temporise. Should the progress be aggressive, local curettage and grafting is advised, making every attempt to conserve the growth plate. A more aggressive policy may be adopted in the upper limb, where growth disturbance is not such a problem (Schuppers & van der Eijken 1998).

CHONDROMYXOID FIBROMA

Definition

This is a rare tumour of young adult life. It is benign and, as its name suggests, contains three elements in its stroma: cartilage with myxomatous and fibromatous tissue (Gherlinzoni et al 1983) (Fig: 13.10).

Clinical features

Characteristically, this lesion, which may be painful, occurs in the metaphyses of long bones, particularly the tibia. There is a slight preponderance in males.

Behaviour

Radiographically, the chondromyxoid fibroma is a benign active lesion. There is usually a sclerotic rim; the cortex may be eroded, with a thin shell of reactive new bone formation. Histologically, the stroma consists of myxoid and fibromatous elements: the cartilage component is usually scant, and the myxoid features dominate.

Most behave as benign active lesions, although occasionally some show aggressive characteristics. Malignant change is not a practical problem. Local staging procedures should be performed and the nature of the disorder confirmed by biopsy.

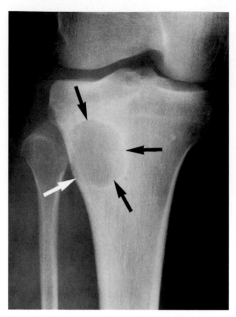

Figure 13.10 Chondromyxoid fibroma of the upper right tibia in a 17-year-old woman, demonstrating a classic geographic boundary, but some expansion and erosion of the cortex – an example of a benign active lesion, Lodwick IB.

Differential diagnosis

This includes aneurysmal bone cyst and giant-cell tumour.

Treatment

Recurrence is a major difficulty, and a wide-margin excision with reconstruction by autografting is advised, although there may be a need to compromise the margin at the growth plate if this is still open. Recurrence is common after simple curettage.

BONE-FORMING LESIONS

OSTEOID OSTEOMA

Definition

Osteoid osteoma is a small, solitary, benign painful lesion with a characteristic radiographic appearance. A central nidus contains osteoid tissue (Fig. 13.11).

Clinical features

Most cases occur between the ages of 5 and 30 years; there is a male predominance. The long bones of the lower limb are particularly susceptible, although any site may be affected. Lesions in the spine are a classic cause of a painful scoliosis. The posterior elements, particularly the region of the pedicle, are particularly prone to involvement (see Ch. 31.1).

Clinically, the patients present with significant pain that is characteristically worse at night and relieved by aspirin. If the affected area is adjacent to a joint, an effusion often forms.

Behaviour

Radiographically, a lesion in the cortex consists of an extensive area of reactive bone formation with a central nidus or

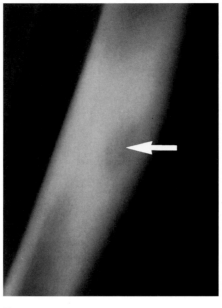

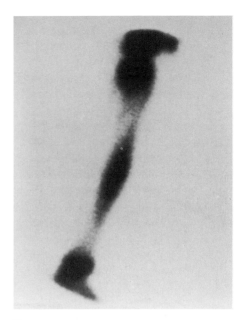

B

C

A

Figure 13.11 This 11-year-old boy had classic nocturnal pain in his left tibial shaft. A The dense sclerotic cortical lesion in the mid-shaft has a central nidus that is better seen in B. The nidus had an increased isotope uptake (C). This is a typical osteoid osteoma.

lucent zone, as seen on tomography or CT. In cancellous bone, the reactive component may be much less prominent or absent, so that identification on plain radiographs may be very difficult. Staging procedures include plain radiology, tomography or CT. A bone scan will demonstrate a hot lesion; this or an MRI scan is a mandatory investigation in any child with painful scoliosis.

Differential diagnosis

The clinical setting and staging procedures usually identify this disorder. The differential diagnosis includes stress fracture, subacute osteomyelitis and the early stages of an osteogenic sarcoma.

Treatment

Although the natural history appears to be one of gradual resolution of pain and ossification of the central nidus with maturity, the symptoms in most patients demand intervention.

One may start conservative therapy with non-steroidal anti-inflammatory drugs. If a more aggressive strategy is necessary because of pain, curettage or electrocoagulation under fluoroscopy is the method of choice. In rare cases, en

block resection is necessary (Rosenthal et al 1992, Ward et al 1993).

OSTEOBLASTOMA

Definition

This resembles osteoid osteoma, but has a central nidus greater than 2 cm in diameter (Fig. 13.12).

Clinical features

In age and sex predilection, osteoblastoma is similar to osteoid osteoma, with the lesions commonly being seen in the long bones, posterior elements of the spine and the talus. Pain is usually less severe than that seen in osteoid osteoma, and the response to salicylates less impressive.

Behaviour

Osteoblastomas are either active or aggressive benign lesions. They may be medullary or cortical in nature and, in general, have less exuberant cortical thickening than osteoid osteoma. In cancellous bone and in the spine, the radiographic appearances may be dramatic, with an expanded soap-bubble appearance, the host having time to form only

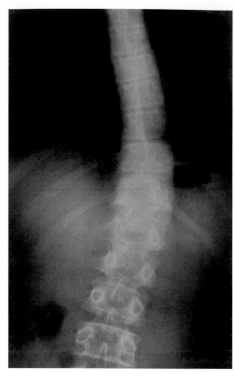

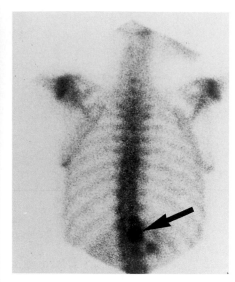

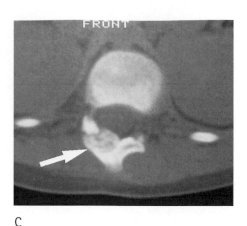

C

B

A

Figure 13.12 This 12-year-old girl presented with a painful scoliosis (A). The lesion is demonstrated by increased uptake on the bone scan (B) and identified on the lamina of T12 on CT (C). This is a classic presentation for osteoblastoma.

a thin periosteal rim. Frank soft tissue invasion is uncommon. The soft-tissue components of the tumour may be very vascular and staging studies should include angiography if excision in a difficult site is anticipated.

Differential diagnosis

This includes aneurysmal bone cyst, giant-cell tumour and in the aggressive forms, osteogenic sarcoma.

Treatment

The natural behaviour of these tumours is to be more aggressive and persistent than osteoid osteoma. Although they do not metastasise, osteoblastomas may lead to a fatal outcome with involvement of the spinal cord.

Depending upon the characteristic nature of the staging studies, the site and size of the lesion, biopsy may or may not be required before one proceeds to definitive surgery. When in doubt, it there is reasonable access and a large lesion, preliminary biopsy is recommended. Active and aggressive lesions in peripheral sites should be treated by a wide-margin excision where possible. In the spine this may not always be feasible, particularly with extensive involvement of the posterior elements. Active lesions will respond well to intracapsular curettage, but aggressive tumours show a significant recurrence rate with this procedure. Radiation has little to offer, but the surgeon may choose to use cement filling or cryosurgery as an adjunct when an aggressive lesion is sited where a wide-margin excision is not feasible. Progression to a fully malignant state is rare.

BENIGN TUMOURS OF UNCERTAIN ORIGIN

ANEURYSMAL BONE CYST

Definition

Aneurysmal bone cyst is a benign, usually solitary expansile lesion of bone, most often seen in the metaphysis of long bones. The cyst contains blood-filled spaces with solid areas formed by a mixed stroma that contains giant cells (Fig. 13.13).

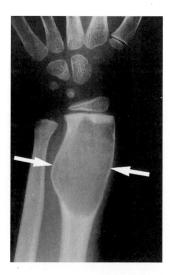

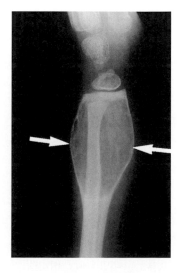

Figure 13.13 This 6-year-old boy demonstrates the features of aneurysmal bone cyst, a benign active lesion, Lodwick IB.

Clinical features

This is a disorder of the young, with lesions being rare beyond the age of 30 years. There is no sex predilection. Clinical presentation may vary between minor aching pain and a swelling to the presence of a rapidly expanding clinical mass. Aneurysmal bone cyst can present anywhere in the body. It is much more common in the ribs, spine, flat bones and pelvis than simple bone cysts. Fracture is uncommon.

Behaviour

Aneurysmal bone cysts epitomise the need to understand the nature of the host–tumour interaction; although this is a benign condition, the behaviour may vary between active and highly aggressive.

The lesions are mostly metaphyseal in the long bones, and may be central and expand the bone uniformly or, characteristically, eccentric with an explosively expansile rim – which, however, almost always contains a reactive rind of periosteal new bone. On some occasions, the lesions may arise in what appears to be a subperiosteal position, with scalloping of the cortex from without and the presence of a thin-banded bone rim separating the lesion from the surrounding soft tissue.

There is great debate concerning the nature of this disorder. Some would hold that all aneurysmal bone cysts arise as haemorrhage within another pathological lesion; others believe that there is a primary disorder of aneurysmal bone cyst, although similar radiographic and histological appearances may be undoubtedly generated by haemorrhage within established lesions. Certainly, osteoblastoma, chondroblastoma, giant-cell tumour, osteosarcoma, simple bone cyst, eosinophilic granuloma and fibrous dysplasia can all present with features similar to those of aneurysmal bone cyst, and the presence of the true underlying pathology may be detected only by careful histological assessment of the soft-tissue margins (Campanacci et al 1986).

Because of the peculiarly aggressive nature of this disorder, full staging procedures, particularly for evaluation of the local lesion, are indicated before biopsy. Angiography may be misleading in that, although there is new vessel formation in the reactive bone shell, much of the main lesion itself will not develop contrast.

The diagnostic radiographic feature is the way in which aneurysmal bone cysts extend to adjacent bones, particularly in the spine, where adjacent vertebrae, ribs, or both, may become involved. No other benign lesion commonly behaves in this way. Another radiologic peculiarity of these cysts is the appearance of fluid levels on CT or MRI.

Differential diagnosis

In the young, the differential diagnosis is with simple bone cyst, and in those who are skeletally mature the giant-cell tumour may have an identical appearance.

Treatment

The surgeon must always be aware of the possibility that an aneurysmal bone cyst is secondary to a high-grade malignancy such as osteosarcoma or one of the other conditions itemised above. Careful study of the bone scan and CT images may indicate a more extensive lesion than that shown on plain radiography, so that judicious biopsy before definitive treatment is strongly advised. It is critically important that all curettings and tissue excised at surgery be thoroughly examined by the pathologist. In the event of an aggressive local recurrence, the surgeon should be cautious.

In the management of aneurysmal bone cyst, the following three problems must be kept in mind:

1. Is this a primary or secondary aneurysmal bone cyst?
2. At what point of the spectrum of aggression does the tumour lie?
3. Does the site impose any particular technical problems with access or the proximity of vital structures?

Bones that can be sacrificed, such as the patella or head of the fibula, should be resected with a marginal margin.

Small active lesions in accessible sites should be treated by careful and thorough curettage; bone grafting is desirable, but it is not essential. Large aggressive lesions should be treated by wide saucerisation to ensure adequate curettage; grafting may be required to secure skeletal stability. The cavity may also be packed with bone cement. The use of liquid nitrogen to reduce the risk of recurrence is advocated by some (Schreuder 1997).

With recurrence, a marginal margins excision is advised, where possible, with appropriate reconstruction with autograft, allograft or cement (Bollini et al 1998).

In the spine or pelvis, where resection may not be technically feasible, adjuvant radiotherapy (30 Gy) is advised. The risk of delayed sarcoma is small.

EOSINOPHILIC GRANULOMA OF BONE

Definition

Eosinophilic granuloma of bone is a benign tumour-like condition characterised by lytic destruction of bone, with an aggregation of histiocytes and eosinophils.

Clinical features

This disorder is common in the young, particularly in the first decade of life. In some series of patients a slight preponderance of males has been recorded. The disorder is usually detected because of deformity; some are discovered incidentally, and some may present with a pathological fracture. Pain, or a palpable mass, are unusual (Makley & Carter 1986).

Behaviour

The condition is essentially a non-neoplastic, self-limiting disorder. Lesions are found characteristically in the flat bones and those containing red marrow, and are particularly common in the skull and in the metaphyses and diaphyses of long bones. Usually, there is a lucent area of destruction of cortex and some periosteal new bone. In the early phase, some lesions may be permeative, with cortical destruction. The vertebral body may be affected and vertebra plana result. On bone scanning, the lesions are hot; they are vascular on angiography.

Most of these granulomas could be classified as benign active lesions and malignant change does not occur. However, up to 20% of patients presenting with a solitary skeletal defect may go on to develop one of the more widespread variants of this disorder: Hand–Schüller–Christian disease or Letterer–Siwe disease; these are characterised by more aggressive behaviour, multifocal deposits and widespread visceral involvement. Solitary lesions of eosinophilic granuloma are self-limiting and eventually heal.

Histologically, the lesions consist of aggregations of histiocytes, some of which are of the Langerhans type and contain a T6 antigen marker. Birbeck granules can be seen on electron microscopy and are characteristic of this cell type. Aggregations of eosinophils are a feature.

Differential diagnosis

It is important to remember that eosinophilic granuloma is the great imitator and should be considered in any bony lesion in the appropriate age group, particularly if the appearances are at all atypical. The differential diagnosis includes chronic or subacute osteomyelitis and Ewing's sarcoma.

Treatment

Eventually, all eosinophilic granulomata heal. When the diagnosis is not clear, a needle biopsy should be performed. Often the lesion heals after biopsy alone. In painful persisting lesions, one may inject with corticosteroids. There is no indication for chemotherapy or radiation for a solitary lesion (Bom 1994).

Children with the more aggressive variants detailed above are candidates for irradiation therapy and chemotherapy.

MALIGNANT LESIONS

OSTEOSARCOMA

Definition

Osteosarcoma has been defined as a primary malignant tumour of bone, characterised by the formation of bone from the tumour cells of the stroma. Many tumours excite the formation of reactive bone. In this latter tissue, the bone is formed from a normal rim of osteoblasts, and the cytology of these cells and the osteocytes enclosed within the bone is essentially normal. In tumour bone, the osseous tissue is formed directly from the malignant cells without the presence of intervening osteoblasts, and the cytology of the cells contained within the bone is abnormal (Fig. 13.14).

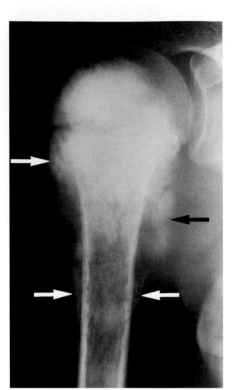

Figure 13.14 Classic osteosarcoma of the upper right humerus in a 14-year-old girl. Note destruction of the cortex, extraosseus soft-tissue mass and the Codman's triangle seen on both sides of the shaft inferiorly; this shows permeative destruction. The lesion is Grade IIB, Lodwick III.

Clinical features

Osteosarcoma is the most common primary malignant tumour of bone other than myeloma. The incidence is approximately 1.7 cases per million in the USA. Half occur in the second decade of life, with a slight male preponderance. Most patients present with a mass, which is sometimes painful. Pathological fracture can occur as a presenting feature or a late event. Sites of predilection include the lower femur, upper tibia, humerus and upper femur.

Behaviour

Conventional osteosarcoma may be classified as osteoblastic, chondroblastic or fibroblastic, depending upon the predominant matrix pattern. Osteosarcoma secondary to radiation or Paget's disease, and parosteal osteosarcoma in general, occur outside the paediatric age group. A true multicentric osteosarcoma is seen rarely, and the telangiectatic variant probably carries the worst prognosis. Attention is drawn to the so-called low-grade central form, which has a better outlook. Tumour size and increased concentrations of alkaline phosphatase are believed to be predictive factors. The hallmark of osteogenic sarcoma is the formation of tumour bone, which classically has a sunray appearance radiologically, with a mass of osseous tissue arising from the cortex of the bone. The periosteum is elevated and often breached, with tumour invading soft tissue. The elevated periosteum at the margins of the tumour may form new bone, giving rise to Codman's triangle. There is a varying degree of destruction of the underlying cortex and cancellous bone. Early metastases occur to the lung and other bones, and late metastases to many sites.

Differential diagnosis

This may include Ewing's sarcoma, and where tumour bone formation is scant, confusion may arise with aggressive benign lesions such as giant-cell tumour.

Treatment

Full staging procedures are required for this tumour, including CT and MRI if available. These determine the extent of the lesion, particularly any intramedullary spread and tissue extension, which is critical where limb salvage surgery is a possibility. Staging should be completed before biopsy. The authors are strongly in favour of needle biopsy.

There is no single correct treatment for osteosarcoma. Rather, there is a range of options and the patient and relatives must be given time and the opportunity to consider the possibilities and reach a conclusion in conjunction with a team of medical advisers, who must include at least the surgeon and an oncologist.

The points to be considered are as follows:

1. Whether the tumour is localised or metastases have already occurred.
2. The stage of the tumour: is it extracompartmental, and to what extent does it involve vital structures such as major vessels and, in particular, major nerves?
3. The desirability of referral to a specialist centre in relation to the local availability of appropriate surgical and oncological skills, bone banking, and custom prostheses. The future accessibility for the patient to orthotic services, particularly for procedures such as a rotationplasty, will need to be determined.

Role of chemotherapy

There are three reasons for treatment with chemotherapy:

1. It can diminish tumour size, and make operative resection easier.
2. Because of tumour necrosis, there is less risk of metastasis and the risk of cell spread during the operation is decreased.
3. Existing micrometastases (for instance in the lungs) may be destroyed.

Chemotherapy is therefore used before and after operation (neo-adjuvant therapy). Doxyrubicin and cisplatinum appear to be the most suitable agents for this purpose (Whelan 1997).

Six weeks after the start of chemotherapy, operation is undertaken. Overall survival is about 60% after 5 years (Souhami et al 1997), and cumulative evidence suggests that radical excision (e.g. hip disarticulation) is associated with a virtually zero local recurrence rate.

Limb salvage procedures in association with chemotherapy with or without radiation therapy are associated with a 5–10% local recurrence rate (Rougraff et al 1994). Limb salvage was found to achieve results comparable to those of amputation for osteosarcoma of the distal end of the femur, in the same long-term oncological, functional and quality-of-life study. However, a radical procedure causes major loss of function. The current view is that through-femur amputation (rotationplasty) or limb salvage surgery is the preferred modality for tumours around the knee.

Limb salvage

Requirements

There must be appropriate surgical expertise. Staging of the tumour must be accurate. A wide margin must be achievable, with preservation of vital structures, particularly the sciatic nerve or its branches. One of the principal complications of limb salvage surgery is necrosis of skin flaps, and soft-tissue cover after resection must be feasible. If motion at a reconstructed knee is to be retained, then there must be sufficient muscle retained to confer stability and to provide adequate power for walking (Simon & Springfield 1998).

Methods of reconstruction

Because about 60% of these malignant tumours are situated around the knee, the following methods of reconstruction are described for tumours in that region.

a. Resection arthrodesis. This technique should be used where widespread muscle excision is required. Fusion is best achieved over a long intramedullary rod using autograft either from the femur, tibia, iliac crest, or both, often in combination with an intercalated segment of allograft bone (Weiner et al 1996).

b. Allograft reconstruction. The affected bone may be resected and reconstructed with a massive allograft. The principal complications of this technique are infection, graft fracture and collapse of the articular surface. The principal advantage is restoration of bone stock for subsequent reconstructive procedures and the ability to reconstruct ligaments and joint capsule for preservation of knee motion. This method is less widely used, because of the unpredictable long-term results. It is more common now to use allografts in combination with prostheses.

c. Prosthetic replacement. Custom prostheses can be fabricated for reconstruction for either femoral or tibial tumours. The principal complications are infection, wound difficulties, and long-term problems with relation to the fixation and therefore the durability of the implant (Unwin et al 1996). Devices that allow for increased lengthening with age are available (Schindler et al 1997).

d. Rotationplasty (van Nes procedure). After resection of a malignant tumour of the proximal tibia or of the distal femur, the lower leg is used to lengthen the femoral stump. The tibial remnant is rotated through 180°, allowing the ankle and foot to function as a new knee. Preservation of the sciatic nerve is essential for this procedure. The procedure is mostly used for tumours of the distal femur.

When there is soft-tissue extension of the tumour into the popliteal fossa, this procedure is oncologically safer than local resection, because the vessels may be resected together with the tumour.

Rotationplasty should be considered for large tumours if the vessels are in contact with tumour tissue and if the sciatic nerve is still free. In young children, rotationplasty is a good alternative to the growing prosthesis. When a prosthesis has failed and amputation seems necessary, rotationplasty may be possible as a salvage procedure.

Function after rotationplasty is comparable to that achieved with prosthetic replacement, and the long-term complications are fewer. The ugly cosmetic appearance seems to cause few major psychological problems (Kotz & Salzer 1982, Gottsauner-Wolf et al 1991, Hillmann et al 1999, Veenstra et al 2000).

The authors' preferred plan of management for reconstruction may be summarised as follows:

1. The goal of treatment is to perform an oncologically safe procedure, with optimal function and a minimum of complications and admissions to hospital. Some patients may choose a radical solution such as amputation or rotationplasty to minimise the risk of complications. Others prefer to save the limb with an endoprosthesis, accepting the increased risk in the long term.
2. When the patient presents with a pathological fracture, an amputation is not always necessary. Limb salvage is possible if the haematoma is shown not to involve the neurovascular structures on MRI. This is often a low-energy fracture and the haematoma remains within the tumour capsule (Hoffman et al 1995).
3. The limb-saving surgery is performed after wide resection of the tumour, and reconstruction achieved with an endoprosthesis (sometimes in combination with an allograft).
4. When there is insufficient musculature left after resection to allow correct function, we prefer an arthrodesis, with allograft and an intramedullary rod. An arthrodesis loses function, but is associated with less risk of complications.
5. Rotationplasty is preferred for children younger than 10 years. This is also considered if there is a large soft-tissue tumour extension into the popliteal fossa. Rotationplasty should be considered as a salvage procedure after failed previous reconstruction.
6. For the patient who presents with metastases, the authors favour local radiation and chemotherapy to determine the pattern of disease behaviour.

It is realistic to expect a 5-year survival of 60% in patients presenting without metastases when chemotherapy is combined with one of these surgical manoeuvres.

EWING'S SARCOMA

Definition
This is a highly aggressive primary tumour of bone characterised by the histological appearance of small, rounded close-packed cells with an indistinct cell membrane (Figs 13.15 and 13.16).

Clinical features
Two-thirds of Ewing's sarcomas occur before 20 years of age; the tumour is slightly less prevalent than osteosarcoma. Approximately 50% of the tumours occur in the long bones, but the ribs, flat bones and the periphery are also involved more frequently than in osteosarcoma. The patients may present with fever, and an increased erythrocyte sedimentation rate.

Differential diagnosis
This includes osteosarcoma, other forms of lymphoma and metastatic deposits. Subacute osteomyelitis may give rise to a similar onion-skin appearance of elevated periosteum.

Behaviour
Whereas osteosarcoma is a lesion of metaphyses, Ewing's tumour tends to be more common in the diaphysis, and is characterised by permeative destruction and, classically, by an 'onion-skin' appearance produced by sequential layers of bone being laid down by an elevated periosteum. Soft-tissue extension of the tumour is common, and best detected on MRI. Metastases are frequent.

Management
The need to discuss biopsy details with a pathologist before surgery has been emphasised; if Ewing's sarcoma is

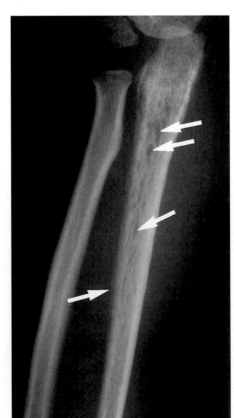

Figure 13.15 Ewing's sarcoma in a 6-year-old boy, demonstrating moth-eaten destruction, with lytic areas of varying size and destruction of part of the cortex. Periosteal new bone can be seen distally. A Lodwick III lesion.

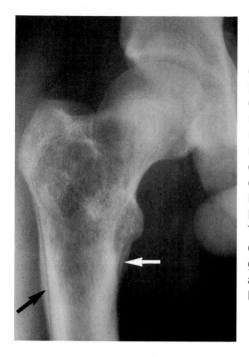

Figure 13.16
Radiograph of a 16-year-old youth, demonstrating permeative destruction of the metaphyseal and neck region of the right femur and onion-skin layering of the periosteum laterally. Diagnosis: Ewing's sarcoma. The medullary disease still has a geographic appearance; this is Lodwick II.

suspected, this is critically important. Lymphoma and other rare tumours such as primitive neuroectodermal tumour of bone, or metastases from neuroblastoma, can have similar appearances on paraffin sections (Triche & Cavazzana 1988).

In Ewing's sarcoma, there is a translocation of the long arms of chromosomes 11 and 22 (Aurias et al 1983). Correct identification of the tumour, in specialist laboratories, will involve electron microscopy, immunocytochemistry, karyotyping, cytogenetics and, possibly, short-term tissue culture.

There is no doubt that all patients with Ewing's sarcoma should have chemotherapy, and modern regimens recommend the use of vincristine, dactinomycin, doxirubicin, cyclophosphamide, with or without ifosfamide and etoposide (Paulussen et al 1999).

The optimal management for the primary lesion is controversial. The use of radiotherapy alone has led to significant rates of local recurrence (up to 30%) and considerable long-term sequelae from radiation damage to skin, soft tissues and growth plates. If a wide excision with limb preservation can be carried out, this should be performed with or without additional radiation. There is increasing acceptance of the value of surgery in the management of all primary lesions (Paulussen et al 1999), hence marginal excision with radiation is better than radiation alone. At the present time, there are insufficient data available to provide accurate guidelines, but it would appear that, in general, surgical attempts to control the primary lesion increase survival. Survival rates of up to 60% at 5 years are being achieved with appropriate operative and chemotherapeutic procedures.

MISCELLANEOUS TUMOURS

Adamantinoma is a rare tumour seen classically in the shaft and upper end of the tibia. The tumour should be considered a possibility in the case of any unusual lesion with extensive bone destruction. The risk of metastases is about 25% (Hazelbag et al 1994). A wide-margin resection is required for most tumours, with appropriate reconstruction.

Leukaemia may present with permeative destruction adjacent to the growth plate on the metaphyseal side. The blood picture should identify the nature of the pathology. In osteogenesis imperfecta, an aggressive *hyperplastic callus* can develop after fracture and may be confused with osteogenic sarcoma unless the pathologist is aware of the underlying disorder.

Myositis ossificans may occur in the paediatric age group and is characterised by the formation of calcified osteoid in soft tissues adjacent to bone (Fig. 13.2). Classically there is a lucent zone radiographically between the bone and the tumour, with calcification being more intense at the periphery of the lesion. In contradistinction, tumours generally ossify and calcify in a centrifugal fashion.

Giant-cell tumour is very rarely seen while the growth plate is open, but can occur in children, when it is a metaphyseal lesion. In the adult, it is classically epiphyseal and extends to the region of the subchondral bone plate.

ACKNOWLEDGEMENTS

We wish to thank Dr H Mankin, Boston, for his guidance and help for many years. I am indebted to Dr W F Enneking whose proposals on tumour behavioural classification and philosophies underlie many of the opinions expressed in this chapter.

REFERENCES

Altman A J, Schwartz A D 1978 Malignant diseases of infancy, childhood and adolescence. W B Saunders, Philadelphia

Aurias A, Rimbaut C, Buffe D, Dubousset J, Mazabraud A 1983 Chromosome translocations in Ewing's sarcoma. New England Journal of Medicine 309: 496–497

Bollini G, Jouve J L, Cottalorda J, Petit P, Panuel M, Jacquemier M 1998 Aneurysmal bone cyst: analysis of twenty-seven children. Journal of Pediatric Orthopaedics 7B: 274–285

Bom L P A 1994 Langerhans cell histiocytosis. Wibro disseratie drukkerij Helmond

Campanacci M, Capanna R, Picci P 1986 Unicameral and aneurysmal bone cysts. Clinical Orthopaedics and Related Research 204: 25–36

Enneking W F 1983 Musculoskeletal tumor surgery. Churchill Livingstone, New York

Enneking W F 1986 A system of staging musculoskeletal neoplasms. Clinical Orthopaedics and Related Research 204: 9–24

Gherlinzoni F, Rick M, Picci P 1983 Chondromyxoid fibroma. Journal of Bone and Joint Surgery 6A: 198–204

Gottsauner-Wolf F, Kotz R, Knahr K, Kristen H, Ritschel P, Salzer M 1991 Rotationplasty for limb salvage in the treatment of malignant tumours at the knee. Journal of Bone and Joint Surgery 73A: 1365–1375

Hazelbag H M, Taminiau A, Fleuren G J, Hoogendoorn P, 1994 Adamantinoma of the long bones. Journal of Bone and Joint Surgery 76A: 1482–1499

Hillmann A, Hoffmann C, Gosheger G, Kraukau H, Winkelmann W 1999 Malignant tumor of the distal part of the femur or proximal part of the tibia: endoprosthetic replacement or rotationplasty. Journal of Bone and Joint Surgery 81A: 462–468

Hoffmann C, Jalar S, Ahrens S et al 1995 Prognosis in Ewing sarcoma patients with initial pathological fractures of the primary tumour site. Klinische Padiatrie 211: 151–157

Kim J H, Chu F C, Woodard H Q, Melamed M R, Huvos A, Cantlin J 1978 Radiation induced soft-tissue and bone sarcoma. Radiology 129: 501–508

Kotz R, Salzer M 1982 Rotation-plasty for childhood osteosarcoma of the distal part of the femur. Journal of Bone and Joint Surgery 64A: 959–969

Lodwick G S, Wilson A J, Farrell C, Virtama P, Dittrich F 1980 Determining growth rates of focal bone lesions from radiographs. Radiology 134: 577–583

Lokiec F, Weintroub S 1998 Simple bone cyst; etiology, classification, pathology, and treatment modalities. Journal of Pediatric Orthopaedics 7B: 262–273

Makley J T, Carter J R 1986 Eosinophilic granuloma of bone. Clinical Orthopaedics and Related Research 204: 37–44

Mankin H, Mankin C J, Simon M A 1996 The hazards of biopsy, revisited. Journal of Bone and Joint Surgery 78A: 656–663

Mulder J D, Schutte B E, Kroon H M, Taconis W K 1993 Radiologic atlas of bone tumours. Elsevier, Amsterdam

Paulussen M, Ahrens S, Braun-Munziger G et al 1999 EICESS 92 (European Intergroup Cooperative Ewing's Sarcoma Study) – Preliminary results. Klinische Padiatrie 211: 276–283

Rosenthal D I, Alexander A, Rosenberg A E, Springfield D 1992 Ablation of osteoid osteoma with a percutaneously placed electrode: a new procedure. Radiology 183: 29–33

Rougraff B T, Simon M, Kneisl J S, Greenberg D B, Mankin H J 1994 Limb salvage compared with amputation for osteosarcoma of the distal end of the femur. A long-term oncological, functional and quality-of-life study. Journal of Bone and Joint Surgery 76A: 649–656

Schindler O, Cannon S, Briggs T, 1997 Stanmore custom-made extendible distal femoral replacements. Journal of Bone and Joint Surgery 78B: 927–937

Schreuder H W B 1997 Aneurysmal bone cysts treated by curettage, cryosurgery and bone grafting. Journal of Bone and Joint Surgery 79B: 20–25

Schuppers H A, van der Eijken J W, 1998 Chondroblastoma during the growing age. Journal of Pediatric Orthopaedics 7B: 293–297

Schwartz H S, Zimmerman N B, Simon M A, Wrobel R R, Millar E A, Bonfiglio M 1987 The malignant potential of enchondromatosis. Journal of Bone and Joint Surgery 69A: 269–274

Simon M A, Springfield D, 1998. Surgery for bone and soft-tissue tumours. Lippincott-Raven, Philadelphia

Skrzynski M C et al, 1996 Diagnostic accuracy and charge savings of out patient core needle biopsy compared with open biopsy musculo-skeletal tumours. Journal of Bone and Joint Surgery 78A: 644–649

Souhami R L, Craft A W, van der Eijken J W et al 1997 Randomised trial of 2 regimens of chemotherapy in operable osteosarcoma: a study of the European Osteosarcoma Intergroup. Lancet 350: 911–917

Springfield D S, Capanna R, Gherlinzoni F, Picci P, Cumpanacci M 1985 Chondroblastoma. Journal of Bone and Joint Surgery 67A: 748–755

Stephanson R B, London M B, Hanlin T M, Kaufer H 1987 Fibrous dysplasia. An analysis of options for treatment. Journal of Bone and Joint Surgery 69A: 400–409

Triche T, Cavazzana A 1988 In: Unni K K (ed) Bone tumours. Churchill Livingstone, Edinburgh, pp 199–223

Unwin P S, Cannon S, Grimer R, Kemp H, Sneath R, Walker P 1996 Aseptic loosening in cemented custom-made prosthetic replacements for bone tumours of the lower limb. Journal of Bone and Joint Surgery 78B: 5–13

Veenstra K M, Sprangers M, van der Eijken J W, Taminiau A H M 2000 Quality of life in survivors with a van Nes-Borggreve rotationplasty after bone tumour resection. Journal of Surgical Oncology 73: 192–197

Walter J B, Israel M S 1987 General pathology, 6th edn. Churchill Livingstone, Edinburgh

Ward W G, Eckhardt J J, Shayenstehfar S, Mirrar J, Cogen T, Oppenheim W 1993 Osteoid osteoma diagnosis and management with low morbidity. Clinical Orthopaedics and Related Research 291: 229–235

Weiner S D, Scarborough M, Van der griend R A 1996 Resection arthrodesis of the knee with an intercallary allograft. Journal of Bone and Joint Surgery 78A: 185–192

Whelan E R 1997 Paediatric update osteosarcoma. European Journal of Cancer 33: 1611–1619

Section III
Neuromuscular disorders

Chapter 14

Neurology overview

J. Wilson

INTRODUCTION

There is an intimate relationship between the practice of orthopaedics and clinical neurology in children. Important prognostic, therapeutic and genetic issues may be involved when the orthopaedic surgeon recognises that there is a neurological component underlying an orthopaedic problem (Fig. 14.1).

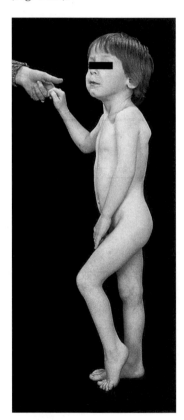

Figure 14.1 Child of 3 years with a left spastic hemiplegia.

HISTORY

A careful history and clinical examination are crucial to neurological evaluation. The family history – especially of consanguinity – and, on occasion, examination of both parents may be very revealing. During gestation, the stage at which fetal movements are perceived, their vigour and character may help to establish if weakness or seizures are of prenatal onset. Primiparous mothers usually recognise fetal movements later, e.g. at 22–24 weeks in contrast to 16–18 weeks for a multiparous mother who has the benefit of

experience. Many mothers of deformed or neurologically abnormal children state that they felt unwell during pregnancy or sensed that 'something was not right'. Sometimes these opinions are well founded, but these doubts are frequent during otherwise normal pregnancies, and tend to be forgotten when a healthy child is born.

Prematurity remains the most common cause of infantile neurological morbidity, especially in infants weighing 1 kg or less at birth. The frequency is greater in those who have low Apgar scores at birth, and if there has been respiratory distress, fits or apnoeic attacks in the neonatal period. The Apgar score, ranging from 1 to 10, is an arbitrary scoring system incorporating measures of colour, heart rate, ventilatory rate, cry and tone in newborns. Although not ideal, it is a useful measure of newborn vigour. Neonatal jaundice, with increased concentrations of unconjugated bilirubin, can be damaging, especially in premature infants. Fetal distress may be a sign of hypoxic–hypotensive insult before or during delivery. Profound hypoxia for a relatively brief period (10–30 minutes) can lead to selective damage to the basal ganglia, whereas prolonged (more than 1 hour) partial hypoxia will cause more diffuse cortical damage, with watershed infarction.

Any infant who is underweight for gestational age has a greater frequency of neurological abnormalities than other infants of comparable maturity but normal weight. Exceptionally small infants have an increased liability to cerebral birth injury, hypoglycaemia, congenital abnormalities and ventilatory problems. Sometimes parents are slow to recognise conditions that were present from birth. In infants with hemiplegic cerebral palsy, the development of the brain and the acquisition of certain developmental skills such as reaching or grasping or voluntary kicking have to reach a certain stage before the contrast in voluntary control between the two sides becomes obvious. Handedness does not usually become clearly defined until after 12 months of age, and strong lateralisation before this suggests that an infant has a hemiplegia unless there is some more obvious explanation. Similarly, in many infants and young children who ultimately prove to have significant degrees of mental handicap or locomotor problems, these are not recognised until developmental progress diverges sufficiently from the normal for this to be noted. It is important to distinguish between what is reported and what is observed. It has been acknowledged that unless the mother has kept a 'baby book' or a health visitor a contemporary record, an infant's developmental milestones are quickly forgotten.

In presenting a history of an evolving condition or one of apparently subacute onset, it is common for parents to relate the condition to trauma or infection. Although often coincidental, it is clear that some conditions, such as Guillain–Barré syndrome (postinfectious polyneuritis), are a complication of a viral infection. In certain degenerative diseases, such as spinal muscular atrophy, infection appears to serve as a 'trigger', but is not the cause. In other conditions, such as spinocerebellar degenerations, there is sometimes a clear history of trauma apparently acting as a trigger. Interpretation of these events becomes particularly important when a medicolegal opinion is sought.

EXAMINATION

HYPOTONIA AND WEAKNESS

Hypotonia is a common component of locomotor dysfunction in infancy and early childhood. It is necessary to decide whether a child is weak or not. This distinction can be difficult in very young children, but if an infant has a lusty cry, is sucking well and its limbs seem active, it is unlikely that there is a significant degree of weakness, however floppy the infant may seem. Hypotonia *per se* may be of peripheral or central origin (Fig. 14.2). The most common peripheral cause is probably congenital ligamentous laxity; when prominent, this may suggest a primary neuromuscular disease. In certain comparatively benign metabolic myopathies, e.g. central core disease, hypotonia may be more obvious than weakness. Both the cerebellum and basal ganglia influence tone, but their contribution may not be immediately obvious in an infant who presents only with delayed motor development and hypotonia, and whose balance and co-ordination problems are not yet established. Many severely mentally handicapped children are also hypotonic.

MUSCLE WASTING

Muscle wasting may be difficult to evaluate in an obese infant. Ultrasound, computed tomography (CT) or magnetic resonance imaging (MRI) examination of the limbs can reveal the extent of the wasting. Fasciculation, signifying lower motor denervation, may also be obscured by subcutaneous fat, but can be seen more easily in the tongue. When present in the interossei, it may cause fine irregular tremor of the fingers, signs worth seeking in infants and young children with suspected Werdnig–Hoffmann disease or the more chronic forms of spinal muscular atrophy.

Disuse atrophy can occur very quickly, and this is presumably the basis of muscle wasting confined to one limb, which may confuse the diagnosis of osteoid osteoma and other tumours. It seems likely that 'reflex' wasting is secondary to pain and may be comparable to the sudden onset of focal weakness and hypotonia associated with the pain of a greenstick fracture or synovitis of a joint. Trophic changes are commonly seen in both upper and lower motor neurone denervation. This is seen most dramatically in poliomyelitis, myelomeningocele and arthrogryposis. Differences in growth velocity occur in hemiplegic limbs, although differential growth rates do not inevitably cause a progressive discrepancy throughout childhood. Trophic differences between the upper limbs, e.g. in hemiplegic cerebral palsy,

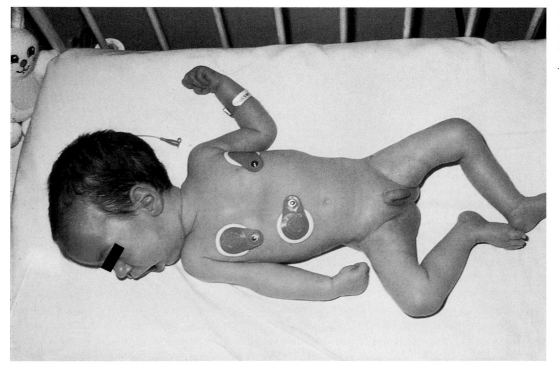

Figure 14.2 Hypotonic (floppy) baby suffering from an X-linked myopathy and joint contractures.

may be very subtle, such as differences in thumb-nail size in a child with minimal hand involvement. Limb hypertrophy may occur in association with hemihypertrophy of the brain, but patterns vary. Many children with cerebral damage or maldevelopment of early onset do not grow normally.

HYPERTONUS

The distinction between voluntary resistance and reflex involuntary hypertonus can be very difficult, especially in a distressed and excited child. Spastic hypertonus is usually associated with hyper-reflexia, unless there is marked contracture or the associated tendon has been the site of previous surgery. Extrapyramidal hypertonus is characteristically variable. It may or may not be associated with increased tendon reflexes, but in the infant and young child it is usually associated with symmetric and asymmetric tonic neck reflexes, increased startle response, and feeding problems, with tongue thrust. Co-ordination of sucking and swallowing are also affected.

EVALUATION OF TENDON REFLEXES

Tendon reflexes tend to be much brisker in infants than in older children. It is well known that the Babinski sign is an unreliable sign of pyramidal dysfunction in this age group. In infants and toddlers up to the age of 18 months to 2 years, an extensor response may be entirely normal; likewise, a few beats of ankle clonus are normal in infancy and early childhood. Conversely, in older children a flexor plantar response may be found despite other compelling evidence of pyramidal dysfunction. Although there is much to commend examining a young child who is sitting quietly on the mother's lap, tendon reflexes in the upper limbs are normally less brisk than in the lower limbs when elicited in the sitting position. Absence or reduction of tendon reflexes usually signifies denervation of either afferent or efferent pathways, but this may also be depressed in myopathic disorders if the muscle stretch receptors are severely involved or if myopathic weakness is very advanced.

ATAXIA

Ataxia means unsteadiness or inco-ordination. Some writers use it to imply a cerebellar disorder, but this is an incorrect restriction of its derivation and usage. Many conditions interfering with proper co-ordination and muscle function will cause ataxia. Thus ataxia may result from weakness, sensory impairment or interference with central regulation – that is, cerebellar or basal ganglia disorders. It may be difficult to distinguish the early stages of cerebellar disorders from denervating or myopathic conditions.

SENSATION

Most children from 3 years of age are able to co-operate in sensory testing. In younger children and infants, and in older mentally handicapped children, the presence of sensory impairment may have to be inferred. Impairment of pain sensation is important, because this may give rise to trophic ulcers and chronic sensory arthropathy (Charcot joints). In children this is relatively rare, being seen mostly in congenital sensory neuropathies (Fig. 14.3), myelomeningocele and other forms of spinal dysraphism.

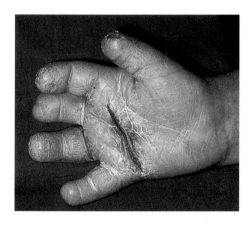

Figure 14.3 The right hand of a child with congenital insensitivity to pain. Note the healing injury to the palm and the loss of the finger tips as a result of repeated trauma, which is often self-inflicted in these children.

CONTRACTURES

Contractures occur relatively easily in children, but there are certain diseases in which they are particularly liable to develop:

- Myopathies, especially:
  - Duchenne muscular dystrophy
  - Emery–Dreifuss sex-linked muscular dystrophy
  - congenital fibre-type disproportion
- Denervating conditions
  - intermediate forms of chronic spinal muscular atrophy
  - traumatic denervation
  - poliomyelitis
  - post-infective polyneuritis
  - prenatal denervation producing arthrogryposis
- Spastic disorders
  - cerebral palsy (hemiplegic, diplegic, quadriplegic)
  - hereditary spastic paraplegia
- Extrapyramidal
  - athetoid/dystonic cerebral palsy
  - torsion dystonia
  - postencephalitic athetosis
  - postanoxic damage to the basal ganglia
  - genetically determined neurometabolic syndromes

PES CAVUS

A neurological basis for pes cavus should always be carefully sought. This involves examination, not only of the patient, but also of the parents and siblings. Remediable conditions such as diastematomyelia, syringomyelia and congenital intramedullary cysts of the spinal cord should always be sought. Progressive conditions, particularly those with genetic implications such as Friedreich's ataxia, ataxia telangiectasia and hereditary motor and sensory neuropathies (Charcot–Marie–Tooth disease), should be considered (Fig. 14.4).

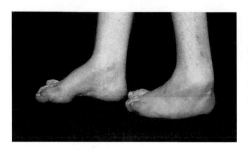

Figure 14.4 Bilateral cavovarus feet in hereditary motor and sensory neuropathy Type I.

TOE-WALKING

Toe-walking may be a purely idiosyncratic phenomenon, seen particularly in tense, excitable, hyperactive children and in some mentally handicapped children. In the early stages the child can be persuaded to bring the heels to the ground. If the habit persists, calf contracture and fixed equinus can develop. If a contracture does not develop, it is possible to demonstrate that there is neither spasticity nor hyper-reflexia; however, once a contracture is present, muscle tone is difficult to evaluate and tendon reflexes may be impossible to elicit. A neurogenic basis for toe-walking should always be looked for in these children.

SPINAL DEFORMITY

Idiopathic thoracic scoliosis is usually convex to the right. Scoliosis in the opposite direction is a feature of syringomyelia associated with the Arnold–Chiari malformation. MRI is particularly helpful in investigating both these conditions.

Scoliosis and torticollis occur in a large number of other neurological disorders. There may be associated vertebral abnormalities and diastematomyelia, or congenital cysts (intramedullary and extramedullary). There is also an association with the Klippel–Feil deformity and Sprengel's shoulder. If there is evidence of osseous malformation with or without neurological abnormality, cord imaging is recommended. MRI is very useful, but may not invariably show significant cord pathology, in which case contrast myelography is necessary. Head tilt may be a manifestation of cerebellar hemisphere tumour before classical cerebellar signs or evidence of increased intracranial pressure are obvious.

INVESTIGATION OF NEUROLOGICAL DISORDERS

DIAGNOSTIC IMAGING

Plain radiology

Although plain radiology of the skull has been largely superseded by CT except in the routine assessment of suspected head injuries, plain radiology of the spine remains very valuable. Vertebral malformations, subluxation (for which views carefully obtained in flexion and extension may be needed), erosion of the pedicles, widening of the vertebral canal or enlargement of the intervertebral foramina (both with space-occupying lesions), scalloping of the vertebral bodies (neurofibromatosis) and beaking of the lumbar vertebrae (mucopolysaccharidoses) can be seen.

Computed tomography

High-resolution CT of the brain is very valuable, but has important limitations. Brain-stem and cord anatomy are not well shown, but contrast myelography in conjunction with CT is very informative. At the level of the foramen magnum and the first cervical vertebra, the technique may show evidence of an Arnold–Chiari malformation and can also demonstrate very well both ventricular size and macroscopic cortical architecture in patients with meningomyelocele. Abnormal calcification is particularly well shown.

Single-photon emission CT (SPECT)

SPECT combines the imaging techniques of CT with a more dynamic and functional localisation of pathology using an injected isotope. It is particularly valuable when an alteration of the permeability of the blood–brain barrier or vascular perfusion is being investigated.

Magnetic resonance imaging

This technique is particularly useful in investigating demyelinating conditions and to demonstrate brain-stem, pituitary and hypothalamic structures. The posterior fossa is also well demonstrated.

Imaging of the spinal cord presents technical difficulties because of the difficulty of obtaining a satisfactory sagittal image if there is more than 1° of spinal deformity. In both the brain and spinal cord, imaging of inflammatory and neoplastic conditions can be markedly enhanced by intravenous injection of gadolinium.

Technical advances have brought much faster imaging than that of 10 years ago, but the need for immobility to ensure optimum imaging requires sedation, or even general anaesthesia, for children who cannot co-operate adequately.

Positron emission tomography (PET)

PET combines the administration of radioactively labelled metabolically active compounds with MRI, and provides a refined form of functional imaging. Mainly a non-invasive research tool, it provides exciting data concerning the localisation of higher cortical function.

Cranial ultrasound

Real-time cranial ultrasound can be a useful investigation in infants, provided that the anterior fontanelle is open. It can be used for suspected intracranial insult and to evaluate malformations such as agenesis of the corpus callosum and hydrocephalus.

Muscle biopsy

Where it is anticipated that muscle disease is patchy, as in autoimmune diseases such as polymyositis or dermatomyositis, muscle MRI or ultrasound examination can be used to locate a site for biopsy at a maximally involved location. Many myopathies are metabolically determined and are characterised by their histochemistry and ultrastructure. Techniques of open biopsy and needle biopsy are simple, but should not be undertaken unless the investigating laboratory has the necessary technical expertise to interpret them; the interpretation of a muscle biopsy is highly skilled. If an open biopsy is required, it is most important to avoid trauma to the specimen from compression, infiltration or previous needling – e.g. electromyography. The fascicle is isolated by blunt dissection, ligatured proximally and distally, and pinned in an extended position on a cork before being sent to the laboratory for investigation.

Nerve biopsy

When peripheral nerve biopsy is required, the sural nerve is usually chosen, as it passes between the lateral malleolus and the calcaneum. The resulting sensory loss along the outer aspect of the foot does not seem to worry children.

Electrophysiological investigation

Electroencephalography is valuable in the investigation of seizure problems, in the evaluation of acute neurological disease, and in certain degenerative disorders. The measurement of sensory evoked potentials is particularly useful during scoliosis surgery for monitoring cord function.

Electroneuromyography is used for the study of peripheral nerve and muscle function. It is usually possible to distinguish between myopathic and denervating conditions. Among the latter, it is possible to distinguish between segmental demyelination, in which conduction in myelinated fibres is markedly slowed, and axonal degeneration, in which denervation characteristics are seen on electromyelography with a reduction in amplitude of nerve action potentials but relatively mild slowing of nerve conduction. In anterior horn cell degeneration, in addition to electromyographic evidence of denervation, giant motor unit potentials are seen.

Electrocardiography and echocardiography

Cardiac function may be seriously affected in certain myopathic disorders such Duchenne muscular dystrophy, and an electrocardiogram should be included in the investigation of suspected myopathic disorders. In Friedreich's ataxia, hypertrophic obstructive cardiomyopathy occurs; for this, electrocardiography is the non-invasive investigation of choice.

Clinical biochemistry

The measurement of plasma creatine kinase (CK) is the most frequently used screening test for muscle damage. This enzyme is crucial in the release of energy from energy-rich phosphocreatinine, and is present in very high concentration in muscle cells. When these are damaged, the enzyme leaks into the blood and urine, and increased concentrations can easily be measured. This is most useful in distinguishing myopathic from denervating disorders. Very large increases in CK concentrations are seen in Duchenne muscular dystrophy and moderate increases in certain metabolic myopathies, whereas in very indolent dystrophic disorders such as facio-scapulo-humeral dystrophy, plasma CK values are normal. The CK should be measured before any potentially damaging procedures such as electromyography or intramuscular injections are performed.

Such have been the advances in molecular genetics in the past decade, that tissue sampling for the identification of gene loci is now part of the investigative process for gentically determined neuromuscular diseases. Tests are expensive, and their discerning application should be guided by clinical geneticists.

DISEASES AND SYNDROMES

Neural tube defects

Neural tube defects can occur at any site in the neuraxis, but only those involving the spinal cord concern us here. The term 'spinal dysraphism' is applied to midline fusion defects, both anterior and posterior, involving the vertebral column and neural tube separately or in combination. There is a wide variation in severity from the spina bifida occulta that is present in approximately 10% of otherwise normal children and without evidence of neural involvement, to the open meningomyelocele with exposed neural tissue leaking spinal fluid. The Arnold–Chiari malformation, with varying degrees of protrusion of the cerebellar tonsils into the upper cervical canal, is commonly associated with spinal dysraphism. This malformation may be asymptomatic, but may cause obstructive hydrocephalus, which requires urgent shunting. Hydrocephalus may only become evident and require shunting when an open neural tube has been closed.

The degree of weakness and secondary deformity in the limb depends, not only on the spinal segmental level of the malformation, but also on the degree of involvement of the cord and nerve roots. At the lower levels, a lipoma is often entangled in the cauda equina, which is also tethered to the vertebral canal. Sphincter involvement is invariable in the most severe forms. A history of disturbance of micturition and bowel function should always be sought.

Fetal ultrasonography can now detect the more severe forms of malformation at a stage of pregnancy at which it is lawful to abort a defective foetus if the parents so wish. Closed neural tube defects, however, with an insignificant meningocele, are difficult to detect prenatally. Clinically, spinal dysraphism is suspected if there is a vascular or pigmented naevus, hairy patch, lipoma or coccygeal pit in or near the midline (Fig. 14.5). However, there may be no

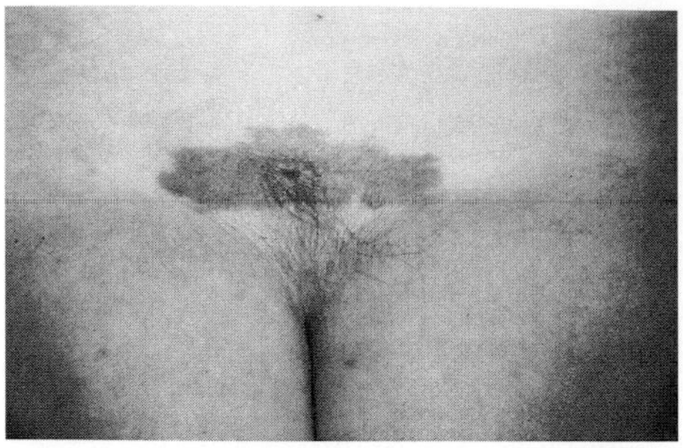

Figure 14.5
Hairy naevus over the lower lumbar spine in a child with spinal dysraphism who presented with club foot and leg wasting.

superficial abnormality, and the clinical manifestation is a foot deformity or trophic changes in one or both feet, with wasting of the calf and, commonly, reduction of the ankle jerk. There may be sensory impairment, particularly in the distribution of S1. Plain radiology of the lumbar spine may be normal, as abnormalities of cord development with or without tethering (myelodysplasia) are not always accompanied by radiological spina bifida or cutaneous abnormalities. It is sound practice to image the entire spine, including the cervical spine, when there is a neurological abnormality or neurogenic deformity in the feet or legs.

Space-occupying lesions

Space-occupying lesions of the central nervous system are common, but do not usually present as orthopaedic problems. Nevertheless, some lesions may present as gait abnormalities, postural abnormalities of the spine, or foot and toe deformities. Slowly growing intracranial lesions usually present as asymmetric spasticity, with or without ataxia. Space-occupying lesions of the cord may present as gait problems with spasticity, often asymmetric, and there may be lower motor neurone signs (wasting, weakness, impaired tendon reflexes), which help to localise the pathology. Sensory involvement is difficult to evaluate in young children, and its clinical use is limited in the younger age group.

A syrinx may present as an asymmetric weakness of one or more upper or lower limbs. It may be difficult to demonstrate any sensory impairment. Scoliosis is often seen. The Arnold–Chiari malformation is commonly associated and sooner or later most, if not all, patients with this malformation and spina bifida cystica develop a syrinx. This may not be symptomatic, but any condition in which there is disturbance of cerebrospinal fluid hydrodynamics in the vertebral canal, particularly at the cervico-medullary junction, can lead to syrinx formation.

Muscular dystrophies and denervating diseases
These are considered in Chapter 15.

Cerebral palsy
This is described in Chapter 18.

Hereditary sensorimotor neuropathies
It is important for the orthopaedic surgeon to be aware of these sensorimotor neuropathies, because they often produce

orthopaedic symptoms and signs. There are at least six clinically and genetically distinct disorders in which abnormalities of sensorimotor nerves are prominent, although not necessarily exclusive. They are distinguished from conditions in which peripheral neuropathy is part of a more generalised neuraxial abnormality (e.g. Friedreich's ataxia and metachromatic leucodystrophy), and from the sensory neuropathies in which motor nerves are spared but can produce important problems for orthopaedic surgeons because of neuropathic joints, neuropathic fractures and ulceration. The predominantly clinical classification of sensorimotor neuropathies shown below has not yet been completely superseded by a molecular genetic classification, although molecular defects have been identified in the majority.

Type I. Charcot–Marie–Tooth disease with demyelinating neuropathy
Type II. Axonal neuropathy
Type III. Dejerine–Sottas disease (hypertrophic interstitial neuropathy)
Type IV. Refsum's disease (heredopathia atactica polyneuritiformis, also known as hereditary areflexia)
Type V. Hereditary sensory neuropathy with spastic paraplegia
Type VI. Hereditary sensorimotor neuropathy with optic atrophy

Types I–III are of most importance to the orthopaedic surgeon. Type I, Charcot–Marie–Tooth disease, is usually inherited as an autosomal dominant and is rarely seriously disabling in childhood. Children may present for the first time in an orthopaedic clinic for advice about pes cavus, equinus deformity and broadening of the forefoot. Kyphosis and scoliosis may present later in childhood. Tendon reflexes tend to be lost early, and sensory impairment, especially of joint position and vibration sense, may be seen in childhood. The classical 'champagne bottle' leg deformity is rarely seen in children. Many affected parents are unaware that they have the disease themselves. It is always worth examining the parent in addition to the child. Among sporadic cases, 30% are believed to represent new dominant mutations, whereas the remainder are believed to be autosomal recessive. Exceptionally, a few patients with a similar but more severe condition show a sex-linked recessive inheritance.

Type II is considered to be similar to Type I both genetically and clinically, but is claimed to be more slowly progressive, and the sensory impairment to be less obvious.

In the type III condition, sensorimotor disturbance tends to be more severe, with club feet, severe muscle wasting and weakness, and peripheral impairment of all sensory modalities. There is also proximal involvement, and scoliosis is commonly seen as the disease advances. There is a hypertrophic interstitial neuropathy with 'onion-skin' formation demonstrable microscopically in the early stages and clinically evident as palpably thickened subcutaneous nerves.

It is important for the orthopaedic surgeon to recognise that these conditions are progressive. Corrective surgery may be indicated and useful, but will inevitably tend to relapse with time. These patients do not tolerate prolonged immobilisation, which should be avoided at all costs. With the identification of molecular genetic defects, genetic counselling is now much more focused than in the days when it was based exclusively on the statistics of Mendelian ratios.

FURTHER READING

Aicardi J 1998 Diseases of the nervous system in childhood, 2nd edn. MacKeith Press, London

Brett E M 1997 Paediatric neurology, 3rd edn. Churchill Livingstone, Edinburgh

Chapter 15

Hereditary and developmental neuromuscular disorders

E. E. Bleck

INTRODUCTION

This chapter does not encompass acquired neuromuscular diseases such as poliomyelitis or developmental disabilities such as arthrogryposis, cerebral palsy and spina bifida, which are described in other chapters. Discussion is confined to those conditions characterised by weakness resulting from pathology primarily in the muscles or the anterior horn cells of the spinal cord. In their later stages these disorders have recognisable clinical features, but in the early stages all share a common set of symptoms and physical signs that merit electromyographic studies, blood tests for muscle enzymes, and muscle biopsies for staining and microscopic analysis. In muscular dystrophies, dystrophin immunoblotting or DNA mutation analysis or both (from a piece of frozen muscle) have been increasingly used to differentiate between the types of muscular dystrophy. Dystrophin testing has enhanced the diagnosis of the muscular dystrophies, the identification of carriers, and the accuracy of prenatal diagnosis in 70–80% of cases (Shapiro & Specht 1993). Furthermore, advances in molecular biology have identified the locus of the specific gene responsible for the disorder in many conditions (see Table 15.3).

In the first part of this chapter, the diagnostic features will be discussed. The second part will describe the characteristics of each disease and the orthopaedic deformities encountered. Some classifications and names for the diseases of muscle have changed since the last edition of this book.

CLINICAL EXAMINATION

SYMPTOMS

Most parents are aware of the normal milestones of development and are concerned if their child is not reaching them. The most common symptoms that cause parents to seek consultation are listed in Table 15.1. It is salutory to remember that Read & Galasko (1986) reported a mean delay of 2 years in making the diagnosis of Duchenne muscular dystrophy, particularly on the part of orthopaedic surgeons.

GAIT

Children should be asked to walk along a well-lit walkway or corridor and their gait observed, so that stance and swing phase in the sagittal plane, and rotation in the transverse plane, can be assessed (Fig. 15.1).

A waddling gait may not necessarily represent hip

Table 15.1 Common symptoms of neuromuscular disease	
Infancy	
	Floppy baby
	Slow development; not sitting unaided at 9 months
	Muscles lack consistency and tone
Childhood	
	Tiptoeing (most common complaint in Duchenne muscular dystrophy)
	Clumsy; awkward
	Cannot keep up with other children
	Runs strangely
	Seems weak and fatigues easily
	Waddling gait
	Posture is poor; stands with 'sway-back and pot-belly' (Fig. 15.1)
	Cannot cut with scissors in kindergarten
	Printing by hand or writing is slow and laboured
	Is he/she 'learning disabled'?

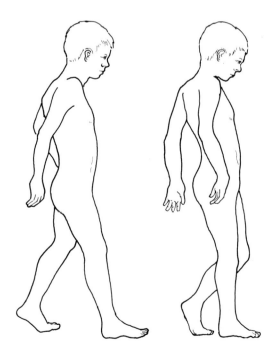

Figure 15.1 Typical gait of a child who has muscular dystrophy.

abductor weakness; dysplasia of the hip will have to be ruled out by radiographs. A high-stepping gait is associated with weakness of ankle dorsiflexion and a toe-drag gait with spasticity.

When asked to run, a child with barely perceptible spastic hemiplegia will often flex the elbow and clench the fist on the involved side in the so-called 'folded wing' position. A child with muscle weakness appears laboured when running, and seems to be in a heel–toe walking race.

POSTURE

Slight degrees of shift of the spine from the midline may be noted in addition to a loin crease, both of which are early signs of scoliosis, an early manifestation of neuromuscular disease. Forward drooping of the shoulders, a prominent abdomen or lumbar lordosis should arouse suspicion (Fig. 15.2). Winging of the scapula can be mistaken for a benign, slumped posture (Fig. 15.3).

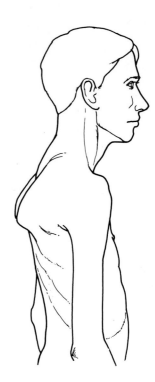

Figure 15.3 Postural 'slump', forward cupping of the shoulders and winged scapulae, characteristic of scapulohumeral muscular dystrophy. (Redrawn from Walton & Gardner-Medwin 1981.)

nine times in sequence. The Trendelenburg test may be difficult to elicit in a normal child younger than 6 or 7 years, because of a lack of fully developed balance reactions.

Manual muscle testing
In children who can co-operate (generally at 7 years or older), manual muscle testing and Medical Research Council (MRC) grading should be performed (Table 15.2).

Muscle tone
Although contemporary physiotherapists commonly use the term 'tone', its meaning is poorly defined. The French use the

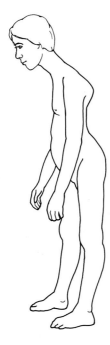

Figure 15.2 Typical standing posture of a child with a myopathy.

MUSCLE TESTING AND OBSERVATION

Manual muscle testing is difficult in a child younger than 6 years.

Activity test
The child should be asked to walk on his heels, sit on the floor and then rise (Gower's sign; Fig. 15.4), stand on one foot, hop, step up and down from a stool, climb stairs and walk on tiptoe. One-sided tiptoeing, while the examiner holds the child's hand for balance, is a most useful way of demonstrating significant gastrocnemius–soleus weakness. Normally, a child should be able to rise on one foot eight to

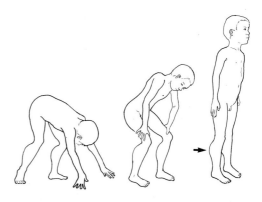

Figure 15.4 Gower's sign: the child arises from the floor by 'walking up' the thighs with his hands – a functional test for quadriceps muscle weakness. Note the bulky calf (arrow).

Table 15.2 Manual muscle testing (MRC grading)	
Power 5 (normal)	The portion of the limb being tested moves through its full range against gravity and maximum resistance
Power 4 (good)	Moves against gravity and moderate resistance
Power 3 (fair)	Moves against gravity, but not against resistance
Power 2 (poor)	Moves only with gravity eliminated
Power 1 (trace)	Flicker of contraction only
Power 0 (zero)	No movement

terms 'extensibilité' – the amount of lengthening permitted by the muscle – and 'passivité' – denoting the lack of resistance to passive movement (André et al 1960). Passivité can be best assessed by flapping the hand after grasping the forearm and moving it up and down rapidly. The real value of the term is in the diagnosis of the 'floppy' or hypotonic infant (Dubowitz 1969); later in childhood, the sign is less useful. The hypotonic infant will form the inverted letter U when suspended by the abdomen (Fig. 15.5), and will tend to slip through the fingers when held vertically under the axillae (Fig. 15.6). Head lag, occurring when the baby is pulled upwards from the supine position, is usual (Fig. 15.7) and the 'scarf sign' demonstrates shoulder girdle weakness (Fig. 15.8).

There are many causes of hypotonia: they may be classified under the broad categories of chemical, endocrine and neuromuscular. The most common causes in infancy are spinal muscular atrophy, congenital myopathies (e.g. central core disease and nemaline myopathy), mental retardation, cerebral palsy, Down's syndrome, and benign congenital

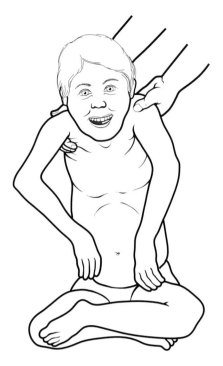

Figure 15.6 When lifted by the hands under the axillae, the hypotonic child slips through the examiner's hands.

hypotonia. Definitive diagnosis of the paralytic type of hypotonia is largely dependent on muscle biopsy.

In 41 of 80 infants who had the floppy infant syndrome electrodiagnostic results were correlated with the nerve and muscle biopsies (David & Jones 1994). Nerve conduction velocities were highly correlated with the biopsies in 93% who had Werdnig-Hoffman disease and 100% with those who had congenital infantile polyneuropathy. The correlation of electromyography with a biopsy proven myopathy was only 40%.

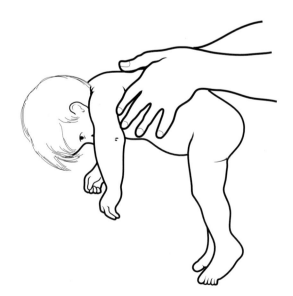

Figure 15.5 A hypotonic infant assumes the inverted 'U' posture when held prone.

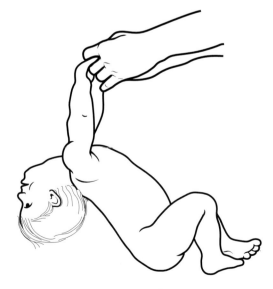

Figure 15.7 When pulled upward by the arms from supine, the hypotonic child has head lag.

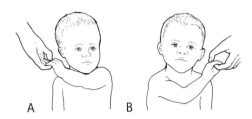

Figure 15.8 Scarf sign. On adduction of the upper limb across the chest, the hypotonic limb can be wrapped around the neck. **A** Affected child. **B** Normal child.

Atrophy and hypertrophy

The degree of atrophy in lower motor neurone disease is generally consistent with the amount of weakness, whereas in primary myopathies it is not.

Hypertrophy is most noticeable in myotonia congenita, in which muscle strength is proportional to bulk. Early in Duchenne muscular dystrophy, the calves, deltoid and vastus lateralis muscles will appear hypertrophied. In later stages 'pseudohypertrophy' occurs as the muscle fibres are replaced by fat.

Three myopathies are characterised by severe weakness, but no atrophy: myasthenia gravis, polymyositis, and periodic paralysis. This observation is very important, because these three myopathies are among the very few that can be treated (Walton 1981a).

Fasciculations

Spontaneous twitching of the muscles, especially in the calf, the intrinsic muscles of the hand and the tongue, characterises a degenerating anterior horn cell disease. However, if fasciculations are not seen, anterior horn cell disease cannot be ruled out, as denervation fibrillation (arrhythmic 'blips' that can be seen only on the electromyograph) may still be present.

Reflexes

The deep tendon reflexes usually disappear early in the neuropathies and diminish in parallel with muscle weakness in the myopathies. They are preserved in polymyositis and myasthenia gravis. The plantar responses are always flexor (negative Babinski sign) in the myopathies and neuropathies, except in the rare case of spinal muscular atrophy with pyramidal tract involvement (Gardner-Medwin et al 1967). If extensor responses occur, upper motor neurone disease should be suspected.

LABORATORY INVESTIGATIONS

SERUM ENZYMES

By far the most sensitive test in the diagnosis of Duchenne muscular dystrophy is the measurement of creatine phosphokinase. Very high concentrations occur before the onset of symptoms and signs, and gradually decrease as the disease progresses, because the muscle is replaced by fat in the later stages. The concentrations of serum aldolase, serum glutamic oxaloacetic transminase (aspartate aminotransferase) and lactic dehydrogenase are increased in muscle wasting disease, but are less reliable indicators than the creatine phosphokinase concentration.

ELECTROMYOGRAPHY

Although the electromyogram reveals quite specific forms of denervation fibrillations and fasciculations in lower motor neurone lesions, it is less diagnostic in muscle fibre diseases (Figs 15.9 and 15.10). In the latter, polyphasic and giant

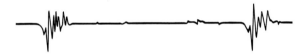

Figure 15.9 Electromyograph of lower motor neurone degenerative disease, depicting positive sharp waves with interspersed denervation fibrillation potentials (neuropathic

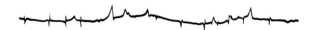

Figure 15.10 Electromyograph demonstrating fasciculations in a patient with spinal muscular atrophy (neuropathic pattern).

motor units are seen, with voluntary contractions of the muscle; however, about 10% of normal individuals will show similar electromyographic patterns (Fig. 15.11).

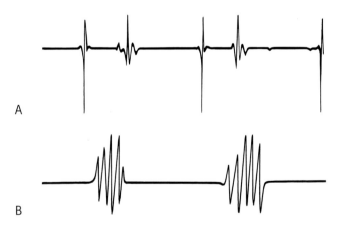

Figure 15.11 A Electromyograph in Duchenne muscular dystrophy, showing the polyphasic motor units of a myopathic pattern. **B** Normal electromyograph pattern, with moderate voluntary effort.

If the recording device is one that emits sound, the myotonias produce the noise of a 'dive-bomber' in response to voluntary contraction or the insertion of a needle electrode. The electromyograph records initial high activity, followed by delayed relaxation, termed 'prolonged trains' (Fig. 15.12).

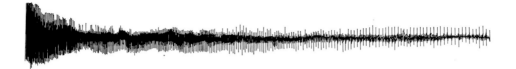

Figure 15.12 Electromyograph showing classic myotonic discharge pattern on voluntary muscle contraction.

Nerve conduction studies in motor neurone disease are normal. However, these are useful in distinguishing muscle weakness resulting from peripheral neuropathies, when they will confirm prolongation of normal velocity times.

Motor and sensory (usually the sural or the median) nerve conduction studies assist in differentiating the hypertrophic type (type I) of Charcot–Marie–Tooth disease from the other four types (Bradley 1981).

MUSCLE BIOPSY

The muscle chosen for biopsy should be abnormal, and should be distant from the site of needle insertion, to avoid distortion of the histology. Biopsies are usually obtained from the vastus lateralis, rectus femoris or the lateral head of the gastrocnemius. In those who have proximal muscle weakness, the vastus lateralis is sampled, but in the case of distal weakness, the gastrocnemius is the preferred site (Shapiro & Specht 1993).

Although local anaesthesia can make the biopsy useless because of muscle fibre distortion, percutaneous Bergstrom needle sampling with local skin anaesthesia and no infiltration of the muscle has been demonstrated to be an effective means of providing samples for histological, histochemical and electron microscopic analysis. Using this needle, several muscle sites can be sampled in sedated infants and children (DiLiberti et al 1983; Heckmatt et al 1984). The tissue obtained is immediately frozen, usually in liquid nitrogen, and then processed for microscopy.

Open biopsy in children requires spinal, regional or general anaesthesia. A 1.4-cm wide clamp is best to hold the muscle fibres. Alternatively, both ends of a 1.5-cm piece of muscle are secured by suture to a wood stick or card before the muscle is severed 2–4 mm from the sutured ends. Cautery should be avoided until a specimen is obtained. *The specimen must not be immersed in formalin, as the muscle will be ruined for histological study.* It should be *fixed immediately in 4% glutaraldehyde for electron microscopy.* If there is delay in fixing the specimen, it should be placed in a Petri dish, on a piece of filter paper dampened with saline, but avoiding excessive wetting. A 15-minute delay is permissible, but a dry specimen is unusable.

HISTOLOGICAL DIAGNOSIS

Although microscopy of muscle biopsies prepared with histochemical stains is unnecessary in Charcot–Marie–Tooth disease, myotonias and myasthenia, histology is essential in the diagnosis of myopathies. Two main histochemical types of muscle fibre are recognized: type I (slow twitch, oxidative) and type II (fast twitch, glycolytic). Type II fibres are further divided into IIa (high glycolytic and high oxidative enzymes) and IIb (predominantly glycolytic). Normal human muscles possess an equal distribution of type I and type II fibres. However, long-distance runners may develop 90% of type I fibres, and some sprinters have a predominance of type IIa fibres (Gamble 1988a). Electron microscopy affords further definition of muscle structure.

Later in this chapter, drawings are presented to depict the particular characteristics of the muscle when processed for histological diagnosis. These examples of the histological patterns in a variety of muscle diseases are not intended as a definitive exposition of the subject. Students who wish to pursue the topic should consult the authoritative text by Walton (1981b).

AETIOLOGY AND INHERITANCE

With the exception of myasthenia, the exact pathogenesis of the neuromuscular disorders is unknown, but almost all, except polymyositis and myasthenia, have defined patterns of inheritance: the dystrophies and myopathies are usually autosomal dominant or sex-linked, whereas the atrophies are generally autosomal recessive (Table 15.3). A positive family history is not invariable, as spontaneous mutations may occur. The responsible gene in Duchenne and Becker muscular dystrophies has been identified on the xp21 region of the X- chromosome, with 65 coding regions (exons), including coding for the 400-kilodalton protein, dystrophin. Dystrophin protein comprises 0.01% of the muscle protein, functioning as a component of the cell membrane exoskeleton. Its distribution correlates well with the clinical findings in Duchenne and Becker muscular dystrophies.

DIFFERENTIAL DIAGNOSIS

Table 15.3 lists the most common neuromuscular disorders that need to be considered in children, showing the relevant clinical, hereditary and laboratory details. Figure 15.13 categorises them anatomically.

MANAGEMENT

PHYSICAL THERAPY

The emphasis in any physical therapy programme should be upon mobility and independence. The child should be moved

Table 15.3 Inheritance, diagnostic criteria, orthopaedic deformity of neuromuscular disorders*

Diagnosis	Inheritance	Gene locus	CPK	EMG	Nerve conduction	Muscle biopsy	Orthopaedic deformity
I. Anterior horn cell							
Spinal Muscular Atrophy	AR	5q13, deletion exon 7 on SMN	Normal to slight Increase	Neuropathic	Normal	Neuropathic	Scoliosis, hip dislocation Flexion contractures
I. Werdnig–Hoffman							
II. Chronic infantile							
III. Kugelberg–Welander							
II. Nerve Fibre							
Charcot–Marie–Tooth (HMSN)							
Type I	AD		Normal	Neuropathic	Decreased	Neuropathic	Cavovarus feet
Type II	AD				Can be normal		Scoliosis
Type III	AR				Decreased		Hip dysplasia
Type IV	AR				Normal		
Type V	AD				Can be normal		
III. Muscle							
A. Dystrophies							
Duchenne (dystrophin absent)	XL	xq21.2	Very increased	Myopathic	Normal	Myopathic	Equinovarus feet Scoliosis, Contractures Heart‡; Intellectual‡
Beckers (dystrophin present)	XL	xq21.2	Very increased	Myopathic	Normal	Myopathic	None
Emery–Dreifuss	XL	xq28	Mild increase	Myopathic	Normal	Myopathic	2nd decade: equinus, flexion contractures elbow, extension contracture neck, stiff back, AV heart block‡
Fascio–scapulo–humeral	AD	4q3.5	Normal to slightly high	Myopathic	Normal	Myopathic	Winged scapulae
Limb–girdle	AR	5q22-q34	Increased	Myopathic	Normal	Myopathic	Late contractures
Infantile fascio–scapular–humeral	AR		Normal	Myopathic	Normal	Myopathic	Facial diplegia, winged scapulae, extreme lumbar lordosis, foot drop, hearing loss‡
Congenital muscular dystrophy							
Merosin neg.	AR	6q2	Normal	Myopathic	Normal	Characteristic	Contractures; CNS involvement‡
Merosin pos.	AR		Normal	Myopathic	Normal	Characteristic	No CNS involvement

Fukuyama	AR	9q31-33	Increased	Myopathic	Normal	Characteristic	Muscle necrosis, CNS involvement‡
B. Myopathies							
Central core	AD		Normal	Myopathic	Normal	Characteristic	Hip dislocation, scoliosis pes valgus, malignant hyperthermia‡
Nemaline	AD		Normal	Myopathic	Normal	Characteristic	Scoliosis
Myotubular	AD, R, XL	xq28	Normal	Myopathic	Normal	Characteristic	Scoliosis, foot
Fibre type disporption	AD		Normal	Myopathic	Normal	Characteristic	Scoliosis
Minicore	AD		Normal	Myopathic	Normal	Characteristic	Rare
Mitochondrial	Unknown; familial		Normal	Myopathic	Normal	Characteristic	None reported
C. Myotonias							
Myotonia Congenita							
Becker	AR	7q	Normal	Typical+	Normal	Muscle hypertrophy	None
Thomsen (Calcium Chloride Disease)	AD		Normal	Typical	Normal	Muscle hypertrophy	Malignant hyperthermia‡
Myotonic dystrophy	AD		Normal	Typical	Normal	Muscle atrophy; type 1 fibres Motor end plate changes	Muscle weakness, atrophy, late frontal baldness, testicular atrophy, cataracts, heart conduction defects‡
(Steinhart Disease; Myotonia dystrophica; Myotonia Atrophica)							
Congenital myotonic dystrophy	AD		Increased or normal	Typical	Normal	Atrophy type 1 fibres	Club foot Mental retardation‡
D. Polymyositis–dematomyositis	No inheritance		Increased or Variable	Myopathic	Normal	Characteristic	Late muscle contractures
E. Myasthenia gravis	AR		Variable	Normal	Repetitive nerve stimulus response	Normal	None; variable weakness

* Adapted from Shapiro & Specht 1993; Aicardi 1998
† Typical=electromyographic pattern of contraction with trailing-off (dive bomber sound)
‡ Other significant involvement
AD, autosomal dominant; AR, autosomal recessive; CNS, central nervous system; HMSN, hereditary motor and sensory neuropathies; SMN, surviving motor neuron; XL, sex-linked

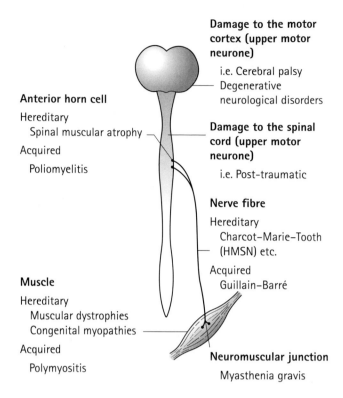

Damage to the motor cortex (upper motor neurone)

    i.e. Cerebral palsy
    Degenerative
    neurological disorders

Anterior horn cell

Hereditary
    Spinal muscular atrophy

Acquired
    Poliomyelitis

Damage to the spinal cord (upper motor neurone)

    i.e. Post-traumatic

Nerve fibre

Hereditary
    Charcot–Marie–Tooth
    (HMSN) etc.

Acquired
    Guillain–Barré

Muscle

Hereditary
    Muscular dystrophies
    Congenital myopathies

Acquired
    Polymyositis

Neuromuscular junction

    Myasthenia gravis

Figure 15.13 Schematic representation of differential diagnosis in muscle weakness.

out of the seated position for 2–3 hours during the day and allowed to roll about and play on a mat. This is more effective than passive stretching by the physiotherapist, although every attempt should be made to counteract the remorseless development of contractures. Walking should be encouraged, but eventually proves impossible when the hip abductor and extensor muscles weaken to grade III or less. Formal ventilatory therapy to maintain and enhance diminishing ventilatory reserve has not been sufficiently rewarding to recommend its routine use. Adaptive physical education and wheelchair games seem to encourage respiratory exchange and avoid repetitive and tedious exercises. Swimming in a heated pool is ideal, as water allows the trunk and limbs to move freely and at the same time provides resistance to maintain muscle strength.

The therapist should select external supports to maintain walking ability. When this is no longer possible, the child should be provided with a wheelchair of appropriate specification.

Occupational therapists are adept in the design and fabrication of eating and grooming utensils. They can suggest clothing adaptations for easier dressing, toiletry and bathing, and instruct both parent and child about wheelchair transfer techniques.

ORTHOTICS

The plastic ankle–foot orthosis has been useful in preventing equinus contracture. However, once a contracture of greater than 5° develops these devices become ineffective. Plastic knee–ankle–foot orthoses are useful as long as the child has the hip muscle power to walk. Attempts to substitute for hip muscle strength by the addition of a pelvic band are fruitless if function is the goal. Orthoses do not prevent hip flexion contractures, because the patient merely develops a greater compensatory lumbar lordosis. Hip flexion contractures greater than 45° lead to loss of standing ability.

Spinal orthotics are ineffective in preventing the progression of scoliosis (Colbert & Craig 1987). The Milwaukee brace has been discarded, although plastic body jackets (thoraco-lumbar spinal orthoses) possibly retard progression slightly and are usually prescribed to 'hold' the curve until the patient is old enough to undergo spinal instrumentation and fusion (Evans et al 1981). Instrumentation without fusion in children younger than 10 years is preferable to the struggle of enforcing orthotic wear that will inevitably fail. A custom-made wheelchair insert appears to be a better and more comfortable spinal support for those patients confined to a wheelchair.

ASSISTIVE TECHNOLOGY

Powered wheelchairs that allow the patient to recline, sit up and stand up are available. Electrically operated beds afford comfort when resting and sleeping. Transportation in specially designed wheelchair vans has expanded the horizon of these unfortunate children outside the home and increased the freedom of the family. Electric toothbrushes and ingenious bath-tub lifts, alteration in shower stall entrances, bidets that attach to toilet seats to obviate the need for laborious and often impossible paper cleansing, have improved independence as well as eased the constant burden on the family and carers. Electronic environmental controls with sensitive pressure switches put the command of much of the household at the fingertips. Patients with impaired breathing can be assisted by a custom Cuirass ventilator powered from the wheelchair batteries. Finally wheelchair accessible residences, public buildings, streets and pavements should provide freedom of movement and improved social contact.

ORTHOPAEDIC SURGERY

Scoliosis

Scoliosis occurs in 90% of the spinal muscular atrophies, Duchenne muscular dystrophy and some of the myopathies. Fortunately in the past 20 years the development of spinal instrumentation has allowed surgical correction before respiratory compromise becomes too great and the operative risk untenable (see Ch. 31.2).

Segmental interlaminar wiring to L-rods, originated by Luque (1982) and modified for pelvic fixation, is currently the preferred method of instrumentation and fusion (Allen & Ferguson 1982). If the patient has large enough vertebrae, 6.5-mm rods can be used rather than the smaller 3.25-mm ones. The unit rod, consisting of two limbs bent in the top as a U, with lower extensions to enter the pelvis, is favoured by most surgeons. Postoperatively, splintage with anteroposterior plastic shells (Kydex R) supports the patient during sitting for approximately 6 months. Anterior disc excision and fusion to mobilise a rigid curve, followed by posterior instrumentation and fusion, should be undertaken infrequently, because of the poor lung vital capacity in these children. Anterior thoraco-lumbar approaches to the spine invariably entail cutting the entire diaphragm from its rib and vertebral attachments, which contributes to increased ventilatory compromise.

The rise of the acquired immunodeficiency syndrome epidemic has stimulated the use of autologous blood transfusion and cell-saver devices in the operating room, to reduce the need for large quantities of donor blood. Freeze-dried bone allografts have also reduced blood loss by eliminating the necessity for harvesting large amounts of bone from the patient to supplement these very long spinal fusions.

In Duchenne muscular dystrophy, spinal fusion and instrumentation should be performed when the child is no longer an independent walker. Usually, the curvature at this stage is 35–40° (Smith et al 1989). Once the curve approaches 70–90° and the vital capacity is less than 30–40%, the patient is likely to retain carbon dioxide, and surgery under general anaesthesia is too great a risk. Blood gases and pulmonary function should always be measured before operation. A patient who retains carbon dioxide will continue to do so after surgery and may never be released from a respirator, and frequently requires a tracheostomy. Therefore there is a strong case for early surgery.

Scoliosis in spinal muscular atrophy develops early and invariably progresses to a severe degree, with accompanying respiratory compromise. Spinal instrumentation should be performed relatively early, before the curve becomes too severe (Aprin et al 1982). Harrington instrumentation according to the method of Moe et al (1984), in which no fusion is performed, would seem to be ideal to prevent further progression of the curve until the child is old enough for fusion (usually older than 10 years). Luque instrumentation without fusion in young children has been abandoned because of unacceptable breakage of instrumentation after surgery (Rinsky et al 1985).

Contractures

Flexion contractures of the hip and knee and equinus and varus of the ankle and foot are common in neuromuscular disorders. In order to prolong walking ability, some surgeons relieve these contractures by tenotomy, lengthening and myotomy (Siegel 1981), although outcome studies suggest that in those treated the mean age of cessation of walking was on average 1 year later than the expected age of 10.5 years. This vigorous surgical and orthotic approach may not be appropriate, as Duchenne muscular dystrophy is inevitably progressive. After surgery the amount of walking is generally brief, and the energy consumed by the patient in trying to walk is considerable. Helping the patient achieve optimal function and independence in a powered wheelchair and with adaptations to other equipment has been more satisfying.

Equinus of the ankle and varus of the foot are exceptions to this limited surgical perspective. Hsu (1990) reported his experience with foot and ankle releases and transfer of the tibialis posterior tendon through the interosseous membrane in 25 children aged between 8 and 13 years with Duchenne muscular dystrophy. The use of knee–ankle–foot orthoses prolong walking by an average of 38 months. Even if the patient cannot walk, an equinus contracture prevents comfortable positioning of the foot in a wheelchair because the toes drag on the ground, with resultant skin breakdown and pain.

In the slowly progressive spinal muscular atrophies, a case can be made for surgical treatment of flexion contractures of the hips and knees if there is some evidence of preservation of motor power in the hip extensors and abductors and knee extensors.

Upper limb contractures in Duchenne muscular dystrophy are almost always in the position of function, and should not be altered.

Hip subluxations and dislocations

These occur frequently in the myopathies and probably account for the failure of maintenance of reduction in some cases of presumed congenital dislocation of the hip. The diagnosis of a myopathy should alert the surgeon and the family to a guarded prognosis and the likely development of contractures despite physiotherapy (Gamble 1988b).

SPINAL MUSCULAR ATROPHY

CLASSIFICATION

Three types of spinal muscular atrophy have been described and classified according to the patient's age at disease onset (Shapiro & Specht 1993). All show muscle weakness, a 90% incidence of scoliosis, serious compromise of ventilatory function, and the need for orthopaedic care.

Type I (acute infantile (Werdnig–Hoffman's) disease)

This presents a characteristic posture, with the upper and lower limbs in the 'pithed frog' posture and diaphragmatic breathing (Fig. 15.14). The mean survival is 6 months and 95% of affected infants are dead by 18 months (Campbell & Liversedge 1981, Gardner-Medwin & Tizard 1981). The onset of the type I form is from birth to 6 months.

Type II (chronic infantile (intermediate group))

The chronic infantile form of spinal muscular atrophy has an onset from 6 months and is usually manifest by the age of 2 years, after which it is slowly progressive. Life expectancy can extend into the third decade of life. Progressive scoliosis, limb contractures and diminished vital capacity are the rule.

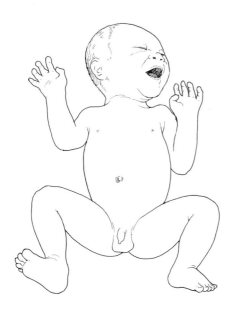

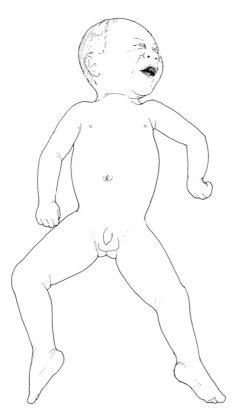

A

B

Figure 15.14 A Typical 'pithed frog' posture of a new-born with spinal muscular atrophy; the upper and lower limbs lie akimbo, with abduction at the hip and shoulder, the knees and elbows flexed, and the hands open. **B** Posture of a new-born with spinal muscular atrophy, type I (Werdnig–Hoffman), showing bloated abdomen, and shoulders internally rotated, giving a 'jug handle' appearance.

Type III (chronic proximal (Kugelberg–Welander))

Type III has its onset in the child older than 2 years and commonly affects young adults. Authorities describe chronic distal, scapulo-peroneal and fascio-scapulo-humeral forms, which can be mistaken for the muscular dystrophies (Campbell & Liversedge 1981).

MUSCLE TESTING

Muscle biopsies show a typical neuropathic pattern (Fig. 15.15). The electromyograph confirms a lower motor neurone disease with characteristic fibrillation and fasciculation potentials (see Fig. 15.10).

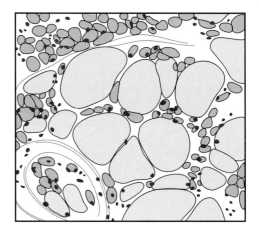

Figure 15.15 Schematic drawing of muscle biopsy in spinal muscular atrophy. There is characteristic atrophy of mixed fibre types, and enlarged fibres that have a similar enzymic (neuropathic) profile. (After haematoxylin & eosin staining; original magnification ×300.) (Redrawn from Dubowitz 1981.)

MUSCULAR DYSTROPHIES

DUCHENNE TYPE

The prevalence of this sex-linked, severe and progressive dystrophy has been estimated as between 1.9 and 3.4 per 100 000 population (Walton & Gardner-Medwin 1981). It is a disease almost entirely exclusive to males. The female carriers can be detected by an increased serum creatine phosphokinase concentration in 70–75% of cases. Detection can be aided by electromyographic examination, followed by muscle biopsy of the abnormal muscle.

Clinical signs

The earliest symptoms are clumsiness, impaired balance and a tiptoe gait. Although present at birth, the disease does not normally manifest itself until the age of 3–4 years. Walking ceases at a median age of 10 years (range 7–11 years) and fatal cardiac failure occurs between the ages of 19 and 21 years, occasionally up to 25 years. The intellect is affected, and approximately 30% of patients have an intelligence quotient less than 75 (Zwelleger & Hanson 1967).

Diagnosis

The diagnosis is confirmed by a creatine phosphokinase concentration 100–300 times greater than normal. The electromyograph demonstrates polyphasic units and shortened duration action potentials on voluntary muscle contraction. The changes are not diagnostic for Duchenne muscular dystrophy, but are characteristic of myopathies (see Fig. 15.11).

Dystrophin testing of a piece of skeletal muscle has advanced the diagnosis and differentiation of the Duchenne type from the Becker and Emery–Dreifuss types (Hoffmann & Kunkel 1989). In Duchenne muscular dystrophy, dystrophins are completely absent, whereas in the other two types they are present, but altered in size or decreased in amount, or both (Shapiro & Specht 1993).

The muscle biopsy shows a dystrophic pattern, with variation in the size of both fibre types, indicating hypertrophy and atrophy (Fig. 15.16).

Treatment

Obesity is common in the muscular dystrophies, and physicians are urged to prevent it by correct nutritional instruction of the parents and child.

Treatment of the dystrophies by means of megavitamins, amino acids, anabolic steroids and other experimental methods has been tried over the years, without any effect on the progress of the disease. Transfer of myoblasts of normal muscle into the muscle of boys who had Duchenne muscular dystrophy was attempted in 10 boys who were implanted with 100 million myoblasts into the anterior tibial muscle of one leg, with the other as a control. Unfortunately, myoblast implantation was not effective in replacing a significant amount of dystrophin in the muscles (Miller et al 1997). This is not surprising, given experimental experience in which massive death of myoblasts recurred after their injection into the dystrophic muscles of female mdx mice (the animal model for Duchenne muscular dystrophy) (Fan et al 1996).

Scoliosis should be treated by early operative correction and fusion. Galasko et al (1992) offered surgical stabilisation of the spine to 58 patients in whom the curve was 20° or more. Thirty-two accepted surgery at a mean age of 14 years. In this group, the mean correction was 30° and there was progression of only 4° after 36 months. In those who rejected surgery, the curve increased to a mean of 93° in 36 months. These authors reported that the peak expiratory flow rate increased in those who had surgery. However, Shapiro et al (1992) did not find lasting improvement in the mean forced vital capacity in 27 patients who underwent scolosis surgery.

Equinovarus deformities of the feet should be treated surgically. Lengthening of tendo-Achilles and transfer of the posterior tibial tendon anteriorly through the interosseous membrane to the midfoot has been useful (Miller et al 1982).

Aggressive release of contractures of muscles and joints to prolong walking beyond the usual age of 10 years (when it ceases in most boys who have Duchenne muscular dystrophy) has to be very selective and individualised. The child and parents have to understand that the goals of the surgery are limited to the maintenance of walking. This may not be restored by surgery or may cease within weeks or months depending upon the progression of the disease. Claims that boys of 14 or 15 years have continued to walk after surgical treatment have to be modified, because these boys may have had undiagnosed Becker muscular dystrophy. Nowadays, this more benign muscular dystrophy can be identified by molecular studies and laboratory confirmation of low dystrophin concentrations.

Electric wheelchairs offer independent and efficient mobility. Motor vans with wheelchair lifts or ramps have enhanced the quality of life for patient and family alike.

BENIGN X-LINKED (BECKER) MUSCULAR DYSTROPHY

Clinical signs

Becker muscular dystrophy is a sex-linked recessive muscle disease that differs from the Duchenne type by its later onset and the relatively benign course; only 10% of those affected become unable to walk before the age of 40 years. Although it cannot be easily differentiated from the Duchenne type in its early presentation, nowadays muscle dystrophin determination will differentiate it from the Duchenne type, because dystrophin is present in the muscles, albeit in decreased amounts. Dystrophin is a protein localised to the muscle cell membrane, but is also present in the brain and other tissues.

Calf enlargement is the most frequent early sign of the disease, and muscle cramps are more common than in the

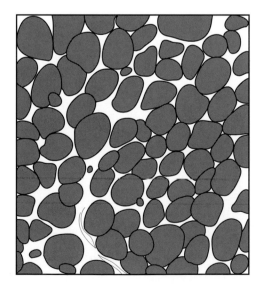

Figure 15.16 Duchenne muscular dystrophy. Schematic drawing of a muscle biopsy shows variation in fibre sizes affecting both type I and II fibres. (After ATPase, pH 9.4.) (Redrawn from Dubowitz 1981.)

other dystrophies and myopathies. Leg pains and cramps are so prevalent in childhood that they can be misconstrued as so-called exercise cramps or growing pains.

Diagnosis

The creatine phosphokinase concentration is high in Becker muscular dystrophy, and a normal finding rules it out in boys who complain of persistent leg pains and cramps. Determination of the dystrophin concentration has become an important means of differentiating it from the Duchenne type.

Prognosis

Contractures are rare, and do not occur until very late in the disease when the patient is already confined to a wheelchair. Cardiac involvement is not a feature of this myopathy and, consequently, life expectancy exceeds that of Duchenne muscular dystrophy (mean age of death 42 years, range 23–63 years).

EMERY–DREIFUSS MUSCULAR DYSTROPHY

Clinical signs

The initial presentation of Emery–Dreifuss muscular dystrophy is a non-specific muscle weakness in the first few years of life, with an awkward gait and, possibly, toe-walking. The dystrophy becomes fully developed in the second decade of life, with fixed equinus, flexion contractures of the elbows, and an extension contracture of the neck. Most importantly, these patients have bradycardia and eventually develop complete heart block. The condition is autosomal recessive.

Diagnosis

Electromyography and a muscle biopsy confirm the myopathy. The creatine phosphokinase concentration is only slightly to moderately increased. If Duchenne or Becker muscular dystrophy (or both) have been ruled out by determination of the dystrophin protein in the muscle, the diagnosis of Emery–Dreifuss muscular dystrophy is confirmed.

Prognosis

Muscle weakness is progressive but slow, so that walking is generally possible into the fifth or sixth decades of life. The ankle equinus can become severe. Elbow contractures appear as early as 7 years, whereas limited flexion of the neck, caused by the extension contracture, may be evident at 5 years and is clearly evident by the 20s. The importance of defining this type of muscular dystrophy is the need for a cardiac assessment. Bradycardia and a first-degree atrio-ventricular heart block can result in sudden death between the ages of 25 and 60 years (Shapiro & Specht 1993).

Orthopaedic management

Lengthening of tendo-Achilles may be indicated for severe equinus. If varus of the foot is present, transfer of the posterior tibial tendon anteriorly to the dorsum of the foot

may be advised. Elbow flexion contracture, even if it is 90°, rarely limits function; consequently, no treatment is necessary. If scoliosis develops, it generally stabilises at an acceptable 40° after spinal growth has ceased, and surgery is probably not indicated.

LIMB–GIRDLE MUSCULAR DYSTROPHIES

Clinical signs

This group of autosomal recessive dystrophies present at variable ages and with varying progression. They represent a heterogeneous disorder that encompasses the slowly progressive muscle weakness that affects either the upper limbs in adolescence (scapulo-humeral type) or the lower limbs (limb-girdle type), without facial weakness, after the age of 20 years. In more severe cases, the distal muscles of the limbs are also affected (Fig. 15.17). The presence of facial weakness changes the term to 'facio-scapulo-humeral' muscular dystrophy. The hallmark of the scapulo-humeral type of limb-girdle muscular dystrophy is winging of the scapula, although the biceps and triceps are affected also (see Fig. 15.3). Strangely, the deltoid seems preserved. Foot drop as a result of anterior tibial muscle weakness occurs in the facio-scapulo-humeral type, but is rare in the scapulo-humeral form. Contractures of muscles and joints are not a prominent feature.

An infantile form of facio-scapulo-humeral muscular dystrophy has now been identified. It is more severe than the adult form and is inherited as an autosomal recessive. Facial diplegia and sensorineural hearing loss are usually diagnosed by the age of 5 years. Scapular winging is

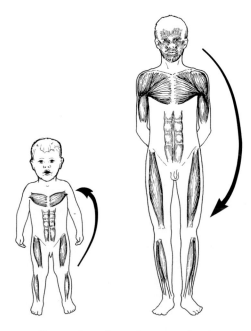

Figure 15.17 Illustration of usual progression in two types of muscular dystrophy. **A** Duchenne progresses from lower limbs to the upper limbs. **B** Facio-scapulo-humeral progresses from the face and upper limbs to the lower limbs.

present. The most striking deformity is marked lumbar lordosis, upon which the patient depends to maintain balance. Walking ability is usually lost in the 20s (Shapiro & Specht 1993).

Diagnosis

The creatine phosphokinase concentration is very high in the limb-girdle muscular dystrophies. Electromyograms confirm a general myopathy. The condition is indistinguishable from the Duchenne or Becker types and acid maltase deficiency in childhood, and a normal dystrophin assay, together with muscle biopsy, is necessary to establish the diagnosis (Arikawa et al 1991).

Orthopaedic management

Scapulo-thoracic fusion is effective in stabilising the winged scapula (Sage 1987, Letournel et al 1990, Bunch & Siegel 1993). Scoliosis can occur in these dystrophies and, when progressive, instrumentation and spinal fusion may be indicated.

Severe lordosis is more common than scoliosis and defies rational treatment. If it becomes too severe and causes intractable back pain, a wheelchair may be the only solution. Attempts to correct the lordosis by spinal fusion will remove the ability to balance so that standing and walking will become impossible.

A plastic ankle–foot orthosis of the posterior 'spring-leaf' type assists in overcoming footdrop when weak hip flexors do not allow sufficient hip flexion during swing phase for the foot to clear the ground.

CONGENITAL MUSCULAR DYSTROPHY

In contrast to Duchenne and Becker muscular dystrophy, congenital muscular dystrophy affects both sexes. The creatine phosphokinase is greatly increased. No involvement of the dystrophin gene or protein is found. The muscle biopsy features a variation of fibre diameter within each fascicle, and perimysial and endomysial fibrosis. Stiffness of joints is present in some, but not in others, whereas joint contractures may occur.

Type I congenital muscular dystrophy can be classified as two types according to the presence or absence in the muscles of merosin (or laminin-M), an extrasarolemmal protein that links with dystrophin through glycoproteins. It is somehow involved in stabilisation of the cell membrane. Children with merosin-negative congenital dystrophy have severe weakness and mental retardation. MRI studies of the brain show extensive areas of low T1-weighted and high T2-weighted signals from the white matter. The merosin-positive type (also called 'occidental') has no central nervous system involvement, and abnormal white-matter signals in brain MRIs are rare. Kobayshi et al (1996) described a merosin-positive form of congenital muscular dystrophy in which 86% of those affected had delayed motor development, but 92% were able to walk after the age of 4 years.

A Japanese variant is type II, the Fukuyama congenital muscular dystrophy. Extensive muscle necrosis is present, and these patients also have joint contractures. Motor and intellectual development are retarded (Shapiro & Specht 1993). Creatine phosphokinase concentrations are high. MRI studies of the brain show extensive white-matter lucencies and a thick, poorly sulcated cortex.

MUSCLE MYOPATHIES

CLINICAL SIGNS

The myopathies are characterised by hypotonia at birth (the floppy infant) and by delay in motor development. In childhood and adolescence, joint contractures, foot deformities and scoliosis are common as the disease progresses. The varieties of myopathy can be diagnosed only by muscle biopsy and histological studies. The serum enzymes are within normal limits, and the electromyogram shows only the non-specific electrical activity of myopathies in general.

Central core myopathy

This disorder may cause alarming repercussions for the orthopaedic surgeon, who can easily miss the underlying diagnosis. Presumed congenital dislocation or subluxation of the hip will redislocate in more than 50% of cases, and recurrent dislocation of the patella is resistant to surgical correction (Gamble 1988b). Pes planus is very common. Scoliosis responds to treatment with instrumentation and fusion. An awareness of this myopathy should lead to definitive diagnosis by muscle biopsy, which reveals the highly specific pathology (Fig. 15.18). Surgeons and anaesthetists

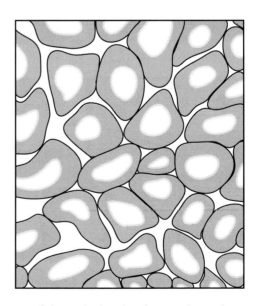

Figure 15.18 Schematic drawing from a photomicrograph of a biopsy in central core myopathy. A single core is within each muscle fibre. (Nicotinamide adenine dinucleotide lactate dehydrogenase-tetrazolium reductase [NADH-TR]; original magnification ×330.) (Redrawn from Dubowitz 1981.)

combination of fibrillation, polyphasic potentials of low amplitude and short duration, and high-frequency discharges evoked by stimulation of the muscle. Muscle biopsy provides a definitive answer when the specimen shows degeneration, regeneration and infiltration with inflammatory cells (Fig. 15.24).

Treatment

Other than myasthenia gravis this is the only muscle disease that responds successfully to corticosteroids.

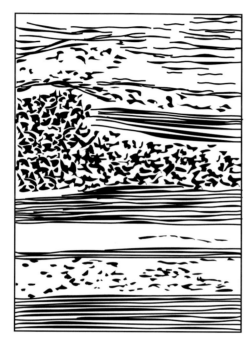

Figure 15.24 Schematic drawing of a photomicrograph of a biopsy in polymyositis–dermatomyositis, showing necrosis of muscle fibres and infiltration of the interstitial portions with lymphocytes. (After haematoxylin & eosin staining; original magnification ×53). (Redrawn from Currie 1981.)

Immunosuppressive therapy has been used in combination with corticosteroids in refractory cases (Mastaglia et al 1997). Regular passive stretching, followed by active exercise, is important to prevent muscle contractures and joint deformity. Tendon lengthening and capsulotomy may be indicated for joint contractures. The articular cartilage of the joints is preserved and no synovitis is present, so that surgery can be rewarding.

MYASTHENIA GRAVIS

Myasthenia, in contrast to myotonia, is weakness after repetitive voluntary muscle action, and tends to recover with rest. The condition shows a positive response to anticholinesterase drugs.

Clinical signs

Females outnumber males in a ratio of 4:1 at the time of onset of the disease, but in later adult life the sexes are equally affected (Simpson 1981). Symptoms are generally insidious in onset, but can start with a sudden crisis. Important to surgeons is the possibly abnormal response to general anaesthesia. Ocular myasthenia and diplopia may be the first symptoms of this. The second stage is characterised by general muscular weakness; third and fourth stages are fulminating and marked by ventilatory arrest that can result in death.

Diagnosis is confirmed by the therapeutic response to anticholinesterase drugs, of which the most common is edrophonium chloride.

Thymic hyperplasia, with T-cell lymphocytes in both the cortex and medulla, develops in 70–80% of the patients. Thymectomy, however, does not afford a cure, although it does arrest a further deterioration. Fortunately, regular, oral anticholinesterase medication is highly effective.

REFERENCES

Aicardi J 1998 Diseases of the Nervous System in Childhood. MacKeith Press and Cambridge University Press, London, pp 699–711 (Spinal muscular atrophies); pp 750–774 (Primary muscle disease)

Allen B L Jr, Ferguson R L, 1982 The Galveston technique for L rod instrumentation of the scoliotic spine. Spine 7: 276–284

André-T, Chesni Y, St Anne-Dargassies A 1960 The neurological examination of the infant. Little Club Clinics in Developmental Medicine, No. 1. Spastics Society, London

Aprin H, Bowen J R, MacEwen G D, Hall J E 1982 Spine fusion in patients with spinal muscular atrophy. Journal of Bone and Joint Surgery. 64A: 1179–1187

Arikawa E, Hoffman E P, Kaido M, Nonaka I, Sugita H, Arahata M D 1991 The frequency of patients with dystrophin abnormalities in a limb-girdle patient population. Neurology 41: 1491–1496

Bleck E E, Nagel D A 1982 Physically handicapped children: a medical atlas for teachers. Grune & Stratton, New York, p 388

Bradley W G 1981 The neuropathies. In: Walton J N (ed) Disorders of voluntary muscle, 4th edn. Churchill Livingstone, Edinburgh, pp 769–771

Bunch W H, Siegel I M 1993 Scapulothoracic arthrodesis in fascioscapulohumeral muscular dystrophy. A review of seventeen procedures with three to twenty-one year follow-up. Journal of Bone and Joint Surgery 75A: 372–376

Campbell M J, Liversedge L A 1981 The lower motor neurone, diseases (including muscular atrophy). In: Walton J N (ed) Disorders of voluntary muscle, 4th edn. Churchill Livingstone, Edinburgh, pp 736–739

Colbert A P, Craig C 1987 Scoliosis management in Duchenne muscular dystrophy: prospective study of modified Jewett hyperextension brace. Archives of Physical Medicine and Rehabilitation 68: 302–304

Currie S 1981 Polymyositis and related disorders. In: Walton J N (ed) Disorders of voluntary muscle, 4th edn. Churchill Livingstone, Edinburgh, pp 525–568

David W S, Jones H R Jr 1994 Electromyography and biopsy correlation with suggested protocol for the evaluation of the floppy infant. Muscle and Nerve 4: 424–430

DiLiberti J H, D'Agostino A N, Cole G 1983 Needle muscle biopsy in infants and children. Journal of Pediatrics 103: 566–570

Dubowitz V 1969 The floppy infant. Clinics in Developmental Medicine, No. 31. Spastics International Medical Publications with William Heinemann, London

Dubowitz V 1981 Histochemical aspects of muscle disease. In: Walton J N (ed) Disorders of voluntary muscle, 4th edn. Churchill Livingstone, Edinburgh, pp 261–295

Evans G A, Drennan J C, Russman B S 1981 Functional classification and orthopaedic management of spinal muscular atrophy. Journal of Bone and Joint Surgery 63B: 516–522

Fan Y, Maley M, Beilharz M, Grounds M 1996 Rapid death of injected myoblasts in myoblast transfer therapy. Muscle and Nerve 19: 853–860

Galasko C S B, Delaney C, Morris P 1992 Spinal stabilisation in Duchenne muscular dystrophy. Journal of Bone and Joint Surgery 74B: 210–214

Gamble J G 1988a The musculoskeletal system. Raven Press, New York, pp 131–132

Gamble J G 1988b Orthopaedic aspects of central core disease. Journal of Bone and Joint Surgery 70A: 1061–1066

Gardner-Medwin D, Tizard J P M 1981 Neuromuscular disorders in infancy and early childhood. In Walton J N (ed) Disorders of voluntary muscle, 4th edn. Churchill Livingstone, Edinburgh, pp 625–663

Gardner-Medwin D, Hudgson P, Walton J N 1967 Benign spinal muscular atrophy arising in childhood and adolescence. Journal of the Neurological Sciences 5: 121–158

Heckmatt J Z, Mossa C, Maunder-Sewry C A, Dubowitz V 1984 Diagnostic needle muscle biopsy. A practical and reliable alternative to open biopsy. Archives of Diseases of Children 59: 528–532

Hoffman E P, Kunkel L M 1989 Dystrophin abnormalities in Duchenne/Becker muscular dystrophy Neuron 2: 1019–1029

Hsu J D 1990 Surgical intervention in the management of the Duchenne muscular dystrophy (DMD) patient. Annual Meeting of the American Orthopaedic Association, Boston

Hudgson P, Mastaglia F L 1981 Ultrastructure studies of diseased muscle. In: Walton J (ed) Disorders of voluntary muscle, 4th edn. Churchill Livingstone, Edinburgh

Kobayshi O, Hayashi Y, Arahata K, Ozawa E, Nonaka I 1996 Congenital muscular dystrophy: clinical and pathologic study of 50 patients with the classical (Occidental) merosin-positive form. Neurology 46: 815–818

Letournel E, Fardeau M, Lytle J O, Serrault M, Gosselin R A 1990 Scapulothoracic arthrodesis for patients who have fascioscapulohumeral muscular dystrophy. Journal of Bone and Joint Surgery 72A: 78–84

Luque E R 1982 Segmental spinal instrumentation for correction of scoliosis. Clinical Orthopaedics and Related Research 163: 192–198

Mastaglia F L, Phillips B A, Zilko P 1997 Treatment of inflammatory myopathies. Muscle and Nerve 20: 651–654

Miller G M, Hsu J D, Hoffer M M, Rentfro R 1982 Posterior tibial tendon transfer: a review of the literature and analysis of 74 procedures. Journal of Pediatric Orthopaedics 2: 363

Miller J J III 1982 Dermatomyositis. In Bleck E E, Nagel D A (eds) Physically handicapped children: a medical atlas for teachers. Allyn & Bacon, Needham Heights, MA, p 265

Miller R G, Sharma K R, Pavlath G K et al 1997 Myoblast implantation in Duchenne muscular dystrophy: the San Francisco study. Muscle and Nerve 20: 469–478

Moe J H, Kharrat K, Winter R B 1984 Harrington instrumentation without fusion plus external orthotic support for the treatment of difficult curves in young children. Clinical Orthopaedics and Related Research 185: 35–45

Read L, Galasko C S B 1986 Delay in diagnosing Duchenne muscular dystrophy in orthopaedic clinics. Journal of Bone and Joint Surgery 68B: 481–482

Rinsky L A, Gamble J G, Bleck E E 1985 Segmental instrumentation without fusion in children with progressive scoliosis. Journal of Pediatric Orthopaedics 5: 687–690

Sage F P 1987 Heritable progressive neuromuscular disorders. In: Crenshaw A H (ed) Campbell's operative orthopaedics. CV Mosby, St Louis, p 3077

Shapiro F, Specht L 1993 Current Concepts Review. The diagnosis and orthopaedic treatment of inherited muscular diseases of childhood. Journal of Bone and Joint Surgery 75A: 439–454

Shapiro F, Specht L 1991 Locomotor problems in infantile fascioscapularhumeral muscular dystrophy. Acta Orthopaedica Scandinavica 62: 367–371

Shapiro F, Sethna N, Colan S, Wohl M E, Sprecht L 1992 Spinal fusion in Duchenne muscular dystrophy: a multidisciplinary approach. Muscle and Nerve 15: 604–614

Siegel I M 1981 Diagnosis, management and orthopaedic treatment of muscular dystrophy. Instructional Course Lectures, vol 30. CV Mosby, St Louis, pp 3–35

Simpson J A 1981 Myasthenia gravis and myasthenic syndromes. In: Walton J N (ed) Disorders of voluntary muscle, 4th edn. Churchill Livingstone, Edinburgh, pp 587–603

Smith A D, Koreska J, Moseley C F 1989 Progression of scoliosis in Duchenne muscular dystrophy. Journal of Bone and Joint Surgery 71A: 1066–1074

Walton J N (ed) 1981a Disorders of voluntary muscle, 4th edn. Churchill Livingstone, Edinburgh

Walton J N 1981b Clinical examination of the neuromuscular system. In: Walton J N (ed) Disorders of voluntary muscle, 4th edn. Churchill Livingstone, Edinburgh, pp 481–524, 486–492

Walton J N, Gardner-Medwin D 1981 Progressive muscular dystrophy and the myotonic disorders. In: Walton J N (ed) Disorders of voluntary muscle, 4th edn. Churchill Livingstone, Edinburgh, pp 497–524

Zwelleger H, Hanson J W 1967 Psychometric studies in muscular dystrophy type IIIa (Duchenne). Developmental Medicine and Child Neurology 9: 576–581

Chapter 16

Neural tube defects, spina bifida and spinal dysraphism

M. B. Menelaus and H. Kerr Graham

INTRODUCTION

Neural tube defects are a varied group of congenital spinal anomalies associated with abnormal closure of the neural tube. *Anencephaly* represents the major abnormality that may occur at the cranial end of the tube. *Spina bifida* belongs to the group of disturbances of development of the vertebral arches. These are often associated with abnormalities of structures derived from the neural tube and the meninges and may be associated with cyst formation. *Spinal dysraphism* refers to a variety of hidden abnormalities affecting the spinal cord or cauda equina, which may produce occult or overt neurological disturbance. The diversity of these conditions suggests that causative factors exert their effects at different periods of fetal development.

ABNORMALITIES ASSOCIATED WITH MYELOMENINGOCELE

Myelomeningocele is the form of neural tube defect that most commonly leads to significant motor and sensory deficit and lower limb and spinal deformity.

In addition to the gross spinal abnormality, other pathology is generally present – the Arnold–Chiari malformation, hydrocephalus, cerebellar hypoplasia, hydromyelia, syringomyelia and diastematomyelia (Fig. 16.1). The majority of patients also have upper limb disabilities as a result of a variety of subtle neurological lesions. Children with myelomeningocele generally have paralysis of the bladder, bowel incontinence, and a propensity for trophic ulceration in areas of skin anaesthesia. Approximately 80% of affected children will develop hydrocephalus and, as a group, they score 10–15 points below average on standardised

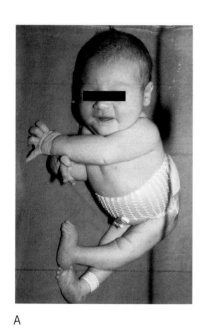

A

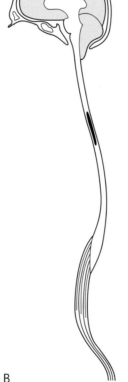

Hydrocephalus

Chiari 2

Syrinx

Tethered cord

B

Figure 16.1 A Newborn child with an open spina bifida lesion and dressing *in situ*. Evidence of congenital deformities and muscle imbalance can be seen by inspection and much more can be gained by careful examination in the neonatal period. **B** The sites of neurological involvement, including hydrocephalus, the Chiari 2 malformation, syringomyelia and tethered cord. In general, the problems of hydrocephalus are seen in the neonatal period, but neurological deterioration from the Chiari 2 malformation, syringomyelia and the tethered cord are seen in later childhood and may present insidiously.

intelligence tests. Neuropsychological testing reveals a consistent profile of learning difficulties and short-term memory problems, in addition to deficits in visuospatial, perceptual, numerical and executive skills.

INCIDENCE OF SPINA BIFIDA

The incidence of spina bifida varies with the geographical area and ethnicity. There are also seasonal variations. During the past 5 years, there has been a significant decrease in the number of children born with spina bifida, and a less dramatic decrease in the incidence of pregnancies with spina bifida. Periconceptual vitamin supplementation, maternal α-fetoprotein testing, routine antenatal ultrasound, and termination of affected pregnancies are some of the factors responsible.

The greatest incidence of spina bifida world-wide has been in Ireland, Wales and the north of England (up to 5 per 1000 live births), but recently a high incidence has been reported in certain regions of China. In North America and Australia, the incidence is fewer than one per 1000 live births.

AETIOLOGY

Multifactorial genetic and environmental factors have been implicated in the aetiology of spinal cord defects. A spectrum of neural tube defects results from similar causes acting at slightly different times during embryogenesis.

Genetic predisposition to neural tube defects

Neural tube defects have been shown to follow a multifactorial pattern of inheritance: a number of genes are believed to have a small additive effect, which may combine with environmental factors. When this compound effect passes a critical threshold there is a liability for the child to have the disorder. There is also an association with chromosomal disorders (trisomy 13, trimsomy 18, triploidy, unbalanced translocations and microdeletion of 22q11), in addition to rare dominant and recessive disorders. The birth of a child with spina bifida also predisposes to subsequent children being born with anencephaly, with extensive congenital vertebral abnormalities or with spinal dysraphism.

Possible environmental influences: diet and drugs

The environmental factors that have been implicated as a cause of neural tube defects include folate deficiency, other vitamin deficiencies, absence of selenium from the regional soil and hence from the diet, poor maternal nutrition, a high maternal intake of alcohol, maternal diabetes mellitus, fever at a critical stage of pregnancy, and a wide variety of other factors (Shurtleff 1986). Drugs that are associated with an increased incidence of neural tube defects include valproic acid, other anticonvulsants, isoretinoin (for the treatment of acne), etritinate (for the treatment of psoriasis), thalidomide and methotrexate.

EMBRYOLOGY AND PATHOLOGY

Spina bifida may be subdivided into spina bifida cystica, when a cyst forms and spina bifida occulta, when the defect is completely or largely hidden from the examining eye. The various forms of spina bifida are illustrated in Fig. 16.2.

SPINA BIFIDA CYSTICA

This may be in one of three forms:

1. *Myeloschisis or myelocele* (Fig. 16.2A). The vertebral arches are deficient and neural plate material is spread out on the surface, sometimes in a shallow depression, but more commonly over a cystic swelling of the meninges.
2. *Myelomeningocele* (Fig. 16.2B). A fluid-filled cystic swelling, lined by dura and arachnoid, protrudes through a defect in the vertebral arches under the skin. The spinal cord and nerve roots are carried out into the fundus of the sac.
3. *Meningocele* (Fig. 16.2C). A cystic swelling of dura and arachnoid protrudes through a defect in the vertebral arches under the skin. The spinal cord is entirely confined within the vertebral arches, but may exhibit abnormalities.

SPINA BIFIDA OCCULTA

In this form of spina bifida (Fig. 16.2D), there is a localised defect in one or more of the vertebral arches, because the respective halves of the arches fail to meet and fuse in the 3rd month. The spinal cord and meninges remain within the vertebral canal. The skin overlying the spina bifida occulta may be normal, or there may be a dimple which may connect with the dura by a fibrous cord, a patch of hair, pigmentation or a lipoma (possibly continuous with a similar intradural lipoma). All these and the rare intramedullary dermoid probably represent abnormalities of separation of presumptive skin from neural tissue during the process of closure of the neural tube. These conditions will be considered under the heading 'spinal dysraphism'.

CAUSES OF DEFORMITY

Muscle imbalance

Muscle imbalance has traditionally been regarded as the major cause of deformity in patients with spina bifida; clearly, it is one of many causes and may be less important than earlier studies suggested. The imbalance is, in large part, caused by the defects in the nerve roots and spinal cord already present at birth. However, further neurological injury (with a change in neurosegmental level) may be produced by prenatal traction on the abnormally tethered cord, direct pressure and longitudinal shearing forces during delivery and postnatal drying, and infection of the neural plate (Shurtleff 1986).

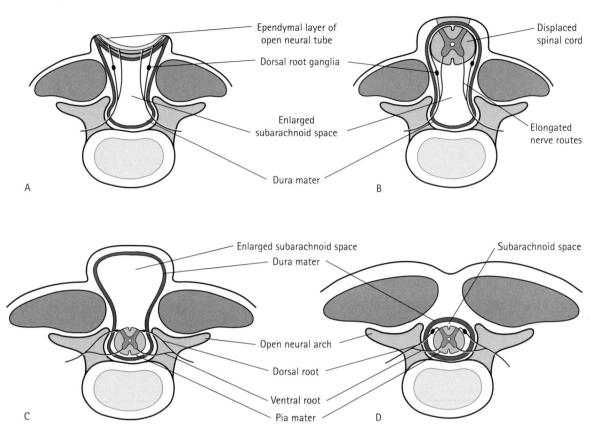

Figure 16.2 Schematic diagrams of the major types of spina bifida. (Based on Patten 1952.) **A** Myeloschisis. **B** Myelomeningocele. **C** Meningocele. **D** Spina bifida occulta.

Lower motor neurone lesions

There is some correlation between the lowest neuroseg-mental level that is functional, the muscles that are acting and the limb posture (as indicated in Table 16.1). This correlation is most pronounced at the foot and ankle, but less obvious at the hip. Patients in whom L5 is spared (Fig. 16.3) almost invariably have a calcaneus deformity of the foot because of activity in the tibialis anterior, the peroneus tertius and the extensor digitorum longus, and no activity in the soleus or gastrocnemius. Such muscle imbalance ultimately leads to fixed deformity.

More recent studies raise some doubt about the influence of muscle imbalance, especially on hip deformity. Flexion contracture at the hip is most severe and progressive in those patients with thoracic-level lesions with no muscle function at the hip (Shurtleff et al 1986). In these children, postural factors related to greatly reduced physical activity are probably the most important factor. There was, furthermore, no evidence of spasticity in those patients with the most severe hip flexion contractures. Further studies (Wright et al 1991, Broughton et al 1993) raise additional doubts about the place of muscle imbalance as the most significant cause of deformity in spina bifida.

Upper motor neurone lesions

Sixty-seven percent of infants with myelomeningocele have an additional upper motor neurone lesion. There is an interruption

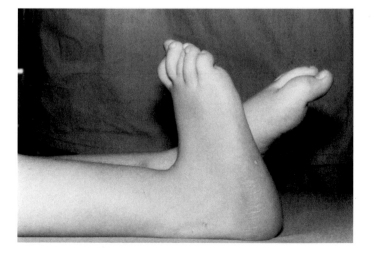

Figure 16.3 The neurological lesion in spina bifida is much more frequently assymetric than symmetric. This boy has an L3 level lesion on the left side, with paralysis of both the calf and the anterior tibial muscles. He has a dropped foot and a mild equinus deformity, because of the effects of gravity. On the right side he has an L4 level lesion, with a strong tibialis anterior working against a paralysed calf. He has a calcaneus deformity, which requires treatment by posterior transfer of tibialis anterior to the os calcis. Muscle imbalance produces much more predictable deformities at the foot and ankle than at the hip.

Table 16.1 Effect of the neurosegmental level of the lesion on muscle activity and limb posture

Lowest neurosegmental level functioning	Muscles acting	Limb posture
T12	–	Dictated by gravity
L1	Sartorius	Flexion and external rotation at hip
	Iliopsoas (weak function)	
L2	As above plus:	Flexion and adduction at hip
	Iliopsoas (strong)	
	Pectineus	
	Gracilis	
	Adductors of the hip	
	Rectus femoris	
L3	As above plus:	Hip flexed and adducted
	Quadriceps (power slightly diminished)	Knee extended or hyperextended
L4	As above plus:	Hip flexed, adducted and externally rotated
	Tibialis anterior (and posterior)	Knee extension and hyperextension
	Medial hamstrings weak	Foot varus
L5	As above plus:	Hip flexion
	Tensor fascie latae	Knee in some flexion
	Gluteus medius and minimus	Feet in calcaneus
	Peroneus tertius	
	Extensor digitorum longus	
S1	As above plus:	Hip and knee in some flexion
	Gluteus maximus	
	Biceps femoris	
	Gastrocnemius	Flattening of the sole and clawing of the toes
	Soleus	
	Flexor digitorum longus and brevis	
	Flexor hallucis longus and brevis	
Lower lumbar level with spastic sacral segment	Spasticity in hamstrings, calf, peronei	Knee flexion deformity
		Foot equinus or valgus or vertical talus

Based on Sharrard (1964); some modifications are indicated in the text.

of long spinal tracts, with preservation of reflex activity in isolated distal segments. Reflex activity is often perceived by parents as voluntary activity. Three subtypes can be recognised.

In the first, cord function is intact down to a certain level where there is flaccid paralysis with loss of sensation and reflexes; more distally there is isolated cord function, evident from exaggerated reflex activity.

In the second, the 'gap' in cord function is narrow, amounting virtually to a cord transection. There is no movement of the lower limbs when the infant is crying, but a wealth of purely reflex activity (including flexion withdrawal) can be elicited by direct stimulation.

In the third subtype, in which transection of the long tracts is incomplete, the child will have a spastic paraplegia, with preservation of some voluntary movement and sensation.

Thus the muscle imbalance producing deformity in spina bifida may be summarised as of three types:

1. Normal muscle/flaccid antagonist.
2. Spastic muscle/normal antagonist.
3. Spastic muscle/flaccid antagonist.

The last type produces the worst deformity.

There is evidence that important upper motor neurone lesions occur around the time of birth. Deformities resulting from spasticity are therefore not present at birth, but develop in the early months of life. Some effects of such lesions are illustrated in Fig. 16.4.

Intrauterine posture

Sometimes deformity is present at birth in totally paralysed lower limbs. In some of these cases the deformity may be fixed, which suggests that muscle power (and imbalance) has been present in fetal life. In others, the pattern of deformity suggests that it has resulted simply from pressure on paralysed limbs.

Habitually assumed posture after birth

Deformity can develop after birth in flaccid legs that are allowed to lie in one particular posture, under the influence of gravity. The classic 'diamond posture' is hip flexion/abduction/external rotation in combination with

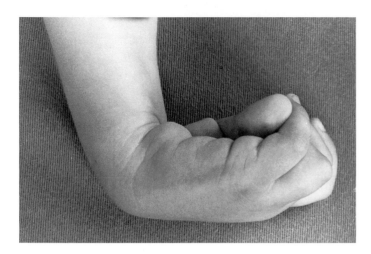

Figure 16.4 This is the left hand of a boy aged 5 years with a thoracic-level myelomeningocele, with no voluntary function in the left upper limb or the left lower limb. Note the marked spasticity of the finger and wrist flexors. Upper limb involvement is common in children with spina bifida, but the effects are usually much more subtle. (Reproduced with permission from Menelaus 1998).

knee flexion and equinus or equinovarus at the ankle and foot.

Coexistent congenital malformation

This is probably not a common cause of deformity in spina bifida, but syndactyly of the second and third toes and renal anomalies are sometimes encountered.

Arthrogryposis

Some of the limb deformities associated with spinal cord defects resemble those seen in arthrogryposis multiplex congenita. There is rigidity and lack of normal flexion creases. Such deformities are very resistant to treatment.

Traction of nerve roots

Some children who have had a myelomeningocele closed at birth present later with progressive foot deformity (usually cavovarus). This should be treated by surgical release of the abnormal tethers. Foot deformity, which develops for the first time in a growing child, should prompt a careful search for spinal cord pathology, including the various manifestations of spinal dysraphism.

PROBLEMS RESULTING FROM SKIN ANAESTHESIA AND BONE FRAGILITY

Pressure sores and chilblains

These result from skin anaesthesia and poor circulation. If serial plasters are necessary to correct deformity, they should be very carefully padded, because there is no pain to warn the surgeon of pressure on the skin. In most instances, plaster casts should be used only to maintain the correction

of deformity that has been achieved by soft-tissue surgery. Hip spicas should include paralysed feet. Varus feet are always unacceptable, and pressure sores are inevitable. Parents should be warned to protect their children from extremes of temperature.

Bone fragility

Pathological fractures occur in approximately 20% of those patients with paralysis in the lower limbs. Epiphyseal displacements and hyperplastic callus formation are common. Osteopenia because of reduced muscle bulk and physical activity is the most obvious reason for bone fragility, but renal rickets and vitamin C or D deficiency are not uncommon.

Pathological fractures in patients with spina bifida are commonly mistaken for bone or joint infection; the patient may present with a painless, red, hot and swollen limb without a history of trauma. Radiographs will often disclose a fracture that has occurred days or weeks previously. In the later stages, if there is a delay in diagnosis and immobilisation of a fracture, the florid callus may be misdiagnosed as a primary bone tumour.

The principle of treatment of pathological fractures is that the immobilisation of the child and the fractured limb should be the minimum compatible with union in a satisfactory position. Well-padded hip spicas, applied with the limbs in an extension posture, may permit early weight bearing with the use of a prone standing frame. These are also useful devices with which to prevent osteopenia in the postoperative period.

Patients who are unable to walk require less perfect reduction of such fractures and simple closed treatment should be adequate.

MANAGEMENT: CONCEPTION TO BIRTH

PRIMARY PREVENTION

Throughout the past two decades, a series of studies have demonstrated that the incidence of neural tube defects can be dramatically reduced by the administration of folic acid in very early pregnancy. Since 1998, all enriched cereals sold in the USA have been fortified with folic acid – the first time food has been fortified for the prevention of birth defects (Watkins 1998). Despite uncertainties regarding the mechanism of action, dose, timing and optimum method of administration of the folic acid, public health policy in all countries should be directed towards this simple and safe method of primary prevention of neural tube defects.

GENETIC COUNSELLING

Genetic counselling should provide the family with sufficient information on which to base a decision about further children, and help them come to terms with the problems they face. It should involve careful discussion of the recurrence risk for further pregnancies, and the availability of antenatal diagnosis. A sympathetic understanding of the burden faced by the parents and child, and explanation of the variability of the condition are essential.

Counselling aims to be non-directive: the family needs time to make decisions about the future. Such decisions should evolve slowly as the family learns to cope with the affected child.

RECURRENCE RISK

Recurrence risk varies from area to area; counselling should be based on local experience. The most detailed guidelines have been established in the UK. In general, the recurrence risk following the birth of an affected baby is approximately 1 in 25, of which half is for anencephaly and half for other neural tube defects. If the parents have had two affected children, the risk increases to approximately 1 chance in 10; after three children it is approximately 1 in 4. The birth of a child with anencephaly, multiple congenital vertebral anomalies, or spinal dysraphism gives families the same predisposition to the occurrence of neural tube defects. Adult survivors with spina bifida who are considering starting a family face the same risk as the parents of a single affected child.

ANTENATAL DIAGNOSIS

Ultrasound

A competent, experienced obstetric ultrasonographer can detect most anencephalies and some spina bifida lesions using vaginal ultrasound at 10–12 weeks of pregnancy. Ultrasound at 16–18 weeks identifies virtually all cases of anencephalies and more than 80% of those with spina bifida. Neural tube defects can usually be identified on ultrasound, but they cannot be excluded with certainty; thus the technique is often used in combination with amniocentesis.

Amniocentesis

Amniocentesis is always undertaken with ultrasound control to localise the placenta, confirm gestation and exclude multiple pregnancy and visible malformations. In experienced hands, the risk of producing a miscarriage is about 1 in 200.

The fluid aspirated is submitted for α-fetoprotein estimation and, in some laboratories, acetylcholinesterase concentrations. The values obtained are compared with the ranges of normal established in that laboratory for each particular week of gestation. In open neural tube defects, the α-fetoprotein concentration is usually two or three times the upper limit of normal. By a combination of ultrasonography and amniocentesis, it is possible to recognise almost all foetuses with anencephaly and at least 90% of those with spina bifida. The neural tube defects that are missed are small, skin-covered lesions. Once a sample of amniotic fluid is taken, it is desirable to look at the chromosomes of cultured amniotic fluid cells, to detect chromosome disorders such as Down's syndrome.

Estimation of α-fetoprotein in maternal serum

This estimation can be performed as a screening test between the 16th and 20th weeks of pregnancy. If the serum concentration is increased, ultrasound and amniocentesis are performed.

SECONDARY PREVENTION

Intrauterine diagnosis allows the termination of pregnancies with neural tube defects when this is acceptable to parents. Thus antenatal diagnosis has the potential to reduce greatly the incidence of this disorder and the recent decline in the frequency of neural tube defects in live births in England and Wales is due, in large part, to an effective antenatal diagnostic programme.

It has been shown that there is a lower incidence of severe neurological deficit in those babies who have been delivered by caesarean section at the 36th week of pregnancy, compared with those delivered vaginally at term. Parents who will not accept abortion may accept the possibility of a less severely disabled child by embracing this option. In 1998, successful fetal surgery for spina bifida was reported. This approach may preserve neurological function and arrest or reverse the development of hydrocephalus and the Arnold–Chiari type 2 malformation.

Prophylaxis in subsequent pregnancies

There is clear evidence that periconceptual vitamin supplementation will reduce the very high risk of a second child being affected, after the birth of a child with a neural tube defect.

MANAGEMENT: LIFETIME

CO-ORDINATED MANAGEMENT: THE SPINA BIFIDA CLINIC

A correct management programme for affected children – involving, as it does, many disciplines and a variety of medical specialists and allied health personnel – can be properly carried out only if there is a formal organisation – a spina bifida clinic. The orthopaedic problems of these children cannot be managed in isolation from their numerous other problems, which should be dealt with at a minimum number of hospital inpatient admissions and outpatient attendances and by staff who have been trained in the special problems created by the condition.

The personnel of the clinic are:

- co-ordinator
- neurosurgeon
- orthopaedic surgeon
- urologist
- psychologist and psychiatrist
- social worker
- physiotherapist and occupational therapist
- orthotist.

Adequate treatment and care of a multiply handicapped child depend upon the recognition that the child is an individual whose needs far exceed the range of the separate specialities listed above. Hence the need for a co-ordinator who is a physician with training and expertise in the management of children with multiple disabilities. The co-ordinator imparts unity to the clinic, is the person to whom the parents may turn as their 'general practitioner' and should possess a good working knowledge of all the specialist treatments, combined with an interest in the interactions of the child and the family.

Such an organisation supports the family to the maximum, by ensuring that treatment is integrated and that admissions to hospital are correctly co-ordinated.

Neonatal management

The orthopaedic surgeon should examine every child with spina bifida at birth or as soon as possible thereafter, not only to record basic information, but also to make it possible to monitor progress over the first few months and to plan orthopaedic treatment, if survival seems likely. The only condition requiring treatment in the neonatal period is talipes equinovarus, which is best treated by serial casts, very well padded to protect the anaesthetic skin.

The mortality rate is high in infancy but, if the child survives the first year of life, long-term survival is now the rule.

ORTHOPAEDIC MANAGEMENT

The reader is referred to Menelaus (1998) and Schafer & Dias (1983) for more detailed consideration of the orthopaedic management of spina bifida and myelomeningocele.

The principal aim of orthopaedic management in spina bifida is to establish a stable extension posture by the correction of fixed deformity (Fig. 16.5). If affected children are to be able to stand for long periods and to remain on their feet in adult life, they must have their centre of gravity directly over their feet, with minimal flexion deformities at the hips and knees. Indeed, it is very desirable that there be some hyperextension at both hips and knees. About 60% of children with spina bifida have neurological deficiencies in their upper limbs and often need to use *both* hands for activities that other children perform with one hand. It is for this reason, also, that we strive, where possible, to encourage standing for long periods without the use of the hands for support.

Orthopaedic surgery has different goals according to the level of the neurosegmental lesion. This level may be ill defined because of skin lesions, other neurological deficits or general disabilities. Furthermore, the neurosegmental level may change because of tethering of the cord. The implications of the level of the lesion with regard to walking are:

- Children with *thoracic* lesions will not continue useful walking in adult life

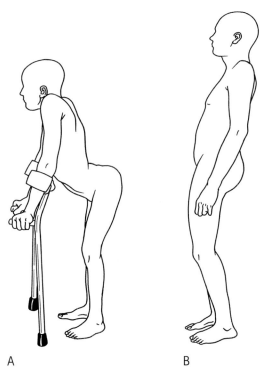

A   B

Figure 16.5 A Flexion posture in the untreated child is common. If there is a flexion deformity at the hips, this results in an anterior pelvic tilt and a lumbar lordosis. The patient must use both arms to use crutches because his centre of gravity is so far in front of the hip, knee, ankle and foot; the arms then lose their other more valuable functions. **B** This is the desired extension posture, which often requires anterior hip releases, posterior knee releases and reconstructive surgery at the level of the foot and ankle in order to permit effective bracing. (Reproduced with permission from Menelaus 1998.)

- Children with *lumbar* lesions may continue useful walking in adult life if they have strong quadriceps muscles and do not develop significant deformity at their hip joints. Those with strong quadriceps require only below-knee orthoses, but may need assistive devices (walking sticks or crutches) in addition
- Children with *sacral* lesions can be expected to be useful walkers, without orthoses, into adult life. Recent studies, however, have revealed a higher level of morbidity and disability in adolescence and early adult life than had previously been anticipated.

Those who will not continue walking require simple surgery to provide them with a stable posture in childhood, whereas those who will continue walking require more sophisticated surgery to meet the increased demands of their way of life.

Because the surgery necessary in children with high lesions is relatively minor, it can and should be performed at several levels and in both limbs under one anaesthetic. Muscle imbalance must be corrected in all circumstances, to minimise recurrent deformity. Radical surgery is necessary to correct rigid, arthrogrypotic-type deformities (notably in the feet),

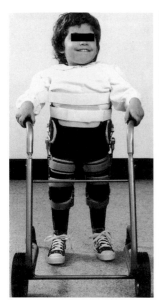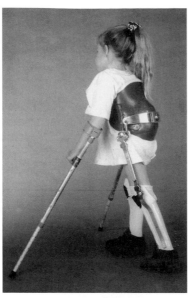

Figure 16.7 High-level bracing and assistive devices are useful in promoting the upright position and walking in younger children with high lesions. These children are using different types of reciprocal gait orthoses, which are probably the most effective type of high bracing; they are certainly the most popular with children and parents. High-level bracing is rarely used in adolescence or adult life, because wheelchair mobility is so much more practical. (Reproduced with permission from Menelaus 1998.)

MANAGEMENT OF DEFORMITIES

THE FOOT

General observations

Fixed varus deformity invariably requires correction by operation, as complications from weight bearing on a small area of the sole are otherwise inevitable. Undercorrection must never be accepted as further surgery will almost certainly be required.

Valgus feet, while they remain mobile, can usually be controlled with appropriate footwear and orthoses until adolescence. Mobile valgus deformity of the subtalar joint is commonly complicated by torsional and valgus deformity of the ankle mortise; the deformity is difficult to control by bracing, and surgery is often necessary to correct this complex deformity. The valgus foot/ankle requires careful clinical and radiological evaluation including standing anteroposterior and lateral X-rays of the foot, in addition to a standing mortise view of the ankle. Correction of the valgus foot will fail if there is unrecognised and therefore untreated ankle valgus.

Calcaneus deformity tends to be progressive, and should be treated surgically.

Whenever possible, operations on the foot and leg should be performed under the same anaesthetic as other limb surgery, urological surgery or neurosurgery.

Although mobile feet are preferable to stiff feet, triple arthrodesis at maturity has a useful place in the management of both varus and valgus deformity, as a long-term follow-up has shown (Olney & Menelaus 1988).

Equinovarus deformity

The rigidity of this deformity varies from that seen in the usual form of talipes equinovarus to the extreme rigidity of arthrogryposis. This is the most troublesome foot deformity, because of its tendency to recur despite apparently adequate initial correction. Unless survival is unlikely, the deformity should be treated from birth. The feet are placed in well-padded plaster casts, which are changed frequently while the baby is still in hospital, and then at intervals of 4–6 weeks. Before treatment, the feet may appear to be purely varus or even calcaneovarus, but, as the varus is corrected, it is usually apparent that there is tightness of the Achilles tendon. In these circumstances, percutaneous tenotomy is indicated. Despite this early management, a soft-tissue release will generally be necessary between the ages of 4 months and 1 year.

The rigid equinovarus foot will inevitably require postero-medial release, the technique of which is described in Chapter 29, but some modifications are necessary. As the calf is not functioning, the skin incision need have no vertical component. Portions of the tendons of the Achilles tendon, tibialis posterior and the long toe flexors are excised, rather than just divided. Only occasionally will the degree of deformity be so mild that conservative treatment will correct the varus and adductus, leaving only equinus to be corrected by posterior release.

Tendon transfers have a limited role in this condition (Fig. 16.8). Should the deformity recur, a repeat soft-tissue release is performed. However, a better option may be correction of deformity by slow distraction, using a circular external fixation frame of the Ilizarov type (Fig. 16.9). This frame is a powerful tool that can achieve complete correction of deformity. The majority of children who present with recurrent foot deformity have reduced or absent sensation, and the fact that this frame allows the limb to remain under inspection throughout the period of correction abolishes the risks of cast sores and is a major advantage in revision surgery. Soft-tissue releases, osteotomies and, occasionally, talectomy can be used in conjunction with circular frame deformity correction.

The management of talipes equinovarus in spina bifida can be summarised thus:

1. *Birth to 3 months.* Serial casting, well padded and carefully monitored.
2. *3–6 months.* Percutaneous tenotomy of the tendo-Achillis and serial casting.
3. *6–12 months.* Posteromedial release.
4. *Late childhood.* Lateral column surgery, heel and midfoot osteotomies, Ilizarov techniques.
5. *Adolescence.* Ilizarov techniques, triple arthrodesis.

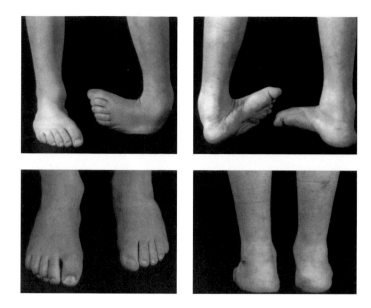

Figure 16.8 Bilateral equinovarus deformities in a five-year-old child who had not had previous treatment. These deformities are managed by posteromedial releases of the contracted muscles and joint capsules and, when necessary, muscle balancing procedures. In this patient, muscle balancing was achieved by lateral transfer of tibialis anterior. Both feet are plantigrade, and required no further surgery. (Reproduced with permission from Menelaus 1998.)

Cavus deformity

The management of this condition depends upon its rigidity, and the age of the child. Open division of the tight plantar structures may correct minor deformity in a young child. If there is heel varus and the child is older than 4 years, osteotomy of the os calcis is appropriate. The efficacy of soft-tissue and bony procedures may be enhanced by the use of an Ilizarov frame, and fewer children may then require salvage by triple arthrodesis at maturity.

Calcaneus deformity

Generally this deformity (see Fig. 16.3) is left untreated until muscle power can be properly assessed when the child has reached the age of 3–5 years. If the strength of the tibialis anterior is normal, this tendon is transferred, through the interosseous membrane, to the heel. Any other active ankle dorsiflexors are divided and, if there is fixed calcaneus deformity, an anterior ankle release is combined with this tenotomy. If the anterior muscles are spastic or if they are weak, they are divided and the Achilles tendon is fixed to the fibular metaphysis by tenodesis. The drill-hole through the fibula stimulates growth at the lower end of the bone, and this may correct valgus deformity at the ankle mortise – a deformity that commonly occurs in combination with calcaneus deformity. The late-developing calcaneus deformity with a 'pistol grip' heel is best treated by osteotomy of the os calcis, removing a wedge based posteriorly so that the tuberosity lies less vertically. At the same time, restoration of

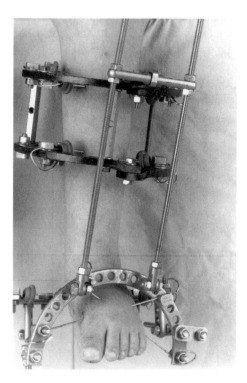
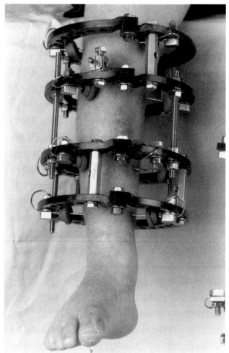

Figure 16.9 Ilizarov frames are invaluable in the management of deformities of the foot and leg in children with spina bifida. The principal indications are revision surgery and the management of complications. There may be an increasing role for the use of circular frames in primary surgery.

Table 16.4 Indications for reduction of hip dislocation in spina bifida

	Bilateral	Unilateral
HIGH LESIONS		SELDOM REDUCE
	NEVER	May do so if:
Weak quadriceps	REDUCE	1) Dislocation is not gross
Require above-knee bracing	DISLOCATION	2) The other leg has a low
Probably short-term walkers		lesion
LOW LESIONS	SELDOM REDUCE	
	May do so if:	ALWAYS
Strong quadriceps	1) Dislocation is not gross	REDUCE
Short bracing	2) Surgery is, in any case,	DISLOCATION
Life-time walkers	necessary for hip flexion	
	contracture	

define. Reduction of the dislocated hip in spina bifida may not improve walking ability. Nevertheless some patients, particularly if the dislocation is unilateral, have a troublesome leg-length discrepancy if the hip remains dislocated. A guide to decision making is outlined in Table 16.4; it is based upon whether the patient has a high or low lesion, and whether the dislocation is bilateral or unilateral.

If the hip is to be reduced, it is important to minimise the duration of plaster immobilisation. Hip reduction should be stabilised by pelvic osteotomy, either Pemberton (1965) or Dega procedures (see Ch. 24). Only 6–8 weeks of plaster immobilisation are necessary postoperatively.

Provision of abductor and extensor power

The absence of functioning hip extensors and abductors at the lumbar level has been considered to be the main reason for hip dislocation and provides the logic for muscle and tendon transfer surgery. Sharrard (1964) stressed the importance of providing abductor and extensor power and depriving the hip of the strong flexor power of the psoas muscle by performing ilio-psoas transfer. It is now clear that dislocation of the hip is most common in patients with flail hips, and there is doubt about the need to correct muscle balance at the hip in the prevention of hip dislocation.

The ilio-psoas transfer has many practical and theoretical flaws. It is a major intervention, with significant complications. Gait analysis studies suggest that the transfer continues to fire during the swing phase of gait, that it makes the key pelvic kinematic deviations worse and, by inference, that it increases energy expenditure (Duffy et al 1996a). None of the tendon transfers that have been described to stabilise the hip in spina bifida has been adequately studied by objective means, and the suspicion remains that they are all flawed by incorrect timing or inadequate strength. The percentage of hips reduced at follow-up is an inadequate measure of success; it is gait and function that are of paramount importance. In addition to the posterior ilio-psoas transfer (Figs 16.11 and 16.12), other transfers

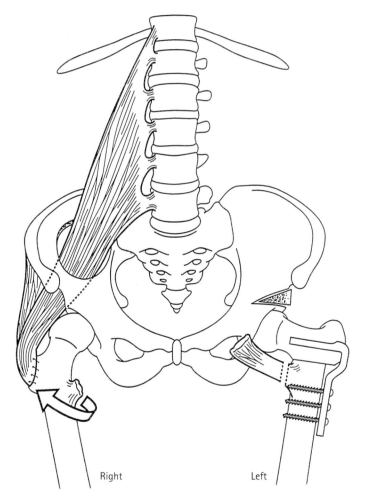

Right Left

Figure 16.11 Options in the management of the dislocated hip in spina bifida include the posterolateral ilio-psoas transfer of Sharrard as shown on the right, or a one-stage open reduction, femoral varus derotation osteotomy, Pemberton acetabuloplasty and lengthening (rather than transfer) of the ilio-psoas as shown on the left. (Reproduced with permission of the American Academy of Orthopaedic Surgeons 2001.)

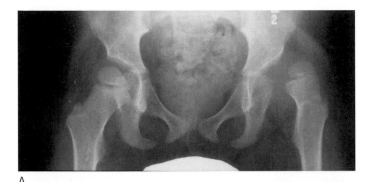

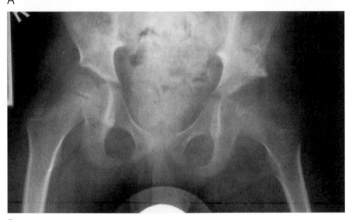

Figure 16.12 **A** Unilateral hip dislocation in a boy with an L4-level lesion. **B** After open reduction, ilio-psoas transfer and Pemberton acetabuloplasty.

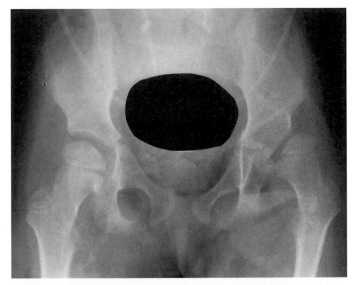

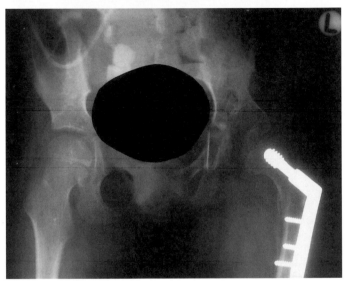

Figure 16.13 Unilateral hip dislocation (top), managed by open reduction, femoral varus derotation osteotomy and Pemberton acetabuloplasty (bottom).

include external oblique transfer to the greater trochanter or transfer of the adductor origin posteriorly (Yngve & Lindseth 1982). Varus derotation osteotomy of the proximal femur may be used to stabilise an open or closed reduction of the hip. Given the current uncertainties as to the value of the individual operations in managing the unstable hip, our current practice is pragmatic rather than scientific (Fig. 16.13; see also Fig. 16.11):

1. The dislocated hip usually requires open reduction, psoas and adductor lengthening, Pemberton or Dega acetabuloplasty and varus derotation osteotomy, as a one-stage hip reconstruction. We no longer use tendon transfers.
2. A reducible hip subluxation is managed by varus derotation osteotomy.
3. Acetabular dysplasia is managed in the younger child by a Pemberton or Dega acetabuloplasty, and in the adolescent by a Chiari osteotomy or Staheli shelf.

THE SPINE

Spinal deformity is frequently too disabling to be ignored, but conservative methods of treatment are seldom applicable.

Spinal deformity impairs not only walking, but also sitting. If the child has such poor sitting balance because of spinal deformity that one hand is needed to maintain

upright posture, spinal deformity has led to a crippling impairment of function (Fig. 16.14). Because of subtle neurological disturbances in the upper limbs, patients with spina bifida commonly need to use both hands for functions that unaffected people can perform with one hand.

In treating the deforming spine surgically, every effort must be made to avoid prolonged immobilisation. Osteoporosis, fractures, genitourinary complications and psychological disturbance are heavy prices to pay for a surgical complication such as infection or pseudoarthrosis. A child with spina bifida who is prevented from mobilising for as little as 3 months may never walk again.

Classification of spinal deformity

Spinal deformities in patients with spina bifida may take one or more of the following forms:

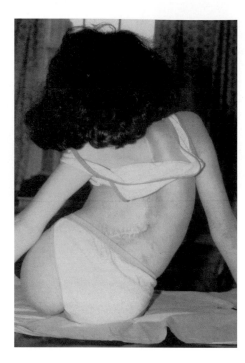

Figure 16.14 Loss of sitting balance because of scoliosis adversely affects sitting, and requires the use of the hands for propping. A level pelvis and balanced spine for comfortable hands-free sitting is an important goal for these children.

1. Defects of the neural arch and wide separation of the pedicles at the level of the neurological and meningeal lesion.
2. The full range of vertebral body anomalies seen in congenital scoliosis and occurring either at the level of the spina bifida or any other level of the spine. These anomalies include defects of segmentation, defects of formation and mixed defects.
3. Diastematomyelia.
4. Spondylolisthesis.
5. Absence of the sacrum – partial or complete.
6. Kyphosis – paralytic and congenital forms.
7. Lordosis – commonly secondary to fixed flexion deformity of the hip and becoming fixed.
8. Scoliosis – the most common form of scoliosis occurring in patients with myelomeningocele is paralytic in type, but congenital, mixed congenital and paralytic curves also occur. The curve may be a lordo-scoliosis or a kypho-scoliosis.

Kyphosis

Children who are born with kyphosis generally have hydrocephalus and are among the most severely affected children. Some of these children do not survive. The kyphosis is generally in the lumbar spine and averages 80° at birth, increasing by an average of 8° per annum. Portions of the erector spinae muscles may lie anterior to the axis of flexion and become spinal flexors, aggravating the tendency to kyphosis. Children born with a lumbar kyphosis generally have complete paralysis of the leg muscles.

Management of kyphosis

The indication for correction is recurrent skin ulceration. A variety of surgical techniques is available and the choice depends upon the age of the child and the severity of the kyphosis. Procedures available include:

- kyphectomy with segmental posterior instrumentation and fusion
- anterior strut graft/fusion
- combinations of anterior and posterior surgery

Scoliosis

The curve in scoliosis is most commonly paralytic in origin, but it may be congenital or mixed. Furthermore, patients who have hydrosyringomyelia may develop scoliosis secondary to this cause and drainage of the syrinx may prevent progression. All children with spina bifida therefore require MRI of the entire cord before spinal surgery.

Severe and progressive scoliosis is most common in patients with thoracic-level lesions. The incidence progressively diminishes with lesser degrees of neurological deficit.

Management of scoliosis

There is a small place for bracing in children with rapidly progressive scoliosis who are considered too young for surgery.

Indications for operative management. These include progressive deformity of over 35° in children between the ages of 8 and 14 years. The size of the child, the growth of the spine, and the flexibility of the curve must be taken into account. The main aims of surgery are to provide:

- a stable fusion that will not be followed by further deformity
- a stable posture for standing and sitting
- a level pelvis and a vertical trunk, without the need for hand support
- maximal length of the trunk
- removal of convexities that may be the site of pressure
- preservation of good ventilatory function and satisfactory cosmesis.

The principles of surgery. Stable fusion by both anterior and posterior approaches should be considered. Anterior instrumentation enables correction of the tight curve at the apex of the primary curve (which is usually at the thoracolumbar junction), and this procedure has a high fusion rate; posterior instrumentation increases the length of spine that can be fused and allows better correction of pelvic obliquity (see Ch. 31.2).

SUMMARY

Orthopaedic management of spina bifida patients must be tailored to meet the future demands of the child. In general, those with high-level lesions and weak quadriceps muscles will place minimal demands on their feet and legs during the period when they are walking and are best served by simple surgery. This will generally take the form of soft-tissue release, to free the patient from fixed deformity.

Children with low-level lesions and strong quadriceps muscles are likely to walk throughout life; they put greater demands on their feet and legs and benefit more from a good range of motion at the hip and knee. The role of tendon transfers to stabilise the hip and surgery for hip dislocation requires more objective study utilising functional outcome measures, including gait analysis. Plantigrade feet are essential, and the role of circular frames to correct resistant or recurrent deformities should increase.

Those with high-level lesions, however, more frequently require radical surgery for scoliosis, preferably by anterior and posterior fusion.

SPINAL DYSRAPHISM

This term is applied to a group of conditions in which the dorsum of the embryo forms abnormally. The condition is of importance to orthopaedic surgeons as a cause of foot deformity and leg weakness.

DEFINITION

Spinal dysraphism refers to all forms of abnormality of formation of midline structures of the future dorsum of the embryo.

INCIDENCE

Between 10% and 30% of the population have a degree of this abnormality, be it only spina bifida occulta affecting one vertebral arch.

Clinically significant spinal dysraphism is comparatively rare although the precise incidence is not known.

DIAGNOSIS AND DIFFERENTIAL DIAGNOSIS

Patients may present to the orthopaedic surgeon at any age from birth to maturity. Most commonly, they will present before the age of 5 years, with one of the following features:

- a short, often wasted, leg
- a small foot
- cavovarus foot deformity
- paralytic valgus
- trophic ulceration.

In addition to the above features, examination may or may not disclose a cutaneous lesion in the form of a patch of hair, a naevus, a lipoma, a scarred area or a sinus or dimple. In a series of 200 cases of spinal dysraphism (James & Lassman 1981), approximately 25% had no external cutaneous manifestation. Thus it is imperative that the clinician has a high level of suspicion and carries out appropriate special investigations.

Differential diagnosis depends to some extent on the presenting features. If the patient presents with a short leg or small foot, it is most commonly the result of hemihypertrophy or hemiatrophy. If, however, neurological features are present, the following must be excluded:

- cerebral palsy in the form of a mild hemiplegia
- spinal cord tumour
- hereditary sensory and motor neuropathy
- polyneuritis.

Patients should be fully investigated (as described below) before a diagnosis of 'idiopathic' pes cavus is accepted.

EMBRYOLOGY AND PATHOLOGY

Spinal dysraphism may affect all or some of the primary embryonic layers to a varying degree. The type of dysplasia and the resultant conditions are listed in Table 16.5. Details of all aspects of the condition have been described by James & Lassman (1972, 1981).

The most common forms of pathology are as follows:

1. Diastematomyelia, in which the spinal cord or filum terminale, or both, are split sagitally by a bony or fibrocartilaginous septum (Fig. 16.15).
2. Lumbosacral lipoma.
3. Meningocele manqué, in which a loop of nerve root or trunk emerges from the spinal cord, cauda equina or filum terminale, becomes adherent to the dura and then returns to the cauda equina or filum near to its point of origin.

Table 16.5 Spina bifida, spinal dysraphism or the spinal dysraphic state

Embryonal origin	Type of dysplasia	Resultant condition
Cutaneous: Somatic Ectodermal	Cutaneous	Cutaneous defect Hypertrichosis Naevus Dermal sinus
Mesodermal	Vertebral	Split in spinous process Laminal defects Rachischisis
	Dural	Non-fusion of dura mater
Neural: Neurectodermal	Neural tube	Myelodysplasia Intramedullary and extramedullary growths associated with dysraphia
	Neural crest	Ectopia of spinal ganglia and of posterior nerve roots

Adapted from Lichtenstein (1940).

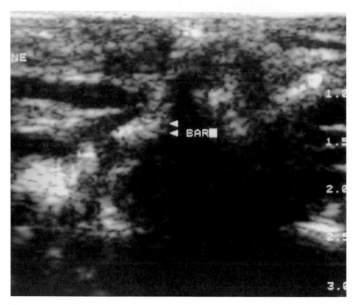
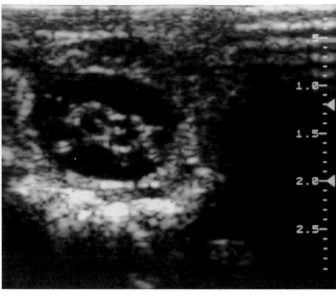

A   B

Figure 16.15 Ultrasound examination of the spinal canal at the lumbar spine in a child with spina bifida occulta. Note the presence of a bony bar on the sagittal image (**A**). On the transverse section (**B**), note the duplicated spinal cord with two sets of nerve roots (diplomyelia). This is an example of diastematomyelia with diplomyelia within the spinal canal. Ultrasound can give detailed information about the status of the spinal cord and spinal canal in an infant younger than 3 months, without the need for sedation or anaesthesia.

4. Dermoid cyst.
5. Tight or tethered filum terminale; this may result in an abnormally distal conus; normally the conus is at the following levels: in the foetus at the coccyx, at birth at the upper border of the 3rd lumbar vertebra, and at the age of 5 years at the upper border of the 2nd lumbar vertebra.
6. Hydromyelia.
7. Atrophic meningocele.
8. Arachnoid cyst.
9. Various forms of myelodysplasia.

Frequently, more than one of these abnormalities is present in combination.

SPECIAL INVESTIGATIONS

The following sequence of special investigations will generally be performed:
• Plain radiographs. These may disclose:
  – varying degrees and extent of spina bifida
  – a wide interpeduncular distance
  – various anomalies of formation and segmentation of vertebrae
  – a bony spur (if diastematomyelia is present)

  It is important that the full length of the spine be X-rayed in all patients.

• Ultrasound (Fig. 16.15). This investigation is useful in patients up to the age of 6 months. Should a patient present with a cutaneous lesion on the back or a foot deformity then this investigation can clarify the nature of the underlying lesion without the need for general anaesthesia
• Plain computed tomography
• Computed tomography and myelography (combined)
• Magnetic resonance imaging (Fig. 16.16).

The last three investigations have increasing sensitivity in defining the precise nature of the lesion.

MANAGEMENT

The sequence of events in the management of patients with spinal dysraphism is:

• recognition that a neurological condition is present
• diagnosis of the cause of the condition, to allow correct management of the underlying spinal lesion and the assessment of prognosis
• management of any foot deformity that is present.

Recognition that the condition has a neurological basis
This is dependent on a high degree of suspicion of a neurological cause for any lower limb abnormality and, in particular, for a foot deformity or discrepancy in limb size. The clinician should look for muscle imbalance, carry out a careful neurological examination, and always examine the spine of the patient.

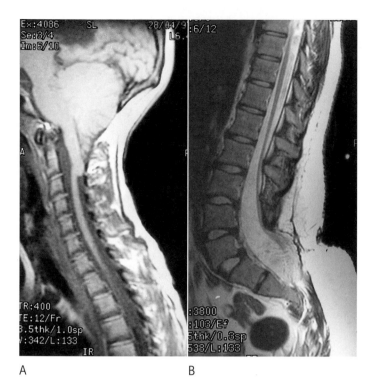

A   B

Figure 16.16 The use of magnetic resonance imaging has transformed our understanding of the spinal pathology and the reasons for late neurological deterioration in the child with spina bifida. **A** the Chiari 2 malformation with caudal displacement of the medulla, fourth ventricle and cerebellar vermis. **B** In this T2-weighted sagittal MRI image, tethering of the cord is noted, with elongation and thinning of the cord, which remains tethered to the dural sac at the site of the original repair. This child presented with back pain, an alteration in bowel and bladder function, and a progressive unilateral foot deformity, all classical features of the tethered cord syndrome.

Diagnosis of the precise cause

Appropriate investigation should allow precise definition of the neural tube defect. In cases in which a neurological defect progresses but the lesion is surgically treatable,

careful liaison between orthopaedic surgeon and neurosurgeon allows the best treatment.

Management of the foot or leg abnormality

Cavus and other foot deformities that may be present will, in general, be managed by:

- correction of muscle imbalance by tendon lengthening and transfer
- soft-tissue release, between birth and age 5 years
- metatarsal and os calcis osteotomy, between 5 and 10 years
- wedge tarsectomy or triple arthrodesis, from 12 years to maturity
- at all ages, circular frame correction may be used as an adjunct to conventional surgery.

COMPLICATIONS

Deformity may recur after soft-tissue releases, as a result of persistence of the causative spinal lesion. Overzealous soft-tissue release may result in reversal of the deformity.

Excessive lengthening of the Achilles tendon may result in calcaneus deformity, which is worse than the original equinus deformity. It is generally wise to correct cavus deformity at one stage and equinus deformity at a second stage.

Postoperative casts should be carefully applied, to avoid pressure on insensitive skin, particularly that overlying prominent metatarsal heads.

SUMMARY

Spinal dysraphism is one cause of abnormality in size, shape or muscle power in leg or foot. In the presence of such abnormalities, the surgeon should invariably examine the lumbar spine, carry out a neurological examination and be aware of the special investigations that are appropriate. It can be assumed at the beginning that all these children have the potential to walk, except those who are severely cognitively impaired or have gross spasticity. Children should be taught to stand and walk as soon as this becomes practicable. The age at which various orthopaedic procedures are carried out is shown in Table 16.2.

REFERENCES

American Academy of Orthopaedic Surgeons 2001 Caring for the Child with Spina Bifida

Broughton N S, Menelaus M B, Cole W G, Shurtleff D B 1993 The natural history of hip deformity in myelomeningocele. Journal of Bone and Joint Surgery 75B: 760–763

Dias L S 1985 Valgus deformity of the ankle joint: pathogenesis of fibular shortening. Journal of Pediatric Orthopaedics 5: 176–180

Duffy C M, Hill A E, Cosgrove A P, Corry I S, Graham H K 1996a. Energy consumption in children with spina bifida and cerebral palsy: a comparative study. Developmental Medicine and Child Neurology 38: 238–243

Duffy C M, Hill A E, Cosgrove A P, Corry I S, Mollan R A B, Graham H K 1996b Three-dimensional gait analysis in spina bifida. Journal of Pediatric Orthopaedics 16: 786–791

Dunteman R C, Vankoski S J, Dias L S 2000 Internal derotation osteotomy of the tibia pre and post operative gait analysis for persons with high sacral myelomeningocele. Journal of Pediatric Orthopaedics 20: 623–628

Evans D 1975 Calcaneo-valgus deformity. The Journal of Bone and Joint Surgery 57B: 270–278

Grice D S 1952 An extra-articular arthrodesis of the subastragalar joint for correction of paralytic flat feet in children. Journal of Bone and Joint Surgery 34A: 927–940

James C C M, Lassman L P 1972 Spinal dysraphism. Spina bifida occulta. Butterworths, London

James C C M, Lassman L P 1981 Spina bifida occulta. Orthopaedic, radiological and neurosurgical aspects. Academic Press, London/Grune & Stratton, New York

Lichtenstein B W 1940 Spinal dysraphism. Spina bifida and myelodysplasia. Archives of Neurology and Psychiatry 44: 792–810

Mazur J M, Shurtleff D, Menelaus M B, Colliver J 1989 Orthopaedic management of high-level spina bifida. Journal of Bone and Joint Surgery 71A: 56–61

Menelaus M B 1998 In: Broughton N S, Menelaus M B (eds) Menelaus' orthopaedic management of spina bifida cystica, 3rd Edn. W B Saunders, London

Mosca V S 1995 Calcaneal lengthening for valgus deformity of the hindfoot. Results in children who had severe, symptomatic flatfoot and skewfoot. Journal of Bone and Joint Surgery 77A: 500–512

Nicol R O, Menelaus M B 1983 Correction of combined tibial torsion and valgus deformity of the foot. Journal of Bone and Joint Surgery 65B: 641–645

Olney B W, Menelaus M B 1988 Triple arthrodesis of the foot in spina bifida patients. Journal of Bone and Joint Surgery 70B: 234–235

Patten B M 1952 Overgrowth of the neural tube in young human embryos. Anatomical Record 113: 381

Pemberton P A 1965 Pericapsular osteotomy of the ilium for treatment of congenital subluxation and dislocation of the hip. Journal of Bone and Joint Surgery 47A: 65–86

Schafer M F, Dias L S 1983 Myelomeningocele; orthopaedic treatment. Williams & Wilkins, Baltimore, London

Sharrard W J W 1964 Posterior iliopsoas transplantation in the treatment of paralytic dislocation of the hip. Journal of Bone and Joint Surgery 46B: 426–444

Shurtleff D B (ed.) 1986 Myelodysplasias and extrophies: significance, prevention and treatment. Grune & Stratton, Orlando

Shurtleff D B, Menelaus M B, Staheli L T et al, 1986 Natural history of flexion deformity of the hip in myelodysplasia. Journal of Pediatric Orthopaedics 6: 666–673

Vankoski S J, Sarwark J F, Moore C, Dias L 1995 Characteristic pelvic, hip and knee kinematic patterns in children with lumbosacral myelomeningocele. Gait and Posture 3: 51–57

Watkins M L 1998 Efficacy of folic acid prophylaxis for the prevention of neural tube defects. Mental Retardation and Developmental Disabilities Research Reviews 4: 282–290

Williams P F, Menelaus M B 1977 Triple arthrodesis by inlay grafting: a method suitable for the underformed or valgus foot. Journal of Bone and Joint Surgery 59B: 333–336

Williams P F 1982 Orthopaedic management in childhood. Blackwell, Oxford.

Wright J G, Menelaus M B, Broughton N S, Shurtleff D 1991 Natural history of knee contractures in myelomeningocele. Journal of Pediatric Orthopaedics 11: 725–730

Yngve D A, Lindseth R E 1982 Effectiveness of muscle transfers in myelomeningocele hips measured by radiographic indices. Journal of Pediatric Orthopaedics 2: 121–125

Chapter 17

Poliomyelitis

E. K. W. Ho and J. C. Y. Leong

INTRODUCTION

The poliomyelitis virus may attack the central nervous system and cause paralysis and subsequent deformities. An effective vaccine and vaccination programme started in North America in 1954. The World Health Organisation statistics demonstrate a dramatic reduction in reported cases in Europe and the North American Continent, but the disease is still endemic in Africa, Southern America and Asia. A survey (Anonymous 1979) showed only a 15% decrease in world-wide incidence.

AETIOLOGY AND IMMUNISATION

The disease is caused by one of the three types of poliomyelitis virus (Brunhilde, Lansing and Leon) belonging to the enterovirus group, which includes Coxsackie C and the ECHO viruses. The last two viruses can produce a clinical picture indistinguishable from that of poliomyelitis. The lack of cross-immunity between each type of polio virus makes reinfection possible.

The virus is most commonly transmitted through the gastrointestinal tract via infected food or faecal matter, although the disease may be contracted via the respiratory tract. The virus is blood-borne to the central nervous system. Epidemics used to occur during summer and autumn; however, with the widespread use of oral vaccine, epidemics are now unusual.

Two types of vaccine are available. The Salk vaccine is a killed vaccine given by injection, whereas the Sabin (1965) vaccine is a live, attenuated oral vaccine. The latter type is cheaper, safe, and effective against all three types of polio virus. Immunity conferred is usually life-long.

PATHOLOGY

ACUTE STAGE

Poliomyelitis starts as a systemic infection. The incubation varies from 1 to 3 weeks. Initial extraneural involvement is mainly in the reticulo-endothelial system, with hyperplasia of the spleen and lymph nodes. Only 1–2% of those affected ultimately suffer from neural damage.

Neural involvement occurs chiefly in the brain stem and anterior horn cells of the spinal cord. However, inflammatory changes may occur in the posterior ganglia and nerve roots.

Initially, the spinal cord shows inflammatory changes, with polymorphonuclear cell infiltration, later replaced by lymphocytes. There are varying degrees of neuronal degeneration, with cell death and disintegration as the worst histological signs after a few days. Glial cell replacement occurs as the chronic stage of the disease appears. Because of anterior horn cell involvement, there is lower motor neurone paralysis, especially of muscles innervated by the cervical and lumbar enlargements. Flaccid paralysis is present, with normal sensation in the extremities. Intramuscular injection during the acute stage may lead to localisation of paralysis in a certain segment of the cord. Similarly, surgery – for example tonsillectomy – may trigger the appearance of bulbar palsy.

CHRONIC STAGE

Residual paralysis is of varying severity and combination. The muscles of the lower limb are affected at least four to five times more often than those of the upper limb. The quadriceps, glutei, tibialis anterior, hamstrings and hip flexors are involved, in descending order of frequency. The intrinsic muscles of the foot are sometimes affected. In the upper limb, the deltoid, triceps and pectoralis muscles are commonly affected. Trunk muscles are weakened less often.

After the initial stage of muscle irritability and spasm, atrophy and fibrosis set in. Muscle imbalance leads to joint deformity, and sometimes dislocation. This is often aggravated by gravity, posture and subsequent growth of the child. Secondary contracture of the tendons, ligaments, joint capsule, and sometimes the skin, all add to the rigidity of the deformity. Because paralysis occurs in a growing limb, shortening will develop. The bones are thin and sometimes osteoporotic, and thus prone to fracture. The joints may show restricted mobility, with possible subluxation or dislocation. Osteoarthritis does not commonly occur, unless there has been previous operation or trauma.

The respiratory system may be affected secondary to bulbar palsy or paralysis of the ventilatory muscles (intercostals or diaphragm). Bulbar palsy usually recovers fully.

RECOVERY PROGNOSIS

Most functional recovery in muscle power occurs within the first few months and is complete by 6 months after the initial illness; theoretically, recovery is possible for up to 2 years. Good prognostic factors for recovery include young age, partial paralysis and upper extremity involvement. Careful muscle charting, followed by serial assessment during the initial few months, is therefore important as a means of assessing the likelihood of recovery.

CLINICAL FEATURES

ACUTE STAGE

Acute symptoms include fever and malaise. Symptoms of encephalomyelitis appear within a week: severe headache, vomiting, neck rigidity, meningism and backache are common. Simultaneously, paralysis of the extremities occurs. Asymmetric involvement of the lower extremities is the most common pattern. Absence of progression of muscle paralysis heralds the end of the acute phase. Signs during the early stage include muscle spasm, with tenderness on palpation. With impending paralysis of the affected limb, the deep tendon reflex is either exaggerated or decreased. The superficial reflexes are usually absent initially. Irritation may be present, but sensation of the limb is normal.

Upper-limb muscle paralysis affects the shoulder girdle more often than the arm. Particular attention must be paid to detecting paralysis of the intercostals and diaphragm. Neck muscle weakness may be associated with difficulty in swallowing. Lower limb muscle paralysis is invariably associated with back and abdominal muscle weakness. The quadriceps are more frequently involved.

The acute stage usually lasts 1–2 weeks.

CONVALESCENT STAGE

This is the stage in which muscle recovery occurs. It lasts for 2 years after the acute illness. Serial muscle charting is necessary, especially in the first few months, when most of the recovery is expected. Initial examination may be difficult because of muscle pain or spasm. Loss of recovery potential in some muscles may occur if excessive activity is allowed in the early convalescent stage. Contractures of fascia, muscle aponeurosis and muscle itself begin during this period.

CHRONIC STAGE

No muscle recovery is expected 2 years after the onset of the disease. By then, the orthopaedic surgeon is best placed to utilise residual motor activity. Deformities may be fixed or mobile: with time, some mobile deformities, if neglected, can become structural. Growth and posture further aggravate the joint deformities. Initially, only the soft tissues are involved, but later secondary changes occur in bone and joint. The younger the patient, the greater the chance of significant deformity.

Common deformities in the chronic phase are shown in Table 17.1.

DIAGNOSIS

The diagnosis of poliomyelitis is largely a clinical one. The prodromal phase is similar to other viral infections of the gastrointestinal or upper respiratory tracts. It may pass unnoticed, especially if it is not followed by neurological problems. The poliomyelitis virus may be found in the throat swab or stool. The diagnosis is usually made at the paralytic stage (differential diagnosis below). Laboratory investigation shows non-specific changes, such as a slight increase in the erythrocyte sedimentation rate and a leucocytosis. Lumbar puncture yields clear, pus-free fluid. There may be an increase in cerebrospinal fluid pressure, together with an increase in the white blood cell count – initially neutrophils, later lymphocytes. The protein content in the cerebrospinal fluid may increase. Attempts at culture of the poliomyelitis virus from the cerebrospinal fluid are rarely useful, and other sophisticated laboratory tests are impractical. Patients in the chronic stage cease to reveal these changes.

DIFFERENTIAL DIAGNOSIS

Acute stage

- any cause of meningitis or encephalitis
- Guillain–Barré polyneuritis
- bone and joint infection
- pseudoparalysis of whatever cause
- myalgia or acute paraplegia of whatever cause
- acute rheumatic fever.

Chronic stage

- tuberculosis/spinal infection
- transverse myelitis
- spinal/spinal cord tumour
- cerebral palsy
- talipes equinovarus.

MANAGEMENT

GENERAL

During the acute stage, the patient is usually under the care of a paediatrician. General supportive treatment is necessary. Ventilatory failure requires active resuscitation and the prevention of complications. Tracheotomy, assisted ventilation, chest physiotherapy and antibiotics may be needed, particularly for patients with bulbar involvement, who need expert ventilatory monitoring. Bed rest and fluid replacement are necessary, but sedatives should be avoided because they cause further depressant effects.

The orthopaedic surgeon should be involved, even in the acute stage. Muscle spasm is relieved by hot packs, and contractures are prevented by early splintage of the joints in a functional position. Particular attention should be paid to prevent equinus contracture of the ankle by using a right-angle board, and deformity of the knee by support with a small roll behind the knee. The hip is protected by keeping the thigh in slight abduction and neutral rotation, and the deltoid by holding the arm in mild abduction and neutral

Table 17.1 Common deformities in the chronic phase of poliomyelitis

Site	Lesion	Effect
Upper Limb		
Shoulder	Deltoid paralysis	Limitation of shoulder abduction
Elbow	Flexor paralysis	Inability to flex the elbow
Forearm	Fixed suppination	Inability to pronate interferes with the position of the hand in normal activities
Wrist	Extensor weakness	Inability to dorsiflex the wrist
Hand	Intrinsic paralysis	Impaired hand function
Thumb	Thenar muscle loss	Lack of opposition of the thumb
Lower limb		
Hip	Paralytic dislocation	Relative overaction of the hip flexors and adductors
	Flexion or flexion–abduction contracture	Contracture of anterior and sometimes lateral structures
	Gluteal paralysis	Usually mixed extension–abduction weakness
	Flail hip	Extensive weakness of muscles around hip
Knee	Flexion contracture	Strong hamstrings
	Genu valgum	Weak quadriceps
	External tibial torsion	Contracted ilio-tibial tract
	Genu recurvatum	Weak quadriceps
		Lax soft tissue at the back of knee
	Flail knee	Extensive paralysis around the knee
Foot and ankle	Equinovalgus contracture	Weak tibialis anterior
		Weak tibialis posterior
	Eversion deformity	Weak tibialis posterior only (rare)
	Equinovarus deformity	Weak tibialis anterior, peronei and toe extensors
	Calcaneus deformity	Weak triceps surae
	Claw toes	Over-active long toe extensors (with weak ankle dorsiflexors)
		Over-active long toe flexors (with weak triceps surae)
	Pes cavus	Imbalance between intrinsic and extrinsic foot muscles
	Leg length discrepancy	Shortened muscles affect bone growth
Trunk		
Spine	Scoliosis	Asymmetric paralysis of paraspinal muscles. Ilio-tibial tract contracture and pelvic obliquity
	Pelvic obliquity	Ilio-tibial tract contracture (hip abductor contracture)
		Leg length discrepancy
		Scoliosis
		Weak abdominal muscles

rotation. Physiotherapy should be started gently (especially while the irritable stage is subsiding), consisting of gradual gentle stretching of spastic muscles by passively putting the joints through the normal range of motion. In the later stage of the acute phase, assisted muscle exercises lead gradually to an active exercise programme.

MANAGEMENT OF ESTABLISHED CONTRACTURES

Basic principles

Secondary factors very often worsen the effects of a primary muscle imbalance, to produce fixed contractures. These secondary factors consist of contractures of the joint capsule, aponeurosis, neurovascular bundle and skin, and deformity of joint surfaces.

Gentle stretching of a joint contracture is very useful, but care must be exercised during manipulation because the osteoporotic bone is prone to fracture or the epiphysis may slip. When the contracture position has been fully stretched, the joint is splinted in an over-corrected position but removed from the splint for mobilisation every day.

Dynamic splintage is preferred to static splintage. If conservative treatment fails, consideration should be given to surgical correction. The following clinical factors must be taken into account:

1. The degree of contracture in the adjacent joints of the ipsilateral limb.
2. The status of the contralateral limb.
3. Residual power of the lower limbs as a predictor of independent walking, with or without calipers.
4. Residual power of the upper limbs (especially triceps function, to enable the patient to use elbow crutches).

As a general rule, older patients with severe deformities respond poorly, but young patients with mild to moderate fixed deformity are suitable candidates for surgery.

Provision of motor power after correction of contractures is important in management. This requires the application of the basic principles of tendon surgery (Mayer 1956), sometimes in combination with bony stabilisation procedures (preferably delayed until bone maturity).

Orthotic splintage is necessary, not only to keep the manipulated joint in the over-corrected position to prevent recurrence of deformity, but also to augment weak muscles and protect paralysed muscle from over-stretching. Tendon transfers should also be protected from over-stretching in the first few months after surgery.

UPPER LIMBS

Shoulder

Deltoid paralysis (Saha 1967). The deltoid is one of the two prime movers of the shoulder, so that dysfunction of this muscle causes difficulty in initiating abduction. Deltoid paralysis is usually partial, with sparing of the posterior portion, and therefore transfer of trapezius is recommended. However, multiple muscle transplantation in stages may be necessary (depending upon the remaining muscle power) using the clavicular fibres of pectoralis major, the remaining posterior portion of deltoid, the origin of the long head of triceps and the short head of biceps, latissimus dorsi and teres major (Saha 1967). The possible transfers are detailed in Table 17.2. The results of these transfers are less certain than after brachial plexus palsy.

Shoulder arthrodesis. Extensive muscle paralysis around the shoulder causes subluxation or dislocation. When this becomes symptomatic, shoulder arthrodesis may be considered, provided that:

1. Good scapulothoracic control by trapezius and serratus anterior compensates for the loss of glenohumeral movement.
2. The limb functions well distal to the shoulder.

The exact position of shoulder arthrodesis is controversial, but there should be approximately 20° of abduction, 30° of flexion and 40° of internal rotation. This position enables the hand to reach the face for feeding and cleaning, and the perineum for toileting. Adjustments must be made to avoid the scapula being unduly prominent after shoulder arthrodesis with the arm at the side of the body. Shoulder arthrodesis may be intra-articular, extra-articular or combined (Rowe 1974) and intraoperative X-ray may be helpful in determining the angle of abduction attained between the humeral shaft and the vertebral border of the scapula.

Elbow

Flexor paralysis. The main indication for treating paralysis of elbow flexion caused by loss of biceps, brachialis and brachio-radialis is the presence of good hand function. Weakness of the muscles around the shoulder and wrist are contraindications to reconstruction.

The most commonly used substitute for the elbow flexors is the wrist flexor mass (Steindler's flexorplasty) (Steindler 1944), in which the medial epicondyle and the origin of the wrist flexors are transferred proximally to the lower humerus. Possible complications include the development of a fixed pronation deformity and a mild flexion contracture of the elbow. Failure of the operation may be due to initially weak wrist flexors or poor fixation of the medial epicondyle to the humerus. A posterior bone block operation may prevent a weak elbow flexor from becoming overstretched.

When Steindler's flexorplasty is not feasible, other muscle transfers may be considered to reconstitute elbow flexion (Table 17.3).

Triceps paralysis. Gravity assists elbow extension and thus partly compensates for loss of triceps function. However, when active forceful elbow extension is needed, as in crutch walking or transferring from bed, strong extension is needed. Possible transfers include brachio-radialis or latissimus dorsi. The latissimus dorsi has a long neurovascular bundle, making mobilisation of the muscle easy.

Forearm

Pronator contracture. Supination is restored by transferring pronator teres and flexor carpi radialis around the ulnar border and the dorsum of the forearm to the radio-volar aspect of the radius.

Supinator contracture. This is usually associated with a strong biceps. When there is insufficient power for tendon transfer, osteotomy of both forearm bones and stabilisation in an over-corrected position is necessary. The alternatives for fixed deformity include interosseous membrane release, release of the radio-ulnar joints, and biceps lengthening.

Table 17.2 Possible substitute by transfer	
Muscle paralysed	Substitution
Subscapularis	Superior portion of serratus anterior
Supraspinatus	Levator scapulae or sterno-cleidomastoid
Subscapularis/infraspinatus	Latissimus dorsi or teres major
Serratus anterior paralysis	Pectoralis minor by posterior transfer

Table 17.3 Transfers to produce elbow flexion

Muscle transfer	Comment
All of pectoralis major muscle (Brooks–Seddon procedure)	Clavicular portion of pectoralis major must be strong. Used when the biceps brachii is completely paralysed. Muscle control of shoulder and scapula must be good
Sternal head of pectoralis major (Clark's procedure)	Used when the clavicular portion of pectoralis major is paralysed
Pectoralis minor	Used when pectoralis major and biceps are paralysed. A fascia lata graft is necesary to bridge the gap
Sterno-clavicular head of sterno-cleidomastoid muscle	Fascia lata graft to bridge the gap; may cause webbing of the neck
Latissimus dorsi muscle (Hovnanian procedure)	Provides good cross-sectional area and strength for the transfer. Origin of latissimus dorsi transplanted into biceps tendon
Triceps anterior transfer	Indicated when other transfers are not feasible. Active extension of the elbow may be weakened.

Wrist. Wrist drop develops if the wrist dorsiflexors are involved; it can be controlled by a splint. If this improves finger function, a wrist arthrodesis may be indicated.

Fingers. Clawing of the fingers is the result of intrinsic muscle paralysis. The thumb lacks active opposition because of involvement of opponens and the short abductor muscles. The classical Bunnell transfer is sometimes helpful in providing opposition, but the flexor digitorum sublimis that is to be transferred from the middle or ring finger must have at least MRC (Medical Research Council) grade 4 power (see Ch. 15, Table 15.2). The remaining profundus muscle must be strong enough to flex the finger.

Flail arm. Usually, no surgery is indicated. A wrist or elbow splint may be helpful to improve cosmesis.

LOWER LIMBS

The aim of surgery in the lower limb is to provide a stable, balanced gait, with or without a caliper. Muscle contracture and imbalance, contracture of intermuscular septa and fasciae, shortened tendons and retardation of bone growth all contribute to difficulty in walking. The patient presents with an abnormal gait. Examination of the lower extremities should concentrate on the presence and extent of fixed or mobile deformity, the range of motion of the joints, residual muscle power, leg length discrepancy (both real and apparent), and concomitant pelvic obliquity. Lower limb deformities are usually multiple, so good initial documentation is necessary, followed by careful planning (Figs 17.1 and 17.2). In general, the hip problems – usually a contracture – should be dealt with first. Sometimes, deformities can inhibit a weakened muscle, and relief of such deformities places the weakened muscle in a mechanically more advantageous position.

Hip

Flexion or flexion–abduction contracture. The offending structure is usually a contracted ilio-tibial tract and lateral intermuscular septum. This tether is very often associated with an anterior soft-tissue contracture (rectus femoris, tensor fasciae latae, sartorius, ilio-psoas and the hip capsule), further aggravated by weakness of hip extension (gluteus maximus) and hip abduction (gluteus medius).

The ilio-tibial tract lies anterior to the hip and posterior to the knee joint, and therefore produces a flexion contracture of the hip and knee. Palpation of the contracture is facilitated by adduction and extension of the hip, revealing the primary fixed abduction flexion deformity and secondary external rotation of the hip, genu valgum, external tibial torsion, occasional varus deformity of the foot, pelvic obliquity, and a short leg.

Surgical release of anterior soft-tissue contracture is achieved preferably via the standard ilio-femoral approach. The contracted muscles that must be released include tensor fasciae latae, gluteus medius and minimus, sartorius, rectus femoris and the anterior hip capsule.

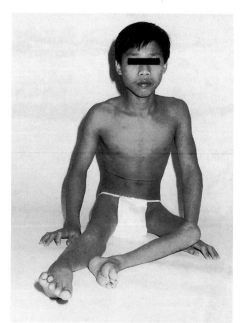

Figure 17.1 This 12 year-old boy contracted poliomyelitis at the age of 6 months, and has never walked.

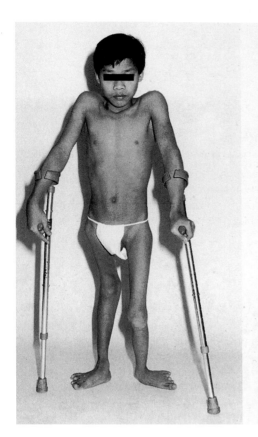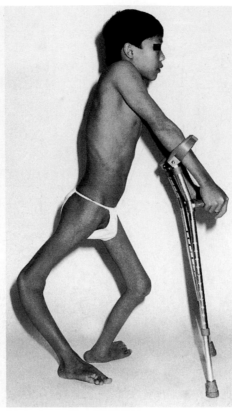

Figure 17.2 His attempt at standing with elbow crutches confirmed the presence of a 50° flexion contracture of the left knee, 70° recurvatum of the right knee, fixed valgus of the left foot, and equinus and pronation of the right foot. (Quadriceps power grade 0 bilaterally, hamstring power grade 4 on the left and grade 0 on the right, and triceps surae grade 3 bilaterally.)

Sectioning of the ilio-tibial tract together with a portion of the lateral intermuscular septum alone is a simple and effective measure for mild contractures. Release must be followed by serial casting, with the hip in progressive adduction and extension and the knee straight.

Gluteal paralysis

Weakness of hip abduction (gluteus medius and minimus) produces a positive Trendelenburg sign. This can be treated by the Mustard procedure (Mustard 1959). When both gluteus medius and maximus are paralysed, hip abduction and extension are weak. There is also forward tilting of the pelvis (backward body lurch) in addition to a Trendelenburg sign. Under such circumstances, the Sharrard transfer of ilio-psoas (Sharrard 1964) is preferred. The ilio-psoas transfer forms part of the treatment of paralytic dislocation of hip in poliomyelitis. It should not be forgotten that hip flexion is weakened by the transfer.

Iliopsoas transfer by the Mustard and Sharrard procedures is useful for patients with partial gluteal paralysis. It will improve stability during walking and thus the gait. Good abdominal muscle strength and a powerful sartorius, which becomes a primary hip flexor later, are important prerequisites.

The aim of the Mustard procedure (Mustard 1959) is to transfer the iliopsoas to augment hip abduction. The iliopsoas, with its bony attachment, is isolated via a standard Smith–Peterson approach. The muscle is passed through a bony notch between the anterior superior and inferior iliac spines, to be attached to the greater trochanter. Postoperative immobilisation of the hip in abduction is necessary.

In the Sharrard procedure (Sharrard 1964), the iliopsoas is transferred posterior and lateral to the hip joint, through a large window in the ilium adjacent to the sacro-iliac joint. The tendon is advanced through a tunnel in the greater trochanter to its anterolateral surface. This procedure is more extensive and technically more difficult than the Mustard procedure, but may be appropriate for patients with weakened hip extension. Prior anterior soft-tissue release, abductor tenotomy and concomitant varus osteotomy of the hip may be required.

External oblique transfer. This muscle may be transferred to the greater trochanter in patients suffering from gluteus medius paralysis in whom the iliopsoas is not suitable for transfer.

Tensor fasciae latae transfer. This muscle can be transferred posteriorly for gluteus medius weakness and hip instability when no other muscles are suitable for transfer.

Erector spinae transfer. This procedure is occasionally used for gluteus maximus weakness.

Paralytic poliomyelitic hip dislocation

Soft-tissue and bony factors contribute to hip subluxation and dislocation in poliomyelitis (Lau et al 1986). Initially, the hip abductors and flexors overpower the abductors and extensors. Subsequently, bony factors develop in the form of femoral neck valgus and increased anteversion. The acetabulum becomes shallow and oblique as the patient begins to bear weight, stretching the capsule and allowing the femoral head to subluxate or dislocate. Pelvic obliquity aggravates this process, the hip on the higher side adducting and displacing.

Both soft-tissue and bony factors have to be dealt with. Concentric reduction of the hip is achieved by either closed or open reduction. Traction is often required for late cases before open reduction, especially after 3 years of age.

The muscle imbalance must be corrected by appropriate tendon transfers, but must be deferred until bony deformities have been corrected. Both upper femoral varising derotation osteotomy (sometimes with shortening of the femur to decrease the tension on the reduced femoral head) and acetabular reconstruction are required; alternatively redirection by innominate osteotomy, or increase in femoral head coverage by the procedure of Chiari osteotomy may be indicated, depending upon the configuration of the acetabular defect. Acetabular reorientation procedures are often inappropriate because the acetabulum has 'wandered' superiorly and laterally. Any associated predisposing cause of subluxation such as pelvic obliquity must be dealt with to prevent recurrence. Hip arthrodesis is seldom indicated for paralytic dislocation, unless there is articular degeneration and painful impingement.

The flail hip

Lack of muscle power around the hip is often associated with major paralysis distally. Multiple orthotic devices may be necessary to allow standing and walking. The flail hip seldom dislocates, and is usually asymptomatic unless other factors such as pelvic obliquity render it prone to subluxation. Arthrodesis is only indicated when there is good surrounding musculature (quadriceps, abdominal and paravertebral), a stable foot and ankle, and a strong ipsilateral knee, free from contracture. Successful arthrodesis will improve gait by providing stability and pain relief, but should be reserved for the patient older than 10 years.

Pelvic obliquity

This can be produced by contracture above the pelvis when lumbar or thoraco-lumbar scoliosis is produced by asymmetric paralysis of the quadratus lumborum and oblique abdominal muscles. Below the pelvis, a contracture of the ilio-tibial tract causes ipsilateral downward tilting of the pelvis, followed by contracture of the trunk muscles on the contralateral side. A lumbar scoliosis and hip subluxation are further aggravated by an adduction contracture with apparent shortening of the opposite leg. The treatment of pelvic obliquity is directed at the cause and any fixed secondary deformities, if present (O'Brien et al 1975a).

The knee

The most common deformity of the knee is fixed flexion deformity of varying severity. Other deformities are genu recurvatum, genu valgum and, rarely, genu varum.

The causes of fixed flexion contracture include ilio-tibial tract contracture and quadriceps paralysis in the presence of normal hamstrings. Genu valgum and external rotation of the tibia coexist because of ilio-tibial tract contracture and a strong biceps femoris with weak medial hamstrings. Posterior subluxation of the tibia may also occur secondary to muscle imbalance. This is one of the factors limiting serial plaster correction of fixed-knee deformities; this technique should be used only in mild cases.

Knee flexion contracture of more than 25–30° places the knee at a mechanical disadvantage, and in order to prevent the knee buckling during walking the patient may require a 'hand on the knee' gait. A Yount fasciotomy of the ilio-tibial tract may be necessary (Yount 1926). Flexion contracture of moderate to severe degree is difficult to treat. Secondary adaptive changes are present in the form of flattening of the articular surface and disproportionate increase in growth of the anterior portion of the tibia and femur compared with the posterior half. This further increases the chance of posterior subluxation of the tibia upon the femur (Fig. 17.3).

Surgical correction of severe flexion contracture may require staged procedures; the results are usually better in children. Initial posterior capsulotomy and ilio-tibial tract release, including division of the posterior cruciate ligament, and skeletal traction or casting may be necessary. A supracondylar osteotomy (Leong et al 1982) with or without shortening of the bone is required in the second stage (Fig. 17.4). A good range of knee flexion is important for success.

Genu recurvatum. Mild genu recurvatum is common and is not disabling. It results from thigh paralysis or stretching of the posterior knee structures.

When the triceps surae is normal in the presence of paralysis of the quadriceps and hamstrings, the knee cannot be

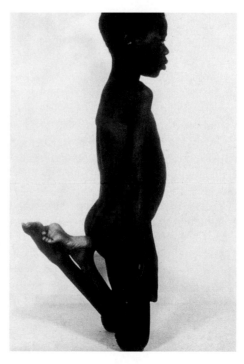

Figure 17.3 Severe flexion contractures of the knees making walking impossible except by kneeling.

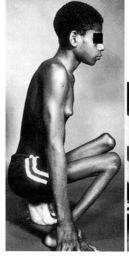
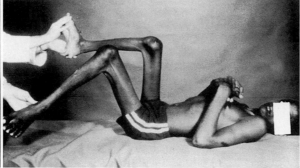
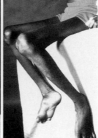

Figure 17.4 A Lower limb contractures in a 14-year-old boy who developed polio at the age of 1 year. B The right knee was corrected by a supracondylar femoral osteotomy and the left knee was arthrodesed. (By kind permission of Professor R. L. Huckstep.)

A

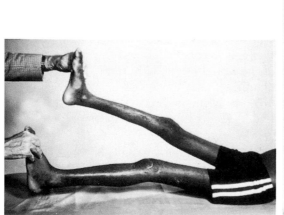
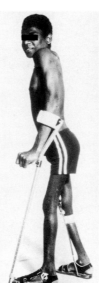
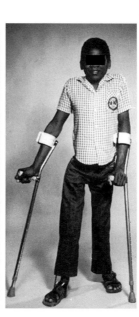

B

locked straight and therefore hyperextends during walking. Secondary bony changes result in progressive flattening of the anterior aspect of both upper tibia and femoral condyles. The tibial plateau slopes downward and forward. Such deformity develops slowly, and is amenable to surgical correction: operative correction of the bony malalignment by a wedge osteotomy of the upper tibia is followed by anterior hamstring transfer to the patella.

When there is weakness in both the triceps surae and hamstrings, the knee hyperextends and the posterior structures stretch. Gait is poor because of lack of push off by the calf muscles. This type of recurvatum progresses more rapidly, and early long-leg bracing is necessary. A posterior tenodesis to block hyperextension of the knee usually stretches, and knee arthrodesis may have to be considered as a salvage procedure. However, an anterior bone block, perhaps using the patella, may prevent this.

Quadriceps paralysis is common. Anterior hamstring transfer is reserved for the potentially brace-free patient with a good gluteus maximus, hamstrings and triceps surae. Lateral dislocation of the patella is a troublesome complication.

Flail knee. Bracing is required. Arthrodesis is indicated only for skeletally mature patients whose work is strenuous.

Foot and ankle

A stable, plantigrade foot is required for normal walking. The foot affected by poliomyelitis may be unstable, and muscle imbalance produces various combinations of deformity, which become structural with time. Plantar flexion/dorsiflexion imbalance produces equinus/calcaneus deformity at the ankle joint, whereas invertor/evertor imbalance produces varus/valgus deformity at the subtalar joint. Tendon release or transfer is useful and is the main method of treatment for a flexible deformity before bony maturity (Fig. 17.5). Bony resection and stabilisation are indicated

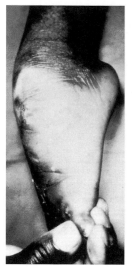
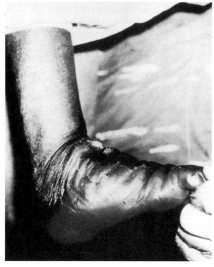

A   B

Figure 17.5 A Calf contracture producing severe equinus and a dorsal callosity of the foot secondary to weight-bearing. **B** Lengthening of the tendo–Achilles produced excellent correction. (By kind permission of Professor R.L. Huckstep.)

after skeletal maturity, and are often best performed just before tendon transfer.

Dorsiflexion: invertor insufficiency. This is caused by tibialis anterior paralysis. The foot assumes an equinovalgus posture. The metatarsal heads are depressed and the proximal phalanges hyperextended. The toes claw during the swing phase as the long extensors attempt to provide ankle dorsiflexion. The calf muscle becomes contracted and passive dorsiflexion is limited. A cavus deformity often coexists because of overaction of peroneus longus and tibialis posterior.

Early treatment of mild cases involves stretching of the tight structures behind the ankle; an ankle orthosis may be useful. Surgery involves posterior ankle capsulotomy and anterior transfer of peroneus longus to the base of second metatarsal. The peroneus brevis is sutured to the distal stump of peroneus longus to preserve its remaining tension on the first metatarsal. Active dorsiflexor power may also be improved by transfer of the extensor digitorum longus to the dorsum of the midfoot, whereas the correction of the claw toes requires transfer of the long toe extensors to the metatarsal necks. The distal stump of extensor hallucis longus is attached to the brevis to prevent recurrence of clawing of the big toe. Additional fixed cavovarus deformity requires plantar fasciotomy and intrinsic muscle release. For structural deformities, a triple arthrodesis (Lambrinudi modification) is necessary before peroneal transfer. The tibialis posterior can also be transferred through the interosseous membrane to provide ankle dorsiflexion.

Paralysis of tibialis anterior and tibialis posterior results in equinovalgus deformity. The peroneus longus is transferred to the base of the second metatarsal to replace the tibialis anterior. One long toe flexor is used to substitute for the tibialis posterior.

Isolated tibialis posterior paralysis is rare. An eversion deformity results. Tendon transfer using flexor hallucis longus, flexor digitorum longus or extensor hallucis longus has been successful.

Evertor insufficiency. Isolated evertor insufficiency is rare. It usually occurs in association with paralysis of the long toe extensors and tibialis anterior.

In pure peroneal palsy, the hindfoot inverts and the forefoot adducts. The deforming force is the tibialis anterior, which produces a dorsal elevation of the distal part of the 1st metatarsal and a dorsal bunion. Lateral transfer of the tibialis anterior to the base of 2nd metatarsal will correct a mild flexible deformity. Fixed 1st metatarsal deformity requires osteotomy at its base, whereas hindfoot deformity requires a triple arthrodesis. Sometimes when the extensor hallucis longus overacts after tibialis anterior transfer, it may need transfer to the 1st metatarsal with interphalangeal fusion or tenodesis (Robert–Jones operation).

Weakness of both peronei and long toe extensors produces a mild equinovarus deformity and treatment is the same as for pure evertor insufficiency. Paralysis of peronei, long toe extensors and tibialis anterior produces a severe equinovarus deformity. The tibialis posterior and triceps surae are the deforming forces and anterior transfer of the tibialis posterior to the base of the 3rd metatarsal is effective. It may be augmented by prior soft-tissue release of the cavus, and anterior transfer of the long toe flexors.

Triceps surae paralysis. Triceps surae paralysis produces a calcaneus deformity. There is lack of push-off during the gait cycle and the weight of the body cannot be transferred effectively to the metatarsal heads. Active ankle dorsiflexion stretches the calf and the posterior ankle capsule. The toe flexors and intrinsic muscles aggravate the deformity by pulling the forefoot into plantaris. The tibialis posterior, peronei and long toe flexors, instead of plantar flexing the hindfoot, cause further depression of the metatarsal heads, and a fixed calcaneo-cavus deformity results, with a plantar aponeurosis contracture and secondary bony changes.

The posterior lever arm of the os calcis decreases as this deformity develops, and the heel becomes shortened, together with the foot. Ultimately, the weakened triceps surae loses function as the axis of the tibia and the os calcis coincide. 'Pistol-grip' graphically describes the deformity (see Ch. 29.4).

Treatment of calcaneal foot and ankle deformities

Early splintage and a muscle exercise programme are used to achieve maximal recovery of muscle power and to prevent the calcaneus deformity. An orthosis may be necessary to assist plantar flexion at the ankle and to limit dorsiflexion.

In the skeletally immature foot 'push-off' power can be helped by multiple tendon transfers such as tibialis posterior, the peronei and, rarely, tibialis anterior to the os calcis. The plantar aponeurosis and intrinsic muscles should be released.

In the skeletally mature foot, bony resection and arthrodesis of the hindfoot are necessary before tendon transfer, usually with an interval of 6 weeks. With gross instability, a pantalar arthrodesis may be indicated. This is usually undertaken in patients with associated paralysis, in order to eliminate the use of a caliper.

Tendon transfer in calcaneal deformities

Invertor and evertor balance must be achieved during tendon transfer for calcaneal deformity. Calcaneo-cavus deformity is controlled by transfer of both peroneus brevis and tibialis posterior to the heel. Calcaneo-cavovalgus deformity requires transfer of both peronei. For mobile calcaneal deformity, translocation of the peroneus longus into a groove on the posterior aspect of the os calcis is sometimes useful. The hamstrings have also been used to replace triceps surae function. Transfer of the tibialis anterior posteriorly through the interosseous membrane is advocated for younger patients with a flexible deformity.

Foot and ankle arthrodesis

The most commonly practiced procedures are extra-articular subtalar arthrodesis and triple arthrodesis. Bone block procedures and ankle arthrodesis are now seldom performed.

Extra-articular subtalar arthrodesis (Grice procedure) (Greene & Grice 1952). The aim is to correct bony deformity in patients between the ages of 3 and 8 years, maintaining growth of the foot, by avoiding injury to preosseous cartilage. The procedure is indicated for subtalar valgus in the presence of a mobile forefoot.

Standing X-rays of the foot and ankle are necessary to determine the site of the valgus deformity, because it may also be present at the ankle. Calcaneo-valgus deformity treated by this procedure is sometimes complicated by postoperative varus and increased ankle valgus. The varus deformity produces a painful callosity over the lateral aspect of the foot. The modification suggested by Dennyson and Fulford (1976) helps to avoid this problem.

Triple arthrodesis. This operation is frequently performed after the child has reached the age of 10 years, for equino-valgus or varus deformity. The subtalar, calcaneo-cuboid and talo-navicular joints are resected and arthrodesed. Bony wedges are taken out to produce a plantigrade foot. Modifications of this procedure include posterior displacement of the foot to improve the mechanical advantage of the weakened triceps surae and the Lambrinudi arthrodesis for fixed equinus deformity (Tang et al 1984). Any limb rotational malalignment must be considered before the triple arthrodesis, in order to avoid malalignment of the foot during the procedure. The talo-navicular joint is prone to non-union and avascular necrosis of the talus may occur because of excessive resection. Late osteoarthritis of the ankle may develop secondary to stiffening of the hindfoot and ankle ligament laxity. Lastly, although recurrence of hindfoot deformity is rare, secondary forefoot deformity may occur because of muscle imbalance.

Ankle and pantalar arthrodesis

Both procedures are seldom performed for poliomyelitis. The flail foot is an indication for such a fusion. A strong gluteus maximus (to extend the hip) and good hamstrings and posterior knee capsule (to prevent hyperextension of the knee) are prerequisites. A preoperative weight-bearing lateral X-ray will demonstrate talar subluxation in cases where pantalar arthrodesis is indicated.

Other procedures for calcaneal foot deformity

Calcaneal osteotomy. Cavovarus deformity in a growing child may benefit from a calcarneal osteotomy. The os calcis can also be displaced posteriorly during the osteotomy.

Talectomy. This is indicated only when arthrodesis cannot be performed. The result is satisfactory for pain relief and cosmesis. Tibio-calcaneal fusion is necessary if talectomy fails.

Elmslie's procedure. This is a two-stage operation. Initially, soft-tissue release and dorsal wedge excision of the talo-navicular and calcaneo-cuboid joints correct the cavus deformity. This is followed by a second-stage posterior wedge excision of the subtalar joint, with the base of the wedge posteriorly to correct the calcaneal deformity. The tendo-Achilles is shortened and tenodesed to the posterior aspect of the tibia. The long toe flexors are cut and sutured to the tendo-Achilles.

Forefoot equinus. A mobile forefoot equinus needs splintage only. Structural forefoot equinus deformity requires release of the plantar aponeurosis and wedge resection of the midfoot, to enable the foot to be fitted with an orthosis.

Toes

There are three common causes for claw toe deformity (hyperextension of the metatarsophalangeal joint and flexion of interphalangeal joints):

1. Loss of ankle dorsiflexion. The clawing is noticeable during the swing phase, as the long toe extensors try to compensate for the loss of ankle dorsiflexion power. Restoration of ankle dorsiflexion cures the clawing if it is still mobile.
2. Loss of ankle plantar flexion. The clawing is noticeable during stance phase, as the long toe flexors try to compensate for loss of ankle plantar flexion power. Restoration of active plantar flexion will eliminate the clawing.
3. Clawing associated with a cavus foot. The prime object is to treat the cavus. Intrinsic weakness is often present.

Clawing of the big toe can be dealt with by transferring the extensor hallucis longus to the neck of the first ray. The interphalangeal joint of the big toe needs to be arthrodesed (Jones 1916).

Clawing of the other toes as a result of the long toe flexors overacting may need a flexor to extensor transfer.

Leg length discrepancy (Macnicol & Catto 1982). This is discussed in Chapter 28.

Spinal deformity

Scoliosis is a common sequel of poliomyelitis (Leong et al 1981, 1990). Kyphosis is relatively rare. Post-poliomyelitic scoliosis is due to imbalance between trunk and intercostal muscles in the growing child. Curvature can be due to asymmetric paralysis of trunk muscles or extensive symmetric paralysis resulting in a collapsing spine. Six types of curves are commonly seen:

1. High thoracic curve. This is extremely unsightly and the prognosis is poor.
2. Thoracic curve. This is usually a long curve associated with an angular rib hump.
3. Lumbar curve. This is usually associated with pelvic obliquity, impaired sitting balance and asymmetric ischial pressure. The hip on the high side subluxates.
4. Double major curve. This is uncommon.
5. Long C curve. The entire trunk is involved, with the apex at the thoraco-lumbar junction.
6. Collapsing spine. The entire trunk sags because of extensive muscle involvement and the effect of gravity. The patient supports himself on the upper limbs, holding onto the bed. Pelvic obliquity may be present.

Indications for surgical treatment

Most moderate to severe curves require surgery. Bracing is poorly tolerated and acts as a passive holding device only. Before surgery, the following should be considered:

Age. The ideal time for surgery is just before the adolescent growth spurt, when most progression is expected. An extensive fusion is usually necessary because of the nature of the curve.

Curve pattern. High thoracic curves need early fusion. The collapsing spine tends to remain flexible, but needs to be fused when flexibility decreases or if upper limb function is grossly impaired and is no longer able to support the trunk. A mild thoracic, thoraco-lumbar, lumbar or double major curve should be treated according to the same principles as idiopathic curves.

Progression. Curves of more than 40–50° that progress despite adequate bracing require surgical correction and fusion.

Pelvic obliquity. Obliquity of more than 30° disturbs sitting balance, and causes hip dislocation and asymmetric ischial pressure. Surgical correction and fusion are indicated.

Method of treatment

Preoperative casting has largely been abandoned because it is uncomfortable and causes further pulmonary dysfunction. The results of spinal surgery in poliomyelitis without internal fixation showed considerable loss of correction at final follow-up and a high pseudoarthrosis rate. Multiple operations were usually required. By contrast, the use of internal fixation has markedly improved correction and maintenance of correction at long-term follow-up. The recent introduction of segmental spinal instrumentation and combined anterior and posterior instrumentation, together with a meticulous spinal fusion, has further improved the results and reduced or made unnecessary the period of postoperative external splintage.

Preoperative halopelvic/femoral traction is very useful in the poliomyelitic spine undergoing corrective surgery, especially when staged anterior and posterior surgery are contemplated. This combined method (O'Brien et al 1975b) is useful for lumbar long C curves, collapsing spines and severe long thoracic curves. Combined anterior and posterior fusion down to the sacrum reduces the chance of pseudoarthrosis. Anterior instrumentation down to L5 provides maximum correction of pelvic obliquity. Curves above 100° or between 80° and 100° with rigidity will benefit from preoperative halopelvic traction. Long C curves, collapsing spines and lumbar curves with pelvic obliquity should be fused to the sacrum.

Operation. The most popular simple posterior instrumentation is still the Harrington system, with or without sublaminar wiring. Segmental spinal instrumentation has become increasingly accepted as a better alternative. Newer systems using multiple hooks/pedicle screws are alternative choices. This can be extended into the ilium if fusion across the lumbo-sacral junction is required. Combined anterior and posterior instrumentation is used in severe curves, especially with severe pelvic obliquity. The anterior Zielke system or modified systems using a stiff rod are often used.

Postoperative care. For fusion extending into the thoracic and cervical areas, postoperative halocast immobilisation is used. Halopelvic immobilisation can also be used postoperatively, but preferably for less than 3–6 months, for fear of cervical complications. The Risser cast is still very useful for thoracic, thoraco-lumbar, lumbar and long curves. Fusion across the lumbo-sacral joint requires a pantaloon cast, immobilising one hip for 3 months. Thereafter, spinal support is continued for a total of 1 year after operation.

REFERENCES

Anonymous 1979 Poliomyelitis in 1977, Notes and News. WHO Chronicle, 33: 63–70

Dennyson W G, Fulford G E 1976 Subtalar arthrodesis by cancellous grafts and metallic internal fixation. Journal of Bone and Joint Surgery 58B: 507–510

Green W T, Grice D S 1952 The management of chronic poliomyelitis. AAOS Instructional Course Lectures 9: 85–90

Jones R 1916 The soldier's foot and the treatment of common deformities of the foot. Part III Claw foot. British Medical Journal 1: 749

Lau J H K, Parker J C, Hsu L C S, Leong J C Y 1986 Paralytic hip instability in poliomyelitis. Journal of Bone and Joint Surgery 68B: 528–533

Leong J C Y, Wilding K, Mok C K, Ma A, Chow S P, Yau A C 1981 Surgical treatment of scoliosis following poliomyelitis. Journal of Bone and Joint Surgery 3A: 726–732

Leong J C Y, Alade C O, Fang D 1982 Supracondylar femoral osteotomy for knee flexion contracture resulting from poliomyelitis. Journal of Bone and Joint Surgery 64B: 198–203

Leong J C Y, Hsu L C S 1990 Poliomyelitis of the spine. In McCollister Evarts C (ed) Surgery of the musculoskeletal system, 2nd edn. Churchill Livingstone, New York, Section 4, 70, pp 2049–2072

Macnicol M F, Catto A M 1982 Twenty-year review of tibial lengthening for poliomyelitis. Journal of Bone and Joint Surgery 64B: 607–610

Mayer L 1956 The physiologic method of tendon transplants. Reviewed after forty years. AAOS Instructional Course Lectures 13: 116–121

Mustard W T 1959 A follow-up study of iliopsoas transfer for hip instability. Journal of Bone and Joint Surgery 41B: 289–293

O'Brien J P, Dwyer A P, Hodgson A R 1975a Paralytic pelvic obliquity. Journal of Bone and Joint Surgery 57A: 626–632

O'Brien J P, Yau A C, Gertzbein S, Hodgson A R 1975b Combined staged anterior and posterior correction and fusion of the spine in scoliosis following poliomyelitis. Clinical Orthopaedics and Related Research 110: 81–111

Rowe C R 1974 Re-evaluation of the position of the arm in arthrodesis of shoulder in the adult. Journal of Bone and Joint Surgery 56A: 913–917

Sabin A B 1965 Oral poliovirus vaccine. History of its development and prospects. Eradication of poliomyelitis. Journal of the American Medical Association 194: 872–881

Saha A K 1967 Surgery of the paralysed and flail shoulder. Acta Orthopaedica Scandinavica Supplement 97: 7–90

Sharrard W J W 1964 Posterior iliopsoas transplantation in the treatment of paralytic dislocation of the hip. Journal of Bone and Joint Surgery 46B: 426–434

Steindler A 1944 Muscle and tendon transplant at the elbow. AAOS Instructional Course Lectures in Reconstructive Surgery 2: 276–282

Tang S C, Leong J C Y, Hsu L C S 1984 Lambrinudi triple arthrodesis for correction of severe rigid drop-foot. Journal of Bone and Joint Surgery 66B: 66–72

Yount C C 1926 The role of the tensor fasciae femoris in certain deformities of the lower extremities. Journal of Bone and Joint Surgery 8: 171–177

Chapter 18

Orthopaedic management of cerebral palsy

J. E. Robb and R. Brunner

DEFINITION

Ingram (1964) has provided a suitable description: 'Cerebral palsy is used as an inclusive term to describe a group of non-progressive disorders occurring in young children in which disease of the brain causes impairment of motor function. Impairment of motor function may be the result of paresis, involuntary movement, or incoordination, but motor dysfunctions which are transient, or are the result of progressive disease of the brain, or attributable to abnormalities of the spinal cord are excluded'. All children with cerebral palsy are 'brain-damaged' and have associated disabilities such as: epilepsy (33%), mental handicap (19–50%), speech disorders (25–80%), behavioural disturbances, specific learning difficulties, or abnormal visual perception (34–58%) (Brown & Minns 1989). Although the neurological damage may be non-progressive, cerebral palsy is certainly a progressive orthopaedic condition that may be influenced by growth, posture or intervention. The condition is rarely manifest at birth, but presents later as developmental delay. As the damage affects the immature brain, symptoms and secondary problems differ significantly from those resulting from brain damage acquired at a later stage.

CLASSIFICATION

This may be:

1. Topographical: hemiplegia, diplegia, and total body involvement (tetraplegia or quadriplegia) or
2. Neurological: spastic, athetoid, ataxic, rigid or mixed.

Classification based on severity is difficult because of the inaccuracy of quantifying the severity of spasticity, athetosis or ataxia. Some children fit into typical patterns, but others do not, and often there is an overlap. The term 'total body involvement' is preferred to 'tetraplegia', as it embraces the concept of impaired head and trunk control.

INCIDENCE

Cerebral palsy occurs in approximately 0.25% of all live births, and in the majority no cause can be identified. It was commonly believed that the disorder resulted from brain asphyxia as a result of problems during labour yet, despite advances in obstetric care, the incidence has remained constant in the past 10 years. The majority of cases do not arise as a result of obstetric problems, and there is a need for

research into the cause of cerebral palsy to focus more on antenatal events (MacLennan 1999). However, the pattern of cerebral palsy has changed, in that there has been a notable decrease in athetosis caused by erythroblastosis fetalis. In a multicentre study that involved approximately 54 000 births, Nelson & Ellenberg (1986) found that only 21% of the 189 children who developed cerebral palsy had any sign of intrapartum asphyxia, and 9% had evidence of asphyxia in the absence of congenital malformation. Maternal mental retardation, a birth weight less than 2 kg and fetal malformation were the leading predictors. Breech presentation was also a predictor, but breech delivery was not. This study showed that a large proportion of the cases of cerebral palsy remain unexplained. Bejar et al (1988) observed periventricular leucomalacia (multifocal necrosis of the white matter) on echo encephalography *in utero*. Their study suggested that there were prenatal antecedents of cerebral palsy, rather than intrapartum and postnatal factors.

PATHOLOGY

Knowledge of the underlying pathology and its consequences is essential for subsequent management. The areas of the brain that control movement are the motor cortex, basal ganglia and cerebellum; spastic cerebral palsy is therefore the result of cerebral cortical damage, dyskinesia from basal ganglia damage, and ataxia from abnormalities of the cerebellum (Brown & Minns 1989). This usually produces a mixed picture of lack of co-ordination, muscle weakness and spasticity. Inappropriate timing of muscle activity results in non-physiological co-contraction, functional weakness and inappropriate tone. It is important to distinguish between spasticity, which is an increasing muscle contraction in response to stretch (Sherrington 1947) and can be abolished by posterior root section, and rigidity, which is not affected by posterior root section. There are two clinical types of spasticity: phasic and tonic. In phasic spasticity, the muscle does not produce a permanent contracture, whereas the tonic system is adapted to postural control and the muscle always resists stretching. This can induce shortening of the muscle and a joint contracture. In rigidity, there is an involuntary sustained contraction of the muscle, which is neither dependent on a stretch being applied to the muscle nor abolished by posterior root section. A clinical example of this is dystonic cerebral palsy, which may be flexor or extensor. In clinical practice, one sees 'dynamic deformities' and an associated full range of movement under general anaesthesia or during slow and gentle examination.

Weakness occurs in cerebral palsy and may arise from brain damage. Reciprocal innervation of joint agonist and antagonist muscle groups provides a mechanism whereby one group relaxes while the other contracts; if only one group is weakened, a secondary and worse deformity may be produced by the unopposed action of the antagonist. Grading by the Medical Research Council scale of strength in cerebral palsy is difficult, for the above reasons.

The brain develops despite the damage, and uses strategies that compensate for the deficits and to optimise function. Brain performance can be improved by retraining motor skills. The peripheral expression of the underlying central damage often changes as the patients grow; compensatory mechanisms may, at first, be advantageous, but may later result in secondary deformities. During growth, muscle has to keep pace with skeletal lengthening. In spastic paralysis there is relative shortening of the musculotendinous unit during growth, and often little stretching of muscle during daily activities. Ziv et al (1984) have shown experimentally that muscle adds sarcomeres in response to constant stretch, but that when muscles are spastic this mechanism does not occur. Tardieu et al (1988) believe that the major factor causing contracture is the maintenance of the muscle in a shortened position, either passively or by sustained contraction. Deformity in cerebral palsy arises in several ways: as a result of brain damage, as an aberration of growth, and as a result of positional deformity. Compensatory mechanisms may produce deformity that can also result from clinical management.

Deformities in cerebral palsy are mobile or fixed, and result from disorganised posture, balance and movement. Developmental delays cause retarded motor skills and the persistence of infantile reactions. Delay in acquiring motor skills means that these appear later than normal and may be fewer than those found in the normal child. There may also be variations and abnormal patterns in the motor skills that are subsequently acquired. It should not be forgotten that there may be other reasons for motor delay, such as visual handicap or learning difficulties. Immobility may be a result of multiple handicaps, blindness and learning difficulties (Levitt 1995). Postural mechanisms are an intrinsic part of motor skills and are linked to voluntary movement mechanisms. If equilibrium is insufficient, a child may not be able to initiate movement, even though voluntary movement is possible. Retarded postural mechanisms may lead to loss of trunk and head control. Abnormal reflexes may manifest as automatic stepping or the asymmetric tonic neck reflex, and recurring stimulation of abnormal reflexes may result in deformity. Abnormal postures may result from deformities as muscles shorten, or as a compensation to maintain equilibrium or its loss; they may also result from asymmetry of muscle function, or from limb length inequality. Spasticity may also be used as a compensation, and the child relies upon this to stand erect. Established contractures of one joint can have a subsequent effect on other joints – for example a hip flexion contracture will cause the knee to flex on the affected side. It should also be remembered that isolated muscle groups are not spastic, but there is co-contraction of agonists and antagonists at any given joint, and it is usually the effect of the weaker antagonist that results in the deformity. This can be seen at the hip, where inadequate control of muscle forces causes joint subluxation or dislocation, and the acetabulum then fails to develop normally.

Cerebral palsy is not a purely motor disorder. Sensory changes might reasonably be expected, but these changes are not easily assessed by simple bedside tests and, if present, do not always correlate with the motor deficit.

PHYSICAL ASSESSMENT

STATIC EXAMINATION

The patient is assessed supine on a couch, which can be replaced by mother's lap in the case of young children. The patient is positioned with the pelvis at the end of the couch and the legs are not supported; this position allows assessment of the range of motion of all joints of the lower extremities without moving the patient. Alternatively, a prone position can be used. The child can then be brought into the sitting position to observe head control, spinal deformity and pelvic obliquity. In a walking child, the upper limbs are examined while the child sits. The assessment should include passive and active movements of the shoulder, elbow, wrist and hand. Stance and gait should be observed in a walker when appropriately undressed. Co-ordination and balance can be assessed simply by asking the child to stand or hop on one leg.

Thomas's test is descriptive enough for clinical purposes, but is less accurate than measuring hip flexion contractures in the prone position as described by Staheli (1977) (Fig. 18.1). The patient is placed so that the pelvis lies off the examining table, and the examiner places one hand on the posterior superior spines while the hip under examination is

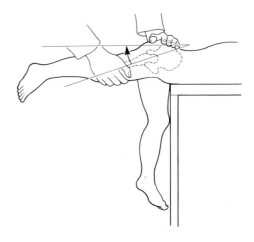

Fig. 18.1 Staheli hip extension test.

extended. The point of contracture is when the pelvis begins to tilt. Whilst the child is supine, internal and external rotation and abduction and adduction can be measured. These are assessed with the hips in extension for a walker and with the hips in flexion for a non-walker, as these are the positions of function in these two circumstances. When assessing abduction and adduction, it is essential to observe and palpate the anterior superior spines, to get an accurate assessment of the amount of abduction. If the spines are not visualised and felt, it is possible to show a 'satisfactory' range of abduction when, in reality, there may be only 5° or 10° of abduction on one side and 30–40° on the opposite side.

The knee is assessed for range of movement and a capsular contracture. Straight leg-raising assesses hamstring spasticity and contracture (Fig. 18.2). An alternative is to use the popliteal angle, which is found by flexing the hip to a right angle and extending the knee to the point of resistance. The angle lies between the extended position of the knee and the tibia at the point of resistance (Fig. 18.3). It is important that the pelvis does not tilt during either of the hamstring tests; if the patient is a walker, the straight leg-raise test probably gives a better indication of functional hamstring length than does the popliteal angle.

The range of dorsiflexion of the ankle is measured with the heel held in inversion; this stabilises the talo-navicular joint and prevents lateral bow-stringing of the tendo-Achilles when the heel is valgus (producing a pseudocorrection). By holding the foot in varus, dorsiflexion of the mid-tarsal joints is prevented. In a varus deformity, however, the heel has to be kept in valgus. Traditionally, Silverskiöld's test is used to differentiate between contracture of the gastrocnemius and soleus. The knee is flexed to 90° and the foot dorsiflexed in inversion as far as possible, and an assessment is made of the foot–shank angle. This is then repeated with the knee fully extended. An unchanged range of ankle dorsiflexion suggests a soleal contracture. Subtalar and mid-tarsal movements can then be assessed, along with toe deformities.

The patient is then moved up the couch and lies prone. Femoral anteversion is determined by palpation of the greater trochanter at its maximally prominent site and by

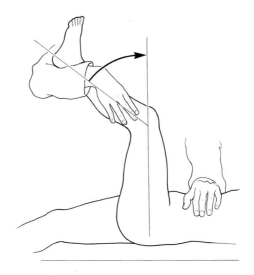

Figure 18.3 Popliteal angle.

measuring the angle between the tibia and the vertical (Ruwe et al 1992). The thigh–foot angle (Staheli & Engel 1972) is then assessed, giving a measurement of tibial torsion. The knee is flexed to 90° and the ankle is dorsiflexed into neutral, but without everting or inverting the foot. The relationship of the heel to the thigh is assessed visually or with a goniometer. The thigh–foot angle is invalid after hindfoot surgery. The examination so far will determine torsions between the femoral shaft and the calcaneum, although rotation may be within the foot itself. Because most patients have a mobile hindfoot, it may be more accurate to assess tibial torsion by measuring the angle between the transmalleolar axis and the femoral condyles. The knee must be flexed to 90° for this measurement.

Traditional stretch tests are inaccurate in cerebral palsy and have limited specificity. The Duncan Ely test (rectus stretch test) also generates action potentials in ilio-psoas (Perry et al 1976) and the Thomas test generates similar electrical activity in the rectus femoris and ilio-psoas. Phelp's (gracilis) test and straight leg-raising induce the same amount of electrical activity in the medial hamstrings. The specificity of Silverskiöld's test has been questioned by Perry et al (1974) because, on the electromyogram (EMG), both gastrocnemius and soleus showed increased action potentials, irrespective of the position of the knee.

EVALUATION OF GAIT

Walking is an extremely complex activity, and it is essential to have an appreciation of the events that occur during normal walking before one can understand aberrations of gait. Events occur in the coronal, sagittal, and transverse planes in reciprocating gait. Descriptions of the gait cycle have been traditionally made in the sagittal plane. The goals of gait are sufficient stability, and progression. The prerequisites are stance phase stability, swing phase clearance, lower extremity preposition in terminal swing, a positive step

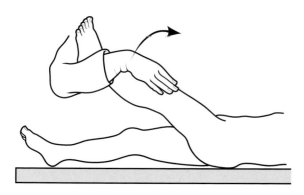

Figure 18.2 Straight leg-raising to assess hamstring length.

length and energy conservation (Gage 1991). The upper body must be supported in both double and single support, and may be challenged by two factors: first by body weight, and second by the alterations of the body segments during walking.

Smooth progression depends upon the maintenance of forward velocity, clearance of the leg in swing and absorption of energy before and at foot contact. During single support, there are two main progressional forces: first, there is the input of energy to stabilise the lower limb and to assist the upward and forward motion of the hip and upper body; this is then followed by a controlled and downward fall of the body from a high point and represents the conversion of potential to kinetic energy, assisted by gravity. The gait cycle is divided into swing and stance phases (Fig. 18.4). Stance is divided into two periods of double support and one of single support (Fig. 18.5). The first period of double support occurs from foot contact to opposite foot-off, and is known as the loading response. Single support occupies about 40% of the cycle, while the opposite leg is in its swing phase. During the phase of single support, the pelvis rises and falls and single support may be divided into two phases, mid-stance and terminal stance. Pelvic high point (Hullin & Robb 1991) corresponds to the point of reversal of fore–aft forces as determined by Sutherland (1984) and can be used to differentiate between mid- and terminal stance. The second period of double support occurs from opposite foot contact to foot-off. In the swing phase, the hip rises and falls, and also represents two important biomechanical phases. The hip rises to allow clearance of the foot and then falls to allow foot contact. Swing can then be divided into initial swing, mid-swing and terminal swing.

Visual observation of gait is used traditionally to assess aberrations in walking patterns. In practice, it is difficult to perform this accurately when there are abnormalities at several anatomical levels: trunk, pelvis, hip, knee, ankle and foot, and in three planes. The resolution in time, however, is not good enough to assess fast movements, as the human eye can only fix on one point at a time. The analysis of complex problems requires knowledge of the position of several joints simultaneously, at any given time. A sagittal and coronal video recording is a cheap and effective tool

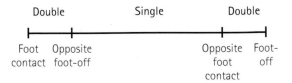

Figure 18.5 Stance phase of gait is divided into two periods of double support or stance and one period of single support or stance.

and will show most of the problems. The recording can be stopped at, for example, heel contact, mid-stance and push-off for both legs. Joint positions can be assessed at these points. However, although video is very helpful for clinical purposes, it does not provide scientifically useful data and the estimation of joint angles is inaccurate, particularly when there are rotational deformities in the limbs.

More detailed and scientifically valuable data can be obtained from semi-automatic systems that measure the kinematics of the legs and, in some systems, the entire body. Kinematics are measurements used to describe the spatial movement of the body; they include linear and angular displacements, velocities and accelerations. If the ground reaction force is measured simultaneously using three-dimensional force plates, the kinetics at the different joint levels can be calculated from inverse dynamics. Kinetics are measurements used to describe the mechanisms that cause movement; these include ground reactions, joint moments and joint powers. These procedures, however, calculate only the resultant external forces and moments acting on the locomotor system. These moments need to be counteracted by an internal moment of the same value but opposite sign to maintain stability. The internal (body) moment counteracting the external moment may arise from muscle activity and the actions of the soft tissues such as ligaments, which are supported by the skeleton. It is also possible to calculate joint powers that can show the generation or absorption of energy. An EMG recorded simultaneously provides information about muscle control. The superficial muscles can easily be assessed with superficial electrodes, whereas the deep muscles such as the tibialis posterior require fine wire electrodes. The assessment of muscle activity can help to determine the source of the internally generated forces and moments. However, EMG activity does not correlate with muscle force, and the abnormal timing of muscle stimulation may result from altered use of the lower extremity. Another approach is to measure energy consumption during walking; several methods are available – for example, tests using heart rate or oxygen consumption before and after exercise.

Knowledge of normal kinetics, kinematics and muscle contraction is helpful to determine gait abnormalities. Muscles work in one of three ways. *Concentric* contraction results in muscle shortening; accelerators work in this way. *Eccentric* or lengthening contraction results in deceleration; an example of this is the action of the hamstrings in decelerating the shank in terminal swing. *Isometric* contraction

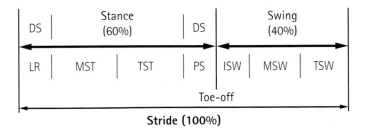

Figure 18.4 The gait cycle. DS, double support; LR, loading response; MST, mid-stance; TST, terminal stance; PS, pre-swing; ISW, initial swing; MSW, mid-swing; TSW, terminal swing; IC, initial contact.

produces a stabilising action and is seen in the postural and antigravity muscles, for example the gluteus medius. Normal ankle kinematics are characterised by an initial plantar flexion (first rocker) controlled by the tibialis anterior and toe extensor muscles, followed by a phase of dorsiflexion. At this time, the triceps surae muscle is first eccentrically and then concentrically active, and controls the position of the shank with respect to the floor. As a result, the tibia is held back while the centre of gravity is advancing, which results in knee extension without the need of knee extensor activity. This period is termed 'second rocker'. At terminal swing, the concentric action of the triceps surae together with the flexor hallucis muscles pushes the leg off and accelerates it, together with the hip flexors, into swing. Third rocker occurs as the foot rotates over the metatarsal heads (Fig. 18.6). In early swing the foot position, which is almost plantigrade, allows the foot to clear the ground and to prepare for loading at the next initial contact. The knee is almost extended at heel strike, then flexes slightly whilst being controlled by the knee extensors. The subsequent knee extension is mainly passive, as the ground reaction force has passed in front of the knee joint centre. The extensor moment stabilises the knee in extension. At push-off, the knee extensors act again to control the knee and to flex the hip through the rectus femoris. The hip joint is externally rotated, abducted and flexed at initial contact and becomes adducted, internally rotated and slightly hyperextended during stance phase. Initially, the adductors and extensors are active to stabilise the hip, and in terminal stance the extensors are active again to accelerate the body. During swing phase, the hip joint movement is inverse and largely controlled by the hip flexors. At mid-swing, however, there is almost no muscle activity.

The ground reaction force is assessed in three dimensions. In the *vertical* direction, a peak at foot strike is followed by a first maximum (120% body weight) indicating the braking force to control the falling centre of gravity. The knee becomes extended and the centre of gravity is pushed up and is shown as a reduction in the vertical force to 80% body weight. The centre of gravity falls again and is accelerated to load the opposite leg, which is reflected by another increase in the vertical force. In the direction of gait (*fore–aft* force), the force is first negative, indicating braking of the limb, then becomes zero at mid-stance, and finally becomes positive during acceleration. While an individual is walking at a self-selected constant speed, the braking force and acceleration reach equal absolute values. The forces in the frontal plane are directed medially at initial contact because, as the leg is being circumducted physiologically, it is decelerated whilst moving from lateral to medial. The leg is then positioned lateral to the ground reaction force, which results in a *laterally* directed force component. At push-off, the force turns medially again because the leg, acting as a pendulum, needs to be accelerated slightly laterally to initiate physiological circumduction. An example of pre- and postoperative data from a diplegic patient is shown in Fig. 18.7.

Gait analysis has become an important investigative tool in cerebral palsy, and in some centres is regarded as essential before surgery. It certainly provides a means of objective audit after intervention, but not all surgeons have access to this complex type of investigation. Gait is only one aspect of function, and should not be viewed in isolation.

Although ungainly, abnormal walking patterns may represent the most efficient method of progression for the child and result from a variety of factors. The walking pattern may be a compensation for deficient control of equilibrium, joint contracture or muscle spasticity. Many children with cerebral palsy are effectively in a state of 'collapse', and cannot support their body weight on one leg so that they walk rapidly to avoid falling over. The common pattern in hemiplegia and diplegia is internal rotation, flexion and adduction of the hip (Fig. 18.8). There may also be flexion of the knee and an equinus posture of the ankle. The knee may extend fully passively, but may tend to lie in valgus when walking, although there may not be a fixed valgus deformity. Secondary deformities may ensue, such as external tibial torsion below excessive internal femoral torsion. A valgus calcaneum and pes valgus are common associated deformities.

PRINCIPLES AND AIMS OF MANAGEMENT

In general, the shape of the locomotor system depends upon function, which depends, in turn, upon activity. This explains why a joint can lose motion if its range is not used. One aim of management of patients with cerebral palsy therefore involves control of posture and daily activities, during which the available range of joint movement and muscle length should be used. Training is an important aspect of physical therapy, optimising muscle strength and central nervous system function (Lin et al 1999).

It is important to distinguish between disturbances of function that are due to the underlying condition, useful adaptations (which may look abnormal), and functional difficulties secondary to deformity. The advantages and disadvantages of any given intervention need to be considered.

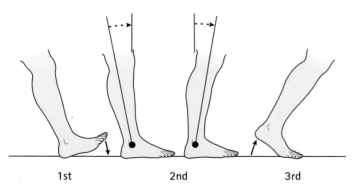

Figure 18.6 Rocker sequence in stance. (Adapted from Gage 1991.)

1st   2nd   3rd

The Anderson Gait Analysis Laboratory
Rehabilitation Engineering Services, Edinburgh
Sagittal Plane

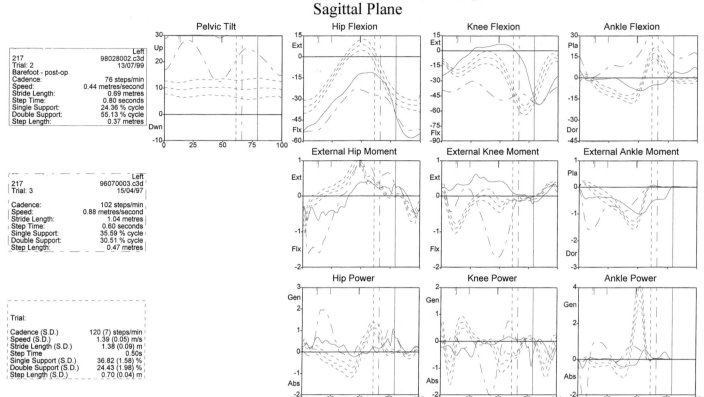

Left	
217	98028002.c3d
Trial: 2	13/07/99
Barefoot - post-op	
Cadence:	76 steps/min
Speed:	0.44 metres/second
Stride Length:	0.69 metres
Step Time:	0.80 seconds
Single Support:	24.36 % cycle
Double Support:	55.13 % cycle
Step Length:	0.37 metres

Left	
217	96070003.c3d
Trial: 3	15/04/97
Cadence:	102 steps/min
Speed:	0.88 metres/second
Stride Length:	1.04 metres
Step Time:	0.60 seconds
Single Support:	35.59 % cycle
Double Support:	30.51 % cycle
Step Length:	0.47 metres

Trial:	
Cadence (S.D.)	120 (7) steps/min
Speed (S.D.)	1.39 (0.05) m/s
Stride Length (S.D.)	1.38 (0.09) m
Step Time	0.50s
Single Support (S.D.)	36.82 (1.58) %
Double Support (S.D.)	24.43 (1.98) %
Step Length (S.D.)	0.70 (0.04) m

The Anderson Gait Analysis Laboratory
Rehabilitation Engineering Services, Edinburgh
Coronal Plane

Left	
217	98028002.c3d
Trial: 2	13/07/99
Barefoot - post-op	
Cadence:	76 steps/min
Speed:	0.44 metres/second
Stride Length:	0.69 metres
Step Time:	0.80 seconds
Single Support:	24.36 % cycle
Double Support:	55.13 % cycle
Step Length:	0.37 metres

Left	
217	96070003.c3d
Trial: 3	15/04/97
Cadence:	102 steps/min
Speed:	0.88 metres/second
Stride Length:	1.04 metres
Step Time:	0.60 seconds
Single Support:	35.59 % cycle
Double Support:	30.51 % cycle
Step Length:	0.47 metres

Trial:	
Cadence (S.D.)	120 (7) steps/min
Speed (S.D.)	1.39 (0.05) m/s
Stride Length (S.D.)	1.38 (0.09) m
Step Time	0.50s
Single Support (S.D.)	36.82 (1.58) %
Double Support (S.D.)	24.43 (1.98) %
Step Length (S.D.)	0.70(0.04) m

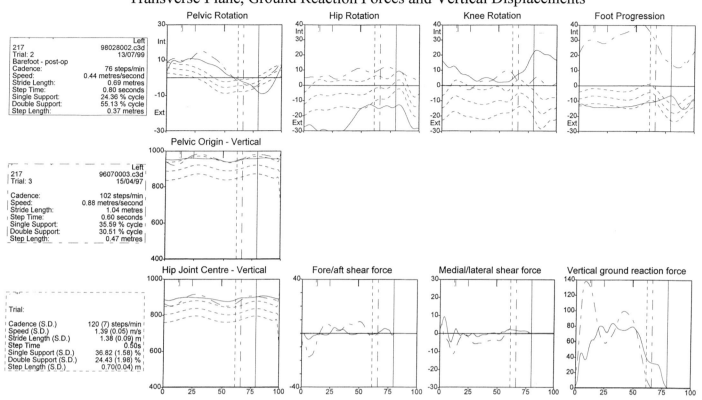

The Anderson Gait Analysis Laboratory
Rehabilitation Engineering Services, Edinburgh
Transverse Plane, Ground Reaction Forces and Vertical Displacements

Figure 18.7 Gait data for the left leg of a 15-year-old diplegic patient who underwent bilateral femoral derotation osteotomies, bilateral intramuscular hamstring lengthenings and bilateral intramuscular gastrocnemius lengthenings. The plots show preoperative data as long and short dashed lines (– - — -), 1 year postoperative data as solid lines, and normal values ± 1 standard deviation as dashed lines (- - - -).

For example, standing with the knees bent places a load on the quadriceps, which is tiring. Straightening the knees can solve this stance phase problem for the patient, but could cause difficulties in the swing phase of gait.

Dynamic instability, or lever arm dysfunction, is a major factor interfering with function and can result in bony deformity and joint dislocations. Joints can be stabilised with orthoses or by arthrodesis; however, absolute stability at a given joint may be a disadvantage in the longer term and can remove some compensatory movement for a deformity at a more proximal level. For example, external rotation in the foot can be a compensation for excessive femoral anteversion. Stabilising the foot and ankle with an orthosis or the subtalar joint by a fusion may remove this compensation at the foot and exacerbate the internal hip rotation.

Some patients with cerebral palsy appear to have strong muscles, but spasticity will often mask an underlying muscle weakness. The imbalance of muscle actions across a joint may be managed by lengthening or weakening the agonist to restore the imbalance. Force and length are related to each other physiologically; lengthening is used to gain length or to reduce muscle force. Muscle tension may decrease after tendon transfers and a reduction of force occurs as a secondary event. Thus reduction of muscle force is a regular consequence of non-operative and operative management. The effect is transient after casting, or aponeurotic (intramuscular) lengthening (Brunner 1998, Jaspers et al 2000), and longer lasting after tendon lengthening (Tardieu et al 1979, Brunner 1998, Bassett et al 1999, Jaspers et al 2000). Force reduction may give the impression of being advantageous, because spasticity seems to be reduced. In reality, however, the output from the central nervous system remains unchanged, but spasticity may be less noticeable because of a decrease in muscle force. The advantage of reducing spasticity may be counteracted by the disadvantage of muscle weakness for postural control and function. Hence, muscle force training may help to improve function, despite concerns about possibly increasing spasticity. The aims of management have to take into account the overall function of the patient and the presence of deformity does not necessarily suggest that its correction is essential.

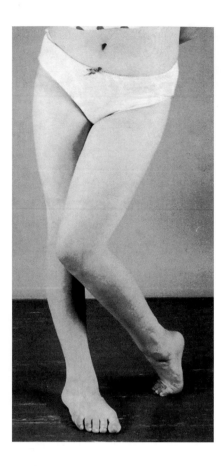

Figure 18.8 Typical posture of adduction and internal rotation at the hip, and flexion of the knee and ankle.

ORTHOTIC MANAGEMENT

THE LOWER LIMB

Orthoses may be prescribed for several reasons: first to maintain posture, second to prevent deformity, and third to obtain a biomechanical effect. A secondary effect may be to compensate for missing muscle activity and strength. The orthoses can be used as aids during walking or as positional devices at night.

Ankle–foot orthoses may be indicated for children with cerebral palsy as part of non-operative and postoperative management. They may be used for walkers and non-walkers. The manufacture of an orthosis depends upon an accurate 'positive plaster' cast of the child's foot and calf, from which a light-weight thermoplastic splint is manufactured. Apart from static function, such as preventing deformity and maintaining posture, the orthosis can be used to alter the biomechanical forces acting on joints. Two clinical examples are illustrated in Figs 18.9 and 18.10. In the first (Fig. 18.9), the child walks with a crouch gait (flexed hips and knees, and excessive ankle dorsiflexion) and has a passive full range of knee extension. In the second (Fig. 18.10), the patient walks with knee hyperextension. An ankle–foot orthosis can be applied in such a way as to correct both of these problems.

When the foot is applied to the ground, an equal and opposite ground reaction force is generated in response to this load (Newton's third law). The ground reaction force has magnitude in three directions and can be measured with a force plate which is akin to bathroom scales. Knowledge of the orientation of the vertical component of the ground reaction force to any given joint, which may be either flexor or extensor, is helpful when changing an orthotic prescription. In the case of the child with crouch gait, in whom the vertical component of the ground reaction force is flexor in relation to the knee, the goal is to change the direction of the ground reaction force to pass through the knee joint. During normal walking there is a smooth progression of the ground reaction force origin from the heel, at foot contact, to the metatarsal heads at foot-off. In the case of crouch gait, the origin of the ground reaction force rests at the heel throughout stance, and forward progression of the upper body over the stationary foot occurs by an excessive amount of tibial progression in relation to the foot, resulting in knee flexion. By means of an ankle–foot orthosis, excessive tibial progression in relation to the foot is prevented (Fig. 18.9) (Hullin et al 1992). This then reorientates the vertical component of the ground reaction force so that it passes through or near to the axis of the knee, and thus the patient walks with a more upright posture. If the orthosis is set in neutral or in plantar flexion, knee hyperextension may result. This is illustrated in Fig. 18.10. Here, the forward progression of the tibia over the stationary foot is prevented by the orthosis, but, if the gastrocnemius and knee flexors are not tight, the femur may continue to progress over the stationary foot, resulting in knee hyperextension, because the ground reaction force passes in front of the knee. In this case there are two solutions: either to readjust the foot–shank angle of the ankle–foot orthosis so that it lies in some dorsiflexion, or to apply a rocker that permits a smoother progression of the ground reaction force along the foot (Fig. 18.11). Ankle–foot orthoses are powerful tools, not just pieces of plastic. They can have dramatic and reversible

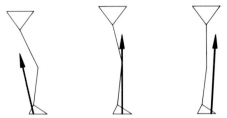

Figure 18.9 Effect of ankle–foot orthosis on crouch gait.

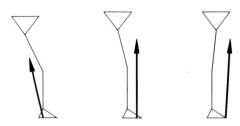

Figure 18.10 Knee hyperextension in ankle–foot orthosis.

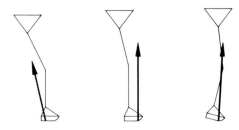

Figure 18.11 Hyperextension prevented by rocker sole.

effects upon the biomechanics of gait and standing posture, and are usually worn inside the shoe. Shoes always have a slight heel raise, so this should be taken into account when considering the angle between the foot and the shank of the ankle–foot orthosis.

Orthoses can be used to modify different phases of the gait cycle. The goal of foot contact is to bring the heel down first on the ground, and an orthosis can be used here to control a drop foot, to permit heel contact rather than toe contact with the ground, or to control varus or valgus alignment of the foot. An analogy is an aircraft landing on its main wheels, not on the nose wheel. During the loading response, the orthosis can substitute for pre-tibial muscle function and prevent excessive inversion or eversion, and an orthotic modification for this phase would be the provision of a solid ankle cushion heel. The aircraft analogy in this case would be to prevent the wheels buckling on landing.

During the first phase of single support, the goal is tibial progression over the stationary foot and control of the ground reaction force in relation to the hip and knee. Here, excessive tibial progression can be prevented by the use of an ankle–foot orthosis or a floor reaction orthosis. Rockers may also allow a smoother progression of the foot along the floor. In terminal stance, the goal is to provide acceleration of the limb before pre-swing. There is no orthotic solution for problems in this phase of the gait cycle at present. In cerebral palsy, the main use of the ankle–foot orthosis is to control or substitute for tibialis anterior and gastrocnemius and soleus activity. In swing, the prerequisites are limb clearance and step length, and in this phase the orthosis will compensate for a foot drop and preposition the foot in terminal swing.

Orthoses should not interfere with knee motion. In the walker, these various demands can be achieved using mobile flexible orthoses with a plantar flexion stop, as they have been shown to improve gait more than the stiffer ankle–foot orthoses (Brunner et al 1998). Resting orthoses may be used at night, to minimise future deformity or to stretch contracted muscles; however, stretching is an uncomfortable sensation and can interfere with sleep, with the result that resting orthoses are often poorly tolerated at night.

A knee–ankle–foot orthosis may be indicated to stretch short hamstrings. It is applied during rest (but not at night) under full tension for 1–2 hours at a time. It can also be used

postoperatively, and has the advantage over plaster of being detachable, preventing potential complications of plaster such as neurological compromise or skin pressure problems.

Underarm orthoses are helpful in controlling upper body posture in the profoundly handicapped child. They can be a useful adjunct for head and upper extremity control during feeding. They do not influence the natural history of spinal deformity in cerebral palsy.

THE UPPER LIMB

Indications for upper limb orthoses are rare; however, there are two groups of patients who may benefit. Spasticity of the wrist flexors turns the hand out of the patient's field of vision, which makes hand function difficult. This can be improved by the application of a splint to stabilise the wrist. An alternative would be a Green transfer of the flexor carpi ulnaris to the extensor carpi radialis brevis for a dynamic deformity. The other group of patients present with progressive flexion deformities of the fingers and wrist, which interferes with hygiene. These muscles often respond well to stretching by a splint worn during the day, and the splint needs to be re-adjusted regularly to maintain the range of motion gained. Splintage for the elbow and shoulder is difficult and usually ineffective.

PHARMACOLOGICAL MANAGEMENT

Excessive muscle tone in cerebral palsy is amenable to reduction by pharmacological means.

INTRATHECAL BACLOFEN

Baclofen has been used orally for the reduction of muscle tone for many years, but the side effects of drowsiness and drooling limit its oral use. Baclofen has poor lipid solubility and, if injected intrathecally, allows the use of much smaller doses than those required orally. Its site of action is believed to be on γ-amino butyric acid receptors (preventing the release of excitatory neurotransmitters) and on polysynaptic pathways (antagonising the actions of glutamate and glycine). There is increasing interest in its use in spastic cerebral palsy (Albright et al 1993, Armstrong et al 1997) and dystonic cerebral palsy (Albright et al 1998). The ideal patient is one with diplegia without contractures, but the method is also effective in those with hemiplegia and tetraplegia.

The advantage of the drug over rhizotomy is that intrathecal baclofen is reversible but the disadvantages are the danger of infection and the need to implant a relatively bulky pump subcutaneously in the anterior abdominal wall of a child who may be cachectic (Armstrong et al 1997). The pump can be programmed to vary the amount of baclofen given intrathecally over 24 hours. Albright (1996) reported complications in almost 20% of children leading to removal of the system in 5%. The procedure has been reported as reducing the need for lower extremity orthopaedic surgery in patients with spastic cerebral palsy (Gerszten et al 1998), and the authors recommended that spasticity be managed first before orthopaedic surgery. There is definite potential benefit from intrathecal baclofen in cerebral palsy, but the procedure does have significant complications. More experience from centres who have not pioneered the technique is required to define the longer-term benefits of the procedure.

BOTULINUM TOXIN A

This drug has gained increasing importance in the management of spastic muscles. The toxin irreversibly blocks release of acetylcholine at the neuromuscular junction, leading to a flaccid paralysis of the muscle. Nevertheless, muscle activity recovers in 2–3 months, without any loss, by forming new endplates. The drug is injected into the target muscle, which then becomes temporarily paralysed. Cosgrove & Graham (1994) reported a beneficial effect on muscle growth in spastic mice. Botulinum toxin A has been introduced for the management of spastic muscles in cerebral palsy and good functional results have been reported for tone-related problems in gait (Koman et al 1994, Garcia et al 1996). The target muscles need to be defined biomechanically; gait analysis is helpful for this (Thompson et al 1998). Botulinum toxin A may also postpone the need for surgery and its effects last for about 2–3 months, or even longer. Muscle lengthening is another indication for its use. The paralysed muscle can be stretched more efficiently, and the method is reported to be as effective as casting (Corry et al 1998). The best effects from botulinum toxin are seen in the lower extremity in the younger child who does not have any muscle shortening.

SURGERY

Orthopaedic surgeons should be clear about what can and cannot be corrected by surgery. Excessive tone, muscle imbalance, contractures and bony deformity are amenable to surgery. Bony deformities and contractures are typical indications for orthopaedic intervention. Muscle balancing procedures, however, can be undertaken for an imbalance of strength or length. Muscle force will be reduced after surgery, which is not always beneficial for the patient. Tone reduction may be achieved surgically by rhizotomy, in addition to pharmacological correction with botulinum toxin and baclofen. There is no surgical solution for hypotonia, which is also seen in cerebral palsy. However, the fundamental injury to the central nervous system, namely loss of selective control and persistent reflex activity, is incurable.

Surgery affords a means of influencing spastic muscle activity. Tardieu et al (1979) have shown that tendon lengthening results in a persistent loss of muscle force. Hence spastic muscle force and activity can be reduced despite there being no change in the central nervous system. It has recently been reported that the frequency of electromyographic potentials was reduced after casting and tendon lengthening, both of which decrease muscle force (Lin et al 1999). In contrast, muscle force is reduced temporarily after intramuscular tendon or aponeurotic lengthening procedures (Brunner 1998).

Orthopaedic operations may also be directed towards muscle or tendon lengthening (Fig. 18.12), tendon transfers, tenotomy, bony operations to improve rotational problems or to relocate joints, and neurectomy. Soft-tissue surgery alone will not correct a fixed skeletal deformity. There is a trend now to perform surgery in one stage where possible, and operations in the mobile child can be designed for both the swing and stance phase problems. In the presence of mobile deformity, the surgeon should think of balancing procedures around joints, whereas rotational and fixed bony deformities require bony surgery.

There are two important steps in assessing a patient for surgery: clinical examination and assessment of gait, where appropriate. A slow and gentle examination technique is necessary to distinguish between tone and contracture, and the findings will reflect the situation in daily life. Confirmation of the physical findings should be carried out under anaesthesia on the day of surgery.

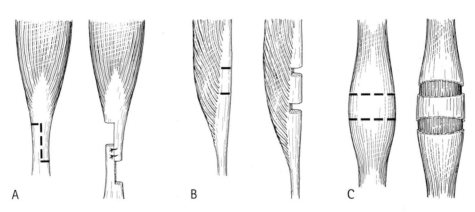

Figure 18.12 Techniques of musculotendinous lengthening: (**A**) Z-lengthening, (**B**) intramuscular tendon lengthening and (**C**) aponeurotomy.

SELECTIVE POSTERIOR RHIZOTOMY

This has been popularised by Peacock et al (1987). Its objective is to obtain a better balance between facilitatory and inhibitory control of the anterior horn cells. They have reported encouraging data in predominantly spastic diplegic patients in whom spasticity of muscle was reduced even to the point of flaccidity. The procedure entails selective sectioning of approximately 25–50% of the L2–S1 nerve rootlets that demonstrate abnormal responses to electrical stimulation at the time of surgery. This does not abolish primitive motor reflexes or fixed contractures of musculo-tendinous units or joints.

The ideal patient for rhizotomy is a walking spastic diplegic who has minimal fixed contractures, but the approach may also be helpful for the non-walker with total body involvement. Other favourable criteria include prematurity, pure spasticity, good trunk control and strength, minimal contractures, motivation and the availability of physiotherapy. Poor indicators are hemiplegia, weakness of antigravity muscles, rigidity, dystonia, athetosis, marked flexion contractures and fixed spinal deformity (Oppenheim 1990). One concern after rhizotomy is the possibility of producing later spinal deformity, which could result from postoperative hypotonia and the laminectomy (Crawford et al 1996). Greene et al (1991) reported rapid progression of hip subluxation in six patients during the year after selective dorsal rhizotomy, which can be explained by reducing sensory input from the joint, necessary for dynamic control. Normally the L1 root is preserved, so the hip flexors may not be as denervated as their antagonists, thus predisposing to dysplasia. Further information and postoperative evaluation over a longer period are necessary to define the place of rhizotomy in the management of cerebral palsy.

SURGERY FOR THE NON-WALKER

It can be very difficult to assess functional ability in the presence of severe impairment, and often the clinician has to rely on the parents, carers or therapist for further information. This information, however, is important for any decision, because the state of the patient at a clinic visit may be very different from usual. One problem in this respect is pain, which may not be a constant feature and hence could be missed during an assessment. For example, assessment of 'hip' pain in the patient with total body involvement can be difficult, as gastrointestinal pain can present as pain in the 'hip' region.

Severe handicap should not rule out treatment. The major cause for restricted function in severely affected patients is the lack of co-ordination and adequate muscle control. One of the major goals for a non-walker is to acquire the ability to transfer either independently or with a helper. Any intervention that may interfere with lower extremity joint stability – for example proximal femoral resection for hip dislocation – may be disadvantageous for this type of patient. Management of severe secondary deformities should not affect existing function either. The goals in this group are different from those in walking patients, and mostly orientated towards pain-free existence, balanced seating, or, if the patient is capable of transfers, to render the feet plantigrade and to reduce knee flexion and hip flexion contractures. Adduction deformities of the hip can be particularly troublesome for seating and nappy changing (Fig. 18.13).

Spinal deformities

The cause of spinal deformity is the lack of dynamic muscle control to counteract the deforming forces resulting from gravity. The greater the deformity, the greater the lever arm of the deforming force and the faster the progression. For this reason, management needs to start early, provided the spinal deformity is not fixed. Under-arm braces of various types can be applied to stabilise the trunk in an upright position, with as little residual deformity as possible. Adapted seating is often less efficient than an under-arm brace, and should not be used as an initial corrective device. Some spinal mobility is possible when using an under-arm brace,

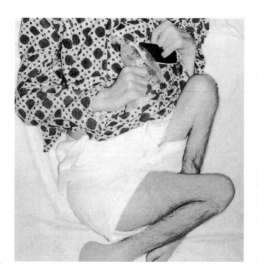
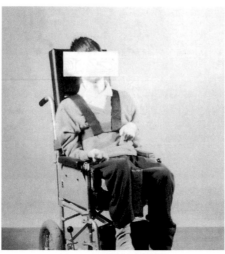

Figure 18.13 Before and after surgical soft-tissue releases for seating.

and this can help to compensate for insufficient hip flexion in sitting, or stiff hips when transferring or walking.

The spine should not be viewed in isolation. Hip dislocation and subluxation and pelvic obliquity often coexist with scoliosis. James (1956) found that muscle release operations beneath the iliac crest did not alter the scoliosis, and Lonstein & Beck (1986) reported no association between hip dislocation, pelvic obliquity and scoliosis in cerebral palsy; the scoliosis developed regardless of the pelvic position. Although single and double thoraco-lumbar curves occur in cerebral palsy, the single C-type curves occur more frequently in the patient in whom the entire body is involved, who usually has absent truncal equilibrium reactions and pelvic obliquity. Curve progression is inevitable, and Madigan & Wallace (1986) found that the greatest progression was in the most severely involved groups. Curves continue to progress even after skeletal maturity (Thomas & Simon 1988).

If a curve is progressive and threatens the child's ability to sit in spite of wheelchair modifications and bracing, surgical stabilisation of the spine should be considered. Recently, there has been greater interest in performing spinal arthrodesis, even in the severely handicapped child who is a wheelchair user (Fig. 18.14). The more severe curves require

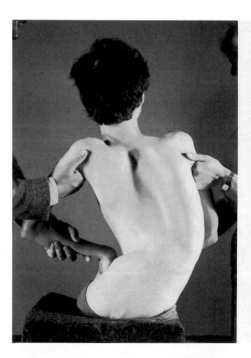
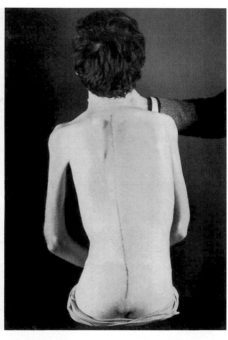
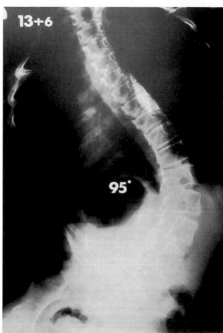
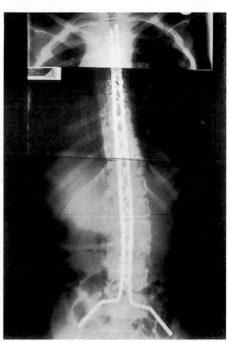

Figure 18.14 Before (left) and after (right) spinal arthrodesis. (Courtesy of Mr M. J. McMaster.)

preliminary anterior release and posterior stabilisation (Gersoff & Renshaw 1988). If there is fixed pelvic obliquity, the fusion should be extended to the sacrum. Leaving the L5–S1 segment free leaves some spinal mobility, but risks instability and the need for further bracing later. This is major surgery, and severe learning difficulties or handicap may present a quandary for the parents or carers and surgeon. However, relieving the patient of discomfort from pelvic obliquity and rib impingement on the iliac crest is advantageous, and the patient may be easier to nurse and to seat.

Kyphosis usually begins as a postural problem in patients who have poor trunk and head control. It is flexible initially, but can become fixed during subsequent growth. Severe kyphosis is a disabling deformity, and in severe cases surgical correction, including ventral release and dorsal correction and fusion, is indicated. Hyperlordosis is usually indicative of hip flexion contractures. The sacrum becomes almost horizontal and back pain often ensues. A constant lordotic sitting posture needs to be avoided, because severe and persistent hyperlordosis can become painful. Changing position from standing, during which the spine may be hyperlordotic, to a supine posture or to a more kyphotic one during sitting, may help to vary spinal posture and relieve back pain.

The hip

The windswept deformity (abduction contracture of one hip and displacement of the other hip in adduction) is a typical finding of the non-walker and causes difficulties with perineal hygiene and seating. In the absence of hip flexion contracture, intramuscular tenotomy of adductor longus and a myotomy of gracilis on the adducted side is usually sufficient, provided symmetry of abduction can be obtained. A more extensive procedure, or complete division of adductor longus, should be avoided, as this produces a secondary abduction contracture that is very disabling and can threaten transfer capabilities and cause seating problems.

As the cause of hip dislocation in cerebral palsy is not clear, an effective prophylaxis is not possible. The hip in cerebral palsy is generally normal at birth. The lack of dynamic control, persisting fetal anteversion, and positioning (Fulford & Brown 1976) lead to a unidirectional acetabular enlargement, which finally results in a dislocation. The hip flexion contracture may then worsen as the centre of rotation of the hip changes with displacement. The more severely affected patient may spend extended periods of time in one position, particularly at night. This can result in one hip being persistently adducted, which increases the pressure against the upper part of the acetabulum, resulting in a dislocation. The role of spasticity in dislocation remains unclear, but is certainly overestimated, because hip dislocations occur with both hypotonia and spasticity.

The clinical diagnosis of hip dislocation is unreliable, as contractures are common and restrict motion. The diagnosis is made from X-rays. Many geometric measurements have been proposed to provide objective criteria, but a critical assessment is important: only the common sagittal dislocation is correctly shown. All geometric indices, such as Reimer's migration index (Fig. 18.15) or the Wiberg centre–edge angle, depend upon the position of the joint and are greatly influenced by rotation and adduction. A hip can be dislocated in neutral rotation and centred in internal rotation (Fig. 18.16). A better indicator is the lateral acetabular edge: a progressive convexity indicates excessive pressure against this structure (Howard & Williams 1984) where the typical dislocation channel starts to form (Brunner et al 1997).

Arthrographic findings (Heinrich et al 1991) show that progressive deformation of the cartilaginous acetabulum and femoral head occur before obvious hip instability. The hip develops a typical deformity during dislocation consisting of a unidirectional enlargement of the acetabulum. Unidirectional instability, joint subluxation, and a femoral deformity consisting of increased anteversion, valgus, or both, develop in association with muscle contractures (Brunner et al 1997). As 91% of the hips dislocate craniolaterally, this deformity is recognised on plain anteroposterior X-rays. Different avenues of dislocation can only be detected by computed tomography scans.

Management of hip dislocation is indicated for three reasons: instability, restriction of motion, and pain, which may already be present in relatively minor subluxations (Brunner & Baumann 1994, Brunner & Döderlein 1996). There is controversy, however, as to whether a dislocated hip is painful, although a study by Cooperman et al (1987) suggested that 50% of a small group of non-institutionalised patients complained of pain in the dislocated hip. They concluded that a dislocation should be reduced. Treatment thus aims at correcting all three problems. After a child has reached the age of 5 years, progressive uncovering of the

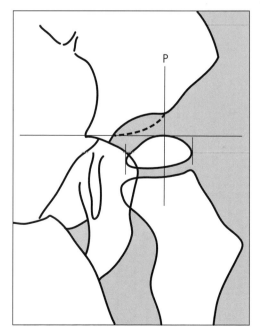

Figure 18.15
Reimer's migration index is the part of the femoral epiphysis extending beyond Perkin's line (P), expressed as a percentage of the entire width of the epiphysis measured in the horizontal plane.

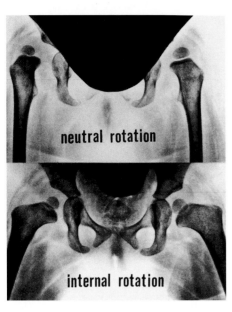

Figure 18.16 The effect of rotation on hip location in a patient with total-body involvement.

femoral head requires the addition of varus derotation osteotomy (Kalen & Bleck 1985). The femoral deformity is either excessive anteversion or valgus, or both. It should be remembered that coxa valga may be a radiographic artefact as a result of femoral torsion, and a femoral correction view (an anteroposterior X-ray with internal rotation to neutralise anteversion) is a prerequisite to show the true femoral pathology. The aim of surgery is to produce a neck–shaft angle of about 120°. A blade plate provides excellent fixation for this purpose. Where there is acetabular dysplasia or a dislocation, the reduction and femoral osteotomy require an additional acetabular procedure. The acetabular pathology consists of a defect of shape and volume, and a reshaping procedure such as the Pemberton or Dega periacetabular osteotomy is indicated to correct the acetabular radius. These procedures bend the elongated part of the acetabulum down over the reduced femoral head (Brunner 2000). Procedures that redirect the acetabulum within the pelvis (the triple or the Ganz osteotomy) or enlarge the coverage (Chiari osteotomy or shelf procedures) are less adequate and they are usually indicated for other acetabular pathologies.

The hip capsule may need to be opened and the ligament teres divided and the transverse ligament incised, to ensure complete reduction. It is certainly wise to perform an open reduction if there is any doubt about a complete reduction of the femoral head. Sufficient femoral shortening at the time of femoral osteotomy is most important to produce a relative lengthening of the contracted muscles and to avoid pressure upon the femoral head. Additional soft-tissue procedures are not usually necessary.

This complex operation is difficult, and has a success rate of about 95% for lateral or posterior dislocations; the anterior dislocation type has a failure rate of up to 30%. A femoral head deformity or loss of cartilage is not a contraindication, as the head will usually remodel to some degree, and the risk of osteoarthritis seems to be small in these patients, who have greatly reduced levels of activity. If a reconstruction is not possible, there is a choice of procedure to obtain reasonable abduction (Gamble et al 1990). A subtrochanteric abduction osteotomy (Schanz osteotomy) can be carried out, which will give sufficient abduction for perineal hygiene and seating. Proximal femoral resection has in the past been plagued by ectopic bone formation, but Castle & Schneider (1978) have described a technique of interposition arthroplasty using the gluteus medius and minimus and vastus lateralis between the resected femur and acetabulum. Proximal femoral resection should not be performed in patients who have transfer capabilities, as hip stability is lost.

The knee

In the non-walker, the goals of treatment for the knee are to obtain a comfortable posture when sitting in a chair, lying in bed, and standing in a standing frame, if such a device is used. Excessive knee flexion can cause skin pressure problems from the edge of the chair. Fractional hamstring lengthening rarely brings complete correction, but often helps. If the result is insufficient, because the contractures are long-standing and involve the posterior capsule of the knee, a closing wedge supracondylar extension osteotomy can be added. This will not give the patient any further range of motion, but will simply change the arc of available movement to a more useful one. In time, femoral remodelling will lead to a recurrence of the flexion deformity.

Foot and ankle deformity

In the non-walker, the goals are a satisfactory foot shape for shoewear, allowing the foot to rest on the footplate of the wheelchair, and for it to be plantigrade when the patient stands in a standing frame. Severe equinus is undesirable, but can be managed with a well-fitted orthosis (in equinus with a heel) and appropriate shoewear, if surgery is not indicated. Fixed deformity may have to be corrected by bony surgery. Arthrodeses are well tolerated and provide long-standing results, whereas there is a high tendency for deformity to recur after soft-tissue procedures alone.

SURGERY FOR THE WALKER

In normal standing, the ground reaction force passes behind the hip joint centre and in front of the knee joint centre, thereby creating a passive external extensor moment. This moment stabilises these joints and is counteracted by the anterior hip joint capsule and the ilio-femoral ligament at the hip level, and by the posterior knee joint capsule and the posterior cruciate ligament at the knee. Hyperextension to some degree is a prerequisite for these joints. The position of the foot is of lesser importance. The shank, however, needs to be balanced perpendicular to the floor (and not to the foot) by the triceps surae muscle, to keep the ground reaction force correctly oriented with respect to the hip and the knee. Gait requires some stability of the leg in stance, but too much stability interferes with walking (stance during gait is less stable than during standing). During swing, the leg must shorten functionally to pass by the opposite leg.

There are surgical solutions for both the stance and swing phases of gait. Correction of deformities should be considered in the sagittal, coronal and transverse planes. Only a small percentage of patients with total-body involvement are mobile, and the following passage relates mainly to those with diplegia and hemiplegia, in whom hip dislocation is unusual.

The hip

Loss of extension of the hip is a disabling problem and is one of the first deformities that should be redressed in the lower extremity, as it can cause secondary flexion of the knee and ankle. Absent extension of the hip may imply that the child has already lost 15–20° of hip extension, and lengthening of the psoas is indicated. This is best performed by an intramuscular psoas tenotomy. It is important to preserve the iliacus muscle to maintain the strength of the hip flexors; a complete tenotomy is usually reserved for the non-walker. Adduction contracture of the hip may be manifested by a short stride length, approximation of the knees and, in more severe cases, scissoring. In walking patients, adductor longus intramuscular tenotomy with gracilis myotomy is the procedure of choice; if there is asymmetry of abduction, adductor longus and gracilis may be tenotomised on one side and the gracilis only on the other. Anterior branch obturator neurectomy is contraindicated in the walking patient because the adductor brevis muscle, which is a hip stabiliser, is denervated.

Internal rotation deformity can be corrected by derotation femoral osteotomy. The intertrochanteric level is preferred and a standard AO blade plate gives excellent fixation. In general, it is better to delay the derotation osteotomy until age 7 or 8 years, as femoral torsion does not change in children after the age of 8 years and may recur if performed at a younger age (Brunner & Baumann 1997, Fabry 1977). When assessing rotational deformity of the legs, it is important that compensatory external tibial torsion is not made more obvious by femoral derotation, and if present this can be corrected at the same operation. Dislocated or subluxed hip joints are treated as for the non-walker, by a joint reconstruction including an open reduction, a corrective femoral and pelvic osteotomy and, rarely, additional soft-tissue procedures. It is preferable to shorten the femur sufficiently to reduce pressure within the joint and hence avoid head necrosis, rather than to preserve leg length.

Internal rotation arising at the hip is a common deformity in walkers. It should be noted, however, that this deformity is functionally advantageous when not excessive. The patients have difficulties in controlling their legs, which can give way during walking. An internal rotation position makes the leg flex underneath the centre of gravity, and compensatory movements to rebalance the body are minimal. In external rotation, however, the patient must position his body over the leg, which manifests as a Duchenne gait pattern in which the upper trunk leans over the affected hip. For this reason, when an internal rotation deformity is being corrected, a slight internal rotation of about 10° should be left.

The knee

There may be extension or flexion deformities at the knee. It is simplistic to consider a flexed knee posture as being due solely to spasticity of the hamstrings, as it could equally be caused by weakness of the quadriceps or a hip flexion contracture. It is essential to evaluate the joints above and below the knee. Egger's procedure of transfer of the distal hamstrings to the femur is known to result in knee hyperextension as a result of the co-spasticity of the quadriceps, which produces an extension deformity and a circumduction gait; this procedure should no longer be used. Fractional lengthening of the hamstrings is the preferred procedure, and allows some choice over the degree of lengthening (Fig. 18.17). The biceps does not always need to be lengthened, and this will depend upon the amount of shortening of the muscle. The problem with co-spasticity of the quadriceps has been addressed by Gage et al (1987) who recommended a medial transfer of the distal part of the rectus to reduce the spasticity of the quadriceps after fractional hamstring lengthening. The rectus femoris tendon is usually transferred to semitendinosus. This procedure increases the dynamic range of motion by about 15–20° (Abel et al 1999). Knee hyperextension may result from previous surgery, if the knee flexors become too weak. If the hyperextension is due to spastic quadriceps, one solution is to perform a distal rectus transfer.

Foot and ankle

These are common deformities associated with cerebral palsy, and a useful guide to their management has been provided by Fulford (1990). Equinus deformity may be primarily caused by a contracture of the gastrocnemius or the soleus, or may be secondary to hip or knee flexion contractures. Whereas a knee flexion contracture requires hip flexion for compensation (and *vice versa*), the foot position, in principle, is independent of the position of the proximal joints of the lower limb. Because hip and knee flexion result in a functional shortening of the leg, a compensatory equinus position is often used to allow foot contact. The ankle, therefore, should not be examined in isolation. The aim of treatment of an equinus deformity is to ensure full contact of the foot, with the shank perpendicular to the floor for standing posture. Thus an equinus can be accepted, but requires a heel raise for compensation. In this case, additional stabilisation may be necessary from orthopaedic shoes or orthoses. An ankle–foot orthosis is especially helpful to correct a drop-foot deformity.

If the equinus deformity is too severe or conservative means are not tolerated, the aim of management is to produce a plantigrade foot. Mild contracture of the calf

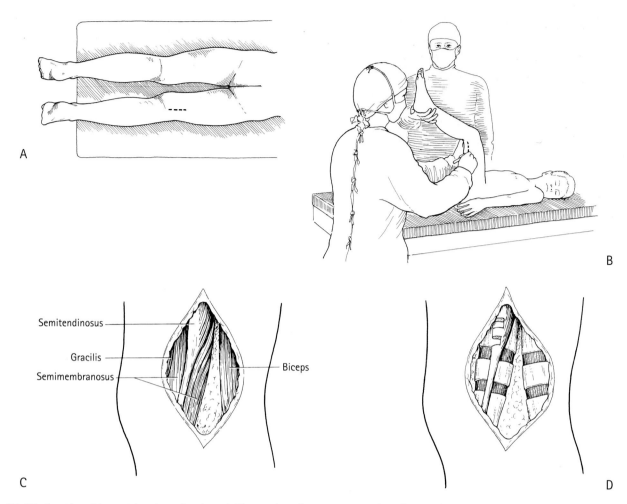

Figure 18.17 Fractional hamstring lengthening. **A** The patient is prone or supine. A tourniquet is not necessary. A mid-line incision is made in the distal third of the thigh and stops at the transverse crease of the knee. **B** Semimembranosis and semitendinosis are identified and lengthened routinely and biceps and gracilis may also be included. **C** Biceps and semimembranosis are lengthened by aponeurotomy, usually at two levels; the edges of these muscles require eversion to identify the aponeurosis fully. Where possible, intramuscular lengthening of the tendon of semitendinosis is performed, but often this is not possible in the younger patient, and Z-lengthening is necessary. A popliteal angle of 20° after lengthening is desirable. A plaster cast or splint is applied for 3 weeks and weight bearing, if appropriate, encouraged as soon as possible.

muscles can respond to serial casting. Resting ankle–foot orthoses are widely used, but if stretching is required to improve dorsiflexion, the acceptance of an orthosis may be poor. Serial casting and correction by splints require diligence and skill, and may postpone the need for surgery; applied injudiciously, they can lead to serious damage if the foot is used as a lever to dorsiflex the ankle, as this may produce a pseudocorrection at the expense of a mid-tarsal or hindfoot break. To apply true stretch to the triceps surae muscle, the subtalar joints must be locked by adduction–inversion in cases of valgus–abduction feet, or the opposite in varus–adduction feet.

If surgical lengthening of the triceps surae (tendo-Achilles lengthening or aponeurotic lengthening) is performed at an early age, there is a likelihood of subsequent lengthening. This has to be balanced against the disadvantage of the social inconvenience of multiple visits for serial casting that

may become less effective. Secondary deformities in the proximal lower limb, and the risk of iatrogenic overlengthening of the triceps muscle, are recognised risks. Flexible ankle–foot orthoses worn during walking can maintain or even slightly improve dorsiflexion if plantiflexion is blocked and only dorsiflexion is free. These orthoses afford a gait that is superior to walking barefoot or with stiff orthoses (Brunner et al 1998).

In the assessment of equinus, it is essential to distinguish, if possible, between tonic and phasic spasticity, because the former is more likely to produce fixed contracture. Most operations are designed to correct tonic spasticity. Intramuscular tendon lengthening of the gastrocmenius or aponeurotic lengthening of the gastrocnemius, soleus, or both (Baumann & Koch 1989) are the procedures of choice for moderate equinus. In the Baumann procedure, the aponeuroses of the gastrocnemii and, if necessary, of the soleus are exposed in the middle one-third of the calf and are divided three or four times, perpendicularly to the fibre direction. This procedure does not produce a direct length gain, and hence intensive physiotherapy is mandatory. The advantage of this procedure is the preservation of muscle force (Brunner 1998, Jaspers et al 2000).

Excessive weakening of the triceps surae can be disastrous. Careful consideration should be given before any surgery to the triceps, because of its biomechanical importance. It controls standing posture, and its strength is necessary for running, jumping, and stair climbing; weakening this muscle might improve gait, but can interfere with many other functions. In the case of severe equinus and associated true shortening of the soleal and gastrocnemius components, judicious lengthening of the tendo-Achilles is helpful and may be performed open or closed. A percutaneous Hoke technique is effective, assuming that this is a primary procedure and that no other lengthenings in that region are required. Tendo-Achilles lengthening can also be achieved percutaneously after previous surgery, providing the skin is not adherent to the underlying tendon. The tendon is tenotomised in three sites: one-half medially and distally, one-half medially and proximally, and one-half laterally between the two medial cuts. The tendon slides apart as the foot is dorsiflexed, to no more than a right-angle when the hind-foot is held in varus. A below-knee cast is then applied while the foot is held at a right-angle, but not beyond, to avoid producing calcaneus.

There are three possible causes for pes varus: spasticity of the tibialis posterior, tibialis anterior, or gastrocnemius-soleus. Gastrocnemius–soleus spasticity causes inversion of the ankle, whereas that of the tibialis posterior causes hind-foot varus, and tibialis anterior, midfoot varus. Indications for surgery in this group are failure of an orthosis to control the foot deformity, which may be difficult if the deformity occurs during swing. Subsequent bony changes must be prevented. A variety of procedures have been advocated for this. If there is no fixed joint deformity, the aim should be to balance the foot by procedures on the deforming musculotendinous units. Inversion at the ankle is corrected by judicious elongation of the triceps surae. Inversion of the hindfoot can be corrected by either an intramuscular tibialis posterior lengthening (Ruda & Frost 1971) or a split tibialis posterior transfer (Green et al 1983). Simple tibialis posterior tenotomy is contraindicated, for fear of producing a valgus deformity.

Inversion of the midfoot is corrected by a split tibialis anterior tendon transfer (Hoffer et al 1985, Barnes & Herring 1991). Alternatively, the entire tendon can be transferred to the mid-dorsum of the foot. The object is to balance muscle action over the medial and lateral sides of the foot. Fixed bony deformity requires a combination of soft-tissue surgery and bony correction. For a fixed varus hindfoot, a lateral closing wedge osteotomy of the calcaneum in addition to soft-tissue surgery is indicated. For a fixed hind- and midfoot, a triple fusion is indicated after soft-tissue release,

but it should be noted that patients who have marginal walking abilities tend to have difficulties in coping with a stiff foot. Pes valgus may be due to spasticity of the peroneal muscles or triceps surae, but a major factor is torsional moments occurring during gait. Unless treated, the deformity will progress from flexible to rigid and produce secondary hallux valgus. The foot deformity can be managed either conservatively, by an ankle–foot orthosis, or surgically. The procedure of choice is a calcaneal lengthening (Evans procedure), which is efficient as long as the foot is flexible. An alternative is the extra-articular subtalar fusion and the Dennyson & Fulford (1976) modification of the Grice technique (Grice 1952) has also proved very reliable.

Hallux valgus may be treated by a metatarsal osteotomy or metatarso-phalangeal fusion. The foot should not be considered in isolation, and it is essential to check that the underlying cause for a foot or toe deformity does not lie more proximally. In older patients, hallux flexus can produce pressure sores at the metatarso-phalangeal joint or on the pulp of toe. This deformity is best managed by a combination of soft tissue and bony procedures.

UPPER LIMB SURGERY

Only a small number of patients are suitable for upper limb surgery and the assessment should be considered along with the overall disability of the child. Surgical procedures usually attempt to position the arm in a more functional or cosmetic position; orthoses are generally poorly tolerated and less effective than in the lower extremities. Important criteria for intervention include intelligence, motivation, motor function, sensibility and age (Koman et al 1990). As with the lower limb, muscle weakness, fixed deformity, dynamic deformity and contractures need to be assessed. Similarly, distinction should be made between phasic and tonic spasticity. Rigidity may produce either flexor or extensor dystonia. There is no reciprocal inhibition associated with dystonia, so both agonists and antagonists grow normally and tendon transfers in this situation can produce the opposite and equally disabling posture. Poor sensibility does not exclude surgery, but poor stereognosis, two-point discrimination greater than 15–20 mm, and the inability to position the hand in space when the eyes are closed, are relative contraindications to procedures designed to improve fine co-ordination (Koman et al 1990). Athetosis may make tendon transfers unreliable.

Operations in the upper limb include joint stabilisation, release of contractures, musculotendinous lengthening, and tendon transfer. Some patients, especially at an older age, develop severe flexion deformities in the upper extremities at the wrist, the elbow or, sometimes, the shoulder. The usual deformity in the shoulder is adduction and internal rotation, and where there is a fixed contracture, derotation humeral osteotomy can improve elbow and forearm position. Painful subluxation of untreated shoulder deformities is rare.

Elbow flexion contractures can cause a severe functional problem. Loss of 30° of extension may not require treatment on its own, but if loss of elbow extension prevents efficient use of crutches or if the patient, who is usually hemiplegic, dislikes the appearance, surgical release can be effective. An anterior elbow release (Z-lengthening of biceps tendon, fractional lengthening of brachialis and release of the flexor–pronator origin) can improve the contracture, but care should be taken to avoid a fixed extension deformity.

The following deformities may occur distal to the elbow: pronation of the forearm, wrist and finger flexion, and thumb adduction or 'thumb-in-palm'. In the forearm, pronation can be dealt with by pronator teres tenotomy if this is an isolated problem, or can be combined with a flexor–pronator release (Page 1923) if there is a severe flexion deformity of the wrist and fingers. This operation produces an unselective release of all the flexors and should be reserved for severe deformity with no prospect of useful hand function; otherwise, selective flexor lengthenings and transfers should be considered. Excessive wrist flexion is a common deformity and inhibits hand grasp.

Zancolli et al (1983) have provided guidelines for the surgical management of wrist and finger flexion deformities, which are summarised here. Wrist flexion is often associated with ulnar deviation, and extension can be improved by tendon transfers. Where there is mild spasticity, a tenotomy of the flexor carpi ulnaris and musculoaponeurotic release of the flexor origins is recommended. If the wrist extensors are weak, the flexor carpi ulnaris is transferred to extensor carpi radialis brevis. Musculoaponeurotic release of the flexors may also be necessary and, where finger extension is only possible with the wrist flexed beyond 50°, an additional pronator release is recommended. Severe flexion of the fingers and an inability to extend the fingers in full wrist flexion may be dealt with by multiple tendon lengthenings in the forearm. Transfer of flexor carpi ulnaris to extensor digitorum communis has the advantage over the Green & Banks (1962) transfer to extensor carpi radialis brevis in that it may not result in extension contractures of the fingers.

Wrist arthrodesis is indicated for cosmesis in the non-functional hand (and is usually requested by those with hemiplegia), for degenerative changes at the wrist with associated pain, or where there is functional finger flexion and extension when the wrist is immobilised in neutral. One technique is to use a semi-tubular plate between the 3rd metacarpal and the radius, after the articular surfaces have been denuded. The plate can be contoured to give an acceptable cosmetic appearance. One pitfall of arthrodesis in a functional hand arises in those patients who rely on crutches or a wheelchair for mobility: they may not be able to do so once the wrist has been fused in the 'optimum' position, because they are unable to transfer body weight to the palm of the hand.

Adduction contracture of the thumb can be treated by myotomy of the adductor muscle in the palm. This is pre-ferred to tenotomy, as it releases the 1st metacarpal but does not allow hyperextension of the metacarpo-phalangeal joint (Matev 1963). The thumb-in-palm deformity is complex, and often difficult to treat. The main deforming force is the flexor pollicis longus, but there may also be spasticity of the adductor pollicis, flexor pollicis brevis or abductor pollicis brevis. To confirm that the flexor pollicis longus is the principal deforming force, thumb flexion should decrease on wrist flexion; conversely, wrist extension will exaggerate the deformity. Several procedures are necessary to deal with the deformity: release of adductor pollicis, flexor pollicis brevis and abductor pollicis brevis, arthrodesis of the metacarpo-phalangeal joint if unstable, lengthening of flexor pollicis longus and re-routing of extensor pollicis longus (Bleck 1987, Goldner et al 1990, Koman et al 1990).

POSTOPERATIVE MANAGEMENT AND COMPLICATIONS

Immediate postoperative management will depend on the type of procedure performed.

Bone and tendon surgery will require a period of immobilisation, to allow tissue healing and to lessen the effects of muscle spasm. In the lower limb, a percutaneous tendo-Achilles lengthening can be undertaken on a day-case basis and immediate weight bearing in a below-knee plaster cast begun within the limits of comfort.

Isolated hamstring and rectus femoris surgery requires the use of either a long leg cast or a light-weight detachable splint. If the hamstrings are particularly tight, the knee is not extended to its limit but is left in a slightly flexed position. Further improvement can be obtained using an orthosis with a variable knee hinge or by serial casting 2 weeks later, after wound healing. Excessive tension has been reported to produce persistent neural damage (Aspen & Porter 1994). Alternatively, an orthosis with an extendible knee hinge can be used. The advantage of this is that the stretch can be applied while the patient is conscious, and adjustments are possible at any time. The splint needs to be fitted before surgery and is worn 23 hours per day until extension is sufficient. It is usually more comfortable for patients undergoing adductor surgery to be immobilised in either broomstick plasters or a double spica until muscle spasms have worn off. Plaster immobilisation is not necessary after isolated psoas surgery or interventions at the muscle belly.

Spicas are used routinely after major skeletal surgery in non-walkers. Careful consideration should be given to the relief of pain and spasm and the maintenance of the desired position of the limb in the immediate postoperative period. In the lower limbs, postoperative epidural anaesthesia is highly desirable, and can be maintained for several days. The child should be mobilised as soon as is practicable.

Rehabilitation after surgery is lengthy, time-consuming and involves both the therapist and parents. Recovery after even a 'minor' procedure can take many months because of the new demands made upon the neuromuscular system. It may take up to 1 year to achieve maximum benefit after multiple-level surgery in the lower limb and the patient, parents, therapist and surgeon can be frustrated by the apparent lack of progress after such procedures. It should not be forgotten that cerebral palsy is an incurable condition, and careful preoperative assessment is essential to avoid exchanging one problem for an even worse one. One should avoid setting unrealistic goals.

The need for surgery may coincide with unfavourable events occurring in the natural history of the child's development, such as diminishing efficiency of walking, so that an indifferent outcome does not necessarily result from the surgery. The present trend to perform multiple-level surgery at one operation is justifiable providing excellent preoperative assessment is made. However, it does increase the possibility of error.

There are several pitfalls in the surgical management of cerebral palsy, apart from the complications common to any surgical procedure. The most serious result from inadequate assessment, operations at the wrong level and failure to allow for the action of muscles that cross two joints. An example of this type of error is a tendo-Achilles lengthening for equinus that is caused by a hip flexion contracture. Over-lengthening of musculotendinous units may produce an even worse deformity; for example, calcaneus after excessive tendo-Achilles lengthening, an excessively broad-based gait or, even worse, an abduction contracture at the hip after excessive adductor surgery. In principle, it is better to correct proximal deformities first and to reassess the influence of this distally. Incorrect assessment of bony deformity can give poor results; for example, significant uncovering of the femoral head is unlikely to be corrected by muscle releases alone, and if relocation is contemplated it should be done before the appearance of significant femoral head deformity. Equally, in considering torsional deformity, neither the femur nor the tibia should be viewed in isolation; correction of excessive femoral internal torsion by external derotation osteotomy in the presence of compensatory external tibial torsion will exaggerate the clinical appearances of an externally rotated lower limb.

Unpredictable results follow surgery for rigidity or phasic spasticity, and after soft-tissue procedures in the presence of fixed bony deformity. Assessment of the child with cerebral palsy is challenging, and surgical intervention will only be effective when properly applied. Surgery should be seen as only one aspect in the overall management of the patient; after all, there is no known disease that surgery cannot make worse (Steel 1980).

REFERENCES

Abel M F, Damiano D L, Pannunzio M, Bush J 1999 Muscle–tendon surgery in diplegic cerebral palsy: functional and mechanical changes. Journal of Pediatric Orthopaedics 19: 366–375

Albright A L 1996 Baclofen in the treatment of cerebral palsy. Journal of Child Neurology 11: 77–83

Albright A L, Barron W B, Fasick M P, Polinko P, Janosky J 1993 Continuous intrathecal baclofen infusion for spasticity of cerebral origin. Journal of the American Medical Association 270: 2475–2477

Albright A L, Barry M J, Painter M J, Schultz B 1998 Infusion of intrathecal baclofen for generalised dystonia in cerebral palsy. Journal of Neurosurgery 88: 73–76

Armstrong R W, Steinbok P, Cochrane D D, Kube S D, Fife S E, Farrell K 1997 Intrathecally administered baclofen for treatment of children with spasticity of cerebral origin. Journal of Neurosurgery 87: 409–414

Aspen R M, Porter R W 1994 Nerve traction during correction of knee flexion deformity. A case report and calculation. Journal of Bone and Joint Surgery 76B: 471–473

Barnes M J, Herring J A 1991 Combined split anterior tibial-tendon transfer and intramuscular lengthening of the posterior tibial tendon. Journal of Bone and Joint Surgery 73A: 734–738

Bassett G S, Engsberg J R, McAlister W H, Gordon J E, Schoenecker P L 1999 Fate of the psoas muscle after open reduction for developmental dislocation of the hip (DDH). Journal of Pediatric Orthopaedics 19: 425–432

Baumann J U, Koch H G 1989 Ventrale aponeurotische Verlängerung des Musculus gastrocnemius. Operative Orthopädie und Traumatologie 1: 254–258

Bejar R, Wozniak P, Allard M et al 1988 Antenatal origin of neurologic damage in newborn infants. Preterm infants. American Journal of Obstetrics and Gynecology 159: 357–363

Bleck E E 1987 Orthopaedic management in cerebral palsy. Clinics in developmental medicine, No. 99/100. MacKeith Press, Oxford

Brown J K, Minns R A 1989 Mechanisms of deformity in children with cerebral palsy. Seminars in Orthopaedics 4: 236–255

Brunner R 1998 Die Auswirkungen der Aponeurosendurchtrennung auf den Muskel. Habilitation-Dissertation, University of Basel, Basel, Switzerland

Brunner R, Baumann J U 2000 Open reduction of hip dislocation in children with cerebral palsy. Orthopaedics and Traumatology 8: 22–36

Brunner R, Baumann J U 1994 Clinical benefit of reconstruction of dislocated and subluxated hip joints in patients with spastic cerebral palsy. Journal of Pediatric Orthopaedics 14: 290–294

Brunner R, Baumann J U 1997 Long term effects of intertrochanteric varus-derotation osteotomy on femur and acetabulum in spastic cerebral palsy. Journal of Pediatric Orthopaedics 17: 585–591

Brunner R, Doderlein L 1996 Pathological fractures in patients with cerebral palsy. Journal of Pediatric Orthopaedics 85: 232–238

Brunner R, Picard C, Robb J E 1997 Morphology of the acetabulum in hip dislocations due to cerebral palsy. Journal of Pediatric Orthopaedics 86: 207–211

Brunner R, Meier G, Ruepp T 1998 Comparison of a stiff and a spring-type ankle–foot orthosis to improve gait in spastic hemiplegic children. Journal of Pediatric Orthopaedics 18: 719–726

Castle M E, Schneider C 1978 Proximal femoral resection-interposition arthroplasty. Journal of Bone and Joint Surgery 60A: 1051–1054

Cooperman D R, Bartucci E, Dierrick E, Millar E A 1987 Hip dislocation in spastic cerebral palsy: long-term consequences. Journal of Pediatric Orthopaedics 7: 268–276

Corry I S, Cosgrove A P, Duffy C M, McNeill S, Taylor T C, Graham H K 1998 Botulinum toxin A compared with stretching casts in the treatment of spastic equinus: a randomised prospective trial. Journal of Pediatric Orthopaedics 18: 304–311

Cosgrove A P, Graham H K 1994 Botulinum toxin A prevents the development of contractures in the hereditary spastic mouse. Developmental Medicine and Child Neurology 36: 379–385

Crawford K, Karol L A, Herring J A 1996 Severe lumbar lordosis after dorsal rhizotomy. Journal of Pediatric Orthopaedics 16: 336–339

Dennyson W G, Fulford G E 1976 Subtalar arthrodesis by cancellous grafts and metallic internal fixation. Journal of Bone and Joint Surgery 58B: 507–510

Fabry G 1977 Torsion of the femur. Acta Orthopaedica Belgica 43: 454–459

Fulford G E 1990 Surgical management of ankle and foot deformities in cerebral palsy. Clinical Orthopaedics and Related Research 253: 55–61

Fulford G E, Brown J K B 1976 Position as a cause of deformity in children with cerebral palsy. Developmental Medicine and Child Neurology 18: 305–314

Gage J R 1991 Gait analysis in cerebral palsy. Clinics in developmental medicine, No. 121. MacKeith Press, Oxford

Gage J R, Perry J, Hicks R R, Koop S, Werntz J R 1987 Rectus femoris transfer to improve knee function of children with cerebral palsy. Developmental Medicine and Child Neurology 29: 159–166

Gamble J G, Rinsky L A, Bleck E E 1990 Established hip dislocation in children with cerebral palsy. Clinical Orthopaedics and Related Research 253: 90–99

Garcia Ruiz P J, Sanchez Bernardos V, Urcelay V et al 1996 Tratamiento de la espasticidad asociada a paralisis infantil con toxina botulinica. Neurologia 11: 34–36

Gersoff W K, Renshaw T S 1988 The treatment of scoliosis in cerebral palsy by posterior spinal fusion with Luque-rod segmental instrumentation. Journal of Bone and Joint Surgery 70A: 41–44

Gerszten P C, Albright A L, Johnstone G F 1998 Intrathecal baclofen infusion and subsequent orthopaedic surgery in patients with spastic cerebral palsy. Journal of Neurosurgery 88: 1009–1013

Goldner J L, Koman A L, Gelberman R, Levin S, Goldner R D 1990 Arthrodesis of the metacarpophalangeal joint in children and adults. Adjunctive treatment of thumb in palm deformity in cerebral palsy. Clinical Orthopaedics and Related Research 253: 75–89

Green N E, Griffen P P, Shiavi P 1983 Split posterior tibial tendon transfer in spastic cerebral palsy. Journal of Bone and Joint Surgery 65A: 748–754

Green W T, Banks H H 1962 Flexor carpi ulnaris transplant and its use in cerebral palsy. Journal of Bone and Joint Surgery 44A: 1343–1352

Greene W B, Dietz F R, Goldberg M J, Gross R H, Miller F, Sussman M D 1991 Rapid progression of hip subluxation in cerebral palsy after selective posterior rhizotomy. Journal of Pediatric Orthopaedics 11: 494–497

Grice D S 1952 An extra articular arthrodesis of the subastragalar joint for correction of paralytic flat feet in children. Journal of Bone and Joint Surgery 34A: 927–940

Heinrich S D, MacEwan G D, Zembo M M 1991 Hip dysplasia, subluxation and dislocation in cerebral palsy: an arthrographic analysis. Journal of Pediatric Orthopaedics 11: 488–493

Hoffer M M, Barakat G, Koffman M 1985 10-Year follow-up of split anterior tibial tendon transfer in cerebral palsied patients with spastic equino-varus deformity. Journal of Pediatric Orthopaedics 5: 432–434

Howard C B, Williams L A 1984 A new radiological sign in the hips of cerebral palsy patients. Clinical Radiology 35: 317–319

Hullin M G, Robb J E 1991 Biomechanical effects of walking in a plaster cast. Journal of Bone and Joint Surgery 73B: 92–95

Hullin M G, Robb J E, Loudon I R 1992 Ankle–foot orthosis function in low-level myelomeningocele. Journal of Pediatric Orthopaedics 12: 518–521

Ingram T T S 1964 Paediatric aspects of cerebral palsy. Churchill Livingstone, Edinburgh

James J I P 1956 Paralytic scoliosis. Journal of Bone and Joint Surgery 38B: 660–685

Jaspers R T, Brunner R, Baan G C, Huijing P A 1999 Acute effects of intramuscular aponeurotomy, tenotomy and intramuscular fasciatomy: evidence for local adaptation of connective tissue. Journal of Biomechanics 32: 71–79

Kalen V, Bleck E E 1985 Prevention of spastic paralytic dislocation of the hip. Developmental Medicine and Child Neurology 27: 17–24

Koman L A, Gelberman R H, Toby E B, Poehling G G 1990 Cerebral palsy: management of the upper extremity. Clinical Orthopaedics and Related Research 253: 62–74

Koman L A, Mooney J F 3rd, Smith B P, Goodman A, Mulvaney T 1994 Management of spasticity in cerebral palsy with botulinum-A toxin: report of a preliminary, randomized, double-blind trial. Journal of Pediatric Orthopaedics 14: 299–303

Levitt S 1995 Treatment of cerebral palsy and motor delay, 3rd edn. Blackwell, Oxford

Lin J-P, Brown J K, Walsh E G 1999 Continuum of reflex excitability in hemiplegia: influence of muscle length and muscular transformation after heel-cord lengthening and immobilization on the pathophysiology of spasticity and clonus. Developmental Medicine and Neurology 41: 534–548

Lonstein J E, Beck K 1986 Hip dislocation and subluxation in cerebral palsy. Journal of Pediatric Orthopaedics 6: 521–526

MacLennan A, for the International Cerebral Palsy Task Force 1999 A template for defining a causal relationship between acute intrapartum events and cerebral palsy: international consensus statement. British Medical Journal 319: 1054–1059

Madigan R R, Wallace S L 1986 Scoliosis in cerebral palsy: short term follow-up and prognosis in untreated institutionalised patients. Orthopaedic Transactions 10: 17

Matev I 1963 Surgical treatment of spastic 'thumb-in-palm' deformity. Journal of Bone and Joint Surgery 45B: 703–708

Nelson K B, Ellenberg J H 1986 Antecedents of cerebral palsy. New England Journal of Medicine 315: 81–86

Oppenheim W L 1990 Selective posterior rhizotomy for spastic cerebral palsy. Clinical Orthopaedics and Related Research 253: 20–29

Page C M 1923 An operation for the relief of flexion-contracture in the forearm. Journal of Bone and Joint Surgery 5: 233–234

Peacock W J, Arens L J, Goldberg M J 1987 Cerebral palsy spasticity. Selective posterior rhizotomy. Paediatric Neurosciences 13: 61–66

Perry J, Hoffer M M, Giovan P, Antonelli D, Greenberg R 1974 Gait analysis of the triceps surae in cerebral palsy. Journal of Bone and Joint Surgery 56A: 511–520

Perry J, Antonelli D, Plur J, Lewis G, Greenberg R 1976 Electromyography before and after surgery for hip deformity in children with cerebral palsy. Journal of Bone and Joint Surgery 58A: 201–208

Ruda R, Frost H M 1971 Cerebral palsy spastic varus and forefoot adductus, treated by intramuscular posterior tibial lengthening. Clinical Orthopaedics and Related Research 79: 61–70

Ruwe P A, Gage J R, Ozonoff M B, DeLuca P A 1992 Clinical determination of femoral anteversion. Journal of Bone and Joint Surgery 74A: 820–830

Sherrington C 1947 The integrative action of the nervous system. Yale University, New Haven

Staheli L T 1977 The prone hip extension test. Clinical Orthopaedics and Related Research 123: 12–15

Staheli L T, Engel M 1972 Tibial torsion. A method of assessment and a survey of normal children. Clinical Orthopaedics and Related Research 86: 183–186

Steel H H 1980 Gluteus medius and minimus insertion advancement for correction of internal rotation gait in spastic cerebral palsy. Journal of Bone and Joint Surgery 62A: 919–927

Sutherland D H 1984 Gait disorders in childhood and adolescence. Williams & Wilkins, Baltimore

Tardieu G, Thuilleux G, Tardieu C, Huet de la Tour E 1979 Long term effects of surgical elongation of the tendo calcaneus in the normal cat. Developmental Medicine and Child Neurology 21: 83–94

Tardieu C, Lespargot A, Tabary C, Bret M D 1988 For how long must the soleus muscle be stretched each day to prevent contracture? Developmental Medicine and Child Neurology 30: 3–10

Thomas K J, Simon S R 1988 Progression of scoliosis after skeletal maturity in institutionalised adults who have cerebral palsy. Journal of Bone and Joint Surgery 70A: 1290–1296

Thompson N S, Baker R J, Cosgrove A P, Corry I S, Graham H K 1998 Musculoskeletal modelling in determining the effect of botulinum toxin on the hamstrings of patients with crouch gait. Developmental Medicine and Child Neurology 9: 622–625

Zancolli E A, Goldner J L, Swanson A B 1983 Surgery of the spastic hand in cerebral palsy; report of the committee on spastic hand evaluation. Journal of Hand Surgery 8: 766–772

Ziv I, Blackburn N, Rang M, Koreska J 1984 Muscle growth in normal and spastic mice. Developmental Medicine and Child Neurology 26: 94–99

Chapter 19

Arthrogryposis multiplex congenita

J. A. Fixsen

INTRODUCTION

Arthrogryposis multiplex congenita literally means multiple curved joints, occurring as a congenital anomaly in the newborn. The first description is ascribed to Otto in 1841. Sheldon in 1932 published the first detailed description in the UK, and called the condition 'amyoplasia congenita', emphasising the lack of muscle development in this condition. It is important to realise that arthrogryposis is a descriptive term, and not an exact diagnosis. Hall (1985) from Vancouver, who has made a special study of the genetics of the disorder, pointed out that there are at least 150 possible diagnoses that can result in multiple curved joint deformities in the newborn child. The reader is referred to Hall (1998) for a comprehensive discussion of the disorder.

The features of the syndrome are multiple rigid joint deformities, with defective muscles but normal sensation (Fig. 19.1). In the classical form, termed amyoplasia congenita by Sheldon, all four limbs are involved, but the condition can also occur only in the upper limbs, or only in the lower limbs. Hall et al (1982) described a distal form in which the hands and feet are severely deformed with only minor contractures more proximally, although the spine may develop scoliosis. This form is important, as it can be inherited as an autosomal dominant, whereas the majority of forms of classic arthrogryposis do not have a genetic background. At birth, the children can look terribly deformed, and the parents are often horrified by the appearance of their child. In addition to the multiple rigid joint contractures, the skin lacks creases, and deep dimples over the joints are very characteristic. The limbs are tubular and featureless, but the trunk is rarely affected. Other congenital anomalies such as cryptorchidism, hernias, gastroschisis and bowel atresia may also occur.

INCIDENCE

The reported incidence varies widely, probably because arthrogryposis is a descriptive term that may be applied to all patients with stiff curved joints or only to those in whom there is no ascertainable cause after careful investigation. In Helsinki, an incidence of 3 per 10 000 live births was reported, but in the Edinburgh birth register, there was only one case in 56 000 live births. Wynne-Davies et al (1981) looked at the incidence in the UK, Australia and the USA, and showed there was an apparent increase in the 1960s, which suggested an infective cause for this unusual condition. Hall (1998) quotes an incidence of classic arthrogryposis multiplex congenita (amyoplasia congenita) of 1 in 10 000 live births.

AETIOLOGY

There are many causes of arthrogryposis. Animal studies have shown that limitation of intrauterine movement can lead to a contracture at birth. Intrauterine infection by the akabane virus in sheep, cows and horses can produce a condition very similar to classical arthrogryposis. Mothers of babies born with multiple contractures often note decreased intrauterine mobility of the foetus. The factors that predispose to decreased intrauterine mobility include neuromuscular and connective tissue disorders, fetal crowding, oligohydramnios, multiple pregnancy and malposition such as breech.

An interesting case is reported of a pregnant mother treated with curare for severe tetanus who gave birth to an arthrogrypotic baby. Wynne-Davies et al (1981) concluded that the best description of the aetiology was 'an environmental disease of early pregnancy associated with one or more unfavourable intrauterine factors'.

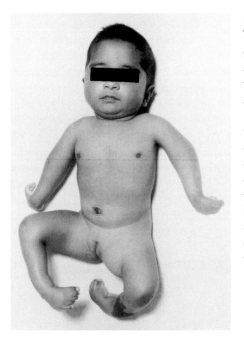

Figure 19.1 Typical appearance of a child with arthrogryposis in all four limbs. Note adduction and internal rotation at the shoulders, extension at the elbows and flexion of the wrist, severe fixed flexion of the knees, and equinovarus deformity of the feet.

DIAGNOSIS

The paediatrician or orthopaedic surgeon presented with a child with arthrogrypotic features must first try to establish the diagnosis. The parents of the child are, not surprisingly, extremely agitated and often want immediate answers to the cause of their child's deformity. However, parental counselling should be approached with caution, particularly with regard to prognosis and possible treatment, until the aetiology has been elucidated. It is not uncommon for anxious parents to be given an extremely pessimistic prognosis before the diagnosis is fully understood. Conversely, an over-optimistic prognosis can also be misleading if the child subsequently proves to have a severe underlying cause for arthrogrypotic deformities.

The following investigations should be considered:

- radiographs of the whole spine and computed tomography of the head
- chromosome analysis
- collagen biochemistry
- plasma creatine kinase estimation, to exclude myopathic disorders
- electromyography and nerve conduction studies
- muscle and nerve biopsy.

Possible *differential diagnoses* can be considered under the following headings:

Neurological disorders
1. Spina bifida and spinal dysraphism in all its forms.
2. Myelodysplasia.
3. Sacral and lumbar agenesis (Fig. 19.2).
4. Spinal muscular atrophy.
5. Fetal neuropathy.

Muscle disorders
1. Dystrophia myotonica.
2. Congenital muscular dystrophy.
3. Fetal myopathy.
4. Fetal myasthenia.

Connective tissue disorders
1. Marfan's syndrome.
2. Ehlers–Danlos syndrome.

Miscellaneous syndromes
1. Freeman–Sheldon syndrome (cranio-carpo-tarsal dystrophy).
2. Turner's syndrome.
3. Edward's syndrome (trisomy 18).
4. The pterygium or popliteal web syndrome.
5. Diastrophic dwarfism.

The help of a paediatrician with an interest in dysmorphology and a geneticist are very important in establishing

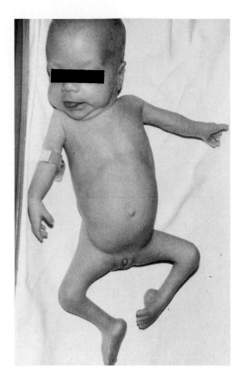

Figure 19.2 Infant with sacral agenesis. Note how similar the lower limbs appear to those of the child in Fig. 19.1. X-rays of the entire spine would establish the diagnosis.

the diagnosis and prognosis. In general, classic amyoplasia congenita is not inherited, except for the distal form (Hall et al 1982) affecting the hands and feet, which is commonly inherited as an autosomal dominant.

ORTHOPAEDIC MANAGEMENT

From the orthopaedic point of view, it is important to see these patients as soon as possible. Although it will take some time to establish the exact diagnosis, it is important to start treating the deformities early, as some of them will respond remarkably well to physiotherapy, stretching and splintage. Some of the patients may be born with fractures and need orthopaedic attention, usually by simple splintage. However intractable a deformity may appear, it is worth trying gentle manipulation and simple splintage, much of which can be done by the parents under the supervision of the physiotherapist (Palmer et al 1985). This strategy can also be very helpful in coping with the understandable parental concern. The parents must be told, however, that simple conservative treatment with stretching and splintage is unlikely to correct the deformities completely. Significant gains are especially likely in the hands, and often the knees and elbows.

In general, the limb deformities tend to be more severe distally. The feet and hands are nearly always involved, but the hips and shoulders may be quite mobile. None the less, if the hips are involved this is often with irreducible dislocation. The application of early splintage to such hips should be avoided, as it may cause avascular necrosis and increase the child's disability. Many of these children are rather weak and floppy in the first few months of life. Robinson (1990) has pointed out that these children have significant problems with feeding, swallowing, sucking, weight gain and recurrent chest infections in the first year of life. Corrective surgery should be delayed until it is clear that the child is thriving and is developing trunk and sitting balance.

If orthopaedic deformities are corrected early, they must be rigorously splinted. There is a very strong tendency for recurrent deformity unless the corrected position can be adequately held by splintage. This can be very difficult in the small, tubular, featureless limbs that characterise this condition. Lower limb deformities that inhibit or prevent standing and walking by the time the child shows evidence of wanting to do so should be corrected at the age of 18 months to 2 years.

In the upper limb, a careful assessment of overall function should be made before any decision regarding surgery. This usually means waiting until the age of 4 or 5 years, and a considerable period of observation and assessment. The use of special tools and utensils, assessment, and education by an occupational therapist are often preferable to a complex operation, which may improve one joint but introduce other problems for the child because of the overall nature of the disorder (Williams 1985, Robinson et al 1992).

ORTHOPAEDIC MANAGEMENT OF THE LOWER LIMBS

The foot

The foot is usually in fixed severe equinovarus (see Fig. 19.1). Less commonly, a congenital vertical talus deformity is present. Serial stretching and strapping or splintage may sometimes produce a degree of correction. However, frequently the foot is completely incorrigible and shows no response to conservative measures. Once it is clear that conservative treatment will not be successful, surgery should be considered, preferably when the child is ready to walk. The foot is likely to require an extensive soft-tissue release involving the medial, posterior and lateral structures, which is best performed through the Cincinnati approach. If the foot fails to correct fully with even the most extensive soft-tissue release or relapses quickly within 2–3 years, talectomy must be considered.

Talectomy has produced good results in these stiff, rigid feet (Green et al 1984, Hsu et al 1984, D'Souza et al 1998). The talus is best approached through a lateral incision, as for a triple arthrodesis. The important details are as follows. First, the entire talus must be removed. This can be difficult, because the normal tissue planes are poorly developed and the anatomy distorted, particularly if previous extensive soft-tissue surgery has been performed. Second, it is important to find the ankle joint early during the operation and work round the talus, avoiding cutting into the talus itself or the tibia and malleoli. The posterior

structures form an inextensile tether, and it is sensible not simply to lengthen the tendo-Achilles, but to excise a 1-cm length of the fibrous cord that represents the tendo-Achilles posteriorly. Once the talus has been removed, the os calcis should be stablised below the tibia by a Kirschner wire, driven up through the heel pad and os calcis into the tibia and retained for 6 weeks. Talectomy produces a plantigrade foot that is inevitably stiff and requires long-term splintage.

Recurrent deformity after talectomy is difficult to treat. The flexor hallucis longus is often tight, and it should be divided distally at the level of the metatarso-phalangeal joint of the big toe to prevent troublesome flexion of the toe. Talectomy cannot influence forefoot adduction, and if this persists and is symptomatic, a later calcaneo-cuboid fusion can be considered. Spontaneous fusion of the os calcis to the tibia occurs in some patients, but does not cause problems provided the os calcis is in a satisfactory neutral position.

The Ilizarov technique and apparatus offer the opportunity of correcting complex foot deformities in three dimensions. Grill & Franke (1987) reported the use of the Ilizarov apparatus in nine severely deformed feet, with satisfactory results in terms of function and appearance; one of their patients suffered from arthrogryposis. More recently, Reinke & Carpenter (1997) reported that Ilizarov applications in the paediatric foot achieved satisfactory results in 21 of 24 feet; three of their patients suffered from arthrogryposis.

The more rare congenital vertical talus is approached through a Cincinnati incision, allowing a posterior release, reduction of the talo-navicular dislocation and lengthening of the tight lateral structures. The corrected position is held with K wires. This operation produces a satisfactory stiff plantigrade foot for walking. Again, there is no urgency to rush into operation, because the child can stand very well on a rocker-bottomed foot and, if necessary, the operation can be deferred until other procedures on the hip and knee have been carried out.

The knee

The knee presents with one of two problems: either severe fixed flexion (see Fig. 19.1) or fixed extension. Both deformities should be treated initially by repeated stretching and splintage, supervised by the physiotherapists. Surprisingly good results can be obtained in apparently rigid deformities. If the deformity does not respond to soft-tissue stretching, surgery must be considered (Murray & Fixsen 1997). It is most important to plan surgery for the knee in relation to treatment of the foot. If the foot requires immobilisation with the knee flexed, then attempts to straighten a flexed knee should wait until the foot has been treated. Conversely, if the knee is in fixed extension, it is often better to correct the knee extension before operation on the foot, so that the foot can be immobilised with a flexed knee.

In general, most joints in arthrogryposis have a fixed arc of movement, and the aim of surgery is to transfer that arc into the most useful range, rather than hoping to gain a significant improvement. Although, occasionally, there is a very gratifying improvement in the overall range, the main aim of treatment is to convert, for instance, a range of movement at the knee from fixed flexion of 90° with further flexion to 130°, to a range of flexion from 5° to 45° – a much more useful range for walking and sitting. The operation for fixed flexion involves an extensive posterior release of all the soft-tissue structures except the neurovascular bundle at the back of the knee. Usually, it is not possible to use a tourniquet, because of the small size of the child's leg. It is essential to divide all the structures that are tight. Medial and lateral incisions, rather than a midline longitudinal incision, should be used, to minimise problems with wound healing when the knee is extended. The heads of the gastrocnemii and the posterior capsule of the knee joint usually constitute the cause of significant deformity, and should be divided. Sometimes the posterior cruciate has to be released. Instability is rarely a problem, because these joints are inherently stiff and the patient will have to wear an orthosis for many years to maintain correction. It is often impossible to extend the knee fully immediately, because of the tightness of the neurovascular bundle; serial plasters over a period of weeks will slowly bring the knee out to the required extension. Once this is gained, splintage for many years is necessary to maintain knee extension. Sometimes, in older children who have not had early soft-tissue surgery, it is not possible to extend the knee without jeopardising the blood supply to the lower leg. In this situation, shortening of the lower end of the femur to produce relative lengthening of the soft tissues can be used to obtain full extension at the knee. Occasionally, if there is gross bony deformity at the knee, fusion to correct the deformity may be considered. It is extremely tempting to consider supracondylar osteotomy to obtain correction and ease the problem of the soft tissues. Unfortunately unless this is delayed until near maturity, the patient may develop, with growth, an extremely ugly and awkward angular deformity at the site of the osteotomy. In general, osteotomies for the correction of deformity in arthrogryposis should be delayed until near maturity, to avoid progressive or recurrent deformity.

Fixed hyperextension of the knee may respond remarkably well to serial stretching and splintage. If there is no response to conservative treatment, a quadricepsplasty comprising an extensive dissection of the scarred and fibrotic quadriceps muscle is necessary to obtain some flexion at the knee. Long-term splintage is likely to be necessary to protect and support the knee after this type of surgery.

The Ilizarov apparatus would appear to be an attractive alternative to difficult surgery with a high recurrence rate in the knee. However, Damsin & Trousseau (1996) and Brunner et al (1997) point out the difficulties and high recurrence rate, particularly in younger children, with this method. Nevertheless, it provides a useful alternative to surgery after failed physiotherapy, particularly in the older patient or the patient in whom previous surgery has failed.

The hip

Frequently, one or both hips are dislocated. The clinical diagnosis can be very difficult. The general stiffness of the joints may make it impossible to perform the clinical tests for hip instability. There is often marked limitation of abduction, and a radiograph or ultrasound of the hips is necessary to decide whether they are displaced. If the hips are dislocated, they are rarely reducible on abduction, and should not be splinted if irreducible. Splinting an unreduced hip is liable to cause avascular necrosis. If one hip is reduced and the other dislocated, it is worth surgically reducing the dislocated hip. If both hips are dislocated, Lloyd-Roberts & Lettin (1970) advised that they should be left alone, as it was rarely possible to get a satisfactory result on both sides and the complication rate, particularly stiffness and recurrent dislocation, was high. In 1987, Staheli et al reported a small series of patients in whom reduction through the medial approach before the age of 1 year had been successful. Szoke et al (1996) have reported the early results of the medial approach in 25 hips, seven of which were unilateral and nine bilateral. The majority of these operations were undertaken in children younger than 1 year. In this series Szoke and colleagues reported only one redislocation and two cases of increased stiffness. In contrast, Akazawa et al (1998) recommend an extensive anterolateral approach to the hip, and report satisfactory results in a small series of patients followed for a mean of 11.8 years. In the author's small experience of the medial approach, when successful, this does not appear to cause increased stiffness, but redislocation can occur, particularly if the hip is very dysplastic. Experience of extensive open reduction with femoral shortening has not always produced a stable, mobile hip. Adult patients with arthrogryposis and bilateral stable but completely dislocated hips tend to manage very well, and the penalties for failing to treat bilateral dislocations successfully on both sides remain high.

Apart from dislocation, the hips may be fixed in a very awkward frog or 'Buddha' position of abduction and external rotation (Fig. 19.3). Fortunately, the conservative measures for the deformities in the lower limb distal to the hip, such as the plasters and splintage necessary for treating the feet and knees, help to stretch the hips, making it unnecessary to perform soft-tissue release or corrective osteotomies to bring the hips into a neutral position. Fixed flexion of the hips is very common. It may require release, but when combined with some flexion at the knee it is often best left alone. As always in arthrogryposis, it is important to consider the treatment of the whole limb, and not a single joint in isolation.

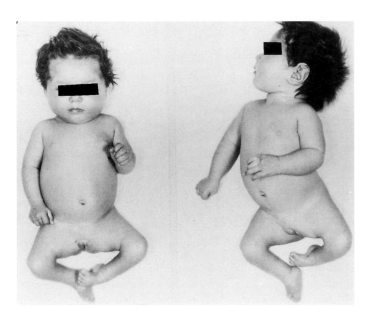

Figure 19.3 Child showing the flexed abducted hips and flexed knees of the so-called 'Buddha position'.

ORTHOPAEDIC MANAGEMENT OF THE UPPER LIMBS

As stated in the introduction, because of the complex inter-actions of all the deformities in the upper limb and the child's ability to develop remarkable trick movements, surgery should be considered very carefully, and probably delayed at least until the child is aged about 4 years (Axt et al 1997). Physiotherapy has a major role in obtaining as much movement as possible at the joints, especially in the fingers and wrists, where stretching and night splintage in the first year of life can be very helpful. Careful assessment by a skilled physiotherapist or occupational therapist should always be undertaken before making decisions about surgery.

The shoulder

Weakness around the shoulder is very common. The charac-teristic position is adduction and internal rotation (see Fig. 19.1). Surgical intervention is rarely indicated, although a simple external rotation osteotomy of the upper humerus will bring the hand and forearm into a more useful func-tional position.

The elbow

At the elbow, the two common positions are fixed extension with little or no flexion (see Fig. 19.1) and fixed flexion with little or no extension. Both deformities respond quite well to physiotherapy, but surgery may have to be considered once the child is established in walking. Activities such as using crutches and reaching the perineum for toileting require active extension of the elbow. The same applies to the ability to push oneself out of a chair, and so it is very important not to jeopardise active extension in the elbows by surgery designed to improve active flexion. If it is clear, once the

child is walking, that it would be valuable to increase flexion in the elbow, there are three methods of gaining active flexion once passive flexion has been achieved.

Passive flexion is achieved by a posterior release of the elbow, lengthening the triceps, releasing the posterior capsule and the collateral ligaments. This can be a very rewarding procedure and produces a useful arc of movement that allows the child to get their hand to their mouth without losing too much extension. Many children find that they can use passive flexion extremely well, and do not particularly want to have an operation to provide active flexion if it means that they will lose active extension.

Once a reasonable range of passive flexion has been established, active motor power can be provided in the following ways:

1. If the forearm flexors and extensors are sufficiently strong, a Steindler flexorplasty advancing the flexor origin up the humerus, and reinforcing this if necessary by advancing the extensor origin, is satisfactory. The problem with this operation is that, often, the muscles are not sufficiently strong to give useful flexion, and it may adversely affect the function of the fingers and wrist.
2. Triceps transfer was popularised by Williams (1985). In this operation, the triceps tendon is transferred to the radius, and is a very strong active flexor. However, there is loss of active extension, which could be devastating for those patients requiring crutches or to push out of a wheelchair. A troublesome complication is increasing fixed flexion, which may develop with time after this transfer.
3. Pectoralis major transfer can be used. Unfortunately, the biceps tendon is often not present and in this situation a modified Clark type of transfer (Lloyd-Roberts & Lettin 1970) will be necessary. This requires mobilising the pectoralis major low down on the chest wall, and produces an extensive and unsightly scar. In practice, many patients find that the passive range of flexion after release of the elbow posteriorly is sufficient, and do not wish to have a further muscle transfer to gain active flexion, because this frequently means the loss of active extension.

The wrist and hand

The wrist is frequently fixed in flexion, and the fingers curved and relatively immobile (Fig. 19.4). Manipulation and splintage in the first year of life can produce remarkable improvement in the range of movement. The thumb is often adducted, and should be stretched out of the palm. Operations to correct wrist deformity have been described, such as partial or complete carpectomy or a dorsal wedge carpectomy. However, with growth, recurrence is very common. Fortunately, the flexed position of the wrist is very functional in these children, and often an advantage rather than a disadvantage.

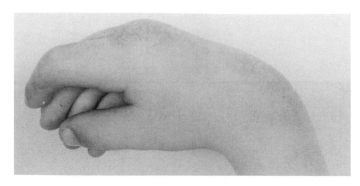

Figure 19.4 This shows a typical hand and wrist position, with flexion of the wrist, stiff, flexed fingers and adducted thumbs

as hooks and 'hangers' on which articles can be hung and manipulated.

At or near maturity, wrist arthrodesis can be considered both for functional and cosmetic gain but, as in rheumatoid arthritis, it is usually wise to fix the wrist in a slight degree of flexion, rather than extension.

These patients cause great distress to their parents when they are born because of their appearance. It is important in the early stages to counsel parents carefully and to be cautious about prognosis until the possible causes of the condition have been elucidated. Those patients who have the classical type of arthrogryposis (amyoplasia congenita) are usually delightful children who are a pleasure to treat because they try so hard and are so adept at finding ways round their physical disabilities. There is a tendency for deformity to recur throughout growth and, as a result, long-term splintage and orthoses are frequently necessary. However, the classical form of the condition is non-progressive, and there is no disorder of sensation, so that the children benefit significantly from surgery and will remain active in adult life.

It is extremely difficult to improve finger function, because of the basic stiffness of the fingers, and operations are rarely indicated. Release of the thumb adductors and enlargement of the first web space can be useful to correct the 'thumb in palm' deformity. These patients become extremely adept at using their stiff, flexed fingers and hands

REFERENCES AND FURTHER READING

Akazawa H, Mitani S, Yoshitaka T, Asaumi K, Inoue H 1998 Surgical management of hip dislocation in children with arthrogryposis multiplex congenita. Journal of Bone and Joint Surgery 80B: 636–640

Axt M W, Niethard F U, Doderlein L, Weber M 1997 Principles of treatment of the upper extremity in arthrogryposis multiplex congenita type 1. Journal of Pediatric Orthopaedics B6: 179–185

Brunner R, Hefti F, Tgetgel J D 1997 Arthrogrypotic joint contracture of the knee and the foot: correction with a circular frame. Journal of Pediatric Orthopaedics B6: 192–197

Damsin J-P, Trousseau A 1996 Treatment of severe flexion deformity of the knee in children and adolescence using the Ilizarov technique. Journal of Bone and Joint Surgery 78B: 140–144

D'Souza H, Aroojis A, Chawara G S 1998 Talectomy in arthrogryposis: analysis of results. Journal of Pediatric Orthopaedics 18: 760–764

Green A D L, Fixsen J A, Lloyd-Roberts G C 1984 Talectomy for arthrogryposis multiplex congenita. Journal of Bone and Joint Surgery 66B: 697–699

Grill F, Franke J 1987 The Ilizarov distractor for the correction of relapsed or neglected clubfoot. Journal of Bone and Joint Surgery 69B: 593–597

Hall J G 1985 Genetic aspects of arthrogryposis multiplex congenita. Clinical Orthopaedics and Related Research 194: 44–53

Hall J G 1998 Overview of arthrogryposis. In: Staheli L T, Hall J G, Jaffe K M, Paholke D O (eds) Arthrogryposis: a text atlas, ch. 1. Cambridge University Press, Cambridge, pp 1–25

Hall J G, Reed S D, Greene G 1982 The distal arthrogryposis; delineation of new entities: review and nosologic discussion. American Journal of Medical Genetics 11: 185–239

Hsu L C S, Jaffray D, Leong J C 1984 Talectomy for club foot in arthrogryposis. Journal of Bone and Joint Surgery 66B: 694–696

Lloyd-Roberts G C, Lettin A W F 1970 Arthrogryposis multiplex congenita. Journal of Bone and Joint Surgery 52B: 494–508

Murray C, Fixsen J A 1997 Management of knee deformity in classical arthrogryposis multiplex congenita (amyoplasia congenita). Journal of Pediatric Orthopaedics B6: 186–191

Otto A W 1841 Monstrum humanum extremitatibus incurvatus. Monstrorum sexcentorum descriptio anatomica in Vratislaviae Museum. Anatomico-Pathologieum, Breslau, p 322

Palmer P M, MacEwen G D, Bowen J R, Matheus P A 1985 Passive motion therapy for infants with arthrogryposis. Clinical Orthopaedics and Related Research 194: 54–59

Reinke K A, Carpenter C T 1997 Ilizarov applications in the paediatric foot. Journal of Pediatric Orthopaedics 17: 796–802

Robinson R O 1990 Arthrogryposis multiplex congenita: feeding, language and other health problems. Neuropaediatrics 21: 177–178

Robinson R O, Cartwright R, Fixsen J A, Jones M 1992 Arthrogryposis. In: McCarthy G T (ed) Physical disability in childhood. Churchill Livingstone, Edinburgh, London, New York

Sheldon W 1932 Amyoplasia congenita (multiple congenital articular rigidity; arthrogryposis multiplex congenita). Archives of Disease in Childhood 7: 117–136

Staheli L T, Chew D E, Elliott J S, Mosea V S 1987 Management of hip dislocation in children with arthrogryposis. Journal of Pediatric Orthopaedics 7: 681–685

Staheli L T, Hall J G, Jaffe K M, Paholke D 1998 Arthrogryposis: a text atlas. Cambridge University Press, Cambridge

Szoke G, Staheli L T, Jaffe K, Hall J G 1996 Medial approach open reduction of hip dislocation in amyoplasia type arthrogryposis. Journal of Pediatric Orthopaedics 16: 127–130

Williams P F 1985 Management of upper limb problems in arthrogryposis. Clinical Orthopaedics and Related Research 194: 60–67

Wynne-Davies R, Williams P F, O'Connor J C B 1981 The 1960's epidemic of arthrogryposis multiplex congenita. A survey from the United Kingdom, Australia and the United States of America. Journal of Bone and Joint Surgery 63B: 76–82

Section IV
Regional disorders

Chapter 20   The upper limb

PART 1 Developmental anomalies of the hand
P. Burge

INCIDENCE

A large study of limb reduction defects in British Columbia gave an incidence of 5.97 per 10 000 live births, with 75% affecting the upper limb (Froster-Iskenius & Baird 1989). Half the cases had associated abnormalities, mostly in the musculoskeletal system, but defects of other organ systems were also common.

LIMB DEVELOPMENT

The upper limb bud appears towards the end of the 4th week and is fully differentiated by the end of the 7th week of intrauterine growth. The developing limb bud is a core of mesenchymal tissue covered with ectoderm. A thickening of the ectoderm, the apical ectodermal ridge (AER), controls the development of the underlying progress zone, an area of undifferentiated mesenchymal tissue. A group of cells at the posterior border of the progress zone constitutes the zone of polarising activity (ZPA). Growth and differentiation of the limb bud are influenced by signals from the AER and ZPA. The AER determines limb outgrowth in a proximal to distal direction by sending signals to the progress zone; its removal results in truncation of the limb. Ectodermal tissue also controls dorsoventral patterning of the limb. The ZPA determines differentiation in the anteroposterior axis. Transplantation of the ZPA to the anterior aspect of the AER of another limb bud produces a symmetric duplication that imitates the rare human malformation of mirror hand. Genes such as sonic hedgehog (SHH) and several fibroblast growth factors are intimately involved in controlling growth of the limb bud.

  The study of developmental biology may eventually explain the occurrence of congenital anomalies of the upper limb, but the cause of most malformations is unknown at present. Genes associated with some inherited anomalies have been localised (e.g. Holt–Oram syndrome, triphalangeal thumb) (Zguricas et al 1998). Many anomalies that are sporadic and unilateral may be the result of vascular or other insults to the limb at a crucial stage of development. The developing limb bud is sensitive to teratogenic agents. The variety of defects that may be produced by a single agent probably reflects the critical effect of timing and concentration on the interaction between components of the limb bud during development. Conversely, defects that are superficially similar, such as transverse deficiencies, may have different causes. For the present, we remain unable to identify the cause of isolated defects or to relate clinical classification to developmental mechanisms.

CLASSIFICATION

The classification adopted by the International Federation for Societies for Surgery of the Hand is widely used (Swanson et al 1983), although some malformations do not sit easily in a system that attempts to give embryological explanations for abnormalities that at present have only morphological descriptions. The classification divides malformations into seven categories. The list below shows how the anomalies described in this chapter fit into the classification:

1. **Failure of formation of parts**
   Transverse arrest
   Proximal forearm
   Digital absence
   Symbrachydactyly
   Longitudinal arrest
   Radial dysplasia
   Ulnar dysplasia
   Cleft hand
   Intercalated defects (phocomelia)

2. **Failure of differentiation (separation) of parts**
   Soft tissue involvement
   Syndactyly
   Clasped thumb
   Absent finger extensors
   Windblown hand
   Camptodactyly
   Trigger digits
   Skeletal involvement
   Radio-ulnar synostosis
   Radial head dislocation
   Clinodactyly

Kirner deformity
Triphalangeal thumb
Congenital tumorous conditions
Neurofibromatosis
Hereditary multiple exostoses

3. **Duplication**
Thumb
Post-axial polydactyly

4. **Overgrowth**
Macrodactyly

5. **Undergrowth**

6. **Congenital constriction band syndrome**

7. **Generalized abnormalities and syndromes**
Madelung's deformity

GENERAL PRINCIPLES OF MANAGEMENT

AIMS OF TREATMENT

The primary aim of treatment of congenital hand anomalies is to achieve the best possible function. Cosmesis is sometimes an indication for operation, but it should not be achieved at the expense of function.

The main requirements for function of the hand are *control of its position* in space, *sensate skin* and motor activity sufficient for *power grasp* and *precision handling*. The function of congenitally deficient hands is remarkable when compared with that of hands that have suffered anatomically similar defects as a result of trauma, because the developing brain 'grows up' with the defective hand and learns the most effective pattern of control. However, the functional needs of the small child are not those of the adult. When considering treatment, we need to consider the future needs of the patient and should aim to maximise function and the options for employment in the longer term. In unilateral defects, regardless of their severity, the presence of a normal limb ensures that most daily activities can be completed without assistance. However, the presence of a simple pinch or grasp in the abnormal limb confers the great benefit of *bimanual* activity and should be provided if possible. Bilateral defects impair function much more severely and consequently justify more extensive procedures.

A sympathetic approach to parents and a realistic prognosis are important aspects of general management. An early consultation with the team responsible for management can do much to allay anxiety and reduce feelings of guilt (Kay 1999). Genetic counselling may be required, and parents should be informed about support groups for patients and their families. Referral to a paediatrician may be appropriate, to exclude anomalies in other systems. Parents should be helped to understand the limitations of surgical reconstruction. It is seldom possible to replace what is missing, only to rearrange what remains. Videotapes of postoperative cases or, even better, meeting a patient with a similar problem, may help them to understand what surgery will achieve.

TIMING

Reconstruction of congenital hand anomalies should, when possible, be completed before school age, bearing in mind that more than one operation is often required. Oedema distal to a constriction band may require operation during the neonatal period. Early surgery (between 6 and 12 months) is needed in those conditions liable to cause progressive deformity (radial dysplasia, syndactyly between digits of different length).

FAILURE OF FORMATION

TRANSVERSE ABSENCE

Proximal forearm
The most common site of terminal transverse absence is the upper one-third of the forearm. It is usually sporadic, not associated with other anomalies and more common on the left side. A light plastic prosthesis fitted in the first few months of life improves cosmesis and accustoms the child to wearing a prosthesis. At about 18 months of age, a gripping device such as a split hook operated by a motivating cord and loop from the opposite shoulder can be fitted. Training in its use by a therapist, regular review, and support of the parents are essential at this stage. When the child has reached the age of $3\frac{1}{2}$ years, a myoelectric prosthesis operated by electrical impulses generated in the forearm muscles may be fitted. Small children can learn to make excellent functional use of a myoelectric prosthesis.

Transverse absence at the level of the carpus is consistent with useful manipulative function using the mobile proximal carpal row, which is usually present. A prosthesis interferes with sensibility and impairs function, but may be worn for cosmesis on social occasions.

Digital absence
Transverse absence of digits is seen in three situations:

1. Transverse absence.
2. Symbrachydactyly.
3. Congenital constriction band syndrome.

The term symbrachydactyly describes a type of terminal absence characterised by digital nubbins containing rudimentary nails that may retain connections to tendons, causing the nubbins to retract with active movement (Fig. 20.1). The appearance suggests an intercalary defect in which the skeleton has failed to develop, leading to secondary failure of development of the soft tissues. Whether this anomaly is truly different from simple transverse absence is unknown. Symbrachydactyly shows a teratogenic sequence that ranges from simple shortness of the middle phalanges to absence of all phalanges, with short metacarpals. The index, middle and ring fingers are most severely affected, and the thumb least affected. Absence of the central digits gives the appearance formerly termed 'atypical cleft hand'.

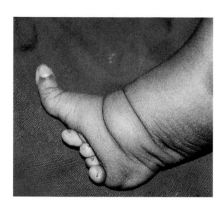

Figure 20.1
Symbrachydactyly.

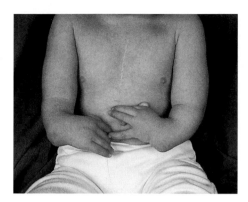

Figure 20.2
Bilateral radial absence with floating thumbs. Note the median sternotomy scar.

Four types of symbrachydactyly are recognised:

1. Short finger type.
2. Cleft hand type.
3. Monodactylous type; a hypoplastic thumb is the only digit.
4. Absence of all five digital rays.

Most cases are unilateral and sporadic. Tendons, nerves and arteries that are useful for reconstruction are usually present in the more distal lesions.

Absence of one or two fingers is consistent with good function. In more extensive anomalies, the aim should be to provide a basic type of grasp. This requires a minimum of two digits, at least one of which must be mobile. Therefore, if a single digit is present, every attempt should be made to provide another digit or post for opposition. Lengthening a short metacarpal or deepening the first web may give side-to-side pinch. Short digits may be lengthened by transfer of toe phalanges, which are more likely to grow if they are transferred extraperiosteally as non-vascularised grafts before the age of 15 months. Microvascular transfer of a second toe is feasible if suitable nerves and tendons can be found in the hand. Loss of the second toe is functionally and cosmetically acceptable. Transfer of one or both second toes can greatly improve function of the severely deficient hand (Kay & McGuiness 1999).

LONGITUDINAL ABSENCE

Radial dysplasia

Radial dysplasia is the most common form of longitudinal deficiency. This ugly deformity results from complete or partial absence of the radius, but the deficiency affects many other tissues in the limb. Although many cases are sporadic, there are important *associations with anomalies in other organ systems*, especially the haemopoietic and cardiovascular systems (Fig. 20.2), which may influence surgical management:

1. *Thrombocytopenia-absent radius (TAR) syndrome* (the thumbs are present whereas they are often absent in other forms of severe radial dysplasia). Thrombocytopenia is usually transient in this autosomal recessive disorder.

2. *Fanconi anaemia* is an autosomal recessive progressive pancytopenia of childhood in which the cells exhibit extreme chromosomal instability.
3. *The Holt–Oram syndrome* is an autosomal dominant disorder that includes radial dysplasia (often comprising triphalangeal thumb) and cardiac anomalies such as septal defects and Fallot's tetralogy.
4. *VACTERL* is a mnemonically useful acronym for vertebral anomalies, anal atresia, cardiac malformations, tracheoesophageal fistula, renal anomalies and limb anomalies (humeral hypoplasia and radial aplasia).

There are also many rare syndromes that may be associated with radial dysplasia (see Online Mendelian Inheritance in Man at www3.ncbi.nlm.nih.gov/omim/).

The skeletal deficiency ranges from mild shortening to absence of the radius. The forms of radial dysplasia are classified as:

- Type 1: short distal radius
- Type 2: hypoplastic radius
- Type 3: partial absence of radius
- Type 4: absent radius.

In cases of complete absence of the radius, the ulna is bowed and typically grows to only 60% of the length of the normal ulna (Fig. 20.3). The carpus articulates with the radial aspect of the distal ulna. The scaphoid and trapezium may be absent. Muscle anomalies tend to be proportional to the skeletal deficiency and chiefly affect the radial side of the limb. The radial flexor and extensor muscles of the wrist are often fused and insert into the carpus via a short tendon. Extensor tendons of the index and middle fingers may be absent or show abnormal insertions. The superficial radial nerve is absent, being represented by a radial branch of the median nerve. The median nerve itself is abnormally situated and at risk of operative injury, lying just beneath the deep fascia on the radial side of the forearm. The radial artery is absent; the hand is supplied by the ulnar artery, which is usually normal, and by the anterior interosseous artery.

The thumb may be absent or hypoplastic. The index and middle fingers often show hypoplasia, contractures and stiffness, reflecting the deficiency that extends widely across the radial side of the limb. The ring and little fingers usually

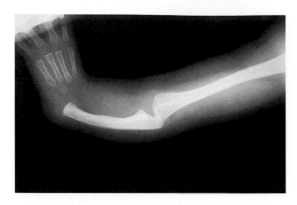

Figure 20.3 Radiograph of radial absence. The ulna is bowed and the thumb is absent.

have normal movement and the child may prefer them for manipulation. The elbow may lack passive flexion at birth, but the range usually improves with growth. However, bilateral lack of elbow flexion is a contraindication to centralisation of the carpus, as the hands may then fail to reach the mouth.

The deformity of radial absence is very unattractive. The power of the finger muscles is dissipated by instability at the wrist. Centralisation of the carpus gives a marked aesthetic improvement and also increases function (Lamb et al 1997).

In the management of the newborn child, other anomalies should be excluded and fixed contractures prevented until centralisation can be performed at the age of 6 months. In most cases of radial absence, the deformity is passively correctable at birth. Regular stretching should be instituted as soon as possible. After each feed, gentle traction and ulnar deviation is applied. Splintage is difficult to maintain in the neonate, but may be useful in the older infant. If the deformity is not correctable, distraction lengthening may be necessary before centralisation.

The surgical treatment of radial absence has a long history, but modern efforts concentrate on centring the carpus on the ulna. Two operations are in common use: *centralisation* places the distal ulna in a slot cut into the carpus (Lamb et al 1997) (Fig. 20.4A); in *radialisation*, the carpus is mobilised extensively and the ulna is placed beneath the radial aspect of the carpus, to maximise the moment arm of the muscles on the ulnar side (Buck-Gramcko 1985) (Fig. 20.4B). Re-balancing the deforming forces by shortening the extensor carpi ulnaris tendon and transferring the deforming radial wrist muscles to the ulnar side of the wrist are essential components of each procedure. In each case, the position is maintained by a longitudinal pin (Fig. 20.5). Osteotomy of a bowed ulna may be performed at the same time. Great care must be taken to avoid damage to the distal ulnar epiphysis and its blood supply. Radialisation requires that the deformity be correctable, and is best performed when the child is aged between 6 and 12 months. Some useful wrist motion is retained from the neutral position into flexion (Fig. 20.6). The skeletal shortening of

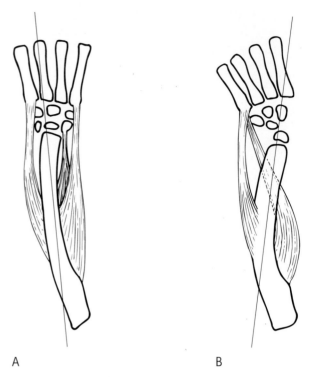

A   B

Figure 20.4 A 'Centralisation' of the carpus. **B** 'Radialisation' of the carpus, preserving carpal bones.

centralisation allows correction of fixed deformities and is more appropriate for older children or those with fixed deformity. Although the aim of centralisation is to maintain some motion between carpus and ulna, long-term maintenance of correction is often associated with spontaneous ulno-carpal fusion. The wrist is stiff, but there may be a little motion at the carpo-metacarpal joints. Skeletal distraction with an external fixation device is being used increasingly to correct fixed deformities before radialisation or centralisation. It appears to be a useful technique, but greater experience is necessary before its place can be defined.

The pin is removed some months later. If necessary, pollicisation of the index finger is performed at a later stage. The wrist is splinted full-time for several months, and at night until skeletal maturity. There is a tendency for radial deviation to recur in some cases, although seldom to the original position. Improved alignment and stability of the wrist appear to improve function in the long term (Lamb et al 1997).

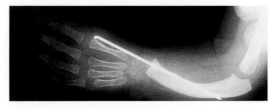

Figure 20.5 Radiograph after radialisation of the carpus.

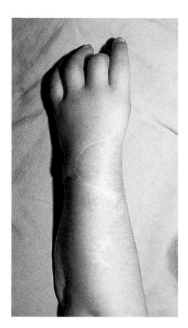

Figure 20.6 Appearance of the forearm 3 years after radialisation.

The complications of centralisation and radialisation include premature closure of the distal ulnar epiphysis, pin breakage and recurrent deformity.

Ulno-carpal fusion may be needed at or near skeletal maturity in cases of persistent deformity or instability. Distraction lengthening of the ulna has been undertaken, but it is questionable whether the gain in length justifies the high complication rate.

Ulnar dysplasia

Ulnar dysplasia is much less common than radial dysplasia. Most cases are sporadic, but may be associated with lower limb anomalies such as fibular deficiency (Schmidt & Neufeld 1998). Unlike radial dysplasia, in ulnar dysplasia associated anomalies in other organ systems are uncommon. *Ulnar dysplasia is classified* thus:

- Type 1: hypoplastic ulna
- Type 2: partial absence of ulna
- Type 3: absent ulna
- Type 4: absent ulna and radio-humeral synostosis.

Hypoplasia of the ulna is associated with bowing of the radius and dislocation of the radial head, but the carpus is supported by the radius and does not show the acute angulation that characterises radial dysplasia (Fig. 20.7).

Deficiencies in the hand tend to be more extensive in ulnar dysplasia than in radial dysplasia (Cole & Manske 1997). Multiple digital absence, syndactyly and camptodactyly are common, but there is no correlation between the extent of hand deformity and the degree of ulnar deficiency.

The main determinants of functional impairment are the severity of the hand deformity and elbow stiffness, rather than bowing of the forearm. Management of the hand deformities may include release of syndactyly and correction of first web-space contractures. Progressive forearm bowing has been treated by excising the fibrous anlage of the ulna, but its value is unclear. Severe instability of the forearm can

Figure 20.7 Ulnar hypoplasia. **A** The ulna is terminally deficient and three rays are absent. **B** The forearm is bowed to the ulnar side.

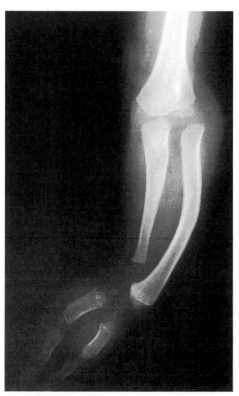

A

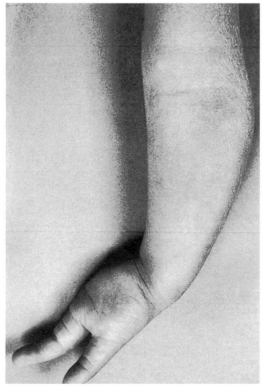

B

be corrected, at the expense of rotation, by creating a one-bone forearm, fusing the ulna proximally to the radius distally. Some patients with associated radio-humeral synostosis have a severe internal rotation or adduction deformity that may be improved by humeral osteotomy.

Cleft hand

Cleft hand is characterised by a central V-shaped cleft, with absence of one or more digits. Unlike radial and ulnar dysplasia, it is not accompanied by deficiency in the forearm. In the past, cleft hand has been grouped with other causes of central deficiency such as symbrachydactyly. True cleft hand is often familial, bilateral and associated with cleft feet. Inheritance is autosomal dominant with variable penetrance. Cleft hand may be part of syndromes such as EEC (ectrodactyly, ectodermal dysplasia, and cleft lip/palate) and the split hand/split foot malformation (SHSM).

The depth of the cleft varies from absence of the phalanges only to a deep cleft extending into the carpus. Syndactyly between the border digits (thumb/index and ring/little) and contracture of the thumb web are common (Fig. 20.8). Skeletal remnants of the missing rays may be aligned transversely or fused with adjacent bones. The term 'lobster claw hand' is disliked by patients and their families: *cleft hand* is neutral and more accurate.

Flatt (1994) has stated that the typical cleft hand is 'a functional triumph and a social disaster'. Functional impairment results more from syndactyly and thumb web contracture than from the cleft itself. Border syndactyly should be released by the age of 6 months, before unequal growth can produce angular deformity of the longer digit. Early removal of transverse bones that are causing deformity may also be needed. In a typical case of first web contracture and absence of the middle ray, simultaneous closure of the cleft and widening of the thumb web is best performed at around 18 months.

FAILURE OF DIFFERENTIATION

SOFT TISSUE INVOLVEMENT

Syndactyly

Syndactyly is a common congenital anomaly of the hand. It is an example of incomplete differentiation of digital rays, which normally occurs by programmed cell death (apoptosis) of interdigital tissue. The process begins distally and proceeds proximally; its failure leads to partial or complete syndactyly.

Simple syndactyly involves skin and soft tissue; in *complex* syndactyly, the digits are also connected by bone. *Complete* syndactyly extends to the fingertips; *partial* syndactyly does not. In *acrosyndactyly*, which occurs in association with the congenital constriction band syndrome and in cranio-facial anomalies such as Apert's syndrome, short digits are fused at the tips and are often separated proximally by fenestrations.

Syndactyly is seen in association with other hand anomalies, such as ulnar dysplasia, cleft hand, or as a feature in several syndromes (Poland's syndrome, cranio-facial syndromes, constriction band syndrome). Simple syndactyly is inherited in at least 10% of cases, usually as an autosomal dominant trait. In half the cases it is bilateral. The distribution of syndactyly between the digital rays is shown in Fig. 20.9.

In syndactyly there is *always* a shortage of skin (Eaton & Lister 1990). Although it might appear that there is *additional* skin joining the digits, simple geometry shows that 22% *less* skin covers the syndactylised digits than covers the surfaces of two separate fingers. Skin is also deficient transversely in the interdigital web, as may be seen by measuring the distance along the web from the tip of one finger to the tip of its neighbour.

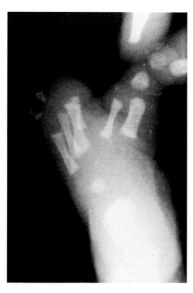

Figure 20.8 Cleft hand with complex syndactyly.

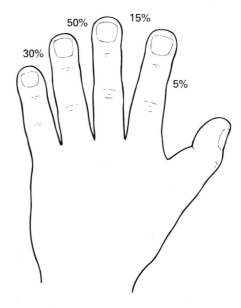

Figure 20.9 The frequency of syndactyly of digital clefts.

Syndactyly between digits of unequal length (thumb/index, ring/little) should be released by the age of 6 months, before unequal growth deforms the longer digit. Otherwise, the timing of release is not critical, but is generally before the age of 3 years. Successful release of syndactyly requires the use of acute zigzag incisions, local flap skin for reconstruction of the web, and full-thickness skin grafts. Skin grafts are best taken from the groin crease, lateral to the femoral pulse (to avoid growth of hair at puberty). If a finger is joined to the digits on both sides, only one surface should be released at one operation.

Congenital clasped thumb

A congenital clasped thumb lies flexed across the palm and cannot be extended actively. Two types of clasped thumb are recognised (McCarroll 1985).

Supple clasped thumb is caused by an isolated deficiency of the thumb extensor tendons. It is often bilateral, and is more common in males. Passive extension is usually normal at birth, but may be lost if the disorder is untreated. The clasped thumb may have loss of extension at the interphalangeal (IP) joint, at the metacarpo-phalangeal (MP) joint, or at both. Differentiation from trigger thumb is straightforward if there is no loss of passive extension. In cases of clasped thumb with flexion contracture, the contracture usually affects the MP joint and other soft tissues, whereas the contracture of trigger finger is confined to the distal joint.

Supple clasped thumb frequently responds to continuous and prolonged splintage in extension, if treatment is started soon after birth. A plaster cast extending to the thumb tip is changed every few weeks to accommodate growth and is retained for 3–6 months. If active extension is not regained, tendon transfer is required.

The term *complex clasped thumb* refers to disorders in which the thumb is part of a more extensive anomaly such as arthrogryposis, thumb hypoplasia, or the Freeman–Sheldon (whistling face) syndrome. The skin, thumb web, adductor pollicis and flexor pollicis longus may require lengthening, in addition to chondrodesis of the MP joint and augmentation of extension by tendon transfer.

The windblown hand

Congenital flexion deformity of the fingers takes several forms and probably has several causes. Less severe types resemble the supple clasped thumb, affecting one or more fingers with deficient active extension but normal passive extension. They are probably due to congenital deficiency of the extensor mechanism, and often respond to prolonged splintage in extension. Reconstruction by tendon transfer is required in some patients.

The combination of flexion contracture of the fingers, ulnar deviation at the MP joints and a flexion/adduction contracture of the thumb is known as 'windblown hand'. It is a feature of distal arthrogryposis and the Freeman–Sheldon (whistling face) syndrome.

Splintage can improve contractures or hold them stable until the child is fit for surgery. Correction of the thumb web contracture is valuable; surgery can improve the fingers, but does not provide full movement. Each component of the deformity requires correction. Releases of skin and fascia at the base of the digits are closed with full-thickness skin grafts. Centralisation of the extensor mechanism at the MP joint requires release of tight ulnar sagittal bands and plication or reconstruction of elongated radial sagittal bands. Release of the thumb web contracture generally creates a defect that requires a transposition flap from the dorsoradial aspect of the index. An unstable thumb MP joint may be stabilised by ligament reconstruction or by chondrodesis. Tendon transfers may augment thumb extension.

Thumb hypoplasia

Hypoplasia of the thumb is frequently associated with radial dysplasia and may, therefore, be accompanied by visceral malformations. The *classification* of Blauth is widely used (Manske & McCarroll 1992):

- Type I: minor hypoplasia, normal function
- Type II: thumb web contracture; thenar muscle hypoplasia; MP joint instability; anomalous flexor tendon
- Type III A: severe skeletal and muscle hypoplasia
            B: + deficient basal joint
- Type IV: floating thumb
- Type V: absent thumb.

Type I hypoplasia is consistent with normal function and requires no treatment. In *type II* (Fig. 20.10), function is impaired by instability of the MP joint, contracture of the thumb web, weakness of opposition and limited motion of the IP joint. Release of the web usually requires lengthening of the web skin by Z-plasty or by a transposition flap from the dorsum of the thumb or index finger. If the ring superficialis tendon is used as an opposition transfer, it may be passed through the metacarpal neck and used to reconstruct the ulnar collateral ligament of the MP joint. Anomalous connections between the long flexor and extensor tendons may limit IP joint flexion or lead to abduction deformity (pollex abductus).

It may be difficult to decide whether a *type III* hypoplastic thumb is worthy of reconstruction (Fig. 20.11), and even

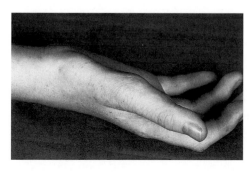

Figure 20.10
Type II hypoplasia of thumb, showing hypoplasia of the thenar muscles.

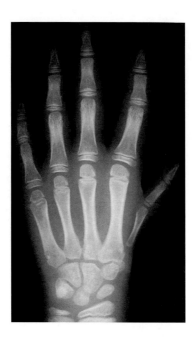

Figure 20.11 Type III hypoplasia of thumb with deficient basal joint.

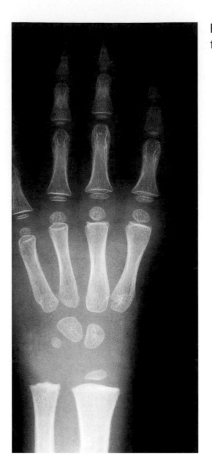

Figure 20.13 Absent thumb.

more difficult to convince parents that it is not. Much depends on the tissues that are available. However, if the basal joint is unstable, pollicisation of the index finger is likely to provide better function.

Attempts at reconstruction of the floating thumb (*type IV*) are fruitless. The digit contains no useful skeleton or tendons and it is attached too far distally and dorsally to be functional (Fig. 20.12). Pollicisation of the index finger provides much better function (Buck-Gramcko 1971). Pollicisation is also the best treatment for the absent thumb (*type V*) (Fig. 20.13). Current techniques of pollicisation are based on the work of many surgeons over the past 50 years, notably Buck-Gramcko (1971). In essence, the index finger is mobilised on its intact digital neurovascular bundles and dorsal veins, excising the shaft of the metacarpal and placing the metacarpal head anterior to the base of the metacarpal. The metacarpal head is sutured into place with the MP joint extended, otherwise the new thumb may exhibit excessive hyperextension at its basal joint. The

digit is rotated 160° into opposition. The first dorsal and first palmar interosseous muscles are sutured into the lateral bands at the level of the proximal interphalangeal (PIP) joint, becoming the short thumb abductor and the adductor pollicis respectively. It is necessary to shorten the extensor tendons, but the flexor tendons will in time accommodate to the shorter skeleton. For the index finger to look like a thumb, skin flaps must be designed so that the new thumb web reaches the digit at the level of the PIP joint (the new MP joint) (Fig. 20.14). When the absent thumb is accompanied by a normal radius, the index finger usually has good musculature and supple joints and will make a satisfactory thumb. The decision to pollicise the index finger should take into account the pattern of prehensile function that the child shows. Children who lack thumbs utilise a 'cigarette' grip between adjacent fingers.

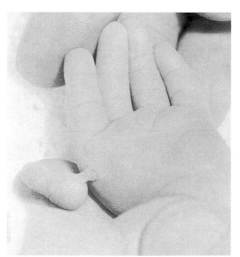

Figure 20.12 Floating thumb (type IV hypoplasia) is not capable of useful reconstruction. It should be excised and replaced by pollicisation of the index finger.

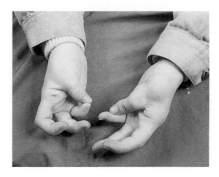

Figure 20.14 Pollicisation of the index fingers for bilateral absent thumb.

When the thumb is missing as part of severe radial dysplasia, the index frequently lacks good motion. Nevertheless, it may still make a satisfactory thumb provided that the child uses the index-middle cleft for prehension. If the child excludes the index finger from hand function, the digit may be ignored after pollicisation.

Camptodactyly

Camptodactyly describes a common painless non-traumatic flexion deformity of the PIP joint, usually affecting the little finger. An autosomal dominant pattern of inheritance is frequently present. Camptodactyly occurs in two age groups that coincide with periods of rapid growth of the hand. In *infants*, it may affect any finger; it is equally common among males and females and it may be associated with other anomalies. In *adolescents*, camptodactyly is more frequent in females and almost invariably affects the little finger. It appears as a fixed flexion contracture of the PIP joint, which is usually at least 30° at the time of presentation (Fig. 20.15). The little finger may adopt the intrinsic-minus posture of hyperextension of the MP joint with increased flexion of the PIP joint when the fingers are extended actively.

Camptodactyly may be distinguished from post-traumatic boutonnière deformity by the absence of swelling and by the presence of full distal joint movement. Ulnar nerve palsy is excluded by the absence of neurological signs.

In an established case of adolescent camptodactyly, examination will demonstrate tightness of the volar PIP joint

capsule, the superficialis tendon and the skin. It is not surprising, therefore, that almost every structure that crosses the palmar aspect of the PIP joint has been implicated in the aetiology of camptodactyly. Imbalance between the extrinsic and the intrinsic muscles of the little finger during periods of growth is the most plausible mechanism. This explanation is consistent with recognised mechanisms of musculoskeletal deformity and is supported by the frequent finding of an abnormal insertion of the lumbrical muscle into the capsule of the MP joint, the superficialis tendon or the extensor expansion of an adjacent finger (McFarlane et al 1992). Shortening of the superficialis muscle is a common, and probably secondary feature that may be demonstrated by the effect of wrist and MP joint position on deformity of the PIP joint.

Treatment

Infancy. As much correction as possible should be obtained by splintage. Static splints such as serial plaster casts are easier to manage at this age than are dynamic splints. Persistent contractures may be managed by release of tight volar soft tissues and tendon transfer to augment extension. However, it may be difficult to restore normal movement. Long-term extension splintage is often required.

Adolescence. It is difficult to restore full extension in adolescent camptodactyly. Static or dynamic splintage, or both, may produce useful improvement, but splintage must be continued until skeletal maturity (Miura et al 1992). As a moderate flexion deformity is consistent with good function, and less disabling than loss of flexion, most patients should be advised to use a splint and accept the deformity unless it is severe or the patient has a specific requirement for good extension. The results of operative treatment of fixed contracture are unsatisfactory. In a series of patients reported by McFarlane et al (1992), contracture was reduced from 49° to 25°, but only one third of patients regained full flexion. Soft-tissue release is contraindicated if there is bony deformity of the PIP joint (Fig. 20.16); dorsal angulation osteotomy through the neck of the proximal phalanx will improve extension at the expense of flexion. The hand of the rare patient who exhibits inadequate active PIP joint extension but who has full passive extension may be improved by transfer of a superficialis tendon or extensor indicis proprius into the extensor mechanism over the PIP joint.

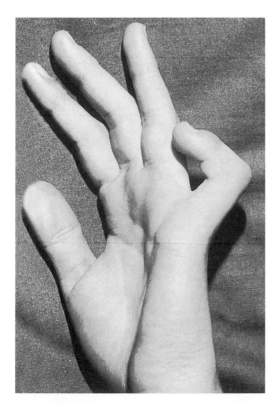

Figure 20.15 Camptodactyly.

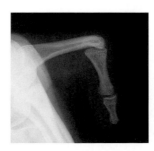

Figure 20.16 Long-standing camptodactyly with secondary deformity of the head of the proximal phalanx, precluding soft-tissue release.

Clinodactyly

The term clinodactyly describes the condition of angulation of a digit to the radial or ulnar side. It occurs in association with a variety of syndromes, but the common isolated form is bilateral radial angulation of the little finger, with autosomal dominant inheritance. Clinodactyly is the result of abnormal growth, usually of the middle phalanx, which may have many causes. Three types of clinodactyly are encountered:

1. Minor angulation, normal length.
2. Minor angulation, short phalanx.
3. Marked angulation, delta phalanx.

Minor degrees of clinodactyly are common, and are consistent with normal function. Corrective osteotomy is indicated if the finger overlaps the adjacent digit on flexion, using a closing wedge osteotomy if the length of the phalanx is normal and an opening wedge if it is short.

Although 'delta' phalanx is named after the triangular Greek letter, the bone is usually trapezoidal. It is a curious anomaly in which the proximal epiphysis extends beyond its normal transverse position to pass along the shorter side of the bone to its distal end (Fig. 20.17). The C-shaped epiphysis effectively constitutes a bony bridge that restricts longitudinal growth and causes progressive angulation. Delta phalanx is frequently found in association with triphalangeal thumb and with polydactyly.

Division of the longitudinal bar and interposition of a free fat graft may permit more normal growth. For later cases, reverse wedge or opening wedge osteotomy is the best option. Great care must be taken to avoid damage to the joint surfaces and to divide the small bone cleanly. The osteotomy is transfixed with a Kirschner wire for 4–6 weeks.

Kirner deformity

In 1927, Kirner described a curvature of the distal phalanx in a radial and palmar direction. It affects females more

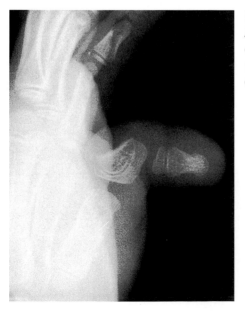

Figure 20.17
Angular deformity of the thumb resulting from a delta phalanx.

commonly than males and may be inherited as an autosomal dominant trait. The onset is between 8 and 12 years, beginning with painless swelling of the distal phalanx and followed by progressive radio-palmar deviation of both little fingers. The age of onset, the presence of swelling and the radiographic appearance of lysis within the growth plate (Fig. 20.18) suggest that the disorder is acquired rather than congenital. Its nature is unknown. A similar deformity may follow epiphyseal damage by frostbite or by an infected open fracture. Severe deformity may be improved by osteotomy of the distal phalanx.

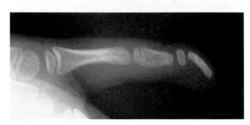

Figure 20.18
Kirner deformity with palmar angulation in the distal phalanx.

Trigger digits

Trigger thumb is the most common hand disorder in children. It presents with painless loss of passive extension of the IP joint. The clicking that characterises trigger thumb in adults is uncommon in children. A nodule may be palpable at the proximal (A1) flexor tendon pulley at the level of the MP joint. It should be distinguished from congenital clasped thumb (see above), in which the deformity usually affects the MP joint.

Trigger thumb is seldom present at birth; no cases were found in a screening study of 4719 neonates (Slakey & Hennrikus 1996). The normal infant tends to hold the thumb flexed into the palm, and it may be some time before the problem is noticed. Approximately 30% of trigger thumbs presenting in infancy resolved spontaneously within 12 months (Dinham & Meggitt 1974). Of those presenting between 6 and 36 months, 12% resolved within 6 months of presentation. A period of observation is appropriate in children presenting in the first year of life. Extension splintage for a mean of 10 months cured 24 of 43 trigger digits in children of average age 2 years, with improvement in seven others (Nemoto et al 1996). If the condition persists, division of the A1 pulley is curative. Permanent IP joint contracture does not seem to occur, provided that the digit is released by the age of 4 years. The skin is incised transversely at the proximal MP joint crease, avoiding the digital nerves that lie immediately beneath the skin. The A1 pulley is incised longitudinally under direct vision, revealing a nodule (Notta's node) or thickening of the flexor tendon. The oblique pulley should be preserved to avoid bowstringing of the flexor tendon.

SKELETAL INVOLVEMENT

Congenital radio-ulnar synostosis

Synostosis may be transverse (e.g. humero-radial synostosis in type IV ulnar dysplasia) or longitudinal. Radio-ulnar synostosis is the most common form (Fig. 20.19). It may be uni-

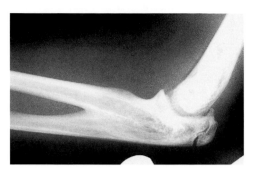

Figure 20.19 Radiograph of congenital radio-ulnar synostosis at the typical proximal site.

lateral or bilateral, and is usually at the proximal end of the forearm. Some compensatory rotation occurs at carpal level.

Disability depends on the rotational alignment of the forearm. Internal rotation and abduction of the shoulder can bring a supinated hand into the palm-down position. Shoulder motion compensates less readily for fixed prona-tion. Unilateral synostosis causes little disability and seldom requires treatment. Bilateral synostoses are often fixed in marked pronation, causing difficulty with accepting coins and holding a glass.

Until recently, attempts to restore rotation had been unsuccessful and operative correction was confined to rota-tional osteotomy, generally through the fusion mass. The technique of Green & Mital (1979) controls alignment with a longitudinal intramedullary pin and rotation with a trans-verse transulnar pin incorporated in a cast. The method allows the correction to be undone easily in the event of neurovascular compromise after surgery. However, Kanaya & Ibaraki (1998) have shown that movement can be restored by excision of the synostosis, interposition of a vascularised fat-fascia flap and relocation of the dislocated radial head by radial shortening osteotomy. A mean of 83° rotation was obtained in four patients.

Congenital radial head dislocation

Dislocation of the radial head may be congenital, traumatic (see Ch. 37) or secondary to diminished growth of the ulna (e.g. ulnar dysplasia, multiple hereditary exostoses). Congenital dislocation is posterior in two thirds of cases; the remainder are lateral or anterior. Differentiation between traumatic and congenital dislocation is sometimes difficult; deformity of the radial head and hypoplasia of the capitellum are features of both types. Dislocation is likely to be congenital if it is bilateral, familial, associated with other malformations, or present in infancy. A healed fracture of the ulna or heterotopic ossification suggests that dislocation was the result of injury.

Congenital dislocation of the radial head is a feature of numerous malformation syndromes, which should be sought during examination. The dislocation causes remarkably little loss of function during childhood, although radial head excision after skeletal maturity may be indicated for pain and prominence of the radial head if these symptoms are clearly attributable to the dislocation.

Dislocation of the radial head is liable to occur whenever growth of the ulna is diminished and radial growth contin-ues. It may be possible to prevent dislocation if the length of the ulna can be maintained by distraction lengthening, with or without radial shortening or epiphyseal stapling. Parents may ask that the radial head be relocated. However, the indi-cation for operative reduction of established congenital radial head dislocation has not been defined. The procedure may involve osteotomy of a bowed ulna and radial shortening in addition to reconstruction of the annular ligament. Considering the minimal symptoms experienced by most patients, such surgery is seldom justified.

DUPLICATION

Duplication may be *radial* (preaxial), *ulnar* (postaxial) or, rarely, *central*. It is probably the most common congenital anomaly in the hand.

Ulnar polydactyly is common as an autosomal recessive con-dition in African Americans, in whom it is seldom associated with other abnormalities. It is 8–10 times less common in white populations, but is more likely to be part of a syndrome.

Radial polydactyly is usually sporadic. Wassel (1969) described a logical classification based on the level of dupli-cation (Fig. 20.20). Almost half the cases are type IV (Fig. 20.21). In types I and II, in which the duplication is symmet-rical, a central wedge may be excised and the defect closed

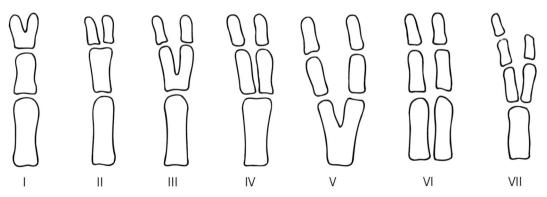

I II III IV V VI VII

Figure 20.20 Wassel classification of thumb duplication. Type IV accounts for almost 50% of cases.

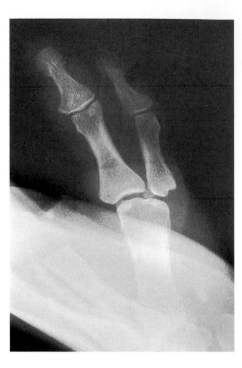

Figure 20.21 Wassel type IV duplication of the thumb.

by apposition of the outer halves of the distal phalanges (Bilhout–Cloquet procedure). Nail-bed deformity and premature epiphyseal closure may mar the final result. Instead of splitting the nail, the entire nail bed may be taken from one thumb and the nail bed of the other discarded.

In considering operative treatment of types III–VII thumb duplication, it is vital to regard the procedure as a reconstruction of a split thumb, and not excision of an extra thumb. A decision on which thumb should be discarded is based on size, deviation, passive joint mobility, stability, and anomalous tendon insertions of the parts. The principles of reconstruction include zigzag incisions (to avoid later scar contracture), preservation or reconstruction of ligaments, alignment of the skeleton and alignment of tendon insertions. It may be necessary to augment the remaining thumb with tissues from the excised segment.

Triphalangeal thumb

Triphalangeal thumb may be part of type VII duplication, when it is an autosomal dominant condition, or an isolated anomaly. The additional bone is interposed between the distal and proximal phalanges. It may be a normal phalanx, a short phalanx or a delta phalanx. As a result, the thumb may be too long, angulated or both. The metacarpal may also be too long.

Triphalangeal thumb is consistent with good function, but many fine precision activities are hampered by excessive length. Excision of a delta phalanx should be performed as early as possible and the soft tissues of the IP joint reconstructed. For cases presenting later in childhood, it may be necessary to fuse the distal phalanx to the proximal phalanx after excision of the intervening delta phalanx. Correction of thumb web narrowing and thenar muscle hypoplasia may also be required.

OVERGROWTH

Macrodactyly

Macrodactyly is congenital enlargement of a digit. It is very rare and is not inherited; 90% of cases are unilateral. In 70% of patients, more than one digit is affected and the involvement corresponds with the territory of one or more peripheral nerves, most frequently the median. The enlargement may be present at birth and grow in proportion with other digits, but more commonly it progresses during childhood. Macrodactyly affects all the tissues in a digit and should be distinguished from other causes of enlargement such as haemangioma, arteriovenous malformations and lymphoedema.

Three types of macrodactyly are seen. *Nerve territory orientated macrodactyly* is associated with enlargement or lipofibromatous hamartoma of a peripheral nerve. The peripheral nerve is thickened by infiltration with fat and fibrous tissue; these changes may extend well proximal to the enlargement of other tissues and, in the case of the median nerve, may lead to its compression within the carpal canal. Skin, nerve and bone are affected more than tendon or blood vessels. Less frequently, macrodactyly is associated with *neurofibromatosis*. In the rare *hyperostotic macrodactyly*, osteocartilaginous protuberances arise around the digital joints and limit motion. In addition to the serious cosmetic impairment, these large digits are likely to be stiff, deformed and prone to ulceration.

Treatment of macrodactyly is difficult. Amputation may be appropriate for digits that are severely deformed, stiff, painful or ulcerated. In childhood, cosmetic considerations often demand attempts at reduction procedures, which should be staged to avoid vascular impairment (Tsuge 1985). The blood supply of the skin is relatively poor, and necrosis of skin flaps is a common complication. Longitudinal growth may be controlled by fusion of the phalangeal epiphyses when the digit has reached its expected adult length; however, circumferential growth may continue.

CONSTRICTION BAND SYNDROME

Constriction band syndrome (also known as amniotic band syndrome and Streeter's dysplasia) occurs sporadically at the rate of around 1 in 15 000 live births. It remains uncertain whether the cause is localised failure of mesodermal development or constriction by intrauterine amniotic bands (Miura 1984). The abnormalities are asymmetric and present at birth. Four types of lesion occur:

1. Simple constriction bands.
2. Constriction rings with distal deformity, lymphoedema, or both.
3. Soft-tissue fusion of distal parts (acrosyndactyly).
4. Amputation.

Constriction band syndrome is distinguished from other types of congenital deformity and amputation by the presence of constriction bands, by the multiple asymmetric defects and by the normality of the part proximal to the band. Deep constriction bands may seriously impair vascular supply and innervation; a temperature gradient across the band and distal lymphoedema are signs of vascular impairment.

Circular constricting bands are excised and the circular scar broken up by Z-plasties. Bands that produce severe distal lymphoedema in the neonate may require urgent release. Syndactyly and intrauterine amputations may also need treatment. The normality of proximal nerves, vessels and tendons is a distinct advantage during reconstruction.

MISCELLANEOUS ABNORMALITIES AND SYNDROMES

MADELUNG'S DEFORMITY

Madelung's deformity is a congenital disorder that affects growth of the distal radius; it is usually bilateral. It is seldom evident before the age of 8 years. Females are affected more often than males. The primary abnormality is failure of normal growth of the ulnar and palmar half of the distal radial physis, leading to curvature in an ulnar and palmar direction (Fig. 20.22). A localised area of radiolucency may appear on the ulnar edge of the distal radius, and the ulnar part of the physis fuses prematurely. The ulna is relatively long and becomes prominent dorsally. The carpus sinks, along with the ulnar half of the distal radial articular surface, into the gap between the two forearm bones. Rotation of the forearm is limited by incongruity of the distal radio-ulnar joint.

The cause of Madelung's deformity is unknown. It may be inherited as part of dyschondrosteosis (Leri–Weill disease). Similar deformities may occur in multiple hereditary exostoses, multiple epiphyseal dysplasia and dyschondroplasia (Ollier's disease), or after damage to the distal radial physis by trauma or infection.

Many patients with Madelung's deformity function well and the problem is chiefly cosmetic. Pain may develop at the wrist or distal radio-ulnar joint as the patient approaches skeletal maturity. Pain may improve after skeletal maturity.

During growth, deformity may be controlled or reduced by physiolysis of the volar/ulnar part of the distal radial physis (Vickers & Nielsen 1992). However, experience with this method is limited. Deformity may be improved by radial osteotomy and ulnar shortening (Ranawat et al 1975) or by radial lengthening with the Ilizarov method (de Billy et al 1997). Wrist fusion and operations such as ulnar head excision and the Sauve–Kapandji procedure are salvage options.

Hereditary multiple exostoses

Hereditary multiple exostoses is an autosomal dominant condition resulting from mutations in the *EXT* family of tumour suppressor genes (Porter et al 2000). It should probably be classed as a familial neoplastic trait rather than as a skeletal dysplasia.

Involvement of the forearm may cause swelling, pain, loss of motion and unequal longitudinal growth. Exostoses that affect the radius seldom produce severe angular deformity. However, exostoses of the distal ulna are associated with restricted ulnar growth, leading to bowing of the forearm and, frequently, to dislocation of the radial head. The end result is a short, bowed forearm with loss of rotation. The dislocated radial head is prominent and may be painful.

Excision of exostoses may be indicated to improve appearance and forearm rotation. Because exostosis size is inversely correlated with ulnar length (Porter et al 2000), it would be logical to remove the exostoses as early as possible. However, the effect on growth is not known.

Distraction lengthening of the ulna can help to correct the length discrepancy, improve bowing and maintain length (Fig. 20.23). Monoaxial fixators or small circular frames can be used (Dahl 1993).

Management of established radial head dislocation associated with multiple exostoses is difficult. Relocation of the radial head requires extensive surgery and may fail to provide a congruent joint or satisfactory forearm rotation. If instability of the forearm is a problem, creation of a one-bone forearm between the ulna proximally and the radius distally may be appropriate.

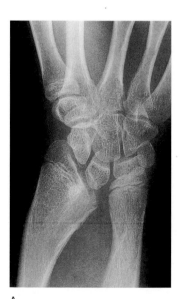

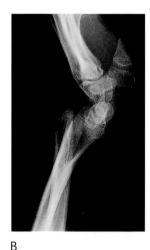

B

A

Figure 20.22 Madelung's deformity. **A** Anteroposterior view: inadequate growth of the ulnar half of the distal radial epiphysis allows the lunate to sink between the forearm bones. **B** Lateral view: the distal radius is angulated palmarwards and the distal ulna is prominent dorsally.

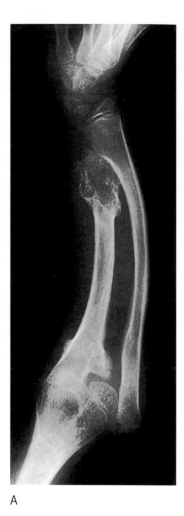
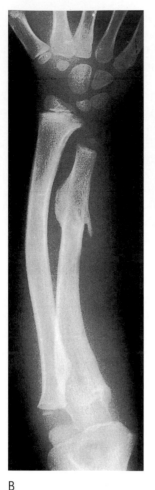
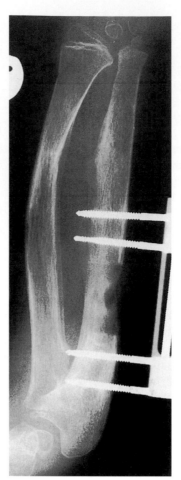

Figure 20.23 A Extensive multiple exostoses associated with diminished growth of the ulna and dislocation of the radial head at the age of 10 years. **B** Distal ulnar exostosis with shortening of the ulna and progressive radial bowing in a boy aged 6 years. The radial head is not dislocated. **C** Lengthening of 2.5 cm was obtained by corticotomy and callus distraction using a monoaxial fixation device. Note over-lengthening of the ulna and early remodelling of the ulnar cortex of the radius.

A   B   C

Congenital pseudarthrosis of the forearm

Congenital pseudarthrosis of the forearm bones is very rare. In many respects it resembles congenital pseudarthrosis of the tibia. One or both bones may be affected (Fig. 20.24). Evidence of neurofibromatosis is present in most cases. Untreated, it produces progressive deformity, instability and loss of rotation. Failure of ulnar growth may lead to dislocation of the radial head.

Conventional orthopaedic techniques such as non-vascularised bone grafts and internal fixation have generally failed to achieve union. Thorough excision of abnormal tissue, free vascularised fibular grafting and stable osteosynthesis offers the best chance of healing. Creation of a one-bone forearm, providing stability at the expense of rotation, is an alternative when only the distal part of the ulna is affected.

Finger-sucking deformities

Radial deviation and supination deformities of the index finger may occur as a result of prolonged finger sucking (Rankin et al 1988) (Fig. 20.25). Deformity is unlikely if the habit ceases by the age of 6 years. Moderate deformities may correct spontaneously once the deforming force is removed. A period of observation of 1–2 years seems appropriate, followed by osteotomy if deformity persists.

Osteochondritis dissecans of the capitellum

This rare lesion presents with aching pain, swelling, clicking and loss of extension of the elbow between the ages of 10 and 14 years. It is much more common in males than females and is frequently bilateral. Repetitive stress in throwing sports has been implicated in the causation. The presenting symptoms are pain, swelling and loss of extension. Initially, the radiographs show irregularity and increase in density of the capitellum; later, lucency and fragmentation are evident. At an early stage, the condition may respond to rest and avoidance of throwing activities. Later, it may produce loose bodies, loss of extension and incongruity of the radio-humeral articulation. Operative treatment is confined to removal of loose bodies.

Arthrogryposis multiplex congenita

Arthrogryposis is derived from the Greek, meaning 'curved joint'. It is a descriptive term for the condition in children presenting with multiple, non-progressive joint contractures at birth. There are at least 150 causes (see Ch. 19).

The typical *clinical* picture comprises multiple contractures of joints in upper and lower limbs. The limbs are atrophic, the skin is waxy and joint creases are absent. Skin dimples may be found over contracted joints. The characteristic

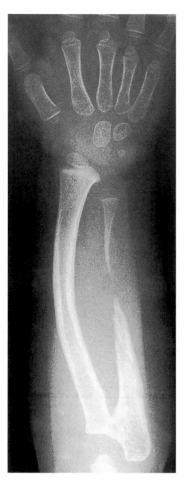

Figure 20.24 Congenital pseudarthrosis of the ulna in a 2-year-old girl with neurofibromatosis.

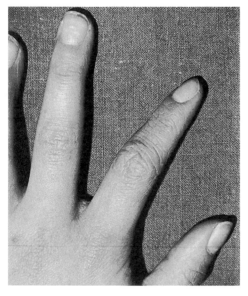

Figure 20.25 Rotational deformity of the index finger caused by finger-sucking.

posture of the upper limbs is shoulder adduction, elbow extension, flexion/ulnar deviation at the wrists, and flexion deformity of the fingers, with flexion/adduction of the thumb (Fig. 20.26).

The *treatment* of arthrogryposis is difficult. As soon as possible after birth, attempts should be made to correct contractures of the hand and wrist by serial splintage and to maintain the correction by static splintage. Correction is usually incomplete. When considering operative correction, provision for independent walking should generally take priority over correction of the upper limbs.

Loss of active and passive flexion of the elbow is a common problem in arthrogryposis. Restoration of active flexion of one hand to the mouth is desirable, but strong extension at the opposite elbow should be preserved for pushing up from the sitting position and for personal hygiene. If passive flexion of the elbow is good or can be restored by serial splintage, an elastic harness will encourage hand–mouth function until the child is old enough for tendon transfer. Posterior soft-tissue release and triceps lengthening may be necessary. The pectoralis major, if well developed, may be transferred into the biceps tendon or into the proximal ulna (Atkins et al 1985).

Flexion deformity of the wrist is managed by splintage. Soft-tissue release or proximal row carpectomy may be considered in severe cases. The aim of treatment of the flexed and adducted thumb is provision of a simple pinch, but the combined deficiency of extensors, abductors and web skin, together with contracture of adductor pollicis and flexor pollicis longus, requires extensive surgery and the results may be disappointing. Function of the fingers may be impaired by flexion and ulnar deviation deformity, but their function is seldom improved by surgery.

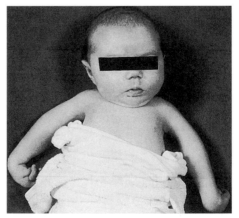

Figure 20.26 The typical posture of arthrogryposis: elbow extension and wrist flexion.

REFERENCES

Atkins R M, Bell M J, Sharrard W J 1985 Pectoralis major transfer for paralysis of elbow flexion in children. Journal of Bone and Joint Surgery 67B: 640–644

de Billy B, Gastaud F, Repetto M, Chataigner H, Clavert J M, Aubert D 1997 Treatment of Madelung's deformity by lengthening and relaxation of the distal extremity of the radius by Ilizarov's technique. European Journal of Pediatric Surgery 7: 296–298

Buck-Gramcko D 1971 Pollicization of the index finger. Method and results in aplasia and hypoplasia of the thumb. Journal of Bone and Joint Surgery 53A: 1605–1617.

Buck-Gramcko D 1985 Radialization as a new treatment for radial club hand. Journal of Hand Surgery 10A: 964–968

Cole R J, Manske P R 1997 Classification of ulnar deficiency according to the thumb and first web. Journal of Hand Surgery 22A: 479–488

Dahl M T 1993 The gradual correction of forearm deformities in multiple hereditary exostoses. Hand Clinics 94: 707–718

Dinham J M, Meggitt B F 1974 Trigger thumbs in children. A review of the natural history and indications for treatment in 105 patients. Journal of Bone and Joint Surgery 56B: 153–155

Eaton C J, Lister G D 1990 Syndactyly. Hand Clinics 64: 555–575

Flatt A E 1994 The care of congenital hand anomalies. Quality Medical Publishing, St Louis

Froster-Iskenius U G, Baird P A 1989 Limb reduction defects in over one million consecutive livebirths. Teratology 39: 127–135

Green W T, Mital M A 1979 Congenital radio-ulnar synostosis: surgical treatment. Journal of Bone and Joint Surgery 61A: 738–743

Kanaya F, Ibaraki K 1998 Mobilization of a congenital proximal radioulnar synostosis with use of a free vascularized fascio-fat graft. Journal of Bone and Joint Surgery 80A: 1186–1192

Kay S P J 1999 Pyschosocial aspects of the child with a congenital hand anomaly. In: Green D P, Hotchkiss R N, Pederson W C (eds) Operative Hand Surgery, 4th edn. Churchill Livingstone, New York

Kay S, McGuiness C 1999 Microsurgical reconstruction in abnormalities of children's hands. Hand Clinics 15: 563–583

Lamb D W, Scott H, Lam W L, Gillespie W J, Hooper G 1997 Operative correction of radial club hand. A long-term follow-up of centralization of the hand on the ulna. Journal of Hand Surgery 22B: 533–536

McCarroll H R Jr 1985 Congenital flexion deformities of the thumb. Hand Clinics 1: 567–575

McFarlane R M, Classen D A, Porte A M, Botz J S 1992 The anatomy and treatment of camptodactyly of the small finger. Journal of Hand Surgery 17A: 35–44

Manske P R, McCarroll H R Jr 1992 Reconstruction of the congenitally deficient thumb. Hand Clinics 8: 177–196

Miura T 1984 Congenital constriction band syndrome. Journal of Hand Surgery 9A: 82–88

Miura T, Nakamura R, Tamura Y 1992 Long-standing extended dynamic splintage and release of an abnormal restraining structure in camptodactyly. Journal of Hand Surgery 17B: 665–672

Nemoto K, Nemoto T, Terada N, Amako M, Kawaguchi M 1996 Splint therapy for trigger thumb and finger in children. Journal of Hand Surgery 21B: 416–418

Porter D E, Emerton M E, Villanueva-Lopez F, Simpson A H 2000 Clinical and radiographic analysis of osteochondromas and growth disturbance in hereditary multiple exostoses. Journal of Pediatric Orthopaedics 20: 246–250

Ranawat C S, DeFiore J, Straub L R 1975 Madelung's deformity. An end-result study of surgical treatment. Journal of Bone and Joint Surgery 57A: 772–775

Rankin E A, Jabalay M E, Blair S J, Fraser K E 1988 Acquired rotational digital deformity in children as a result of finger sucking. Journal of Hand Surgery 13A: 535–539

Schmidt C C, Neufeld S K 1998 Ulnar ray deficiency. Hand Clinics 14: 65–76

Slakey J B, Hennrikus W L 1996 Acquired thumb flexion contracture in children: congenital trigger thumb. Journal of Bone and Joint Surgery 78B: 481–483

Swanson A B, Swanson G D, Tada K 1983 A classification for congenital limb malformation. Journal of Hand Surgery 8A: 693–702

Tsuge K 1985 Treatment of macrodactyly. Journal of Hand Surgery 10A: 968–969

Vickers D, Nielsen G 1992 Madelung deformity: surgical prophylaxis (physiolysis) during the late growth period by resection of the dyschondrosteosis lesion. Journal of Hand Surgery 17B: 401–407

Wassel H D 1969 The results of surgery for polydactyly of the thumb. Clinical Orthopaedics and Related Research 64: 175–193

Zguricas J, Bakker W F, Heus H, Lindhout D, Heutink P, Hovius S E 1998 Genetics of limb development and congenital hand malformations. Plastic and Reconstructive Surgery 101: 1126–1135

PART 2   The Shoulder
J. A. Fixsen

CONGENITAL AND ACQUIRED DISLOCATION OF THE SHOULDER

Congenital dislocation of the shoulder is very rare. It is usually associated with other significant congenital anomalies in the upper limb, such as absence of the radius and deficiency or absence of part of the humerus. On examination, the humerus is unstable in all directions and the condition is normally painless. The shoulder is small, with deficiency of the deltoid, the pectorals and other periscapular muscles. Radiographs show a small scapula, with underdevelopment of the glenoid. The proximal portion of the humerus may be deficient. There is no satisfactory surgical treatment for this condition, but function of the rudimentary shoulder and abnormal upper limb is often surprisingly good, despite the inherent instability.

Acquired dislocation of the shoulder occurring at birth in association with obstetrical brachial plexus palsy is more common, but frequently remains unrecognised for several months. The arm is flail, and only when the fixed abduction deformity persists is the diagnosis of an anterior subglenoid dislocation made, as pointed out by Babbitt & Cassidy (1968). The clinical findings were reported as fixed abduction of the shoulder with winging of the scapula. The humeral head was palpable in the subglenoid position. Closed reduction failed and open reduction was necessary to reduce the dislocation. Dunkerton (1989) reported four patients who presented late

with posterior dislocation and associated birth palsy. In the past, this has been considered to be the result of abnormal muscle pull after birth (Wickstrom et al 1955) or subscapularis contracture (Narakas 1987). However, Dunkerton felt that true posterior dislocation at birth was due to the brachial plexus injury (see Ch. 21.2).

Recurrent dislocation, although common in adults, is rare in children, but may be seen in association with marked familial joint laxity in those younger than 2 years. The child is usually brought to the clinic by the parents, who are alarmed by the shoulder apparently 'slipping' or 'snapping' in and out of joint when the child is being dressed or undressed. The condition is usually pain-free, and the shoulder reduces spontaneously. Carter & Sweetnam (1960) reported this type of joint dislocation in association with familial joint laxity. Fortunately, the shoulder usually stabilises with time. Manoeuvres that cause the shoulder to displace should be avoided. Recurrent dislocation is also seen in other conditions with excessive joint laxity, such as osteogenesis imperfecta and the Ehlers–Danlos syndrome, and should be treated conservatively if possible. More recently, Hamner & Hall (1995) reported two patients with multidirectional shoulder instability in association with Sprengel's deformity, which they believed was caused by repetitive stretching of the shoulder capsule as a result of the relative immobility of the scapula in this condition. Wood et al (1995) reported progressive instability of the shoulder in Apert's syndrome, which could occur both at the shoulder and at the elbow; they suggested it was due to ligamentous laxity leading to progressive bone dysplasia.

Traumatic dislocation of the shoulder in the newborn with normal musculature is extremely rare, if it occurs at all. In experimental attempts to produce traumatic dislocation, epiphyseal separation occurs, rather than dislocation of the joint (Bateman 1978). The capsule forms a stout layer over the joint continuous with the periosteum of the humerus, which protects the joint. The epiphyseal plate or physis is the weakest zone and as a result traumatic epiphyseal separation, as in the hip joint, is more likely than dislocation to occur in the normal child (see Ch. 35).

CONGENITAL PSEUDARTHROSIS OF THE CLAVICLE

This condition is rare: approximately 100 cases have been reported (Grogan et al 1991). It presents as a non-tender lump lateral to the midpoint of the clavicle (Fig. 20.27), usually at or soon after birth. It is almost invariably on the right side,

and has only been described on the left side in association with dextrocardia (Gibson & Carroll 1970). It may be mistaken for a clavicular fracture at birth, but it is not associated with birth injury or obstetrical palsy and, unlike a fracture, does not form callus. It should be differentiated from cleido-cranial dysostosis, in which all or part of both clavicles are deficient and associated anomalies are seen in the skull, facial bones, pelvis and upper femora (Fig. 20.28). The

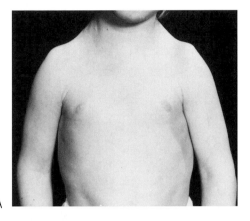

A

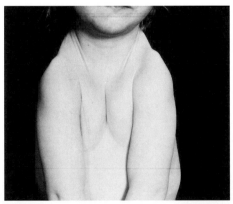

B

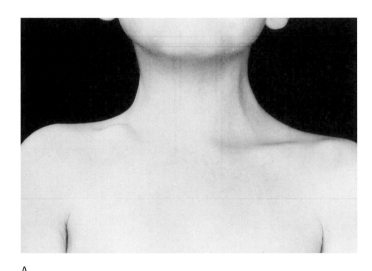

A

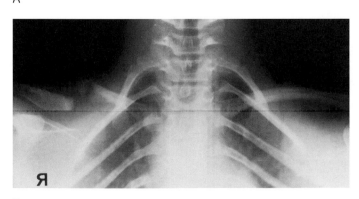

B

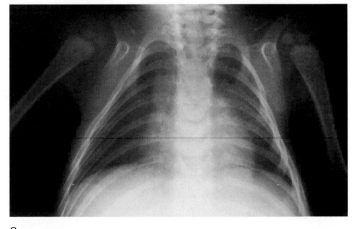

C

Figure 20.27 A Clinical appearance of congenital pseudarthrosis of the clavicle. Note the prominent lump on the right side. B X-ray of clavicles. The pseudarthrosis is on the right side.

Figure 20.28 Clinical photographs of cleido-cranial dysostosis. A With the shoulders in normal position. B With the shoulders approximated. C Radiograph of the chest and shoulders, showing only rudimentary clavicles in cleido-cranial dysostosis.

clavicle is the first bone to undergo primary ossification. This is believed to start in membrane but, subsequently, cartilaginous growth areas develop at both acromial and sternal ends. Alldred (1963) suggested that pseudarthrosis of the clavicle was the result of failure of the two centres of ossification to fuse. Lloyd-Roberts et al (1975) suggested that pressure attrition from the subclavian artery may be responsible for the pseudarthrosis. They noted that the right subclavian artery normally lies higher than the left, and that this may explain the right-sided predominance of the condition. They also noted that one of the very rare left-sided cases was associated with dextrocardia and an abnormally high left subclavian artery. A significant proportion of their patients also had abnormally high first ribs or cervical ribs. In the bilateral deficiencies seen in cleido-cranial dysostosis, abnormal elevation of the upper ribs is characteristic of the condition.

Spontaneous union of the pseudarthrosis does not occur. Radiologically, there is an established pseudarthrosis, with a bulbous lateral end of the sternal half of the clavicle overlying a tapering medial end of the acromial half. Shoulder and upper limb function is good on the affected side, but the prominent lump is unsightly. Unlike congenital pseudarthrosis of the tibia, the condition normally responds well to excision of the pseudarthrosis and bone grafting, using a block of iliac bone to bridge the gap and internal fixation with an intramedullary threaded pin to prevent migration. Alldred (1963) suggested that union was easier to obtain before the child was 8 years of age, and that operation was best performed around the age of 4 years. Grogan et al (1991) reported excellent results in eight children in whom the fibrous pseudarthrosis was resected early, carefully preserving the continuity of the periosteal sleeve and approximating the bone ends without grafting. All their patients healed solidly by 14 weeks after operation; they were aged from 7 months to 6 years at the time of surgery. After the age of 8 years, it appears to be more difficult to obtain fusion, and an alternative to bone grafting is excision of the prominent lateral end of the sternal half of the clavicle. This addresses the major cosmetic deformity, but ignores the pseudarthrosis, which rarely impairs function.

CONGENITAL ELEVATION OF THE SCAPULA (SPRENGEL'S SHOULDER)

The limb bud for the arm appears during the 4th week of intrauterine life, between the 5th cervical and 1st thoracic vertebrae. The scapula develops within the limb bud during the 5th week of intrauterine life, and descends over the next 3 weeks to its normal position alongside the 2nd to the 7th thoracic vertebrae. Failure to descend fully during this period gives rise to congenital elevation of the scapula, so-called Sprengel's deformity (Sprengel 1891). Occasionally the condition is familial, inherited as an autosomal dominant. Clinically, the scapula is elevated and rotated so that the superomedial angle is high and prominent, and the glenoid and acromium are rotated downwards and forwards (Fig. 20.29). In the past, the scapula was believed to be hypoplastic, but a recent three-dimensional computed tomography study by Cho et al (2000) has shown that affected scapulae have a characteristic shape, with a decrease in the height: width ratio, but were larger than the

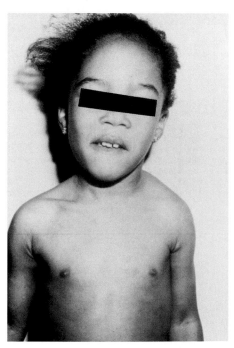
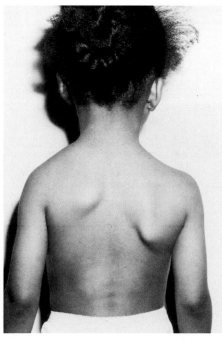

Figure 20.29 Clinical photographs of a child with a left Sprengel's shoulder. **A** Anterior view. **B** Posterior view. Note the elevation and rotation of the scapula.

A   B

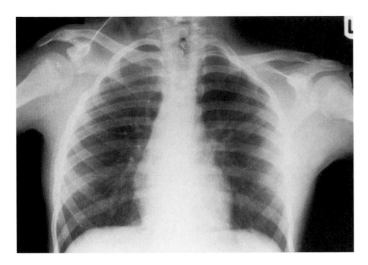

Figure 20.30 Anteroposterior radiograph of the chest, showing both shoulders in a patient with right congenital elevation of the shoulder. Note anomalies in the lower cervical and upper thoracic spine. An X-ray showing the entire cervical spine should be taken.

contralateral normal scapulae. The condition may be bilateral, and is often associated with brevicollis and cervical abnormalities (the Klippel–Feil deformity; see Ch. 30).

The superomedial angle of the scapula may be joined to the cervical spine by a fibrous or bony omovertebral bar, first described by Willet & Walsham (1880). The bar arises from the superomedial angle or upper one-third of the medial border of the scapula, to which it may be fused by bone or joined by a fibrous band, cartilage, or even a true joint. The medial end is attached to a spinous process, lamina or transverse process in the lower half of the cervical spine between the level C4–C7. The muscles of the shoulder girdle are often weak and defective, particularly the trapezius, which may be absent. The rhomboids and levator scapulae are hypoplastic and often partially fibrotic. The serratus anterior, pectorals, latissimus dorsi and sternomastoid may also be affected. Other bony anomalies are frequently seen, in particular: absent or fused ribs, cervical ribs, brevicollis with vertebral anomalies, and spina bifida occulta in the cervical and upper thoracic region. The arm itself may also be short and hypoplastic. The condition is not always noticed at birth, but usually becomes obvious when the child starts to stand. In bilateral cases, the neck appears unusually short and the shoulders hunched. The sexes are equally affected, but in the unilateral form the condition is more common on the left. Abduction and external rotation of the arm are limited to some extent on the affected side, partly as a result of the lack of mobility of the scapula on the thorax, and also because the glenoid is rotated abnormally downwards and forwards in association with the position of the scapula. An anteroposterior radiograph showing both shoulders confirms the diagnosis (Fig. 20.30), and radiographs of the cervical spine and chest should be taken because of the commonly associated spinal and rib anomalies.

TREATMENT

The major problem is usually the cosmetic appearance, rather than the limitation of movement of the shoulder. This is the basis of the well-known Cavendish classification of the deformity (1972). A programme of exercises develops the maximum range of movement, but does not alter the position of the scapula. From the surgical point of view, the surgeon may simply confine himself to a cosmetic procedure in which the prominent superomedial angle of the scapula is removed, together with the omovertebral bar if it is present. The bone should be removed extraperiosteally to avoid reformation. The patient must be told of the extensive scar posteriorly, because a wide dissection is required; the surgeon should be aware of the close proximity of the superomedial corner of the elevated scapula to the brachial plexus. This type of surgery produces an acceptable cosmetic result, but in no way alters the position of the scapula or the range of movement of the shoulder.

A more radical approach is to try to alter the position of the scapula and pull it down into its normal position. Green (1957) described an extensive procedure in which the muscles connecting the scapula to the trunk are divided at their insertion along the medial border and spine of the scapula through a long posterior incision. The omovertebral bar and the superomedial angle of the scapula are removed extraperiosteally. The attachments of the latissimus dorsi muscle to the scapula are divided extraperiosteally and, by blunt dissection, a large pocket is created deep to the superior part of the latissimus dorsi. The scapula is displaced distally and secured by a traction wire, which passes from the scapula subcutaneously down to the iliac region on the opposite side and then out to be incorporated in an external plaster spica. Woodward (1961) suggested the method in which the scapular muscles are divided from their origins on the spinous processes, rather than the scapula itself, and the deformity corrected by moving the muscle origins downwards. This procedure requires a long posterior incision and may be modified by excision of the medial border of the scapula and part of the supraspinous portion (Borges et al 1996). Both procedures involve extensive dissection and can leave large and ugly scars. There is a well-reported incidence of damage to the brachial plexus if the scapula is displaced downwards too forcefully.

Campbell & Wilkinson (1979) popularised an attractive procedure, originally described by Konig in 1914, in which a vertical osteotomy of the scapula 2 cm from its medial border is performed. This is combined with excision of the superomedial angle and the omovertebral bar, together with any fibrous tethering bands. The portion of the scapula lateral to the osteotomy is then rotated, correcting the abnormal downward inclination of the glenoid, improving the range of abduction at the shoulder, and the two portions are sutured together through offset drill holes, pre-drilled before the osteotomy, to maintain the corrected position.

This is a less extensive procedure than either the Green or Woodward operations. Despite this, among the 11 patients reported, one developed mild brachial plexus palsy, but recovered, and slight winging of the scapula occurred in another patient.

ABDUCTION CONTRACTURE OF THE SHOULDER

Bhattacharyya (1966) reported three patients with abduction contracture of the shoulder resulting from fibrosis of the intermediate part of the deltoid. Clinically, the skin was indrawn over the contracted portion of the muscle and the arm was held in approximately 30° of abduction. In two patients this was bilateral; excision of the fibrotic muscle improved the range of movement in all three patients. There was no definite history of trauma or injection, but the condition appeared analogous to that described in the quadriceps muscle after repeated intramuscular injections. Since that time, a number of further cases have been reported in children and young adults (Hill et al 1967, Goodfellow & Wade 1969, Wolbrink et al 1973). The cause of the fibrosis is not usually known, but it seems likely that it follows injections into the muscle and responds satisfactorily to excision of the fibrous contracted area.

REFERENCES

Alldred A J 1963 Congenital pseudarthrosis of the clavicle. Journal of Bone and Joint Surgery 45B: 312–319

Babbitt D P, Cassidy P H 1968 Obstetrical paralysis and dislocation of the shoulder in infancy. Journal of Bone and Joint Surgery 50A: 1447–1452

Bateman J E 1978 The shoulder and neck, 2nd edn. W B Saunders, Philadelphia, p 37

Bhattacharyya S 1966 Abduction contracture of the shoulder from contracture of the intermediate part of the deltoid. Journal of Bone and Joint Surgery 48B: 127–131

Borges K L P, Shah A, Cobo Torres B, Bowen J R, 1996 Modified Woodward procedure for Sprengel's deformity of the shoulder. Journal of Pediatric Orthopaedics 16: 508–513

Campbell D, Wilkinson J A 1979 Scapular osteotomy for the treatment of Sprengel's shoulder. Journal of Bone and Joint Surgery 61B: 514

Carter C, Sweetnam R 1960 Recurrent dislocation of the patella and shoulder: their association with familial joint laxity. Journal of Bone and Joint Surgery 42B: 721–727

Cavendish M E 1972 Congenital elevation of the shoulder. Journal of Bone and Joint Surgery 54B: 395–408

Cho T-J, Choi I H, Chung C Y, Hwang J K 2000 The Sprengel's deformity. Journal of Bone and Joint Surgery 82B: 711–718

Dunkerton M C 1989 Posterior dislocation of the shoulder associated with obstetric brachial plexus palsy. Journal of Bone and Joint Surgery 71B: 764–766

Gibson D A, Carroll N 1970 Congenital pseudarthrosis of the clavicle. Journal of Bone and Joint Surgery 52B: 629–643

Goodfellow J W, Wade S 1969 Flexion contracture of the shoulder joint from the anterior part of the deltoid muscle. Journal of Bone and Joint Surgery 51B: 356–358

Green W T 1957 The surgical correction of elevation of the scapula (Sprengel's deformity). Journal of Bone and Joint Surgery 39A: 1439

Grogan D P, Love S M, Guideria K J, Ogden J A 1991 Operative treatment of congenital pseudarthrosis of the clavicle. Journal of Pediatric Orthopaedics 11: 176–180

Hamner D L, Hall J E 1995 Sprengel's deformity associated with multi directional shoulder instability. Journal of Pediatric Orthopaedics 15: 641–643

Hill N A, Liebler W A, Wilson J H, Rosenthal E 1967 Abduction contractures of both glenohumeral joints and extension contracture of one knee secondary to partial muscle fibrosis. Journal of Bone and Joint Surgery 49A: 961–964

Konig F 1914 Eine Neue operation def angeborenen schulterblatthochstandes. Beitrage Klinische Chirurg 94: 530–537

Lloyd-Roberts G C, Apley A G, Owen R 1975 Reflections upon the aetiology of congenital pseudarthrosis of the clavicle. Journal of Bone and Joint Surgery 57B: 24–29

Narakas A O 1987 Obstetrical brachial plexus injuries. In: Lamb D W (ed) The paralysed hand. The hand and upper limb. Churchill Livingstone, Edinburgh, vol 2, pp 116–135

Sprengel O 1891 Die Angeborene verschiebung des schulterblattes nach oben. Langenbecks Arch Klin Chir 42: 545–549

Wickstrom J, Haslam E T, Hutchinson R H 1955 The surgical management of residual deformities of the shoulder following birth injuries with a brachial plexus. Journal of Bone and Joint Surgery 37A: 27–36

Willet A, Walsham W J 1880 An account of the dissection of the parts removed after death from the body of a woman the subject of congenital malformation of the spinal column, thorax and left scapular arch with remarks on the probable nature of the defects in development producing the deformities. Medical and Surgical Transactions, London 63: 256

Wolbrink A J, Hsu Z, Bianco A J 1973 Abduction contracture of the shoulders and hips secondary to fibrous bands. Journal of Bone and Joint Surgery 55A: 844–846

Wood D E, Sauser D D, O'Hara R C 1995 Shoulder and elbow in Apert's syndrome. Journal of Pediatric Orthopaedics 15: 648–651

Woodward J W 1961 Congenital elevation of the scapula: correction by release and transplantation of the muscle origin. Journal of Bone and Joint Surgery 43A: 219–228

Chapter 21

Obstetrical brachial plexus injuries

PART 1   Management of the injury
A. Gilbert

INTRODUCTION

The evolution of microsurgical methods has significantly changed our attitude towards surgical reconstruction in peripheral nerve lesions, including brachial plexus lesions. However, because of the distance that the nerves have to regenerate after restoration of anatomical continuity in the brachial plexus, the results in adults have been modest, despite the more sophisticated methods available. In contrast, the same methods in children give better results because of their superior capacity for regeneration. The potential for regeneration diminishes gradually after birth, remaining fairly good until adolescence, and then deteriorating rapidly after the cessation of growth. Obstetrical lesions occurring at birth are best considered separately, because they represent a uniform group for patient's age and type of lesion, whereas lesions occurring during childhood are more heterogeneous.

AETIOLOGY AND PATHOGENESIS

Obstetrical birth palsy has been recognised since the late 19th century, although some controversy has existed until recently. Modern series in which operative exploration has been carried out have confirmed the pathology.

The aetiology is always a tearing force caused by traction on the head or arm. There are two basic types of lesion:

1. Overweight babies (more than 4 kg) with vertex presentation and shoulder dystocia who require excess force by traction, often with forceps or ventouse extraction for delivery. This results in upper plexus injury, most commonly to the C5 and C6, and occasionally the C7 roots, but never the lower roots (Fig. 21.1).
2. Breech presentation, usually of small babies (less than 3 kg) requiring excessive extension of the head and, often, manipulation of the hand and arm in a fashion that exerts traction on both the upper roots and the lower roots. This may cause rupture or avulsion of any, or occasionally all, of the roots (Fig. 21.2).

CLINICAL PRESENTATION

The initial diagnosis is obvious at birth. After a difficult delivery of an obese baby by the vertex presentation or a small baby by the breech, the upper extremity is flail and dangling. A more detailed analysis of the pattern of paralysis of the various muscles of the upper extremity is not necessary, as the picture will change rapidly. Examination of the other extremities is important, to exclude neonatal quadriplegia or diplegia. Occasionally, birth palsy may be bilateral. Forty-eight hours later, a more accurate examination and muscle testing can be performed. At this stage it is usually possible to differentiate two types of paresis:

1. The *Erb–Duchenne* type paralysis of the upper roots. The arm is held in internal rotation and pronation. There is no active shoulder abduction or elbow flexion (Fig. 21.3). The elbow may be slightly flexed (lesion of C5–C7) or in complete extension (lesion of C5–C6). The thumb is in flexion, and sometimes the fingers will not extend. As a rule, the thumb flexor and the flexors of the fingers are functioning. The pectoralis major is usually active, giving an appearance of forward flexion of the shoulder. There are no vasomotor changes or gross impairment of distal sensation.
2. Complete paralysis (*Dejerine–Klumpke*). The entire arm is flail and the hand clenched (Fig. 21.4). Sensation is diminished, and there is vasomotor impairment, giving a pale or even 'marbled' appearance to the extremity. Often, Horner's sign is present on the affected side.

A shoulder X-ray should be taken to eliminate fracture of the clavicle or the upper humerus, which can occur in association with the paresis. Occasionally, a phrenic nerve palsy can be detected by fluoroscopy.

The clinical development during the first month is variable, and many pareses will recover during this stage

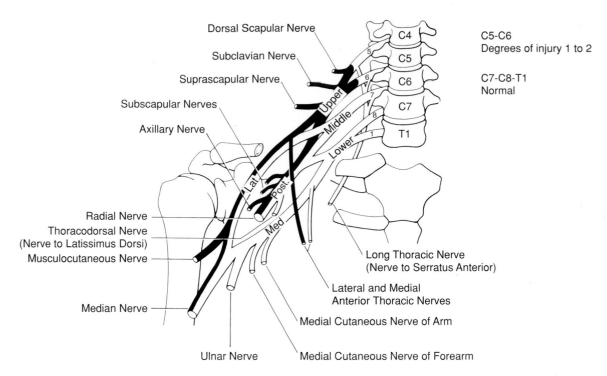

Figure 21.1 C5/6 brachial plexus lesion: paralysed fibres are shaded. (Reproduced with permission from Lamb 1987.)

(Bennet & Harrold 1976). However, Wickstrom et al (1958) reported that only 10% of total palsies recover to any useful extent. These patients should be carefully evaluated at the age of 3 months, clinically, electromyographically and by cervical myelography. Gentle physiotherapy should be used during this recovery period, to minimise the development of contractures while awaiting spontaneous recovery. At this stage, complete paralysis with Horner's sign will remain

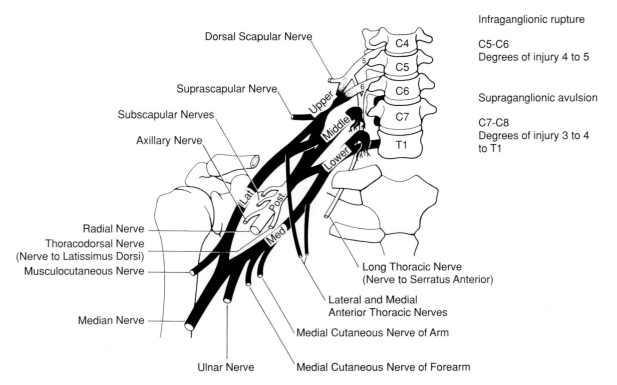

Figure 21.2 Entire brachial plexus lesion. Rupture of the upper trunk, supraganglionic avulsion of C7 and C8, severe damage to T1. (Reproduced with permission from Lamb 1987.)

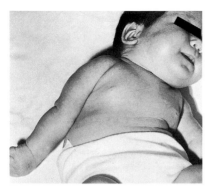

Figure 21.3 C5/C6 lesion at 3 months of age. (Reproduced with permission from Lamb 1987.)

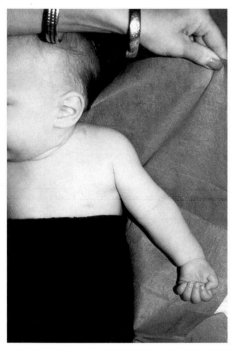

Figure 21.4 Complete paralysis.

unchanged, and early operation should be considered in these babies at 3 months.

Paralysis of the upper roots may show spontaneous recovery during the first 3 months. These babies should be treated with physiotherapy, and assessed clinically and electromyographically by the age of 3 months.

SPONTANEOUS RECOVERY

The literature reports varying rates of spontaneous recovery, from 7 to 80%. Useful guidelines are given in the thesis of Tassin (1984), who came to the following conclusions:

1. Complete recovery is seen in those infants showing some contraction of the biceps and the deltoid by the end of the 1st month and a normal contraction by the 2nd month.
2. No infant in whom neither the deltoid nor the biceps contract by the 3rd month can be expected to obtain a good result. Testing the deltoid can be difficult. As a result, assessment of the biceps is the most reliable

indicator for operative intervention. If there is no evidence of any recovery in the biceps by the end of the 3rd month, operation is indicated. Clinical assessment is more reliable than electrical testing. If surgery is not undertaken, some recovery will continue to take place spontaneously, but it is likely to be less satisfactory than that after surgery.

INDICATIONS FOR OPERATION

If recovery of the biceps has not begun by 3 months, the prognosis is poor and surgical repair of the plexus is indicated (Gilbert & Tassin 1984, Gilbert et al 1989, Gilbert & Whitaker 1991). The following clinical situations pose particular problems:

1. Complete palsy with a flail arm after 1 month, particularly with a Horner's syndrome, will not recover spontaneously and is a prime candidate for surgery. These babies are best treated by early operation at the age of 12 weeks.
2. Complete palsy of C5 and C6 occurring after breech delivery with no sign of recovery by the 3rd month.
3. The most common C5, C6 and sometimes C7 palsies almost always show some sign of recovery, which can be misleading, and which has in the past encouraged a conservative approach. If, however, after careful examination recovery of the biceps is completely absent at 3 months, surgery should be considered. Great difficulty arises when infants are seen late – towards the 6th to 8th month – and show minimal recovery of biceps function. The parents are often encouraged by the early signs of recovery and will not accept the idea of an unsatisfactory final result. Under these conditions, it is difficult for the surgeon to advise surgery that cannot promise a definitive result. In order to avoid this situation, it is important to try to make decisions by the 3rd month.

Several centres have been unable to show good correlation between electromyographic changes and the final prognosis. Frequently, the preoperative electromyogram (EMG) gives cause for overoptimism, because it takes only a few fibres to provoke an electrical response that is not associated with subsequent clinical recovery. However, a negative EMG with complete absence of signs of regeneration at the age of 3 months almost invariably signifies root avulsion.

Myelography has been used extensively in the past, but is unpredictable and associated with false negative and false positive results. Computed tomography with myelography has improved the quality of the results considerably.

The recent use of MRI, although promising, does not give sufficiently precise information to be used routinely.

Myelography involves general anesthesia for the baby, and should be used only if there is doubt as to the condition of the roots (breech presentation, lower root avulsion).

SURGICAL INTERVENTION

Surgery is performed under general anaesthesia. Usually a supraclavicular approach is sufficient, but this can be extended transclavicularly to expose the lower plexus if necessary. The neuroma usually lies between C5 and C6 and the divisions of the upper trunk at the level of the clavicle. The nerves may be ruptured totally or avulsed. The neuroma is resected back to normal tissue and one to two sural nerves are used as grafts between the sectioned nerve ends. The nerve anastomosis can be performed either by suture or by fibrin glue (Tissucol). If avulsions are present, reconstruction must be tailor-made to the situation and the expertise of the surgeon. As a rule, children seem to have a far greater capacity to accommodate to differential neurotisations from, for example, the accessory, long thoracic, thoraco-dorsal or pectoral nerves as donors and to different kinds of internal neurotisations, for example, from C5 to the upper trunk as a whole or even from C7 to the upper trunk. It is best to concentrate on reconstruction of the upper roots, to gain useful elbow and shoulder movement. Until now, even the most painstaking reconstruction of the lower roots has produced disappointing results with regard to finger flexion and extension. For the time being, these sequelae should be treated by later muscle transfer.

ANATOMICAL LESIONS

The anatomical lesions observed at surgery correspond to those described by Taylor in 1920. These include rupture at the level of the primary trunk or root, or avulsion of the roots. Contrary to the reports of lesions in the adult, we have never seen a double-level lesion or lesions of the secondary trunk of two branches of the plexus. Associated vascular lesions are exceptional, and we have seen only one rupture of the axillary artery, which was treated by vein graft. The upper roots are more often ruptured and the lower roots avulsed (Fig. 21.5). The results in 436 cases operated on up to 1996 showed the following distribution of root lesions (Gilbert 1988, 1995):

1. C5 and C6:   48%
2. C5 to C7:   29%
3. Complete involvement: 23%, of which almost all were avulsions.

POSTOPERATIVE CARE

Stretching the reconstructed area must be avoided in the first 3 weeks after operation. This can be achieved by a plaster cast. Physical therapy is then resumed by gentle passive exercises and encouraging voluntary movement. Every effort should be made to counteract retraction and internal rotation of the shoulder and flexion of the elbow. Physiotherapy should be continued throughout the recovery period, usually for 2 years, but regular physiotherapy should

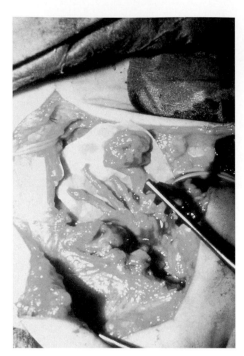

Figure 21.5
Rupture of the two upper roots and avulsion of three lower roots, with spinal ganglia.

then be discontinued. Recovery is slow. It can be seen 4–6 months after direct suture and at 6–10 months after graft reconstruction. It can continue in upper plexus lesions for more than 2 years and in complete lesions for more than 3 years.

RESULTS OF SURGERY

Four hundred and thirty-six patients operated on between 1976 and 1995 have been reviewed, with more than 4 years of follow-up. The results in the shoulder, using the Mallet (1972) scale, are summarised here.

C5 and C6
At 2 years the results were:

- grade IV+ (good–excellent): 52%
- grade III: 40%
- grade II: 8%

After 2 years, 30% of the patients required secondary surgery:

- subscapularis releases: 13
- latissimus dorsi transfers: 33
- trapezius transfers: 6

A further evaluation at 4 years (after tendon transfers) showed the following results:

- grade IV+:   80%
- grade III: 20%
- grade II: 0%

An example of the results of successful graft repair of C5/C6 rupture is shown in Fig. 21.6.

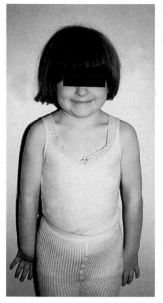
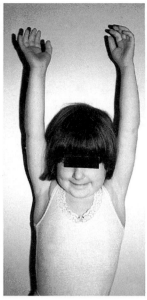
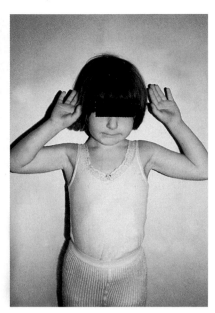

Figure 21.6 Clinical result 6 years after graft repair of C5/6 rupture.

C5, C6 and C7

At 2 years the results were:

- grade IV+:   36%
- grade III: 46%
- grade II: 18%

Within 2 years, some patients required secondary surgery:

- subscapularis releases: 7%
- latissimus dorsi transfers: 24%
- trapezius transfers: 1%

The results were evaluated again at 4 years:

- grade IV+:   61%
- grade III: 29%
- grade II: 10%

Complete paralysis

The results in the shoulder in complete paralysis are less satisfactory, because part of the upper roots destined for the shoulder and elbow must be sacrificed in order to obtain function in the hand. The shoulder results at 4 years are as follows:

- class IV: 22.5%
- class III: 42%
- class II: 35.5%

In the hand, however, for which the prognosis is very poor for spontaneous recovery, the results showed some function in 83% and useful function in 75% of patients, 8 years after a neurotisation.

COMPLICATIONS

In the series reviewed, there have been no operative deaths. The overall complication rate was 1%, including phrenic nerve lesions, lesions of the thoracic duct, wound infections and vascular lesions, all of which have been managed satisfactorily, without late sequelae.

RECOMMENDATIONS

On the basis of the results of the author's series of patients, the following recommendations can be made:

1. Babies who do not recover biceps function by the age of 3 months should be considered for immediate operation.
2. Primary suture without tension is rarely possible. Nerve grafting is usually necessary for root or trunk ruptures.
3. In the presence of root avulsions, an internal neurotisation should be attempted between different roots, particularly as children seem to have a far greater capacity to accommodate to differential neurotisations.
4. When it is not possible to perform an internal neurotisation, an external neurotisation can be performed, using one or more of the following donor nerves in the following order of preference: the pectoral nerves, the intercostal nerves, the accessory nerve.
5. The reconstruction should be protected from excessive motion for the first 3 weeks.
6. Physiotherapy should be continued up to 2 years of age, but then continued by the parents in the form of play and activities of daily living.
7. Secondary surgery can be considered when it is clear that recovery after reconstruction has failed.

MANAGEMENT OF LATE DEFORMITY

The sequelae of obstetrical palsy are due to a combination of paralysis, muscle contracture, cross-innervation and joint deformity. They may occur in the shoulder, elbow, forearm, wrist and hand. Physiotherapy should be started as soon as possible after diagnosis, to try to prevent contractures occurring and becoming established.

THE SHOULDER

Imbalance at the shoulder, especially in the upper type of plexus lesion, rapidly produces increasing internal rotation as a result of progressive contracture of the subscapularis muscle. This may become fixed within a few months. If there is no improvement with physiotherapy, early release of the subscapularis muscle is advised. It is important to verify that the shoulder joint is not deformed before performing this release, and computed tomography combined with arthrography is the most accurate method of assessing the state of the shoulder joint. The simple release operation can be performed through an axillary approach and can restore up to 70–80° external rotation. The arm is kept externally rotated in a plaster for 3 weeks after operation. If this operation is performed early, it is unlikely to relapse, and secondary transfers to reinforce the rotator muscles are rarely necessary. When all the contractures have been treated, the strength and activity of the shoulder muscles can be assessed. Weakness of abduction and external rotation are the most common.

Several tendon transfers are available and may be used sometimes in combination. For moderate palsies with abduction of around 90° and lack of external rotation, the isolated transfer of latissimus dorsi to the rotator cuff gives an average of 30° improvement in abduction and good external rotation. When paralysis is severe and the shoulder almost flaccid, it is necessary to combine the latissimus transfer with trapezius transfer from the acromium to the humeral head. Some authors add a third transfer of either the levator scapulae or pectoralis major. The results of these combined transfers is not so predictable, but can give excellent function on occasion (Gilbert et al 1988b).

In late cases in which the shoulder joint is deformed, external rotation osteotomy of the humerus should be used. This operation is best undertaken after the child has reached the age of 7–9 years.

THE ELBOW

In the elbow, the following problems may occur:

1. Paralysis of flexion or extension.
2. Progressive bone and joint deformity.

Paralysis of elbow flexion is rare but should, if possible, be treated. The best transfers are the latissimus dorsi transfer and the Steindler's flexorplasty. The latissimus dorsi transfer is strong and gives good function, but the muscle may be needed for shoulder reconstruction.

Steindler's flexorplasty is easy and effective. We prefer not to transfer the finger flexors. The flexor carpi ulnaris is completely released and attached to the humerus more proximally. Active wrist extension is necessary, and if there is no wrist extension this can be helped by dorsal transfer of the flexor carpi ulnaris tendon.

Paralysis of elbow extension is rare, but troublesome. Reconstruction is difficult, but the latissimus dorsi transfer can give acceptable results.

A fixed flexion deformity at the elbow is common. In our series of patients, 25% showed an extension lag varying from 5 to 70°, with an average of 16°. Night splintage is helpful in managing this condition. If significant loss of extension at the elbow (more than 40°) persists, an anterior release can be undertaken; all muscles are detached, the brachialis lengthened, and the articular capsule opened. The biceps tendon is left untouched, although it participates in the contracture. If it is lengthened, the patient may lose active flexion. There are very few indications for extension osteotomy of the humerus.

THE FOREARM

Pronation is rarely a problem that needs treatment. It is usually the supination deformity that follows lower root involvement for which the patient seeks treatment. With time, this paralytic deformity leads to bony deformation and dislocation of the radial head. It is possible to treat the early case with supple joints by rerouting the biceps tendon as described by Grilli (1959) and Zancolli (1967). It is sometimes necessary to add a substantial soft-tissue release of the interosseus membrane. If the radial head is dislocated, it has been our experience that reduction is useless, and the only effective treatment is distal rotation osteotomy of the radius.

THE WRIST AND HAND

Wrist drop is one of the main sequelae of obstetrical palsy. Our preferred treatment, when possible, has been to transfer the flexor carpi ulnaris to the extensor carpi radialis brevis through the interosseus membrane. Unfortunately, the results of this usually excellent procedure can be quite disappointing in obstetrical palsy. In the hand, the sequelae of obstetrical palsy are very severe and transfers are rarely indicated or successful. Tenodesis utilising wrist extension may be of some help to finger flexion, but will never give a good grasp. The severity of these hand and finger sequelae justify any attempt to re-innervate the lower roots during the original plexus operation.

REFERENCES

Bennet G C, Harrold A J 1976 Prognosis and early management of birth injuries to the brachial plexus. British Medical Journal 1: 1520–1521

Gilbert A 1995 Long-term evaluation of brachial plexus surgery in obstetrical palsy. Hand Clinics 11: 583–587

Gilbert A, Duclos L 1995 Obstetrical palsy: early treatment and secondary procedures. Ann Acad Med Singapore 24: 841–845

Gilbert A, Tassin J L 1984 Réparation chirurgicale du plexus brachial dans la paralysie obstétricale. Chirurgie 110: 70–75

Gilbert A, Whitaker I 1991 Obstetrical brachial plexus lesions. Journal of Hand Surgery 16B: 489–491

Gilbert A, Brockman R, Carlioz H 1989 Surgical treatment of brachial plexus birth palsy. Clin Orth 264: 39–47

Gilbert A, Razaboni R, Amar-Khodja S 1988 Indications and results of brachial plexus surgery in obstetrical palsy. Orthopedic Clinics of North America 19: 91–105

Gilbert A, Romana C, Ayatti R 1988 Tendon transfers for shoulder paralysis in children. Hand Clinics 4: 633–642

Grilli F P 1959 Il fupianto del bicipite brachiale in funzione Dronatona. Archivo Putti 12: 359–371

Lamb D W 1987 The paralysed hand. Churchill Livingstone, Edinburgh

Mallet J 1972 Paralysie obstetricale. Revue de Chirurgie Orthopedique 58 (suppl 1): 115

Tassin J L 1984 Paralysies obstétricales du plexus brachial, evolution spontanée, resultats des interventions reparatrices precrées. Thèse, Université Paris VIII

Taylor A S 1920 Brachial birth palsy and injuries of similar type in adults. Surgery, Gynecology and Obstetrics 30: 494–502

Wickstrom J, Haslam E T, Hutchinson R H 1958 The surgical management of residual deformities of the shoulder following birth injuries of the brachial plexus. Journal of Bone and Joint Surgery 47A: 27–36

Zancolli E A 1967 Paralytic supination contracture of the forearm. Journal of Bone and Joint Surgery 49A: 1275–1284

PART 2   Late sequelae
R. Birch

INTRODUCTION

Medial rotation contracture and posterior dislocation of the shoulder is the most common and significant secondary deformity in obstetrical brachial plexus palsy (Birch et al 1998). Operations to correct the deformity were necessary in more than 30% of the 1200 children seen in our Unit from 1986. Diagnosis is often delayed. Treatment in the late adolescent or young adult is difficult, and at times impossible. The untreated deformity has severe consequences for the function of the upper limb as a whole. By late adolescence or early adult life, movements of the shoulder girdle are greatly restricted. The upper limb lies in fixed medial rotation. There is pain from the disorganised gleno-humeral joint, and a flexion–pronation posture of the elbow and forearm, often complicated by subluxation of the head of the radius.

It is important that orthopaedic surgeons understand that, with early detection and appropriate treatment, most children with obstetrical brachial plexus palsy progress to good or at least useful neurological recovery (Fig. 21.7)

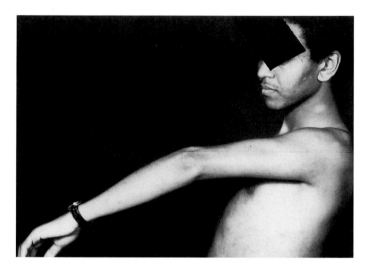

Figure 21.7 Complex dislocation in a 21-year-old man. The shoulder was stiff and painful. The head of the radius was dislocated. Function throughout the upper limb was substantially marred, in spite of good neurological recovery.

HISTORICAL BACKGROUND

The causation, course, skeletal consequences and logical methods of treatment were set out by workers more than 60 years ago. It seems that their work has been neglected, in spite of the recent resurgence of interest in the neurological lesion itself. Fairbank (1913) was of the opinion that the subscapularis muscle was the major impediment to free lateral rotation of the shoulder. He described results of operation in 18 patients in whom a technique was used in which the subscapularis tendon and capsule, and the coraco-humeral ligament were divided. In three patients the coracoid was sectioned. The radiological features of the deformity were fully described by Sever (1925) in his analysis of a series of 1100 children with obstetrical brachial plexus palsy. He recognised delayed ossification of the head of the humerus, progressive deformation of the glenoid and, in later stages, overgrowth of the acromion and 'marked elongation of the coracoid process, due probably to the pull of the contracted coraco-brachialis muscle'. Sever was

unable to demonstrate any case of epiphyseal separation or of dislocation caused during delivery. Scaglietti (1938), reporting Putti's work, believed that the deformity was caused by direct injury to the proximal humerus, resulting in retroversion of the head of the humerus on the shaft. The controversy continues. Zancolli & Zancolli (1993) believed that damage to the growth plate (epiphysiolysis) was the major factor in causation of the deformity, but in the same volume Gilbert (1993) wrote: 'posterior subluxation deformity of the humeral head, permanently worsens the prognosis. These anomalies have long been considered the result of obstetrical palsy are, in fact, in consequence of untreated contractures'. Our experience suggests that both views are correct and represent important contributions.

CAUSATION

Posterior dislocation occurred at or very shortly after birth in about 5% of the 450 patients studied at our hospital clinic.

One father gave a clear description of the mechanism of injury: evidently, during a difficult vertex delivery, the affected arm was pulled into abduction and then across the chest, into forced flexion with medial rotation. In a few children in whom neurological recovery was good, it was found that the subscapularis muscle was densely fibrosed, which may represent a post-ischaemic or compartment syndrome lesion analogous to that described in an adult by Landi et al (1992). However, in most children the deformity developed or progressed whilst under observation; in some, the deformity occurred after repair of the upper trunk and progressed in spite of continuing observation and assiduous exercises. More than 80% of these 450 children had good hand function and useful recovery in C5, C6 and C7, either spontaneously or after surgical repair. Birch & Chen (1996), in their analysis of 120 consecutive cases, made the alarming observation that the shoulder in no fewer than 12 children, awaiting treatment for uncomplicated medial rotation contracture, had progressed to dislocation whilst awaiting admission. This suggests that the primary cause is, in most cases, the neurological lesion, which invariably afflicts C5 and C6 irrespective of whether the remainder of the plexus is damaged or not. There is paralysis of the lateral rotator muscles, of infraspinatus and teres minor, innervated by the 5th cervical nerve. The medial rotators, particularly the subscapularis muscle, innervated by the 7th and 8th cervical nerves, are never paralysed, or are weakened only for a short time, so that their action is unopposed. Muscular imbalance is a potent cause of deformity in the growing limb, and shoulder deformity reflects this general principle. The author has not encountered a single instance of anterior dislocation of the gleno-humeral joint.

CLASSIFICATION OF THE DEFORMITY

The rate of progression of the deformity varies from child to child. It is not necessarily related to age: advanced secondary bone changes have been seen in children aged 3 years or less, whereas dislocation in the presence of only minor deformity has been seen in children aged 11 or 12 years. The deformity is progressive, and there is a spectrum from medial rotation contracture to complex dislocation of the shoulder (Table 21.1).

Table 21.1 A clinical classification of shoulder deformity

Type	Relation of head of humerus to glenoid	Clinical evidence	Radiological evidence	Supplementary investigations
Medial rotation contracture	Congruent	Loss of passive lateral rotation of 30° or more	Normal: coracoid may be elongated	Ultrasound congruent. MRI scan may show retroversion of head upon shaft of humerus
Posterior subluxation (simple)	Head of humerus in false glenoid	Lateral rotation to neutral. Head palpable posteriorly	Incongruent. No other skeletal abnormality	Ultrasound, CT and MRI scans confirm incongruency. Retroversion and 'double facet' glenoid may be seen
Posterior dislocation (simple)	Head of humerus posterior to glenoid	Fixed medial rotation contracture at about 30° Head evidently lying behind glenoid	Head of humerus behind glenoid. No other skeletal deformity	Ultrasound, CT and MRI scans confirm. Retroversion maybe seen
Complex subluxation	Head of humerus in false glenoid. Secondary bone deformity	Lateral rotation to neutral or less. Overgrowth of coracoid and acromion palpable	Extent of coracoid and acromion abnormality seen: 'double facet' of glenoid	Confirm incongruency and skeletal abnormality, but may mislead about glenoid shape
Complex dislocation	Head of humerus behind glenoid. Secondary bone deformity	Fixed medial rotation contracture of 30° or more. Obvious secondary bone changes	Head of humerus behind glenoid. Overgrowth of coracoid and acromion. Abnormality of glenoid	Confirms dislocation and extent of skeletal abnormality

Note 1: In all cases, a flexion–pronation posture of elbow and forearm is seen. In advanced cases, this deformity becomes fixed, and may be associated with dislocation of the head of the radius.
Note 2: The extent of retroversion of the head upon the shaft of the humerus cannot be measured accurately by any ancillary investigation, and it is best determined during open reduction.
MRI, magnetic resonance imaging; CT, computed tomography.
(Based on observations made by Dr Liang Chen (Birch et al 1998).)

MEDIAL ROTATION CONTRACTURE

The only abnormality associated with medial rotation contracture is restriction of passive lateral rotation, which is diminished by 30–40°. There is a mild flexion–pronation posture of the forearm, but this is not fixed. Radiographs show delayed ossification. An uncommon cause of medial rotation contracture is overgrowth of the coracoid, which abuts against the head of the humerus, blocking lateral rotation.

POSTERIOR SUBLUXATION (SIMPLE)

The head of the humerus is prominent posteriorly to palpation, passive lateral rotation is restricted to about 10°, and there is a flexion–pronation posture of the forearm. There is no radiological evidence of secondary deformity affecting the acromion, the coracoid, or the glenoid (Fig. 21.8).

POSTERIOR DISLOCATION (SIMPLE)

There is obvious abnormality of the contour of the shoulder, and the head of the humerus can be seen and palpated behind the glenoid. There is a fixed medial rotation contracture, and there may be a fixed flexion–pronation posture of the forearm. There is no active supination beyond the neutral position. Radiographs confirm displacement without evidence of secondary skeletal change.

COMPLEX SUBLUXATION–DISLOCATION

Marked secondary skeletal abnormalities are now apparent clinically and radiologically. The coracoid is elongated and inclined posteriorly – an abnormality easily detectable by palpation. The acromion is elongated and hooked downwards. The glenoid appears as two facets: the true glenoid

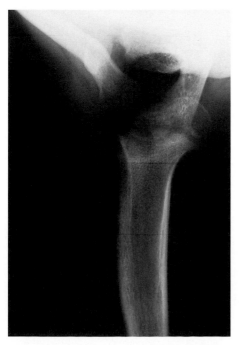

Figure 21.8 Simple subluxation in a 3-year-old boy. There is still contact between the deformation and the glenoid.

lying above and anterior, and the false glenoid lying below and inferior. In *complex subluxation*, the articulation is between the head of the humerus and the false glenoid (Fig. 21.9). In *complex dislocation*, the articulation is between the lesser tuberosity and the false glenoid (Figs 21.10–21.12). The extent of retroversion of the head of the humerus can be detected only at operation.

DIAGNOSIS

The diagnosis is made by physical examination. Babies are best examined supine. The examiner holds both upper limbs with the elbows flexed to 90°. *The arms are held adducted against the chest, and the upper limbs are gently rotated into lateral rotation.* Any diminution in the range of passive lateral rotation in the affected upper limb is significant. Serious errors in diagnosis are caused by incorrect examination and the practice of examining one limb in isolation or of estimating passive range for rotation within the arm in abduction is unsatisfactory. The examination is performed gently, and if the infant protests, the examiner must suspect incongruity at the gleno-humeral joint.

In older children, the posture of the upper limb is characteristic, lying in medial rotation with flexion and pronation at the elbow. The contour of the shoulder is abnormal, as the head is prominent behind the glenoid. Palpation reveals abnormalities of the coracoid and of the acromion (Figs 21.13 and 21.14).

In almost every case, a clear impression of the extent of bone deformity can be formed from the physical examination supplemented by plain anteroposterior and axial radiographs. Arthrograms, computed tomography and magnetic resonance imaging (MRI) have been used in diagnosis (Pearl & Edgerton 1998, Waters et al 1998), and preliminary findings suggest that ultrasound examination may help diagnosis in the first 12 months of life when the clinician suspects an incongruity at the shoulder.

RECORDING SHOULDER FUNCTION

Three systems are used to record shoulder function in our Unit. Nearly all children aged 1 year or more willingly demonstrate these exercises, using coloured crayons or small toys as lures. Observation of the infant gives useful information about the range of active movements and, of course, the passive range can be measured. Records are made at each clinic attendance and the three systems, taken together, provide useful information about shoulder function.

The first method (Table 21.2) is derived from the system proposed by Gilbert (1993). It has been modified to record the presence of functional medial rotation. The child with fixed medial rotation contracture such that the passive range of lateral rotation is restricted to the neutral position or less is, by convention, given a grade of Stage 1 and no more. Mallet's system (Fig. 21.15) records five shoulder functions, according a maximum of three points to each. A child with

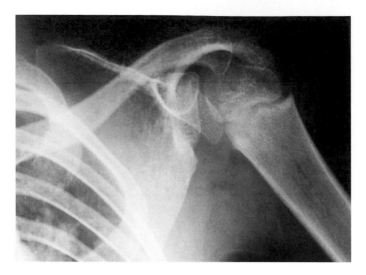

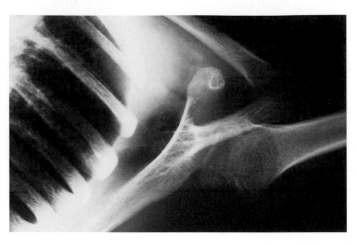

Figure 21.9 Complex subluxation in a 15-year-old boy, showing advanced bone changes. Significant overgrowth of coracoid and of the acromion are demonstrated.

Figure 21.10 Complex dislocation in a 14-year-old girl. The deformed anterior part of the head of the humerus articulates with the false glenoid.

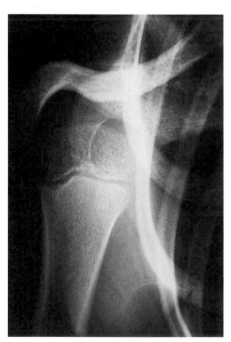

Figure 21.11 Complex dislocation in a 9-year-old boy. The coracoid and the acromion are overgrown. The 'double facet' deformation of the glenoid is seen. The head of the humerus is scarcely deformed.

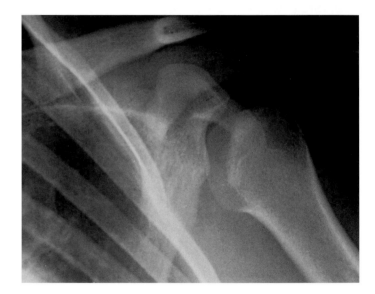

Figure 21.12 Complex dislocation in a 17-year-old man. The true and false glenoids are well developed. The lesser tuberosity articulates with the true glenoid. There is a 'trench' in the anterior part of the head of the humerus, which has been rocking between the true and the false glenoid cavities.

15 points has a good shoulder, but by no means a normal one. The system of recording the active and passive range of movements of the shoulder is set out in Table 21.3; it includes measurement of the range of active pronation–supination, which usually improves after successful re-location of a dislocated joint. This system recognises that loss of active range may arise from paralysis or weakness of muscles, but also from fixed contracture. The following two specific measures merit description.

The inferior gleno-humeral angle
This is the angle between the axes of the humerus and the lateral border of the scapula with the arm in abduction. In the normal shoulder this is at least 150°. In some children, contracture of the inferior capsule and of latissimus dorsi and teres major is so tight that the active and the passive angle is diminished to 30–40°. Weakness of the abductor muscles of the shoulder is shown by substantial discrepancy between the passive and the active range.

Table 21.2 A method of staging shoulder function in obstetrical brachial plexus palsy

Stage 0	Flail shoulder
Stage I	Abduction or flexion to 45°. No active lateral rotation
Stage II	Abduction <90°. Lateral rotation to neutral
Stage III	Abduction = 90°. Weak lateral rotation
Stage IV	Abduction <120°. Incomplete lateral rotation
Stage V	Abduction >120°. Active lateral rotation
Stage VI	Normal

The suffix + is added to indicate the presence of sufficient medial rotation to permit the hand to come against the opposite shoulder.
Our convention restricts children with no lateral rotation beyond neutral to Stage I; usually I +, because adequate medial rotation is maintatined.
(Reproduced from Gilbert 1993.)

The posterior gleno-humeral contracture

This is measured as follows. The affected hand is placed on to the opposite shoulder, with the axis of the humerus parallel to the ground. The angle between the axes of the humerus and of the blade of the scapula is measured. In a normal shoulder this should be 70°, whereas in a severe contracture it may be reduced to 0°. Some of this contracture arises from capsular tightness, and it can be overcome by firm depression of the scapula onto the chest wall while the arm is held in the position described. However, most of the contracture is caused by retroversion of the neck of the humerus. It is commonly seen after successful re-location of dislocation. The treatment is straightforward and outlined below.

TREATMENT

Obviously, the best treatment is prevention. It is possible to overcome an uncomplicated medial rotation contracture by

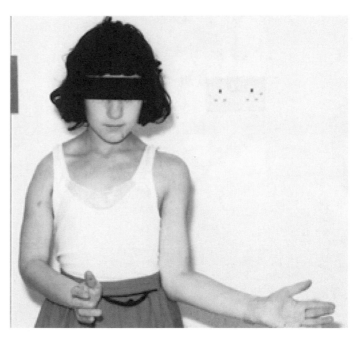

Figure 21.14 Posterior dislocation in a 7-year-old girl. Note the limitation of lateral rotation, the flattening of the contour of the shoulder, and the elevation of the spine of the scapula.

assiduous, but gentle, stretching of both limbs into lateral rotation *with the arms adducted against the side*. The clinician should teach the parents this exercise and insist that physiotherapists perform the stretch correctly. Close monitoring is essential: the author expects to review such children at least every 6 weeks. The exercises are performed four or five times before every feed, in the case of infants. The arms are held in the position of lateral rotation for 4 or 5 seconds. If the exercise provokes pain then the clinician should assume that the shoulder is incongruent. Persisting with these exercises when the shoulder is plainly incongruent is damaging.

TREATMENT BY OPERATION

Subscapularis recession

This was described by Carlioz & Brahimi in 1986. Gilbert (1993) emphasised that the operation should be performed only if the shoulder is congruent. This operation was undertaken in 86 children during the years 1987 to 1992 and, although initial results were promising, the deformity recurred in 41 of them (48%). Each year sees a steady flow of further failures. My colleagues and I are no longer of the opinion that subscapularis recession has any place in treatment and it has been abandoned in our Unit.

Lateral rotation osteotomy of the shaft of the humerus

This operation also has no place in the treatment of the deformity. It does nothing to secure congruent reduction of the head of the humerus into the true glenoid, and it increases retroversion of the humeral head. Results have

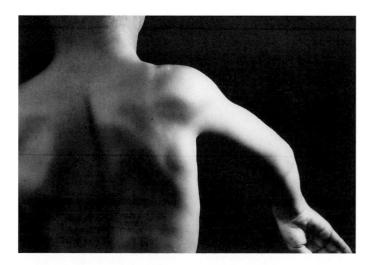

Figure 21.13 Posterior subluxation in a 5-year-old boy. The head of the humerus is prominent, and there is a flexion–pronation posture at the elbow. Radiographs showed no significant secondary bone deformity.

Table 21.3 The Hospital Peripheral Nerve Injury Unit system for recording active and passive ranges of movement in the shoulder of patients with obstetrical brachial plexus palsy (OBPP)

Peripheral nerve injury unit operative and follow up chart in OBPP

Name	
Hospital number	

Shoulder pathology	1. Dislocation
	  a. Simple or complex
	  b. Overgrowth of coracoid
	2. Subluxation
	  a. Simple
	  b. Complex
	
	3. Contracture
	  a. Internal rotation
	  b. Posterior contracture
	  c. Abduction contracture
	  d. Abduction and posterior contraction
	4. Flail
	NB: Abd. Contracture signifies inferior GH contracture and internal rotation signifies medial rotation

Operative history	Operation on shoulder 1. Subscapularis recession 2. Anterior release 3. Posterior release 4. Anterior release with bone work 5. Simple muscle transfer 6. SMT LD to cuff 7. SMT pec major 8. ERO 9. CMT 10. CMT for abduction 11. CMT for abduction and ER 12. Relocation shoulder simple 13. Relocation shoulder complex 14. Elongation LD 15. Lengthening subscapularis 16. Simple muscle release 17. MRO
Date	Date
Date	Date

Pre and post operative scores

Date	Mallett	Gilbert	Raimondi	Elbow

page 2 (OBPP shoulder)

Range of movement

Date	Forward flexion		Lateral rotation		Inferior GH angle		Post GH angle		Abduction		Medial rotation		Rotation forearm	
	Active	Passive	Active	Passive	Active	Passive	Active	Passive	Active	Passive	Active	Passive	Active	Passive

been singularly unimpressive in those patients in whom it was used as a palliation for the irreducible shoulder.

Correction of deformity by the anterior approach

The purpose of this operation is to secure congruent re-location of the head of the humerus into the true glenoid. The obstacles to reduction include overgrowth of the cora-coid process, contracture of the coraco-humeral ligament, and contracture of the subscapularis muscle. Significant retroversion of the neck of the humerus must also be corrected.

RESULTS OF TREATMENT

There have been no major complications in 450 operations for correction of medial rotation contracture or subluxation–dislocation. However, re-dislocation has occurred in 12 cases of complex dislocation and in these a posterior bone block proved necessary. The precise indication for this technique has yet to be clarified, but it is probably necessary in long-standing cases with marked abnormality of the posterior lip of the glenoid. It is in these cases that an MRI scan has a place in defining glenoid morphology.

Medial de-rotation osteotomy of the humerus is necessary

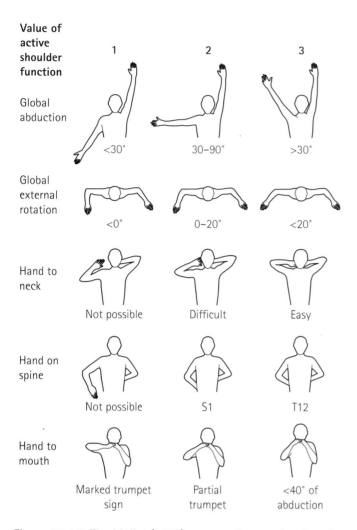

Value of active shoulder function	1	2	3
Global abduction	<30°	30–90°	>30°
Global external rotation	<0°	0–20°	<20°
Hand to neck	Not possible	Difficult	Easy
Hand on spine	Not possible	S1	T12
Hand to mouth	Marked trumpet sign	Partial trumpet	<40° of abduction

Figure 21.15 The Mallet (1972) system of measuring function at the shoulder.

in about 30% of cases. The long-term outcome from this intervention will not be known for a number of years. It is likely that later reconstructive operations will prove neces-

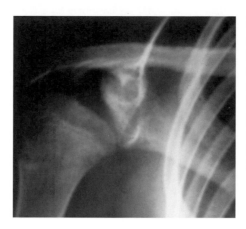

Figure 21.17 Anteroposterior radiograph of the shoulder of the girl despicted in Fig. 21.16, showing persisting deformation of the head of the humerus.

sary in some of these children when they reach adult life. We hope that, by improving the anatomical relation of the gleno-humeral joint, it will render subsequent arthroplasty or even arthrodesis a practical proposition.

The improvement in function at the elbow and in the forearm is, at times, remarkable. Birch & Chen (1996) found that the range of active forearm rotation was increased by, on average, 50°. In a small number of children, improvement of active extension of the wrist was seen. The observations of parents and our functional assessments in these children suggest that successful re-location of the shoulder brings about marked improvement, not only at the shoulder but also in the function of the limb as a whole (Figs 21.16–21.18).

ACKNOWLEDGEMENTS

Mr George Bonney MS kindly gave permission for use of the photographs in this chapter, drawn from *Surgical Disorders of the Peripheral Nerves* (Birch et al 1998). The copyright is held by him and his co-authors. Mrs Margaret Taggart was responsible for collating all clinical records and preparation of the manuscript.

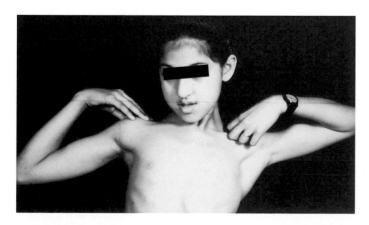

Figure 21.16 Shoulder movements in a 12-year-old girl, 6 years after reduction of complex dislocation of her shoulder. Her range of shoulder movement was virtually normal.

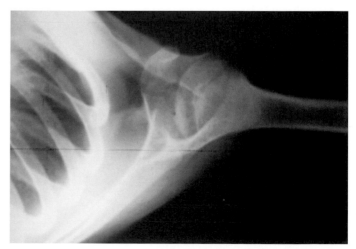

Figure 21.18 Axial radiograph of the shoulder of the girl depicted in Fig. 21.16, showing good re-modelling of the glenoid, but the head of the humerus appears broad and flattened.

REFERENCES AND FURTHER READING

Birch R, Chen L 1996 The medial rotation contracture of the shoulder in obstetric brachial plexus palsy. Journal of Bone and Joint Surgery 73B (Suppl): 68

Birch R, Bonney G, Wynn Parry C B 1998 Birth lesions of the brachial plexus. In: Birch R, Bonney G, Wynn Parry C B (eds) Surgical Disorders of the Peripheral Nerves, Churchill Livingstone, London

Carlioz H, Brahimi L 1986 La place de la désinsertion interne du sous-scapulaire dans le traitement de la paralysie obstétricale du membre supérieur chez l'enfant. Annales de Chirurgie de l'infant 12: 159

Fairbank H A T 1913 Subluxation of shoulder joint in infants and young children. Lancet 1: 1217–1223

Gilbert A 1993 Obstetrical brachial plexus palsy. In: Tubiana R (ed) The Hand, vol 4, Ch. 38. W B Saunders, Philadelphia, pp 576–601 (English translation)

Gilbert A 1995 Paralysie obstétricale du plexus brachial. In: Alnot J-Y, Narakas A (eds) Les Paralysies du Plexus Brachial, 2nd edn. Monographie de la Société Français de Chirurgie de la Main. Expansion Scientifique Français, 270–281

Landi A, Schoenhuber R, Funicello R, Rasio G, Esposito M 1992 Compartment syndrome of the scapula. Annals of Hand Surgery 11: 383–388

Mallet J 1972 Paralysie obstetricle. Revue de Chirurgie Orthopedique 58 (suppl 1): 115

Pearl M L, Edgerton B W 1998 Glenoid deformity secondary to brachial plexus birth palsy. Journal of Bone and Joint Surgery 80A: 659–667

Scaglietti O 1938 The obstetrical shoulder trauma. Surgery, Gynecology and Obstetrics 66: 868–877

Sever J W 1925 Obstetrical paralysis. Report of eleven hundred cases. Journal of The American Medical Association 85: 1862–1865

Waters P M, Smith G R, Jaramillo D 1998 Gleno-humeral deformity secondary to brachial plexus birth palsy. Journal of Bone and Joint Surgery 80A: 668–677

Zancolli E A, Zancolli E R 1993 Palliative surgical procedures in sequelae of obstetrical palsy. In: Tubiana R (ed) The Hand, vol 4. W B Saunders, Philadelphia, pp 602–623 (English translation)

Chapter 22

Classification and management of lower limb reduction anomalies

J. A. Fixsen

INTRODUCTION

Congenital limb deficiencies or reduction anomalies in the lower limbs are the result of failure of formation of parts in the first trimester of pregnancy. They can also result from the constriction band syndrome sometimes known as Streeter's dysplasia.

Two types of abnormal development can occur, causing transverse and longitudinal deficiency. In *transverse deficiency*, the proximodistal development is normal until the level of the deficiency, although there is nearly always some attempt at development of rudimentary digits (digital buds) on the end of the limb, which may vary from puckering of the skin to small but formed digits (Fig. 22.1). In *longitudinal deficiency*, there is a reduction or absence of a bone or bones in the long axis of the limb. However, there are often normal or near normal elements distal to the affected bone or bones (see Fig. 22.6A). It is most important to remember that the deficiency is not simply of bone, but also of muscles and soft tissues.

CLASSIFICATION

In the past, many classifications have been suggested, often using Greco-Latin terms such as fibular hemimelia, dysmelia or amelia. However, in 1989, the International Standards Organisation published ISO 8548/1 'Method of Describing Limb Deficiencies Present at Birth' (Day 1991). This has now been generally accepted by the International Society for Prosthetics and Orthotics (ISPO) and other national organisations. It uses a simple anatomical system based on whether the deficiency is transverse or longitudinal.

Transverse deficiencies in the lower limb are described by the segment at which the limb terminates and then the level within that segment beyond which there are no skeletal elements, disregarding digital buds. The segments defined in the lower limb are the pelvis, thigh, leg, tarsal, metatarsal, phalangeal (note metatarsal and phalangeal can be combined, when they are termed a 'ray'). Thus a transverse deficiency at upper third tibial level would be termed 'transverse leg upper third' (Fig. 22.1).

Longitudinal deficiency is described by naming the affected bones in a proximodistal sequence and whether each affected bone is partially or totally absent. If a bone is partially absent, its position and the approximate fraction missing can be described. The bones are named as ilium,

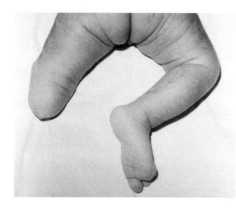

Figure 22.1
Transverse deficiency. Transverse leg upper third.

ischium, pubis, femur, tibia, fibula, tarsals, metatarsals, and phalanges; the last two can be described together as a ray. Thus a case of proximal femoral focal deficiency with partial absence of the fibula and a four-ray foot (see Fig. 22.6) would be described as femur, partial upper two thirds, fibula, partial upper quarter, ray 5 total.

AETIOLOGY

The orthopaedic surgeon dealing with children should be familiar with the three main forms of congenital shortening of the lower limb:

1. Shortening of the femur or femoral dysplasia in all its forms, encompassing idiopathic coxa vara, congenital short femur and proximal femoral focal deficiency (PFFD).
2. Congenital short tibia with absent or hypoplastic fibula.
3. Congenital dysplasia or absence of the tibia with intact fibula.

The lower limb bud appears at 28 days of intrauterine life and major development of the limb is complete in 10–14 days, after which growth and enlargement occur. A number of agents, of which the drug thalidomide is the best known, can cause abnormalities of development during this early vital period. The majority of major congenital limb deficiencies occur sporadically; a few, such as tibial dysplasia and some instances of idiopathic coxa vara, have an unequivocal genetic background. In the chick embryo, it has been possible to reproduce all the various limb deficiencies by insults to the limb bud; however, the cause in the great majority of children remains unknown. Abnormality in development of the normal vascular pattern in the limb has been suggested by Morgan & Somerville (1960), Hootnick et al (1980) and, more recently, by Szeizel et al (1994), who looked at the association between smoking during pregnancy and congenital limb deficiency. Although the major deficiency is usually in one segment of the limb, a lesser degree of shortening in the other segments of the limb, which adds to the overall length discrepancy is extremely common and must be recognised.

The parents of a child with a major limb deficiency are always extremely upset by the deformity and want to know the cause and the treatment as soon as possible. Unfortunately, apart from the few inherited forms, the cause, is almost invariably unknown. Treatment should never be rushed, and it is most important to reassure parents that these children will be able to walk despite their major limb deficiency. It is usually most unwise to rush into any surgical treatment in the first year of life, although physiotherapy to stretch and mobilise deformities may be useful. Many of these children will require extension prostheses, and sometimes amputation. It is important to introduce the parents gently to the idea of an extension prosthesis, and possibly an amputation, as most will find this very hard to accept in the first instance. A visit to the prosthetic surgeon and the prosthetic unit where they can see another child with the same or similar condition is very helpful in reassuring them with regard to the child's future walking ability and function with a prosthesis. An important report by the working party of the Amputee Medical Rehabilitation Society on recommended standards of care for the child with congenital limb deficiency was published in 1997 and reviews the subject, recommending that there should be special limb deficiency clinics to which the child and the parents could be referred as soon as possible after birth – certainly within 3 months of birth. This would be a major advance in the management of these children and their families.

THE FEMUR

IDIOPATHIC COXA VARA (DEVELOPMENTAL COXA VARA, INFANTILE COXA VARA)

This condition is the most minor form of femoral dysplasia. It involves the inferior portion of the capital femoral epiphysis and adjacent metaphysis. It is rarely, if ever, diagnosed at birth, but becomes apparent as the child grows and the leg appears short, with the development of a Trendelenburg gait, limitation of abduction and increased external rotation of the affected side. The cause is unknown, although there are reports of families in which there appears to be a genetic influence. The child normally presents, after walking age, with a limp and shortening. On examination, there is limitation of abduction and usually an increased range of external rotation at the affected hip. The majority of cases are unilateral, but the condition can occur bilaterally. Its incidence is not clearly known. When first discovered, idiopathic coxa vara is sometimes mistaken for congenital dislocation of the

hip and it is important to consider other causes of coxa vara such as trauma, infection, bone dysplasia, metabolic disease and the common association with other forms of limb dysplasia to be described later. The important point in idiopathic coxa vara is that the X-ray changes are confined entirely to the femoral neck.

X-ray changes

Radiological changes are typical once they appear. In the first year of life, they may be difficult to distinguish. Until proximal femoral ossification occurs, the femur may appear relatively normal. As the femoral head and neck ossify, the classical triangular fragment (Fairbanks' triangle) on the inferior surface of the femoral neck becomes apparent, together with varus deformity of the femoral neck. The epiphyseal plate lies vertical and appears irregular. An inverted Y delineates the triangular fragment in the inferior part of the femoral neck (Fig. 22.2). If the condition is untreated, dysplasia of the femoral neck increases with growth and the varus increases, with proximal migration of the greater trochanter relative to the femoral head, giving rise to the so-called 'shepherd's crook' deformity. When considering differential diagnoses, it is important to remember cleido-cranial dysostosis, which can give rise to bilateral coxa vara associated with absence or poor development of the clavicles, and delayed fusion of the skull suture lines and symphysis pubis (Fig. 22.3). Osteogenesis imperfecta and metaphyseal dysostosis can also give rise to coxa vara.

Management

Once the condition has been diagnosed, correction of the coxa vara should be considered. A varus deformity greater than 110° should be observed and may resolve. However, once the varus of the neck decreases to less than 110°, progession of the deformity is likely to occur. In the early stages, a simple shoe raise can be used, but if varus progresses to less than 100°, surgery should be considered to prevent inevitable deterioration. The aim of surgery is to

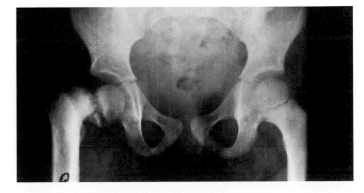

Figure 22.2 Anteroposterior X-ray of the pelvis of a patient with idiopathic coxa vara affecting the right hip. Note the severe reduction of the neck–shaft angle, the clear-cut Fairbanks' triangle and the inverted Y appearance of the epiphyseal plate.

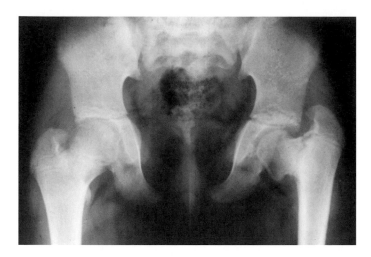

Figure 22.3 Anteroposterior X-ray of the pelvis of a patient with cleido-cranial dysostosis. Note the bilateral coxa vara, the proximal migration of the greater trochanters, the shepherd's crook deformity on the left and the absence of ossification at the public symphysis.

correct the neck–shaft angle to 140° by an abduction osteotomy. Many techniques have been described, but provided the operation achieves 140° of neck–shaft angle and a more horizontal position of the epiphyseal plate, the changes in the femoral neck should heal and recover. Repeat valgus osteotomy may be necessary, particularly if the initial osteotomy is performed early in childhood. Leg length discrepancy is rarely sufficient to require leg lengthening. Occasionally, in a neglected case, there is significant overgrowth of the greater trochanter and trochanteric transfer may be necessary.

CONGENITAL SHORT FEMUR AND PROXIMAL FOCAL FEMORAL DEFICIENCY (PFFD)

It is customary to classify major congenital shortening of the femur into these two groups. In reality, when one looks at the entire spectrum of the disorder there is a steady progression from congenital short femur, in which the femur is virtually normally formed but short, to almost total absence of the femur, with only the distal femoral condyles appearing in bone some years after birth. Ring (1959, 1961) made the important observation that the proportional shortening remains the same throughout growth, provided further displacement as a result of coxa vara or hip subluxation does not occur. Therefore if the femur is 20% short at birth, it is likely to be 20% short in the adult, and so a reasonable estimate of the overall shortening at maturity can be made in the first year of life. It is important to remember that the abnormality is not confined to the femur. The knee is nearly always to some extent unstable, and there may be congenital absence of the cruciates (Thomas et al 1985, Sanpera et al 1995). The lower leg is nearly always to some degree short, and there may be absence or hypoplasia of the fibula. The foot is often remarkably normal.

Classifications have been published by Amstutz & Wilson (1962), Hamanishi (1980) (Fig. 22.4) and Pappas (1983). On the basis of data from the Edinburgh birth registry, Hamanishi suggested that the incidence of this condition was around 1 in 50 000 live births.

The cause of this disorder is unknown. It can be associated with abnormalities not only in the lower limb, but also in the upper limb, and with facial abnormalities as in the congenital short femur abnormal facies syndrome.

Embryologically, the hip and upper femur develop from the same anlage and so it is not surprising that, the more dysplastic the upper end of the femur, the more dysplastic the hip. Clinically, the leg appears short, although minor degrees of congenital short femur may not be noted at birth. Subsequently, as the legs grow, the shortening becomes obvious. It is also associated with some flexion and external rotation at the hip as a result of retroversion of the femoral neck. X-rays show a shortened femoral shaft or, in the most severe forms, no femoral shaft. The acetabulum may be normally developed or virtually absent in the most severe forms.

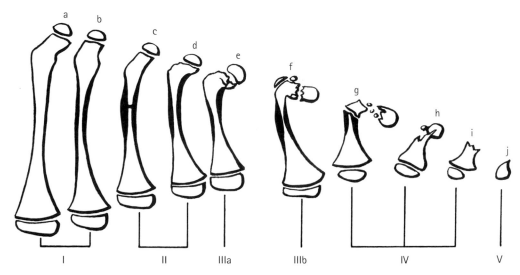

Figure 22.4 Classification of femoral dysplasia as described by Hamanishi in 1980. (© Journal of Bone and Joint Surgery.)

Fixsen & Lloyd-Roberts (1974) pointed out the importance of the appearance of the acetabulum and upper end of the femur in the early X-ray. The X-ray at birth can be difficult to assess, but that at 1 year is more reliable (Fig. 22.5). If the acetabulum is well formed, a femoral head is likely to appear. If the upper end of the femoral shaft is rounded and bulbous without sclerosis, spontaneous ossification of the cartilaginous femoral neck is likely to occur with time. If, however, the proximal end of the femur is sclerosed or pointed and migrates proximal to the acetabulum, there is established instability of the unossified femoral neck, which justifies surgical correction if the femoral head is developing satisfactorily. Sanpera & Sparks (1994) concluded that this was the most reliable classification among five they tested. In the future, magnetic resonance imaging may give us a much better picture of what is happening in the proximal femur.

Congenital short femur

Congenital short femur is the mildest form of femoral dysplasia, in which the femur is short, with an average growth retardation of about 10%. Affected patients (Fig. 22.6) have typically a rather bulky thigh, with a fixed external rotation deformity at the hip and a mildly unstable knee. They are good candidates for femoral lengthening. However, care must be taken not to increase instability of the knee. It is also possible to displace the hip during lengthening, if it is in any way dysplastic.

Proximal femoral focal deficiency (PFFD)

Proximal femoral focal deficiency (PFFD) was initially defined by Aitken in 1969. He defined four types, A–D (Fig. 22.7). He pointed out the importance of the appearance of the acetabulum with reference to the appearance of the femoral head, and the increasing coxa vara that occurs with increasing severity. These patients are likely to have major shortening, and in some cases the foot will be at the level of

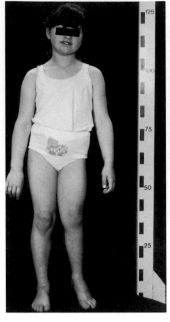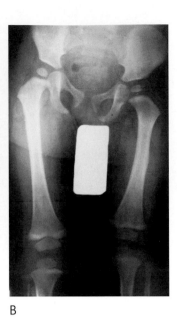

A

B

Figure 22.6 A Clinical photograph of a patient aged 8 years, with left congenital short femur. Note the bulky thigh, slight external rotation of the leg and valgus knee. The girl has a four-ray foot that is in equinus; she can reach the floor easily by tilting the pelvis down on the left and putting her foot in equinus. B Anteroposterior X-ray of both femora and pelvis in the same patient. Note that the femur is short and slightly laterally bowed, with some sclerosis in the diaphysis.

the opposite knee (Fig. 22.8). In those patients who develop a reasonable femoral head, it seems logical to stabilise the femoral shaft on the femoral head by abduction osteotomy in the less severe forms and by the King procedure (King 1969), in which the proximal end of the ossified femur is

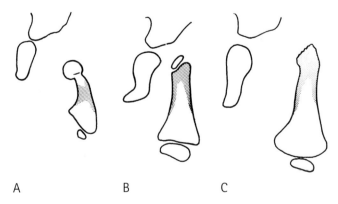

A   B   C

Fig. 22.5 Classification described by Fixsen & Lloyd-Roberts (1974), relating the appearance of the acetabulum and upper end of the femur in the early X-ray to the future development of stability of the upper end of the femur. A Type 1 (stable). B Type 2 (unstable). C Type 3 (unstable). (© Journal of Bone and Joint Surgery.)

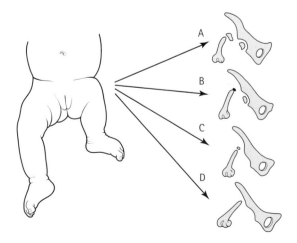

Figure 22.7 The classification of proximal femoral focal deficiency described by Aitken in 1969. (Reproduced with permission.)

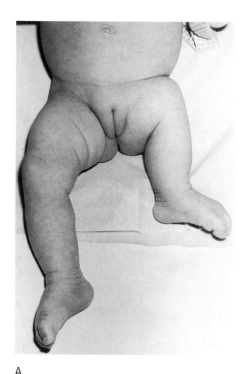

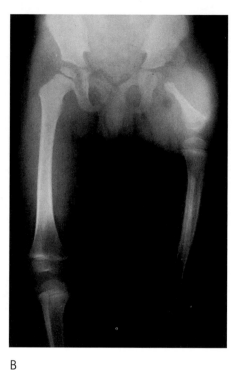

Figure 22.8 **A** Clinical photograph of a child aged 1 year with proximal femoral focal deficiency. Note the very short femoral segment, which is held flexed and externally rotated. The foot is almost at the level of the opposite knee. **B** Anteroposterior X-ray of a similar patient. Note again the very short femoral segment and that there is abnormality below the knee, with hypoplasia of the fibula.

A

B

implanted into the cartilaginous head and neck, in the more severe forms.

Goddard et al 1995 reviewed the natural history and treatment of instability of the hip in proximal femoral focal deficiency in 67 patients. These patients will all have a degree of shortening that requires a prosthetic extension leg early in life. Lengthening, even by modern methods, becomes increasingly difficult because of the severe shortening and the abnormality of the hip and knee. Damsin et al (1995) published an excellent review of the problems of management of major congenital limb shortening, in which they divided the problems into three types: a) the type in which equalisation by leg lengthening and overall stability of the limb was possible, b) the type in which leg lengthening and equalisation were possible, but stability was not, and c) the type in which successful leg equalisation by leg lengthening was not possible.

If the foot is at the level of the opposite knee, two possible approaches are advocated. The knee may be fused and the foot amputated to provide an adequate above-knee stump so that a good above-knee prosthesis can be fitted (Panting & Williams 1978). Alternatively, the Van Nes rotationplasty described by Borggreve in 1930 and reviewed by Gillespie & Torode (1983) may be advised. In this procedure, the limb is rotated 180° and the knee fused. The foot faces backwards, and acts as a new knee. There is considerable dispute between these two schools of thought, but the Van Nes rotationplasty is suitable only if the foot and ankle that are to be rotated are virtually normal, with the ability of the foot to plantarflex to 180°.

In the most severe forms, in which the hip has not formed satisfactorily, it has been suggested that fusing the remnant

of the femur to the ilium and using the knee as a primitive hinge hip would be useful. However, the majority of prosthetic surgeons find the limb easier to fit and manage if the femoral remnant is allowed to remain freely mobile.

CONGENITAL SHORT TIBIA WITH ABSENT OR HYPOPLASTIC FIBULA

This condition, like femoral dysplasia, can vary in severity from complete absence of the fibula, with a short bowed tibia and a major reduction deformity of the foot, to simple shortening of the tibia and fibula, with reduction deformity in the foot and a relatively minor shortening at maturity. It is the most common form of major congenital shortening in the lower limb, occurring in approximately 1 in 25 000 live births. It does not appear to be inherited, but may be associated with other abnormalities in the same limb or the upper limb.

The clinical appearance in the classical form is typical, with marked anterior bowing of the tibia, and a dimple over the skin at the apex of the tibial kyphosis (Fig. 22.9); this dimple is also seen over the lateral side of the femur in congenital short and dysplastic femur. The foot is usually in valgus, with absence of one or more of the lateral rays. X-rays show marked anterior bowing of the tibia with some sclerosis; it is very important not to mistake this condition for congenital pseudarthrosis of the tibia, which also shows sclerosis at the site of bowing, but not the other features of this condition. The fibula may be totally absent or hypoplastic, being represented by a short or very small distal remnant of ossification. A classification of the condition that is most widely used is that of Achterman & Kalamchi

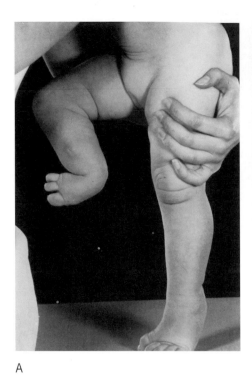

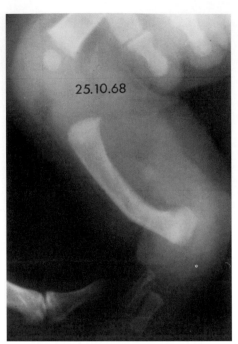

A

B

Figure 22.9 A Clinical appearance of congenital short tibia with absent fibula and deficient lateral two rays of the foot. Note the dimple over the apex of the tibial bow and severe valgus and everted position of the foot, which lacks the lateral two rays. B Radiograph in the first year of life, showing the anterior bowing of the tibia. There appears to be a small degree of ossification in the line of the fibula, and a three-ray foot. At this age, the tarsal coalition cannot be seen because the bones are not yet ossified.

(1979), who divided the deformity into types IA and IB, in which some of the fibula was present, and type II in which the fibula was completely or virtually completely absent on X-ray (Fig. 22.10). The anterior bowing of the tibia usually corrects spontaneously and does not require correction by osteotomy. If, however, the tibia is osteotomised it will, unlike congenital pseudarthrosis, heal satisfactorily. The position of the foot in severe cases is nearly always in valgus. If the fibula is completely absent, a fibrous

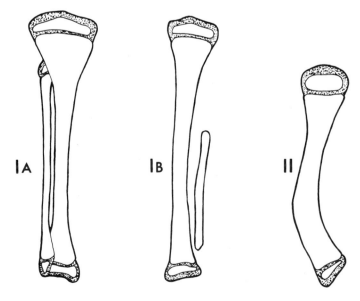

Figure 22.10 Classification of congenital short tibia with absent or hypoplastic fibula. (From Achterman & Kalamchi 1979 © Journal of Bone and Joint Surgery.)

Thompson's band may be found. It is important to realise that, in addition to having a deficient ray or rays in the foot, there is frequently tarsal coalition, and so release of the lateral structures will not completely correct the valgus deformity of the foot. The knee often shows both cruciate deficiency and a valgus deformity. Hootnick et al (1977) showed that the proportional shortening of the lower limb obeyed the same rules as that described by Ring in 1959, and so it is possible in the first year of life to estimate the expected shortening at maturity. Subsequently, Hootnick et al (1980) demonstrated vascular abnormalities as the possible cause of the deformity.

If the foot is reasonably intact, with modern leg lengthening techniques it is possible to consider retaining the foot and lengthening the leg. To correct the equinovalgus deformity of the foot, removal of the lateral fibrocartilaginous band should be considered by the time the child wants to walk. Serafin (1967) described the Gruca operation, in which a bony ankle mortice is made from the lower end of the tibia. However, Thomas & Williams (1987) reported mediocre results in the long term from this ingenious procedure. If the foot is grossly abnormal and the tibia significantly short, amputation of the foot through the ankle joint is still the best operation and gives excellent functional results (Wood et al 1965). The important features of this amputation are that the flaps are kept very long and that the heel pad, which is drawn posteriorly by the equinus position of the foot, should be positioned squarely on the end of the tibia and held with a K wire for the first 2 weeks, to ensure that the weight-bearing heel pad remains in position over the distal end of the tibia.

If lengthening is undertaken in the severe deformity with

a reasonable foot, the Ilizarov apparatus, which has the ability both to correct deformity in the foot and to lengthen the leg, offers an excellent method of correcting this complicated deformity (Gibbons & Bradish, 1996).

In its more minor form, the condition may not be recognised because the fibula is present and the most obvious anomaly is the reduction deformity in the foot (Fig. 22.11). These patients are often believed to have simply a reduction deformity in the foot, and only present later with variable shortening of the lower leg. X-rays confirm the reduction deformity in the foot, and also tarsal coalition. With the latter, there is usually a ball and socket ankle joint. The fibula is present, though it may be slightly hypoplastic and, interestingly, the foot deformity is usually one of equinovarus rather than valgus. These children may require leg equalisation, either by epiphyseodesis or by leg lengthening (Maffuli & Fixsen 1991).

CONGENITAL DYSPLASIA OR ABSENCE OF THE TIBIA WITH INTACT FIBULA

This is the rarest of the major congenital anomalies of the lower leg. It occurs in 1 in 1 000 000 live births. It may be inherited and associated with medial duplication of both the hands and feet. Jones et al (1978) proposed a classification into four groups, based on the initial radiograph (Fig. 22.12A). This has subsequently been modified into three types by Kalamchi & Dawe (1985) (Fig. 22.12B). However, Schoenecker et al (1989), in a major review of 71 limbs in 57 patients, felt that the Jones classification into four groups was preferable.

The clinical appearance is typical, with gross equinovarus deformity of the foot, which may show medial duplication (Fig. 22.13A and B). The fibula is intact, and there may be severe varus at the knee. As in femoral dysplasia, the X-ray at 1 year gives a clearer picture of the dysplasia than the X-ray at birth.

Type 1a

There is no evidence of ossification in the tibia, and no tibial cartilaginous remnant is present. The distal end of the femur is hypoplastic, and the ossific nucleus small or absent. In these patients there is usually no quadriceps apparatus, or it is only very poorly developed, and the best treatment is disarticulation through the knee. The alternative is the procedure described by Brown (1965), in which the intact fibula is placed under the femur and held there with K wires. The problem concerning this reconstruction is the inherent instability of the knee and the lack of the quadriceps apparatus. Brown advises that the operation is best performed before the child reaches the age of 1 year, usually around 6 months. Long-term review of this procedure by Loder & Herring (1987) suggested that it is rarely satisfactory, because of ligamentous instability, poor active range of movement and a progressive flexion contracture, so that the patient functions as a through-knee amputee, despite retention of the fibula. However, it is an alternative in patients whose parents refuse amputation.

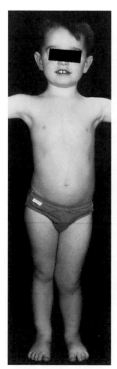

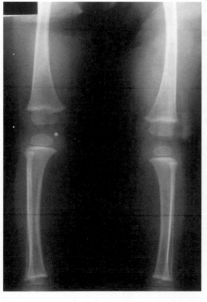

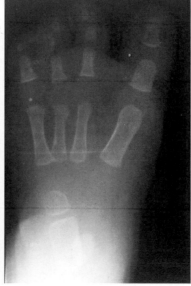

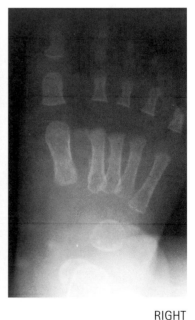

B   C   LEFT   RIGHT

Figure 22.11 A Clinical photograph of the minor form of congenital short tibia with hypoplastic fibula and absence of the lateral ray of the foot. Note there is still a degree of valgus at the knee. **B** Anteroposterior X-ray of the same patient. Note that the fibula is present on both sides. **C** Anteroposterior X-ray of the feet of the same patient. Note the absent fifth ray on the left.

A

Type	Radiological description		No. of limbs
1a		• Tibia not seen • Hypoplastic lower femoral epiphysis	6
1b		• Tibia not seen • Normal lower femoral epiphysis	12
2		• Distal tibia not seen	5
3		• Proximal tibia not seen	2
4		• Diastasis	4

A

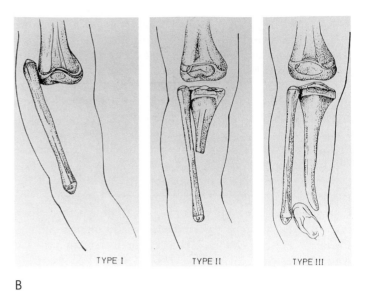

B

Figure 22.12 **A** The classification of congenital dysplasia of the tibia with intact fibula as described by Jones et al (1978). **B** Classification of congenital dysplasia of the tibia with intact fibula as modified by Kalamchi & Dawe (1985). (© Journal of Bone and Joint Surgery.)

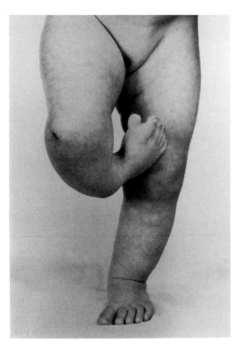

A

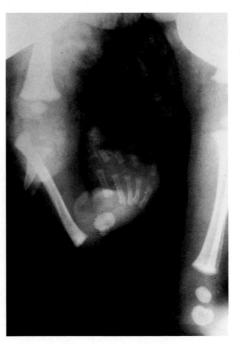

B

Figure 22.13 Type 2 tibial dysplasia with intact fibula. **A** Clinical appearance. Note the severe equinovarus of the foot, which shows duplication of the big toe only in this child. **B** Anteroposterior X-ray of the leg. Note that the upper end of the tibia is present in bone, and the fibula in marked varus at the knee, with severe equinovarus of the foot.

Type 1b

The distal end of the femur is well developed with a normal or near normal ossific nucleus. The proximal tibia is present in cartilage, but not visible on the early X-ray. The quadriceps apparatus is also present. As a result of these features, these children can be treated as type II patients, in whom the upper end of the tibia is ossified on the X-ray.

Type 2

The upper end of the tibia and the quadriceps apparatus are present, and it is reasonable to preserve the leg below the knee. Because of the foot deformity, amputation of the foot is still advised, and the fibula is fused to the tibial remnant to obtain a longer below-knee stump. As this is a through-joint amputation, there should be no problems with overgrowth of the end of the stump during growth. It is interesting that, in children, through-joint amputations do not overgrow and require revision, whereas through-bone amputations inevitably overgrow and often require repeated revision during growth. These patients do well with a prosthesis, and if their knee control is satisfactory they can manage with a below-knee patellar-tendon-bearing prosthesis. De Sanctis & Nunziata Rega (1996) have reported a maturity review of three patients in whom the foot had been retained in type II tibial dysplasia, although this required repeated surgery for recurrent deformity of the foot and limb lengthening.

Type 3

The tibia is represented by a typically amorphous segment of bone, which is present more distally than proximally. This is the rarest type, representing only two cases in the series of Jones et al (1978), and seven in that of Schoenecker et al (1989). All were treated by amputation.

Type 4

The tibia is present, but short, and there is diastasis between the lower end of the tibia and the fibula. The foot is in equinovarus, and may be mistaken for a severe club foot deformity (Fig. 22.14A and B). However, the talus articulates not with the lower end of the tibia but with the fibula, and it is extremely difficult to correct the foot deformity. In the past, amputation for this, the mildest form of tibial dysplasia, has been advocated; however, parents find this difficult to accept, particularly with modern leg-lengthening techniques. The Ilizarov apparatus, which allows control of the foot and lengthening of the limb, would appear to be the most suitable technique to use if the foot is to be retained.

CONGENITAL PSEUDARTHROSIS OF THE TIBIA

Congenital pseudarthrosis of the tibia is rare. Its estimated incidence is 1 in 140 000 live births. Its aetiology is unknown and its management difficult. The name is confusing, in that fracture at birth is rare; the condition is better called infantile pseudarthrosis of the tibia. Fracture commonly occurs in the first 2 years after birth, but may be delayed until very much later.

CLINICAL AND RADIOLOGICAL APPEARANCES

The tibia is bowed anteriorly, and commonly laterally, often with shortening (Fig. 22.15). The most common site of the deformity is at the junction of the proximal two-thirds with the distal one-third of the tibia. A number of classifications based on the clinical and radiological appearances have been described, of which the best known is that of Boyd (1982), who describes six different types. Radiologically, however, there are two main types of deformity. The more common one shows narrowing, and often

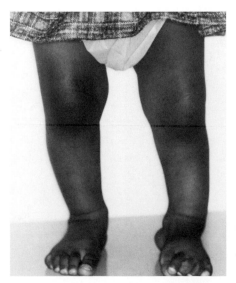

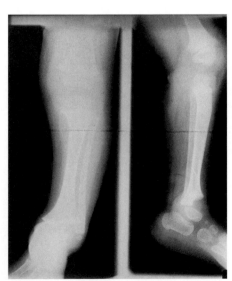

Figure 22.14 Type 4 tibial dysplasia. **A** Clinical photograph. Note the inversion of the foot and broadening of the ankle caused by the diastasis between the short dysplastic tibia and the fibula. **B** Anteroposterior and lateral X-rays of the same patient. Note the shortening of the tibia and the lack of development of a proper ankle joint.

A   B

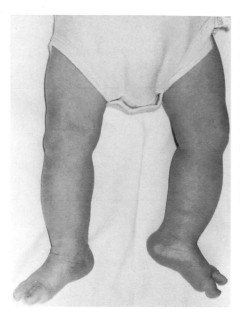

Figure 22.15 Clinical photograph of a child aged 9 months with congenital pseudarthrosis of the left tibia. Note the anterior bowing and slight shortening. At this stage the tibia is not fractured.

later. The characteristic 'cafe au lait' spots of pigmentation in the skin often do not appear until the age of 2 years. Other members of the family should be examined, because relatives very reasonably do not relate their child's bowed tibia to the occurrence of skin nodules, pigmentation or nerve tumours in other members of the family.

MANAGEMENT

Management is complex. Once fracture has occurred, union is very difficult to obtain. It is most important to recognise the condition in the prepseudarthrotic stage if possible, and not to consider osteotomy for the deformity and to precipitate non-union. Prophylactic bracing from the time the child is first diagnosed seems very worthwhile if compliance can be maintained. Murray & Lovell (1982), in an important long-term study, reported good results in a small group of patients treated by bracing alone. Prophylactic bypass grafting using graft from the fibula or tibia of the opposite leg was suggested by Lloyd-Roberts & Shaw in 1969. This method was first described by McFarland in 1951, and seems particularly appropriate in those cases with neurofibromatosis. Strong & Wong-Chung (1991) reported good results in six of nine patients treated this way with a variety of graft materials; the three patients who failed required further procedures to obtain union. Once pseudarthrosis becomes established, it is extremely difficult to heal. Many methods of grafting have been described, in a condition that is so rare that most experience is of small numbers and tends to be anecdotal. In a large review by Hardinge (1972), an amputation rate of 29% was reported; more recently, Baker et al (1992) reported four amputations (22%) in a review of 18 consecutive patients from a large American centre.

obliteration, of the marrow cavity, with surrounding sclerosis related to the apex of the anterior bowing, usually at the junction of the middle and lower thirds of the tibia (Fig. 22.16). The less common type shows a cystic lesion at the site of deformity in the tibia; it is important not to confuse this with fibrous dysplasia, which can cause a similar deformity and fracture, but responds much better to treatment in the form of curettage, grafting and intramedullary rodding. The fibula can also be involved in the disease process, either on its own or in association with changes in the tibia. Between 40 and 80% of patients will show neurofibromatosis, and it is important to look for the stigmata of this condition, which may be present when the pseudarthrosis is diagnosed, or may develop

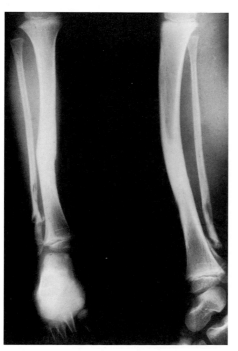

Figure 22.16 Anteroposterior and lateral radiographs of a patient with congenital pseudarthrosis of the tibia. Note the sclerosis, loss of the marrow cavity and bowing. In this patient, the fibula is involved and has already fractured.

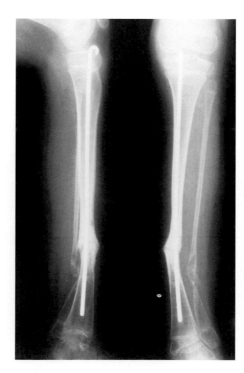

Figure 22.17 Anteroposterior and lateral radiographs showing intramedullary rodding using a Rush nail, for congenital pseudarthrosis of the tibia. At insertion, the rod was passed across the ankle joint into the talus to stabilise the lower end of the tibia, but as the tibia has grown, the rod has shortened relatively.

Three methods seem to have emerged as the best way of obtaining union in this difficult condition:

1. *Intramedullary rodding*, as described by Charnley in 1956, in which the rod is passed across the ankle into the hindfoot and combined with excision of the pseudarthrosis and autologous bone grafting (Fig. 22.17). In 1992 Anderson et al reported union in 10 of 10 patients treated in this manner, but subsequent refracture required further grafting or re-rodding in five. Paterson & Simonis (1985) used electrical stimulation from an implanted stimulator (osteostim) in addition to intramedullary rodding and obtained union in 20 of 27 tibiae. Again, these authors emphasised the importance of not removing the intramedullary rod until maturity, to avoid the danger of re-fracture.
2. *Free vascularized fibula graft*. Gilbert (1983), Pho et al (1985) and Simonis et al (1991) have reported satisfactory results using free vascularised fibula grafting from the opposite leg. This is particularly useful for a large defect and where there has been failure of previous operations.
3. *Bone transport*. Grill (1996) reported good results with a modification of the Ilizarov technique in a series of nine patients, seven of whom had several previous failed operations. This technique appears to be particularly useful in bridging large bony gaps in congenital pseudarthrosis of the tibia and in other difficult problems of bone loss in the tibia. Ilizarov first described the technique using his apparatus in 1971.

By means of one of these three methods, union can usually be obtained in at least 75–80% of patients. In view of the rarity of this condition, it is important that in any one geographical area a particular individual surgeon or group of surgeons specialises in its management and collects a sufficient number of cases to enable them to become expert in the use of one or more of these methods, and to have enough experience to provide authoritative reports on its management. The results of the European Pediatric Orthopaedic Society (EPOS) multicentre study of congenital pseudarthrosis of the tibia were recently published and are an important addition to our knowledge of this rare and difficult condition (Grill et al 2000).

TIBIA RECURVATUM (POSTEROMEDIAL ANGULATION OF THE TIBIA)

This is a very rare deformity. The tibia is bowed posteriorly and, commonly, medially at the junction of the middle and lower thirds. It occurs in association with marked calcaneus of the foot (Fig. 22.18). The appearance is alarming, but the prognosis benign. The majority of cases respond

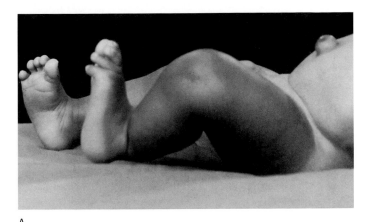

A

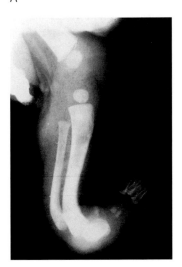

B

Figure 22.18 A Clinical photograph of a child age 5 months, with left tibia recurvata. Note the calcaneum position of the left foot. B Lateral radiograph of the same patient. Note the marked posterior bowing of both the tibia and fibula.

readily to stretching and splintage of the foot into equinus. If the surgeon is prepared to wait long enough, probably all cases will correct with time. Pappas (1984) reviewed a large group of 33 patients with this rare condition. He pointed out that, in general, the greater the initial bowing the greater the ultimate leg length discrepancy, and that the proportionate length differences between the normal and bowed tibiae remain stable after the child had reached 12 months of age. The maximum leg length discrepancy seen in his series of patients was 6.9 cm. However, if there is persistent deformity when the child starts to walk, corrective osteotomy can be undertaken. Unlike congenital pseudarthrosis of the tibia, the osteotomy will heal, despite the sclerosis at the site of angulation. However, union may take some time, and an intramedullary rod is a useful way of splinting the tibia while awaiting union. Once the deformity has corrected, the child normally manages extremely well, but should be followed up as he or she is liable to be left with some residual shortening, which may require leg equalisation procedures near maturity (Heyman et al 1959).

REFERENCES

Achterman C, Kalamchi A 1979 Longenital deficiency of the fibula. Journal of Bone and Joint Surgery 61B: 133–137

Aitken G T 1969 In: Aitken G T (ed) Proximal femoral focal deficiency. A congenital anomaly. Symposium held in Washington, 3 June 1968. National Academy of Sciences, Washington DC, pp 1–22

Amputee Medical Rehabilitation Society 1997 Congenital Limb Deficiency Recommended Standards of Care. A report by the working party of the Amputee Medical Rehabilitation Society published December 1997. Available from the Amputee Medical Rehabilitation Society c/o the Royal College of Physicians, 11 St Andrew's Place, Regents Park, London NW1 4LE, UK

Amstutz H C, Wilson P D Jr 1962 Dysgenesis of the proximal femur (coxa vara) and its surgical management. Journal of Bone and Joint Surgery 44A: 1

Anderson D J, Schoenecker P L, Sheridan J J, Rich M M 1992 Use of an intramedullary rod for treatment of congenitial pseudarthrosis of the tibia. Journal of Bone and Joint Surgery 74A: 161–168

Baker J K, Cain T E, Tullos H S 1992 Intramedullary fixation for congenital pseudarthrosis of the tibia. Journal of Bone and Joint Surgery 74A: 169–178

Borggreve J 1930 Kniegelenksersatz durch das in der Beinlängsachse um 180 Grad gedrehte Fussgelenk. Archiv der orthopädischen und Unfallchirurgie 28: 175–178

Boyd H B 1982 Pathology and natural history of congenital pseudarthrosis of the tibia. Clinical Orthopaedics and Related Research 166: 5–13

Brown F W 1965 Construction of a knee joint in congenital total absence of the tibia (paraxial hemimelia tibia) – a preliminary report. Journal of Bone and Joint Surgery 47A: 695–704

Charnley J 1956 Congenital pseudarthrosis of the tibia treated by the intramedullary nail. Journal of Bone and Joint Surgery 38A: 283–290

Damsin J B, Pous J G, Ghanem I 1995 Therapeutic approach to severe congenital lower limb length discrepancies, surgical treatment versus prosthetic management. Journal of Pediatric Orthopaedics B4: 164–170

Day H J B 1991 The ISPO/ISO classification of congenital limb deficiency. Prosthetics and Orthotics International 15: 67–69

de Sanctis N, Nunziata Rega A 1996 New rationale in management of tibial agenesis type II: a maturity review of its functional, psychological and economic value. Journal of Pediatric Orthopaedics B5: 1–5

Fixsen J A, Lloyd-Roberts G C 1974 The natural history and early treatment of proximal femoral dysplasia. Journal of Bone and Joint Surgery 56B: 86–95

Gibbons T J, Bradish C F 1996 Fibular hemimelia: a preliminary report on management of the severe abnormality. Journal of Pediatric Orthopaedics B5: 20–26

Gilbert A 1983 Vascularised fibula transfer for treatment of congenital pseudarthrosis. Annual Meeting of the American Academy of Orthopedic Surgeons, Anahein, California, 14 March 1983

Gillespie R, Torode I P 1983 Rotationplasty of the lower limb for congenital defects of the femur. Journal of Bone and Joint Surgery 65B: 569–573

Goddard N J, Hashemi-Nejad A, Fixsen J A 1995 Natural history and treatment of instability of the hip in proximal femoral focal deficiency. Journal of Pediatric Orthopaedics B4: 145–149

Grill F 1996 Treatment of congenital pseudarthrosis of tibia with the circular frame technique. Journal of Pediatric Orthopaedics Part B, 5: 6–16

Grill F et al 2000 Results of the EPOS multicentre study. Journal of Pediatric Orthopaedics Part B, 9: 1–15, 69–107

Hamanishi C 1980 Congenital short femur. Journal of Bone and Joint Surgery 62B: 307–320

Hardinge K 1972 Congenital anterior bowing of the tibia. Annals of the Royal College of Surgeons of England 51: 17–30

Heyman C H, Herndon C H, Heiple K G 1959 Congenital posterior angulation of the tibia with talipes calcaneus. Journal of Bone and Joint Surgery 41A: 476–488

Hootnick D R, Boyd N A, Fixsen J A, Lloyd-Roberts G C 1977 The natural history and management of congenital short tibia with dysplasia or absence of the fibula. A preliminary report. Journal of Bone and Joint Surgery 59B: 267–271

Hootnick D R, Levinsohn E M, Randall P A, Packard D S Jr 1980 Vascular dysgenesis associated with skeletal dysplasia of the lower limb. Journal of Bone and Joint Surgery 62A: 1123–1129

Ilizarov G A 1971 Basic principles of transosseous compression and distraction osteosynthesis. Ortopedia Travmatologiial i Protezirovanie 32: 7–15

Jones D, Barnes J, Lloyd-Roberts G C 1978 Congenital aplasia and dysplasia of the tibia with intact fibula. Journal of Bone and Joint Surgery 60B: 31–39

Kalamchi A, Dawe R B 1985 Congenital deficiency of the tibia. Journal of Bone and Joint Surgery 67B: 581–584

King R E 1969 In: Aitken G T (ed) Proximal femoral focal deficiency. A congenital anomaly. A symposium held in Washington, 3 June 1968. National Academy for Sciences, Washington DC, pp 23–49

Lloyd-Roberts G C, Shaw N E 1969 The prevention of pseudarthrosis of the tibia and congenital kyphosis of the tibia. Journal of Bone and Joint Surgery 51B: 100–105

Loder R T, Herring J A 1987 Fibular transfer for congenital absence of the tibia; a reassessment. Journal of Pediatric Orthopaedics 7: 8–13

McFarland B 1951 Pseudarthrosis of the tibia in children. Journal of Bone and Joint Surgery 43B: 36–46

Maffuli N, Fixsen J A 1991 Fibular hypoplasia with absent lateral rays of the foot. Journal of Bone and Joint Surgery 73B: 1002–1004

Morgan J D, Somerville E W 1960 Normal and abnormal growth at the upper end of the femur. Journal of Bone and Joint Surgery 42B: 264–272

Murray H H, Lovell W W 1982 Congenital pseudarthrosis of the tibia, a long term follow up study. Clinical Orthopaedics and Related Research 166: 14–20

Panting A L, Williams P F 1978 Proximal femoral focal deficiency. Journal of Bone and Joint Surgery 60B: 46–52

Pappas A M 1983 Congenital abnormalities of the femur and related lower extremity malfunction; classification and treatment. Journal of Pediatric Orthopaedics 3: 45–60

Pappas A M 1984 Congenital posteromedial bowing of the tibia and fibula. Journal of Pediatric Orthopaedics 4: 525–531

Paterson D C, Simonis R B 1985 Electrical stimulation in the treatment of congenital pseudarthrosis of the tibia. Journal of Bone and Joint Surgery 67B: 454–462

Pho R W H, Levack B, Satku K, Patradul A 1985 Free vascularised fibulograft in the treatment of congenital pseudarthrosis of the tibia. Journal of Bone and Joint Surgery 67B: 64–70

Ring P A 1959 Congenital short femur. Journal of Bone and Joint Surgery 41B: 73–79

Ring P A 1961 Congenital abnormalities of the femur. Archives of Diseases of Childhood 36: 410

Sanpera I Jr, Sparks L T 1994 Proximal femoral focal deficiency: does a radiological classification exist? Journal of Pediatric Orthopaedics 14: 34–38

Sanpera I Jr, Fixsen J A, Hill R A 1995 The knee in congenital short femur. Journal of Pediatric Orthopaedics Part B, 4: 159–163

Schoenecker P L, Kapelli A M, Millar E A et al 1989 Congenital longitudinal deficiency of the tibia. Journal of Bone and Joint Surgery 71A: 278–287

Serafin J 1967 A new operation for congenital absence of the fibula. Journal of Bone and Joint Surgery 49B: 59–65

Simonis R B, Scirali H R, Mayou B 1991 Free vascularised fibular grafts for congenital pseudarthrosis of the tibia. Journal of Bone and Joint Surgery 73B: 211–215

Strong M L, Wong-Chung J 1991 Prophylactic bypass grafting of the prepseudarthrotic tibia in neurofibromatosis. Journal of Pediatric Orthopaedics 11: 757–764

Szeizel A E, Codaj I, Lenz W 1994 Smoking during pregnancy and congenital limb deficiency. British Medical Journal 308: 1473–1476

Thomas I H, Williams P F 1987 The Gruca operation for congenital absence of the fibula. Journal of Bone and Joint Surgery 69B: 587–592

Thomas M P, Jackson A M, Aicroth P M 1985 Congenital absence of the anterior cruciate ligaments. Journal of Bone and Joint Surgery 67B: 572–575

Wood W L, Zlotsky N, Westin G W 1965 Congenital absence of the fibula. Journal of Bone and Joint Surgery 47A: 1159–1169

Chapter 23

The limping child

G. Hansson and F. S. Jacobsen

INTRODUCTION

The evaluation of a limp in a growing child is a problem that paediatricians, Accident and Emergency department doctors, general practitioners and orthopaedic surgeons frequently face. There are many causes, ranging from surgical emergencies to children who need observation only (Lawrence 1998). It is often not possible to know with certainty the seriousness of the condition at the initial examination, which is why it is important to adopt a systematic approach when evaluating the problem.

The aim of this chapter is to give an overview of the limping child, to discuss important points in the history and physical examination, to suggest appropriate imaging and laboratory tests, and to describe the most common causes. Treatment will be dealt with in the relevant chapters.

HISTORY

The history of a limp is just as important as the findings on physical examination. If the right questions are asked, a provisional diagnosis can be made, in most cases, at the primary examination. Although the history may be difficult to obtain from a toddler, it is usually possible to identify the specific anatomical area involved. The majority of limping children have symptoms related to the hip (34%), followed by the knee (19%), the remainder of the leg (18%) and the spine (fewer than 2%) (Fischer & Beattie 1999). Most children presenting with a limp have pain (Fischer & Beattie 1999). The probability of referred pain is greater in children than in adults (Hensinger 1986): pain from the spine may be referred to the thigh or the abdomen, and hip pain is very often referred to the thigh or the knee.

The patient's age is important. Fractures and infection are seen in all age-groups, but some conditions are more age-specific (Table 23.1). Child abuse is usually seen in children younger than 2 years, Legg–Calvé–Perthes' disease between 4 and 8 years and a slipped capital femoral epiphysis is more frequent in adolescence.

A family history, past medical history and details of previous treatment must be obtained, together with an assessment of the child's general health.

The onset of fever should be noted, when it started, its variability, and whether the patient is receiving any antipyretic medication or antibiotics. A preceding illness

Table 23.1 Age-specific conditions that cause a limp	
1–3 years	Developmental dysplasia of the hip
	Child abuse
	Neuromuscular disease
	Juvenile idiopathic arthritis
	Leg length discrepancy
	Infections
4–10 years	Transient synovitis
	Legg–Calvé–Perthes' disease
	Leg length discrepancy
	Juvenile idiopathic arthritis
	Infections
>10 years:	Slipped capital femoral epiphysis
	Overuse syndrome such as
	Anterior knee pain
	Osgood–Schlatter's disease
	Shin splints
	Tarsal coalition
	Heel pain
	Köhler's disease
All age groupes	Trauma
	Tumour

was found by Fischer & Beattie (1999) in about 40% of children presenting with an acute limp.

It is important to determine whether the onset of the limp was sudden, as in trauma, or whether it came on gradually – typical of a more chronic disease. A history of trauma or change in activity may prompt suspicion of a fracture or stress reaction. It is essential to ask about the duration of the limp, and any aggravating factors. Juvenile idiopathic arthritis usually presents with limping and stiffness that are more marked at the beginning of the day when the child is getting out of bed. Neuromuscular problems usually get worse towards the end of the day, because of muscle fatigue. Constant pain during the entire day and night should raise concern about a tumour.

GAIT ANALYSIS

Physical examination should start with observation of gait. The physician must, therefore, be familiar with normal patterns of gait and motor development in children.

NORMAL GAIT

Gait is a repeated cycle of limb motion controlled by muscle activity that carries the body forward. The gait cycle is traditionally described as starting when one heel strikes the ground and ending when it strikes the ground again (Fig. 23.1).

The gait cycle is divided into *stance phase*, which starts with heel strike and ends at toe-off, when *swing phase* starts.

The stance phase occupies 60% of the gait cycle and the swing phase 40%. Opposite legs have toe-off and heel strike at 10% and 50% of the gait cycle (Fig 23.1). The two periods when both feet are on the ground at the same time are called double support; each lasts for about 10% of the gait cycle. Normal gait is symmetrical, and the double support time of each leg is identical.

Neuromuscular maturation is characterised by suppression of the primitive reflexes and the gradual appearance of the postural reflexes. If these reflexes do not appear at the right time, late motor development can occur such as is seen in cerebral palsy.

Most children are able to stand unassisted and cruise under 1 year of age and are able to walk at about 1 year. The young toddler, however, has an immature gait different from that of the adult (Sutherland 1997) and walks in an abrupt and choppy fashion, with a faster cadence (steps/minute) but a slower velocity (cm/second) than the adult. The heel strike (first rocker) is usually absent, and the feet are externally rotated. There is increased hip and knee flexion, and the gait is wide-based. The arms are abducted and the elbows extended. Single stance time is decreased and double stance increased in comparison with adult gait, in order to obtain better stability.

By 18 months, most children have developed heel strike, a narrower support base and smoother movements. Fully mature gait is usually attained by 4 years of age, and all subsequent changes in gait are related to change in height (Sutherland 1997).

When the child's gait is examined, he or she must be wearing a minimum of clothing and must walk bare-footed. It is important to observe the patient walking unassisted in a large room or a corridor, and running; running accentuates any pathological features of gait. It is also helpful to watch the child climbing stairs, to detect muscle weakness.

Gait should be observed several times, focusing on a different component of gait each time: for instance, the feet, followed by the knees and hips. All phases of gait should be observed. Often the child will try to imitate a normal gait, and the genuine walk can then be seen only when the child thinks he or she is unobserved.

PATHOLOGICAL GAIT

A child's limp may be caused by *pain, structural change, weakness,* or a combination of these.

Antalgic gait

The most common form of limp is an antalgic (anti-pain) gait, in which the child limits the time spent on the painful leg in the stance phase (Dabney & Lipton 1995). This is associated with a shorter swing phase on the opposite leg, and a decreased stride length. The child thereby attempts to reduce the duration of weight bearing on the affected leg (Phillips 1987). An antalgic gait is seen in trauma, transient synovitis, and infection.

If the spine is affected, the child walks carefully and slowly, avoiding the trunk rotation that exacerbates pain.

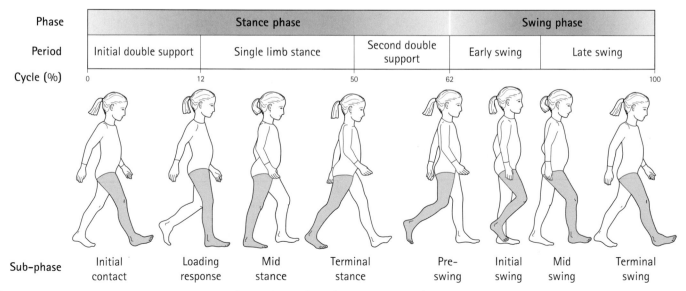

Phase	Stance phase				Swing phase	
Period	Initial double support	Single limb stance		Second double support	Early swing	Late swing
Cycle (%)	0 12		50	62		100
Sub-phase	Initial contact	Loading response	Mid stance	Terminal stance	Pre-swing	Initial swing	Mid swing	Terminal swing

Figure 23.1 Phases of the normal gait cycle. (Reproduced from Sutherland 1988.)

Leg length discrepancy gait

The patient with a leg length discrepancy can compensate by walking on tip-toe on the short side and with slight hip and knee flexion on the long side, in an endeavour to equalise leg lengths.

Trendelenburg gait

A Trendelenburg gait is a painless limp in a patient with weakened hip abductor muscles or an unstable hip fulcrum. During stance phase, the opposite side of the pelvis drops. To compensate, the child leans over the affected hip. Bilateral involvement causes a waddling gait. The time spent in the stance phase on the affected extremity is normal, as pain is often absent. A typical Trendelenburg gait is seen in developmental dysplasia of the hip or in those hip problems in which an overgrowth of the greater trochanter weakens the hip abductors.

Gait in cerebral palsy (see Ch. 18)

The gait pattern in cerebral palsy depends on the specific brain lesion, secondary muscle contractures, and compensatory movements. Tightness in the gastrocnemius–soleus complex and the hamstrings often causes toe walking and secondary flexion of the knee during stance. Rotational malalignment will create in- or out-toeing and tight adductors scissoring. Relative weakness of the gastrocnemius–soleus complex gives a typical crouched gait, with increased flexion of the hips and the knees. A spastic rectus femoris muscle can give rise to a stiff knee gait, with difficulties of foot clearance during the swing phase.

Gait in muscular dystrophy (see Ch. 15)

The muscle weakness in many muscular dystrophy patients causes a very characteristic posture and gait. Duchenne's muscular dystrophy, with early and striking proximal hip extensor weakness, leads to hip flexion contracture and a secondary lumbar lordosis to bring the centre of gravity over the hip joint. The child walks on the toes because of tightness in the gastrocnemius–soleus complex, with a wide, waddling Trendelenburg gait.

PHYSICAL EXAMINATION

STANDING

With the patient standing, the back should be examined for scoliosis, local tenderness and range of motion. If a pelvic tilt is present, it can be measured by placing blocks under the shorter leg until the pelvis is level. A positive Trendelenburg test may indicate hip dysplasia, the sequelae of Legg–Calvé–Perthes' disease or slipped capital femoral epiphysis.

Cutaneous changes such as skin dimples and hairy patches over the lumbar spine, erythema or heat over joints should be noted. Café au lait spots, particularly in the axillae, should lead to the suspicion of fibrous dysplasia or neurofibromatosis.

SUPINE

With the patient supine, each joint should be examined separately. Look for swelling, feel for tenderness, and assess movement. Hip flexion contracture can be judged by Thomas's test. The abdomen should always be examined, as conditions such as appendicitis can occasionally be the cause of a limp (Renshaw 1995).

A full neurological examination should be performed to assess atrophy, muscle strength and tone, sensation and reflexes. Atrophy of the quadriceps muscle is often associated with a painful hip, and correlates with the duration of symptoms.

The examiner should check for leg length discrepancy by measuring the distance from the anterior superior spine to the medial malleolus, in addition to examining the patient standing. A short leg must be distinguished from apparent shortening that is caused by scoliosis with pelvic obliquity or joint contracture.

PRONE

Hip rotation in extension is best tested with the patient prone. The knees should be flexed to 90°, and the tibiae used as lever arms. The amount of internal and external rotation can easily be measured and any asymmetry detected. Limited painful internal rotation of the hip suggests synovitis of the hip joint or a slipped capital femoral epiphysis. Further, with the patient prone, femoral anteversion can be measured, and tibial torsion evaluated by measuring the foot–thigh angle.

DIAGNOSTIC INVESTIGATIONS

BLOOD TESTS

Diagnostic blood tests, in most cases, are non-specific. Appropriate blood tests depend on the patient's history and physical examination. Any patient with fever or possible infection should have a complete blood count, white blood count, erythrocyte sedimentation rate (ESR) and C-reactive protein tests performed. An ESR of 50 mm/hour or more strongly suggests serious disease in patients who present with a limp (Huttenlocher & Newman 1997). In a patient with an infection, the C-reactive protein concentration is usually increased, and subsequently decreases more rapidly than the ESR; it is, therefore, more useful for assessing the efficacy of treatment (Unkila-Kallio et al 1994). In children in whom an arthritic aetiology is suspected, rheumatoid factor, antinuclear antibodies, HLA B27 and Lyme titre should be checked, although many of these tests may be negative in the early stages of disease. If fever is present, blood cultures, together with aspiration of the infected area, should be performed at the initial examination.

JOINT ASPIRATION

Joint effusions should always be aspirated when infection is suspected. The aspirate should be sent for: 1) Gram staining,

2) aerobic and anaerobic culture, 3) a cell count and 4) glucose determination.

RADIOGRAPHIC EXAMINATIONS

Plain radiographs

Radiographs are readily accessible, inexpensive, and specific for a whole range of disorders such as tumour, infection or fracture (Myers & Thompson 1997). Although they give information on bone pathology, they may not show early changes, and give limited information about soft tissue and cartilage. They are, therefore, not very specific for screening purposes in a limping child (Blatt et al 1991).

Simple radiological examinations should be undertaken first. An anteroposterior and a lateral view are always necessary. A comparative view of the contralateral limb can be useful in some cases. Specific X-rays may be necessary, e.g. oblique X-ray of the lumbar spine can show a pars defect; a lateral view of the hip is always necessary in slipped capital femoral epiphysis, a tunnel view for osteochondritis of the knee, and oblique radiographs of the foot to show calcaneonavicular tarsal coalition.

Bone scintigraphy

Bone scintigraphy uses as a tracer, technetium-99m-labelled methylene diphosphate, which is concentrated by areas of osteoblastic activity. It is a non-specific test that focuses only on areas of increased bone metabolism.

Bone scintigraphy can detect subtle abnormalities such as a stress fracture before it is evident on plain X-ray. It cannot differentiate between different diseases, but can be helpful by indicating the anatomical area involved (Connolly & Treves 1998). Aronson et al (1992) found bone scans of great value in a group of limping children in whom the diagnosis was difficult to establish.

A bone scan does not always need to show increased activity to be positive. A photon-deficient (cold) scan may be seen in osteomyelitis. The rapid progression of bacterial infection in bone and subperiosteum can cause increased intraosseous pressure, with decreased blood flow. Affected patients have an aggressive form of osteomyelitis that needs immediate medical and surgical treatment (Pennington et al 1999).

Ultrasound imaging

Ultrasound of the hip shows the relationship of the cartilaginous femoral head to the acetabulum. It can also provide a dynamic evaluation of hip stability without irradiation. The child does not require sedation.

Ultrasound can also be used to assess hip effusion or synovitis, or both, as seen in transient synovitis, Legg–Calvé–Perthes' disease or juvenile idiopathic arthritis. The normal hip capsule is concave, but in the presence of an effusion it balloons out and becomes convex. The diagnostic criterion for a joint effusion is a 2-mm separation between the femoral neck and the joint capsule (Fig. 23.2) (Terjesen & Osthus 1991).

Ultrasonography can also be used in the assessment of other

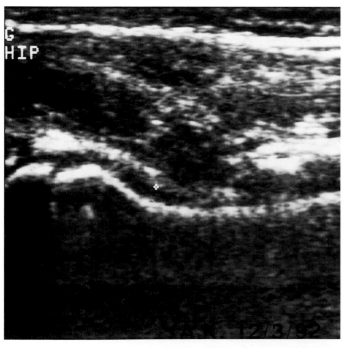

A

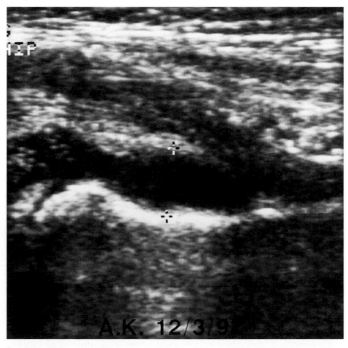

B

Figure 23.2 Ultrasonography of the hips in a 3-year-old patient presenting with a right antalgic limp. A The image of the left hip shows normal joint space between the two markers. B Ultrasonography of the right (painful) hip shows a hip effusion with a distended and bulging joint capsule between the two markers.

infected joints and bones, to reveal a joint effusion or sub-periosteal pus. It is also a very useful guide during aspiration.

Computed tomography

Computed tomography (CT) is helpful in determining more precisely the anatomy of an area. It is also very useful in determining the exact location of an osteoid osteoma, and in evaluating a tarsal coalition or the patellofemoral joint.

Magnetic resonance imaging

Magnetic resonance imaging (MRI) is an expensive and highly sophisticated tool capable of providing a great deal of information. It can be useful in the early diagnosis of Legg–Calvé–Perthes' disease and avascular necrosis, and in the assessment of tumours and infections. However, most young children will require sedation or anaesthesia.

CAUSES OF LIMPING

Trauma is by far the most common cause of limping in a child. The aetiology of non-traumatic causes of limping varies, but is often inflammatory (Table 23.2). In one review, 23% of children younger than 5 years who presented with a limp or refusal to bear weight proved to have a severe bacterial infection (Choban & Killian 1990).

After the initial clinical assessment has been made and the anatomical site of the limp determined, it is important to bear in mind that some diagnoses are typical of certain ages (see Table 23.1).

TRAUMA

Trauma is the most common cause of limping in a child.

Fractures

Fractures are usually apparent clinically and radiologically. They require appropriate treatment by reduction if necessary, and immobilisation.

Stress fractures

Stress fractures are a common cause of limping in children especially in adolescence. When seen in otherwise normal

bone, they are the result of increased or repetitive muscle action, rather than direct impact (Ogden 1982). Bone responds to excessive stress by remodelling and resorption, and eventual increased bone formation. A stress fracture occurs when the fatigue process exceeds the bone repair process. The fatigue of a muscle, decreasing its ability to protect the bone may also contibute to stress fracture.

Fractures can also occur as a result of normal physiological stresses in bones with deficient elastic resistance (Ogden 1982). These insufficiency stress fractures may occur in bone tumours, osteogenesis imperfecta, rickets or the osteoporosis that is associated with immobilisation or cerebral palsy. Anatomical conditions can also predispose to stress fracture; for instance, a rigid cavus or flat foot may fail to absorb energy normally.

The most common site for a stress fracture is the tibia, which accounts for up to 50% of all cases (Walker et al 1996). The fractures, which occur usually in 10–15-year-olds, are usually located in the proximal part of the tibia, between the metaphysis and the diaphysis, either on the posteromedial or on the posterolateral corner. The fibula is the second most common site of stress fracture, usually in a younger age group (see Fig. 23.3). Other sites of stress fractures include the metatarsals, calcaneum, pelvis and femur (see Ch. 33).

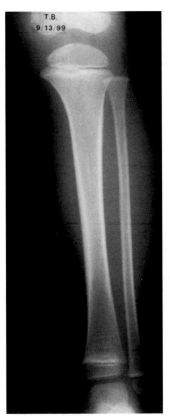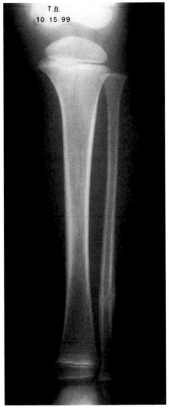

A   B

Figure 23.3 A Normal radiograph of the lower leg in a 4-year-old boy presenting with a limp and slight tenderness over the lateral aspect of the lower extremity. He was treated in a cast on suspicion of a fracture. B Radiograph 4 weeks later, showing a healing stress fracture in the lower part of the fibula.

Table 23.2 Reasons for acute atraumatic limp	
Cause	Frequency (%)
Inflammatory	
Toxic synovitis (transient synovitis)	39.5
Juvenile chronic arthritis + viral illness + other	3.2
Infection	3.6
Developmental	4.1
Tumours	0.8
Overuse	17.7
Diagnosis unknown	31.1

Data from Fischer & Beattie (1999).

Stress fractures are most common in younger children in the spring, when activity levels increase after an inactive winter. In the adolescent, in whom the elasticity of the bone is decreased compared with that of younger children, stress fractures are often seen during or after athletic activities.

The symptoms depend on the site of the stress fracture, but the most common complaint is pain related to activity, relieved by rest and associated with an antalgic gait. Local swelling and tenderness may be present. The patient often gives a history of increased or changed activity, or change of shoes or running surface. Radiographs will initially show a small cortical lucency, followed by a gradual increase in periosteal and endosteal bone formation. These findings can take up to 3 weeks to appear depending on the patient's age.

A bone scan is useful in the early detection of a stress fracture before other radiological changes occur. MRI and CT can also be helpful in establishing the diagnosis. The differential diagnoses include tumours such as osteoid osteoma and Ewing's sarcoma. Biopsy can be misleading because of changes associated with fracture repair seen in a stress fractures, which might be difficult to differentiate from tumour.

Overuse syndromes

The number of children participating in organised sports has increased dramatically during the past few years. This increase is matched by the increased number of patients presenting with overuse syndromes, often with a painful limp. Overuse injuries often occur where different tissues – such as tendon, ligament, muscle, bone – meet. Children who have very recently undergone a significant growth spurt have less joint flexibility and are more prone to injury.

The following overuse syndromes can give rise to a limp:

1. *Spondylolysis*, frequently a stress fracture of the pars inter-articularis, is particularly common in female gymnasts.
2. *Iliac apophysitis* may be seen in adolescent runners. It is also called a 'hip pointer' and presents with pain over the iliac crest one handsbreadth posterior to the anterior superior iliac spine (Lombardo et al 1983). Avulsion of the pelvic apophysis is usually caused by sudden violent contraction of hamstrings, adductors or the ilio-psoas, and is seen in sports such as jumping and sprinting. The pain is localised in the groin or buttock and diagnosed by X-ray. Non-weight-bearing with crutches is usually the treatment indicated.
3. *Osgood–Schlatter's disease*. This is the most common condition around the knee. It is a stress-related partial avulsion injury of the tibial tubercle, with inflammatory changes and swelling. It occurs most commonly in boys between 10 and 15 years of age, with symptoms of local pain and discomfort with activity. Radiology shows soft-tissue swelling and fragmentation of the tibial tubercle.

4. *Sinding–Larsen–Johansson disease* similarly causes anterior knee pain and is probably caused by excessive traction on the inferior pole of the patella. It may also be seen in patients with cerebral palsy and a 'crouch gait'.
5. *Patellofemoral pain* is frequent in females, and often occurs in association with increased femoral anteversion, knee valgus, external tibial torsion, etc.
6. *Sever's disease* (Haglund's disease) is characterised by pain at the calcaneal apophysis, usually chronic or related to activity. Plain X-rays may show fragmentation of the calcaneal apophysis. However, this can be a normal finding in this age group and therefore not specific for this condition.

When the correct diagnosis of an overuse syndrome is made, the treatment is usually pain control and modification of activity, followed by rehabilitation.

Child abuse

An important cause of limping or fracture in a child, particularly in those younger than 2 years, is child abuse. This should be considered in a child with a questionable history of trauma or a delay in presenting to the physician. It is important to look for skin manifestations such as bruises and burns, which are not uncommon. The matter is considered in detail in Chapter 36.

No single lesion is specific for child abuse, but certain fracture patterns are suggestive of it. Metaphyseal corner fractures are typical of child abuse, as the pull and twist that create these fractures are rarely accidental. Multiple fractures in different stages of healing are also commonly seen. The most common sites of fractures are the humerus, the femur and the tibia. Spiral fractures in these bones warrant great concern. If child abuse is suspected, a skeletal survey should be performed, to look for other fractures. It is, of course, important to rule out other causes of fracture such as fibrous dysplasia, osteogenesis imperfecta, etc.

In the case of suspected child abuse, the hospital's child abuse team must be contacted.

INFLAMMATORY SYNOVITIS

Transient synovitis of the hip

Transient synovitis is the most common cause of hip pain in children (Bickerstaff et al 1991). It is a non-pyogenic synovitis of the hip that is also called irritable hip, observation hip, and coxalgia fugax or toxic synovitis. It is characterised by a sudden onset of hip pain and limping in a child who is not systemically ill. The most common age range is from 3 to 8 years, and it is more common in boys. The accumulated risk of contracting transient synovitis before 14 years of age has been shown to be 3% (Landin et al 1987). Repeated episodes of transient synovitis occur in 10% of cases, usually within 6 months of the first episode (Illingworth 1983).

Aetiology

The aetiology is unknown, but trauma, infection and allergy have been suggested. The concept of an infectious aetiology is supported by the finding that these children often have had a preceding viral upper respiratory tract infection, and by the fact that transient synovitis is seen most frequently in the autumn, when the incidence of viral infection is high.

The patient usually presents with an antalgic gait and pain in the hip or referred pain down to the thigh and knee. The pain is variable from a slight limp to a completely stiff and painful joint on which the patient avoids weight bearing.

The patient is usually afebrile, but may have a temperature of up to 38–39°C without being systemically ill. The clinical findings include a hip joint that is held in flexion and abduction to reduce pressure in the joint. The patient is best examined prone when internal rotation of the hip is limited and painful – the most consistent finding in transient synovitis (Haueisen et al 1986).

The synovitis usually lasts only for a few days, and there is usually complete resolution of the symptoms. The long-term effects of transient synovitis are probably benign (Sharwood 1981). In a long-term follow-up of 23 patients, De Valderrama (1963) found that up to 50% developed coxa magna, with a slight risk of developing arthritis in the involved hip. However, 67% of his patients spent an average 3–5 months in hospital, which suggests a more severe disorder than what we now call 'transient synovitis'.

It has been postulated that transient synovitis can cause Legg–Calvé–Perthes' disease. Kallio et al (1986), however, found no cases of Legg–Calvé–Perthes' disease after 1 year in their study of 119 children with transient synovitis. Their opinion was that the cases described in the literature were examples of Legg–Calvé–Perthes' disease at an early stage. Some practitioners recommend that an X-ray of the hip be performed 3 months after the onset of transient synovitis, to check for Legg–Calvé–Perthes' disease. However, a routine follow-up X-ray is probably not indicated in a patient with no hip symptoms.

Radiography

Conventional *radiographs* are normal in typical transient synovitis. Capsular distension and loss of fat planes may be seen, but these changes are non-specific and dependent on rotation of the leg.

Ultrasound is the method of choice for diagnosing a joint effusion. Intracapsular synovitis and fluid can be directly visualised and measured. The child is positioned supine with the leg in the neutral position. Anterior ultrasonography shows the distance between the femoral neck and the anterior joint capsule (see Fig. 23.2).

Treatment

The treatment of transient synovitis is symptomatic and usually consists of bed rest with the leg flexed or, in minor cases, non-weight-bearing with crutches with anti-inflammatory drugs. Treatment can be managed on an outpatient basis with frequent follow-up, except in cases with a high suspicion of septic arthritis in which case the patient should be admitted. A reduction in the synovitis is associated with decreased pain and increased internal rotation of the hip.

Differential diagnosis

The differential diagnosis between transient synovitis and other hip disorders can be difficult.

Legg–Calvé–Perthes' disease in the early stages is clinically similar to transient synovitis. The clinical and radiological course will differ between the two entities, but if an early diagnosis is required, a bone scan or MRI may help to distinguish them.

Juvenile idiopathic arthritis, if seronegative, may be difficult to diagnose. Other differential diagnoses to be considered include osteoid osteoma of the proximal femur, slipped capital femoral epiphysis in its early stages, or bone or soft tissue infections in the pelvis. Plain X-ray is rarely diagnostic, and MRI or, sometimes, bone scintigraphy may be useful (Fig. 23.4).

The most difficult and important differential diagnosis of transient synovitis is *septic arthritis* in the hip. It is extremely important to distinguish between the two, as septic arthritis must be treated urgently by open drainage and antibiotics, whereas transient synovitis can be treated symptomatically. The clinical findings may be similar, but a

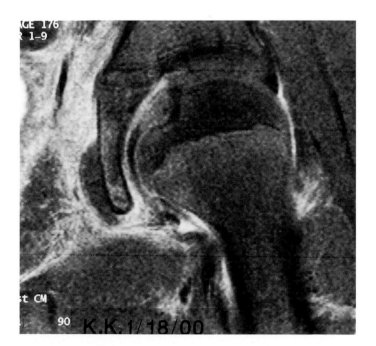

Figure 23.4 MRI of an 11-year-old patient presenting with a limp and a temperature of 38°C. There was slight tenderness over the left hip, but a normal range of motion. Radiographs and ultrasound images were normal, but MRI shows an abscess on the inner side of the acetabulum.

high temperature is uncommon in transient synovitis. In one study, 97% of children with septic arthritis had an ESR greater than 20 mm/hour, a temperature of more than 37.5°C, or both (Del Beccaro et al 1992). There is, however, an overlap in the parameters and, in the same study, 47% of the patients with transient synovitis had similar positive parameters. The C-reactive protein value guides the clinician better, but the general rule is that any child with a fever and an increased ESR should be suspected of having septic arthritis.

In a recent study (Kocher et al 1999), four independent parameters were used to distinguish between the two entities:

1. Fever (temperature more than 38.5°C).
2. Non weight-bearing.
3. ESR greater than 40 mm/hour.
4. Serum white blood count more than 12 000 cells/mm³.

and an algorithm was constructed for the probability of the patient having septic arthritis (Table 23.3).

The consequences of overlooking septic arthritis can be devastating: patients with two or more positive parameters should have the affected joint aspirated and the remainder should be treated expectantly.

JUVENILE IDIOPATHIC ARTHRITIS

The juvenile form of idiopathic arthritis is a generalised systemic arthritis that differs from adult rheumatoid arthritis in both course and prognosis. Subgroups are described on the basis of joint involvement and systemic disease. The condition is considered in detail in Chapter 12.

Juvenile idiopathic arthritis often presents with single joint involvement. The onset is usually gradual and less severe than that seen with infectious processes. The child may present with joint swelling, slight discomfort, and an antalgic gait if the lower extremity is involved.

The diagnosis is often made by exclusion. Initial blood tests include complete blood count, ESR, antinuclear antibodies and rheumatoid factor. If the joint is aspirated, the cell count is usually in the range 2000–50 000 cells/mm³,

Table 23.3 The use of four parameters[†] in the assessment of a patient having a septic arthritis	
Numbers of parameters present	Probability for septic arthritis (%)
0	0.2
1	3.0
2	40.0
3	93.1
4	99.6

[†] Fever >38.5°C; non-weight bearing; ESR >40 mm/hour; white count >12 000/cells/mm³.
(Data from Kocher et al 1999.)

whereas if there is an infectious process the count is usually more than 50 000. However, there is a considerable degree of overlap.

REACTIVE ARTHRITIS

The term 'reactive arthritis' is applied to a systemic disease that is not limited to joints alone, despite its name. Reactive arthritis is commonly triggered as a response to infection elsewhere in the body, such as the upper airway or gastrointestinal or urogenital tracts. It is probably autoimmune and results from a crossover reaction between synovial and infectious antigens. The knee, ankle or hip are usually involved, and the patient feels unwell and feverish. The arthritis is characterised by an acute onset with severe pain, and there is often a migratory polyarthritis.

If the condition follows a group A streptococcal pharyngitis, it can be diagnosed by the presence of an antibody response to group A streptococcus, usually 1–2 weeks after the infection.

The clinical presentation can mimic septic arthritis (Birdi et al 1995) and may warrant joint aspiration. The joint fluid is sterile, but the white blood cell count in the joint fluid is frequently increased.

The reactive arthritis group of diseases merges with others such as Reiter's syndrome and ankylosing spondylitis. In the spondyloarthropathies, the sacro-iliac joint is frequently involved and peripheral joint symptoms occur in most of these children. An early manifestation in addition to arthritis is an enthesopathy, with pain and tenderness at the tendon–bone interface. Inflammation at these sites is often quite painful, and the patient presents with a significant limp. The strong association with HLA B27 positivity suggests a genetic factor; conversely, patients with the HLA B27 antigen have an increased risk of developing reactive arthritis.

Reactive arthritis may also be seen with acute rheumatic fever and after enteric infections from bacteria such as *Shigella*, *Salmonella* and *Yersinia*.

Virus infections also may give rise to reactive arthritis or arthralgia. The duration is usually 1–2 weeks, and the condition is often migratory. It may follow rubella infection or immunisation, alphavirus infection, or herpes virus infection. Reactive arthritis is difficult to diagnose and often is a diagnosis of exclusion.

INFECTIONS

Osteomyelitis

Osteomyelitis occurs throughout childhood (see Ch. 9). It results from haematological spread of bacteria and usually seeds in the metaphysis of the long bone: the most frequent location is the femoral metaphysis, followed by the pelvis and tibia (Scott et al 1990). Osteomyelitis in the pelvis is often adjacent to the hip joint and can present with hip pain and gait disturbance (Mustafa et al 1990). Established infections in bone can spread into the joint, either through the epiphysis in very young children or into the hip joint, as the metaphysis is intracapsular. It is important always to examine the adjacent joints, as 30% of patients also have adjacent septic joint involvement (Perlman et al 2000).

Pelvic osteomyelitis presents with fever, pain and limping. Most patients have pain, and a reduced range of motion in the hip, which is nevertheless less than that in septic arthritis. There is also point tenderness over the infected area. If the abscess is located in the obturator internus muscle, it can easily be mistaken for septic arthritis of the hip (see Fig. 23.4) (Viani et al 1999). The diagnosis is based on swelling, tenderness and fever. Radiological changes occur within 7–10 days, but before that a bone scan can be of value. Ultrasound will show an accumulation of subperiosteal pus, and MRI is also often helpful.

Septic arthritis

Prompt, accurate diagnosis is essential in septic arthritis, to allow early treatment and obtain optimal results (see Ch. 9). Septic arthritis of the hip, knee and ankle accounts for more than 90% of all cases (Lawrence 1998).

The patient is usually febrile, with a temperature greater than 38°C, and presents with a painful joint that is warm and red and with a limited, painful movement. In early childhood, the fever can be absent or mild. The child who has received antibiotics or is immunodeficient may lack typical symptoms and signs. If the hip joint is involved, it is held flexed, abducted and externally rotated. All movement is resisted and painful (pseudoparalysis). Groin or proximal thigh swelling will often be present.

The differential diagnoses include transient synovitis, juvenile idiopathic arthritis, osteomyelitis, Lyme disease, Legg–Calvé–Perthes' disease and slipped capital femoral epiphysis in the adolescent age group. Plain X-rays are usually normal in early septic arthritis and are positive only in cases of osteomyelitis of more than 2 weeks standing. The definitive test for septic arthritis of the hip is aspiration, usually guided by ultrasound; the knee and ankle can be aspirated without any aids.

If infection is present, the joint fluid is usually cloudy, with a cell count of more than 50 000 cells/mm^3, the majority being polymorphonuclear cells. In joint infections or acute rheumatoid arthritis, the synovial fluid glucose level is characteristically lowered. The incidence of positive synovial fluid culture ranges from 30 to 80%. Patients in whom cultures are negative appear to run a clinical course similar to that in patients with positive cultures and should, therefore, receive the same aggressive treatment (Lyon & Evanich 1999).

The treatment of septic arthritis in the hip is immediate open drainage and irrigation. The infected hip represents an orthopaedic emergency, because of the possibility of severe sequelae. These include avascular necrosis of the femoral head, subluxation or dislocation, and growth plate injury. A good outcome is dependent on a prompt surgical response.

Factors that increase the risk of complications are age of less than 6 months, delay in treatment by more than 4 days, and adjacent osteomyelitis of the proximal femur. The knee and ankle must be treated, according to the duration of the disease and the patient's response to antibiotics, with multiple aspirations, arthroscopic drainage, or arthrotomy.

Discitis

Discitis is an inflammation of the disc space that ranges from a benign self-limiting inflammation to a true osteomyelitis involving adjacent bone (Ring et al 1995). It is usually seen in the younger age group, from 2 to 6 years (see Ch. 31.1). The cause of infection is probably bacterial but may, in milder cases, be viral.

In the young child, the presenting symptoms are often limping or refusal to walk or to sit, whereas in the older child, back or neck pain are more common. If the patient is walking, the gait is stiff and guarded.

Physical examination shows rigidity of the spine with muscle spasm and limitation of straight leg-raising, with a loss of lumbar lordosis. The ESR is usually increased, as is the white blood count. Plain X-rays are negative in the first 3–6 weeks of the disease. After that, disc narrowing and, later, erosion into the vertebral bodies can develop. Bone scintigraphy can be helpful but MRI seems to be more reliable in establishing an early diagnosis.

Pyogenic sacro-iliitis can present with back or hip pain, and the patient may have a limp (Hollingworth 1995). A spinal epidural abscess will, in the early stages, present with similar symptoms.

Psoas abscess

A psoas abscess is uncommon in countries where tuberculosis is no longer endemic, but can be seen in association with infection in the spine or abdomen. The child presents with a painful limp and a hip flexion contracture. A psoas mass may be caused by a haematoma, especially in patients with haemophilia or those receiving anticoagulation treatment. Diagnosis is helped by ultrasound and MRI (Malhotra et al 1992).

Lyme disease

Lyme disease is caused by a spirochete, *Borrelia burgdorferi*, and should always be considered as a cause of acute arthritis in an area where the disease is endemic (Rose et al 1994).

The disease starts with a red rash and erythema migrans, followed by cardiac, neurological and joint problems. The large joints such as the knee and ankle are usually affected. Systemic symptoms such as myalgia and fatigue are often seen. If the hip is involved, patients with a more chronic onset of disease have symptoms resembling those of pauci-articular juvenile idiopathic arthritis. The patient with an acute form of Lyme disease may be suspected of having septic arthritis or transient synovitis. A positive enzyme-linked immunosorbent assay test can be helpful in the diagnosis.

OTHER CAUSES OF A LIMP

Many common childhood hip problems present with a limp. A simplistic but valuable observation is that a healthy child with a limp may, until proven otherwise, be assumed to have hip dysplasia if younger than 4 years, Legg–Calvé–Perthes' disease if 4–9 years old, and a slipped upper femoral epiphysis if older than 9 years. These are discussed in detail in Chapters 24, 25 and 26 respectively.

Many 'knee' symptoms are referred from the hip, but there are mechanical disorders of the knee that cause a child to limp. These include patellar instability, dislocations and osteochondritic lesions. Because the growth plates around the knee are among those most actively involved in the rapid growth of a child, they are the most vulnerable to benign and malignant tumours.

At the foot and ankle, limping in an otherwise healthy child may be the result of osteochondritis dissecans, typically of the talar dome. Recurrent sprains, limping and peroneal spasm with exercise are complications of a tarsal coalition. Osteochondritis of the navicular (Kohler's disease) and osteochondrosis of the head of the 2nd metatarsal (Freiberg's disease) present with a limp and localised pain and tenderness. It is well to remember also that limping is sometimes caused by a foreign body in either the shoe or the soft tissues of the foot. Pseudomonas infection should be suspected if the child was wearing sneakers at the time of a puncture injury to the foot (Jacobs et al 1989).

Köhler's disease is an avascular necrosis of the tarsal navicular, seen mainly in boys between 3 and 8 years of age. Patients present with a limp and pain over the medial arch of the foot, with local tenderness. Radiographs show a small sclerotic navicular. Fragmentation may be seen, but in the absence of symptoms this is a normal variant.

Tumours

Fisher & Beattie (1999) reported tumours as the cause of limp in fewer than 1% of children. However, it is essential to consider the diagnosis in the child with a limp, as the consequences of a 'missed' or late diagnosis can be very serious (see Ch. 13).

It is important to remember that a tumour causing a painful limp may not be located in the lower extremity or pelvis. Cerebral and spinal cord tumours can primarily present with a limp resulting from weakness (Skaggs et al 2000).

Two tumours that often present with a limp are leukaemia and osteoid osteoma. Patients with suspected tumours should have anteroposterior and lateral X-rays performed. Further studies such as bone scintigraphy, CT and MRI might be necessary to establish a diagnosis and to stage the tumour.

Leukaemia

Leukaemia is the most common malignancy in childhood and may present at any age. The orthopaedic surgeon may be the first to see the patient before the diagnosis is made as some will present with a limp (Tuten et al 1998). Clinical signs are vague, but include fever, lethargy, bruising and infection. Bone aches and joint pains are frequent and often present asymmetrically in the hips or knees. The symptoms may resemble those of juvenile idiopathic arthritis.

Radiological signs are non-specific and include osteoporosis, periosteal reaction, sclerosis or lytic lesions. Metaphyseal lucency (leukaemic lines) is often the first radiological change, commonly around the knee. However, this banding is a non-specific sign that can also be seen in malnutrition, juvenile idiopathic arthritis and septicaemia. Bone pain is caused by proliferation of the haemopoietic tissue within the medullary canal, and may occur without any obvious radiological changes.

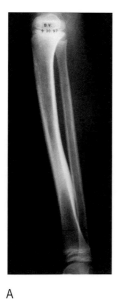
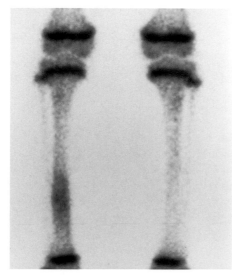
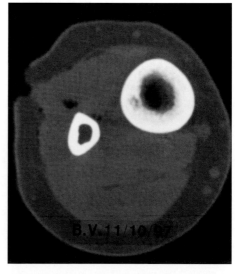

A   B   C

Figure 23.5 Radiographs of a 7-year-old girl presenting with a limp and pain over the right tibia. **A** Plain radiograph, showing posterolateral cortical thickening of the tibia. **B** Bone scintigraphy, showing increased uptake over the lower part of the tibia. **C** CT scan, illustrating a typical osteoid osteoma in the tibia.

The patient will have anaemia, thrombocytopenia and an increased ESR. Surprisingly, about 50% have a low leucocyte count. The diagnosis is confirmed by bone marrow aspiration.

Osteoid osteoma

Osteoid osteoma presents as a painful bone lesion in children who are usually older than 5 years. Most osteoid osteomas are located in the lower limbs and the child presents with pain and a limp. The pain occurs after activity and typically also as pain at night, relieved by aspirin.

On physical examination, the patient may occasionally have tenderness, increased warmth and swelling over the tumour.

The diagnosis can sometimes be made on plain radiographs, where periosteal thickening and endosteal sclerosis are seen. Bone scintigraphy demonstrates increased uptake, and the nidus can also be visualised very precisely with a CT scan (Fig. 23.5).

Histiocytosis-X (Langerhans' cell histiocytosis, LCH)

Eosinophil granuloma is the most common of these disorders. It usually appears as a lytic lesion that is painful and, if present in the lower-extremity, can create a limp. Spinal involvement can cause collapse of a vertebral body (vertebra plana). Systemic and visceral involvement is not infrequent. Up to 20% of those affected may have pulmonary involvement.

The radiographic appearance is that of a destructive lesion with periosteal reaction and can thus mimic other tumours. Sometimes CT scan and MRI are helpful, but an unequivocal diagnosis can only be made by biopsy.

REFERENCES AND FURTHER READING

Aronson J, Garvin K, Seibert J et al 1992 Efficiency of the bone scan for occult limping toddlers. Journal of Pediatric Orthopaedics 12: 38–44

Bickerstaff D R, Neal L M, Brennan P O, Bell M J 1991 An investigation into the aetiology of irritable hip. Clinical Pediatrics 30: 353–356

Birdi N, Allen U, D'Astous J 1995 Poststreptococcal reactive arthritis mimicking acute septic arthritis: a hospital-based study. Journal of Pediatric Orthopaedics 15: 661–665

Blatt S D, Rosenthal B M, Barnhart D C 1991 Diagnostic utility of lower extremity radiographs of young children with gait disturbance. Pediatrics 87: 138–140

Choban S, Killian J T 1990 Evaluation of acute gait abnormalities in preschool children. Journal of Pediatric Orthopaedics 10: 74–78

Connolly L P, Treves S T 1998 Assessing the limping child with skeletal scintigraphy. Journal of Nuclear Medicine 39: 1056–1061

Dabney K W, Lipton G 1995 Evaluation of limp in children. Current Opinion in Pediatrics 7: 88–94

Del Beccaro M A, Campoux A N, Bockers T, Mendelman P M 1992 Septic arthritis versus transient synovitis of the hip: the value of screening laboratory tests. Annals of Emergency Medicine 21: 1418–1422

De Valderrama J A F 1963 The 'observation hip' syndrome and its late sequelae. Journal of Bone and Joint Surgery 45B: 462–470

Fischer S U, Beattie T F 1999 The limping child: epidemiology, assessment and outcome. Journal of Bone and Joint Surgery 81B: 1029–1034

Haueisen D C, Weiner D S, Weiner S D 1986 The characterization of 'transient synovitis of the hip' in children. Journal of Pediatric Orthopaedics 6: 11–17

Hensinger R N 1986 Limp. Pediatric Clinics of North America 33: 1355–1362

Hollingworth P 1995 Differential diagnosis and management of hip pain in childhood. British Journal of Rheumatology 34: 78–82

Huttenlocher A, Newman T B 1997 Evaluation of the erythrocyte sedimentation rate in children presenting with limp, fever or abdominal pain. Clinical Pediatrics 36: 339–344

Illingworth C M 1983 Recurrences of transient synovitis. Archives of Disease in Childhood 58: 620–623

Jacobs R F, McCarthy R E, Elser J M 1989 Pseudomonas osteochondritis complicating puncture wounds of the foot in children: a ten year evaluation. Journal of Infectious Diseases 160: 657–661

Jacobsen F S, Crawford A H, Broste S 1992 Hip involvement in juvenile chronic arthritis. Journal of Pediatric Orthopaedics 12: 45–53

Kallio P, Ryöppy S, Kunnamo I 1986 Transient synovitis and Perthes' disease. Journal of Bone and Joint Surgery 68B: 808–811

Kocher M S, Zurakowski D, Kasser J R 1999 Differentiating between septic arthritis and transient synovitis of the hip in children: an evidence based clinical prediction algorithm. Journal of Bone and Joint Surgery 81A: 1662–1670

Landin L A, Danielsson L G, Wattsgård C 1987 Transient synovitis of the hip. Journal of Bone and Joint Surgery 69B: 238–242

Lawrence L L 1998 The limping child. Emergency Medicine Clinics of North America 16: 911–929

Lombardo S J, Retting A C, Kerlan R K 1983 Radiographic abnormalities of the iliac apophysis in adolescent athletes. Journal of Bone and Joint Surgery 65A: 444–455

Lyon R M, Evanich J D 1999 Culture-negative septic arthritis in children. Journal of Pediatric Orthopaedics 19: 655–659

Malhotra R, Singh K D, Bhan S, Dave P K 1992 Primary pyogenic abscess of the psoas muscle. Journal of Bone and Joint Surgery 74A: 278–284

Mustafa M M, Sáez-Llorens X, McCracken G H, Nelson J D 1990 Acute hematogenous pelvic osteomyelitis in infants and children. Pediatric Infectious Disease Journal 9: 416–421

Myers M T, Thompson G H 1997 Imaging the child with a limp. Pediatric Clinics of North America 44: 637–658

Ogden J A 1982 Skeletal injury in a child. Lee & Febiger, Philadelphia

Pennington W T, Mott M P, Thometz J G, Sty J R, Metz D 1999 Photopenic bone scan osteomyelitis: a clinical perspective. Journal of Pediatric Orthopaedics 19: 695–698

Perlman M H, Patzakis M J, Kumar P J, Holtom P 2000 The incidence of joint involvement with adjacent osteomyelitis in pediatric patients. Journal of Pediatric Orthopaedics 20: 40–43

Phillips W A 1987 The child with a limp. Orthopedic Clinics of North America 18: 489–501

Renshaw T S 1995 The child who has a limp. Pediatrics in Review 16: 458–465

Ring D, Johnson C E, Wenger D R 1995 Pyogenic infectious spondylitis in children: the convergence of discitis and vertebral osteomyelitis. Journal of Pediatric Orthopaedics 15: 652–660

Robben S G, Lequin M H, Meradji M, Diepstraten A F, Hop W C 1999 Atrophy of the quadriceps muscle in children with a painful hip. Clinical Physiology 19: 385–393

Rose C D, Fawcett P T, Eppes S C, Klein J D, Gibney K, Doughty R A 1994 Pediatric Lyme arthritis: clinical spectrum and outcome. Journal of Pediatric Orthopaedics 14: 238–241

Scott R J, Christofersen M R, Robertson W W, Davidson R S, Rankin L, Drummond D S 1990 Acute osteomyelitis in children: a review of 116 cases. Journal of Pediatric Orthopaedics 10: 649–652

Sharwood P F 1981 The irritable hip syndrome in children. Acta Orthopaedica Scandinavica 52: 633–638

Skaggs D L, Roberts J M, Codsi M J, Meyer B C, Moral L A, Masso P D 2000 Mild gait abnormality and leg discomfort in a child secondary to extradural ganglioneuroma. American Journal of Orthopaedics 29: 111–114

Sutherland D, Olshen R, Biden E, Wyatt M 1988 The Development of Mature Walking. Cambridge University Press, Cambridge

Sutherland D H 1997 The development of mature gait. Gait and Posture 6: 163–170

Terjesen T, Osthus P 1991 Ultrasound in the diagnosis and follow-up of transient synovitis of the hip. Journal of Pediatric Orthopaedics 11: 608–613

Tuten H R, Gabos P G, Kumar S J, Harter G D 1998 The limping child: a manifestation of acute leukemia. Journal of Pediatric Orthopaedics 18: 625–629

Unkila-Kallio L, Kallio M J T, Eskola J, Peltola H 1994 Serum C-reactive protein, erythrocyte sedimentation rate and white blood cell count in acute hematogenous osteomyelitis of children. Pediatrics 93: 59–62

Viani R M, Bromberg K, Bradley J S 1999 Obturator internus muscle abscess in children: report of seven cases and review. Clinical Infectious Diseases 28: 117–122

Walker R N, Green N E, Spindler K P 1996 Stress fractures in skeletally immature patients. Journal of Pediatric Orthopaedics 16: 578–584

Wingstrand H 1986 Transient synovitis of the hip in the child. Acta Orthopaedica Scandinavica Supplement no. 219; 57: 219

Chapter 24

Developmental dysplasia of the hip

M. K. D. Benson and M. F. Macnicol

EMBRYOLOGY AND DEVELOPMENT

An understanding of hip development allows an insight into the dysplasias and vascular insults to which it is prone. Within *3 weeks* of fertilisation, the primitive limb buds are already beginning to form. They are initially filled with mesenchyme, but this differentiates with time, to form all joint components except for the blood vessels and nerves (Strayer 1971).

The *6-week* embryo is 12 mm long. Condensations within the mesenchyme outline the ilium, ischium, pubis and femoral shaft. Thereafter, rapid differentiation occurs. The femoral head appears slightly later than the femoral shaft but by *7 weeks*, when the embryo is 17 mm long, an interzone develops between the head and acetabulum. Three separate layers develop within this interzone and come to form the perichondrium of the acetabulum and the femoral head, together with the synovial membrane.

By *8 weeks* the embryo is 30 mm long and blood vessels have grown into the ligamentum teres. It is possible to detect the beginning of angulation of the femoral neck upon the femoral shaft. The cleft that heralds the true joint cavity begins to develop, and the acetabular labrum can be seen as a separate entity.

At *11 weeks*, the embryo is 50 mm long. The femoral head is spherical and measures nearly 2 mm in diameter. It is clearly separate from the acetabulum, and Watanabe (1974) has shown that it is possible experimentally to dislocate the hip at this stage of maturity. The neck shaft angle measures 130–150°, femoral anteversion is already detectable at between 5 and 10°, and the vascular supply to the hip is established.

The *16-week* foetus measures 120 mm. Hip muscles are individually recognisable and well developed, so that the foetus may kick and move. The femoral shaft shows early ossification, but the femoral head and trochanters remain cartilaginous until well after birth (Fig. 24.1). The fetal hip lies typically in flexion, abduction and lateral rotation, with the left hip usually being the more rotated. Blood supply to the femoral head is predominantly through the epiphyseal and metaphyseal vessels. The vessels in the ligamentum teres are insignificant at this stage, but contribute more to the blood supply of the femoral head in the later stages of gestation.

The hip joint enlarges and matures during the last 20 weeks of intrauterine life. Le Damany (1912) showed elegantly that the relative capacity of the acetabulum decreases in the last 3 months of gestation; recent studies have shown that acetabular capacity and depth are probably least at birth (Ralis & McKibbin 1973).

Neck–shaft angulation, femoral neck anteversion and acetabular orientation have been interpreted widely by different authors. The flexed posture of the pelvis upon the lumbar spine contributes to this confusion, because the anatomical position is not achieved until the neonatal lumbar kyphosis and fixed flexion deformity are lost. Watanabe (1974) suggested that femoral anteversion varies in the normal neonate from –30° to +40°. Most authors believe that anteversion increases during the second half of fetal life, reaching an average of 35° at birth. The neck–shaft angle probably changes little; it averages 135–140° at birth.

At birth, the femoral shaft is usually ossified to just above the lesser trochanter. The femoral head and greater trochanter combine in a common proximal chondro-epiphysis (Fig. 24.1). The ossific nucleus is occasionally present within the femoral head at birth, but usually does not appear

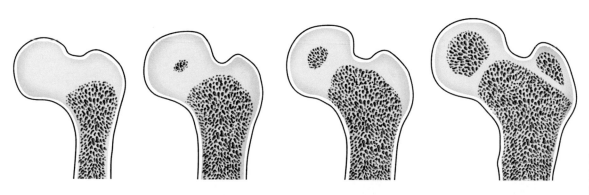

| Birth | 3 months | 6 months | 5 years |

Figure 24.1
Maturation of the femoral head in the first 5 years.

for 3–6 months. Ossification of the pelvis is also well advanced, although the pubis lags behind the ischium and ilium.

HIP GROWTH AFTER BIRTH

Acetabular growth is complex. The triradiate cartilage contributes 70%, enlarging both the diameter and the depth. Double growth plates at the junctions of the three components of the acetabulum allow circumferential enlargement of the cavity to accommodate the growing femoral head. Growth plates under the entire acetabular articular surface replicate head shape. The ring epiphysis, which surrounds the acetabular margin, contributes nearly 30% to acetabular depth. It ossifies at about 12 years and usually fuses in adolescence. The triradiate cartilage closes at about the age 11 years in girls, and a year later in boys.

Although the upper femoral ossific nucleus should be seen radiologically by 6 months, its appearance is often delayed for several months if the hip is dislocated. The greater trochanter does not start to ossify until the fourth year.

BLOOD SUPPLY

Despite its rich blood supply, the femoral head is vulnerable to infarction. This is the consequence partly of its deformable cartilaginous structure and partly of its end-arterial supply. The two main sources of blood supply to the proximal femur stem from the medial and lateral circumflex vessels, each of which usually arises from the profunda femoris artery (Fig. 24.2). The medial circumflex artery passes posteriorly and supplies most of the medial and posterior part of the proximal chondro-epiphysis. The lateral

circumflex artery and its ramifications supply the lateral and anterior part of the chondro-epiphysis, which is largely the greater trochanter. The artery of the ligamentum teres supplies only a small area around the fovea. Although each vessel branches extensively in the proximal epiphysis, there is no intercommunication because each is an end-arterial system (Trueta 1957). With the passing months, the postero-superior branches of the medial circumflex artery contribute the bulk of the intracapsular blood supply to the femoral head.

The vascular ring around the hip joint arises from both medial and lateral circumflex arteries, with additional contributions from the superior gluteal artery and an ascending branch from the first perforating artery. There is a second, often smaller and incomplete, subsynovial vascular anastomosis. The dominant posterior supply perforates the capsule posteriorly and passes proximally, with the synovial reflection, to the epiphyseal plate. The vessels are bound firmly to the femoral neck by the reflected retinacular portion of the capsule and the periosteum. The epiphyseal and metaphyseal arteries of the femoral head arise directly from the posterior vessels. The epiphyseal plate acts as an absolute barrier between the epiphyseal and metaphyseal blood supply, although there is a limited incomplete anastomosis at the periphery.

Ramifying through the cartilage of the femoral head lies an extensive cartilage canal and vascular network. Direct pressure may occlude these canals and render the femoral head ischaemic. If the hip is forced into extreme flexion and abduction, the posterior vessels may be compressed between the short femoral neck and the acetabular margin. Full extension and internal rotation may also wring out the retinacular vessels and lead to avascular necrosis.

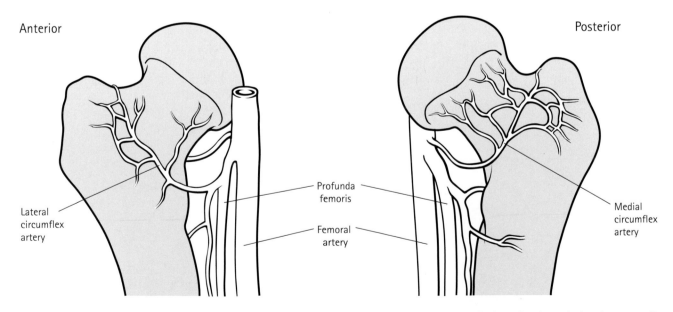

Figure 24.2 The vascular supply of the hip at 6 months. Note that the femoral head is supplied predominantly by the ascending branches of the medial circumflex artery.

DISLOCATION OF THE HIP

The umbrella term 'developmental dysplasia of the hip' is now preferred to 'congenital dislocation of the hip'. While cumbersome and repetitive, it embraces the concepts of instability and imperfect formation. It has the further advantage of not specifying *when* displacement or dysplasia occur. It is, of course, accepted that congenital factors may predispose to the developmental abnormalities.

The hip joint during early infancy is vulnerable to displacement, for the ball and socket articulation is far less stable than that in the adult. Although the signs of instability are subtle, they are usually detectable by careful examination. Therefore, treatment in the neonatal period may prevent progressive subluxation and dislocation or varying degrees of dysplasia, and the hip joint is encouraged to grow normally. If untreated, instability may progress to deformation, loss of function and eventual osteoarthritis.

AETIOLOGY

The position of the foetus *in utero* and the events surrounding birth influence the stability of the otherwise normal hip joint. An extended breech position in the last month of pregnancy (Wilkinson 1963) or a prolonged and difficult labour may displace the femoral head, and this will occur more readily if the capsule is lax or the muscles are hypotonic. Carter & Wilkinson (1960) suggested that increased maternal concentrations of oestrogen, progesterone and the polypeptide, relaxin, may be the cause of pathologically lax tissues in some newborn infants. Other studies have failed to demonstrate consistently high concentrations of maternal hormones; irrespective of this, it is not possible to measure the end-organ sensitivity. Girls are affected at least five times more often than boys.

Joint laxity may also be inherited and account for the familial form of hip dislocation (Wynne-Davies 1970). However, in many patients with hip instability, the hips are not hypermobile and other factors must play a role. The hip that is relatively adducted in flexion is more prone to dislocate, so that hip instability is much more common on the left side as the baby presents typically with the left occiput anterior at birth. A deficiency of liquor, oligohydramnios, allows less freedom of foetal movement and increases the risk of dislocation. Firstborn children are more vulnerable and this is explicable partly on the basis of greater abdominal and uterine muscle tone. Breech presentation, particularly the frank breech, increases the risk of dislocation by a factor of 10 (Dunn 1976).

Hip dysplasia occurs more frequently in association with a variety of other disorders, which have in common a cramped intrauterine environment. These include sterno-mastoid tumour and torticollis, foot deformities especially calcaneovalgus, knee dislocation and scoliosis, It is important to remember that hip anomalies are part of many syndromes: one abnormality should always prompt a search for others.

Neuromuscular imbalance (Bado 1963) may cause the atypical congenital hip displacement seen in association with arthrogryposis, major chromosomal defects and a wide variety of syndromes such as Down's and the 'thrombocytopenia, absent radius' syndrome. Fortunately, such atypical 'teratological' dislocation is rare; it usually develops *in utero*. When it occurs, the hip is almost invariably irreducible and requires an entirely different therapeutic approach. Standard neonatal splintage is both fruitless and potentially dangerous, so that open reduction later in the first year of life is preferable.

PATHOLOGY

Several studies have shown that, in typical hip dislocation of the newborn, the only anatomical abnormalities appear to be elongation of the hip capsule and the ligamentum teres. The acetabulum and its labrum, the femoral head and the orientation of femur and acetabulum are usually normal (McKibbin 1970).

If the hip is not reduced, it may become permanently subluxated or dislocated. Eccentric pressure upon the head leads to segmental flattening, uneven growth and increased anteversion. The acetabulum, lacking the normal stimulus of a contained femoral head, fails to develop anterosuperiorly, particularly if the rim is directly compressed by the displaced femoral head. This leads to lack of sphericity, shallowness and apparent anteversion. In the subluxating hip, the labrum is typically stretched and everted. The capsule of the hip is invaginated in front and below by the ilio-psoas tendon, which may adaptively shorten. In time, a secondary acetabulum develops – within the anterosuperior part of the roof of the true acetabulum if the hip is subluxated, or above the acetabulum with complete dislocation.

Subluxation blends almost imperceptibly into dislocation. Where the hip is dislocated, the everted labrum squashes and distorts. Part of this distorted labrum may fold into the joint, carrying with it a sleeve of capsule and part of the acetabular ring epiphysis. This complex is called the 'limbus'. It may prevent reduction (Fig. 24.3).

The floor of the acetabulum thickens when the head is not concentrically placed. The fibro-fatty pulvinar also hypertrophies and the transverse acetabular ligament and inferior capsule encroach upon the inferior joint space. The muscles that span the hip – particularly the ilio-psoas but also the adductors, abductors and hip extensors – shorten and contribute to the maintenance of hip displacement (Fig. 24.4).

In spite of this displacement, the articular cartilage of the femoral head and acetabulum remains viable, and will remodel if the hip is adequately reduced. The capacity for remodelling decreases with time and by the age of 3 years it is poor. Nonetheless, the potential for improvement can be surprisingly good if the femoral head remains engaged and stable after reduction. Avascular necrosis, which is almost unknown in the untreated hip, adversely affects subsequent development after reduction.

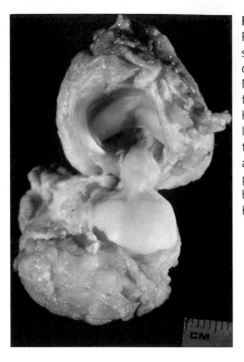

Figure 24.3
Pathological
specimen of a
dislocated hip.
Note the flattened
femoral head, the
hypertrophic
ligamentum teres,
the inverted limbus
and the eccentric
position occupied
by the femoral
head.

INCIDENCE

An enormous variation in the incidence of typical neonatal hip instability is reported, reflecting not only true social and geographical differences, but also different interpretation of the clinical signs. Barlow (1962) showed that 1 in 60 neonates had hip instability demonstrable clinically at birth. In most affected children, this slight capsular laxity tightens spontaneously, and Macnicol's (1990) value of 1 in 400 is probably closer to the British incidence. In the North American Indian, instability has been reported to be as high as 1 in 5, but the condition is virtually absent in the African Negro.

If the diagnosis of hip instability is not made at birth, children may present at walking age with a painless limp and leg shortening. Some, with partially displaced hips, will present as painful dysplasias in adolescence or early adult life. Finally, it should be noted that, in 30% of patients who

undergo hip replacement, acetabular dysplasia is the precursor of secondary arthritis.

SCREENING

Roser noted in 1879 that some children's hips could be "dislocated by adduction of the leg and then reduced again by abduction". Little was made of this observation until Ortolani, in 1937, described his test and the 'snap of entry' of the dislocated hip as it reduced. Von Rosen introduced routine clinical screening of newborns in Sweden in 1957 (von Rosen 1962). Prevention of the late-presenting dislocation remains the aim of neonatal screening programmes (Hadlow 1988, Macnicol 1990), despite the disappointments encountered by some (MacKenzie & Wilson 1981, Catford et al 1982). Examination of the hip should be carried out, not only at birth, but also later during the first year of life (Palmén 1984), preferably at 6 weeks and 6–10 months of age. The efficiency of screening depends upon paediatricians, health visitors and general practitioners to a greater extent than upon orthopaedic personnel, but their combined enthusiasm and team work needs close co-operation and regular communication with those who manage the child with an established dislocation.

Suspicion that the hips may be unstable should be aroused, particularly in the firstborn, after breech delivery and where pregnancy has been complicated by oligohydramnios or maternal hypertension. Girls are four to five times more likely to present with hip displacement, and the left hip is more commonly unstable. If the mother or a close relative has suffered from hip dislocation, the child should be presumed to have abnormal hips until proven otherwise. Other clinical abnormalities should alert the examiner: plagiocephaly, torticollis, scoliosis, foot deformities, herniae and congenital lesions such as skin tags, anal pits and supernumerary nipples.

EXAMINATION

The infant should be relaxed and warm, preferably after a feed. The nappy should be removed and the baby placed on a firm surface that allows easy access. General examination

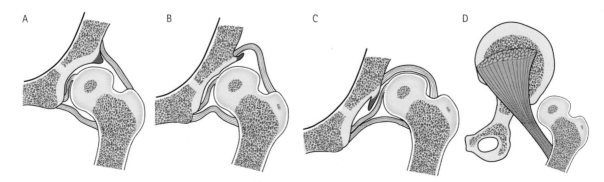

Figure 24.4 A Anatomy of the *normal* hip: the labrum envelops the head, so deepening the acetabulum. **B** In the *subluxating* hip, the labrum everts but the cartilage of the acetabulum deforms and the head occupies an eccentric position. **C** In the *dislocated* hip, the cartilaginous margin of the acetabulum is deformed and the labrum inverts. The capsule may adhere to the outer ilium. **D** In the *displaced* hip, the ilio-psoas tendon invaginates the hip capsule anteriorly.

of the skull, trunk, arms and legs should be thorough but gentle, looking for asymmetry and malformation. When examining the hips, it should be remembered that all newborns have a flexion deformity, as measured by the Thomas test, of 40–50° and it may take several months for this fixed flexion to be lost.

Although there is no set routine for assessing the hips, the following methods seem straightforward:

1. Look for thigh asymmetry. Are the skin creases level and of equal depth, particularly as they extend posteriorly? Is one leg more externally rotated than the other? Note any reduction of active movement.
2. Measure the range of movement of each hip, paying particular attention to abduction in flexion.
3. Attempt to dislocate the femoral head posteriorly (Fig. 24.5): with the infant's hip and knee flexed, the examiner's thumb in the groin presses gently backwards

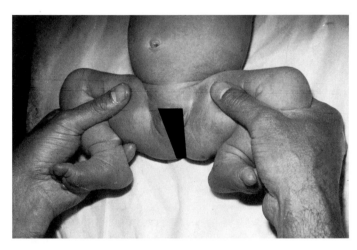

A

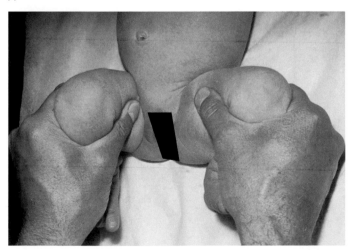

B

Figure 24.5 A Ortolani's test: when the hip is reduced, full abduction of the flexed hip is possible. **B** Barlow's test: with the hip flexed and adducted, lateral pressure from the thumb on the proximal femur will demonstrate instability if it is present.

upon the femoral head. This test was first described by Le Damany (1912), although it has become known as Barlow's (1962) test.

4. The exit clunk of a dislocatable hip can be demonstrated more readily if the thigh is abducted; it is felt more easily if the other hand is placed behind the pelvis.
5. An entry clunk is tested for next, using the middle finger to pull the greater trochanter forward. The sensation of reduction is muffled if a soft-tissue obstruction blocks complete reduction of the femoral head. Occasionally, circumduction may reduce the displaced head (Ortolani 1937).

Asymmetry and limitation of abduction should alert the clinician as much as the presence of a clunk. The 'click' is usually of little consequence, and may represent either a transient vacuum phenomenon within the joint, or muscle or tendon snapping at either hip or knee. However, about 10% of clicks can be associated with hip abnormality.

If there is uncertainty during the initial examination, it should be repeated before the infant is discharged home. Any child suspected of a hip anomaly should be examined by an expert in the treatment of hip displacement.

ULTRASOUND

Although careful clinical examination of the infant should reliably detect instability, it is clear that a proportion of children are not diagnosed by initial clinical screening. This may reflect inexperience of the examiner, an inadequate screening programme, or a hip in which the abnormality is not detectable at birth.

The neonatal hip is largely cartilaginous and although X-rays may help, they are sometimes difficult to interpret. Graf (1984) has delineated the different appearances of the infantile hip as 'seen' ultrasonographically. The investigation is non-invasive and gives both a static and potentially dynamic portrayal of the hip joint and any soft-tissue distortions. A linear scanner should be used, and the images are produced graphically upon a screen or as hard copies. A variety of different projections and views has been defined.

Graf has shown that a mid-sagittal scan of the hip allows the contour of the femoral head and acetabulum to be gauged. Figure 24.6 illustrates his technique for measuring the bony (α) and cartilaginous (β) angles upon the scan. An analysis of these angles allows quantification of the maturity of the hip and any dysplasia present. Figure 24.7 illustrates a normal and a dislocated hip, and Table 24.1 lists Graf's classification and recommendations for treatment.

Other systems for classifying the ultrasonographic appearances have evolved. The Morin (Morin et al 1985) classification assesses acetabular depth relative to head size: this gives a measure of head coverage. It is simpler than Graf's technique. The Suzuki (Suzuki et al 1991) method scans from the front, but the images obtained are more difficult to interpret. Adequate statistical analyses of the systems have not been compared.

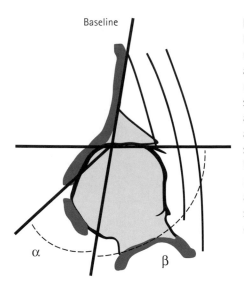

Figure 24.6
Diagram of the ultrasonographic appearance of a reduced hip with a shallow acetabulum. An α angle less than 60° suggests a poor bony acetabular roof. A large β angle, as here, suggests a poor cartilaginous roof.

Baseline

α   β

Table 24.1 Graf's ultrasonographic classification of hip dysplasia

Type	α and β angles	Dynamic stress	Treatment
I	α >60°	Stable	Discharge
IIa	α 50–60° β >77°	Stable	Review if infant under 3 months
IIb	α 50–60°	Stable	Pavlik if infant over 3 months
IIc	α 43–49°	Stable	Pavlik
IId	α 43–49°	Subluxated	Pavlik
III	α < 43°	Low dislocation Labrum everted	Pavlik
IV	α very small	High dislocation Labrum inverted	Pavlik likely to fail; open reduction likely

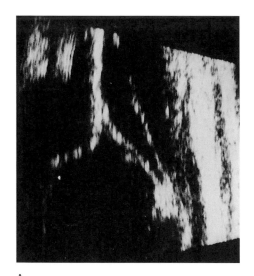

A

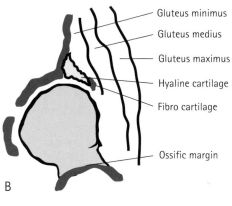

Gluteus minimus
Gluteus medius
Gluteus maximus
Hyaline cartilage
Fibro cartilage
Ossific margin

B

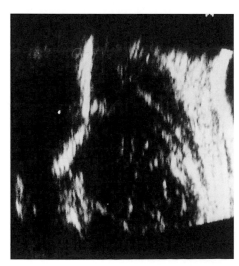

C

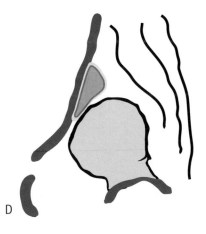

D

Fig. 24.7 A Ultrasonogram of normal hip. **B** Graphic interpretation of ultrasonographic appearance. **C** Ultrasonogram of a dislocated hip with a poor bony roof. **D** Graphic illustration of the dislocated hip.

Ultrasound has increased considerably our understanding of the morphology of hip development. The natural history of each type of hip appearance is, however, difficult to evaluate. Not surprisingly, investigators have been tempted to treat hips that appear to be morphologically dysplastic. It is not always clear whether treatment or simple maturation has allowed such hips to improve.

Ultrasound may be used not only statically but also dynamically. If the examiner attempts gently to displace the hip, graphic images of the manoeuvre are easily obtained. Clarke et al (1985) focused attention on this hip instability and, more recently, Engesaeter et al (1990) suggested that dynamic instability was of greater prognostic significance than morphological appearance (Fig. 24.7).

In Austria and Germany, it has become a national requirement that all babies should undergo ultrasound examination at birth. In Britain and the USA, ultrasound examination is reserved for those children who are suspected of a clinical anomaly or to be at high risk by virtue of family history or breech presentation. Clegg et al (1999) have shown that universal ultrasound screening may prove cheaper than treating late those children with a missed diagnosis of developmental dysplasia of the hip. It remains to be seen whether the routine neonatal use of ultrasound will become the norm.

Ultrasound has established itself securely for monitoring the progress of treatment. In the first few months of life, before the developing ossific nucleus obscures the view of the acetabulum, it allows the surgeon to assess the quality of reduction and to monitor increasing stability and acetabular quality. It has the great advantage over other imaging techniques that it is non-invasive and, if the equipment is available, it is inexpensive. The danger is that it may lead the unwary to overtreat a condition that often resolves.

RADIOGRAPHY

Where ultrasonographic equipment is not available a standardised anteroposterior pelvic radiograph is of great value. Clearly, it is impractical to investigate all babies in this manner but, in suspicious cases, particularly if there is a suggestion of skeletal deformation or asymmetry (Dunn 1976), a carefully taken film adds to the precision of neonatal diagnosis (Bertol et al 1982).

It should be remembered that the *bony* contours demonstrable radiographically give an imperfect indication of the quality of the *cartilaginous* acetabular roof. Nonetheless, the bony acetabular contour can be assessed by the acetabular index (Fig. 24.8), although this is prone to some error. The 'medial gap' (Bertol et al 1982) should not measure more than 5 mm on a standardised radiograph. A smoothly curved line produced along the lower border of the superior pubic

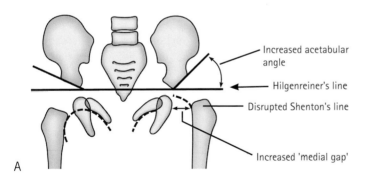

Increased acetabular angle

Hilgenreiner's line

Disrupted Shenton's line

Increased 'medial gap'

A

Figure 24.8 A Features of an infant's radiograph that are used to determine the acetabular index. The right hip shows the normal relationships. **B** The change of acetabular index with time.

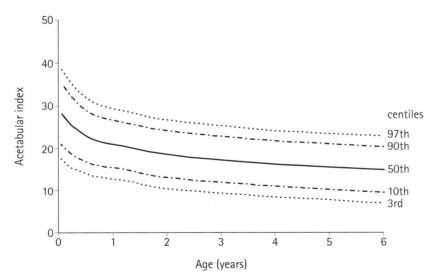

B

ramus should follow the curve of the lower border of the medial femoral neck (Shenton's line). Once the ossific nucleus appears in the femoral head (between 3 and 6 months), radiological assessment becomes easier. The ossific nucleus should lie wholly beneath the triradiate cartilage in infancy and early childhood. It should also lie medial to the perpendicular dropped from the lateral acetabular margin.

Because the reliability and accuracy of radiographs increase with age, it has been proposed that all children should undergo X-ray examination at 6 or 9 months. However, the practical difficulties and expense of this would be considerable.

After a child has been treated for hip instability, sequential review with serial ultrasonograms and later radiographs is important, to ensure that the hips develop normally. When it becomes possible, the child should stand for a weight-bearing film. In the younger child, the acetabular index should be measured at each review and compared with expected development (Fig. 24.8B).

Hip displacement causes the ossific nucleus of the femoral head to appear later and to be smaller than its normal counterpart. Furthermore, the ossific nucleus may be eccentric within the femoral head. As the child grows older and the ossific nucleus enlarges, the centre of the femoral head can be estimated by using Mose's concentric rings. Once the centre of the femoral head is known, the acetabular cover of the femoral head may be measured, the so-called 'centre-edge' angle of Wiberg (1939). In the child, this should measure at least 15°; in the adult is should be 25° (Fig. 24.9). Severin (1941) produced a scheme of classification of hip dysplasia based on the radiological appearance and the centre-edge angle (Table 24.2). Although poorly reproducible, it remains the most widely used system.

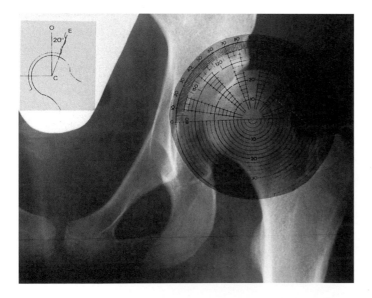

Figure 24.9 Radiograph with Mose's rings superimposed. The centre of the femoral head is delineated and the centre–edge (CE) angle may be measured. The angle in the insert measures 20°; on the X-ray it measures 0°.

Table 24.2 Severin's radiographic classification of hip dysplasia

	X-ray appearance	Centre–edge angle (after Wiberg)
Class 1	Normal	
Ia		6–13 years: >19°
		Over 14 years: >25°
Ib		6–13 years: >15–19°
		Over 14 years: 20–25°
Class II	Moderate deformity of head, neck or socket	
IIa		6–13 years: >19°
		Over 14 years: >25°
IIb		6–13 years: 15–19°
		Over 14 years: 20–25°
Class III	Dysplasia without subluxation	6–13 years: <15°
		Over 14 years: <20°
Class IV		
IVa	Moderate subluxation	>0°
IVb	Severe subluxation	<0°
Class V	Head lies in false socket in upper true acetabulum	
Class VI	Re-dislocation	

When a decision is being taken as to whether additional radiographs of the child's hip should be taken, the risk of irradiation should not be forgotten; unnecessary films and views should be avoided. Gonadal shields should be used.

TREATMENT

AT BIRTH

Barlow (1962) showed that 50% of the hips he considered to be unstable at the time of birth became clinically normal within two weeks and that 80% had stabilised by 2 months. Unfortunately, there is no absolute means of predicting at birth which hip will remain unstable, although the hip that is dislocated rather than dislocatable is more likely to remain displaced. As many mothers are discharged from hospital within 48 hours of delivery, it is often difficult for the same examiner to reassess the hip a week or two later. Knowing the high spontaneous resolution of neonatal instability, it seems sensible to pursue a policy of splintage only for those children at risk of long-term instability. Overzealous screening programmes, whether manual or ultrasound, may encourage splintage rates of as much as 10%. Some practitioners, indeed, recommend that all children should be treated in abduction splintage, to minimise the risk of missing an affected child. If splintage were entirely safe, it would not be unreasonable to treat large numbers of babies unnecessarily. However, it carries a recognised risk of avascular necrosis, and should therefore be reserved for those children in whom it is necessary. If selection for splintage is not rigorously carried out, the screening process itself will be called into question. There is no universal screening and treatment programme. Figure 24.12 outlines the schema used in Oxford.

For the reducibly dislocated hip or the hip that is readily dislocatable, the hip should be held in a reduced position in flexion and abduction. If an inflexible splint such as the Malmo (or von Rosen) splint (Fig. 24.10A) is used, great care must be taken to ensure that at least 30° of freedom in abduction is available beyond the confines of the splint. It is important to remember that the range of abduction varies considerably from child to child: if only 60° of abduction are present, the splint should hold the child's hip in only 30° of abduction (Bradley et al 1987). The hip should not be splinted in extreme abduction.

There are many types of less rigid splint available and the Pavlik harness is perhaps the most widely used (Fig. 24.10B) (Macnicol 1987).

Each splint must be applied carefully and the fit must be checked regularly. No child must ever be splinted in a rigid splint with the hip dislocated. It may be reasonable to attempt a trial of reduction in a Pavlik harness for an apparently irreducible hip, but if reduction is not achieved in a few days its use should be discontinued. Either an ultrasonogram or radiograph should be taken to ensure that the hip is reduced within the splint. At 6 weeks, hip stability can be assessed both clinically and, if possible, ultrasonographically. If acetabular development is satisfactory and the hip is stable, splintage may be discarded. In the presence of poor acetabular development or persistent instability, a longer period of splintage is essential.

Both the Malmo splint and the Pavlik harness demand certain restrictions in bathing and clothing, and help from a health visitor, district nurse or 'mothers' club' is useful. Splintage rarely affects bonding between mother and child, but other complications of splintage may occur (Bradley et al 1987). Avascular necrosis, skin rashes, temporary injury to the femoral nerve and foot deformities have been reported

as occasional complications. It should be noted that earlier advice to nurse children prone in splints has been set aside after investigation of 'cot deaths', as it is clear that children are safer when lying supine or on their side.

Alternative splints, such as the Craig splint and the Frejka pillow, are positioned over the nappy and are regularly removed. There is little evidence to allow comparison between splints, and it is probably best to use carefully the most familiar. Double nappies between the thighs may be useful when a Pavlik harness is in place, but are not adequate to treat a displaced hip on their own.

In addition to the problems of missed diagnosis at birth and the possible failure of splintage, there is the major complication of iatrogenic avascular necrosis. This may be produced by failure to reduce the hip properly or by excessive pressure upon the vulnerable cartilaginous femoral head, particularly when it is placed in extreme abduction in splintage. If the epiphysis alone is injured, the ossific nucleus will be delayed in appearance and may be mottled or fragmented when it does so. When the ossific nucleus has not appeared by 1 year, it is likely that avascular necrosis has occurred. Such avascular femoral heads often flatten and distort with continuing growth. Occasionally, of course, other disorders such as thyroid deficiency, neurological deficit or epiphyseal dysplasia may be the cause of the delayed appearance.

The avascular insult may affect not only the epiphysis but also the growth plate. When it does so, the damage may be complete or incomplete. Kalamchi & MacEwan (1980) described lateral, central and complete injuries to the physis which produce deformities of the head and neck that become more apparent with growth (Fig. 24.11). The deformity of femoral head and neck growth is accompanied by secondary adaptive acetabular changes. The incidence of such iatrogenic avascular change ranges from 0 to 15%. The risk should concern all who treat developmental dysplasia of the hip, and dictate the need for careful supervision of neonatal splintage, the avoidance of unnecessary splintage, and the importance of long-term review of children splinted in infancy.

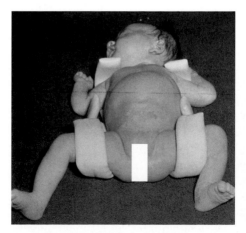

A

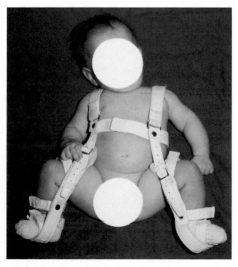

B

Figure 24.10 A Von Rosen splint, maintaining hip flexion and abduction. It is easy to see how the abduction may be too extreme. **B** The Pavlik harness, maintaining hip flexion but allowing considerable freedom of rotation and adduction.

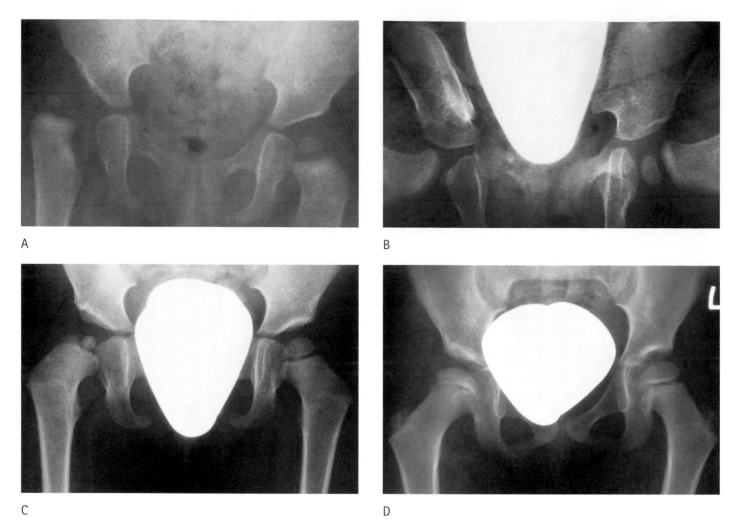

A

B

C

D

Figure 24.11 Avascular necrosis complicating Pavlik harness treatment. **A** 8-month-old girl with right developmental dysplasia of the hip. **B** Position after 3 months of splintage. **C** By 2 years, the right ossific nucleus has grown imperfectly, with the development of a secondary ossific centre. **D** At 5½ years, there is flattening of the femoral head and mild residual subluxation.

TREATMENT BEFORE WALKING AGE

The ideal age for treatment of the unstable hip is at birth, but failed primary screening, failed primary splintage and secondary screening still lead to an appreciable number of infants presenting with dislocation later in the first year of life (Fig 24.12). Although the cartilaginous femoral head is extremely sensitive to pressure, careful reduction of the hip is usually advised when the displacement is first apparent, although in atypical cases it may be wise to delay at least until the ossific nucleus has appeared within the femoral head. Segal et al (1999) have shown experimentally in a porcine model that the presence of the ossific nucleus appears to protect the cartilaginous femoral epiphysis from compressive ischaemic injury.

Although, in the neonate, it is exceptional for the dislocated hip to be irreducible, the situation changes rapidly in the first few months of life. The hip that is dislocated at birth usually becomes irreducible within a matter of weeks. The hip that fails to stabilise may well occupy an intermediate

position of subluxation that becomes fixed. For both the subluxated and dislocated hip, the clinical signs are similar: there is often thigh crease asymmetry and the affected leg is shortened and externally rotated. Flexion and extension are full, but abduction in both flexion and extension is restricted because the hip does not reduce completely.

It is important to be aware of the postural asymmetry that may develop as a consequence of the child lying exclusively upon one side (Fig. 24.13). Under these circumstances plagiocephaly, torticollis, a correctable thoraco-lumbar scoliosis and asymmetric hip abduction may develop in the 'skew' baby (Macnicol 1987). On the habitually dependent side, hip abduction is greater and hip adduction less than that of the opposite hip. In contrast, the habitually upper hip shows restricted abduction in flexion, which may lead the unwary into believing that the hip is subluxated. The difference in abduction is emphasised by examining the legs with the baby lying prone. Radiography, ultrasonography or arthrography usually separate such children with skeletal skew and avoid inappropriate abduction splintage. In the hip

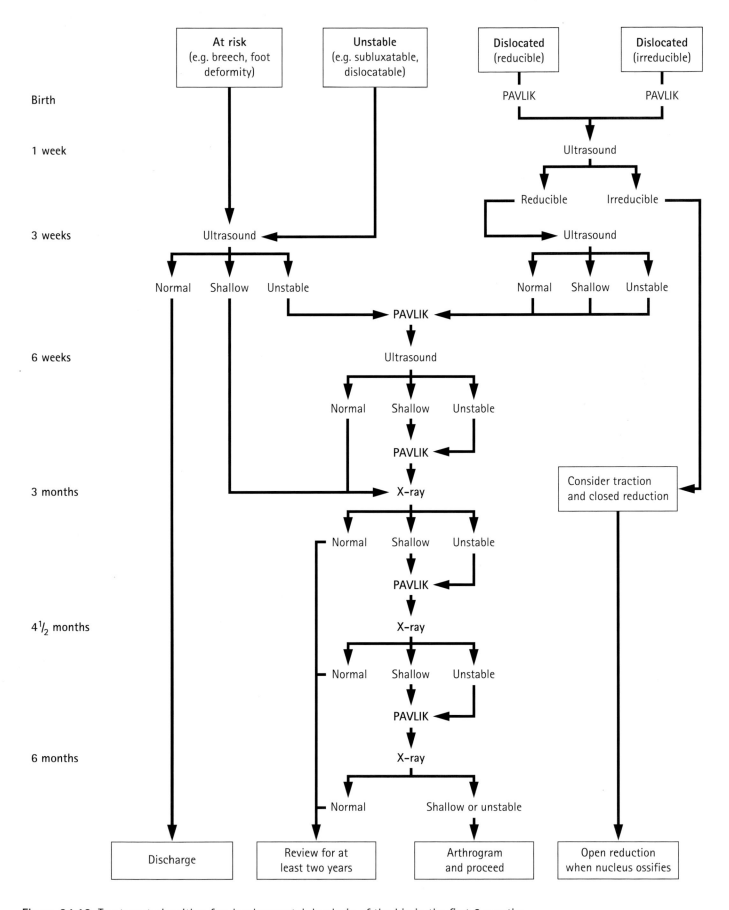

Figure 24.12 Treatment algorithm for developmental dysplasia of the hip in the first 6 months.

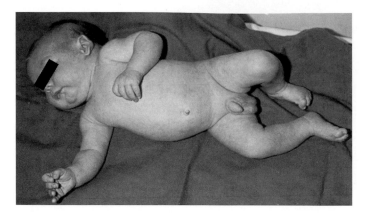

Figure 24.13 Postural asymmetry in the side-lying child.

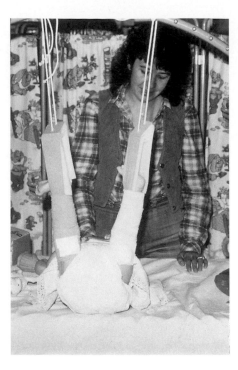

Figure 24.14
Gallows traction.
The baby's bottom
should hang just
free of the bed;
progressive
abduction is
possible when the
hip is reduced.

that is truly subluxated or dislocated, the proximal femur
lies more laterally and proximally than it should. Ossific
nuclear development is typically delayed and the acetabular
index is greater than 30°.

In the child younger than 6 months and whose hip is subluxated only, it is reasonable to pursue a course of abduction
splintage to allow the femoral head to reduce. This splintage
should not be rigid, as forced abduction may compress both
the retinacular vessels posteriorly and the vascular channels
in the cartilaginous femoral head. By the use of a check strap
between the knees, the position of forced abduction is
avoided when the Pavlik harness is in place. It is usually clear
within a week or two whether this harness will allow complete hip reduction, as the lost abduction is rapidly regained
and complete reduction assured. Serial X-rays should chart
the progress of hip development. It should be stressed again
that abduction splintage should not be used for the child
whose hip is completely dislocated and irreducible.

For the irreducible hip or for the hip with less than 30° of
abduction, preliminary traction may be advisable, although
Weinstein & Ponseti (1979) argue that it confers little additional safety. Skin traction in the 'gallows' position (Fig.
24.14) is safe to use in the child younger than 2 years,
provided they weigh less than 12.7 kg (28 lb). Here again,
the hips should not be abducted until the femoral head lies
opposite the acetabulum. After 1–3 weeks of such traction,
the child's hips should be examined under anaesthetic, with
the aid of arthrography, as the relationship between the
femoral head and acetabulum must be defined precisely.

Arthrography

The injection of contrast medium into the hip defines any
obstacles to reduction and the arthrogram, which should be
carried out under a general anaesthetic, defines the treatment
that follows. Injection into the joint may be made anterolaterally, anteriorly, laterally over the greater trochanter, or infer-
omedially. The needle should be guided into the joint under
fluoroscopic control. The joint should not be overdistended
with contrast medium, because this obscures the very features
one hopes to demonstrate; it is best if the contrast medium is
diluted with saline, as this is less likely to obscure detail. The

advantage of arthrography is that the hip may be examined
in a variety of positions and the optimum 'fit' may be assessed.

In the normal hip (Fig. 24.15A), the spherical head sits
within a spherical acetabulum. The cartilaginous roof covers
the femoral head and the labrum extends clearly beyond
this. The limbic 'thorn', representing the recess lateral to the
labrum, indicates that the head is correctly enveloped. The
zona orbicularis is produced by capsular laxity adjacent to
the Y-shaped ligament. The acetabular fossa and the transverse ligament indentation can clearly be seen. The contrast
medium extends well down the neck and delineates the
extent of the normal hip capsule.

With subluxation, a crescent of dye may be seen centrally.
When, as often happens, subluxation is associated with
acetabular insufficiency, this crescent may shift from central
to superior as the hip is moved from anatomical alignment
into flexion and abduction.

Progressive degrees of subluxation and dislocation
deform and entrap the labrum within the joint (Fig. 24.15B
and C). The ligamentum teres (often hypertrophic) is easily
visible, and the transverse ligament encroaches upon the
inferior aspect of the joint. The ilio-psoas tendon indents the
capsule and gives the illusion of an hour-glass constriction
when the hip is completely dislocated.

Assessment

A combination of clinical examination and arthrographic
appearances allows the child's hips to be considered:

1. Normal.
2. Subluxated or subluxating, but with no block to
   reduction.
3. Dislocating but fully reducible.
4. Dislocated with an obstacle to reduction.

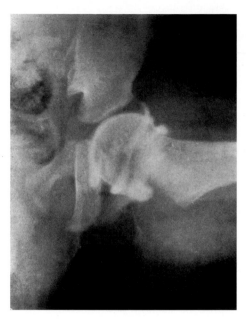

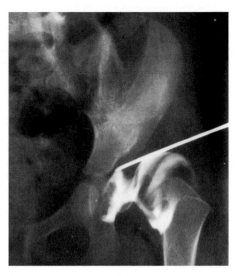

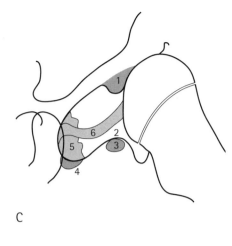

A

B

C

Figure 24.15 A Arthrogram of reduced hip in frog lateral position. Although the bony acetabulum is deficient, the spherical head sits deeply in the acetabulum. **B** Arthrogram of a dislocated left hip. The injecting needle is superolateral. The infolded labrum and superior cartilaginous acetabulum are clearly seen. The deep inferior indentation is made by the tendon of ilio-psoas. **C** Arthrogram interpretation. (1) Deformed cartilaginous rim and infolded labrum. (2) Capsular 'waisting' caused by invaginating ilio-psoas tendon (3). (4) Inferior transverse acetabular ligament. (5) Fibro-fatty pulvinar. (6) Ligamentum teres.

The subluxated hip has modest fixed displacement and exhibits lost abduction in flexion. The subluxating or 'wandering' hip may appear clinically normal as it glides imperceptibly from reduction to displacement. When the hip shows either of these or a fully reducible dislocation, a closed reduction is possible and the child should be treated in a hip spica. If the hip is irreducible, an open reduction is necessary.

Reduction

Closed reduction

A preliminary adductor tenotomy ensures that pressure upon the reduced femoral head is kept to a minimum, although it is unnecessary if the reduced hip abducts widely, with no adductor longus tension. The plaster should be applied in the 'human' position, as advocated by Salter (1969): the hips should be flexed at least to a right angle, but not abducted to more than 45°. This plaster is difficult to apply well, and careful moulding about the greater trochanter is necessary, to ensure that posterior subluxation or re-dislocation cannot occur within the plaster. The entirety of the affected leg should be incorporated in plaster for better femoral control, and the upper edge should extend to the lower thorax (Fig. 24.16).

It is important to confirm reduction. Plain radiographs are not adequate as they may fail to show the posteriorly displaced femoral head. McNally et al (1998) have shown that magnetic resonance imaging is ideal to confirm a satisfactory position. Computed tomography also allows excellent

images, but with some radiation risk. There is currently no available technique to evaluate whether the vascularity of the head has been compromised.

The hip spica should be removed after 6 weeks and the hip re-evaluated, preferably under anaesthetic. When stability remains in doubt, a further plaster should be applied. If the hip seems stable, a period of Pavlik harnessing or abduction bracing allows the gradual re-establishment of hip movement within a limited range. Careful follow-up is necessary to monitor acetabular development. When the hip appears stable and acetabular development is sufficiently advanced,

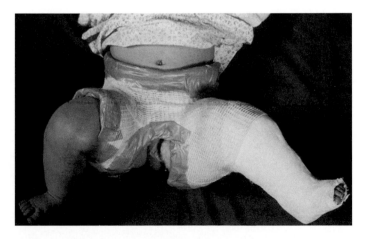

Figure 24.16 One-and-a-half hip spica to maintain reduction of left hip.

the child may be weaned gradually from the harness. Careful prolonged follow-up is essential to ensure that secondary displacement or dysplasia does not occur.

Open reduction

Open reduction is necessary when closed reduction is not possible. It is also needed when an infant's teratological dislocation has delayed treatment until the ossific nucleus has appeared in the cartilaginous femoral head. When there is a defined obstruction, such as an inverted limbus or an encroaching transverse acetabular ligament, surgical reduction is mandatory. The hip may be approached by the medial, anterolateral or posterior routes.

Medial approach. The incision is made parallel to adductor longus or transversely below the groin crease (Fig. 24.17); the transverse scar does not lengthen with growth and is cosmetically preferable. The femoral neurovascular bundle is retracted laterally. The lesser trochanter and its attached psoas tendon is approached from in front or behind adductor brevis. Care should be taken to protect the vessels adjacent to it. The psoas tendon is released from its insertion and allowed to retract proximally. This exposes the inferomedial hip capsule. Through a T-incision, with its long limb along the femoral neck, the transverse acetabular ligament, the pulvinar and the ligamentum teres may be inspected; the labrum is rarely seen because it lies posterior and superior. The approach allows release of the inferior capsule, division of the transverse acetabular ligament and, if need be, excision of the ligamentum teres. This combination usually allows the femoral head to reduce deeply (Ludloff 1913, Weinstein & Ponseti 1979).

In general, the medial approach is appropriate for the child under walking age. It is contraindicated when there is a large inverted limbus. A capsulorrhaphy cannot be performed. There is some risk of injury to the medial circumflex artery, which may lead to proximal femoral avascular necrosis, although the extent of this depends at least in part upon the preoperative management of the child and the type of subsequent splintage. The approach is relatively bloodless, and the recovery of hip movement is usually excellent. Damage to the iliac apophysis is avoided.

Anterolateral approach. This was originally achieved through a Smith–Petersen approach, but this leaves a cosmetically ugly scar. A 'bikini' transverse incision below the iliac crest centred upon the anterior superior spine is preferred (Fig. 24.18). The space between sartorius and tensor fasciae latae is developed after identifying, protecting and retracting the lateral femoral cutaneous nerve. The anterior one-third of the iliac apophysis is split by incising sharply through cartilage to bone. The apophysis with the abductor muscle and periosteum in one sheet are stripped from the outer surface of the ilium. The straight and reflected heads of rectus femoris are divided and reflected distally, exposing the superior and anterior hip capsule. The psoas tendon within the iliacus at the pelvic brim is identified, rolled forward and divided to provide lengthening without loss of continuity.

A T-shaped incision is made in the hip capsule. The capsulotomy should skirt the capsular attachment to the pelvis, and the long arm of the T should pass along the anterior neck. Hip dislocation is completed by adducting, extending and externally rotating the leg. The femoral head is almost invariably slightly flattened and oval. Inspection of the acetabulum may be difficult. The ligamentum teres is the guide to the acetabular depths; it may be excised if it is hypertrophic, because it supplies a negligible area of bone about the fovea. The transverse ligament, which impinges

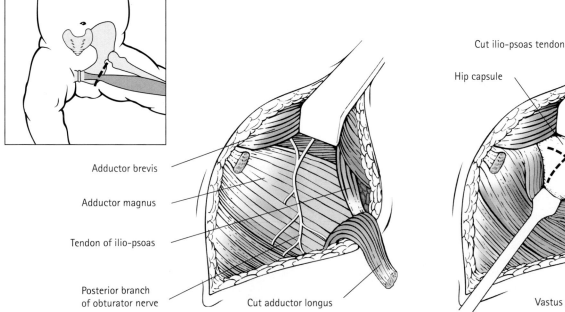
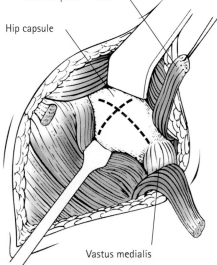

Adductor brevis

Adductor magnus

Tendon of ilio-psoas

Posterior branch of obturator nerve

Cut adductor longus

Cut ilio-psoas tendon

Hip capsule

Vastus medialis

Figure 24.17 The medial adductor approach to the hip.

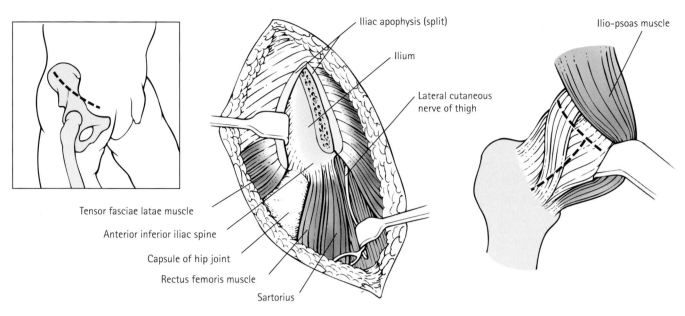

Figure 24.18 The anterolateral approach to the hip.

inferiorly, should be divided. If a limbus is present and inverted, it should be removed only if it cannot be everted by making it more pliant with radial cuts. There is a risk of damaging the preosseous cartilage at the periphery of the socket if the limbus is excised.

The acetabulum should be palpated to ensure that no other obstacle prevents reduction, as adhesions and capsular bands often extend below the femoral head. Image intensification helps to ensure the head is deeply reduced. Often, a thickened acetabular floor appears to 'lateralise' the head. If in doubt, a small pledget soaked in radio-opaque dye may be inserted between head and socket to determine radiologically the adequacy of reduction. As neither femoral head nor acetabulum is spherical, it is inaccurate to describe the reduction as a 'concentric', but this does allow the position of 'best fit' to be judged. Because of secondary femoral anteversion, this is usually with the hip flexed and internally rotated 30–40°. A capsulorrhaphy is performed by excising the redundant capsule superiorly (removing the superior triangle from the T-shaped incision), or by reefing the capsular margins. Rectus femoris is re-attached and the iliac apophysis is carefully repaired, to ensure that it does not become deformed. The hip is maintained in a hip spica in sufficient flexion, abduction and internal rotation for the head to be fully contained by the acetabulum.

In the infant before walking age, it is unlikely that secondary femoral or acetabular procedures will be necessary, and 3 months of plaster immobilisation is usually sufficient, followed by a period of abduction bracing if the acetabular response is slow. In the older child, secondary procedures become progressively more likely and, indeed, it is often advisable to consider them coincidently with open reduction.

Posterior approach. The hip may be approached posteriorly, either through a curved posterolateral or a simple transverse posterior incision. The approach has not gained wide popularity because, although theoretically attractive in giving good access to the limbus, it does not allow an effective capsulorrhaphy, psoas tenotomy has to be performed distally, and there is a significant risk of interfering with the posterior blood supply. Furthermore, if a later pelvic procedure is required, a second incision has to be made.

TREATMENT OF THE TODDLER

The toddler with a hip dislocation presents typically with an abnormal gait. On average, children with a dislocated hip walk only 1–2 months later than their normal counterparts. The gait is a mixture of a Trendelenburg lurch and a short-leg gait. The child walks on tip-toe on the affected side, with truncal asymmetry and external rotation of the leg. Clinical signs include elevation of the greater trochanter, flattening of the buttock, and hollowing below the femoral triangle. A groin lump may be palpable with the hip extended, where the femoral head lies extruded anterosuperiorly. True shortening is demonstrable when the dislocation is unilateral. It is very rare to be able to reduce the dislocated hip of a child of walking age. Characteristically, abduction in flexion is markedly restricted. When both hips are dislocated, the child walks with a bilateral Trendelenburg lurch and develops hyperlordosis of the lumbar spine.

As in the younger infant, the principles of management in the toddler are straightforward: the hip should be concentrically reduced as atraumatically as possible. Reduction should be maintained for the minimum time necessary for stability to be assured.

At one time, treatment of late congenital hip dislocation was by forcible manipulation under anaesthesia and splintage of the hip in the fully abducted position, sometimes for up to 2 years. There can be no doubt that many hips were successfully reduced by this technique, but avascular necrosis of the femoral head occurred in over 50%. Nowadays, preliminary limb traction and adductor tenotomy have reduced the incidence of avascular change, as has the avoidance of extreme positioning of the hip after reduction.

Traction

Fifteen years ago, few surgeons would have considered operating on an older child unless the soft-tissue contractures associated with dislocation had been at least partly overcome by preliminary traction. Although many continue to advise traction, including a period of home treatment, an increasing number do not, believing that shortened muscles may be lengthened at operation by tenotomy. Inevitably financial considerations cloud the picture. For the child older than 2–3 years with a high dislocation, femoral shortening is often necessary to achieve reduction and preoperative traction is clearly inappropriate.

Traction has been applied with the hips in 90° of flexion, in 45° of flexion, or in extension. It may be of simple 'gallows' type (see Fig. 24.14), or progressive abduction in flexion may be achieved if a hoop is placed over the bed. Traction in extension is particularly suitable for the older child, and modified Pugh's traction on a 45° tilted mattress is valuable, as the child may lie either prone or supine and is easier to entertain.

Skin traction needs careful supervision, because blistering may develop unless the tapes and bandaging are regularly changed and carefully applied. It is for this reason that many surgeons prefer to treat children in hospital. With escalating costs, however, home traction is becoming more common. It is unusual now for traction to be continued for longer than 3 weeks, by which time a hip that was irreducible may have become reducible. At this stage, examination under anaesthesia and arthrography will allow the surgeon to plan future treatment.

The reducible hip

Where the hip is fully reducible, it should be held in a hip spica. Care must be taken to avoid the extremes of positioning. In the younger child the so-called 'human' position of more-than 90° flexion and no more than 45° of abduction may be most appropriate, although lesser degrees of flexion are equally effective if the plaster is moulded posteriorly. As the child gets older, the hip is reduced fully in 45° of flexion, 30° of abduction and 30° of internal rotation. It is wise to perform a percutaneous tenotomy of adductor longus before spica application.

Splintage needs to be maintained until adaptive capsular shortening has occurred. The deformed articular cartilage of the acetabular roof should begin to ossify before unsupported walking is permitted.

The irreducible hip

Arthrography will frequently demonstrate that the hip is irreducible, and obstacles to reduction may be defined. Under these circumstances, open reduction should be performed and we prefer the anterolateral approach for these older children. The principles of this reduction are no different from those in the younger child, although femoral head deformity is more pronounced. Femoral anteversion and valgus may be marked, and the acetabulum is shallow and anteverted. If the labrum has been inverted, it becomes more rigid, making it difficult to evert.

In children younger than 2 years, careful reduction of the hip and capsular plication usually promote satisfactory development. In older children, a secondary bony procedure, either to realign the acetabulum or the femur, becomes increasingly necessary. After the age of 3 years, it is almost mandatory to redirect the acetabulum by the Salter innominate osteotomy, or to reshape it by Pemberton osteotomy.

Great care should be taken peroperatively to ensure that the femoral head will reduce without undue pressure. If the femoral head appears to reduce too tightly, release of the adductors and ilio-psoas may have been inadequate. If the femoral head dislocates as the knee is straightened, despite this release, the hamstrings are shortened and may prevent a stable reduction. For children older than 3 years, therefore, it is safest to advise concurrent femoral shortening. This operation was first described by Hey-Groves (1928), but was more recently advocated by Klisic (1976). Femoral shortening prevents proximal epiphyseal compression, which is otherwise inevitable when the hip is reduced.

It is important to mobilise the child for a few days in hospital once a hip spica has been removed, because the osteoporotic femur may fracture. A graduated approach to splintage should reduce this risk, and a progression from full-length hip spicas to pantaloon casts and then removable abduction braces is recommended.

While every optimism may be felt for the promptly recognised and treated neonatal unstable hip, the surgeon should be cautious of promising normal outcomes for older children. There is little doubt that the quality of the long-term result is poorer (Gibson & Benson 1982), and each child who has been treated for hip dislocation needs to be followed at least to skeletal maturity.

TREATMENT IN LATER CHILDHOOD

The majority of children over toddler age who present with congenital hip dislocation represent the failures of earlier management. It is rare for the untreated child with congenital hip dysplasia to develop pain before adolescence. Even then, pain is likely to be experienced as discomfort or fatigue after exercise. In contrast, the child who has been treated unsuccessfully is likely to develop pain in early childhood.

The long-term results of treatment in the older child deteriorate for a variety of reasons; femoral head and acetabular deformity become more marked, femoral anteversion increases, the acetabulum fails to develop anteriorly, and the capacity for remodelling decreases rapidly after the age of 3 years.

Where bilateral dislocation is present, the child stands with a hyperlordotic lumbar spine, which is not present in unilateral dislocation. Shortening becomes more pronounced. Palpation of the groin, beneath the inguinal ligament reveals an 'empty' acetabulum. The trochanter is high and proximal, and may be felt deeply in the buttock, where it is carried by the increasing anteversion of the femoral head and neck.

The principles of treatment for the older child remain exactly the same as before: the hip needs to be reduced atraumatically, preventing abnormal pressure upon the reduced femoral head. To accomplish this, skin traction may be used for a few weeks before surgery, but its value becomes progressively less in the older child. Peroperative femoral shortening reduces the pressure upon the reduced femoral head, and is almost always advisable in the child over the age of 2½ years. Such femoral shortening may with profit be combined with rotation sufficient to counter-act the excessive anteversion. It is prudent to lengthen the ilio-psoas peroperatively, to further minimise femoral head pressure.

Femoral osteotomy

Osteotomy of the proximal femur is readily carried out through a lateral thigh incision. An L-shaped incision in vastus lateralis allows this to be reflected forwards, just below the level of the greater trochanter; the trochanteric growth plate should not be injured. It is sensible to insert wires into the proximal femur so that, after rotation or varus, parallel alignment of the wires confirms that the desired alteration has been achieved. Image intensification should be used if possible. Ideally, the osteotomy should be performed above the level of the lesser trochanter, but this may not be possible if shortening is required. In tiny children the osteotomy is held with a staple or a small plate as a 'bone suture' (Fig. 24.19). In the older child a blade plate is preferable, and from the age of 5 or 6 years compression at the osteotomy site obviates the need for plaster fixation.

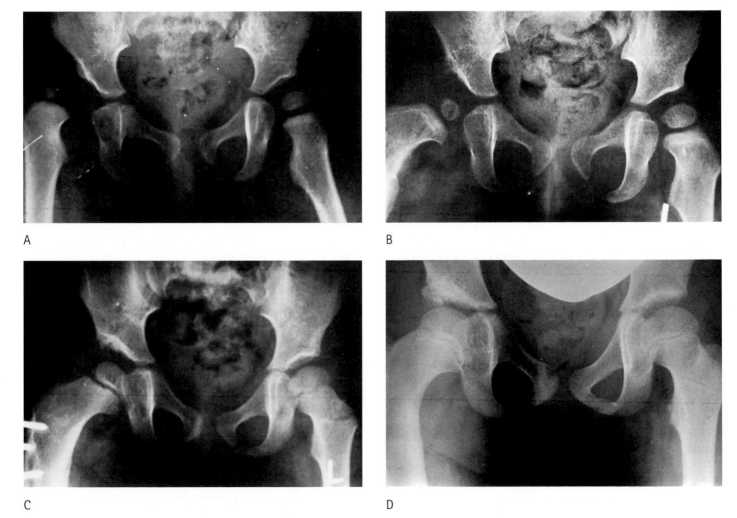

A

B

C

D

Figure 24.19 18-month-old girl with congenital dislocation of the right hip and dysplasia of the left hip. **A** Initial appearance. **B** After open reduction, the lines of temporary growth arrest show symmetrical epiphyseal growth. **C** One year after derotation varus femoral osteotomy. **D** Six years later the acetabular cartilage has ossified and head containment is satisfactory.

Although femoral osteotomy may be necessary, there is a tendency to use it less often than in the past. Typically, the varus introduced at osteotomy resolves 3 years later (Sangavi et al 1996) and the shortening corrects by relative overgrowth within the same time.

It is now uncommon for the child with hip dislocation who is older than 2 years to be treated non-operatively. The surgical approach favoured is almost always by the antero-lateral approach, which provides the best exposure of the hip joint and its contents. In established dislocation, the superior capsule is usually firmly adherent to the side wall of the ilium above the true acetabulum and needs to be elevated and mobilised superiorly and posteriorly if the labrum is to be everted from the joint. The redundant superior capsule should be excised and a careful capsulorrhaphy performed when the head has been fully reduced.

The femoral head and acetabulum are always deformed in the long-established dislocation, but it is important to ensure that the femoral head is seated as deeply as possible in the true acetabulum. If it is impossible to evert the labrum, it should be resected as sparingly as possible to ensure that the lateral acetabular epiphysis is not damaged. It is probably unnecessary to remove the acetabular fat pad (pulvinar), but the transverse ligament should be divided. The inferior capsule may need to be carefully released to allow the femoral head to descend fully. The posterior capsule should not be divided but in some circumstances, particularly after previous failed surgery, it cannot be avoided; great care should then be taken to divide the capsule at the acetabular margin. The procedure is most likely to be necessary where the hip has dislocated posteriorly as a consequence of excessive internal rotation at previous open reduction.

Pelvic osteotomy

Careful preoperative analysis and peroperative assessment should aid the decision as to whether pelvic osteotomy should be performed. The capacity for acetabular remodelling around the femoral head is maximal in infancy and decreases steadily during the first 6 or 7 years of life. If, therefore, the acetabulum contains the femoral head poorly, attempts should be made to improve this acetabular cover.

In the typical dislocation, the anterior limb of the triradiate cartilage is not adequately stimulated and the anterior acetabulum fails to develop. This produces a shallow and apparently anteverted acetabulum. If the acetabulum is flat and oval, its shape may be improved by Pemberton's pericapsular osteotomy (1965). This is described below, but in essence a curvilinear osteotomy is made, following the contour of the acetabular roof, curving downwards and medially to the triradiate cartilage. By levering the roof downwards, anterolateral acetabular cover may be improved and the shape of the acetabulum altered.

If the femoral head and the acetabulum fit well but the acetabulum is too open, Salter's (1961) innominate osteotomy, which rotates the whole acetabulum forwards and laterally, is to be preferred. Klisic (1976) made popular the simultaneous performance of open reduction, femoral shortening and pelvic osteotomy. Some surgeons, however, prefer to reserve pelvic osteotomy for those children in whom it may be seen that the acetabulum is failing to develop adequately after reduction. The stress to the child and family of multiple hip surgery in childhood and the disadvantages of repetitive plaster immobilisation should not be underestimated, and where expertise and facilities allow, the surgeon should attempt both to reduce and stabilise the hip at the time of the first operation. However, the risk of re-dislocation is increased.

Wherever possible, it is best to reshape and reorientate the acetabulum so that articular cartilage covers the femoral head. In the child older than 4 or 5 years, acetabular and femoral head deformity may be such that this is impracticable. Under these circumstances, when irreversible subluxation is present, a salvage procedure such as the medial displacement osteotomy of Chiari (1953) or a shelf procedure may be a better solution.

Although shortening, rotational and varus osteotomy may be necessary both to decrease pressure upon the femoral head and to reorientate the proximal femur, it has been shown (Williamson & Benson 1988) that femoral osteotomy alone in later childhood is inadequate treatment for the subluxated hip.

It has become increasingly rare for children to present with a previously unrecognised hip dislocation after the age of 3 or 4 years. Because of the deteriorating results of treatment with age, many authors suggest that the child older than 7 years with bilateral hip dislocation should be left untreated because operation has a high chance of increasing the likelihood of adolescent hip pain. Where the dislocation is unilateral, however, most surgeons continue to advocate reduction and reconstruction in order to preserve leg length and spinal symmetry.

The innominate osteotomy

The innominate osteotomy of Salter (1961) is suitable for the child between the ages of 2 and 6 years with a dislocated hip, and may be appropriate for the subluxating hip in the older child and adolescent. Certain criteria are necessary for the osteotomy to be undertaken. The hip should reduce concentrically and preserve a virtually normal range of movement. If open reduction is performed at the same time, hip reduction should be congruous and confirmed radiologically. It should be apparent that subluxation of the internally rotated hip occurs as the hip is drawn from flexion into extension and the instability should be anterosuperior. It is precisely this maldirectional instability that the innominate osteotomy is designed to correct.

The innominate osteotomy lengthens the leg; avoidance of this lengthening is possible by combining it with a varus rotational osteotomy (Morscher 1978) or by notching the upper pelvic segment in the older child. Overzealous femoral internal rotation or derotational osteotomy may allow the femoral head to displace posteriorly, as the innominate osteotomy achieves improved anterolateral cover at the expense of posterior support. As already noted, in the child older than 3 years it may be wise to shorten the femur in order to lessen pressure upon the reduced femoral head. Theoretically, the innominate osteotomy in isolation may increase pressure upon the femoral head, but Salter has argued that the pressure increase is trivial. However, the femoral head may remain poorly covered if the limb is lengthened, because the child stands with the hip adducted.

The innominate osteotomy (Fig. 24.20) is best performed through a transverse incision just below the iliac crest. The iliac apophysis is split and the split halves are elevated, in continuity with the gluteal muscles externally and the iliac muscles internally, subperiosteally from the iliac wing. Great care should be taken in exposing the sciatic notch, and the retractors placed through this notch should be clearly seen and felt to be subperiosteal. The psoas tendon should be divided intramuscularly by rolling it at the level of the iliac brim. A curved introducer passed through the sciatic notch allows the Gigli saw to be introduced subperiosteally through the notch.

A transverse pelvic osteotomy is then performed at the level of the anterior inferior iliac spine. Where the hip joint has not been opened the thigh is placed in flexion, abduction and external rotation. Downward leverage upon the knee allows the distal pelvic fragment to rotate anterolaterally. Its direction may be helped by gentle downwards traction using a towel clip placed through the anterior inferior spine or by pulling the posterior edge of the lower fragment forwards with a small Lambotte hook. A wedge of bone taken from the anterior superior iliac spine is trimmed and fashioned to fit

into the triangular gap so created. It is important to keep the osteotomy closed posteriorly. A wedge of bone may be taken from the proximal ilium to minimise lengthening of the leg. Once the bone graft is safely placed, two threaded wires should be passed across the osteotomy and screened radiographically to ensure that joint penetration has not occurred. The implants are cut short, but should be left slightly proud of the closed iliac apophysis.

The wound is closed in layers, taking care to re-appose the iliac apophysis carefully. A one-and-a-half hip spica is applied with the hip in 20–30° of flexion and abduction and neutral rotation. The osteotomy unites in 6 weeks and the pins are removed when the graft has consolidated.

Complications that may occur with this procedure are often the result of faulty technique. The operation should not be performed unless it is possible to reduce the hip satisfactorily. Re-dislocation may occur if open reduction is performed simultaneously. The bone graft may slip or resorb, wires may penetrate the joint or extrude, the sciatic, femoral or lateral femoral cutaneous nerves may be injured, and there may be deformity of the ilium consequent upon splitting the iliac apophysis.

The Pemberton acetabuloplasty

Where the femoral head and acetabulum do not 'match', and where arthrography has demonstrated a bilocular acetabulum in association with subluxation, it may be wiser to reshape rather than to redirect the acetabulum, in the manner described by Pemberton (1965).

Pemberton's procedure allows an incomplete iliac osteotomy to hinge through the triradiate cartilage. This hinge alters the volume of the acetabulum and is therefore applicable for the grossly dysplastic socket. The triradiate cartilage must be open for the procedure to be accomplished, and therefore the osteotomy finds its greatest use in children between the ages of 3 and 11 years. The approach is similar to that described for an innominate osteotomy. Careful preoperative radiographic checking is essential. A series of curved osteotomes is passed above the hip joint, curving medially and posteriorly to the triradiate cartilage, usually at a distance of about 1 cm from the joint proper. Extreme care must be taken to ensure that articular penetration does not occur. A curved bone graft is taken from the anterosuperior iliac spine and inserted into the gap created as the acetabular margin is levered down with the osteotome. When the bone graft is tapped into place the position is usually stable and additional internal fixation is not necessary (Fig. 24.21).

The risks of joint penetration are real in this procedure, and there is a slight increase in the risk of avascular necrosis from pressure directed upon the femoral head by the levered-down acetabular roof. The triradiate cartilage may rarely also be injured and cease to grow.

The Pemberton acetabuloplasty, just like the innominate osteotomy, may be performed in isolation or as part of a complex open reduction in the older child, in whom it may

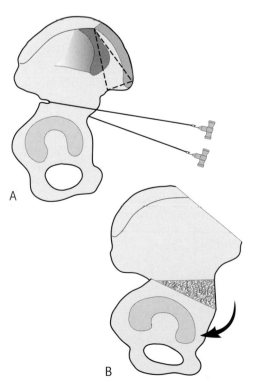

Figure 24.20 A The innominate osteotomy of Salter. The Gigli saw transects the pelvis at the level of the anterior inferior iliac spine and the wedge of bone from the ilac crest (B) is inserted into the osteotomy, allowing the distal fragment to rotate forwards and laterally.

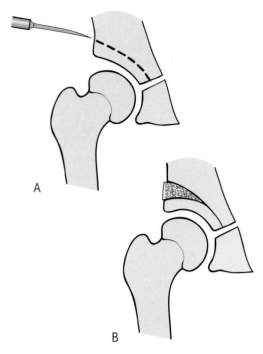

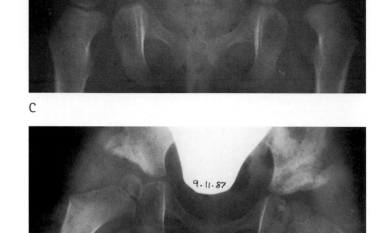

Figure 24.21 A The pelvic osteotomy of Pemberton. The osteotomy curves about 1 cm from the acetabular margin into the triradiate cartilage. **B** Hinging is through the triradiate cartilage as the roof of the acetabulum is brought down and held with a bone graft. **C** 2¼-year-old girl with right hip subluxation and left hip dislocation. **D** The same little girl after open reduction of the left hip and bilateral Pemberton acetabuloplasty.

be combined with femoral shortening and rotation, open reduction and capsulorrhaphy.

The Dega pelvic osteotomy is similar to the Pemberton, except that the pelvic cut is not curved, but directed obliquely downwards and medially to the tri-radiate cartilage from an anteroposterior axis 2 cm above the acetabular margin. It similarly reduces acetabular size, but increases lateral rather than anterior cover.

A variety of more complex acetabular osteotomies has been described (Macnicol 1995). As skeletal maturity approaches, Salter's osteotomy in isolation may not allow as much rotation about the axis from symphysis pubis to greater sciatic notch, unless osteotomies of superior pubic ramus and ischium are performed co-incidentally. This triple innominate osteotomy allows greater displacement of the acetabular complex.

Residual dysplasia often needs treatment after maturity. When an adolescent or young adult develops discomfort with exercise and radiographs demonstrate marked uncovering of the femoral head, a periacetabular osteotomy should be considered. A careful history and examination may suggest the 'rim syndrome' described by Klaue et al (1988). The patient describes sudden sharp groin pain that accompanies twisting movements. There is often a feeling that the

hip may 'give way'. Although the hip may appear to move freely at examination, pain is typically produced when the flexed hip is snapped into adduction. The cause is usually a torn labrum, which may be associated with a ganglionic cyst in the labrum itself or in the bony pelvis. The tear is best demonstrated by gadolinium-enhanced magnetic resonance imaging.

If a complex periacetabular osteotomy is considered, careful preoperative planning is essential. A three-dimensional computed tomography scan best allows three-dimensional reconstruction of the hip and permits a rational assessment of the correction necessary. Significant head deformity or arthritis should preclude the operation. A description is outside the scope of this book.

SALVAGE PROCEDURES

Capsuloplasty

Femoral head and acetabular deformity may become so pronounced, particularly after failed surgery, that congruous reduction cannot be achieved. When this discrepancy is pronounced, the Colonna (1965) procedure should not be forgotten. A circumferential acetabular capsulotomy is performed and the capsule sewn as an envelope over the femoral head. Using serial reamers, the acetabulum is enlarged to accept the femoral head enveloped in its capsular mantle. Where necessary, the femur may be shortened and rotated appropriately (Fig. 24.22). The Colonna arthroplasty provides a stable articulation, but mobility is clearly less satisfactory and discomfort more likely than in a more optimally reduced hip. Nonetheless, the restoration of anatomical alignment makes secondary surgery in adult life a great deal more straightforward. Pozo et al (1987) found 70% of 44 hips so treated had good function at a mean of 20 years.

The Chiari osteotomy

Where subluxation is fixed and the femoral head is uncovered, the Chiari medial displacement osteotomy should be considered. Although Chiari (1953) first envisaged his procedure as being most applicable to the child of 4 or 5 years, it has become increasingly utilised for the older child, adolescent and young adult for treatment of symptomatic dysplasia and subluxation.

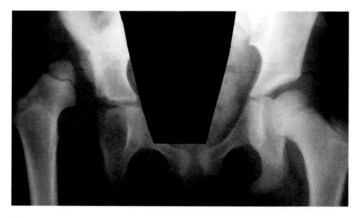

A

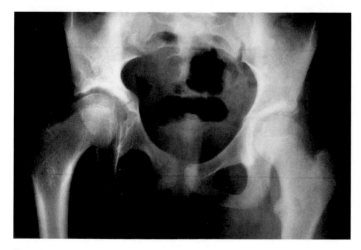

B

Figure 24.22 The Colonna procedure. Where deformity of femoral head and acetabulum are profound, Colonna's procedure may still find a place. **A** This 4-year-old was treated by Colonna arthroplasty. **B** The result, 5 years later, shows the acetabulum has developed with protrusion.

The management of hip dysplasia and the increasing growth deformity is technically demanding in the older child and adolescent. When the femoral head is irreversibly subluxated, the articulation with the abnormal acetabulum has to be accepted, but femoral head cover improved. A shelf procedure affords good support if acetabular insufficiency is mild to moderate, but when the hip joint is lateralised by marked thickening of the acetabular floor, medialisation of the femoral head is advisable. Greater degrees of hip deformity (Fig. 24.23) merit the salvaging effects of the Chiari osteotomy, which produces an iliac bone buttress.

The procedure reduces loading through the femoral head both by increasing the area of contact and by medialising the fulcrum of the hip. The operation should be carried out using an orthopaedic table and image intensifier control. A skin-crease 'bikini' incision affords adequate exposure and heals well (Högh & Macnicol 1987).

The iliac osteotomy should be made just above the hip capsule. The osteotomy level must be checked radiographically, as the reflected fibres of the hip capsule are often well above the elective site for osteotomy. Ideally, the osteotomy should be gently curved from front to back, to follow the contour of femoral head and capsule. The angle of the osteotomy should be almost transverse or slightly cephalad. Increasing obliquity of iliac division imperils the sacro-iliac joint and, by functionally weakening the abductor muscles, makes a persistent Trendelenburg gait more likely.

Displacement of 1 or 2 cm is possible, because the iliac thickness is about 3 cm at this level (Benson & Jameson-Evans 1976). The osteotomy must not be allowed to hinge like a book posteriorly as this causes an *illusory* radiographic appearance of good femoral head cover Anterior femoral head support can be increased by additional bone grafting although this may restrict hip flexion.

If the osteotomy is fixed with a compression screw, the leg can be moved freely in the postoperative period, allowing the patient to return home using crutches after 1 week. Weight bearing is progressively increased over the first 2 months and the limp usually disappears or lessens by 1 year. Because the hip is effectively stabilised, pain relief is significant and lasting. There is a concurrent halt in femoral head migration, and a gratifying degree of pelvic remodelling accompanies technical success. Early complications include too low an osteotomy, with breaching of the joint, excessive or inadequate displacement, injury to adjoining nerves and vessels, and problems with wound healing. Late complications are rare, but delayed union has been reported if internal fixation is inadequate, and pelvic ligamentous pain may retard early progress. Damage to the joint may hasten ankylosis, and numbness in the distribution of the lateral femoral cutaneous nerve may be remarked upon. The osteotomy is contraindicated in the presence of arthritis (Reynolds 1986), particularly if there is significant impingement pain and stiffening. Bilateral procedures may make childbirth per vaginam hazardous, and Caesarean section is recommended.

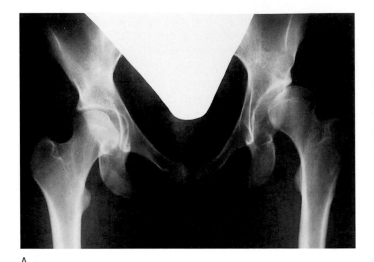

A

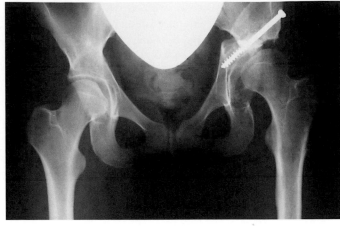

B

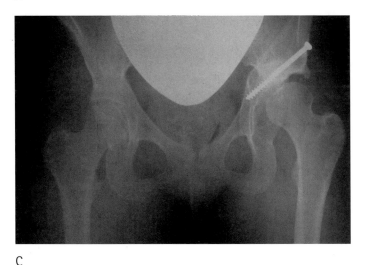

C

Figure 24.23 The Chiari osteotomy. When, as here (**A**), subluxation is marked and secondary acetabular changes are beginning to develop, the Chiari osteotomy allows medialisation of the femoral head and provides a superior bony buttress (**B** and **C**).

As with pelvic osteotomy at an earlier age, it may be appropriate to carry out a concomitant femoral realignment osteotomy, incorporating varus, valgus, rotation or extension, depending upon the resultant congruency of the joint.

In children in whom acetabular development is satisfactory but limp and pain are present, the mechanics of the hip may be improved by correcting marked degrees of femoral anteversion, by shortening the femur if there is a 'long leg dysplasia', and by distal transfer of the greater trochanter (Fig. 24.24) if the femoral neck is short and the abductor mechanism abnormal (Macnicol & Makris 1991). Although these surgical adjustments may seem small, they offer considerable improvement in function, endurance and pain relief if they allow the coaptive relationship between the femoral head and the acetabulum to improve.

OUTCOMES

Provided the hip is reducible and avascular necrosis is avoided, neonates and young infants treated promptly should develop a nearly normal hip.

Children with an irreducible hip at birth do less well. Attempts to reduce the hip neonatally may fail and lead to avascular necrosis. Teratological dislocations often present with considerable head deformity, and it is not surprising to find that long-term outcomes are less satisfactory.

Malvitz & Weinstein (1994) reviewed 152 young adults after they had been treated by closed reduction at an average age of 21 months. In 60% there was evidence of some proximal femoral growth disturbance; 43% of the treated hips were developing degenerative arthritis, and 36% were still subluxated.

Morcuende et al (1997) reviewed the Iowa experience with open reduction via a medial approach. A total of 93 hips in 76 children (average age 14 months) were followed up for 4–23 years. There was some avascular necrotic change in 43%, and 29% had residual dysplasia. The patients were too young to assess the incidence of premature arthritis.

All follow-up studies confirm that later treatment leads to poorer results because it is more difficult to achieve and maintain an excellent reduction. The acetabulum often fails to develop sufficiently, and residual subluxation almost

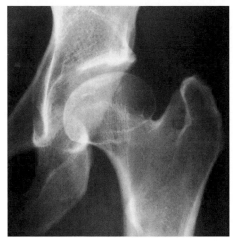

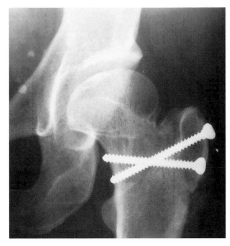

A

B

Figure 24.24 Distal transfer of greater trochanter. **A** After treatment for congenital displacement of the hip, there has been some avascular change in the head and premature closure of the proximal femoral epiphysis. There has been relative overgrowth of the greater trochanter. **B** More effective abduction has been achieved by lateral and distal transfer of the greater trochanter, here stabilised by two screws.

always becomes worse with time. Any hip that is imperfect develops premature osteoarthritis. Joint replacement becomes increasingly necessary after early adult life. It is not possible to predict outcome accurately for many years after treatment, because the subtle changes of growth disturbance in the proximal femur, especially of premature lateral growth arrest, may not appear until adolescence. It is imperative that all children treated for developmental dysplasia of the hip should be followed by serial radiographs at least until skeletal maturity, and that residual instability is recognised and treated as early as possible.

CONCLUSION

In dealing with displacement and developmental dysplasia of the hip, the overriding principle is to achieve a stable reduction of the femoral head. Treatment is therefore most effective in the neonatal period. With increasing age, there is a greater reliance upon surgery. The surgeon must be constantly alert to the dangers of pressure necrosis of the proximal femur and re-displacement. Irrevocable changes occur in the older child, particularly after failed or inadequate surgery, so that their prognosis becomes increasingly poor.

REFERENCES

Bado J L 1963 Le deviazioni dalla normal nella embriogenesi del musculo e nella patogenesis di alcune malformazione congenite. Archivo 'Putti' de Chirugie degli organi dimoviments 8: 37

Barlow T G 1962 Early diagnosis and treatment of congenital dislocation of the hip. Journal of Bone and Joint Surgery 44B: 242–301

Benson M K D, Jameson-Evans D C 1976 The pelvic osteotomy of Chiari: an anatomical study of the hazards and misleading radiological appearances. Journal of Bone and Joint Surgery 58B: 164–168

Bertol P, Macnicol M F, Mitchell G P 1982 Radiographic features of neonatal congenital dislocation of the hip. Journal of Bone and Joint Surgery 64B: 176–179

Bradley J, Weatherill M, Benson M K D 1987 Splintage for congenital dislocation of the hip. Is it safe and reliable? Journal of Bone and Joint Surgery 69B: 259–263

Carter C O, Wilkinson J 1960 Genetic and environmental factors in the etiology of congenital dislocation of the hip. Clinical Orthopaedics and Related Research 33: 119–128

Catford J C, Bennet G C, Wilkinson J A 1982 Congenital dislocation of the hip: an increasing and still uncontrolled disability? British Medical Journal 285: 1527–1530

Chiari K 1953 Beckenosteotomie zur Pfannendachplastik. Wiener Medizinische Wochenschrift 103: 707–713

Clarke N M P, Harcke H T, McHugh P, Lee M S, Borns P F, MacEwan G D 1985 Real-time ultrasound in the diagnosis of congenital dislocation and dysplasia of the hip. Journal of Bone and Joint Surgery 67B: 406

Clegg J, Bache C E, Raut VV 1999 Financial justification for routine ultrasound screening of the neonatal hip. Journal of Bone and Joint Surgery 81B: 852–857

Colonna P C 1965 Capsular arthroplasty for congenital dislocation of the hip: indications and technique. Journal of Bone and Joint Surgery 47A: 437

Dunn P M 1976 Perinatal observations on the aetiology of congenital dislocation of the hip. Clinical Orthopaedics and Related Research 119: 11

Engesaeter L B, Wilson D J, Nag D, Benson M K 1990 Ultrasound and congenital dislocation of the hip. Journal of Bone and Joint Surgery 72B: 197–200

Gibson P H, Benson M K D 1982 Congenital dislocation of the hip. Review at maturity of 147 hips treated by excision of the limbus and derotation osteotomy. Journal of Bone and Joint Surgery 64B: 169–175

Graf R 1984 Classification of hip joint dysplasia by means of sonography. Archives of Orthopaedic and Trauma Surgery 102: 248–255

Hadlow V 1988 Neonatal screening for congenital dislocation of the hip: a prospective 21-year survey. Journal of Bone and Joint Surgery 70B: 740–743

Hey-Groves E 1928 The treatment of congenital dislocation of the hip. 1928 Robert Jones Birthday Volume. Oxford University Press, Oxford

Högh J, Macnicol M F 1987 The Chiari pelvic osteotomy. A long-term review of clinical and radiographic results. Journal of Bone and Joint Surgery 69B: 365–373

Kalamchi A, MacEwan G D 1980 Avascular necrosis following treatment of congenital dislocation of the hip. Journal of Bone and Joint Surgery 62A: 876–888

Klaue K, Durnin C W, Ganz R 1991 The acetabular rim syndrome. A clinical presentation of dysplasia of the hip. British Journal of Bone and Joint Surgery 73B: 423–429

Klisic P 1976 Combined procedure of open reduction and shortening of the femur in treatment of congenital dislocation of the hip in older children. Clinical Orthopaedics and Related Research 119: 60

Le Damany P 1912 Variation en potordeur du cotyle humain aux divers ages. Bulletin Société des Sciences et Médicine d'Ouex 12: 410

Ludloff K 1913 The open reduction of congenital hip dislocation by an anterior incision. American Journal of Orthopedic Surgery 10: 438–454

MacKenzie I G, Wilson J G 1981 Problems encountered in the early diagnosis and management of congenital dislocation of the hip. Journal of Bone and Joint Surgery 63B: 38–42

McKibbin B 1970 Anatomical factors in the stability of the hip in the newborn. Journal of Bone and Joint Surgery 52B: 148–159

McNally E G, Tasker A, Benson M K 1998 MRI after operative reduction for developmental dysplasia of the hip. Journal of Bone and Joint Surgery 80: 556

Macnicol M F 1987 Congenital dislocation of the hip. In: Bennet G C (ed) Paediatric hip disorders. Blackwell, Oxford, pp 64–113

Macnicol M F 1990 Results of a 25-year screening programme for neonatal hip instability. Journal of Bone and Joint Surgery 72B: 1057–1060

Macnicol M F 1995 Color atlas and text of osteotomy of the hip. Mosby-Wolfe, London

Macnicol M F, Makris D 1991 Distal transfer of the greater trochanter. Journal of Bone and Joint Surgery 73B: 838–841

Malvitz T A, Weinstein S L 1994 Closed reduction for congenital dysplasia of the hip. Functional and radiographic results after an average of 30 years. Journal of Bone and Joint Surgery 76A: 1777–1792

Morcuende J A, Meyer M D, Dolan L A, Weinstein S L 1997 Long-term outcome after open reduction through an anteromedial approach for congenital dislocation of the hip. Journal of Bone and Joint Surgery 79A: 810–817

Morin C, Harcke H T, MacEwen G D 1985 The infant hip: real-time US assessment of acetabular development. Radiology 157: 673–677

Morscher E 1978 Our experience with Salter's innominate osteotomy in the treatment of hip dysplasia. In: Weil U H (ed.) Progress in orthopaedic surgery, vol 2. Springer, Berlin

Ortolani M 1937 Un segno poco noto e sua importanza par la diagnosi di preluzzione congenitale dell'ance. Pediatria 45: 129

Palmén K 1984 Prevention of congenital dislocation of the hip. The Swedish experience of neonatal treatment of hip joint instability. Acta Orthopaedica Scandinavica 55 (Suppl 208): 1–107

Pemberton P A 1965 Pericapsular osteotomy of the ilium for treatment of congenital subluxation and dislocation of the hip. Journal of Bone and Joint Surgery 47A: 65–86

Pozo J L, Cannon S R, Catterall A 1987 The Colonna-Hey Groves arthroplasty in the late treatment of congenital dislocation of the hip. A long-term review. Journal of Bone and Joint Surgery 69B: 220–228

Ralis Z A, McKibbin B 1973 Changes in shape of the human hip joint during its development and their relationship to its stability. Journal of Bone and Joint Surgery 55B: 780–785

Reynolds D A 1986 Chiari innominate osteotomy in adults: technique, indications and contraindications. Journal of Bone and Joint Surgery 68B: 45–54

von Rosen S 1962 Diagnosis and treatment of congenital dislocation of the hip in the new-born. Journal of Bone and Joint Surgery 44B: 284–291

Roser W 1879 Ueber angeborene Hueftverrenkung. Langenbeck's Archiv fuer klinische Chirurgie 24: 309–313

Salter R B 1961 Innominate osteotomy in the treatment of congenital dislocation and subluxation of the hip. Journal of Bone and Joint Surgery 43B: 518–539

Salter R B, Kostuik J, Dallas S 1969 Avascular necrosis of the femoral head as a complication of treatment of congenital dislocation in young children: a clinical and experimental study. Can J Surg 12: 44

Sangavi S M, Szoke G, Murray D W, Benson M K 1996 Femoral remodelling after subtrochanteric osteotomy for developmental dysplasia of the hip. Journal of Bone and Joint Surgery 78B: 917–923

Segal L S, Schneider D J, Berlin J M, Bruno A, Davis B R, Jacobs C R 1999 The contribution of the ossific nucleus to the structural stiffness of the capital femoral epiphysis: a porcine model for DDH. Journal of Pediatric Orthopaedics 19: 433–437

Severin E 1941 Contribution to the knowledge of congenital dislocation of the hip joint. Acta Chir Scandinavica 84: Supplement 63

Strayer L M 1971 The embryology of the human hip. Clinical Orthopaedics and Related Research 74: 221–240

Suzuki S, Kasahara Y, Futami T, Ushikubo S, Tsruchiya T 1991 Ultrasonography in congenital dislocation of the hip. Simultaneous imaging of both hips from in front. Journal of Bone and Joint Surgery 73B: 879–83

Tonnis D 1986 Congenital dysplasia and dislocation of the hip. Springer, Berlin

Trueta J 1957 The normal vascular anatomy of the human femoral head during growth. Journal of Bone and Joint Surgery 39B: 358–394

Watanabe R S 1974 Embryology of the human hip. Clinical Orthopaedics and Related Research 98: 8–26

Weinstein S L, Ponseti I V 1979 Congenital dislocation of the hip. Open reduction through a medial approach. Journal of Bone and Joint Surgery 61A: 119–124

Wiberg C 1939 Studies on dyplastic acetabulae and congenital subluxation of the hip joint. Acta Chirurgica Scandinavica Suppl 58

Wilkinson J A 1963 Prime factors in the aetiology of congenital dislocation of the hip. Journal of Bone and Joint Surgery 45B: 268–283

Williamson D M, Benson M K D 1988 Late femoral osteotomy in congenital dislocation of the hip. Journal of Bone and Joint Surgery 70B: 614–618

Wynne-Davies R W 1970 Acetabular dysplasia and familial joint laxity: two aetiological factors in congenital dislocation of the hip. A review of 589 patients and their families. Journal of Bone and Joint Surgery 52B: 704–716

Chapter 25

Legg–Calvé–Perthes' disease

A. Catterall

INTRODUCTION

The intitial descriptions of Legg–Calvé–Perthes' disease were made in 1910 by Legg in Boston, Perthes in Germany and Calvé in France. Despite an ever enlarging literature, its cause remains unclear and treatment for the most part empirical. The early sections of this chapter outline the aetiology, morbid anatomy and natural history. The later sections will develop a scheme of management for the care of the child with Perthes' disease.

AETIOLOGY

The incidence of Perthes' disease varies (Barker et al 1978, Hall et al 1983, Barker & Hall 1986, Hall & Barker 1989). It affects approximately 1 in 9000 children (1 in 8000 boys and 1 in 30 000 girls), 80% of whom are between the ages of 4 and 9 years at the onset of the disease (Table 25.1). The cause is unknown. A working hypothesis for further investigation of the aetiology (Catterall 1982) suggests that "in the susceptible child, the radiological changes which are called Perthes' disease are the consequence of epiphyseal infarction of variable extent, complicated by trabecular fracture and associated with a process of repair. This growth disturbance, if uncontrolled, leads to femoral head deformity and subsequent arthritis." This suggests that there are four aspects to the aetiology and pathology of this condition, namely a susceptible child, recurrent infarction associated with trabecular fracture, a process of repair resulting in a growth disturbance, and subsequent femoral head deformity. Hall's group (Hall et al 1979, Hall 1987), in an extensive review of the aetiology, have shown that the susceptible child is usually a boy between the ages of 4 and 9 years, who comes

Table 25.1 Incidence of Perthes' disease in relation to age and Catterall group†

	Age (months)	Sex ratio (male:female)
All cases	72	3.67:1
Group I	60	14:1
Group II	75	3.7:1
Group III	80	2.5:1
Group IV	59	2.9:1

†The Catterall groups are defined later in this chapter (see also Table 25.4, and Figs 25.2 and 25.3).

from a family of social class 4 or 5. The child is often of short stature, with delayed bone age (Harrison et al 1976); the short stature is disproportionate, with the shortening involving the distal limb segments, but not the spine and pelvis (Burwell et al 1978, 1986). This may explain the delayed bone age noted on X-rays of the wrists and hands.

Recurrent infarction has been suggested by several authors (McKibbin & Ralis 1974, Inoue et al 1976, Catterall et al 1982 a, b). Evidence that this may happen before the condition becomes established is seen in bone scans that show no uptake in the opposite uninvolved hip of a unilateral case. Further scanning reveals that this subsequently recovers, without later evidence of progressive changes. Experimental evidence (Freeman & England 1969, Inoue et al 1976, Calvert et al 1984) has shown that, after interruption of the blood flow the femoral head may show complete recovery in a period of 4–6 weeks, with no radiological stigmata of infarction. The cause of the recurrent infarction has yet to be established.

In 1996, Glueck et al published evidence that there was an abnormality in a number of clotting factors, in particular protein S and protein C, and that these changes could result in thrombophilia, with its increased risk of coagulopathy. More recently, this concept has been challenged in the light of more critical review of the data (Hayek et al 1999, Liesner 1999, Thomas et al 1999). It may be that this is further evidence for a 'susceptible child', rather than the cause of the recurrent infarction.

The trabecular fracture is the incident that dictates that progressive changes will occur. This fracture in avascular bone will not unite until the bone is revascularised. It is this repair process that results in the growth disturbance that is recognised by typical radiological changes. It must be appreciated, therefore, that the changes observed radiologically are a consequence of this repair process and growth disturbance, but do not identify the cause of the condition. The onset of the disease probably occurs some weeks or months before the radiological changes become evident.

MORBID ANATOMY

THE INITIAL STATE OF THE EPIPHYSIS

The architecture of the femoral head varies with age, and hence the changes associated with Perthes' disease develop against a background of changing anatomy. In the younger child, the bony epiphysis is small and much of the femoral head is cartilaginous. In addition, children with Perthes' disease have delayed bone age, which reduces the size of the ossified epiphysis within the femoral head. In contrast, in the older child, the major portion of the femoral head is bone, and trabecular fracture will produce an early and rapid loss of epiphyseal height. In the younger child with a longer period of growth, the repair process after infarction results in a growth disturbance in cartilage, leading to coxa magna.

ESTABLISHED CONDITION

Early stages

The paucity of pathological material has permitted very few accounts of the pathology of this disease, and fewer still in which the sequential changes observed radiologically have been correlated with the morphology. In the early stages after infarction there is overgrowth of the articular cartilage, particularly on the medial and lateral side of the femoral head, resulting in coxa magna (Table 25.2). Infarction is present within the bony epiphysis and there is

Table 25.2 Pathology: early stages

	Phases of onset and sclerosis
Articular cartilage	Thickening of the articular cartilage on both sides of the joint
Acetabulum	Loss of normal lateral curvature because of change in contract shape of the lateral aspect of the femoral head
Femoral head	Overgrowth more pronounced on the lateral side of the femoral head
Bony epiphysis	Variable degree of infarction, with trabecular fracture in subchondral area of the dome of the epiphysis producing loss of epiphyseal height Group I: No infarct Group II and III: Incomplete infarction, greater in group III than II Group IV: Repeated total infarction. Density on radiographs is due to calcification of the necrotic marrow
Growth plate and metaphysis	Distortion of normal columns of cells Excess calcified cartilage in primary spongiosa Formation of localised metaphyseal cysts from unossified columns of cells
Conclusion	There is growth disturbance in cartilage associated with loss of epiphyseal height caused by trabecular fracture. This changes the shape of the femoral head from round to oval or flat, depending on the amount of bone infarcted

an early loss of epiphyseal height as a result of trabecular fracture. The amount of infarction is variable, being absent in Catterall group I disease in which there is only a growth disturbance, and total in Catterall group IV. During this stage of sclerosis (Waldenström 1938), the density noted on fine detail radiography is due partly to the trabecular fracture and appositional new bone formation, but mainly to calcification of the necrotic marrow. The growth plate is also abnormal, with distortion of the cell columns and an increase in the quantity of calcified cartilage in the primary spongiosa.

Intermediate stages

Once the infarction has occurred, a process of repair becomes established to revascularise the intact avascular trabeculae by 'creeping substitution'. Loose necrotic bone in the femoral head is removed and replaced by fibrocartilage (Table 25.3). This repair process produces the appearances of fragmentation. In the thickened articular cartilage, repair is by endochondral ossification, occurring as a natural growth process from the subchondral bone plate of the viable portion of the epiphysis and as islands of new bone formation in the thickened anterior and lateral cartilage. These areas gradually enlarge and then fuse with the bony epiphysis. Radiologically, in the early stages these small islands appear as areas of calcification lateral to the epiphysis. In the growth plate, areas of unossified cartilage are seen streaming down from the growth plate into the metaphyseal region, producing a metaphyseal cyst. Where these are large, the normal architecture of the growth plate is lost, and as a result no further growth takes place in this part of the femoral neck. Because the lesions are usually anterior and lateral, this causes a growth disturbance, with the femoral head tilting forwards on the neck.

Healing and late phases

In the healing phase of Perthes' disease (Table 25.3) most of the loose necrotic trabeculae will have been removed and the fibrocartilage so formed is progressively re-ossified, with the establishment of a new subchondral bone plate. The last portion to reform is the anterosuperior portion of the epiphysis, and hence the pathological process will have converted an initially round head to one that is oval in shape, particularly on its anterior and lateral aspects.

THE PROCESS OF FEMORAL HEAD DEFORMITY

The preceding descriptions have suggested that, in the early phases of this disease, there is a change of head shape as a result of overgrowth of the articular cartilage and loss of epiphyseal height after trabecular fracture. This leads the femoral head to change shape from round to oval. It does not, however, account for the severe deformity that develops in some hips. In the older child there is an early and often serious loss of epiphyseal height as a result of the trabecular fracture. In this situation, a true subluxation can occur, with

Table 25.3 Pathology: intermediate and late stages

	Phases of fragmentation and healing
Articular cartilage Acetabulum	Persisting deformity in cartilage, particularly laterally, with delay in ossification resulting in a secondary acetabular dysplasia, particularly if there is uncovering of the femoral head
Femoral head	Persisting overgrowth beyond the confines of the bony acetabulum. Repair occurs by islands of endochondral ossification forming in the thickened articular cartilage laterally (calcification lateral to the epiphysis), and from the surface of viable bone medially. A 'dent' may be present on the anterolateral aspect if serious uncovering is present
Bony epiphysis	Repair proportional to trabecular structure. Trabeculae intact: creeping substitution Trabeculae fractured: removal and replacement by fibrocartilage (These appearances account for the radiological features of fragmentations)
Growth plate and metaphysis	Progressive disorganisation of growth plate architecture in areas of previous metaphyseal lesion. This leads to differential rates of growth between the anterior and posterior aspects of the femoral neck. (This produces a tilt deformity of the femoral head on the femoral neck)

an upward and lateral movement of the femoral head so that it displaces partly from the acetabulum. This uncovering is further exacerbated by overgrowth of the anterolateral aspect of the femoral head in cartilage.

In the long term, it is important to realise that two types of end result may be encountered; where the femoral head is round or oval, a 'ball and socket' type of joint will persist; where progressive flattening of the femoral head occurs, a 'roller bearing' shape will evolve, referred to by Stulberg et al (1981) as 'aspherical incongruity'. In the roller bearing joint, clinical examination will show that the leg appears to be short because of postural or fixed adduction. The plane of movement is in flexion and extension only, with almost no rotation. As the leg flexes, it moves into abduction rather then the normal neutral plane, the varus deformity of the neck accounting for this change in axis as the hip flexes. The sign of 'flexion with abduction' is seen early in hips in which serious femoral head deformity is occurring. It is one of the earliest signs, therefore, of the 'head at risk'.

Once the growth disturbance becomes associated with an abnormal rhythm of movement, the lateral aspect of the femoral head becomes uncovered by the bony acetabulum. Attempted abduction in these circumstances will produce lateral impingement, resulting in a dent on the superior and lateral surface of the femoral head. Clinically and arthrographically, it is observed that abduction is progressively lost in the early phases of the disease and pure rotation alters to rotation with hinging at the lateral aspect of the bony acetabulum. As overgrowth continues, the head impinges further against the lateral edge of the acetabulum, the subluxation becomes fixed, and a roller bearing joint is the inevitable sequel. This process is called 'hinge abduction' (Fig. 25.1) (Grossbard 1981, Quain & Catterall 1986).

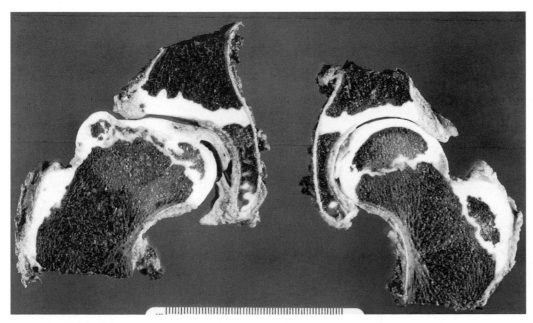

Figure 25.1 Photograph of transverse slab sections taken through the centre of the femoral heads in a child of 8 years who died from lymphocytic lymphoma but was also known to have Perthes' disease. On the involved side there is obvious femoral head deformity, with impingement between the lateral aspect of the acetabulum and the femoral head, producing a dent. On the opposite, normal side there is abnormal thickening of the articular cartilage, particularly on the medial and lateral aspects. (Reproduced from Catterall et al 1982b Perthes' disease: is the epiphysial infarction complete? Journal of Bone and Joint Surgery 64B: 276–281.)

CLINICAL RECOGNITION OF PROGRESSIVE DEFORMITY OF THE FEMORAL HEAD

THE 'HEAD AT RISK'

Clinical recognition of the early stages of progressive deformity of the femoral head is important. If treatment is to be effective, it should be started as early as possible in these patients. The concept of the 'head at risk' was introduced to identify affected patients (Catterall 1971). The preceding discussion has suggested a number of clinical and radiological signs that identify children in whom serious deformity may occur (Table 25.4). The clinical signs reflect the progressive loss of movement, particularly abduction, and the change in the axis of flexion as the femoral head begins to flatten.

The radiological signs depict changes in both the epiphysis and metaphysis (Fig. 25.2). The epiphyseal signs are Gage's sign – a lytic area on the lateral aspect of the epiphysis and adjacent metaphysis – and calcification lateral to the epiphysis. This suggests overgrowth of the articular cartilage laterally. The metaphyseal signs reflect the growth disturbance present within the femoral neck and the tilt of the femoral head on the neck that occurs with time. The horizontal growth plate is seen when the femoral head lies in abduction and external rotation, and is another early sign of the roller bearing joint. In a review of the value of these signs, it has been shown that the presence of two or more adversely affects the prognosis in untreated cases (Catterall 1971, 1981, 1982). Widening of the medial joint 'space' also reflects the increasing deformity of the cartilaginous femoral head.

CATTERALL GROUPING

The Catterall groups (Fig. 25.3) correspond to the extent of infarction present within the epiphysis on radiology (Catterall et al 1982 a,b). Good-quality anteroposterior and lateral radiography, taken if necessary after movement has been restored to the hip, are essential. The clinician attempts to ascertain the extent of the infarction using a number of observable radiological signs in the epiphysis and metaphysis (Tables 25.5 and 25.6).

FACTORS INFLUENCING THE NATURAL HISTORY OF THE DISEASE

In a disease in which approximately 60% of children do well without treatment, is it important to identify those factors associated with the 40% who are likely to do badly and in whom treatment is required (Table 25.7; Catterall 1971). It has been accepted for many years that there are a number of factors that the clinician may find useful in the assessment, some of which he may be able to influence, but most of which he cannot. These may be subdivided into *short-term* and *long-term factors*:

Table 25.4 Signs of the 'head at risk'	
Clinical	Progressive loss of movement
	Adduction contracture
	Flexion with abduction
	The heavy child
Radiogical	Gage's sign
	Calcification lateral to the epiphysis
	A diffuse metaphyseal reaction
	Lateral subluxation
	Horizontal growth plate

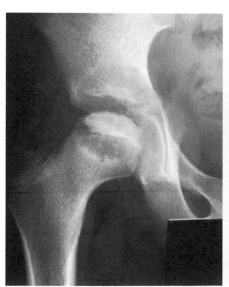

A

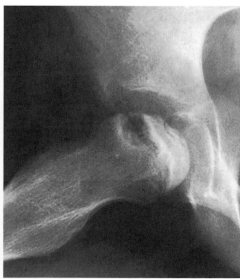

B

Fig. 25.2 Example of 'head at risk'. Radiographs of a child of 6 years with Perthes' disease of 6 months duration. The anteroposterior X-ray (A) shows a horizontal growth plate with a large metaphyseal lesion, which is seen to be anterior on the lateral view (B). There is a small amount of calcification lateral to the epiphysis and widening of the inferomedial joint space. The alteration in shape of the obturator foramen suggests that there is a flexion deformity present. The lateral X-ray confirms a large anterior metaphyseal lesion and the subchondral fracture line passing from the anterior margin into the posterior third of the epiphysis. This is a group III case, with radiological signs of the 'head at risk'.

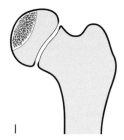
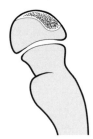
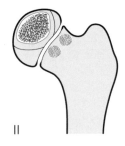
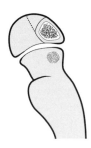
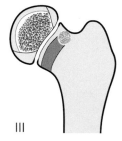
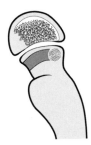
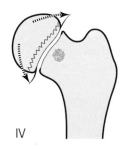
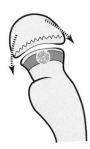

Figure 25.3 Diagrammatic representation of Catterall groups I–IV, which are classified according to radiographic features of the epiphysis and metaphysis (Tables 25.5 and 25.6).

Table 25.5 Epiphyseal signs				
	Group			
Radiological signs	I	II	III	IV
Sclerosis	No	Yes	Yes	Yes
Subchondral fracture line	No	Anterior half	Posterior half	Complete
Junction involved	Clear	Clear	Sclerotic	No
Uninvolved segments		Often 'V'		
Viable bone at growth	Anterior margin	Anterior half	Posterior half	None
Triangular appearance to medial/lateral aspects	No	No	Occasional	Yes

- Short-term prognosis
  - Age and sex
  - Stage of disease at diagnosis
  - Catterall group
  - Signs of the 'head at risk'
  - Restriction of movement

- Long-term prognosis
  - Favourable
    age at time of healing
  - Unfavourable
    persistent lateral uncovering of the femoral head
    a deformed femoral head
    premature closure of the growth plate
    limited abduction

These are considered in more detail below:

Table 25.6 Metaphyseal signs				
	Group			
Radiological signs	I	II	III	IV
Localized	No	Anterior	Anterior	Anterior or central
Diffuse	No	Yes	Yes	Yes
Posterior remodelling	No	No	No	Yes

Table 25.7 Results in untreated patients			
	Good	Fair	Poor
Group I	27	1	0
Group II	23	6	2
Group III	4	7	11
Group IV	0	4	10
Total	54 (57%)	18 (19%)	23 (24%)

SHORT-TERM FACTORS

Age and sex

The prognosis for the younger child is better than for the older, and is more favourable in boys than girls. This is not true in every case, particularly in some of the younger group IV patients in whom a poor result may ensue even with adequate treatment (Snyder 1975). The less favourable prognosis for girls is due to the fact that they have a more severe form of the disease. Over the age of 8 years, rapid deterioration in head shape may occur as a result of trabecular fracture, and early treatment should be considered.

Stage of the disease at diagnosis

It is accepted that the earlier in the disease process treatment is started, the better the prognosis because less deformity has occurred. It must also be added that, once healing has been established radiologically, there will be no further deterioration in the shape of the femoral head (Thompson & Westin 1979). The signs of healing are an increase in the height and size of viable bone on the medial side of the epiphysis and the height and quality of new bone formed laterally. Treatment is indicated at this stage of the disease only if it can be shown to improve congruity of the femoral head. Arthrography is essential to prove this point.

Catterall grouping

The prognosis for an individual case is proportional to the degree of radiological involvement of the epiphysis; this forms the basis of the four groups defined by Catterall (1971). The results at maturity of a series of untreated patients, related to their Catterall grouping, were shown in Table 25.7. The most important observations are that 57% do well without any treatment, and that those in groups I and II fare best.

The Herring classification

In 1992 Herring et al introduced a further classification of Perthes' disease, based on the height and quality of the lateral segment of the bony epiphysis (Fig. 25.4). In group A,

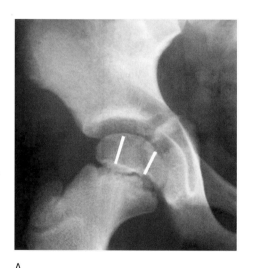

A

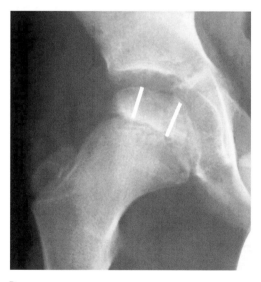

B

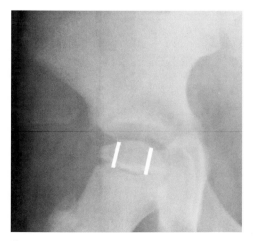

C

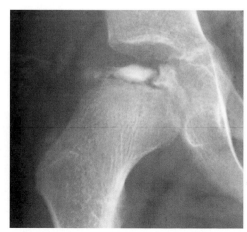

D

Figure 25.4 The Herring classification. **A** Radiograph showing the femoral epiphysis divided into lateral, central and medial segments. **B** Herring group A, with no involvement of the lateral segment. **C** Herring group B, with less than 50% loss of height of the lateral segment. **D** Herring group C, with more than 50% loss of height of the lateral segment. (Reproduced with permission, from Ismail & Macnicol 1998.)

the height of the lateral segment is maintained; in group B, the lateral segment is half its normal height, and in group C its structure is lost. The prognosis deteriorates with increasing involvement of the lateral segment. This classification has the advantage that it requires only a single anteroposterior radiograph, but the classification may change if the results are assessed during the 'early' or 'healing' phases of the disease process. Reports using this classification suggest that the most useful time to apply this method is during the 'fragmentation' phase of the disease (Farsetti et al 1995). It may be less useful, therefore, in the very early stages of the disease. It is another aid to management and should influence the surgeon's selection of definitive treatment, in association with other clinical and radiological considerations.

Signs of the 'head at risk'

These have already been discussed with reference to progressive deformity in the femoral head (Table 25.4). The author considers that the presence of two or more of these radiological signs, together with the clinical sign of flexion with abduction, should be regarded as an absolute indication for treatment.

THE LONG-TERM PROGNOSIS

There are still relatively few good reports of the long-term consequences of this disease, but their conclusions are clear: 86% of patients will develop osteoarthritis by the age of 65 years but in the majority symptoms will not become a problem until the fifth or sixth decade (Mose et al 1977, McAndrew & Weinstein 1984); 30% of patients will improve after healing of the disease, but a small proportion will deteriorate. Nine per cent will require reconstructive surgery by the age of 35 years (Catterall 1986). A further review of the cases from Iowa City (McAndrew & Weinstein 1984) has shown that 45% will require a hip replacement by the age of 45 years. All the patients in that series had been treated on an abduction frame, unlike those in the Mose series who had been treated by bed rest, traction or were, in fact, untreated.

The child who is likely to develop symptoms of early osteoarthritis has disease of late onset – usually after the age of 9 years – which results in an irregular, uncovered femoral head (aspherical incongruity). There is often a premature growth plate arrest and a reduced range of movement. Some hips have an oval femoral head deformity that allows congruity between the femoral head and acetabulum with the leg in the neutral weight-bearing position. This has been called 'congruous incongruity' by Burr Curtis and 'aspherical congruity' by Stulberg et al (1981). Such hips do not deteriorate quickly in the long term. It follows from this observation that, where femoral head deformity is present, the aim of treatment should be to realign the leg so that there is maximum contact between the femoral head and acetabulum with the leg in the neutral position. Abduction of more than 20° without hinging is required to prevent the development of secondary acetabular dysplasia.

It will be appreciated that there are only a few factors in this preceding discussion that the clinician is in a position to control. The age, sex and group are already decided by the time the patient presents. Public education and awareness of early symptoms can encourage early presentation and, when necessary, treatment. Clinical recognition of the child with a poor prognosis as a result of the concept of the 'head at risk' may also provide a better opportunity for effective treatment.

INDICATIONS FOR AND PRINCIPLES OF TREATMENT

Because of the benign natural history of Perthes' disease, it is important to have indications for treatment so that unnecessary therapy can be avoided in these patients. In terms of the described pathology and the short- and long-term prognostic factors, the indications and contraindications for treatment are set out in Tables 25.8 and 25.9. Conservative treatment in which the child is allowed to be free of any restrictive therapy will be indicated if the growth disturbance is mild or if it has already occurred in patients presenting late in the disease. Definitive treatment will be required if the growth disturbance is likely to be severe (all 'head at risk' cases and the older child) or if deformity in the late stages is associated with pain and the phenomenon of hinge abduction.

A knowledge of the natural history and morbid anatomical changes allows us to define four objectives in treatment:

1. To restore and maintain free movement.
2. To reduce abnormal forces through the hip.
3. To correct or prevent subluxation.
4. To accelerate revascularisation of necrotic bone and union of the subchondral fracture.

Normal movement is required to prevent progressive deformity of the femoral head and to encourage remodelling.

Table 25.8 Indications for conservative treatment

Early stages	Group I patients Group II; group III not 'head at risk'
Late stages	Patients in whom healing is established Patients in whom serious femoral head deformity is present without 'hinge abduction'

Table 25.9 Indications for definitive treatment

Early stages	All 'head at risk' patients Group II; group III older than 7 years Group IV patients in whom serious deformity has not occurred
Late stages	Hinge abduction

Abduction of the leg has two effects on the hip: first, to reduce the forces through the joint (Heikkinen & Puranen 1980), and second, to reposition the uncovered anterolateral aspect of the femoral head within the remodelling influence of the acetabulum. This reduction of forces through the joint should promote revascularisation of the infarcted bone and the re-establishment of normal growth. In addition, removing the abnormal forces from the lateral cartilaginous aspect of the acetabulum will allow it to resume a more normal appearance with growth. Where the volume of

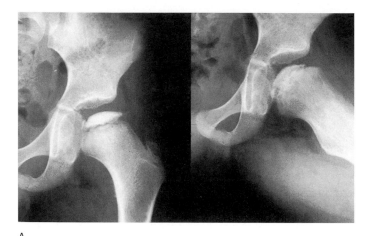

A

27 JUL 73

B

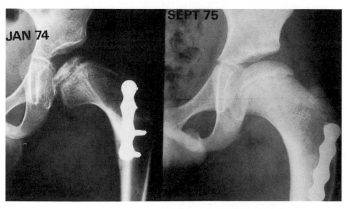

JAN 74   SEPT 75

C

necrotic bone is large, as in the older child, a period of immobilisation may be required to allow revascularisation and prevent further trabecular fracture and therefore collapse of the femoral head. Subluxation, which is a major problem in the older child, must be prevented or corrected. Its persistence will lead to progressive loss of movement and a fixed flexion and adduction deformity of the hip.

When these principles are applied in the early and late stages of the disease, different methods of treatment should be used. In the early stages, where the predominant pathology is cartilage overgrowth, restoration of movement with the femoral head repositioned or contained within the acetabulum should be the method of choice (Fig. 25.5). In the later stages, when serious deformity of the femoral head has occurred or healing is already established, restoration of movement with the joint congruous in the neutral position of weight bearing should allow the best long-term remodeling and prevent the long-term effects of hinge abduction.

MANAGEMENT

The flow chart shown in Fig. 25.6 outlines a scheme of management. This initially may appear rather complex but, if followed through, should answer the clinician's questions stage by stage as he attempts to chart a course through the management of this difficult and often contentious condition.

THE STAGE OF DIAGNOSIS

Children present to the doctor either with symptoms suggestive of hip disease or because their parents become concerned by the persistence of a limp. The symptoms are often chronic, with pain felt in the groin, hip or knee and a limp of variable severity. Some patients present with acute symptoms or with an 'irritable' hip that fails to settle satisfactorily in a short period of time. Radiographs taken at this time are nearly always abnormal; if, however, they are

Figure 25.5 Radiographs of a child aged 5 years with Catterall group IV Perthes' disease treated by femoral osteotomy. **A** July 1973: anteroposterior and lateral radiographs of the left hip. There are changes involving the entire epiphysis, typical of group IV disease. On the lateral view, there is beaking of the posterior metaphysis. There is lateral uncovering of the femoral head and a horizontal growth plate. **B** Radiographs taken at the time of arthrography. The neutral view shows considerable uncovering and flattening of the cartilaginous portion of the femoral head, particularly of its lateral cartilaginous aspect. The position of abduction and internal rotation shows containment of the femoral head within the mould of the acetabulum. **C** Radiographs taken in January 1974 and September 1975. These show that the containment of the femoral head after femoral osteotomy has been maintained. The final result is very satisfactory, with good remodelling of the femoral neck angle.

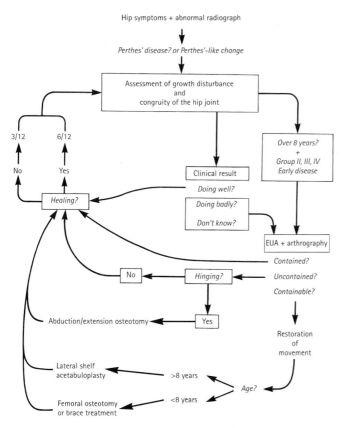

Figure 25.6 Flow chart showing scheme of management of Perthes' disease. EUA, examination under anaesthesia.

changes. The earliest radiological signs are a small epiphysis showing increased density, a subchondral fracture line that is often better seen in the frog lateral view, and widening of the inferomedial joint space. If there is doubt about a case at an early stage, either a bone scan (Tachdjian 1980, Paterson & Savage 1986) or magnetic resonance imaging (MRI) should be undertaken.

ASSESSMENT OF THE GROWTH DISTURBANCE AND CONGRUITY OF THE JOINT

As there is no preventive treatment available, it is helpful to assess the child at each visit to decide whether he or she is 'doing well' or 'doing badly'. Between these two extremes there are patients in whom there is clinical doubt – 'don't know'; such children require further investigation. The assessment must initially be clinical, supported by radiological examination where appropriate (Table 25.10). At each assessment, the stage of the disease must be recognised. Containment treatment will not help, and is contraindicated once healing is established, unless the congruity of the joint can be shown to be improved by a change in position.

Early disease in the older child, for reasons that have already been discussed, demands separate and early arthrographic assessment, because rapid deterioration in the shape of the femoral head may occur in these children. It must also be appreciated that some continuing intermittent discomfort is present during the active phase of the disease in children who are simply being followed conservatively without treatment. Recurrent acute symptoms or increasing discomfort, however, may suggest deterioration. The parents must understand the natural history of the process, and careful explanation and discussion are essential if they are to understand the management and accept the continuing intermittent discomfort their child may suffer during the period of observation.

CLINICAL EXAMINATION

As the child lies on the bed, the position and relative lengths of the legs should be noted. Many patients have a few degrees of fixed flexion, but fixed adduction or external rotation implies that femoral head deformity is present. As

normal, a bone scan is often diagnostic, and shows a characteristic failure of uptake of the isotope in the epiphysis. The possible differential diagnoses must always be considered. If the signs are unilateral, the late sequelae of septic arthritis, growth disturbance after treatment for developmental dysplasia of the hip, sickle-cell disease, lymphoma and Gaucher's disease must be considered. If the changes are bilateral, hypothyroidism, multiple epiphyseal dysplasia and spondyloepiphyseal dysplasia should always be considered. In bilateral disease it is rare for Perthes' disease to have identical appearances on both sides, whereas symmetry is commonly seen in the other causes of bilateral Perthes'-like

Table 25.10 Clinical assessment			
	'Doing well'	'Doing badly'	'Don't know'
Clinical			
Leg length	Equal	Short	?Short
Fixed deformity	Nil	Adduction/flexion	Flexion
Movement	Abduction >20°	Abduction <5°	Abduction <10°
	Flexion in neutral	'Flexion with abduction'	Flexion (? neutral)
Radiological			
Stage of disease	All stages	Active stages	All stages
Group	All	II, III, IV	II, III, IV
Signs 'head at risk'	Absent	Present	Present

the hip is moved into flexion, it should do so in the neutral position. The normal hip has approximately 20–30° adduction with the hip flexed, but this is always reduced in children with Perthes' disease. The sign of 'flexion with abduction' implies femoral head deformity. The range of abduction is now assessed, care being taken to identify the position of the pelvis as the leg is moved. It is seldom that full abduction is present during the active stages of the disease. However, if 20° of abduction in extension is maintained, the result is likely to be satisfactory.

GAIT

In all phases of the disease, the child will limp. There is a short stride on the involved side, suggesting discomfort and stiffness. The Trendelenburg test is commonly positive.

RADIOLOGICAL EXAMINATION

The importance of good-quality radiographs cannot be overestimated. If necessary, these should be taken after a period of rest. An anteroposterior pelvic radiograph including both hips should be taken with the patellae in the neutral position, and a lateral one with the legs in approximately 60° of abduction and flexion (frog lateral). If the radiograph is difficult to interpret, the hips should be screened in various positions of abduction and flexion until a clear lateral view is obtained, and this position recorded. Using this technique, it is often easy to identify the extent of the subchondral fracture line (Salter & Thompson 1984) and the amount of the femoral epiphysis involved in the infarct. The clinician should ask several questions:

1. Is the disease in the early, established or healing stage?
2. Can the extent of the radiological involvement be identified and hence the group established?
3. Is there evidence of fixed deformity?
4. Are signs of the 'head at risk' present?

Femoral head deformity is suggested by the presence of pelvic obliquity, a change in the shape of the obturator foramen, or the appearance or prominence of the ischial spine by comparison with the opposite side. If any of these signs are present and clinical examination has not demonstrated fixed deformity, re-examination of the patient is required. At the end of this assessment, the clinician should be able to decide whether the patient can be described as 'doing well', 'doing badly' or 'don't know' (Table 25.10).

OTHER INVESTIGATIONS

Magnetic resonance imaging

MRI, which is an expensive and time-consuming investigation, is often used in the assessment of these children. Its value as an investigation is difficult to define. As with many scanning techniques, it gives information on a 'slice' of tissue, hence both bone and cartilage can be visualised. It must be realised that, particularly in the late stages of the disease process, there is a three-dimensional change in the shape of the femoral head. Slices that may be vertical in one part of the femoral head and tangential in another cannot easily represent this. In addition, none of the present scanning techniques are real-time and they cannot provide the quality of information obtained by the 'dynamic arthrogram'. MRI can, however, be of great help in recognising avascular necrosis before radiological signs become apparent. It will also confirm, to some extent, the degree of anterolateral deformity. Until its images become real-time and more clear, it is the author's view that MRI remains an expensive investigation that rarely adds to the management of Perthes' disease (Fig. 25.7).

Bone scanning

Technetium polyphosphate bone scans do have a more defined place in management. In the early stages, a 'cold scan' showing no uptake in the epiphysis is diagnostic of early Perthes' disease (Fig. 25.7A). Conway (1993) has undertaken sequential scans in patients with Perthes' disease. In the benign form, there is early revascularisation of the lateral aspect of the epiphysis, whereas in the more aggressive form the lateral column fails to revascularise. This information can be very helpful in an individual patient, to decide whether definitive treatment will be required.

The dynamic arthrogram

If the patient is 'doing badly' or the conclusion after assessment is 'don't know', further investigation by examination of the hip under anaesthesia, screening and arthrograms are required. A dynamic arthrogram is performed: radio-opaque contrast is injected into the joint and the movements of the hip are carefully screened under the image intensifier. This demonstrates not only the cartilaginous shape of the femoral head, but also the way the hip moves and whether unstable movement is present. In the majority of patients examined under anaesthesia, no fixed deformity is present and there is an increased range of both abduction and flexion, suggesting that muscle spasm has limited the movement. This can be treated by simple passive stretching using a broomstick plaster, rather than by soft-tissue release. As the hip is moved, changes in congruity are noted and the position of 'best fit' identified. This movement is ideally recorded on a video and static radiographs then taken to confirm the position. This assessment differentiates the hip that is contained from one that is containable, in which an uncovered femoral head will centre within the acetabulum in abduction, internal rotation and flexion. Finally, there is the uncontainable hip, which hinges on abduction (Fig. 25.8). The stable position for this type of hip is in flexion and adduction. The optimal position must be carefully identified, as it represents the size of the abduction and extension wedge, which must be removed at operation. The contained hip may be observed, whereas the remainder merit active treatment.

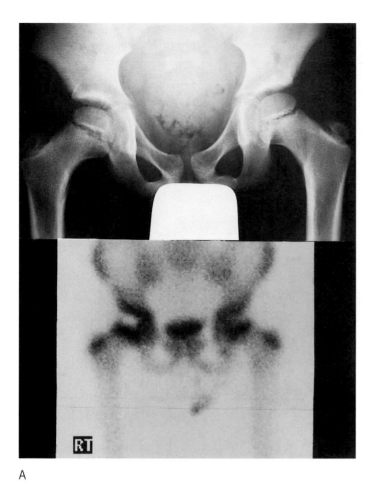

A

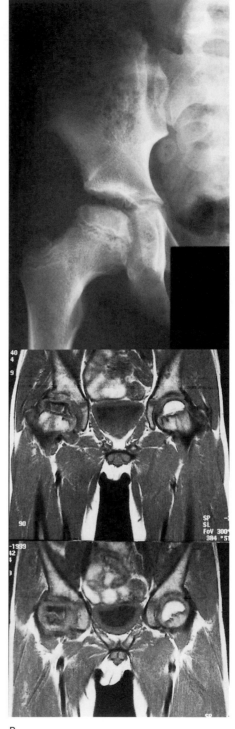

B

Figure 25.7 Radiographs of a child aged 9 years 10 months who presented initially with an irritable right hip. **A** Radiograph and bone scan at presentation. The radiographs were reported as normal, but do show and increase in the inferomedial joint space. The bone scan shows a characteristic lack of uptake of isotope in the upper femoral epiphysis. This is very suggestive of early Perthes' disease. **B** Radiographs and MRI taken 6 months after initial presentation. The X-ray appearances are at the stage of late sclerosis. The MRI taken at this time shows the central area of sclerosis that is also clearly seen on the plain radiographs.

TREATMENT

If a child is 'doing well', no definitive treatment is required, but follow-up is necessary. The frequency of this depends on the stage of the disease. During the early active stage, initial re-assessment at 2 months and subsequently at 3-monthly intervals is required. Care should be taken in the older child, because rapid deterioration can occur in this early stage of the disease. When healing is established, follow-up can be at 6–12-month intervals, to monitor the remodelling of the hip and to check that the range of abduction is preserved. If abduction is restricted, a secondary acetabular dysplasia may occur, which can prejudice the long-term results.

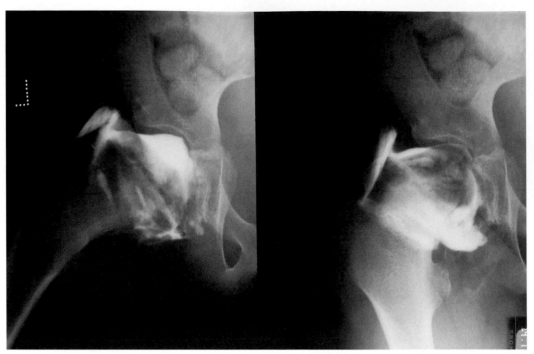

Figure 25.8 Hinge abduction. Appearances on a dynamic arthrogram of typical hinge abduction in a child of 10 years who presented 2 years from the onset of her disease with pain, shortening and limp. The position of best fit or congruency is in adduction and flexion. It was this position that was selected for the subsequent valgus extension femoral osteotomy. (Reproduced from Quain S, Catterall A 1986 Hinge abduction of the hip. Diagnosis and treatment. Journal of Bone and Joint Surgery 68B: 61–64.)

THE CONTAINABLE HIP

Arthrography performed during the early and active phases of the disease has shown that, if the hip is containable, definitive treatment should be considered. The majority of these hips have restricted movement and it is important that movement is restored in order to demonstrate that movement can be maintained with the hip in the 'best-fit' position. This can be undertaken using an adjustable broomstick plaster. In this technique, cylinder plasters are applied to the legs with the knees 30° flexed and a bar is then applied between the cylinders to hold the involved hips in maximum abduction. The child is encouraged to move. The next day, increased abduction is possible and the bar can be adjusted accordingly, both for abduction and for internal rotation. At the end of approximately 2–3 weeks, the desired position of abduction and rotation will have been achieved, with the child moving freely in bed or a wheelchair, but not allowed to stand. Failure to achieve mobility in the contained or best-fit position requires a complete reassessment of management. It is a contraindication to realignment surgery by femoral or innominate osteotomy.

Definitive treatment

The clinician is now faced with the dilemma as to whether the contained position should be maintained by operation or conservative treatment with splintage. In an important review, Wenger et al (1991) concluded that the less complicated and cumbersome braces such as the Scottish Rite orthosis cannot maintain abduction in older children who have more severely affected hips, because hip rotation cannot be controlled with an above-knee brace. This has been

supported in other reports (Martinez et al 1992, Meehan et al 1992). If non-operative treatment is selected for these patients, a long abduction brace is necessary; however, compliance is difficult to obtain. In the younger child up to the age of 6 years who requires definitive treatment, the results of femoral osteotomy or containment braces are almost identical (Curtis et al 1974, Canario et al 1980, Harrison et al 1982, Muirhead-Allwood & Catterall 1982, Coates et al 1990). Hence either can be advised. The advantages and disadvantages of both approaches are shown in Table 25.11. The main advantage of operation is that the treatment is of short duration, effective in maintaining the concentric position, and allows better long-term remodelling while the varus of the femoral neck is correcting. The disadvantage is that, in children older than 8–9 years, the varus will not remodel with time, and this leads to persistent shortening, which may require further reconstructive surgery by trochanteric advancement with contralateral distal femoral epiphysiodesis or a valgus osteotomy.

Salter (1966) reported the use of *innominate osteotomy* in the treatment of Perthes' disease. He recommended that operation should not be considered unless the patient had a full or almost full range of hip movement, and a round or almost round femoral head, with reasonable congruence in abduction. He also recommended that the child should be more than 6 years old with greater than 50% femoral head involvement by the disease (Salter group B). Fourteen years later (1980), Salter reported his results, which were satisfactory in 77% and poor in only 6% of the patients. Other authors, however, have been unable to obtain results as successful with the innominate osteotomy, reporting only 40–55% good results and 27% poor results (Canale et al

Table 25.11 Comparison of operative and non-operative treatment

		Operative	Non-operative
Effective in maintaining reduction	Up to 7 years	Yes	Yes
	7–9 years	Yes	?
	Over 10 years	?	No
Duration of treatment		Short	Long, varies with age and group
Varus in long-term remodelling		Yes	No
Residual shortening	Up to 8 years	Resolves	No
	Over 9 years	Persists	If non-weight-bearing
End-point of treatment		Removal of plaster	? At time of healing
Psychological problems		Of operation	Of child-in-a-splint

1972, Stevens et al 1981). These latter results show no improvement over those obtained with a femoral osteotomy in group III and IV hips as reported by Canario et al in 1980 and Coates et al in 1990. It is also accepted that innominate osteotomy will not control the progressive subluxation occurring in the child presenting after the age of 8 years.

Containment splints, which are of many kinds, have the immediate advantage of no operation, but they are tedious to use, with no precise endpoint to treatment, and problems with compliance. All have the psychological problems of 'the child in the brace' and no long-term varus to encourage good remodelling. In addition, if full movement is not maintained, pelvic obliquity may occur, resulting in a flexion – abduction contracture that prejudices the long-term result. This often occurs in the older child and, as a result, many surgeons consider bracing an unsatisfactory method of treatment for the child older than 7 years. This was confirmed in the follow-up studies by Martinez et al (1992) and Meehan et al (1992).

The long-term results of *femoral osteotomy* have been reported by Coates et al (1990). The operation is effective in maintaining good function and femoral head shape in all ages. After the age of 8 years, however, there may be persisting varus and shortening after femoral osteotomy, and therefore lateral shelf acetabuloplasty may be considered (Willett et al 1992). The long-term results of this procedure have been reported by Daly et al (1999).

The results of *lateral shelf acetabuloplasty* are in general satisfactory for the child up to the age of 11 years. It must, however, be stressed that, once epiphyseal height is lost, it is never regained in the long term, although considerable remodelling of the hip joint may occur over time. It is important, therefore, to operate early in these older children, and not to pursue an expectant policy until such a time that the opportunity to improve the prognosis is lost.

Recently, *arthrodiastasis* or *arthrochondrodiastasis with an external fixator* has been suggested for Perthes' disease. Kocaoglu et al (1999), using the Ilizarov apparatus in a small series of 11 patients followed up for an average of 3 years,

reported that the low success rate in eight of their 11 patients and problems with pin-track infections did not justify the routine use of this method. Guaniero et al, in a paper read to the European Paediatric Orthopaedic Society in Milan in 2000, compared 18 patients treated with arthrochondrodiastasis with a similar group treated by femoral varus osteotomy. They reported satisfactory results in both groups, with more rapid healing in the group treated by arthrochondrodiastasis. However, the follow-up in this series was also short. This novel method of treatment remains unproven at present.

THE UNCONTAINABLE HIP

When a child presents with established femoral head deformity and pain, hinge abduction is usually demonstrable at arthrography. In flexion and adduction, the congruity of the joint is re-established, with no instability on attempted rotation. Abduction extension osteotomy will realign such a hip so that there is maximal congruency and therefore stability in the neutral position of weight bearing. The satisfactory results of this procedure have been reported by Quain & Catterall (1986) and confirmed in the long-term follow-up reported by Bankes (2000). Although, initially, the femoral head is more uncovered after operation, the subsequent remodelling of the hip joint is such that further treatment by lateral shelf acetabuloplasty is seldom required.

POST-TREATMENT FOLLOW-UP

Once the programme of treatment has been completed, the child is free to mobilise. Games, with the exclusion of jumping sports, are permitted as activity increases. The cycle of follow-up now continues, initially on a 3-month and later a 6-month basis. Varus femoral osteotomy may produce moderate restriction of abduction for a 6–9 month period. Limp during this time is often marked, and the family should be reassured that this will lessen progressively with time.

REFERENCES

Bankes M J, Catterall A, Hashemi-Nejad A 2000 Valgus extension osteotomy for 'hinge abduction' in Perthes' disease. Results at maturity and factors influencing the radiological outcome. Journal of Bone and Joint Surgery 82B: 548–554

Barker D J, Dixon E, Taylor J F 1978 Perthes' disease of the hip in three regions of England. Journal of Bone and Joint Surgery 60B: 478–480

Barker D J, Hall A J 1986 The epidemiology of Perthes' disease. Clinical Orthopaedics and Related Research 209: 89–94

Burwell R G, Dangerfield P H, Hall D J, Vernon C L, Harrison H M M 1978 Perthes' disease. An anthropometric study revealing impaired and disproportionate growth. Journal of Bone and Joint Surgery 60B: 461–477

Burwell R G, Vernon C L, Dangerfield P H, Hall D J, Kristmundsdottir F 1986 Raised somatomedin activity in the serum of young boys with Perthes' disease revealed by bioassay. A disease of growth transition? Clinical Orthopaedics and Related Research 209: 129–138

Calvé J 1910 Sur une forme de pseudo-coxalgia greffe e surdes deformation carateristique de l'extremité superieure du femur. Revue de Chirugie 30: 54–84

Calvert P T, Kernohan J G, Sayers D C, Catterall A 1984 Effect of vascular occlusion on the femoral head in growing rabbits. Journal of Bone and Joint Surgery 55B: 526–530

Canale S T, D'Anca A F, Cotler J M, Sneddon H E 1972 Innominate osteotomy in Legg-Calvé-Perthes' disease. Journal of Bone and Joint Surgery 54A: 25–40

Canario A T, Williams L, Wientroub S, Catterall A, Lloyd-Roberts G C 1980 A controlled study of the results of femoral osteotomy in severe Perthes' disease. Journal of Bone and Joint Surgery 62B: 438–440

Catterall A 1971 The natural history of Perthes' disease. Journal of Bone and Joint Surgery 53B: 37–53

Catterall A 1981 Legg-Calvé-Perthes syndrome. Clinical Orthopaedics and Related Research 158: 41–52

Catterall A 1982 Legg-Calvé-Perthes' Disease. Churchill Livingstone, Edinburgh

Catterall A 1986 Adolescent hip pain after Perthes' disease. Clinical Orthopaedics and Related Research 209: 65–69

Catterall A, Pringle J, Byers P D et al 1982a A review of the morphology of Perthes' disease. Journal of Bone and Joint Surgery 64B: 269–275

Catterall A J, Pringle J, Byers P D, Fulford G E, Kemp H B 1982b Perthes' disease: is the epiphyseal infarction complete? Journal of Bone and Joint Surgery 64B: 276–281

Coates C J, Paterson J M H, Woods K R, Catterall A, Fixsen J A 1990 Femoral osteotomy in Perthes' disease. Results at maturity. Journal of Bone and Joint Surgery 72B: 581–585

Conway J J 1993 A scintigraphic classification of Legg-Calvé-Perthes disease. Seminars in Nuclear Medicine 23: 274–295

Curtis B H, Gunther S F, Gossling H R, Paul S W 1974 Treatment for Legg-Perthes disease with the Newington ambulation–abduction brace. Journal of Bone and Joint Surgery 56A: 1135–1146

Daly K, Bruce C, Catterall A 1999 The results of lateral shelf acetabuloplasty in the management of Perthes Disease in the older child – a maturity review. Journal of Bone and Joint Surgery 81B: 380–384

Farsetti P, Tudisco C, Caterini R, Potenza V, Ippolito E 1995 The Herring lateral pillar classification for prognosis in Perthes disease. Late results in 49 patients treated conservatively. Journal of Bone and Joint Surgery 77B: 739–742

Freeman M A R, England P S 1969 Experimental infarction of the cannine femoral head. Proceedings of the Royal Society of Medicine 62: 431–433

Glueck C J, Crawford A et al 1996 Association of antithrombotic factor deficiencies and hypofibrinolysis with Legg-Perthes disease [see comments]. Journal of Bone and Joint Surgery 78A: 3–13

Grossbard G D 1981 Hip pain during adolescence after Perthes' disease. Journal of Bone and Joint Surgery 4B: 572–574

Guaniero R, Luzo C A M, Montenegro N B, Godoy R M 2000 Legg-Calvé-Perthes disease: a comparative study between two types of treatment – femoral varus osteotomy and arthrodiastasis with external fixator. Presented at the 19th meeting of the European Paediatric Orthopaedic Society, Milan

Hall A J 1987 Perthes disease: progress in aetiological research. In: Catterall A (ed) Recent Advances in Orthopaedics 5. Churchill Livingstone, Edinburgh, pp 187–199

Hall A J, Barker D J 1989 Perthes' disease in Yorkshire. Journal of Bone and Joint Surgery 71B: 229–233

Hall D J, Harrison M H, Burwell R G 1979 Congenital abnormalities and Perthes' disease. Clinical evidence that children with Perthes' disease may have a major congenital defect. Journal of Bone and Joint Surgery 61B: 18–25

Hall A J, Barker D J, Dangerfield P H, Taylor J F 1983 Perthes' disease of the hip in Liverpool. British Medical Journal 287: 1757–1759

Harrison M H, Turner M H, Jacobs P 1976 Skeletal immaturity in Perthes' disease. Journal of Bone and Joint Surgery 58B: 37–40

Harrison M H, Turner M H, Smith D N 1982 Perthes' disease. Treatment with the Birmingham splint. Journal of Bone and Joint Surgery 64B: 3–11

Hayek S, Kenet G et al 1999 Does thrombophilia play an aetiological role in Legg-Calvé-Perthes disease? [see comments]. Journal of Bone and Joint Surgery 81B: 686–690

Heikkinen E, Puranen J 1980 Evaluation of femoral osteotomy in the treatment of Legg-Calvé-Perthes' disease. Clinical Orthopaedics and Related Research 150: 60–68

Herring J A, Neustadt J B, Williams J J, Early J S, Browne R H 1992 The lateral pillar classification of Legg-Calvé-Perthes disease. Journal of Pediatric Orthopaedics 12: 143–150

Inoue A, Freeman M A R, Vernon–Roberts B, Mizuno S 1976 The pathogenesis of Perthes' disease. Journal of Bone and Joint Surgery 58B: 453–461

Ismail A M, Macnicol M F 1998 Prognosis in Perthes' disease. A comparison of radiological predictors. Journal of Bone and Joint Surgery 80B: 310–314

Kocaoglu M, Kilicoglu O I, Goksan S B, Cakmak M 1999 Ilizarov fixator for treatment of Legg-Calvé-Perthes' disease. Journal of Pediatric Orthopaedics B8: 276–281

Legg A T 1910 An obscure condition of the hip joint. Boston Medical and Surgical Journal 162: 202–204

Liesner R J 1999 Does thrombophilia cause Perthes' disease in children? Journal of Bone and Joint Surgery 81B: 565–566

McAndrew M P, Weinstein S L 1984 A long-term follow-up of Legg-Calvé-Perthes disease. Journal of Bone and Joint Surgery 66A: 860–869

McKibbin B, Ralis Z 1974 Pathological changes in a case of Perthes' disease. Journal of Bone and Joint Surgery 56B: 438–447

Martinez A G, Weinstein S L et al 1992 The weight-bearing abduction brace for the treatment of Legg-Perthes disease. Journal of Bone and Joint Surgery 74A: 12–21

Meehan P L, Angel D et al 1992 The Scottish Rite abduction orthosis for the treatment of Legg-Perthes disease. A radiographic analysis. Journal of Bone and Joint Surgery 74A: 2–12

Mose K, Hjorth L, Ulfeldt M, Christensen E R, Jensen A 1977 Legg Calve Perthes disease. The late occurrence of coxarthrosis. Acta Orthopaedica Scandinavica Supplementum 169: 1–39

Muirhead-Allwood W, Catterall A 1982 The treatment of Perthes' disease. The results of a trial of management. Journal of Bone and Joint Surgery 64B: 282–285

Paterson D, Savage J P 1986 The nuclide bone scan in the diagnosis of Perthes' disease. Clinical Orthopaedics and Related Research 209: 23–29

Perthes G C 1910 Uber arthritis deformans juvenilis. Deutsche zeitschrift fur Chirugie 107: 11–59

Quain S, Catterall A 1986 Hinge abduction of the hip. Diagnosis and treatment. Journal of Bone and Joint Surgery 68B: 61–64

Salter R B 1966 Experimental and clinical aspects of Perthes' disease. In: Proceedings of the Joint Meeting of the American Physicians' Fellowship and the Israeli Orthopaedic Society. Journal of Bone and Joint Surgery 48B: 393–394

Salter R B 1980 Legg-Perthes disease: the scientific basis for the methods of treatment and their indications. Clinical Orthopaedics and Related Research 150: 8–11

Salter R B, Thompson G H 1984 Legg-Calvé-Perthes disease. The prognostic significance of the subchondral fracture and a two-group classification of the femoral head involvement. Journal of Bone and Joint Surgery 66A: 479–489.

Snyder C R 1975 Legg-Perthes disease in the young hip – does it necessarily do well? Journal of Bone and Joint Surgery 57: 751–759

Stevens P M, Williams P, Menelaus M 1981 Innominate osteotomy for Perthes' disease. Journal of Pediatric Orthopaedics 1: 47–54

Stulberg S D, Cooperman D R, Wallensten R 1981 The natural history of Legg-Calvé-Perthes disease. Journal of Bone and Joint Surgery 63A: 1095–1108

Tachdjian M 1980 99 m technetium diphosphonate bone imaging in Legg-Calvé-Perthes' disease. Acta Orthopaedica Belgica 46: 366–370

Thomas D P, Morgan G et al 1999 Perthes' disease and the relevance of thrombophilia [see comments]. Journal of Bone and Joint Surgery 81B: 691–695

Thompson G H, Westin G W 1979 Legg-Calvé-Perthes disease: results of discontinuing treatment in the early reossification phase. Clinical Orthopaedics and Related Research 139: 70–80

Waldenström H 1938 The first stages of coxa plana. Journal of Bone and Joint Surgery 20B: 559–566

Wenger D R, Ward W T, Herring J A 1991 Legg-Calvé-Perthes disease. Journal of Bone and Joint Surgery 73A: 778–788

Willett K, Hudson I, Catterall A 1992 Lateral shelf acetabuloplasty: an operation for older children with Perthes' disease. Journal of Pediatric Orthopaedics 12: 563–568

Chapter 26

Slipped capital femoral epiphysis

M. F. Macnicol and M. K. D. Benson

INTRODUCTION

Slipping of the upper femoral epiphysis is the most common cause of hip disability in adolescence. Many factors contribute to a relative weakness of the growth plate that culminates in a shearing displacement through the zone of hypertrophic cartilage. The patient's symptoms may be trivial or profound. Treatment is directed at preventing progressive slippage, minimising deformity, and avoiding the major complications of avascular necrosis and chondrolysis.

INCIDENCE

Between 2 and 3 per 100 000 children and adolescents suffer a slipped capital femoral epiphysis. It is three times more common in boys, and they are usually affected between the ages of 14 and 16 years, whereas girls present between 11 and 13 years. After the menarche, girls are almost immune to slipped epiphysis.

The adolescents at greatest risk appear to be those who are skeletally immature and obese, although slipped epiphysis may occur in those with normal physique, especially during a growth spurt. Tall, slender adolescent boys with delayed skeletal maturity may also be at risk.

The left hip is more frequently involved, but in approximately 30% of cases the opposite hip will slip also. There may be subtle changes of pre-slipping in the opposite hip in a further 40%. Both epiphyses may displace simultaneously, but the contralateral event may well be separated both in time and severity, with slipping occuring 6–18 months later (Sorensen 1968, Hagglund et al 1984, Knight et al 1987, Loder et al 1993).

There are racial variations: epiphysiolysis is very rare in Southern Asia and in the black population of Africa. It is at least two or three times more common in black Americans and Puerto Ricans. The disorder appears to be an autosomal dominant with variable penetrance, and there is a 7% risk of a second family member being affected (Rennie 1982).

AETIOLOGY

The interplay of factors that contribute to epiphysiolysis is intriguing: mechanical stress, trauma, endocrine and immunological abnormalities have been considered separately and together as aetiologically important.

MECHANICAL FACTORS

Chung et al (1976) showed that the perichondrial fibrocartilaginous ring surrounding the growth plate contributes significantly to the ability of the epiphysis to withstand shear forces. It is powerfully bound to the subperiosteal metaphyseal bone and is strongest in infancy, but decreases in volume and strength, particularly in adolescence. Coincidentally, the epiphyseal plate widens with the adolescent growth spurt, just as the perichondrial ring thins.

Shear force across the epiphyseal plate is least when the growth plate is horizontal and the femoral neck anteverted. Gelberman et al (1986) have shown relative retroversion in those with epiphyseal slipping. Once displacement occurs, stress through the epiphyseal plate becomes more vertical and the risk of further slipping is increased. Because five to six times body weight may be delivered as shear force during running, it is clear that body weight and repetitive trauma contribute to the risk of slip.

ENDOCRINE FACTORS

Because epiphyseal slipping occurs at a time of maximal growth, and as a significant number of children are either overweight or abnormally lean, it seems logical to suppose that endocrine factors are contributory. Sex hormones increase the shear strength of the epiphyseal plate, whereas growth hormone decreases it. When children with hypopituitarism are treated with growth hormone, there is a significant risk of epiphyseal slip, particularly if sex hormones are not given concurrently. A deficiency of sex hormones also delays epiphyseal closure and increases the time span during which slipping may occur. Furthermore, sex hormone deficiency is associated with obesity, so adding a mechanical factor to the problem.

Other endocrinopathies have been described in association with slipping. Hypothyroidism, whether in isolation or as part of pan-hypopituitarism, has a clear association. Both primary hyperparathyroidism and the secondary hyperparathyroidism complicating renal failure may uniquely alter many physes, and slips may occur not only at the hip but also at the distal radius and ulna. This should be remembered when a child in chronic renal failure presents with a limp or musculoskeletal problems.

It should be stressed that the majority of children with epiphyseal slipping do not have a recognisable endocrine abnormality, and it is probably reasonable only to investigate those whose physique suggests that such an abnormality may be present, particularly those of short stature. Clearly, children younger than 10 years or those over 16 years should be investigated endocrinologically.

IMMUNOLOGICAL FACTORS

Eisenstein & Rothschild (1976) studied a group of patients with epiphysiolysis, finding a significant increase in serum immunoglobulins, particularly of IgA. Patients with complicating chondrolysis showed a greater increase in IgM. The investigators suggested that epiphyseal slipping was therefore either a local manifestation of a generalised inflammatory disorder or, more probably, that the slip exposed a tissue proteoglycan that served as an antigenic stimulus for immunoglobulin and complement production.

Whether the immune complex so produced plays any part in the development of chondrolysis remains obscure. It seems possible, however, that the synovitis associated with acute slipped epiphysis may be caused, at least in part, by local synovial cell production of immunoglobulin. Cell death and the production of tissue breakdown products also promote the inflammatory response.

PATHOPHYSIOLOGY

The growth plate has been assessed mainly by core biopsy specimens, and the histology, histochemistry and ultrastructural appearances are well described. The slip occurs through the zone of hypertrophic cartilage, where chondrocytes lie in irregular clusters with a paucity of collagen fibrils in the ground substance. An abnormal accumulation and distribution of glycoproteins and proteoglycans in the matrix may inhibit normal chondrocyte degeneration and matrix calcification.

In the pre-slipping stage, the synovium is oedematous and hyperaemic. There may be softening and decalcification of the femoral metaphysis, which produces juxta-epiphysial osteopenia radiographically.

In the second stage of true displacement, the slip progresses typically in multiple minute increments, although an acute sudden shear force may lead to the so-called 'acute-on-chronic' slip. Rarely, there may be an acute, catastrophic slip that leads to complete discontinuity between head and neck.

Posteriorly and inferiorly, where the periosteum is stripped up from the neck of the femur, callus forms, leading to remodelling and stability of the displaced epiphysis. The posterior epiphyseal vessels are stripped up with the periosteum and are rarely stretched in the untreated case (although avascular necrosis has been reported).

The synovial membrane and periosteum remain oedematous and hyperaemic throughout the slipping phase, but the inflammatory reaction then subsides. The epiphyseal plate usually closes prematurely, fusion occurring on average 19 months after the onset of symptoms in the untreated case.

THE DIRECTION OF SLIP

The complex three-directional anatomy of the hip and the epiphysis has led to confusion in interpreting the direction of slip. The epiphysis itself is usually held in place in the acetabulum by the ligamentum teres and surface tension. The femoral neck displaces from the femoral head, rotating laterally and upwards. However, if we consider the displacement of head upon neck, the displacement is almost invariably truly posterior. Griffiths (1976) showed neatly, by simply rotating the femur, that anteroposterior radiographs may grossly mislead their unwary interpreter.

As the epiphysis slips, the periosteum remains attached to the posteromedial margin of the head (its growth keeping pace with displacement). The uncovered anterior portion of the metaphysis appears blue with small islands of bone; the cells of this buttress convert gradually to fibrocartilage and may impinge on the acetabular margin and limit movement.

PREDISPOSING FACTORS

As mentioned above, predisposing factors include endocrinopathies such as hypopituitarism, hypogonadism, hypothyroidism and the effects of craniopharyngioma. Growth hormone deficiency and the hyperparathyroidism secondary to renal failure (osteodystrophy) may also cause a slip, and these atypical slips account for between 5 and 10% of the total. Irradiation, chemotherapy and Down's syndrome increase the likelihood of a slip, as may rare metabolic conditions such as the Bartter syndrome. Many of the affected children are shorter than normal (in the shortest 10th percentile) and a predisposing medical condition should be suspected in the stunted child who presents with a slipped epiphysis before the age of 10 years, or after 16 years (Fig. 26.1).

CLINICAL FEATURES

The symptoms typically start insidiously. An adolescent complains of aching in the groin, thigh or often the knee. Despite a limp and external rotation of the leg, symptoms have often been present for weeks or months before medical attention is sought. Most commonly, it is the slow increase in chronic symptoms that leads to further investigation, and delays in diagnosis often result if the hip is not examined radiographically.

In the acute slip, whether this occurs primarily or, more commonly, as a complication of a chronic slip, sudden severe pain may make weight bearing impossible. Fifty percent of the children who present will recollect an injury, although this usually is trivial.

Loder et al (1993) introduced the important concept of the 'unstable' slip. The child is unable to bear weight through the affected leg, even when using crutches. Active straight leg raising is also impossible when an acute, major slip has occurred.

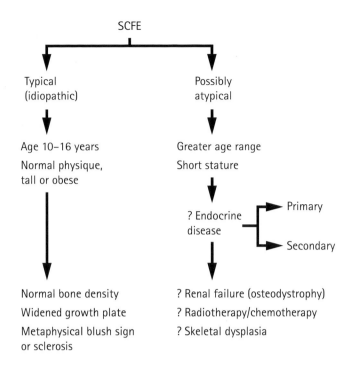

Figure 26.1 Clinical differences between typical and atypical cases of slipped epiphysis.

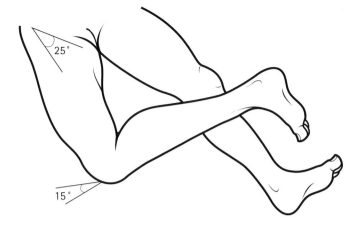

Figure 26.2 The position of the leg that demonstrates the displacement of the epiphysis.

The gait may be antalgic or waddling if both hips are affected. The involved limb lies in external rotation and in adduction when displacement is severe. With a mild slip, internal rotation is the movement most likely to be restricted. In more marked slipping, abduction, flexion and internal rotation will all be decreased. As the examiner flexes the affected hip, the thigh rolls typically into external rotation, producing the 'figure 4' position. It is striking that flexion may be more limited than extension. Restricted mobility is more marked in the acute slip, probably as the result of the greater effusion and more pronounced reactive muscle spasm. Shortening is seldom greater than 2 cm.

As the condition is progressive and may produce chronic disability, it is mandatory that adolescents who complain of hip or knee pain should be investigated, with radiographic views of both hips.

RADIOLOGICAL SIGNS

Both anteroposterior and frog lateral radiographs are essential when the child with a limp is being investigated. The characteristic radiographic changes on the anteroposterior projection may be subtle, and therefore a frog lateral view is more informative, although marked spasm or a significant effusion may make this projection difficult to take. The leg should not be forcibly manipulated to obtain the frog lateral view; it is wiser to take a cross-table lateral if spasm prevents the standard leg positioning.

Radiographic imaging of the slip at operation is difficult, and may be misleading. When the leg is externally rotated, the epiphysis appears to be tilted medially; when the hip is

internally rotated, the tilt is posterolateral. To demonstrate the displacement best, the hip should be flexed 20–30°, the knee flexed 90° and the thigh allowed to rotate externally 15° (Fig. 26.2), as this reduces the parallax effect (Billing & Severin 1959, Griffiths 1976).

PRE-SLIPPING

In the pre-slipping phase, when synovitis and an effusion are present, the metaphysis adjacent to the epiphyseal plate may appear osteoporotic. The growth plate becomes slightly widened, but there is no displacement. The effusion may be confirmed ultrasonographically and the increased metaphyseal blood supply causes increased uptake on a technetium-99m bone scan. Bone changes will also be seen on magnetic resonance imaging (MRI).

THE SLIP

As the epiphysis slips backwards, the epiphyseal height decreases on the anteroposterior film. A line drawn along the upper border of the neck (Trethowan's or Klein's line) will, in the normal hip, cut off a segment of the superior epiphysis (Fig. 26.3). When a minor slip has occurred, the line will skirt the lateral margin of the epiphysis. Note also

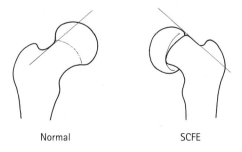

Figure 26.3 Trethowan's or Klein's sign: when slipping occurs, a line drawn along the upper femoral neck fails to cut off a segment of epiphysis laterally.

that the medial edge of the metaphysis no longer overlaps the pelvis and that the growth plate appears even wider. Bone density of the affected side is reduced, but the metaphysis adjacent to the growth plate appears sclerotic (the 'blush sign').

The lateral X-ray gives a more precise indication of the extent of the slip. In the normal hip, the epiphysis should lie at right angles to the long axis of the femoral neck; in the abnormal hip, the angle of slip may be calculated by producing a line at 90° to the line between the anterior and posterior borders of the epiphysis, measuring its transection with the long axis of the femoral neck. It has become the norm to measure the percentage of slip: less than 30° is regarded as mild; 30–60° as moderate, and greater than 60° as severe (Fig. 26.4). These grades correspond to less than one-third femoral head diameter displacement, between one-third and one-half displacement, and more than one-half displacement. The displacement may be more accurately assessed by computed tomography (CT) or MRI scan.

The stages in slipping of the epiphysis are conventionally described as:

- acute (approximately 20% of cases)
- chronic (approximately 30% of cases)
- acute-on-chronic (approximately 50% of cases).

It is not entirely clear why some epiphyses slip minimally and then stabilise, and why others displace either catastrophically, or slowly and progressively. The acute, major slips are rare and may be considered to be transepiphyseal fractures (Ratcliff 1968), as they follow significant trauma and the patient is unable to weight bear on the affected leg. Of the 30% who present with a chronic slip, 50% have displaced less than 30° (Knight et al 1987). The history indicates a more gradual process, often without an obvious precipitant; radiographs reveal that the femoral neck has remodelled and the growth plate may be closing. Acute episodes of slipping superimposed upon chronic mild displacement result in an irritable hip in which deformity is variable. Remodelling of the femoral neck is usually evident radiographically, but the epiphysis overhangs the neck to a greater degree.

A history of a sudden episode of pain, usually after exertion, and an inability to bear weight suggest an acute-on-chronic pathological process, if symptoms have been present before the acute presentation. The sudden change in function suggests that the slip is unstable, and possibly open to gentle early reduction by manipulation. Loder et al (1993) have suggested that an inability to weight bear upon the affected leg indicates that the slip is unstable.

SECONDARY CHANGES

Adaptive changes develop quickly after the epiphysis has slipped. New bone is laid down under the posterior cortex of the neck where the periosteum is stripped up. Remodelling of the anterior buttress occurs and may progress to such an extent that the initial convexity may eventually become concave. These structural changes are evident on the radiograph and if the hip joint is explored surgically.

The major complications of epiphyseal slip, which are much more common after surgery, are avascular necrosis and chondrolysis (Carney et al 1991). Both appear to be more likely in black American children and Hawaiian females. The earliest signs of avascular necrosis are stiffness and muscle spasm with a relative increase in femoral head density some months after treatment. This is followed by fragmentation and collapse of the epiphysis, although the subchondral fracture line noted in Perthes' disease is rarely seen. Narrowing of the joint space indicates avascular necrosis and chondrolysis. This may be present at the time of diagnosis or may appear from a few weeks to 1 year later (Fig. 26.5).

TREATMENT

Treatment depends upon the preference and skills of the surgeon as much as the nature and chronicity of the slip. Minor slips at the end of a growth spurt may be managed conservatively, provided that regular review can be ensured. However, it is generally preferable to pin or screw the epiphysis *in situ*, and plaster cast (spica) fixation is rarely indicated.

Percutaneous procedures using the image intensifier should be relatively safe, provided that the epiphysis is clearly visualised and the tip of the device does not penetrate the joint. However, Greenhough et al (1985) recorded that a complication occurred in up to 50% of the hips in which pins were inserted, and therefore the procedure must be carefully executed, preferably with a single cannulated screw (Fig. 26.6). Epiphysiodesis with a bone graft is unnecessary if the epiphysis is stabilised.

If pins are used, a minimum of two will be required for the unstable slip, in order to control the epiphysis against twisting and shear stresses (Aronsson & Loder 1996). A single cannulated screw is considered sufficient if it has been inserted with compression, but augmentation with another implant, such as a cancellous AO screw, is advised in the heavier and more active patient (Macnicol & Macindoe 1996).

To some extent, the nature of the epiphyseal slip determines the treatment (Fig. 26.7):

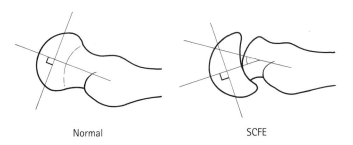

Normal   SCFE

Figure 26.4 The extent of epiphysial displacement is expressed in degrees.

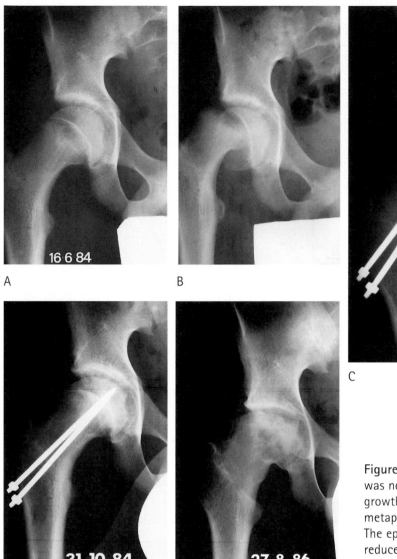

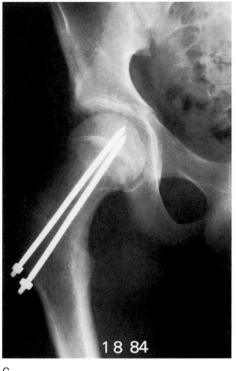

A

B

C

D

E

Figure 26.5 A minor slip of the right upper femoral epiphysis was not appreciated, although Trethowan's sign is positive, the growth plate appears widened, and the proximal, medial metaphysis no longer overlaps the pelvis (**A**).
The epiphysis slipped significantly a few days later (**B**) and was reduced anatomically by manipulation under anaesthesia (**C**). Unfortunately, avascular necrosis and loss of joint space became progressively more obvious (**D, E**).

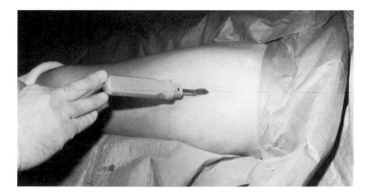

Figure 26.6 Percutaneous screw fixation is carried out using an image intensifier, and is made easier if the affected leg is free to move, allowing accurate positioning of the cannulated screw in the centre of the epiphysis.

- Acute slip
  - *mild*: internally fix *in situ*
  - *moderate*: either accept and pin *in situ* or gently internally rotate the extended leg, and internally fix
  - *severe*: gentle internal rotation of the leg may improve the position, with the leg extended, but manipulation of the flexed hip under general anaesthesia must be avoided; the epiphysis can usually then be stabilised with a cannulated screw(s); later, corrective osteotomy may be indicated

- Chronic slip
  - *mild*: fix *in situ* or ignore if the child is reaching maturity
  - *moderate*: fix *in situ* or consider a realignment osteotomy
  - *severe*: very rare because most of these cases are from an acute slip superimposed upon chronic deformity

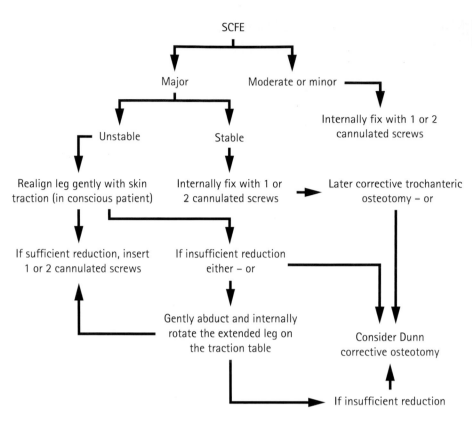

Figure 26.7 Flow diagram to outline the surgical approach for slipped epiphysis.

- Acute-on-chronic
  - *mild*: fix *in situ*
  - *moderate*: attempt a gentle correction by skin traction or by internal rotation under anaesthesia followed by screw fixation, or carry out a corrective osteotomy
  - *severe*: undertake a Dunn & Angel osteotomy (1978) or a Fish procedure (1984) if the growth plate is still open, or a corrective intertrochanteric osteotomy.

With slips of greater than 30°, the *in situ* insertion of implants becomes more difficult. The medullary aperture closes off progressively (Fig. 26.8) and the practice of placing pins or screws across the posterior aspect of the femoral neck cannot be condoned, because the vascularity of the epiphysis is endangered. Furthermore, the extraosseous segment of the implant may break. Effective insertion of the device requires an anterior approach, through the front of the femoral neck (Figs 26.9–26.11).

A perioperative arthrogram has been recommended after pinning (Bennet et al 1984) or cannulated screw insertion (Lehman et al 1984). However, this does not exclude penetration into the joint (Shaw 1984), and therefore whenever possible the pin tips should be placed in the foveal (inferomedial) segment of the epiphysis (Brodetti 1960). The tips of the pins should be kept apart, because there is some evidence that crowding of the tips may produce an avascular segment.

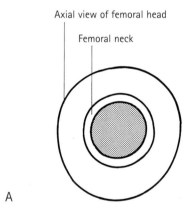

Axial view of femoral head

Femoral neck

A

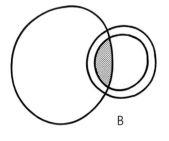

B

Figure 26.8 The aperture shared by the femoral neck and epiphysis (A) gradually closes off as the slip increases (B).

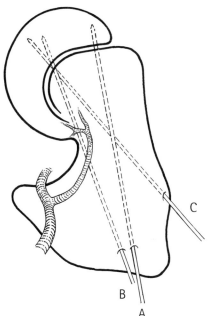

Figure 26.9 The trajectory of the guidewire is important. A lateral guidewire insertion may either result in a poor fix in the anterior epiphysis (A) or, if directed more posteriorly, may breach the posterior surface of the neck and thus injure the vital retinacular vessels (B). A more anterior starting point with the wire will allow the neck to be traversed within the medulla, and the centre of the epiphysis to be secured (C).

Viewing the epiphysis by fluoroscopy is improved if the leg is draped separately, allowing the limb to be moved into various positions between internal rotation and external rotation in the frog lateral posture. Manipulation of the leg in this way may not be possible if the child is very large, but is the preferred method if the cannulated screw or pins are to be viewed from all angles. The operation is facilitated by the

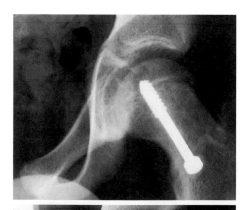

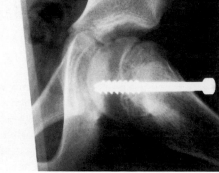

Figure 26.10 Radiographs to show the cannulated screw fixation of a moderate slip.

use of a fracture table, so that an assistant can hold the leg in these varying positions, including extension.

Because image intensification is liable to errors of interpretation, standard anteroposterior and frog lateral radiographs should be obtained before the child is returned to the recovery area after anaesthesia.

The risk of stretching the posterior retinacular vessels is considerable when the leg is manipulated under general anaesthesia in an attempt to reduce the displacement of the epiphysis. If manipulation is attempted under anaesthesia, it must be gentle and consist of no more than internal rotation and partial abduction of the affected limb when supported on an orthopaedic table. Vigorous rotation of the flexed hip is to be condemned. Preoperative traction in flexion may occasionally replace the acutely slipped epiphysis, but it is generally ineffective because spasm of the hip muscles prevents the internal rotation necessary to reduce the slip.

In the younger child – a girl younger than 11 years or a boy younger than 12 or 13 years – the opposite, normal hip may slip at a later date, perhaps in 30% of cases. It is therefore advisable to fix the contralateral hip, particularly if the child is very heavy, the growth plates are widely open, or when the family is felt to be unreliable. Conversely, if the parents and child can be expected to make contact immediately any contralateral symptoms are experienced, and particularly if the child is nearing the end of the adolescent growth spurt, prophylactic pinning can be avoided. However, the child must be observed regularly, at 3–6-monthly intervals, with radiographs to check both the pathological hip and the normal side.

Bilateral epiphyseal slips are more common in children with hormonal abnormalities, such as renal rickets, Cushing's syndrome or hypopituitarism, short stature treated by growth hormone, or in those who have undergone irradiation. A milder, bilateral form, causing femoral head 'tilts' is often seen in athletic young men who have played football and other energetic sports to a high level during adolescence (Fig. 26.12).

OSTEOTOMY

When the epiphysis proves to be irreducibly and severely displaced, an osteotomy of the femoral neck at the level of the physis should be considered. The growth plate must be open. If it is still open, the Dunn procedure (Dunn & Angel 1978) allows the slip to be corrected fully. It is imperative to obtain good access, either by means of a greater trochanteric osteotomy or by careful soft-tissue dissection to expose the femoral neck superiorly and anteriorly (Fig. 26.13). The operation may be carried out with the patient either supine (Macnicol 1996) or lying on the unaffected side with fluoroscopic imaging available. The posterior retinacular vessels of the femoral neck must not be damaged, and this is ensured by:

1. Leaving the soft tissues over the back of the neck undissected.
2. Shortening the femoral neck to allow repositioning of the epiphysis without tensioning the vessels.

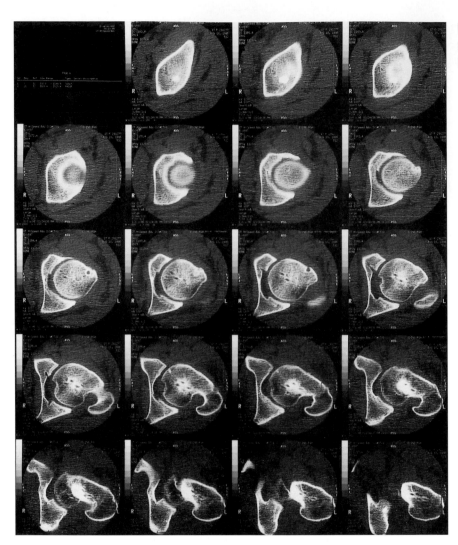

Figure 26.11 A CT scan demonstrates the posterior epiphyseal slip and three artefacts produced by the fixation pins.

Excision of the proximal femoral neck must be conducted with extreme caution, avoiding injury to the epiphysis and its posterior blood supply (Fig. 26.14). The curved line of the femoral neck and the saucer-shaped inferior epiphysial surface must be gradually defined by removing callus, and the posterior retinacular vessels must not be stretched.

The epiphysis is reduced by gently positioning the leg in abduction, mild internal rotation and flexion; if there is any difficulty with reduction, the neck should be shortened further. Eventually, the epiphysis will sit centrally upon the metaphysis and pins or a cannulated screw can be inserted up the neck from the lateral femoral cortex (Fig. 26.15). The tip of the pins or screw should be inferocentral, and double fixation is preferable if rotational instability persists. As with pinning *in situ*, great care must be taken to avoid joint penetration, and the hip should be screened carefully with the image intensifier before closing the wound.

Postoperative mobilisation of the hip depends upon the security of the fixation achieved, and whether a greater trochanteric osteotomy has been used to achieve success. Hip spasm is rapidly lost and the return of a normal range of movement is gratifying. However, this does not guarantee

that the epiphysis will survive with no evidence of avascular necrosis. Partial weight bearing can be permitted after 3 weeks, and full weight bearing by 2 months after operation. Avascular necrosis may occur in 20–40% of patients, even in skilled hands (Szypryt et al 1987), but in complete slips there is no other effective surgical correction. The leg length discrepancy produced by shortening the femoral neck is approximately 1 cm, much less than the initial shortening caused by the displacement and secondary adduction deformity. However, in the younger patient the leg length discrepancy may increase during the years of skeletal growth, so that a contralateral distal epiphysiodesis may be indicated.

In more chronic cases of severe displacement, Fish (1984, 1994) has described a similar cervical procedure. Provided that the growth plate is still open, and this can be checked by (computed) tomography, correction is possible by the removal of bone adjacent to the physis. An anterolateral approach is used and the growth plate is defined with a needle. As with the Dunn procedure, the epiphysis is relocated after shortening of the neck, by appropriate positioning of the leg, and internal fixation permits early mobilisation with crutches.

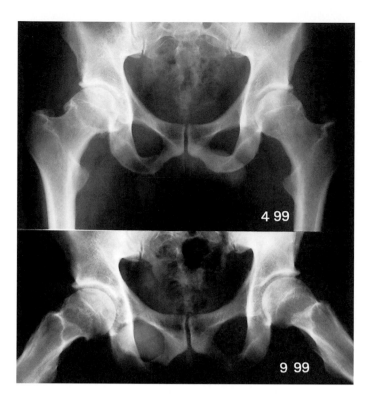

Figure 26.12 Bilateral femoral head tilts (pistol grip deformity).

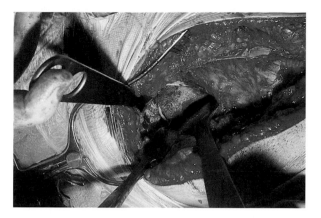

Figure 26.13 Exposure of the femoral neck anterosuperiorly.

When the slip angle measures 30–60°, correction of the deformity can be partially achieved by a de-rotation proximal femoral osteotomy (internally rotating the distal segment), an intertrochanteric osteotomy (Fig. 26.16) (Griffiths 1976) or a Southwick (1967) biplane or triplane osteotomy at the level of the lesser trochanter. Fixation of the epiphysis is usually advisable at a first-stage operation, although Southwick found that realignment resulted in early closure of the plate, possibly stimulated by the subsequent axial compression, so that pinning across the growth plate was unnecessary. Certainly, once the shearing forces across

the plate have been reduced by the realignment, further slipping, in the acute-on-chronic or chronic case, is less likely.

Additional procedures such as epiphysiodesis with bone graft and osteoplasty by removal of the prominent neck bump (Heyman et al 1957) are rarely required, and have no effect upon the underlying deformity. However, like the Southwick osteotomy, they rarely if ever produce epiphyseal avascular necrosis or chondrolysis. In the younger patient, further remodelling of the upper femur can be anticipated after surgery, although closure of the growth plate significantly reduces this potential.

When an avascular segment becomes apparent after the surgical treatment of slipped epiphysis, the treatment depends upon the extent of the femoral head collapse. For the smaller, anterolateral segmental collapse it is sometimes appropriate to undertake a valgus-extension proximal femoral osteotomy (Maistrelli et al 1988) in order to tilt the head posteriorly. However, it is more logical to combine valgus with flexion for the anterosuperior lesions (Scher & Jakim 1993), reserving extension for the rare, posterior lesion. A frog lateral radiograph will define the position of the avascular segment. Mapping of the area of involvement

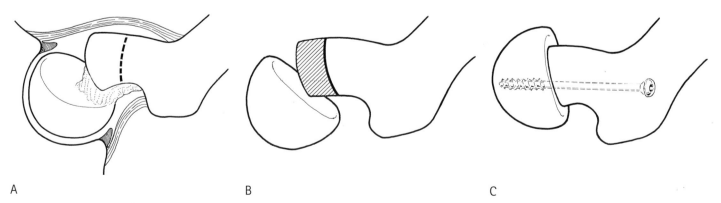

A   B   C

Figure 26.14 A When the epiphysis is being reduced, the femoral neck must be shortened and posterior callus gently removed without damaging the retinacular vessels. B The epiphysis can then be positioned on the shortened neck and one or more cannulated screws inserted (C).

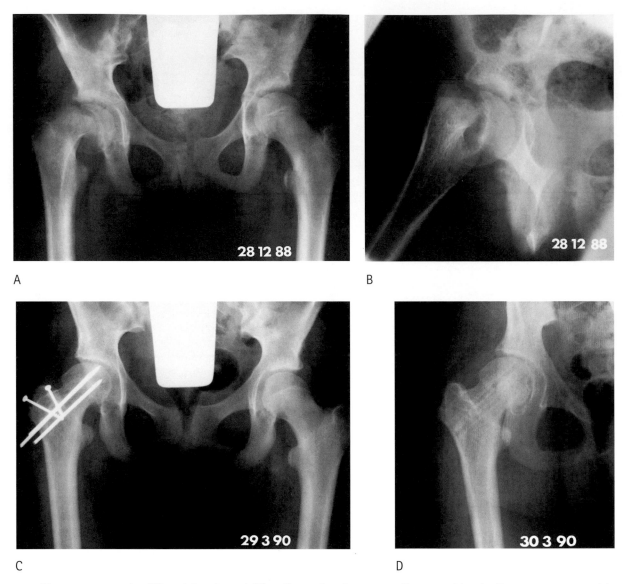

A B

C D

Figure 26.15 The anteroposterior (**A**) and frog lateral (**B**) radiographs of a severe slip treated by the Dunn osteotomy, with exposure using a greater trochanteric osteotomy (**C**) and subsequent removal of the implants (**D**).

can be made more precisely with CT or MRI.

Sugioka (1984) has promoted the transtrochanteric rotational femoral osteotomy. This procedure rotates the head and neck anteriorly; good results have been reported after a minimum of 10 years (Ineo & Sugioka 1999), although other surgeons have not found the results to be satisfactory (Dean & Cabanela 1993).

If the hip stiffens significantly as a result of either chondrolysis or avascular necrosis, there is a limited place for conventional, intertrochanteric realignment proximal femoral osteotomy. This is usually required to correct the flexion, adduction and external rotation deformities that develop. In the younger patient, the salvage of a hip by means of arthrodesis is usually more appropriate than a total hip replacement, but this decision can only be made after careful consideration of the options with the patient and the family.

COMPLICATIONS

In few other orthopaedic conditions are complications more frequently seen than after operation for slipped epiphysis. Avascular necrosis of part or all or the epiphysis may infrequently develop in the untreated case. Most commonly, it is directly related to forced manipulation of the hip under general anaesthesia, or to stretching of the retinacular vessels at the time of cervical excision osteotomy. Clustering of pins may also produce segmental necrosis (Brodetti 1960). Penetration of pin tips into the joint correlates closely with chondrolysis (Bennet et al 1984, Shaw 1984). Other reported complications include breakage of implants (Fig. 26.17), inadequate fixation from short pins, migration of the pins, or the embedding of the implants. The epiphysis may slip further and a fracture may occur at the stress riser where the pins have been inserted. Lastly, the standard operative

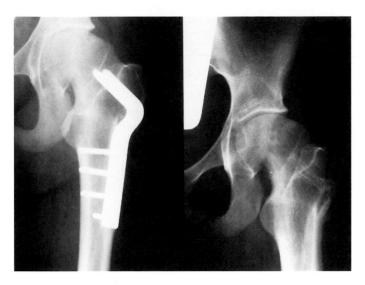

Figure 26.16 A valgus de-rotation (biplanar) proximal femoral osteotomy corrects leg alignment, but the femoral neck deformity persists.

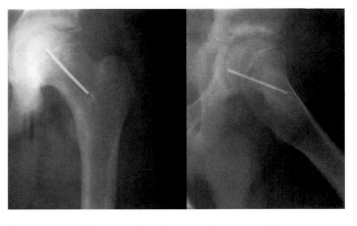

Figure 26.17 The cannulated reamer has severed the guidewire.

complications of infection, nerve and vessel injury and hypertrophic scarring may occur.

For these reasons, a conservative approach to the slipped capital epiphysis is still acceptable if the surgeon is technically inexperienced. However, the use of a plaster spica or prolonged traction is unattractive clinically and socially, so that referral of these children to a centre with experience in this relatively rare condition seems a rational approach to a demanding orthopaedic problem.

CONCLUSION

Failure to diagnose the slipped capital femoral epiphysis remains the main concern in this condition. As a cause of limp in childhood, it accounts for only 0.5% of the total number of hip conditions that are encountered. It is this relative rarity that makes slipped epiphysis difficult to diagnose, coupled with its insidious onset in some children and adolescents, and the fact that pain may be referred to the ipsilateral knee. In any child of short stature, or in whom the medical history is complex, and particularly in the later stages of childhood and in adolescence, the possibility of slipped upper femoral epiphysis must be entertained.

REFERENCES

Aronsson D D, Loder R T 1996 Treatment of the unstable (acute) slipped capital femoral epiphysis. Clinical Orthopaedics and Related Research 322: 99–110

Bennet G C, Koreska J, Rang M 1984 Pin placement in slipped capital femoral epiphysis. Journal of Pediatric Orthopaedics 4: 574–578

Billing, Severin E 1959 Slipping epiphysis of the hip: a roentgenological and clinical study based on a new roentgen technique. Acta Radiologica (Stockholm) (Suppl) 174: 1–76

Brodetti A 1960 The blood supply of the femoral neck and head in relation to the damaging effects of nails and screws. Journal of Bone and Joint Surgery 42B: 794–801

Carney B T, Weinstein S L, Noble J 1991 Long-term follow-up of slipped capital femoral epiphysis. Journal of Bone and Joint Surgery 73A: 667–674

Chung S M K, Batterman S C, Brighton C T 1976 Shear strength of the human capital epiphyseal plate. Journal of Bone and Joint Surgery 58A: 94–103

Dean M T, Cabanela M E 1993 Transtrochanteric anterior rotational osteotomy for avascular necrosis of the femoral head. Long-term results. Journal of Bone and Joint Surgery 75B: 597–600

Dunn D M, Angel J C 1978 Replacement of the femoral head by open operation in severe adolescent slipping of the upper femoral epiphysis. Journal of Bone and Joint Surgery 60B: 394–403

Eisenstein A, Rothschild S 1976 Biochemical abnormalities in patients with slipped capital femoral epiphysis and chondrolysis. Journal of Bone and Joint Surgery 58A: 459–467

Fish J 1984 Cuneiform osteotomy of the femoral neck in the treatment of slipped capital femoral epiphysis. Journal of Bone and Joint Surgery 66A: 1153–1168

Fish J 1994 Cuneiform osteotomy of the femoral neck in the treatment of slipped capital femoral epiphysis. Journal of Bone and Joint Surgery 76A: 46–59

Gelberman R H, Cohen M S, Shaw B A, Kasser J R, Griffin P P, Wilkinson R H 1986 The association of femoral retroversion with slipped capital femoral epiphysis. Journal of Bone and Joint Surgery 68A: 1000–1007

Griffiths M J 1976 Slipping of the upper femoral epiphysis. Annals of the Royal College of Surgeons 58: 34–42

Greenhough C G, Bromage J D, Jackson A M 1985 Pinning of the slipped upper femoral epiphysis – a trouble-free procedure. Pediatric Orthopedics 5: 657–660

Hagglund G, Hanson L I, Ordeberg G 1984 Epidemiology of slipped capital femoral epiphysis in Southern Sweden. Clinical Orthopaedics and Related Research 191: 82–94

Heyman S, Herndon C, Strong J 1957 Slipped femoral epiphysis with severe displacement: a conservative operative technique. Journal of Bone and Joint Surgery 39A: 293–303

Ineo S, Sugioka Y 1999 Minimum 10-year results of Sugioka's osteotomy for femoral head osteonecrosis. Clinical Orthopaedics and Related Research 368: 141–148

Knight D J, Dreghorn C, Main S C 1987 Slipped capital femoral epiphysis in Glasgow. Journal of Pediatric Orthopaedics 7: 283–287

Lehman W B, Menche D, Grant A, Normal A, Pugh J 1984 The problem of evaluating in situ pinning of slipped capital femoral epiphysis. An experimental model and a review of 63 consecutive cases. Journal of Pediatric Orthopaedics 4: 297–303

Loder R T, Richards B S, Shapiro P S, Resnick L R, Aronsson D D 1993 Acute slipped capital femoral epiphysis: the importance of physeal stability. Journal of Bone and Joint Surgery 75A: 1134–1140

Macnicol M F (ed) 1996 Color atlas and text of osteotomy of the hip. Mosby Wolfe (Times Mirror International Publishers Ltd), London

Macnicol M F, Macindoe N 1996 Management of severe slippage of the capital femoral epiphysis. Current Orthopaedics 10: 180–184

Maistrelli G L, Fusco V, Avai A, Bombelli R 1988 Osteonecrosis of the hip treated by intertrochanteric osteotomy: a four-to-15-year follow-up. Journal of Bone and Joint Surgery 70B: 761–766

Ratcliff A H C 1968 Traumatic separation of the upper femoral epiphysis in young children. Journal of Bone and Joint Surgery 50B: 757–761

Rennie A M 1982 The inheritance of slipped upper femoral epiphysis. Journal of Bone and Joint Surgery 64B: 180–184

Scher M A, Jakim I 1993 Intertrochanteric osteotomy and autogenous bone-grafting for avascular necrosis of the femoral head. Journal of Bone and Joint Surgery 75A: 1119–1133

Shaw J A 1984 Preventing unrecognised pin penetration into the hip joint. Orthopaedic Review 13: 142–152

Sorensen K H 1968 Slipped upper femoral epiphysis. Clinical study on aetiology. Acta Orthopaedica Scandinavica 39: 499–517

Southwick W O 1967 Osteotomy through the lesser trochanter for slipped capital femoral epiphysis. Journal of Bone and Joint Surgery 49A: 807–834

Sugioka Y 1984 Transtrochanteric rotational osteotomy in the treatment of idiopathic and steroid-induced femoral head necrosis, Perthes' disease, slipped capital femoral epiphysis, and osteoarthritis of the hip: indication and results. Clinical Orthopaedics and Related Research 184: 12–23

Szypryt E P, Clement D A, Colton C L 1987 Open reduction or epiphysiodesis for slipped upper femoral epiphysis. Journal of Bone and Joint Surgery 69: 737–742

Chapter 27

The knee

M. F. Macnicol and A. M. Jackson

INTRODUCTION

The child's knee is vulnerable to mechanical problems, although the relative frequency of complaints varies with age. For example, instability of the knee in a child is more likely to result from a patello-femoral problem than from a torn meniscus. Isolated congenital abnormalities are often of minor degree, whereas more severe problems are usually found in association with lower limb dysplasias and syndromes. The stiff, congenital knee dislocation that is seen in Larsen's syndrome is an example. Because the growth plates above and below the knee make such a major contribution to longitudinal growth, trauma and infection at these sites in early life can have disastrous consequences, causing leg length discrepancy and deformity. Primary tumours found about the knee, both benign and malignant, are specific for age.

Referred pain from the hip and lumbar spine can sometimes be confusing; in such conditions as slipped capital femoral epiphysis, the first X-ray in the patient's file is invariably one of the knee. Further difficulty and confusion become apparent when a psychological cause for knee pain or bizarre gait is suspected. It is a mistake to focus so much on the knee as to forget the child and the parents. Great caution and diplomacy should be exercised in this area.

KNEE DEFORMITY

GENU RECURVATUM

Familial joint laxity is the common cause of symmetric physiological genu recurvatum, usually seen in girls. Such laxity may predispose the child to ligament sprains and strains and may be associated with patellar instability. When unilateral or severe, recurvatum is more likely to be pathological. One must distinguish between congruous hyperextension, anterior subluxation of the tibia and complete anterior dislocation of the tibia on the femur.

CONGENITAL DISLOCATION OF THE KNEE

Congenital dislocation of the knee is rare; unlike the analogous situation in the hip, it is very obvious. Invariably the child presents at birth in the extended breech position with the feet tucked up around the ears. At birth, the knee looks 'back to front', with an obvious anterior skin crease (Fig. 27.1) and the femoral condyles prominent posteriorly

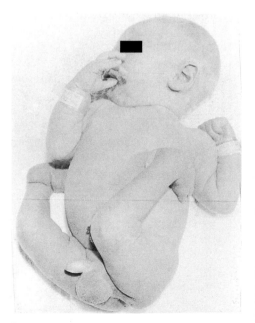

A

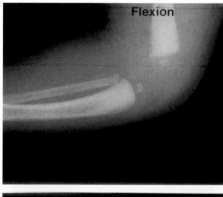

Flexion

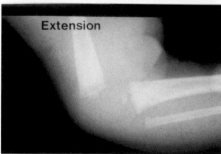

Extension

B

Figure 27.1 A Congenital subluxation and dislocation of the knee produce varying degrees of hyperextension. The knees look 'back to front'. Note the associated club foot deformities. **B** This knee hyperextends to nearly 90°, with subluxation of the tibia on the femur, and it flexes to nearly 90°. With such mobility, the outlook is good with conservative treatment.

because the tibia is displaced forwards. The hamstring tendons subluxate forwards in front of the axis of knee flexion, so that they become extensors of the recurvatum knee and potentiate the deformity.

Most commonly, this deformity is the result of intrauterine moulding of a normal foetus and perhaps this group is analogous to the more common phenomenon of neonatal instability of the hip in an otherwise normal child. In these babies, the knee reduces with a clunk as it is flexed, and the hamstrings and ilio-tibial band move to the flexor side of the knee axis. Usually the knees can be flexed 30–40° at birth. Treatment with anterior plaster slabs that gradually increase knee flexion is easy and rewarding, and usually the splintage can be discontinued at the age of 6 or 8 weeks, with the knee returning to a normal shape and no longer hyperextending.

The second group of patients with congenital dislocation of the knee are recalcitrant to such simple treatment and invariably there are other significant abnormalities affecting the knee and the child as a whole. The patella is often dysplastic and tethered proximally by a shortened fibrotic quadriceps tendon, and the suprapatellar pouch may be obliterated. Perhaps the dislocation is due to abnormalities of the cruciate ligaments (Katz et al 1967). Associated anomalies include developmental displacement of the hip, club foot, calcaneo-valgus and dislocation of the elbow. Arthrogryposis (Curtis & Fisher 1969) and a variety of other soft-tissue anomalies have been reported in patients with this condition (Fig. 27.2).

Skeletal traction is not advised for the recalcitrant case. Curtis & Fisher (1969) have given a good account of the operative technique, in which the quadriceps is lengthened, anterior capsulotomy is performed and the collateral ligaments are mobilised. The menisci usually have a normal appearance. The anterior oruciate ligament, if present, is often elongated and incompetent, in which case a procedure

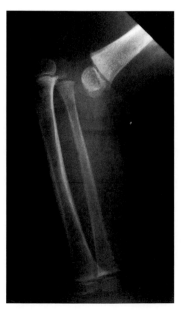

Figure 27.2 Congenital dislocation of the knee in a child with Larsen's syndrome.

to tighten this structure seems a sensible addition to the operation. Early treatment offers a greater chance of achieving reduction before secondary changes affect the tibia. Delay in treatment leads to a progressive sloping deformity of the back of the tibial plateau, and this makes it much more difficult to maintain stability at the time of open reduction.

A rare type of congenital snapping knee resulting from habitual forward subluxation of the tibia in extension has been described (Curtis & Fisher 1970, Ferris & Jackson 1990). The anterior cruciate ligament is usually deficient and the subluxation occurs at about 30° of flexion, with a disturbing clunk. These knees are usually part of a syndrome (e.g. Catel–Manzke or Larsen's syndrome), and the dysmorphic nature of the joints becomes obvious as the child gets older. Division of the ilio-tibial band, perhaps with re-routing, can be helpful. More common causes of snapping knee include patellar problems, discoid meniscus, unstable superior tibio-fibular joint, and osteochondromas.

SECONDARY GENU RECURVATUM

The hyperextended knee is a common feature of several neurological conditions. The usual mechanism is muscle imbalance, in which strong or spastic quadriceps overcome the action of weak hamstrings. Very occasionally, the hamstring deficit may be due to excessive and inappropriate release in patients with cerebral palsy

In poliomyelitis, hamstring paralysis in the presence of active quadriceps can produce stretching of the posterior soft tissues of the knee, and eventually a gross recurvatum that is extremely difficult to control without a calliper. Posterior soft-tissue reefing procedures are not successful, and probably the best surgical option at maturity is the anterior patellar bone block, fixing the patella to the upper tibia so that it acts as a 'doorstop' in extension.

In the totally flail knee, it is well to remember that slight hyperextension enables the patient to lock out and therefore stablise the knee when walking.

A second cause of neurological recurvatum arises when the knee is forced into hyperextension by an equinus foot, this is seen in cerebral palsy and sometimes after head injury. Early lengthening of the tendo-Achilles will prevent progression of knee deformity and improve gait.

Spina bifida patients with a neurological level of L3/4 can present with recurvatum, but this is seldom a problem unless the knee becomes stiff in extension: the stiff, extended knee causes problems with sitting as the child increases in size. A quadriceps tenotomy can achieve knee flexion with ease, but it should be remembered that the skin over the front of the stiff extended knee will not tolerate sudden stretching, and flexion should be gradually regained.

Growth plate damage on either side of the knee can cause genu recurvatum and the most common injury here is to the tibial tubercle, sometimes iatrogenic and sometimes as a result of trauma. In tibia recurvatum, the gain in hyperextension of the knee is equal to the loss in flexion. The correction of tibial recurvatum is best left until skeletal maturity, when a gradual distraction opening wedge anterior osteotomy using the Orthofix or Ilizarov frame gives good control (Choi et al 1999). The osteotomy should traverse from just below the tibial tubercle slanting upwards and outwards; in this way, patella height is not compromised by the surgical correction. (Fig. 27.3). This hemicallotasis technique avoids the need for bone graft, allows knee movement during correction, and gives finger-tip control as the correction proceeds. An alternative is to carry out an opening wedge proximal tibial osteotomy above the tubercle, if a lack of anterior tibial growth has produced a relative patella alta.

FLEXION DEFORMITY OF THE KNEE

During the first few days of life, a mild physiological flexion deformity of the knee is commonplace and rapidly resolves. More obvious and permanent fixed flexion may be seen at birth in arthrogryposis and spina bifida, whereas in cerebral palsy, myopathic and infective conditions, and juvenile idiopathic arthritis the deformity appears later. Serial plaster splints or slabs applied over the first few weeks of life can be effective, but attention needs to be paid to the skin, especially in children who have impaired sensation. The chief shortcoming of serial splintage is that, although the knee may indeed straighten, the correction is often spurious, with the knee hinging open at the back and the tibia impacting against the femoral condyles and failing to glide forwards in a normal and congruous fashion. To overcome this problem, reverse dynamic slings (Stein & Dickson 1975) have been used in haemophilia and are certainly applicable in the older child.

As a rule, however, the surgical correction of flexion deformity is by soft-tissue release in the child and by supracondylar osteotomy of the femur at maturity. When undertaking a posterior release of the knee, it is well to remember that the best surgical approach to the posterior capsule is from the sides. Invariably, the hamstrings must be lengthened, and sometimes the posterior cruciate ligament divided. The common peroneal nerve should always be identified, and one should be aware of the anatomy of the posterior tibial nerve and popliteal vessels. The nerves must be protected from rapid stretching by correcting the flexion deformity slowly. The same principle applies to the correction of severe valgus. In the younger child, soft-tissue release surgery can be supplemented by serial plasters, but once puberty is reached this seems to be much less effective.

In severe flexion deformity, the principle of shortening the bone when the soft tissues cannot be lengthened any further must sometimes be used. In this situation it is difficult to predict, after excision of perhaps 1 cm of bone from the lower femur, whether the resulting extension will occur at the knee joint itself, or only at the osteotomy site. Good results in treating difficult flexion deformities have been achieved using the Ilizarov frame. Perhaps this is a safer

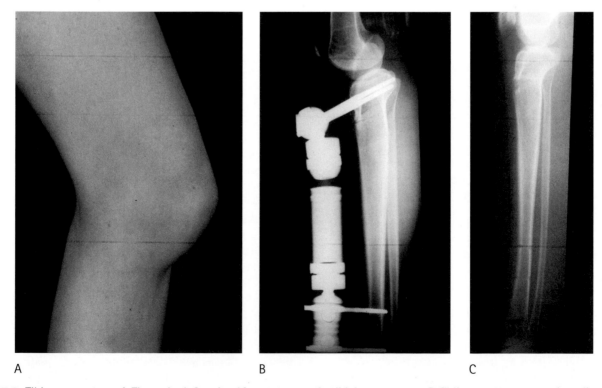

A　　　　　B　　　　　C

Figure 27.3 Tibia recurvatum. **A** The ugly deformity of post-traumatic tibial recurvatum. **B** Oblique osteotomy and application of orthofix. **C** Correction by hemicallotasis.

technique, although a careful eye must be kept on joint congruity. Some of the most severe fixed flexion deformities are seen in thrombocytopenia absent radius syndrome, and before surgery some of these children are so severely affected that they can only walk on their knees.

Congenital knee flexion deformities with popliteal web (pterygium syndrome) are difficult to treat because the neurovascular structures tend to lie in the free edge of the web and are resistant to stretching. Abnormal tendinous bands may run from the ischium to the os calcis and often other serious abnormalities coexist. Soft-tissue release and wound closure with Z-plasties can be helpful, and if a shortage of skin is anticipated it is wise to seek the help of a plastic surgeon in advance of surgery. Once correction of the flexion deformity has been achieved, further growth can lead to recurrence, so that a programme of postoperative splintage is often necessary.

Most flexion deformities are caused by tightness of posterior structures, but an intra-articular obstruction to extension can occur when an anterior cruciate insertion pull-off injury is not properly reduced and the avulsed intercondylar eminence blocks extension of the knee. Occasionally, a major osteochondritic lesion will also produce a chronic, pathological impingement. Early recognition and treatment of these two conditions is obviously important, but unfortunately they are sometimes ignored.

KNOCK KNEE AND BOW LEG

Salenius & Vankka (1975) have provided data on the normal alignment of the legs in childhood (Fig. 27.4). Babies are born with bow legs, and this generally persists through the toddler stage; by the age of 2 years, alignment is neutral and by 3 years physiological knock knee is common (Fig. 27.4). Bow leg may be accentuated by internal tibial torsion. The exaggerated case and 'the late corrector' can be a cause of great anxiety to parents.

Resolution or progression of the deformity can be monitored using photographs, by measuring the intercondylar and intermalleolar gaps, and by radiographs in severe cases. The gaps should be consistently measured in a standard fashion with the patient lying flat on the couch with legs extended. The femoral condyles should be touching when the intermalleolar gap is to be measured for knock knee, and *vice versa* for bow leg (Morley 1957).

Before making a diagnosis of physiological deformity, the clinician should always ask five questions in order to exclude the possibility of pathological deformity:

1. Is the child short or disproportioned, e.g. bone dysplasia/endocrine disturbance?
2. Is the deformity asymmetric or unilateral, e.g. growth plate damage caused by trauma or infection?
3. Is there a family history of a syndrome, e.g. Fanconi, Ellis van Creveld, familial hypophosphataemic rickets?
4. Is the deformity of such a degree that it is unlikely to

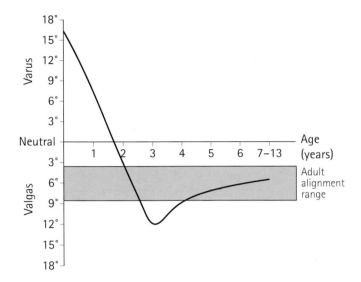

Figure 27.4 Graph constructed from the data of Salenius & Vankka (1975) to show the mean tibio–femoral angle in childhood, plotted against age. (Reproduced from Jackson 1990, with permission.)

be physiological? (E.g. progressive bow legs at age 3 years could well be Blount's disease; a knock knee deformity with an intermalleolar gap greater than 9 cm in an older child is suspicious.)
5. Is the deformity in step with the expected physiological pattern for age? (E.g. a newborn child with a knock knee deformity could not be regarded as normal.)

The most common diagnostic problem is the severe bow leg first seen between the age of 2 and 3 years: is this physiological, or is it Blount's disease? Measurement of the upper tibial metaphyseal–diaphyseal angle of Levene & Drennan (1982) helps with the prediction. The angle between the long axis of the tibia and a line joining the most distal ossified peak of the medial and lateral beaks of the tibial metaphysis is measured. An angle greater than 11° makes Blount's disease extremely likely. In the final analysis, all such patients require follow-up until the diagnostic dilemma is resolved. Many of these patients need firm advice to lose weight.

In the older child physiological knock knee rarely persists, but if the deformity is in excess of 10 cm within 2 years of skeletal maturity, stapling of the inner side of the lower femoral epiphysis is usually recommended. A standing film will demonstrate any obliquity of the knee joint and confirm that staples should be placed above rather than below the knee. Strong staples are required and experience has shown that a 10-cm gap will close in approximately 1 year. Obviously, there must be sufficient potential growth to effect the correction, and the staples must be removed as soon as the correction is achieved; failure to do so, with consequent conversion of a knock knee to a bow leg deformity, will cause immense dissatisfaction. Regular follow-up is therefore mandatory after any stapling procedure.

BLOUNT'S DISEASE (TIBIA VARA)

The aetiology of Blount's disease (Fig. 27.5) is uncertain. Possibly body weight, level of activity and angular deformity combine to exceed a critical point and, as a result, the posteromedial corner of the growth plate fails. In severe cases there is also a mild lateral bow to the femur. The condition is rare, with an estimated incidence of 0.05 per 1000 live births, although this may vary from population to population. The incidence is said to be greatest in children of West African origin and by comparison with white populations, these children are early walkers (Bateson 1968). However, Langenskiöld (1981) has reported a large series from Finland.

Juvenile/adolescent Blount's disease is first noticed between the ages of 6 and 13 years, and in some of these patients, trauma and low-grade infection may be incriminated. Progressive tibia vara may present during infancy or later childhood. A growth failure on the medial side of the upper tibial physis results in a sharp angular deformity at this site.

Infantile Blount's disease

The first definite sign that a physiological bow leg has progressed to Blount's disease is the radiological appearance of fragmentation of the medial metaphyseal beak. Once the diagnosis is established, the prognosis is poor if the condition is left untreated, and the deformity will inevitably increase, with stretching of the lateral ligaments and deformity of the medial side of joint. The early metaphyseal change progresses so that the medial end of the growth plate assumes a step-like appearance. Premature medial fusion as a result of formation of a medial bone bridge will follow, usually by the age of 6 years. Once a bone bridge has been formed, a simple corrective osteotomy will be incapable of

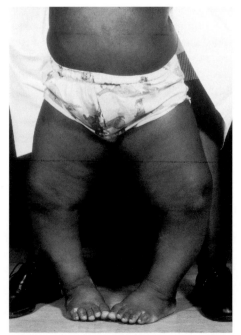

Figure 27.5 Note the internal tibial torsion in this 3½-year-old boy who has bilateral Blount's disease.

achieving lasting correction. In the severe case, the medial femoral condyle may overgrow and the medial meniscus hypertrophy in a vain attempt to counteract deformity.

Langenskiöld (1981) has shown that, if the patient is seen early, single osteotomy of the tibia and fibula, correcting the rotation in addition to the varus into the normal physiological valgus position, will usually effect a cure. Recurrence is most likely if a medial bone bar is missed, but even in the best hands these operations are somewhat unpredictable, and parents should be warned of this.

If a bone bar is demonstrated, its extent can be mapped out from information gleaned from a magnetic resonance imaging (MRI) scan. In patients younger than 10 years, an attempt should probably be made to excise the bone bridge, in addition to performing a corrective osteotomy. In those older than 10 years, corrective osteotomy and complete epiphysiodesis of the upper tibial growth plate may be advisable. The decision will be influenced if the deformity is unilateral. Limb length discrepancy may require correction by means of a contralateral proximal tibial epiphysiodesis.

In the late, neglected case, complex reconstruction with elevation of the medial plateau (Siffert 1982) combined with tibial osteotomy and lateral epiphysiodesis is indicated.

Adolescent Blount's disease

In adolescent patients, the deformity is usually unilateral and less severe than in infantile Blount's disease. Pain may precede deformity. Internal tibial torsion is less obvious, but shortening of up to 2 cm may be present. Corrective osteotomy with lateral epiphysiodesis is probably the most reliable method of achieving and maintaining correction. Leg length discrepancy is corrected by epiphysiodesis above and below the opposite, normal knee at the appropriate time.

AXIAL MALALIGNMENT

Axial or torsional deformity occurs commonly in the child and affects the whole limb, not just one joint or segment. The worst example is the so-called 'miserable malalignment' or 'triple deformity', in which there is excessive anteversion of the femoral neck, inward squinting patellae and compensatory external tibial torsion, often with pronated feet. Patello-femoral pain is common in these children, especially if they are keen on sport. If the pain is persistent, a lateral retinacular release may be appropriate in selected cases. Complex rotational osteotomies and realignment procedures are very rarely indicated.

SECONDARY BOW LEGS

Tibia vara in achondroplasia seldom requires treatment. Rickets of any type tends to cause bow leg rather than knock knee deformity. In nutritional rickets, correction of the diet is usually followed by spontaneous improvement of the angulation, but in resistant rickets the deformity may persist and require operation. These deformities are often complex, requiring osteotomies at more than one site. Metaphyseal dysplasia has a radiological appearance similar to that of rickets, but in these patients the biochemistry is normal.

Always consider the effect of osteotomies on the soft tissues. Correction of a mid-shaft deformity will lengthen the bone and shorten the soft tissues that span the concavity. Soft tissue release and tendon lengthening are therefore sometimes required, particularly when there has been relative shortening of a muscle–tendon unit of such a degree as to cause a contracture.

ANTERIOR KNEE PAIN

Much of the anterior knee pain seen in children is caused by overuse, especially in adolescence when adult demands are placed on a still-growing skeleton. An accompanying father in a tracksuit is sometimes a clue to excessive sporting aspirations and vicarious ambitions. In other patients, the symptoms are vague and unaccompanied by any positive physical sign. Sometimes adolescent girls who feel they should no longer suffer the indignity of organised physical activity use 'painful knees' as a convenient excuse to avoid it.

The anterior knee pain symptom complex has been well described (Insall 1982). In essence, the pain is worse when the patello-femoral joint is under load, as when descending stairs, and better at rest when the knee is held straight; the 'cinema' sign when pain is produced by prolonged sitting with the knee in the flexed position is often positive. Crepitus is a sign of variable significance. A thorough search for a proper diagnosis can be rewarding, but if the diagnosis remains obscure, treatment must be empirical.

It is convenient to consider the causes of anterior knee pain under the headings of 'distinct' and 'obscure'. The first group is made up mainly of focal pathological lesions, for which logical treatment can be applied and outcome predicted. The second group is a spectrum of conditions ranging from anterior knee pain of unknown cause through chondromalacia to dynamic problems of maltracking, subluxation and lateral hyperpression.

DISTINCT CAUSES OF ANTERIOR KNEE PAIN

Osgood–Schlatter disease

This condition is often seen in boys aged between 12 and 14 years. Less commonly, it is seen in girls and at a slightly younger age. The diagnosis is easy if the patient points with one finger precisely to the tibial tubercle and if the prominence is already obvious, making kneeling painful. The adult tendon is firmly anchored to bone by Sharpey's fibres, but in the growing child the anchorage is more tenuous (Fig. 27.6). Repeated micro-avulsion injuries accompanied by half-hearted fibro-osseous repair result in tubercle prominence. Very rarely, infection, trauma or an osteochondroma can masquerade as Osgood–Schlatter disease, so plain radiographs are advisable, especially in the unilateral case. The fragmented appearance of the tubercle is due to partial

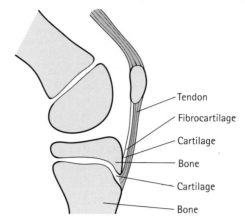

Figure 27.6 The tenuous anchorage of the patellar tendon in the immature skeleton. (Reproduced from Jackson 1994, with permission.)

Tendon
Fibrocartilage
Cartilage
Bone
Cartilage
Bone

separation of chondro-osseous fragments. Treatment is always conservative in the first instance, reducing activities to a level at which symptoms become manageable. Cast treatment is contraindicated because it causes greater disability and inconvenience than the condition itself. The natural history is for the symptoms to resolve within 1–2 years, leaving the prominent tubercle as a permanent marker of the condition. If symptoms remain troublesome into the mid-teens, radiographs may show an ossicle within the substance of the tendon adjacent to the tubercle. Operative removal of the ossicle is usually curative.

Sinding Larsen Johannsson disease

This occurs in the same age group of children, but the point of tenderness and pathology are located at the lower pole of the patella, and very occasionally at the upper pole also. The lateral radiograph of the patella may be normal, or there may be speckled calcification at the lower pole. Treatment is along the same lines as for Osgood–Schlatter disease.

Bipartite patellae

Bipartite patellae are common in childhood, often bilateral and usually regarded as variations of normal ossification. The two centres may proceed to fusion. Very rarely, in response to overuse or acute injury the synchondrosis may become painful and the site of local tenderness. There are three sites at which bipartite patellae are found and each site has its important soft-tissue attachment:

1. The distal pole of the patella – the patella tendon attachment.
2. The lateral margin of the patella – the lateral retinaculum attachment.
3. Superolateral pole – the vastus lateralis insertion.

The boy of approximately 12 years of age who presents with a bipartite lower pole of the patella and who complains of pain and tenderness is of particular interest because this presentation should perhaps be regarded as a sleeve fracture waiting to happen. Activities should be strictly curtailed. The fracture, when it does occur, is along the line of the synchondrosis (Fig. 27.7). The avulsed distal pole is always

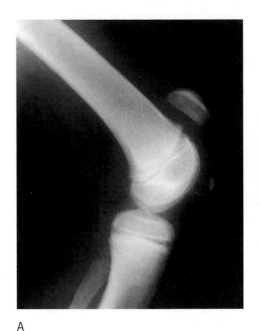 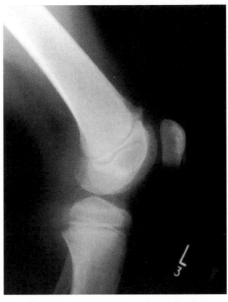

A   B

Figure 27.7 A Widely displaced sleeve fracture of the patella. B Inverted radiograph of the opposite knee, showing the bipartite lower pole. Presumably, separation can occur through the line of the synchondrosis.

much bigger than the radiographs suggest, and must be re-attached (Houghton & Ackroyd 1979).

Stress fractures

Stress fractures of the lower pole of the patella occur in spastic children with a flexed knee gait, and are a cause of pain and further deterioration in walking (Lloyd-Roberts et al 1985). These fractures cannot heal unless steps are taken to correct the fixed flexion deformity of the knees. Transverse stress fractures are also seen in athletes (Devas 1960). The line of a stress fracture passes vertically through the patella, at 90° to the patellar surface, whereas that of a synchondrosis or bipartite patella runs obliquely, and this may help to make the distinction. Histologically, the presence of callus is proof positive of a genuine stress lesion.

Osteochondritis dissecans

Osteochondritis dissecans of the patella is rare, but is occasionally seen in the second decade. The lesion is usually located in the distal half of the patella on the median ridge or medial facet. Studies of patello-femoral loading have demonstrated a contact band sweeping up from the inferior to superior aspects of the articular surface as the knee flexes from full extension to 90° of flexion (Goodfellow et al 1976); it is easy to understand why this localised lesion presents as a painful arc syndrome. Because of the considerable compression and shear forces that are transmitted through the patello-femoral joint, the prognosis for any kind of re-attachment procedure is guarded. Very rarely, osteochondritis dissecans will affect the trochlear groove.

Plicae

Plicae are found at four sites within the knee (Fig. 27.8). They are infolded shelves or partitions formed by the synovial lining of the joint and have a core of fibrous tissue. They are inconsistent, vary in size, and should be regarded as anatomical variants. Only rarely do they cause symptoms. The medial plica, in particular, has become a much overrated focus of attention and many innocent plicae have been removed for want of something better to do. If there is local tenderness at the correct site and perhaps a synovial snap between 30 and 60° of flexion, combined with arthroscopic findings of a frayed, swollen or fibrotic plica adjacent to an erosion on the femoral condyle, then the diagnosis should be regarded as genuine. Surgery in such cases may be rewarding (Johnson et al 1993).

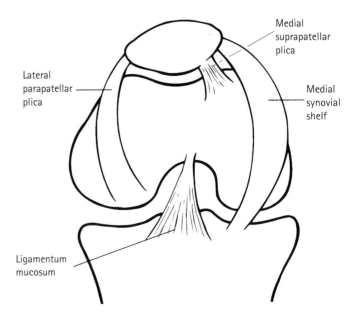

Figure 27.8 The sites of plicae in the knee. They are rarely of much consequence in the child.

Reflex sympathetic dystrophy

This condition presents as severe intractable pain, out of proportion to the original injury or much greater than one would expect after surgery. The knee joint is commonly involved, but the entire lower limb can be affected. Autonomic dysfunction is manifest by cyanosis or mottling of the skin, which is most easily seen when the legs are dependent. There may be a noticeable temperature difference between the affected area and the opposite side, in addition to hypersensitivity of the skin. In late cases, trophic changes involve the skin, the thigh muscle becomes wasted, and the knee joint becomes stiff.

The dysfunction leads to radiological osteoporosis. A three-phase technetium bone scan may be helpful in diagnosis, although less so in the younger patient.

Early diagnosis is important for successful treatment. The first line of treatment includes intensive physiotherapy, possibly on an inpatient basis. Transcutaneous nerve stimulation anti-inflammatory drugs, psychological help, behavioural therapy and, possibly, antidepressants have a role to play in selected patients. The next move is a therapeutic sympathetic block, for which a team approach with the pain specialist is essential. This problem is far from solved. It should be distinguished from focal myotonia, in which there is persistent and unremitting muscular contraction for example of the quadriceps, which may lead to a subluxed, recurvatum knee.

Severe bone dysplasia

This is seen, for example, in Stickler's syndrome (arthro-ophthalmopathy) and can lead to degenerative arthritic symptoms, even in the young.

Hoffa's syndrome

Sometimes, Hoffa's syndrome is diagnosed in patients who have an enlarged infrapatellar fat pad that bulges out on either side of the patella tendon when the knee is extended. Arthroscopically, if viewed from above, the fat pad may seem to protrude more than usual into the distended knee; fibro-fatty areas have also been described. It is not absolutely certain that the fat pad is ever pathological.

Other causes

Miscellaneous and rare causes of anterior knee pain include neuroma, foreign body – which in the child is usually a needle – and tumours. Whenever anterior knee pain is associated with an effusion, one should consider the causes of synovitis.

OBSCURE CAUSES OF ANTERIOR KNEE PAIN

A search for patello-femoral malalignment and the definition of any chondral damage are important, and often these two are related.

Malalignment

Patello-femoral malalignment can be studied clinically, radiologically and at arthroscopy. Several different patterns will become apparent. Obviously, the more extreme cases of maltracking will predispose to recurrent dislocation of the patella, and this can be particularly damaging to the patello-femoral joint. The clinical features to look for are varus or valgus angulation of the knee, recurvatum, triple deformity, patella alta and an increased Q angle (the angle formed by a line drawn from the anterior superior iliac spine of the pelvis to the centre of the patella and from it to the centre of the tibial tubercle (Fig. 27.9)). A Q angle greater than 10° is considered abnormal; however, the measurement is not a very reliable indicator of patella malalignment. Factors such as external tibial torsion may increase the Q angle, and when the patella is subluxed laterally in extension, a spurious normal reading will be obtained. Some advise measurement of the Q angle in slight flexion.

Lateral subluxation in extension is a phenomenon that is best demonstrated by clinical examination. The patient, sitting on the edge of the couch, extends the knee against gravity and, as the patella disengages from a position of bony stability in the trochlear groove, it shifts laterally. This physical sign is usually seen as the knee extends from 20° of flexion up to full extension, and may be associated with and inhibited by pain. This pattern of maltracking when mild may be a cause of anterior knee pain, and when more severe is quite often a feature of recurrent dislocation of the patella, especially in childhood and adolescence. The principal cause of this problem is malalignment of the quadriceps mechanism, which produces a bow-string effect between its mean point of origin and insertion as the knee is extended. The

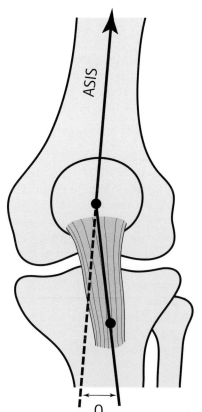

Figure 27.9 The angle between the quadriceps tendon and the patellar tendon forms the Q angle and exerts a valgus force on the patella. In practice, the Q angle is measured from the anterior superior iliac spine (ASIS) to the centre of the patella and then to the centre of the tibial tubercle. (Reproduced from Fox J, Del Pizzo W 1993 Patello-Femoral Joint. McGraw-Hill Inc, Health Professions Division. © The McGraw-Hill Companies Inc.)

lateral retinaculum is not tight and surgical correction, when indicated, must include some type of distal re-alignment. Most patients in this group, whose symptoms are limited to pain and the feeling of instability, respond to physiotherapy.

In contrast, maltracking in flexion is difficult to see clinically, but can be radiologically defined on skyline radiographs taken at 30, 60 and 90° of flexion. Fulkerson & Shea (1990) have emphasised the importance of tilt and subluxation, and have described three pathological patterns (Fig. 27.10). Tilt is produced by a tight lateral retinaculum and can be recognised by drawing Lauren's line (Lauren et al 1978) on the skyline views. This connects the tips of the medial and lateral femoral condyles as a reference line. Subluxation exists when the patella moves laterally from its central position in the groove. After a radiological study of this nature, the clinician should be able to recognise subluxation, subluxation with tilt, and tilt alone, and distinguish them from normal.

Patellar tracking can be studied arthroscopically. In the distended knee, the patella should settle into the trochlear groove at 45° of knee flexion.

Chondral damage

Chondromalacia patellae remains a difficult subject. The cause may be idiopathic, post-traumatic or secondary to maltracking. The term describes a pathological lesion of articular cartilage which, when mild, may be reversible, but when severe merges with osteoarthritis. As chondromalacia is most often seen on the medial facet of the patella and osteoarthritis on the lateral, it is concluded that the one does not necessarily lead to the other. As with osteoarthritis, the symptoms are not always proportional to the macroscopic appearance. Standard radiographs may appear normal when the malacic changes are relatively advanced. MRI scanning can be helpful, but the most valuable assessment is arthroscopic, when one should bear in mind that malacic change on the odd facet on the medial edge of the patella is a normal finding.

A modified Outerbridge classification (1961) will suit the arthroscopist:

- Grade I: closed disease. The articular surface is intact. There may be a slightly blistered appearance, or a soft 'boggy' feel when the area is probed with the hook.
- Grade II: open disease. The probe will now reveal fissures that may or may not be obvious at first sight.
- Grade III: widespread fibrillation or a 'cauliflower' appearance.
- Grade IV: the fibrillation is full thickness, and the erosive changes extend down to bone, which may be exposed.

The size of the lesion should also be recorded, using the hook of the probe as a measure.

Management

Obscure anterior knee pain is best managed with a trial of conservative treatment for 4–6 months. An avoidance of overuse should be combined with a programme of isometric and inner-range quadriceps exercises. Patellar mobilisation may help to stretch the lateral retinaculum and the ilio-tibial band. Taping, a patellar brace, and orthoses for the pronated foot can also be helpful.

Surgery should never be performed in the absence of demonstrable abnormality. When a procedure is indicated, the choice lies between the correction of maltracking if this has been demonstrated, a local operation to repair or improve the articular surface of the patella, or tubercle advancement aimed at reducing load on the patello-femoral joint. Re-alignment procedures involving the tibial tubercle should never be performed before skeletal maturity because of the risk of producing genu recurvatum. Patellectomy is indicated only very rarely in the adolescent, when the symptoms are severe and the articular surface of the patella is severely damaged over a wide area.

PATELLAR DISLOCATION AND INSTABILITY

In the younger child, recurrent dislocation is usually associated with an underlying dysplasia of the patella and condylar surfaces. There is frequently a positive family history and sometimes the instability is associated with a neuromuscular weakness or syndrome (e.g. nail-patella, Down's, or Marfan's syndrome). It is a curious paradox that the more obvious the problem, the less the symptoms.

Acute dislocation is more common in the adolescent. In non-contact injuries, the mechanism is a valgus, external rotation force on the knee and in addition to rupture of the medial retinaculum, MRI scans frequently show damage to the medial ligament and bone bruising of the lateral femoral condyle. Direct injuries to the knee often involve greater force and the 'at risk' factors predisposing to dislocation may be less obvious. In both groups, osteochondral fractures are common.

The standard classification of acute, recurrent, habitual and congenital dislocation of the patella simply state how often the dislocation occurs, and are no help at all in planning surgery. Of much greater importance is a study of the

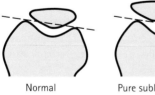

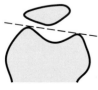

Normal · Pure subluxation · Subluxation + tilt · Pure tilt

Figure 27.10 The concept of tilt, subluxation/tilt and subluxation as different entities.

dynamics of patellar tracking, and clear definition of the factors that predispose to dislocation in each individual case. In the absence of a major maltracking problem, a conservative approach is usually the first line of treatment. Surgery is likely to be required for chronic problems.

CONGENITAL DISLOCATION

Because the entire quadriceps mechanism has dislocated laterally, children with this condition tend to present with knee flexion deformity and a tendency towards valgus and external rotation of the tibia. There are likely to be other less obvious congenital abnormalities of the knee, including patella alta, severe dysplasia of the femoral groove, discoid menisci and absent cruciates. There may also be other abnormalities to suggest a more generalised skeletal dysplasia, and walking will be delayed. The treatment of these knees is open to some debate because, obviously, function cannot be made normal. Some have advocated that the more severe cases should be left alone. Familial cases with prominent dislocation have been noted to function fairly well over a long period if left untreated (Robinson et al 1998).

However, neglect can lead to an increase in deformity, and if walking is the goal an aggressive approach is justified (Goa et al 1990). The operations tend to be *ad hoc* procedures, depending upon the findings. Tight lateral bands (Jeffreys 1963) are invariably found, and an extensive lateral release is the first requirement. The vastus lateralis muscle must be slid proximally along the rectus tendon. Once the patella can be centralised in extension, the knee flexion test must be performed. As a rule, it is impossible to maintain the patella in the groove with increasing flexion until the contracted quadriceps mechanism has been lengthened, usually by a rectus snip. The medial structures are double-breasted over the patella with advancement of the oblique fibres of vastus medialis, and a Roux–Goldthwaite procedure is performed distally by re-routing the lateral half of the patella tendon medially and fixing it under the pes anserinus. Staple fixation is advisable, as loss of tension in the transposed patellar tendon is a recognised cause of failure. A Campbell sling may be required to reinforce the medial side. Significant external rotation can be controlled by a pes anserinus tendon transfer.

ACUTE DISLOCATION

Acute dislocation can be difficult to diagnosis if it is a momentary event with spontaneous reduction. In such a case the management is that of an acute haemarthrosis. Plain radiographs should always include a skyline view, to search for an osteochondral fracture (Fig. 27.11) and investigations must recruit an MRI scan or arthroscopic assessment. After acute dislocation of the patella, patients can do well with conservative treatment alone in perhaps 50% of cases. The exact rate of recurrence after acute dislocation is difficult to estimate, because there is such wide variation reported in the literature.

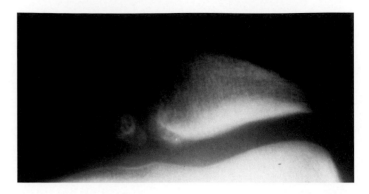

Figure 27.11 An avulsion fracture from the medial border of the patella is indicative of previous patella dislocation.

Patients with established recurrent dislocation have an increased incidence of osteoarthritis. A case has been made for acute repair of the medial retinaculum and medial patello-femoral ligament, sometimes with added lateral release, in a selected group of children who are considered to be 'at risk' of recurrent dislocation. At risk features include minimal precipitating trauma, ligamentous laxity, a positive family history, maltracking in the opposite knee, a Wiberg III patella, and patellar subluxation or tilt seen on the skyline view after reduction. Re-dislocation is more likely if high athletic demands are placed on the knee, and in the overweight patient.

RECURRENT AND HABITUAL DISLOCATION

These two variants are impossible to separate, because the underlying cause of habitual dislocation may be exactly the same as that of recurrent dislocation, only more severe. For example, some patients with extreme lateral subluxation of the patella in extension will present as habitual dislocation of the patella. In these patients, if the patella is nudged into the trochlear groove by the examiner at the beginning of flexion, tracking will proceed in a normal fashion until the patient extends the knee and the patella flips laterally at the point of disengagement.

Generalised joint laxity (Carter 1960) and a family history of patello-femoral problems are common in those with habitual and recurrent dislocation. Abnormalities of the knee itself are often discussed under the headings of soft-tissue problems, bony abnormalities and malalignment. The soft-tissue abnormalities include genu recurvatum and a deficient vastus medialis muscle. Sometimes the vastus medialis can be inhibited, and biofeedback techniques will be helpful in the conservative management of the less severe case. Malalignment includes those with excessive anteversion of the femoral neck, external torsion of the tibia and a Q angle greater than 10°. The bony abnormalities include patella alta, a shallow trochlear groove, and flattening of the normal triangular cross section of the patella. Genu valgum occasionally contributes to malalignment; if this is the case, corrective osteotomy should precede any soft-tissue realignment procedure, which may then sometimes become unnecessary.

Medial subluxation and dislocation are extremely rare and are usually the result of inappropriate or excessive lateral release and distal realignment.

The diagnosis of recurrent lateral subluxation can be subtle, and is easily confused with a torn medial meniscus (Macnicol 1995). The child presents with episodes of the knee giving way without effusions and is often unaware that the patella is unstable. Discomfort is localised over the medial retinaculum and medial fat pad. The apprehension sign is positive and patellar manipulation is painful. There may be a history of problems with the other knee.

Complete dislocation of the patella is easier to diagnose, because the knee is locked in flexion, with the patella standing proud on the lateral aspect of the joint. The morbidity of dislocation varies. A dislocation that produces acute pain and requires 3 or 4 weeks of rehabilitation is quite different from a momentary displacement with symptoms that have worn off in 10 minutes. Minor symptoms in sportsmen may assume major proportions because their demands and expectations are greater. Three groups of recurrent instability can be distinguished.

Lateral subluxation of the patella in extension

This condition (Dandy 1971) is the most common maltracking problem associated with recurrent dislocation in childhood and adolescence. The physical sign is the knee extension test against gravity, when the patella disengages and shifts laterally, sometimes producing pain and a click. The principal cause is malalignment of the quadriceps, producing a bow-string effect between its main origin and insertion. A few children with this condition walk with the knee flexed, to avoid the position of patellar instability. Surgical treatment must include some sort of distal realignment. Lateral release alone is illogical and ineffective, as the lateral retinaculum is loose and redundant and not the cause of the lateral displacement (Fig. 27.12). It must be emphasised that the problem in these patients is the unstable

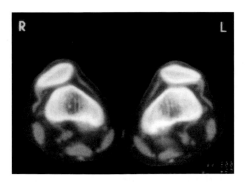

Figure 27.12 Obvious lateral subluxation of the patella in extension. The lateral retinaculum is loose and redundant, and therefore lateral release is illogical treatment for this form of maltracking.

engagement of the patella in the trochlear groove. Mild patella alta and perhaps a Wiberg III patella are common in this group, but otherwise the bony anatomy is often satisfactory. For these reasons, standard skyline radiographs are usually unhelpful. If patella alta is severe it should be investigated, and when tibial tubercle surgery is indicated it is best to wait until skeletal maturity.

Lateral subluxation in flexion

This form of instability is more difficult to identify on clinical examination, and here the skyline radiograph assumes great importance. It will show subluxation or tilt and inform about the patellar shape, the sulcus angle and the joint space (Carson et al 1984). In this group of patients, the lateral retinaculum is invariably tight and lateral release alone may cure moderate symptoms that have failed to respond to physiotherapy.

Dislocation with no evidence of patellar maltracking

Dislocations of this nature are rare. Such patients often have ligamentous laxity, a reduced sulcus angle, and excessive external tibial rotation, which displaces the tibial tubercle laterally. These patients often respond to physiotherapy and may be helped by a brace worn during sporting activities.

TREATMENT

For many patients, the initial management should be conservative with a well supervised exercise programme, in order to develop good quadriceps bulk and muscle tone. If this programme fails, or if the child presents with severe malalignment or subluxation and with repeated episodes of disability, surgery will be necessary.

Surgery has a number of drawbacks. It may leave an ugly scar; it may not altogether prevent subluxations or dislocations from occurring; furthermore, because of the complication of growth plate damage, the tibial tubercle is a 'no go area' in the skeletally immature patient. However, most operations yield better than 80% good results. Many procedures have been designed to stabilise the patella. The three main components are lateral release, medial reefing (Insall et al 1976), and distal realignment, with occasional additional procedures to correct patella alta and to modify the bony anatomy (Fig. 27.13).

Lateral retinacular release may be performed arthroscopically, openly through a small lateral incision, or through the main incision if a major procedure is being performed. The chief complication is swelling and haemarthrosis as a result of bleeding from the lateral superior geniculate artery. Occasionally, lateral subluxation is converted to medial instability because the release is too extreme and has detached the vastus lateralis from the patella. The Roux–Goldthwaite distal re-alignment is appropriate for use in children because it does not disturb the tibial tubercle. This operation can fail if the transposed limb of the patellar

DISCOID MENISCUS

The discoid lateral meniscus occurs in about 5% of the population as judged in a cadaver study (Noble & Hamblen 1975) and this incidence seems slightly greater than clinical experience would now suggest from arthroscopy. A much greater incidence has been reported in the Japanese (Ikeuchi 1982). Discoid lateral menisci are often bilateral, and it is most unusual to see this abnormality on the medial side of the joint. The distinguishing features of a discoid lateral meniscus are its shape and posterior ligamentous attachments. A classification of the abnormality based on that of Watanabe et al (1979) is suggested:

1. *Incomplete discoid meniscus*. This is the mildest form, which is simply a wider form of the normal lateral meniscus. The tapered free margin is interposed between the femoral and tibial condyles, but it does not completely cover the tibial plateau.
2. *Complete discoid meniscus* appears as a biconcave disc or slab with a rolled medial edge, and totally covers the lateral tibial plateau, cushioning the lateral femoral condyle. The complete discoid meniscus does have a stable attachment to the tibia posteriorly. In addition, the anterior menisco-femoral ligament of Humphry and the posterior menisco-femoral ligament of Wrisberg embrace the posterior cruciate ligament and insert into the medial femoral condyle.
3. *The Wrisberg type* of meniscus has the same shape as the complete discoid meniscus, but its posterior ligament attachment is by the menisco-femoral ligaments alone. The normal tibial attachment of the posterior horn of the meniscus is missing, so that this type of meniscus is attached anteriorly to the tibia and posteriorly to the femur. This renders the posterior horn unstable and liable to attrition, and as the knee extends from the flexed position the poorly attached meniscus may sublux into the intercondylar area with a jolt. This is the usual explanation for the classical presenting symptom of the 'clunking' knee found in some patients. This 'clunk', however, is variable and often the presenting symptoms may be vague pain with catching or an effusion. An MRI scan will demonstrate the discoid anomaly clearly and it can be confirmed at arthroscopy if symptoms justify this procedure.

If a diagnosis of discoid meniscus is suspected, the first arthroscopy portal should be anteromedial and the rolled edge can be seen and examined with a hook. If the posterior horn is rounded and can be elevated from the tibia, the Wrisberg configuration is confirmed, even though it may be difficult to see the ligament of Wrisberg itself.

A discoid meniscus should not be removed simply because it exists; treatment of the symptomatic discoid meniscus depends upon its type (Dickhaut & Delee 1982). In the symptomatic Wrisberg type, a complete lateral meniscectomy is advocated as this anomaly is so severe that it cannot be converted to normal. If, however, the posterior horn is stable and a tear is seen, usually involving the inferior surface, it may be possible to trim the meniscus down to a more normal shape (Bellier et al 1989). In a difficult case, distinction between complete and Wrisberg types of discoid menisci may not be possible until trimming has commenced.

SYNOVIAL PATHOLOGY

Synovial chondromatosis in childhood is extremely rare, and when it does occur there may be hundreds of tiny cartilaginous 'rice' particles within the knee (Carey 1983). As these loose bodies are not ossified, the diagnosis will not be made radiologically and the multiple tiny loose bodies may come as a something of a surprise at arthroscopy. They must all be washed out; repeat arthroscopy is sometimes required. The synovial metaplasia may well settle down with time, as it is a curiosity in the older patient that the loose bodies are always of the same generation: immature rice particles are not encountered alongside established and mature loose bodies.

Children are prone to fall on their knees, and whereas metallic *foreign bodies* such as needles are obvious on X-ray, penetrating bits of wood and other radiographically less obvious material may gain access to the knee. In the acute stage, air may be seen within the joint, and this can give a clue to the depth of injury. In the chronic case, a low-grade infective arthritis resembling tuberculosis may occur.

An *acute and transient synovitis* is quite common in the juvenile knee as a response to trauma, and one should also always consider the possibility of missed patellar instability. Synovitis may accompany influenza and other viral illnesses. A chronic swollen knee, often with some fixed flexion, is seen in juvenile idiopathic arthritis, and one should not forget chronic infections such as tuberculosis. When faced with a knee that is warm, boggy and intermittently swollen in a child who may have juvenile arthritis, it is important to examine the child completely. All other joints should be examined for reduced range of movement and synovitis, and the spine should be assessed, together with the sterno-clavicular joints. Slit-lamp examination of the eyes is important, and the thyroid, nails and feet should not be forgotten. Appropriate blood tests should be carried out (see Ch. 12). A second opinion from a rheumatologist is essential, particularly if drug therapy is being considered. In selected cases intra-articular injection of a steroid preparation such as triamcinolone hexacetamide is indicated. Intermittent arthroscopic irrigation and late synovectomy with a powered shaver may also provide symptomatic relief.

Pigmented villo-nodular synovitis is an inflammatory process of unknown cause, although an autoimmune reaction seems likely. The knee is painful, swollen and stiff. Locking and crepitus may be present if the synovial proliferation is exuberant. The synovium is brown, thickened and nodular. Subchondral erosions develop secondary to the release of proteolytic enzymes, and these erosions are seen on both sides of the joint. Histological examination reveals multinuclear giant cells and deposits of haemosiderin, which give the tissue its colour. The treatment is synovectomy.

POPLITEAL CYSTS

Popliteal cysts are twice as common in boys and usually present before the child has reached the age of 10 years, as an asymptomatic fluctuant swelling just to the medial side of the popliteal fossa (Fig. 27.15). If there is doubt about the cystic nature of the lesion, transillumination will settle the issue; this technique is a great deal less expensive than ultrasound and MRI scanning, which are unnecessary. The cyst is probably the semimembranosus bursa; on examination, it is better felt in extension that in flexion. The knee is otherwise normal. Dinham (1975) has drawn attention to the very high recurrence rate after surgical removal, and the natural tendency of these cysts to disappear spontaneously. Operation without very good reason is unjustified and reassurance is all that is required.

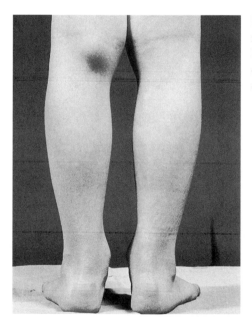

Figure 27.15 A semimembranosus bursa usually disappears in later childhood.

SEPTIC ARTHRITIS (See Ch. 9)

Septic arthritis should be recognised and drained early if articular damage is to be minimised. The diagnosis depends upon the history, the appearance of the child who is pyrexial and unwell, and a swollen and tender knee that is too painful to move. Immunodeficiency and sickle-cell disease should not be forgotten, and the vaccination history should be checked. The initial radiograph is usually unhelpful, but may show a pre-existing osteomyelitic focus. Late in the disease, articular changes may become apparent. Arthroscopy offers a most effective method of obtaining synovial fluid and tissue for bacteriological culture and histological review. The joint can be thoroughly inspected and irrigated, and the procedure produces only a minor degree of morbidity.

Although at first the knee should be splinted and the child rested in bed, gentle movement of the knee and protected weight bearing should soon be encouraged. Systemic antibiotics remain the mainstay of early treatment, depending upon culture and the sensitivity of the organism identified. *Staphylococcus aureus* remains the most common organism, and good initial cover for both staphylococci and streptococci would be flucloxacillin 200 mg/kg per day (given as four equal doses) and ceftriaxone 80 mg/kg per day.

TUMOURS

Tumours in childhood show a predilection for the knee, perhaps because the knee is frequently injured. One should therefore have a low threshold for requesting X-rays, especially when the history is short and the symptoms unexplained. As cancer is the second most common cause of death in childhood, bone and soft-tissue tumours are of considerable concern, particularly as their presentation may be mistaken for other conditions (see Ch. 13).

Gebhardt et al (1990) reviewed 199 cases of tumours affecting the knee in childhood and found that neoplasia was more common the older the child. Benign bone tumours comprise 50% of referrals, and the most common lesion is the osteochondroma, which can cause a variety of problems. A large posterior swelling will limit knee flexion, whereas medial and lateral excrescences can be a cause of snapping knee and attrition of the hamstring tendons. Multiple lesions may be associated with a growth disturbance and consequent knee deformity of a degree that requires correction. Large lesions may be painful because they are always being knocked during games.

The risk of malignant change in an osteochondroma is probably no more than 1%, and is not in itself considered a reason for excision. Other lesions, in decreasing order of frequency are: non-ossifying fibroma, chondroblastoma, osteoid osteoma, aneurysmal bone cyst, giant-cell tumour, chondromyxoid fibroma, simple bone cyst and fibrous dysplasia. Osteosarcoma and Ewing's tumour are the principal malignant tumours, and infiltrative conditions such as leukaemia and histiocytosis can occasionally affect the knee. Soft-tissue tumours should always be considered as potentially malignant but, fortunately, they are rare and easy to distinguish from popliteal and meniscal cysts.

LIGAMENT PROBLEMS

Congenital absence of the anterior cruciate ligament is rare and usually seen only in association with lower limb dysplasias such as congenital short femur or short tibia with dysplastic fibula and absent lateral rays of the foot (Thomas et al 1985). On X-ray, the absence of tibial spines gives rise to a rectangular upper tibial epiphysis. Perhaps because the problem is present from birth, patients tolerate the instability surprisingly well, but if a leg lengthening procedure is undertaken great caution is required to prevent the problem becoming worse.

Collateral ligament injury is rare in childhood because 'the ligaments are stronger than the bones'. A typical injury that may cause the ligaments to rupture in an adult will more probably result in a fracture separation through the lower femoral, or rarely the upper tibial, growth plates in childhood. The proximal tibial epiphysis is relatively protected by the collateral ligaments, which cross the growth plate, giving support, whereas the femoral growth plate is more vulnerable.

Mid-ligament disruption of the anterior cruciate ligament is encountered with increasing frequency throughout adolescence (Lipscomb & Anderson 1986), often in association with meniscal injury. This no doubt reflects a gradual increase in the sporting activities and ambitions of the young. Adolescent boys, who by their nature have reached the age of non-compliance, do not do well with conservative treatment. Fear of damaging the physis led to a trial of extra-articular and non-anatomical reconstructive operations, which were not rewarding. A hamstring reconstruction technique using standard bone tunnels is certainly permissible in the 2 or 3 years before skeletal maturity, as long as the graft fits tightly in the tunnels. Obviously, bone blocks and staples astride the growth plate must be avoided. Anterior cruciate reconstruction is especially important if a meniscal repair is to be protected.

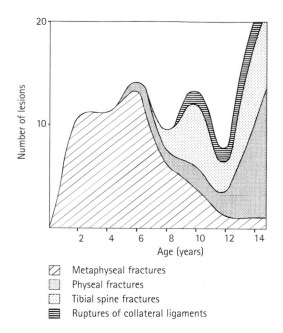

Figure 27.16 The incidence of fracture types related to age.

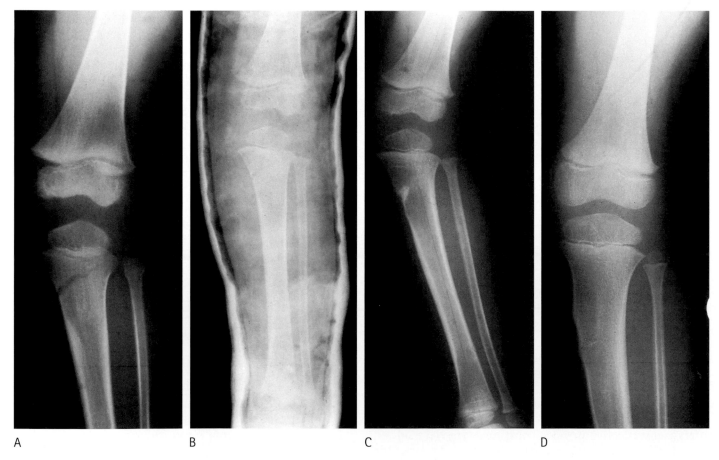

A   B   C   D

Figure 27.17 Metaphyseal fracture of childhood. A Typical fracture. B Fracture reduced and held in a cast. C Delayed valgus deformity at 9 months. D Spontaneous correction with no treatment at 2½ years.

FRACTURES

Injuries of the knee become more common as the child grows. Metaphyseal and buckle fractures give way to greenstick fractures or complete displacements in the older child (Fig. 27.16) Fracture sites, in decreasing order of frequency are:

- proximal tibial metaphysis
- tibial intercondylar eminence
- distal femur (metaphysis and growth plate)
- tibial growth plate and tuberosity.

Of particular interest in the child are the sleeve fracture described in the section on anterior knee pain, bipartite patella, the avulsed insertion of the anterior cruciate ligament, which must always be accurately reduced and fixed if necessary, and the oblique upper metaphyseal fracture, which may lead to delayed valgus deformity as growth proceeds in the 18 months after injury (Fig. 27.17) (Jackson & Cozen 1971). This deformity may improve spontaneously with the further passage of time (Zionts & MacEwan 1986).

PSYCHOSOMATIC SYMPTOMS

No discussion of knee pain is complete without alerting the reader to the problem of psychosomatic pain. In a typical example, pain and disability are completely out of proportion to a minor event or trauma that supposedly triggered the onset of dysfunction. The problem is seen especially at the start of adolescence and the disability may be considerable. The patient may present in a wheelchair, unable to walk and sometimes with an entire term's absence from school. These children must be scrutinised extremely carefully and thoroughly investigated, because the diagnosis of psychosomatic symptoms is one of exclusion.

Inconsistent features are often a clue to diagnosis. An entirely different range of joint movements may be found when the patient is lying horizontal as opposed to when they are standing. The limping child, when asked to walk backwards, may not be able to respond in an appropriate way. Skin hypersensitivity is often a feature, and this can make direct palpation and examination of the joint almost impossible. The possibility of a dysfunctional family background should not be ignored. Although time consuming, it is usually easiest to bring these children into hospital for a team approach involving a physiotherapist, child psychiatrist, pain specialist, neurologist and rheumatologist as required. Video techniques can be useful in showing a young patient the sort of image that they are projecting at this sensitive time in their development. Hysterical patients will have great difficulty in controlling their symptoms, whereas others are more manipulative. Factitious bruising (Fig. 27.18) and the perpetuation of symptoms are seen in those for whom this behaviour may have some perceived advantage.

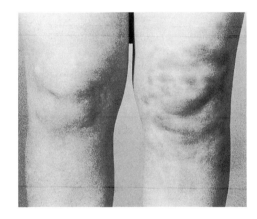

Figure 27.18 Factitious bruising that exactly marks out the anterior window of a canvas knee splint.

REFERENCES AND FURTHER READING

Aichroth P M 1971 Osteochondritis dissecans of the knee: a clinical survey. Journal of Bone and Joint Surgery 53B: 440–447

Arnoczky S P, Warren R F 1982 Microvasculature of the human meniscus. American Journal of Sports Medicine 10: 90–95

Baker R F, Carroll N, Dewar P, Hall J E 1972 Semitendinosus tenodesis for recurrent dislocation of the patella. Journal of Bone and Joint Surgery 54B: 508–517

Bateson E M 1968 The relationship between Blount's disease and bow legs. British Journal of Radiology 41: 107–114

Bellier G, Dupont J Y, Larrain M, Caudrone C, Carlioz H 1989 Lateral discoid menisci in children. Journal of Arthroscopic and Related Surgery 5: 52–56

Caffey J, Madell S H, Roter C, Morales P 1958 Ossification of the distal femoral epiphysis. Journal of Bone and Joint Surgery 40A: 647–654

Cahill B R, Berg B C 1983 99m-Technetium phosphate compound joint scintigraphy in the management of juvenile osteochondritis dissecans of the femoral condyles. American Journal of Sports Medicine 11: 329–335

Carey R P L 1983 Synovial chondromatosis of the knee in childhood. Journal of Bone and Joint Surgery 65B: 444–447

Carson W G, James S L, Larson R L, Singer K M, Winternitz W W 1984 Patello femoral disorders: physical and radiographic evaluation. Part II. Clinical Orthopaedics 185: 178–186

Carter C O 1960 Recurrent dislocation of the patella and of the shoulder. Journal of Bone and Joint Surgery 42B: 721–727

Choi I H, Chung C Y, Cho J J, Park S S 1999 Correction of genu recurvatum by the Ilizarov method. Journal of Bone and Joint Surgery 81B: 769–774

Curtis B H, Fisher R L 1969 Congenital hyperextension with anterior subluxation of the knee. Journal of Bone and Joint Surgery 51A: 255–258

Curtis B H, Fisher R L 1970 Heritable congenital tibiofemoral subluxation: clinical features and surgical treatment. Journal of Bone and Joint Surgery 52A: 1104–1114

Dandy D J 1971 Recurrent subluxation of the patella on extension of the knee. Journal of Bone and Joint Surgery 53B: 483–487

De Haven K E, Hales W 1981 Peripheral meniscal repair: an alternative to meniscectomy. Orthopaedic Transactions 5: 399–400

Devas M B 1960 Stress fractures of the patella. Journal of Bone and Joint Surgery 42B: 71–74

Dickhaut S C, Delee J C 1982 The discoid lateral meniscus syndrome. Journal of Bone and Joint Surgery 64A: 1068–1073

Dinham J M 1975 Popliteal cysts in children. Journal of Bone and Joint Surgery 57B: 69–71

Enneking W F 1990 Clinical musculoskeletal pathology, 3rd edn. University of Florida Press, Gainsville, Florida, p. 166

Fairbank H A 1933 Osteochondritis dissecans. British Journal of Surgery 21: 67–82

Fairbank T J 1948 Knee joint changes after meniscectomy. Journal of Bone and Joint Surgery 30B: 664–670

Ferris B D, Jackson A M 1990 Congenital snapping knee (habitual anterior subluxation of the tibia in extension). Journal of Bone and Joint Surgery 72B: 453–456

Ferris B, Walker C, Jackson A M, Kirman E 1991 The orthopaedic management of hypophosphataemic rickets. Journal of Paediatric Orthopaedics 11: 367–373

Fulkerson J P, Shea K P 1990 Disorders of patello femoral alignment. Journal of Bone and Joint Surgery 72A: 1424–1429

Gebhardt M C, Ready J E, Mankin H J 1990 Tumours about the knee in children. Clinical Orthopaedics and Related Research 255: 86–110

Goa G X, Lee E H, Bose K 1990 Surgical management of congenital and habitual dislocation of the patella. Journal of Pediatric Orthopaedics 10: 255–260

Goodfellow J, Hungerford D S, Woods C 1976 Patello femoral joint mechanics and pathology 2: chondromalacia patellae. Journal of Bone and Joint Surgery 58B: 291–299

Houghton G R, Ackroyd C E 1979 Sleeve fractures of the patella in children. Journal of Bone and Joint Surgery 61B: 165–168

Ikeuchi H 1982 Arthroscopic treatment of discoid lateral meniscus: technique and long-term results. Clinical Orthopaedics and Related Research 167: 19–28

Insall J 1982 Current Concepts Review: patellae pain. Journal of Bone and Joint Surgery 64A: 147–151

Insall J, Falvo K A, Wise P W 1976 Chondromalacia patellae. Journal of Bone and Joint Surgery 58A: 1–8

Jackson A M 1990 Knock knee and bow leg. Current Orthopaedics 4: 47

Jackson A M 1992 Knock knee and bow leg in children. In: Aichroth P M, Dilworth-Cannon W Jr (eds) Knee surgery current practice. Martin Dunitz Ltd, London, p 509

Jackson A M 1994 Anterior knee pain. Current Orthopaedics 8: 84

Jackson D W, Cozen L 1971 Genu Valgum as a complication of proximal tibial metaphyseal fracture in children. Journal of Bone and Joint Surgery 53A: 1571–1578

Jeffreys T E 1963 Recurrent dislocation of the patella due to abnormal attachment of the iliotibial tract. Journal of Bone and Joint Surgery 45B: 740–743

Johnson D P, Eastwood D, Witherow P J 1993 Symptomatic synovial plicae of the knee. Journal of Bone and Joint Surgery 75A: 1485–1495

Katz M P, Grogono B J S, Soper K C 1967 The aetiology and treatment of congenital dislocation of the knee. Journal of Bone and Joint Surgery 49B: 112–120

Kelly M A, Flock T J, Kimmel J A et al 1991 MR imaging of the knee: clarification of its role. Arthroscopy 7: 78–85

King D 1936 The healing of semilunar cartilages. Journal of Bone and Joint Surgery 18B: 333–342

Langenskiöld A 1981 Tibia vara: osteochondrosis deformans tibiae. Clinical Orthopaedics and Related Research 158: 77–82.

Lauren C A, Levasque H P, Dussault R, Labelle H, Peides J P 1978 The abnormal lateral patello femoral angle. Journal of Bone and Joint Surgery 60A: 55–60

Levene A M, Drennan I C 1982 Physiological bowing and tibia vara. Journal of Bone and Joint Surgery 64A: 1158–1163

Linden B 1977 Osteochondritis dissecans of the femoral condyles: a long term follow-up study. Journal of Bone and Joint Surgery 59A: 769–776

Lipscomb A B, Anderson A F 1986 Tears of the anterior cruciate ligament in adolescents. Journal of Bone and Joint Surgery 68A: 19–28

Lloyd-Roberts G C, Jackson A M, Albert J S 1985 Avulsion of the distal pole of the patella in cerebral palsy. Journal of Bone and Joint Surgery 67B: 252–254

Macnicol M F 1995 The problem knee, 2nd edn. Butterworth Heninmen, Oxford, pp 8–13

Merchant A C 1993 The lateral patellar compression syndrome. In: Fox J M, del Pizzo W (eds) The patello-femoral joint. McGraw-Hill Inc., New York

Morley M 1957 Knock knee in children. British Medical Journal 2: 976

Noble J, Hamblen D L 1975 The pathology of the degenerate meniscus. Journal of Bone and Joint Surgery 57B: 180–186

Outerbridge R E 1961 The aetiology of chondromalacia patellae. Journal of Joint and Bone Surgery 43B: 752–757

Robinson A H N, Aladin A, Green A J, Dandy D J 1998 Congenital dislocation of the patella – the genetics and conservative management. Knee 5: 235–237

Salenius P, Vankka E 1975 The development of the tibio-femoral angle in children. Journal of Bone and Joint Surgery 57A: 259–261

Siffert R S 1982 Intra-epiphyseal osteotomy for progressive tibia vara: a case report and rationale of management. Journal of Paediatric Orthopaedics 2: 81

Stein H, Dickson R A 1975 Reversed dynamic slings for knee flexion contractures in the haemophiliac. Journal of Bone and Joint Surgery 57A: 282–283

Thomas N P, Jackson A M, Aichroth P M 1985 Congenital absence of the anterior cruciate ligament. Journal of Bone and Joint Surgery 67B: 572–575

Twyman R S, Desai K, Aichroth P M 1991 Osteochondritis dissecans of the knee. A long-term study. Journal of Bone and Joint Surgery 73B: 461–464

Watanabe M, Takeda S, Kieuchi H 1979 Atlas of arthroscopy. Igakushon, Tokyo

Wilson J N 1967 A diagnostic sign in osteochondritis dissecans of the knee. Journal of Bone and Joint Surgery 49A: 477–480

Zaman M, Leonard M A 1978 Meniscectomy in children: a study of fifty-nine knees. Journal of Bone and Joint Surgery 60B: 436–437

Zionts L E, MacEwan G D 1986 Spontaneous improvement of post-traumatic tibia valga. Journal of Bone and Joint Surgery 68A: 680–687

Chapter 28

Leg length discrepancy

A. M. Jackson, M. F. Macnicol and M. Saleh

INTRODUCTION

Over the past few years the spotlight has focused more on exciting developments in the technique of bone lengthening than on the overall management of the patient with a leg length discrepancy. Selecting the best treatment for the individual patient has perhaps been neglected.

Leg length discrepancies of less than 2 cm are commonplace, seldom cause a problem and, if they do, a small shoe raise is the treatment. Often, the raise can be accommodated within the shoe. A greater difference in leg length will cause a postural imbalance in standing and an uneven gait. Patients seek primarily a cosmetic improvement and invariably reject a cumbersome shoe raise or extension orthosis if there is a more attractive alternative. However, there are also good orthopaedic reasons that justify the correction of significant leg length discrepancies. The avoidance of back ache in later life and osteoarthritis of the hip and knee of the longer leg are obvious. Scoliosis often becomes fixed with age. Stiffness in the spine combined with muscle weakness makes it difficult for some patients to compensate for even a minor discrepancy. Such problems are commonly associated with spinal dysraphism.

AETIOLOGY

Congenital causes of limb length discrepancy include the entire spectrum of lower limb dysplasias, hemiatrophy, hemihypertrophy, vascular malformations and a variety of syndromes such as neurofibromatosis, Ollier's disease, Klippel–Trenaunay syndrome and Russell–Silver dwarfism (Table 28.1). The dysplasias are presumably caused by an insult to the limb bud as it forms and matures between the 32nd and 42nd day of intrauterine life. The trigger may be viral, traumatic, drug-induced or some kind of focal ischaemic event. Most syndromes, in contrast, have a genetic basis and a positive family history can be helpful for early diagnosis. For example, in neurofibromatosis, the leg length discrepancy may be obvious long before the café au lait spots or the plexiform nature of the soft tissues become apparent.

Premature growth plate arrest is the most common cause of *acquired* shortening. The damage may be secondary to trauma, infection or radiotherapy (Fig. 28.1). Sadly, the trauma is sometimes iatrogenic, as when avascular necrosis complicates treatment for congenital dislocation of the hip or when overenthusiastic manipulation of a club foot

Table 28.1 Causes of limb length discrepancy	
Congenital	**Acquired**
Longitudinal defects	Trauma
Proximal femoral focal deficiency	Diaphyseal fracture
Tibia/fibula deficiency	Growth plate injury
Radial/ulnar club hand	Infection
Madelung's deformity	Osteomyelitis
	Septic arthritis
	Inflammation
	Juvenile idiopathic arthritis
	Scleroderma
	Haemophilia
Developmental dysplasia of the hip	Neoplasia
Talipes equinovarus	Haemangioma
	Childhood malignancy
Hemihypertrophy/hemiatrophy	Neurological deficit
	Myelodysplasia
	Hemiplegia
	Cerebral palsy
	Poliomyelitis
	Nerve injury
Osteodysplasias	Miscellaneous
Diaphyseal aclasis	Irradiation
Enchondromatosis (Ollier's disease etc.)	Perthes' disease
	Neurofibromatosis
	Drugs (e.g. thalidomide)
	Arteriovenous malformation
	Fibrous dysplasia

damages the lower tibial physis. If the growth plate is damaged unevenly, progressive deformity and shortening will go hand in hand.

Rarely, mid-shaft fractures heal with excessive shortening, sometimes combined with angular and rotational deformities. Such patients have invariably been victims of polytrauma and exemplify how quickly malunion can occur whilst other more grievous injuries receive attention. Overgrowth of the fractured limb is also recognised, although the resultant discrepancy is rarely more than 2 cm.

Neurological disorders, such as spina bifida, spinal dysraphism and cerebral palsy, account for a large number

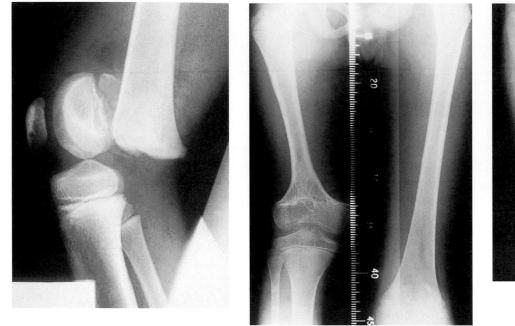

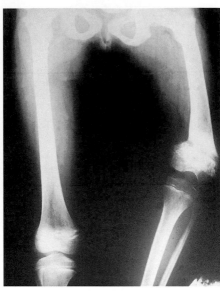

A B C

Figure 28.1 Damage to the lower femoral physis by **(A)** trauma, **(B)** neonatal osteomyelitis, and **(C)** radiotherapy are all potent causes of femoral shortening.

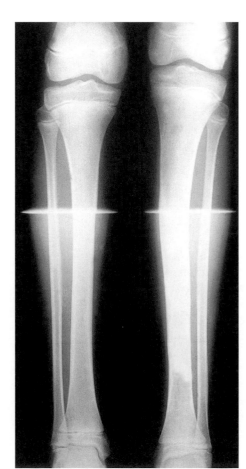

Figure 28.2 Tibial overgrowth caused by chronic diaphyseal osteomyelitis.

of patients with limb length discrepancies, but relatively few of those affected are candidates for equalisation procedures. The short, paralytic limb of poliomyelitis is much less common than it used to be. Two or three centimetres of shortening in a paralysed limb can actually be advantageous when associated with weak hip flexors and a foot drop, because the shortening enables the foot to clear the ground easily during the swing phase of gait. In such patients, larger discrepancies can be reduced, but they should not be totally corrected.

There are relatively few causes for overgrowth of a limb. These include hemihypertrophy, neurofibromatosis, vascular malformation and fibrous dysplasia. Trauma and infection can cause shortening or overgrowth (Fig. 28.2), depending on whether the epiphysis or the diaphysis is involved. More than 4 cm of tibial overgrowth has been seen in a child with chronic salmonella osteomyelitis and sickle-cell disease, and a similar spectacular overgrowth has been observed after a compound tibial fracture that was treated by a free flap.

ASSESSMENT OF THE PATIENT

HISTORY

The history is obviously important in any acquired discrepancy, and a positive family history may indicate a syndrome. Parental height should be recorded and associated congenital abnormalities noted.

TRUE OR APPARENT SHORTENING

It is fundamental to distinguish between true and apparent shortening, and to bear in mind that some patients have both. Apparent shortening is caused by obliquity of the pelvis when standing. This in turn is the result of fixed deformity of one or more of the three lever arms attached to the pelvic ring. Fixed adduction and abduction of the hip are relatively easy to correct, but pelvic obliquity associated with a structural lumbar spinal curve may have to be accepted. Fixed deformities of the hips should be corrected before other equalisation procedures are considered.

If the postural deformity is out of proportion to the measured leg length discrepancy, always look for evidence of scoliosis. True shortening in association with scoliosis and pelvic obliquity needs to be regarded with caution. It may well be to the patient's advantage to have a short leg on the 'down-hill' side of the pelvis. Correction of true leg length in such a patient may render it difficult for them to compensate for an unbalanced scoliosis, and may interfere with walking.

MEASUREMENT OF THE DISCREPANCY

Tape

It is traditional to measure true leg length with a tape measure as the distance from the anterior superior iliac spine to the medial malleolus, but this can be misleading. First, pelvic asymmetry occurs if the triradiate cartilage is damaged early in life – for example by infection or radiotherapy – and the anterior superior spines may lie at different levels. Second, in patients treated for congenital dislocation of the hip, the anterior spine may have been removed. Third, hindfoot height, which is the distance between the medial malleolus and the sole, will be increased if the hindfoot is in calcaneus, or decreased if there is a congenital hindfoot coalition or valgus.

Blocks

The estimation of leg length discrepancy using blocks may seem crude, but in the absence of fixed hip deformity it is the most accurate guide to the amount of correction required (Fig. 28.3). The patient can usually judge precisely whether they feel comfortable with the correction. With the appropriate block, standing radiographs of the pelvis and spine will confirm the correction and show what effect it will have on the hips and how it will influence the scoliosis. The patient should be viewed from behind, flexing forward so that the presence of spinal tilt and rotation can be included in the assessment.

Scanogram

When surgery for complex deformities is being planned, the traditional pelvis-to-ankle radiographic scanogram showing all of both lower limbs in detail on one film remains very helpful. For monitoring limb growth and discrepancy and

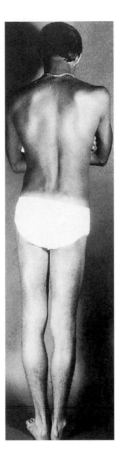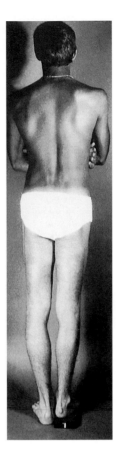

Figure 28.3 In the absence of fixed joint deformities, the 'block' method of estimating leg length discrepancy is extremely useful.

determining exactly how much shortening is in the femur and how much is in the tibia, computed tomography (CT) has become the method of choice. The dose of radiation is reduced and the measurements are automatically written on much smaller films, which are easily stored. By externally rotating the hips some 30°, which turns the feet out, it is possible to measure hindfoot height also. Fixed flexion of the knee will compromise the results of these measurements. In the future, ultrasound methods may gain popularity.

In practice, tape, blocks and scanogram are all used; should there be a discrepancy in the results obtained from these methods, a satisfactory explanation must be sought.

ASSESSMENT OF ASSOCIATED ABNORMALITIES

A systematic list of all the features that adversely affect the patient's stance and gait is required (see Table 28.2). If leg length discrepancy alone does not stand out as a major contributor to the problem, an equalisation procedure will not, on its own, result in much improvement. Furthermore, there are some specific abnormalities that will rule out or modify one or more of the treatment options. For example, dysplasia or subluxation of the hip precludes femoral lengthening: unless an initial stabilisation procedure is performed, the hip is almost certain to dislocate. Great care is required with femoral lengthening if the knee exhibits a positive Lachman test. Congenital absence of the anterior cruciate ligament is commonly encountered in the limb dysplasias (Thomas et al 1985). Sometimes, as in hemiplegia

Table 28.2 Some associated abnormalities to be looked for in the spine and involved leg

Site	Problem	Comment
Spine	Structural scoliosis	Spinal fusion may restrict mobility that is essential for walking In dysraphism, there may be a neurological component to shortening
Pelvis	Fixed pelvic obliquity Asymmetry	Compensatory or compounding the shortening? e.g. caused by premature fusion of triradiate cartilage
Hip	Soft-tissue contracture Bone deformity Dysplasia Muscle weakness	e.g. tight tensor fasciae latae in polio e.g. coxa vara/high trochanter → abductor incompetence Beware femoral lengthening → dislocation Trendelenburg positive will not be altered by lengthening
Femur	Deformity	Angular or rotational Can deformity be corrected at time of lengthening?
Knee	Soft-tissue contracture Bone deformity Ligamentous instability Patella subluxation/dislocation	e.g. pterygium Knee dysplasia as part of lower limb dysplasia e.g. congenital absent cruciate Caution with lengthening Often associated with valgus knee
Tibia	Deformity	Angular or rotational
Foot	Soft-tissue contracture Bone deformity/dysplasia Sensation	e.g. tight heel cord Tarsal coalition
General	Skin problems Muscle Neurovascular abnormalities Bone quality	e.g. tissue paper skin in juvenile scleroderma Wasting, weakness, fibrosis e.g. single embryological axial artery in some tibial dysplasias Avoid lengthening in areas of old osteomyelitis or irradiated bone

for example, the postural and balance problems stemming from a more central cause will complicate the picture.

MONITORING THE PATIENT AND PREDICTING THE DISCREPANCY AT MATURITY

If patients are referred early, which is to be preferred, their maturation and leg length discrepancy can be monitored on an annual basis. Shoe raises can be prescribed as an interim measure and, should limb deformity develop, it will be noticed and dealt with early, as appropriate. The seeds can be sown to prepare the patient and parents for limb equalisation surgery in the future if this is likely.

Several methods of predicting the shortening at maturity and the effect of epiphysiodesis have been published. The child's standing height on the normal leg is recorded on a growth chart. Skeletal age is determined from a radiograph of the left hand and wrist using the atlas of Greulich & Pyle (1959). This atlas allows the estimation of skeletal age by comparing the radiographic appearances of ossification centres with those of standards for various age groups. Bearing in mind the accuracy of this method is probably not greater than ± 18 months, its use will only draw notice to serious abnormalities of skeletal development. When there is

a major discrepancy between chronological and skeletal age, referral to a growth clinic is essential. Surprise diagnoses are not uncommon in these patients, for example, we have seen a very tall individual being followed for old septic arthritis of the hip who was found to have Klinefelter's syndrome in adolescence, and a small girl with neurofibromatosis was found to be a pituitary dwarf. Predicting the patient's overall height at maturity is necessary if a sensible choice is to be made between lengthening and shortening and it is fundamental to the timing of epiphysiodesis.

Most methods of prediction require at least three annual recordings of limb length and assume that growth proceeds in a linear fashion. This is not always the case. Congenital short limbs and those where infection or trauma are to blame are even less predictable. Damage to the lower femoral physis which is the site of 70% of femoral growth is notorious. If the damage is not complete, growth may continue at a slower rate and the unpredictability is caused by premature closure of the growth plate and a consequent rapid increase of discrepancy at the end of growth.

From longitudinal studies in normal children, Anderson et al (1963) published charts assessing residual growth in the lower limb. They stressed the importance of looking for a pattern of discrepancy before recommending surgery.

Moseley's straight line graph (1977) takes into account not only the degree of growth inhibition in the short leg but also the growth percentile. However, Moseley's graph is derived from data compiled from a group of North American children and may not apply to all populations. It also requires data to be compiled over a 3–4 year period and presumes a pattern of linear growth while offering an accuracy to within 0.6 cms.

Eastwood & Cole (1995) modified the arithmetic methods of White & Stubbins (1944) and Menelaus (1966). They incorporated the observed pattern of growth in accordance with the Shapiro (1982) patterns of discrepancy, rather than presuming that the discrepancy would increase at a constant increment annually. Only 8 of the 20 children, monitored prospectively, followed the Type 1 Shapiro pattern of a linear increase in the discrepancy. Their modification was therefore considered to reduce the risk of overcorrection and they rightly questioned the assumption that all growth inhibition occurs in a progressive, incremental fashion.

Westh & Menelaus (1981) describe a simpler method of timing the epiphysiodesis correctly which is particularly useful for children who present late without documentation of the progression of their leg length discrepancy. Their aim was to leave a discrepancy of between half an inch and three quarters of an inch and they assumed that growth stops at the age of 16 years in boys and 14 years in girls (Fig 28.4).

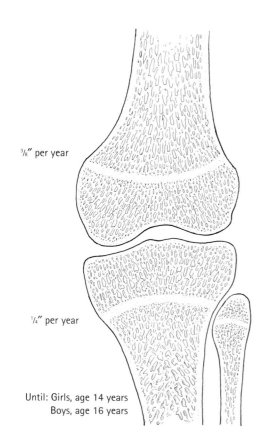

³/₈″ per year

¼″ per year

Until: Girls, age 14 years
Boys, age 16 years

Figure 28.4 Estimation of 'growth to come' at the knee, using the method of Menelaus (1966).

They assume a straight-line relationship between rate of growth and age from the onset of puberty until maturity. The lower femoral epiphysis provides three eighths of an inch and the upper tibial epiphysis one quarter of an inch of growth per year. Their method corrected legs to within half an inch of predicted discrepancy in 85% of their patients.

Macnicol et al (1993) used the same calculation and reported that all their patients achieved a limb length disparity of less than one centimetre.

The chart of anthropometric values, developed by Aldegheri & Agostini (1983) adds a further method for determining remaining growth in the patient who presents late and is applicable to the upper limb as much as to the lower limb.

As a rule of thumb it is worth remembering that the tibia is approximately half its adult length at the age of three years and if one assumes that the percentage discrepancy remains the same throughout growth then the discrepancy at that age will be doubled by maturity.

TREATMENT

The approach to treatment of leg length discrepancy falls into two general categories: limb equalisation, or long-term management of disparate limbs. With respect to the former, the long and the short leg will be considered separately here, but it should be borne in mind that management often involves treatment of both legs: lengthening on one side and shortening on the other, for instance, is a valid combination. Compromise is an inevitable feature of much treatment. For example, after equalisation of leg length, it sometimes occurs that the knees are not at the same level; although this is cosmetically undesirable, it seldom detracts from function. Furthermore, leg equalisation is inappropriate for both the very minor and the very severe discrepancy, and it is for these patients that the second approach to treatment is more suitable.

SHOE RAISE, ORTHOSIS, AMPUTATION/PROSTHESIS

For a small difference in leg length, a shoe raise may be accepted as a permanent solution. In severe congenital abnormalities, it is often clear in the first months of life that either the foot will be functionally useless or the leg length discrepancy will be beyond the capabilities of any lengthening procedure. An extension orthosis or amputation plus prosthesis may be the solution. Remember that the worst outcome is to produce a painful, ugly, unsatisfactory limb at the end of a complex programme of lengthening. An early definitive amputation with subsequent 'operations' on the prosthesis to keep up with growth is preferable.

The spectrum of congenitally short tibia with absent fibula exemplifies the problem. Choi et al (1990) found 88% satisfactory results in their group of patients who underwent amputation, compared with 55% satisfactory results in those

return to normal function within 2 weeks. The correct position of the bone tunnel can be confirmed radiographically and effective epiphysiodesis is apparent when growth arrest lines do not appear subsequently at the operation site. Snyder et al (1994), using serial magnetic resonance imaging (MRI), have also demonstrated the absence of growth arrest lines as indicative of epiphysiodesis. This technique is equally applicable in upper limb epiphysiodesis, although a smaller tube saw would be required for the narrower forearm bones.

Proximal fibular growth plate arrest is necessary when the upper tibial epiphsiodesis is planned to produce more than 2 cm of arrest. The lateral incision allows access to the fibula, and the physis can be excised or drilled.

Complications

Complications were rare in the published series. They include infection and failure of epiphysiodesis, usually because of technical error. Partial arrest of the physis may lead to an angular or recurvatum deformity at the knee. Although fracture through the physis is rare, protective splintage of the limb is recommended, particularly with the more open operative techniques. With the percutaneous tube saw technique, the perichondrial ring and cortex remain largely intact and the operative site resists angulatory and axial stress. The limb can therefore be left unsplinted, encouraging immediate motion, but protected weight bearing for 2 weeks, followed by normal walking.

Morrissy (1992) has abandoned the percutaneous technique, returning to the open Phemister method, for the following reasons:

1. Haemorrhage and swelling appear to be worse than with the open technique.
2. Irradiation is increased to both the patient and the surgeon, because direct vision is no longer possible with the percutaneous approach.
3. The incisions required to remove blocks of bone and to carry out curettage of the growth plate are little greater than that required for the percutaneous technique.

The tube saw technique reduces the amount of haemorrhage because bone is replaced into the defect; irradiation is limited to no more than approximately six pulses of the image intensifier; finally, only a single incision of 1–2 cm is required, and undoubtedly the cosmetic effect improves upon that of the larger double incision of the Phemister approach (Macnicol & Gupta 1997). The ablation of the growth plate becomes apparent in 3–6 months and can be demonstrated more readily with MRI or CT scanning than with conventional radiography. It is customary to monitor the correction of leg length discrepancy with leg-length films or CT scanograms after operation, although the principal assessment is clinical, using blocks.

In summary, the *advantages* of percutaneous epiphysiodesis are:

1. A relatively minor surgical procedure with few complications.

2. Reduced surgical morbidity, hospital stay and rehabilitation period.
3. Cosmetically acceptable results.
4. Reproducible technique.
5. Relatively simple equipment.
6. Combination with lengthening for larger discrepancies.

The *disadvantages* include:

1. A slight reduction in overall limb length (in the lower limb, this means shorter stature).
2. Surgery to the contralateral 'normal' limb in many cases.
3. Limited application in younger children or in the adolescent in whom the remaining growth is insufficient.

The reliability, safety and acceptable cosmetic results make percutaneous epiphysiodesis the method of choice for managing discrepancies of between 2 and 5 cm in the lower limb. Now that more information is available about proportional upper limb growth, epiphysiodesis also offers an attractive option in reconstructive surgery of the arm (Bortel & Pritchett 1993).

Femoral and tibial shortening

The procedures of femoral and tibial shortening are precise if applied once skeletal maturity has been reached. Proximal femoral shortening (Wagner 1977) is favoured for a number of reasons. The short limb is usually thinner than the long and shortening the longer side increases this difference in girth. It is preferable to keep the scarring and bulkiness where it can easily be hidden by normal clothes. In one extreme case, considerable improvement in the post-equalisation girth problem was achieved by liposuction.

If the operative instructions for femoral shortening are followed carefully, the union rate is high, and full weight bearing should be achieved by 8–10 weeks. Muscle weakness is not a problem, and internal fixation allows early mobilisation. Femoral shortening is indicated if:

1. The patient is skeletally mature.
2. The discrepancy is less than 6 cm.
3. The discrepancy is principally in the femur.
4. The patient's height is at or above the 50th centile.

There are some important points in the operative technique (Fig. 28.8). The proximal cut must not be made too low. The lesser trochanter with its ilio-psoas insertion must remain attached to the proximal fragment. Once the segment to be removed has been marked out, the distal cut should be made first and the proximal fragment abducted into the wound, to facilitate the proximal cut. The choice of internal fixation is important: an AO compression blade plate places a tension band across the distraction side of the osteotomy; a dynamic hip screw is not a suitable alternative, and is prone to produce non-union in this situation.

There are many other femoral shortening methods. The reader should be aware of Küntscher's (1965) intramedullary femoral shortening technique, which uses a cam saw. Blair et

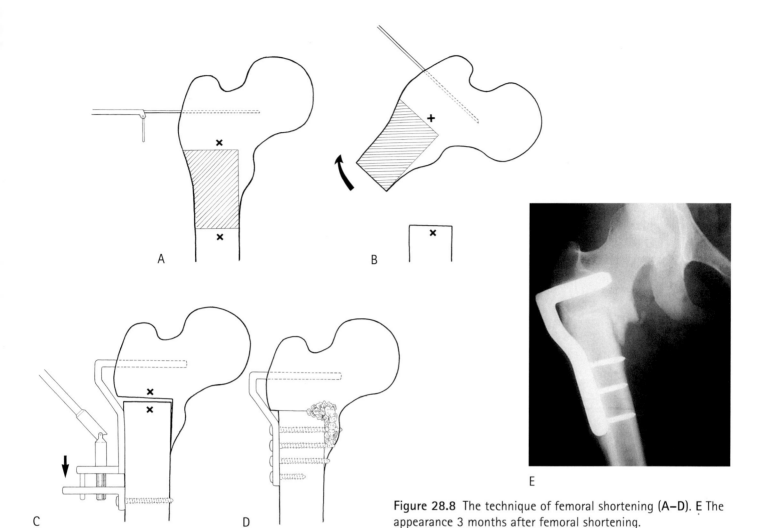

Figure 28.8 The technique of femoral shortening (**A–D**). E The appearance 3 months after femoral shortening.

al (1989) have recently reviewed this procedure, which requires considerable attention to detail. The saws are manufactured in different diameters (13–17 mm), in accordance with the thickness of the femoral cortex. The proximal osteotomy is carried out after the medullary cavity has been reamed wider than the distal osteotomy site. An unscrubbed assistant manipulates the thigh to break the femur at the distal osteotomy. Reverse cutting chisels are inserted down the shaft and hooked upon the free bone segment, which is then split, using a slotted hammer applied to the proximal chisel attachment. Larger segments may need to be weakened with an expander or even split through a short, lateral incision. The proximal and distal femoral segments are approximated with an intramedullary guide wire in place, allowing the insertion of a nail of appropriate size. Distal and proximal locking are advised after the femoral segments have been impacted. Partial weight bearing is possible immediately, and the femur unites in 3 months.

Tibial shortening has a poor reputation. Problems with skin closure, cosmesis and vascularity of the limb are well documented, and there can be few indications for this procedure. Nevertheless, Broughton et al (1989) have described a long step-cut osteotomy at the mid-shaft of the tibia; the length of bone excised from each end of the step equals the shortening required. The osteotomy is secured with two interfragmentary screws, which is preferable to an AO plate where the bulk of the implant may lead to vascular compromise. Shortening of more than 5 cm is risky.

LIMB EQUALISATION: LENGTHENING THE SHORT LEG

Physiological procedures

Growth stimulation in the shorter leg is an intriguing concept, and has given rise to a host of experimental procedures. Venous occlusion, the creation of arteriovenous fistulae, sympathectomy, forage, assorted metaphyseal implants, ultrasound and pulsed electromagnetic fields have all had their advocates, but they have so far failed to produce therapeutically useful and predictable results.

Circumferential periosteal release is still practised in some centres. This manoeuvre does stimulate growth. The mechanism may be a vascular response to trauma, stimulation of metaphyseal blood flow, or the release of periosteal tension. Practically, the gain in leg length is small, not easily predictable and the stimulation effect may continue for 2–3 years. Wilde & Baker (1987) have shown that the response is greater in children younger than 6 years. Perhaps there is a small place for this operation as a 'holding procedure' in the younger child but, in minor discrepancies, epiphysiodesis is probably more accurate and cosmetically more attractive.

Restoration of growth: the Langenskiöld (1981) procedure

When a localised growth-plate arrest occurs – for example at the knee – it is reasonable to excise the bone bridge if less than 50% of the physis is involved (Kasser 1990). Some growth, at least, can be restored in 80% of these patients. Simultaneous corrective osteotomy (see Ch. 27) is required if the angular deformity exceeds 20°. A peripheral bone bridge can be approached directly, whereas a central bar is approached through the metaphysis. Jackson (1993) has described a modification of the Langenskiöld procedure in which a pre-drilled triangular wedge of metaphysis is resected in order to gain access to a central bar. After resection of the bar, the wedge is replaced, locking the free fat graft in place. The risks include fracture of the epiphysis, if it is seriously undermined, and recurrent bridge formation. Epiphyseal mapping from MRI scans is an important part of operative planning. There is still uncertainty as to the best interposition material, although the free fat graft is probably still the most common choice.

Lengthening procedures

Reference has already been made to abduction osteotomy and its use in correcting apparent shortening in addition to slightly increasing the true leg length. The Salter osteotomy can produce 1 cm or so of lengthening and Millis & Hall (1979) have increased this effect by distracting the innominate osteotomy site and inserting a trapezoidal bone graft. Using this transiliac lengthening technique, they were able to produce about 2.5 cm of increased leg length. The major dangers are disruption of the ipsilateral sacro-iliac joint, and sciatic nerve injury. The risk of damage to the hip joint is reduced by ilio-psoas tenotomy. This procedure may be indicated in pelvic asymmetry, or when there is a simultaneous need for acetabular redirection and ipsilateral limb lengthening.

Femoral and tibial lengthening

Since Codivilla's first account of limb lengthening in 1905, interest has waxed and waned. A few spectacular successes were paid for by a greater number of equally spectacular disasters. The increase in length was often combined with a decrease in functional ability, so that patients sometimes completed 18 months or more of treatment to find themselves debilitated, demoralised and deformed. However, in the UK, Abbott (1927) and then Anderson (1972) pioneered safe and carefully graduated lengthening that led to a sustained improvement in gait with no loss of muscle function (Macnicol & Catto 1982). In Russia, Ilizarov (1991) designed the circular frame which gave all-round support and allowed immediate weight bearing.

With increased understanding of the biological process, leg lengthening no longer deserves a poor reputation, and the past two decades have seen a resurgence of interest. Paley (1988) reviewed the basic choice between osteotomy followed by lengthening or distraction of the physis, the former now being preferred. Knowledge that a bone gap can consistently be bridged with callus, without the need for bone grafting and internal fixation (Anderson 1972), together with improvements to external fixators, have revolutionised the approach. Lengthening by callus distraction (callotasis) has fewer complications, requires fewer surgical interventions and is quicker than the Wagner (1977) method, which invariably required bone graft and internal fixation (Fig. 28.9).

The remainder of this chapter is devoted to the subject of limb lengthening.

LIMB LENGTHENING

THE PRINCIPLES OF BONE LENGTHENING

Bone lengthening is a biological event that can be controlled by a mechanical apparatus. Credit must go to Ilizarov (1990) for the discovery of the 'tension-stress' phenomenon whereby a 'mechanical signal' can be sent to the tissues and growth stimulated even after maturity. Indeed, successful callus distraction has been achieved well into the fourth decade. Success in this kind of venture demands attention to detail.

The bone division

As the lengthened segment depends on periosteal and medullary callus, these tissues must be treated with care. In retrospect, it is surprising that bone used to be divided with a power saw: today's purists will try to preserve the integrity of both periosteal and medullary blood supply by performing a subcutaneous or closed corticotomy. This technique is most easily applied in the upper tibial metaphysis. A 5-mm osteotome with a depth guard is passed through a small anterior incision and as much of the cortex as possible is divided under image intensifier control. The inaccessible posterior cortex, perhaps a quarter of the total circumference, is cracked, either by twisting the handle of the osteotome to lever it apart or by applying a twisting force across the corticotomy site itself until the bone gives. Experimental work has shown that, if this is carefully performed, the periosteal sleeve will remain intact, as will the medullary blood supply. In the clinical situation, however, it is not possible to know whether the medullary blood supply has been damaged.

Alternatively, an open procedure may be adopted. The periosteum is split longitudinally and carefully peeled back. The corticotomy site is mapped out with a number of small cortex-only drill holes, which are then joined together by means of a small osteotome. Once again, the posterior cortex must be gently cracked open, then the periosteal tube is reconstituted. One of the advantages of the open procedure is that it may be combined with a limited fascial soft-tissue release.

A true corticotomy can be easily undertaken only at the

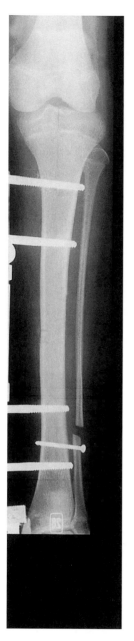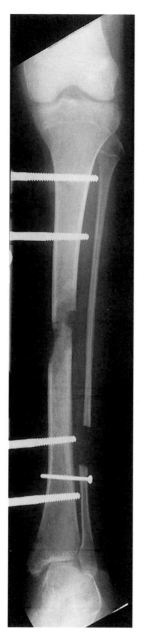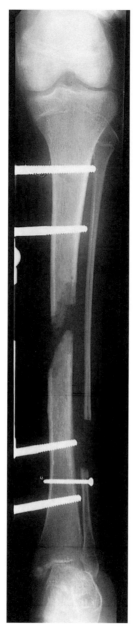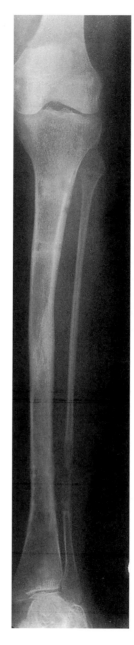

Figure 28.9
Achievement of a 5-cm diaphyseal lengthening of the tibia by callus distraction, starting 2 weeks after corticotomy.

metaphysis, because the force required to break the diaphyseal cortex is so great that a complete fracture is almost certain. In practice, this seems to matter little, as the blood supply across such a low-energy fracture will quickly re-establish itself, given the right conditions. After 10 days in a child and 2 weeks in an adult as De Bastiani et al (1987) have shown, the medullary blood supply is re-established. Delaying the lengthening until early callus formation has occurred is seen as beneficial.

The optimum level for osteotomy is open to debate. The advantage of metaphyseal osteotomy is that the medulla contains more active osteoblasts, and the greater cross-sectional area means that a larger mass of new bone is formed. Mechanically, the wider the bone, the greater the resistance to bending forces, and it may be possible to remove the fixator earlier. Conversely, the larger pins do not

hold as well in cancellous bone, and for this reason it may be advisable to use a mid-shaft osteotomy if a single bar fixator is to be used. In the mid-shaft, a long oblique osteotomy increases its surface area, and allows considerable overlap of the new bone by existing cortex as the distraction proceeds. It may prove possible to increase the amount of callus by interposing a resorbable spacer between the cortex and periosteum in order to elevate the periosteum and increase the size of the periosteal tube. In practice, variations in bone quality, bony deformity and soft-tissue considerations may influence the choice of corticotomy site.

For greater lengthening, a two-level or bifocal lengthening can be considered. Theoretically, this doubles the rate at which the bone can be lengthened and spreads out the stresses on the soft tissues. Bell et al (1990) have shown that hindfoot equinus can be prevented by including the foot in the apparatus, but there are likely to be increased soft-tissue complications about the knee if the femur is lengthened in this manner. Flexion contracture of the knee such as is encountered in poliomyelitis, should be released before lengthening (Leong et al 1982). Vilarrubias et al (1990) appreciated that soft-tissue tension both impaired the lengthening process and endangered joints. Percutaneous tendon releases and splintage of joints in a stable configuration allowed more extensive lengthening, at the expense of injury to tendon and articular cartilage.

The distraction apparatus

In order to produce the distraction-stress phenomenon, the external fixator must provide stability. Undesirable angular and shearing movements will result in the formation of fibrous tissue and not fibrocartilage. In contrast, there is good reason to believe that axial micromovements are beneficial or even essential components in producing the correct tissue response. The exact magnitude of micromovement that one might regard as favourable has yet to be determined. An unstable frame also leads to wire or pin sepsis, loosening and pain.

The current choice of distraction device lies between the single-sided bar with large pin fixation such as the Wagner (1977) or Orthofix (De Bastiani et al 1987) device and the all-round fixators using tensioned wires to hold the bone as popularised by Ilizarov (1990) (considered in more detail later in this chapter). The circumferential frames do have a number of advantages that are appreciated when dealing with the special situation, such as the correction of rotational and angular deformities, bone transport and double-segment or bilevel lengthening. The smaller wires cause less injury to the bone than do pins, and fracture through a wire track is extremely rare. During distraction, the wires pass through the skin more easily, without causing the skin to heap up at the advancing edge as occurs with larger pins, and hence the incidence of wire track infection is low. All-round frames are strong enough to allow partial weight bearing throughout the lengthening period; indeed, this is encouraged. This reduces the well-known complications of disuse in addition to improving the quality of callus formation by inducing axial micromovement. When placing the pins, the surgeon is well advised to have a cross-sectional atlas of limb anatomy to hand: in some areas, placement of the wires is very critical. The disadvantage of the all-round frames is that they are complex and time consuming to apply. They are currently more expensive than the single-bar fixators, the patients may find them bulky, and they are difficult to apply to a short femur, in which one has to resort to a hybrid construction using pins and wires – this compromises the concept of an all-round support.

The single-bar fixators, however, are much less bulky, easier to apply, and easier to lengthen. In the tibia, for example, the pins do not transfix muscle at all, which makes it easier to maintain mobility. The bar must always be placed parallel to the diaphysis of the bone. Even so, loss of alignment is the main problem and this tends to occur towards the end of a reasonably ambitious lengthening. The cantilever configuration of the fixator tends to cause the bones to angle away from the bar, and in the case of the tibia the tight soft tissues are usually on the side of the bone that is opposite to the distractor. The single-bar fixators are difficult to adjust once in place. In a femur with bulky soft tissues or where there is considerable postoperative swelling, the distance from the fixator to the proximal cortex may be so great as to place excessive force on the pins.

The rate and rhythm of lengthening

After a 10–14-day interval from corticotomy, the distraction is commenced. Experience has shown that a distraction rate of 0.5 mm per day may be associated with premature fusion at the distraction site, and 2 mm per day may result in suboptimal new bone formation; most practitioners have found 1 mm per day to be about right. In order to smooth out the distraction forces, it is best to perform the distraction in 0.25- or 0.5-mm, increments. The lengthening is performed by the patient, who charts his own progress.

Early on in the distraction, a physis-like structure forms between the bone ends and remains in the middle of the lengthened segment. Ossification occurs on both sides of this structure and columns of osteoid appear, similar to the process in membrane bone formation. Radiologically, these columns give a striated appearance in the line of the distraction force.

Radiographs or ultrasound can be used at 1–2-week intervals, to check alignment and the quality of callus formation. The findings may influence the supervision of distraction. Deficient callus requires a reduced rate of distraction or a temporary rest before proceeding. If a significant gap appears in the newly formed callus it may be best to stop the distraction, wind the fixator back, wait a few days and then proceed again, slowly, as before.

The soft tissues

It is invariably the soft tissues that determine the limit of lengthening. When problems are anticipated, preoperative soft-tissue release is essential. Most often it is the biarticular muscles that prove troublesome. It is most unwise, for example, to commence tibial lengthening if steps have not been taken to correct fixed equinus at the ankle first. Whether or not preoperative soft-tissue release is required, appropriate joint splintage and physiotherapy are important aspects of limb care during lengthening. We prefer rigid, removable splints to dynamic splints and springs, which require patient compliance and are often poorly tolerated.

Knee stiffness at the end of femoral lengthening is a common problem but, usually, function slowly returns with appropriate physiotherapy. If fixed flexion of the knee greater than 40° occurs during femoral lengthening, a real danger of progressive external rotation of the tibia, subluxation, and ultimately dislocation exists. This must not be allowed to happen. If it seems necessary, after lengthening, to perform a posterior release, remember that the problem is not the same as cerebral palsy; the neurovascular bundle may be just as tight as the hamstrings.

The soft tissues of the congenital short limb seem to present more resistance to lengthening than those of any other group, making it difficult to achieve a significant percentage lengthening in these patients.

Dynamisation and judging the end-point

At the termination of lengthening De Bastiani et al (1987), using the Orthofix device, suggest full weight bearing, with the body-locking screw tight, until radiographs demonstrate good callus. This is usually at about 6 weeks. The bone is then dynamised and the fixator removed, once the callus is seen to consolidate into a tubular structure with cortex and medulla clearly differentiated. It is wise to leave the pins in place for a few days after the frame has been removed so that the bone can be re-secured if necessary. On average, the duration of treatment is approximately 30–40 days per 1 cm of length gained.

The micromovements possible in the Ilizarov frame probably mean that the bone is dynamised throughout the lengthening process, depending on the activity of the patient. Whatever method is used, the timing of frame removal remains a clinical and radiological decision. Early removal risks deformity and fracture, and late removal delays rehabilitation. A simple objective method of measuring bone stiffness by using a strain gauge has been described by Richardson et al (1994) for tibial fractures but it can equally well be applied to limb lengthening and bone transplant.

Early removal of the external fixator followed by intramedullary nailing is possible as soon as the callus is mature enough to resist compression forces. After pin removal, a few days on traction are required whilst the pin tracks heal, and the bone is then secured by an unreamed intramedullary nail. The advantage of this is that it gives immediate whole-bone protection and allows early and vigorous rehabilitation, without fear of fracture. This has proved a useful technique when soft-tissue problems dominate the picture, as in the congenitally short limb, and as a salvage procedure if the femur fractures after removal of the fixator (Fig. 28.10).

Complications

A thorough knowledge of the possible complications is essential when monitoring leg lengthening. To some extent, the complications may be related to the initial clinical problem.

Early complications

Pin-track infection can be largely prevented by regular cleaning, the prevention of skin tension with relieving incisions when necessary, and the use of dressings that stabilise the skin around the pin. Muscle contracture of a dominant muscle group must be recognised early, and appropriate counter-

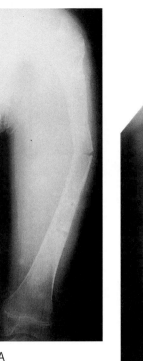

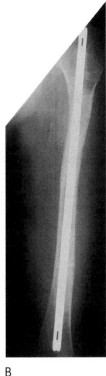

A

B

Figure 28.10 A 'Plastic' failure of the lengthened segment in a patient with congenital short femur. **B** This was salvaged by closed, unreamed femoral nailing.

measures include splintage, physiotherapy and even temporary cessation of lengthening. Loss of alignment must be corrected early, as it has a strong tendency to get worse. If it is associated with pin bending, the pins will need to be replaced. Premature consolidation will occur if the lengthening is too slow. Poor bone formation may be improved by slowing the distraction rate or even back-tracking. Occasionally, supplementary bone grafting is required. Poor patient compliance is not uncommon. The apparatus must be checked to detect overwinding or sudden release. Rapid lengthening can induce hypertension and pain develops as the tissues are progressively tensioned or if the pins become infected or loosened.

In the face of a major problem, never compromise limb function in order to achieve length. Preoperative counselling must condition the patient to the complexity of these procedures, and to the fact that bone length cannot be 'bought off the shelf'. Joint subluxation is only one step from dislocation.

A lateral X-ray of a stiff, flexed knee that shows the tibia in the anteroposterior projection is an impending disaster (Fig. 28.11). Permanent joint damage and stiffness are likely to follow.

Compartment syndromes are rare, and usually present in the period immediately after application of the lengthening device. Early recognition and treatment are essential. Pins and screws may cause vascular injury, but this is less likely with wires. Arteriovenous fistulae and damage to free pedicle grafts have been reported.

Premature consolidation of the corticotomy may occur, requiring osteoclasis or percutaneous division of the regenerate. The fibular osteotomy may also join occasionally

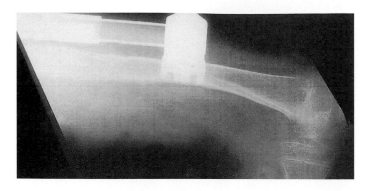

Figure 28.11 Congenital short femur at the end of lengthening. A 90° fixed flexion on X-ray caused great concern. A posterior release was required and full extension was eventually regained.

during tibial lengthening; this is less likely if the fibula has been anchored distally to the tibia with a screw that maintains the malleolar relationship.

Serious nerve injury is rare, but is a sure indication to stop lengthening. The common peroneal nerve is especially at risk if femoral lengthenings in excess of 10 cm are performed. Electromyographic studies by Galardi et al (1990) suggest that subclinical nerve damage is a surprisingly common event, so paraesthesiae in the foot indicate that lengthening must cease immediately.

Late complications

Late complications occur after removal of the external fixator. If soft-tissue flexion deformities do not improve, they generally respond to further surgery. Delayed union and malunion are the price that may be paid if control is lost. The usual cause of this is fracture after removal of the fixator (Simpson & Kenwright 2000) and it is a great pity if leg length is lost at this stage. Non-union is rare, but is likely if the regenerate narrows or forms cysts. Bone mineralisation of the gap tissue can be monitored before removal of the fixator by ultrasonography (Eyres et al 1993) or by dual-energy X-ray absorptiometry.

The distal fibular length must be maintained by a screw, reinforced by a tibio-fibular synostosis between the lower fibular segment at its proximal end and the tibia (Anderson 1972). This ensures that a valgus hindfoot does not develop (Macnicol & Catto 1982) and minimises the risk of worsening foot deformity described by Sofield et al (1958).

EPIPHYSEAL DISTRACTION

In practical terms, it is unlikely that growth plate distraction can be achieved without fracturing the growth plate (Kenwright et al 1989). The separation is believed to occur through the hypertrophic zone, between the proliferating cells and the zone of provisional calcification. Nevertheless, experience shows a real risk of premature closure of the physis after epiphyseal distraction. It is therefore preferable

to use this method in an individual who is approaching skeletal maturity (Fig. 28.12).

Rupture of the physis can be documented by a sudden decrease in the peak load across the physis; it is manifest clinically by the acute onset of pain. Indeed, this may be the most painful method of achieving lengthening. The force required depends largely on the cross-sectional area of the physis.

De Bastiani et al (1986a,b) described a method of epiphyseal distraction (chondrodiastasis) and achieved lengthenings of up to 36% in non-achondroplastic and 64.5% in achondroplastic patients. The redundant soft tissues in the latter seem to adapt remarkably well to lengthening procedures.

Whatever the method chosen, leg lengthening requires complete confidence and co-operation on the part of the patient. A good rapport between doctor, patient and parents is essential. These procedures are not suitable for the faint-hearted and the non-complaint.

THE ILIZAROV TECHNIQUE

The Ilizarov technique incorporates a philosophy of bone and soft-tissue management that offers radically different solutions for the treatment of many paediatric conditions. The ring fixator is an essential part of this method and is preferred for some conditions and mandatory in others. More comprehensive descriptions of the method may be found in other works (Bianchi Maiocchi & Aronson 1991, Ilizarov & Deviatov 1971).

In 1951, Gavril Abramovich Ilizarov developed an interest

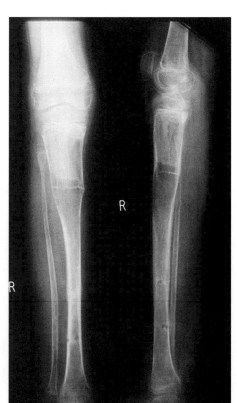

Figure 28.12 Result of proximal epiphyseal lengthening in a 12-year-old boy with congenital short tibia, using the Monticelli frame. Note the wide, strong, straight segment.

in limb injuries and evolved a method of treatment with a basic circular external fixation frame. This consisted of two rings fixed to the bone by a pair of crossed and tensioned Kirschner wires, each controlling one side of the fracture. The rings were connected together by threaded rods and the device was capable of supporting a long bone fracture or non-union to full healing. This simple concept developed into an extremely sophisticated system of external fixation capable of providing varying degrees of circumferential fracture support, based on the following principles:

- precise amount of fracture support
- minimal surgical intervention
- immediate weight bearing
- mobilisation of joints.

The patient was encouraged to weight bear fully and to mobilise adjacent joints. The tensioned Kirschner wires deformed under load, allowing some axial movement. During the healing phase, the stability of the frame could be reduced by removing supporting bars, rings or wires, further stimulating the fracture to take load. Thus all the criteria for an 'ideal' fracture healing environment were fulfilled, without intruding upon the fracture site and producing further surgical trauma and ischaemia. Even in osteoporotic or comminuted fractures, the wire configuration was capable of conferring better long-term support.

Circular frames have the advantage that they provide circumferential support for the bone. By appropriate adjustment of the connecting threaded rods gradual correction of deformity in the sagittal, coronal and transverse planes can be achieved, in addition to lengthening. The rings are fixed to bone with fine wires, usually 1.5–1.8 mm in diameter. Wires should be crossed at as near to 90° as possible (Fig. 28.13A); occasionally, this is prevented by the position of the neurovascular structures. The risk of complications may be minimised by a careful technique and, in particular, by the avoidance of drilling with the wire point free in the soft tissues. With the muscles stretched, a wire is pushed through the skin and soft tissues and onto the bone. The wire is drilled through both cortices and then tapped with a mallet through the tensioned soft tissues and out of the skin on the far side. It is necessary to position the rings in pairs through at least one of the bone ends. In fractures, the rings are

positioned at either end of each bone fragment (Fig. 28.13B), whereas in bone lengthening the rings are kept apart as much as possible. The rings are linked with rods, allowing slow correction. Hinges may be utilised to provide an axis for angular correction, joint movement and to produce (if necessary) translations and rotations (Paley et al 1994). These devices are most applicable in the tibia (Stanitski et al 1996), but are also of value in the upper limb. Fixation in the proximal femur and humerus is precarious and the device is cumbersome, so it is poorly tolerated by the patient.

The psychological and social difficulties attendant upon the prolonged treatment time of bone lengthening and realignment are not overcome by this technique any more than with the unilateral bar. Pain may still limit the full application of the technique (Young et al 1994), and the surgeon must remain vigilant during the all-important monitoring of the lengthening process (Paley 1990).

By the 1960s, the technique had evolved to incorporate the general biological principles that govern the stimulation of tissue growth and regeneration during distraction. Ilizarov noted that gradual distraction of certain living tissues created stresses that stimulated and maintained active regeneration. This concept is perhaps a more specialised statement of Wolff's law (1892) and has been termed the 'tension-stress effect' (Ilizarov 1989a,b 1990). The use of the circular frame techniques developed to lengthen bones and correct soft tissue and bony deformities has modified the approach to treatment of conditions as diverse as congenital fibula hemimelia, Blount's disease, congenital pseudarthrosis of the tibia, club foot and radial club hand (Ghoneem et al 1996).

Choice of frame

The basic principles of limb lengthening have been described. Callus formation in distraction is a well-established technique and may be performed as easily with a monolateral as with a circular frame (Ilizarov & Deviatov 1971, Ilizarov & Trokhava 1973, De Bastiani et al 1987, Aronson et al 1989). Paley (1990) has examined the stability of the Ilizarov frame in comparison with monolateral frames. In most modes, the circular frame is less stiff than the monolateral frame. Axially, the circular frame stiffness is determined by the wire diameter, wire tension and the

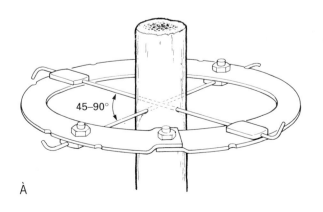

A

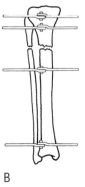
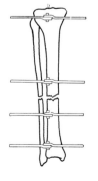
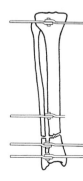

B

Figure 28.13 The Ilizarov technique. **A** Tensioned Kirschner wires are fixed to the ring, and cross within the bone. **B** Standard mounting for a tibial fracture. Note the ring pair configurations.

45–90°

number of rings. Axial stiffness, however, has not been compared with the Orthofix monolateral frame in the dynamic mode or with a dynamisation ring. Coronal and sagittal stiffness vary according to the number of wires and also to the use of olive wires. Stiffness would appear to be a virtue in controlling axial deviation, but systems with axial elasticity generate bone better. The circular frame technique, however, confers certain distinct advantages, as it offers finer control of the lengthening. Analysis of a case may indicate the type of lengthening technique required for the best results, and a working classification (Saleh & Hamer 1993) that could be adopted is suggested in Table 28.4.

Circular frames are indicated in and are useful for progressive correction of pre-existing angular deformities or angulation occurring during lengthening. They are also indicated for unstable joints because the fixation may be extended across a joint to prevent subluxation, and for co-existing soft-tissue contractures such as equinus associated with fibular hemimelia. As circular frames with transfixation wires are less well tolerated and carry an increased risk of nerve or vessel injury, it seems appropriate to reserve their use for lengthenings of types 2, 3 and 4. They are an unnecessary burden for both the patient and surgeon in more simple cases in which a predictable result can be achieved with a monolateral frame (Saleh 1992a,b, Saleh & Scott 1992). The use of circular frames in the femur is much more demanding (Stanitski et al 1995), and many authors now use half rings.

Procedures

Four broad indications for lengthening with deformity correction are described.

Lengthening with angular correction

A straight lengthening is performed, and hinges are placed at the apex of a deformity or at the level of a proposed angular correction. Adjacent threaded rods are compressed or distracted to produce the required correction (Fig. 28.14). Post-traumatic genu recurvatum (Choi et al 1999) and congenital malalignment can thus be corrected.

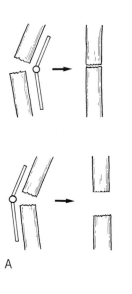

A

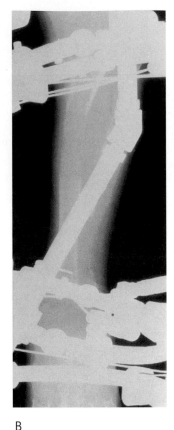

Figure 28.14 Diagram (**A**) and radiograph (**B**) showing hinge placed at the desired position for angular correction.   B

Lengthening with angulation and translation

If the hinges are placed to one side, a degree of translation may be induced (Fig. 28.15).

Lengthening with joint contracture

Extending the frame across a joint will protect it and permit progressive correction to take place either before or during lengthening. Equinus deformity associated with fibular hemimelia may be corrected in stages, using hinges at the level of the ankle and distraction rods to push the os calcis down and pull the forefoot up (Fig. 28.16). Knee flexion deformity may also be amenable to this approach, but not in arthropathies or where the bone is osteoporotic in juvenile idiopathic arthritis.

Lengthening with multilevel corrections

In bifocal lengthening, both metaphyses within the segment may be lengthened simultaneously. This technique has certain theoretical advantages: shorter lengthened segments and better frame stability lead to more rapid consolidation with fewer soft-tissue problems and less bony deformity (Saleh & Hamer 1993). Diaphyseal osteotomies may also be used to correct deformity. Complicated multilevel, multiplanar corrections with lengthening may be performed satisfactorily only with a circular frame (Ghoneem et al 1996) (Fig. 28.17).

Table 28.4 Leg lengthening techniques	
Type 1: low-risk linear	Straight lengthening of less than 20%
Type 2: high-risk linear	Straight lengthening with joint instability or other 'at-risk features' such as lengthening greater than 20%
Type 3: low-risk complex	Lengthening of less than 20% with no 'at-risk features' but soft-tissue or bony correction required
Type 4: high-risk complex	Lengthening with joint instability or other 'at-risk features' such as lengthening greater than 20% and soft-tissue or bony correction required

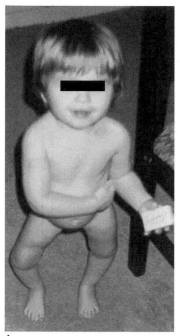

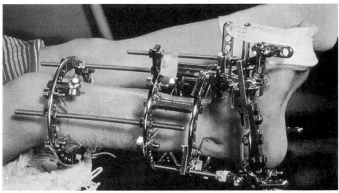

Figure 28.15 A–D Clinical and radiographic appearances in the use of an Ilizarov frame to correct genu varum in Blount's disease. Note the use of radiolucent carbon fibre rings.

Figure 28.16 Short tibia combined with an unstable ankle and equinus deformity in fibular hemimelia. Correction is achieved in two stages: the equinus deformity first, followed by a neutralisation period for the calf muscles before a short tibial lengthening. The frame remains across the ankle until at least the late consolidation phase.

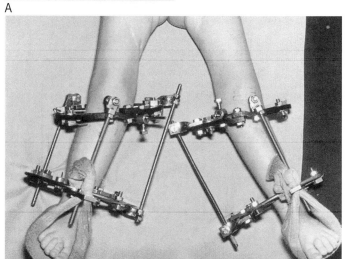

B

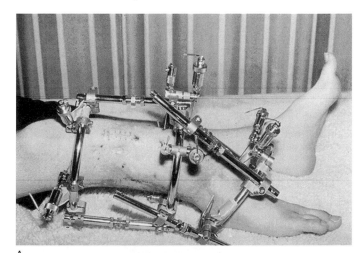

A

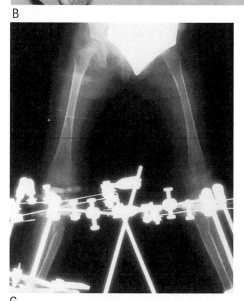

C

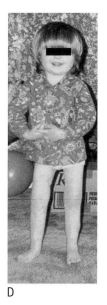

D

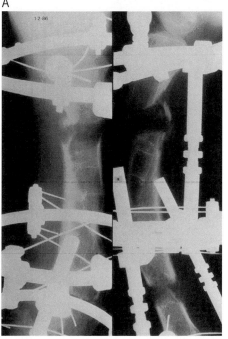

B

Figure 28.17 A & B Bifocal lengthening with correction of two planes of angulation, rotation and equinus, using a Sequoia circular external fixator.

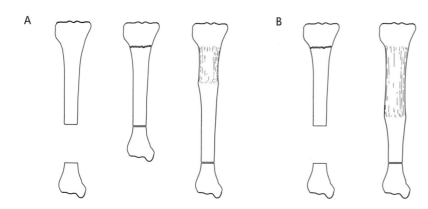

Figure 28.18 Line drawings depicting two techniques for closing bone defects.
A Immediate shortening followed by metaphyseal lengthening (compression/distraction).
B Metaphyseal lengthening and bone transport.

Use in other conditions

Bone defects

Bone defects may be the result of acute bone loss as a result of trauma or surgical resection for disease. Ilizarov described a technique of internal movement of bone known as transport (Ilizarov & Ledyaev 1969). New bone is generated by distraction, but the bone is encouraged to move relative to the soft-tissue envelope, maintaining length but closing a bone gap. Shorter gaps may be closed by immediate shortening, followed by lengthening at a healthy metaphysis – a technique known as compression–distraction (Fig. 28.18) (Ribbans et al 1992).

In congenital pseudarthrosis of the tibia, the Ilizarov method may be used in preference to more conventional methods (Paley et al 1992). In younger patients, overlapping of the fracture fragments and horizontal compression, distraction or invagination may be used to increase the surface area in contact. If these techniques fail or if the patient is elderly, the abnormal segment may be resected and closed by transport or compression–distraction. Whichever method is selected, overall length and alignment may be adjusted by appropriate osteotomies with lengthening and angular correction (Fig. 28.19).

Complex foot deformities

Severe foot deformities caused by relapsed or resistant club foot, arthrogryposis, spina bifida, poliomyelitis, trauma, or congenital origin (such as fibular hemimelia) may be corrected using the Ilizarov technique (Grill & Franke 1987, Grant et al 1992, O'Doherty et al 1992). Fixation is applied in the lower tibia, hindfoot, forefoot and, occasionally, the midfoot (Fig. 28.20). In this way, each part of the foot may be moved separately, enabling each component of the deformity to be corrected by distraction of scars and contractures. Sequential adjustments to the frame configuration are necessary (Fig. 28.21). Slight overcorrection and a period of neutralisation both in the frame and with an ankle–foot orthosis are necessary to reduce the potential for relapse. In young children (younger than 8 years), correction of the soft tissues alone is usually adequate, because some bone remodelling will take place. In older children and adolescents, osteotomies with distraction are usually required (Figs 28.22

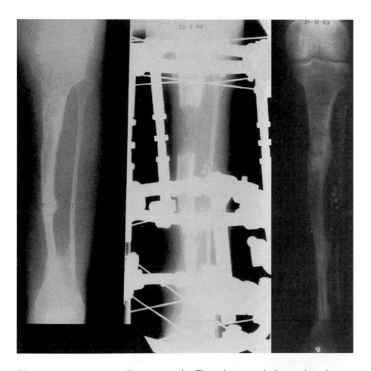

Figure 28.19 Neurofibromatosis. The abnormal tissue has been resected and replaced by a free vascularised fibular graft. The distal end of the graft formed a hypertrophic non-union. Length, alignment and fracture healing were achieved by bifocal lengthening using a Sequoia circular external fixator.

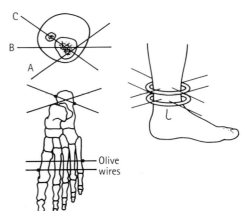

Figure 28.20 Diagram showing wire positioning for foot corrections. A, medial face wire; B, transverse wire; C, fibulo-tibial wire.

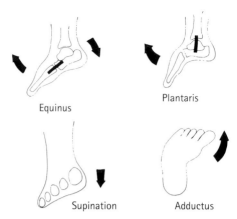

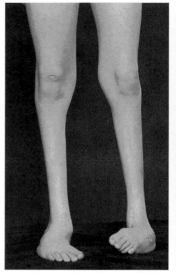

Equinus   Plantaris

Supination   Adductus

Figure 28.21
Diagram illustrating the correct sequence for correction of complex foot deformities.

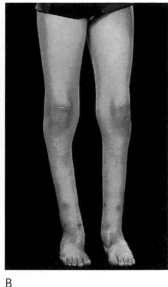

A   B

Figure 28.23 Clinical photographs of an adolescent before (**A**) and after (**B**) correction of severe deformity of the feet.

and 28.23). In severe cases with ankylosis, arthrodesis or coalition, osteotomies may be performed to alter the relationship of the foot to the tibia in addition to that of the hind-foot to the forefoot (Fig. 28.24). The foot often remains small and the calf wasted. Lengthening of the foot through either the midfoot or the metatarsals is possible, but may well lead to intractable stiffness and pain. Ilizarov has also described

a complex tibial widening operation, which appears to offer improved calf cosmesis. Similar corrective operations may be carried out in the forearm, wrist and hand.

CONCLUSION

The Ilizarov technique offers many advantages over conventional unilateral frame lengthening when complex deformity is associated with the limb shortening. Outcome studies in the child (Ghoneen et al 1996) and the adult (McKee et al 1998) confirm the improvement in health that follows successful reconstruction, but also stress that the complication rate remains high and that the method should be confined to resourced and experienced centres.

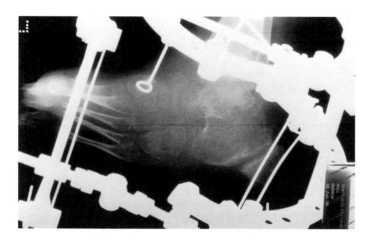

Figure 28.22 Severe talipes equinovarus. Seven operations on each foot have only partially reduced the severe deformity. This 11-year-old boy had never worn normal shoes. Heel height was restored by oblique osteotomy and lengthening of the os calcis. After correction of adductus, the medial arch was restored with an osteotomy of the medial cuneiform.

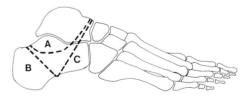

Figure 28.24 'U' and 'V' osteotomies for the correction of severe foot deformities.

REFERENCES

Abbott L C 1927 The operative lengthening of the tibia and fibula. Journal of Bone and Joint Surgery 9: 128–152

Aldegheri R, Agostini S 1983 A chart of anthropometric values. Journal of Bone and Joint Surgery 75B: 86–88

Anderson W V 1972 Lengthening of the lower limb: its place in the problem of limb length discrepancy. Modern Trends in Orthopaedics 5: 1

Anderson M, Green W T, Messner M B 1963 Growth and prediction of growth in the lower extremities. Journal of Bone and Joint Surgery 45A: 1–14

Aronson J, Harrison B H, Stewart C L, Harp J H 1989 The histology of distraction osteogenesis using different external fixators. Clinical Orthopaedics and Related Research 241: 106–116

Bell D F, Armstrong P, Paley D 1990 Extensive two-level limb lengthening: early results, utilizing the Ilizarov technique. Journal of Bone and Joint Surgery 72B: 538

Bianchi Maiocchi A, Aronson J (eds) 1991 Operative principles of Ilizarov. Fracture treatment, nonunion, osteomyelitis, lengthening, deformity correction. Williams & Wilkins, Baltimore

Blair V P, Schoenecker P L, Sheridan J J, Capelli A M 1989 Closed shortening of the femur. Journal of Bone and Joint Surgery 71A: 1440–1447

Blount W P, Clark G R 1949 Control of bone growth by epiphyseal stapling. Preliminary report. Journal of Bone and Joint Surgery 31A: 464–478

Bortel D T, Pritchett J W 1993 Straight line graphs for the prediction of growth of the upper extremities. Journal of Bone and Joint Surgery 75A: 885–892

Bowen J R, Johnson W J 1984 Percutaneous epiphysiodesis. Clinical Orthopaedics and Related Research 190: 170–173

Broughton N S, Olney B W, Menelaus M B 1989 Tibial shortening for leg length discrepancy. Journal of Bone and Joint Surgery 71B: 242–245

Canale S T, Christian C A 1990 Techniques for epiphysiodesis about the knee. Clinical Orthopaedics and Related Research 255: 81

Choi I H, Kumar S J, Bowen R J 1990 Amputation or limb lengthening for partial or total absence of the fibula. Journal of Bone and Joint Surgery 72A: 1391–1399

Choi I H, Chung C Y, Cho T-J, Park S S 1999 Correction of genu recurvatum by the Ilizarov method. Journal of Bone and Joint Surgery 81B: 769–774

Codivilla A 1905 On the means of lengthening in the lower limbs, the muscles and the tissues which are shortened through deformity. American Journal of Orthopedic Surgery 2: 353–369

De Bastiani G, Aldegheri R, Renzi-Brivio L, Trivella G 1986a Limb lengthening by distraction of the epiphyseal plate: a comparison of two techniques in the rabbit. Journal of Bone and Joint Surgery 68B: 545–549

De Bastiani G, Aldegheri R, Renzi-Brivio L, Trivella G 1986b Chondrodiatasis – controlled symmetrical distraction of the epiphyseal plate: limb lengthening in children. Journal of Bone and Joint Surgery 68B: 550–556

De Bastiani G, Aldegheri R, Renzio-Brivio L, Trivella G 1987 Limb lengthening by callus distraction (callotasis). Journal of Pediatric Orthopaedics 7: 129–134

Eastwood D M, Cole W G 1995 A graphic method for timing the correction of leg-length discrepancy. Journal of Bone and Joint Surgery 77B: 743–748

Eyres K S, Bell M J, Kanis J A 1993 New bone formation during leg lengthening. Journal of Bone and Joint Surgery 75B: 96–106

Ferguson C M, Morrison J D, Kenwright J 1987 Leg length inequality in children treated by Syme's amputation. Journal of Bone and Joint Surgery 69B: 433–436

Fixsen J A 1983 Editorial: rotation-plasty. Journal of Bone and Joint Surgery 65B: 529–530

Galardi G, Comi G, Lozza L et al 1990 Peripheral nerve damage during limb lengthening. Journal of Bone and Joint Surgery 72B: 121–124

Ghoneem H F, Wright J G, Cole W G, Rang M 1996 The Ilizarov method for correction of complex deformities. Journal of Bone and Joint Surgery 78A: 1480–1485

Grant A D, Atar D, Lehman W B 1992 The Ilizarov technique in the correction of complex foot deformities. Clinical Orthopaedics and Related Research 280: 94–103

Green W T, Anderson M 1957 Epiphyseal arrest for the correction of discrepancies in length of the lower extremities. Journal of Bone and Joint Surgery 39A: 853–872

Greulich W W, Pyle S I 1959 Radiographic atlas of skeletal development of the hand and wrist, 2nd edn. Stanford University Press, Stanford, California

Grill F, Franke J 1987 The Ilizarov distractor for the correction of relapsed or neglected club foot. Journal of Bone and Joint Surgery 69B: 593–597

Haas S L 1945 Restriction of bone growth by a wire loop. Journal of Bone and Joint Surgery 27A: 25–30

Haas S L 1950 Restriction of bone growth by pins through the epiphyseal cartilaginous plate. Journal of Bone and Joint Surgery 32A: 338–342

Ilizarov G A 1989a The tension-stress effect on the genesis and growth of tissues. Part I: The influence of stability of fixation and soft-tissue preservation. Clinical Orthopaedics and Related Research 238: 249–281

Ilizarov G A 1989b The tension-stress effect on the genesis and growth of tissues. Part II: The influence of the rate and frequency of distraction. Clinical Orthopaedics and Related Research 239: 263–285

Ilizarov G A 1990 Clinical application of the tension-stress effect for limb lengthening. Clinical Orthopaedics and Related Research 250: 8

Ilizarov G A 1991 Transosseous osteosynthesis: theoretical and clinical aspects of the regeneration and growth of tissue. Springer, Berlin

Ilizarov G A, Deviatov A A 1971 Operative elongation of the leg. Ortopediia Travmatologiia Protezirovanie 32: 20–25

Ilizarov G A, Ledyaev V L 1969 The replacement of long tubular defects by lengthening distraction osteotomy of one of the fragments. Vestnik Khirurgii 6: 78

Illzarov G A, Trokhova C G 1973 Operative elongation of the femur. Ortopediia Travmatologiia: Protezirovanie 34: 51–55

Jackson A M 1993 Excision of the central physeal bar: a modification of Langenskiöld's procedure. Journal of Bone and Joint Surgery 75B: 664–665

Kasser J R 1990 Physeal bar resections after growth arrest about the knee. Clinical Orthopaedics and Related Research 255: 68

Kenwright J, Spriggins A J, Cunningham J L 1989 Response of the growth plate to distraction close to skeletal maturity. Clinical Orthopaedics and Related Research 250: 61

Küntscher G 1965 Intramedullary surgical technique and its place in orthopaedic surgery. My current concept. Journal of Bone and Joint Surgery 47A: 809

Langenskiöld A 1981 Surgical treatment of partial closure of the growth plate. Journal of Pediatric Orthopaedics 1: 3

Leong J C Y Alade C O, Fang D 1982 Supracondylar femoral osteotomy for knee flexion contracture resulting from poliomyelitis. Journal of Bone and Joint Surgery 64B: 198–201

Liotta F J, Ambrose T A, Eilert R E 1992 Fluoroscopic technique versus Phemister technique for epiphysiodesis. Journal of Pediatric Orthopaedics 12: 248–251

McKee M D, Yoo D, Schemitsch E H 1998 Health status after Ilizarov reconstruction of post-traumatic lower-limb deformity. Journal of Bone and Joint Surgery 80B: 360–364

Macnicol M F 1994 Tubesaw epiphysiodesis. In: Tachdjian M O (ed.) Atlas of Pediatric Orthopaedic Surgery. W B Saunders, Philadelphia

Macnicol M F, Catto A M 1982 Twenty-year review of tibial lengthening for poliomyelitis. Journal of Bone and Joint Surgery 64B: 607–611

Macnicol M F, Gupta M 1997 Epiphysiodesis using a cannulated tubesaw. Journal of Bone and Joint Surgery 97B: 307–309

Macnicol M F, Krishnan J, Draper E R C 1993 Epiphysiodesis using a cannulated tube saw: comparison with the Phemister technique. Journal of Pediatric Orthopaedics B2: 72–74

May V R Jr, Clemens E L 1965 Epiphyseal stapling: with special reference to the complications. Southern Medical Journal 58: 1203–1208

Menelaus M B 1966 Correction of leg length discrepancy by epiphyseal arrest. Journal of Bone and Joint Surgery 48B: 336–339

Millis M B, Hall J E 1979 Transiliac lengthening of the lower extremity. Journal of Bone and Joint Surgery 61A: 1182–1194

Morrissy R T 1992 Distal femoral epiphysiodesis, Phemister technique. In: Atlas of Pediatric Orthopaedic Surgery. J B Lippincott, Philadelphia, p 405

Moseley C F 1977 A straight line graph for leg length discrepancies. Journal of Bone and Joint Surgery 59A: 174–179

O'Doherty D P, Street R, Saleh M 1992 The use of circular external fixators in the management of complex disorders of the foot and ankle. Foot 2: 135–142

Paley D 1988 Current techniques of limb lengthening. Journal of Pediatric Orthopaedics 8: 73–92

Paley D 1990 Problems, obstacles and complications of limb lengthening by the Ilizarov technique. Clinical Orthopaedics and Related Research 250: 81–104

Paley D, Catagni M, Argnani F, Prevot J, Bell D, Armstrong P 1992 Treatment of congenital pseudarthrosis of the tibia using the Ilizarov technique. Clinical Orthopaedics and Related Research 280: 81–93

Paley D, Herzenberg J E, Tetsworth K, McKie J, Bhare A 1994 Deformity planning for frontal and sagittal plane corrective osteotomies. Orthopedic Clinics of North America 25: 425–465

Phemister D B 1933 Operative arrestment of longitudinal growth of bones in the treatment of deformities. Journal of Bone and Joint Surgery 15: 1–15

Pritchett J W 1988 Growth and predictions of growth in the upper extremity. Journal of Bone and Joint Surgery 70A: 520–522

Ribbans W J, Stubbs D A, Saleh M 1992 Nonunion surgery Part II. The Sheffield experience: 100 consecutive cases. Results and lessons. International Journal of Orthopedic Trauma 2: 19–24

Richardson J B, Cunningham J L, Goodship A E, O'Connor B T, Kenright J 1994 Measuring stiffness can define healing of tibial fractures. Journal of Bone and Joint Surgery 76B: 389–394

Saleh M 1992a Technique selection in leg lengthening: the Sheffield practice. Seminars in Orthopedics 7: 137–151

Saleh M 1992b Nonunion surgery Part I. Basic principles of management. International Journal of Orthopedic Trauma 2: 4–18

Saleh M, Hamer A J 1993 Bifocal lengthening – a preliminary report. Journal of Pediatric Orthopaedics B2: 42–48

Saleh M, Scott B W 1992 Pitfalls and complications in leg lengthening: the Sheffield experience. Seminars in Orthopedics 7: 207–222

Serafin J 1967 Operation for congenital absent fibula. Journal of Bone and Joint Surgery 49B: 59

Shapiro F 1982 Developmental patterns in lower extremity length discrepancies. Journal of Bone and Joint Surgery 64A: 639–651

Shapiro F 1987 Longitudinal growth of the femur and tibia. Journal of Bone and Joint Surgery 69A: 684

Simpson A H R, Kenwright J 2000 Fracture after distraction osteogenesis. Journal of Bone and Joint Surgery 82B: 659–665

Snyder M, Harcke H T, Bowen J R, Caro P A 1994 Evaluation of physeal behaviour in response to epiphysiodesis with the use of serial magnetic resonance imaging. Journal of Bone and Joint Surgery 76A: 224–229

Sofield H A, Blair S J, Millar E A 1958 Leg lengthening: a personal follow-up of forty patients some twenty years after the operation. Journal of Bone and Joint Surgery 40A: 311–322

Stahl E J, Karpmann R 1986 Normal growth and growth predictions in the upper extremity. Journal of Hand Surgery 11A: 593–596

Stanitski D F, Bullard M, Armstrong P, Stanitski C I 1995 Results of femoral lengthening using the Ilizarov technique. Journal of Pediatric Orthopaedics 15: 224–231

Stanitski D F, Shahcheraghi H, Nicker D A, Armstrong P F 1996 Results of tibial lengthening with the Ilizarov technique. Journal of Pediatric Orthopaedics 6: 168–172

Thomas N P, Williams P F 1987 The Gruca operation for congenital absence of the fibula. Journal of Bone and Joint Surgery 69B: 587–592

Thomas N P, Jackson A M, Aichroth P M 1985 Congenital absence of the anterior cruciate ligament. Journal of Bone and Joint Surgery 67B: 572–574

Timperlake R W, Bowen J R, Guile J T et al 1991 Prospective evaluation of 53 consecutive percutaneous epiphysiodeses of the distal femur and proximal tibia and fibula. Journal of Pediatric Orthopaedics 11: 350–357

Vilarrubias J M, Ginebreda I, Jimeno E 1990 Lengthening of the lower limbs and correction of lumbar hyperlordosis in achondroplasia. Clinical Orthopedics and Related Research 250: 143

Wagner H 1977 Surgical lengthening or shortening of femur and tibia; technique and indications. In: Hungerford D S (ed) Progress in orthopaedic surgery. Springer, Berlin

Westh R W, Menelaus M B 1981 A simple calculation for the timing of epiphyseal arrest. Journal of Bone and Joint Surgery 63B: 117–119

White J W, Stubbins S G Jr 1944 Growth arrest for equalising leg lengths. Journal of the American Medical Association 126: 1146–1148

Wilde G P, Baker G C W 1987 Circumferential periosteal release in the treatment of children with leg-length inequality. Journal of Bone and Joint Surgery 60B: 817–821

Wolff J 1892 Das Gesetz der Transformation der Knochen. Verlag von August Hirschwald, Berlin

Young N, Bell D F, Anthony A 1994 Pediatric pain patterns during Ilizarov treatment of limb length discrepancy and angular deformity. Journal of Pediatric Orthopaedics 14: 352–357

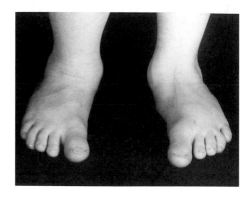
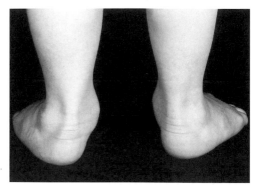

A   B

Figure 29.2 Clinical photographs showing anterior (A) and posterior (B) of a child of 4 years with serpentine or 'Z-feet'.

obvious in the first few months of life or when the child starts to walk. The forefoot is in varus or adduction, very often with some supination but no equinus. The hindfoot is in neutral or valgus. The deformity is often best seen from the sole of the foot, and in mild and moderate cases is easily correctable by simple finger pressure on the first ray. It is essential to examine the whole child carefully, because metatarsus varus can be associated with neurological conditions such as spina bifida occulta or spinal muscular atrophy, in which case there is usually evidence of muscle wasting and lack of normal movements in the lower limb. There is a very rare rigid form of the condition called the serpentine or 'Z-foot' (see below), in which the forefoot adduction and varus deformity is fixed and the hindfoot is in fixed valgus (Fig. 29.2).

The aetiology of metatarsus varus is unknown, although Harris (1972) suggested it could be associated with the persistent prone-lying sleeping position. Recently, prone lying for infants has been associated with the 'cot death' syndrome; supine lying has therefore been encouraged, and the incidence of metatarsus varus appears to have reduced considerably.

X-rays show that the metatarsals are adducted relative to the mid- and hindfoot and the talo-calcaneal angles are normal or increased in the anteroposterior view (Fig. 29.3). In the rare serpentine or 'skew' foot, the navicular and cuboid are laterally displaced on the talus and the calcaneum (Fig. 29.4).

Treatment

There is considerable argument about the treatment of this common condition. The natural history has been reported by Ponseti & Becker (1966) and by Rushforth (1978), who both found that in the majority of patients the condition corrected spontaneously with or without treatment. The former investigators reported that approximately 1 in 9 patients needed treatment. They used plasters, which they pointed out were difficult to apply, and because they were a special centre for children's orthopaedics they probably had a greater number of difficult cases than average. In Rushforth's series, 130 feet – which received no treatment – were followed up for 7

years; 86% corrected completely, 10% showed mild persistence of the deformity, which did not worry the patient or their parents in any way, and only 4% showed persistence of the deformity. Rushforth was unable to predict until the child reached an age of 3–4 years, which feet were not going to correct. This puts the orthopaedic surgeon in a considerable

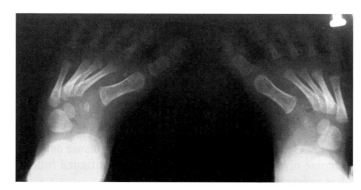

A

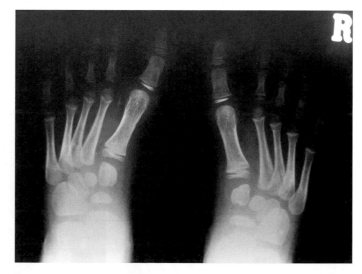

B

Figure 29.3 Anteroposterior radiographs of metatarsus varus. A At 9 months. B 2½ years later, at the age of 3 years and 3 months, with no treatment.

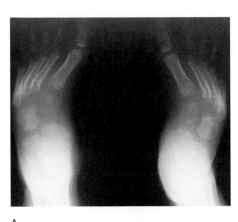

A

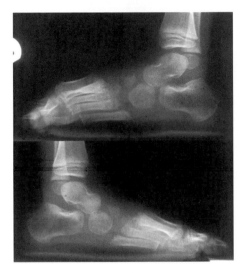

B

Figure 29.4
Anteroposterior (**A**) and lateral (**B**) radiographs of true serpentine or 'Z-feet' in a boy of 5 years and 4 months. Note the lateral shift of the mid-tarsus on the hindfoot and the varus, and supination of the forefoot.

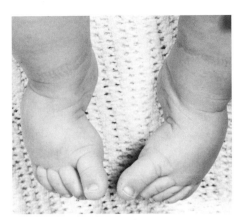

Figure 29.5
Clinical photograph of a child aged 9 months with the severe type of metatarsus varus, showing a significant medial crease. This deformity was rigid, and not passively correctable.

dilemma: at least four in five feet will correct spontaneously without any treatment, and it is very difficult to identify those patients requiring treatment. In general, any patient in whom the foot corrects easily to neutral or beyond will probably correct spontaneously. The child with a very rigid deformity and a deep medial crease should be treated, probably initially by stretching applied by the mother (Fig. 29.5). Ponseti & Becker (1966) advised that plastering above the knee was necessary, to control the whole leg. They emphasised the difficulty of applying these plasters. They advised that the plasters were changed every 2–3 weeks and that correction was usually obtained within 8–10 weeks, but in some patients relapse occurred after the plasters were removed. Farsetti et al (1994) published a long-term follow-up of untreated and non-surgically treated metatarsus adductus that reported good results in all 16 untreated feet and 90% of those treated with long leg plasters. Recently, Katz et al (1999) reported treating 85 inflexible feet with below-knee plasters, with satisfactory results.

In order to avoid excessive over-treatment of this generally benign condition, the vast majority of these feet should be left alone or, if inflexible, treated with plasters. If, at the age of 3–4 years, there is a persistent deformity, operative correction can be considered. Browne & Paton (1979) described an anomalous insertion of the tibialis posterior, and noted that the main bulk of the tendon did not attach to the navicular bone, but extended into the forefoot. This was released together with the abductor hallucis, and the deformity corrected by plaster. Heyman et al (1985) recommended the more extensive procedure of tarso-metatarsal capsulotomies. Stark et al (1987) reported a 41% overall failure rate and a 50% incidence of a painful dorsal prominence at the site of the surgical scar, in a review of this procedure performed over an 18-year period. The author's own limited experience of this operation is similar to that described by Stark et al. After the child has reached the age of 6 years, multiple metatarsal osteotomies described by Berman & Gartland (1971) can be used. Again, there are significant complications associated with this operation, with failure of correction and damage, particularly to the epiphyseal plate of the first metatarsal, causing shortening and progressive deformity, indicating that this operation should be used with great care. It is extremely rare to see an adult with persistent symptomatic metatarsus varus. On this basis, and the evidence that the majority of these feet correct with time, it is important not to overtreat this condition – in particular, not to operate on it unless it is absolutely necessary, because it is quite clear that operation can produce symptoms and deformity of a greater severity than the condition itself.

Bleck (1983) advocated a more radical early approach to conservative treatment with serial plasters, accepting that the results of his study did not make it possible to predict with certainty which feet must be treated, and acknowledging the influence of 'the public attitude toward deformity' amongst his treatment population.

SERPENTINE OR 'Z-FOOT'

A true serpentine or 'Z-foot' is a very rare entity. Kite (1967) described 12 cases among a total of 2818 cases of metatarsus varus – an incidence of 0.43%. In this condition the forefoot varus and adduction is fixed; the hindfoot is in fixed valgus. The X-rays show that the navicular and cuboid bones are laterally displaced on the talus and calcaneum with the metatarsals in varus, giving rise to the classical 'Z- or S-shaped' foot (Figs 29. 2 and 29. 3). This is extremely difficult to treat, because all three components of the deformity require correction. Lloyd-Roberts & Clark (1973) pointed out that this rare condition may be associated with a ball-and-socket ankle joint, so that fusing the subtalar joint will not correct the valgus. It is important to look at the whole patient, as this condition may be associated with other anomalies such as Larsen's syndrome (Fig. 29.6). Mosca (1995), in an important review of skew foot, suggested that, in infants and young children, management should follow that of metatarsus adductus; in older children and adults, only those with symptoms should be treated. In 1995, he described satisfactory short-term results in 10 symptomatic skew feet operated on to correct all three components of the deformity. The operation was performed in children of an average age of 10 years. The operation combined a reversed Dillwyn Evans (1975) type of calcaneal lengthening procedure to correct the hindfoot and midfoot, and a medial cuneiform opening wedge osteotomy, as described by Fowler et al (1959), to correct the forefoot. The tendo-Achilles, which was always short, was also lengthened.

CONGENITAL TALIPES CALCANEO-VALGUS

Postural calcaneo-valgus is the most common position of the foot in the newborn (Fig. 29.7). It is normal to be able to dorsiflex the foot of the neonate so that the dorsum touches the anterior aspect of the tibia; however, there should be a full range of plantarflexion. In congenital talipes calcaneo-valgus, the foot is markedly dorsiflexed and everted, but plantarflexion is limited, often to only the neutral position. The condition is more common in first-born children. It is associated with oligohydramnios and the 'moulded baby syndrome' (Lloyd-Roberts & Pilcher 1965). It is said to be associated with congenital dislocation of the hip in 5% of cases, and instability of the hip must be looked for in patients with this deformity. It is very important to seek any suggestion of neuromuscular abnormality, both in the spine of the infant and in the leg in the form of wasting or a difference in size between the two legs. The condition must be distinguished from congenital vertical talus (congenital convex pes valgus), in which the forefoot is in calcaneus and valgus, but the hindfoot is in fixed equinus.

If there is no evidence of an underlying abnormality, this condition nearly always responds to simple stretching applied by the mother. She is shown by the physiotherapist how to stretch the foot into plantarflexion and inversion. This should be done regularly several times a day, probably when the baby is being fed and the nappy changed. In the vast majority of patients, the condition will correct by the age of 3 months. If there is failure to correct by this age, the patient should be looked at very carefully for evidence of any underlying neuromuscular abnormality or generalised condition. It is probably wise to follow-up the child until walking is established.

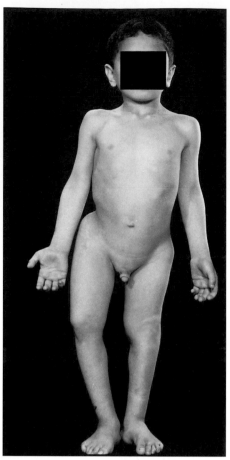

Figure 29.6 A Clinical photograph of a patient with Larsen's syndrome, showing dislocations of the elbows, hips and knees, with serpentine feet. **B** Lateral radiograph of the feet in Larsen's syndrome, showing the characteristic double ossification centre for the os calcis.

A

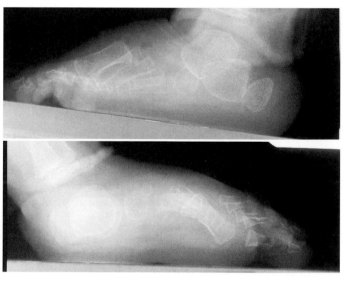

B

Parents are often very worried by this condition and believe that their child will have an abnormal foot or difficulty with walking. Some orthopaedic surgeons such as Giannestras (1973) advocate a more aggressive policy, with serial plasters followed by modifications to shoewear. In the author's experience, this type of treatment has not been necessary unless the

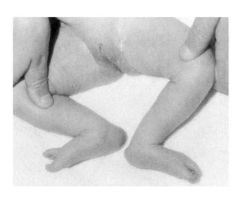

Figure 29.7 Clinical photograph of typical calcaneo-valgus feet in the newborn infant.

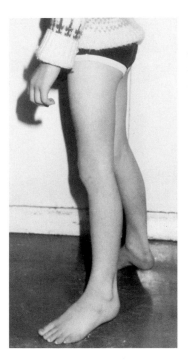

Figure 29.8 Clinical photograph of a child aged 7 years who was a persistent tiptoe walker as a result of true short tendo-Achilles. Note that the heels are well off the ground, with a characteristic broad-based stance.

deformity has been associated with an underlying neuro-muscular or skeletal problem.

TIP-TOE WALKING

PERSISTENT TIP-TOE WALKING OR PERSISTENT EQUINUS

The mature heel–toe pattern of gait should normally be adopted by the age of 2 years (Sutherland et al 1980). One of the most important things for an orthopaedic surgeon to recognise is the child who had developed a mature heel–toe pattern of gait but then reverted to a toe–heel or a toe–toe gait. This is nearly always pathological, and conditions such as muscular dystrophy, spinal dysraphism, peroneal muscular atrophy (hereditary motor and sensory neuropathy) and spinal tumour must be looked for.

IDIOPATHIC TIP-TOE WALKING

In this situation the child persistently walks up on the toes, although when standing may bring the heels to the ground. They may stand with a degree of hyperextension of the knee and also externally rotate their feet in order to get their heels to the ground more easily. Typically, their tip-toe gait is more noticeable in bare feet than when wearing shoes. On the couch, dorsiflexion of the foot with the knee extended is sometimes limited, but can be normal with no evidence of tendo-Achilles shortening. Occasionally, true shortening of the tendo-Achilles with fixed equinus is present. Hall et al (1967) described this as idiopathic shortening of the tendo-Achilles. They pointed out that this condition often was not recognised until the child was at school, as it had been accepted that the child habitually walked like this, and that it would correct with time (Fig. 29.8). They advised surgical lengthening of the tendo-Achilles.

Idiopathic tip-toe walking is a diagnosis of exclusion. Neuromucular disorders such as spastic diplegia and other forms of cerebral palsy should be considered. For a period, all patients referred to the orthopaedic department at The Hospital for Sick Children, London, were referred to a paediatric neurologist, to determine if it was possible to make a neurological diagnosis in every case of tip-toe walking. However, a skilled paediatric neurologist was able to find some underlying neurological cause in only approximately

50% of tip-toe walkers. This gait is also associated with hyper-active children, learning disorders, autism and schizophrenia.

In the past, physiotherapy in the form of stretching by the mother or under the supervision of the physiotherapist, plaster cast, and braces have been advised for the treatment of persistent idiopathic tip-toe walking. However, Eastwood et al (1996) showed that surgery was significantly better than conservative forms of treatment. In their series of patients, 16% had a positive family history of tip-toe walking and 50% had suffered significant neonatal jaundice. In 20% of them, muscle biopsies were performed and these showed features suggestive of a neuropathic process, including a predominance of type I muscle fibres. In 1998, Stricker & Angulo also showed that casts and bracing were really no better than no treatment, and that surgery gave better results. It was interesting that 32% of their 80 patients had a family history of toe walking, 28% were born prematurely, 16% reported delay in psychomotor development or speech, and 31% had perinatal hyperbilirubinaemia. Muscle biopsy was not performed in this series. The investigators concluded that the origin of idiopathic tip-toe walking was unclear in the majority of cases. In those children who showed persistent heel cord contracture, surgical treatment was more effective than conservative methods.

THE PAINFUL HEEL

KOHLER'S DISEASE (OSTEOCHONDRITIS OF THE NAVICULAR)

Kohler (1908) described a painful self-limiting disease of the tarsal navicular that showed flattening, sclerosis and frag-mentation of the navicular on X-ray (Fig. 29.9). The tarsal navicular appears between the ages of 2.5 and 3.5 years. There are

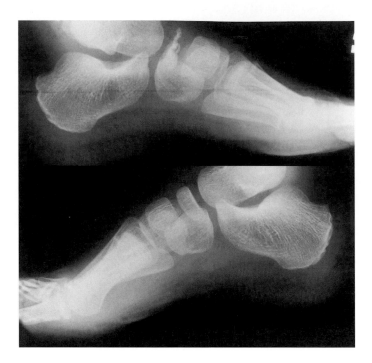

Figure 29.9 Lateral radiograph of the right foot (top) and left foot (bottom), showing Kohler's disease of the right tarsal navicular, with flattening, fragmentation and sclerosis.

considerable variations in the development and pattern of its ossification, so the X-ray appearances may be irrelevant unless the child also has symptoms and local signs. The condition commonly occurs between the ages of 4 and 7 years and in up to 33% of patients, both feet may be involved. The patient presents with pain, limp and tenderness over the tarsal navicular. Sometimes there is sufficient local swelling, redness and warmth for the diagnosis of infection to be considered. Waugh (1958), in a careful study of 52 feet, showed that ossification of the tarsal navicular occurred later in boys than in girls. Abnormalities of ossification were more frequent in boys. He was of the opnion that abnormal ossification resulted from compression of the bony nucleus at the critical phase of growth of the navicular bone. Biopsy performed when the question of infection or tumour had been raised showed areas of necrosis and resorption of dead bone, with the formation of new bone similar to that seen in Perthes' disease. Waugh also showed that, within 2–3 years, the appearances of the navicular had returned to normal. Cox (1958), in a long-term review of 55 patients attending The Hospital for Sick Children, found no evidence of permanent deformity or disability after this disease.

Treatment depends on the severity of the symptoms. Often, no treatment is necessary and the child will recover spontaneously. Occasionally, pain is sufficiently severe to require immobilisation of the foot in a below-knee walking plaster or orthosis for 6 weeks.

CALCANEAL APOPHYSITIS (SEVER'S DISEASE)

Sever described this condition in 1912. He believed it to be a form of osteochondritis of the calcaneal apophysis. However, the appearance of increased density and fragmentation of the calcaneal apophysis is now known to be a normal radiological finding in the age group concerned (Fig. 29.10).

The child, usually between the ages of 7 and 12 years and more commonly a boy than a girl, presents with pain and tenderness over the insertion of the tendo-Achilles into the os calcis. The patient commonly finds it more comfortable to wear a shoe with a heel than to walk barefoot. The child is often a keen footballer or gymnast, and the tenderness is accurately localised to the insertion of the tendo-Achilles. This condition is now believed to be a strain of the insertion of the tendo-Achilles. It must be distinguished from Achilles' tendonitis, which can also occur in children, particularly keen sportsmen, but is associated with pain and swelling over the tendo-Achilles above the os calcis. It is also possible to develop a bursitis in which the small bursa between the posterosuperior corner of the os calcis and the tendo-Achilles becomes inflamed. The rare subacute osteomyelitis of the os calcis should also be considered (see below: under other causes of pain in the heel).

Treatment usually consists of fitting a lift on the heel of the shoe and reducing activity. If this is not sufficient, a short period in plaster may be necessary. However, it is important to regulate activity carefully when the plaster is removed, otherwise the condition will recur. This condition can be a considerable nuisance in children who are keen on sport, particularly football and gymnastics.

CALCANEAL BOSS

This condition is almost entirely confined to adolescent girls, who develop a painful bony swelling over the superolateral corner of the os calcis. This is almost always associated with wearing a high-heeled court shoe, which causes pressure over this area that results in a bursa over the normal prominence of the os calcis at this site. With time, the feet become accustomed to the pressure of the shoes and the condition

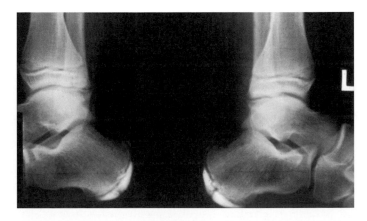

Figure 29.10 Lateral radiograph of both heels of a child aged 11 years with so-called Sever's disease. The sclerosis and fragmentation of the calcaneal apophysis are normal X-ray appearances at this age. The patient was complaining of pain at the insertion of the tendo-Achilles on the right heel only.

settles. However, sometimes there is sufficient anxiety and pressure to do something about it that the surgeon may be persuaded to operate; it is much better to change the design of shoe and take the pressure off the heel, or pad the heel well and wait for the condition to subside. If the surgeon is persuaded to remove the bony lump that underlies the swelling, this involves removing a substantial portion of the posterosuperior corner of the os calcis. Great care must be taken not to damage the terminal branches of the sural nerve and to avoid a painful neuroma, which can cause more troublesome symptoms than the original lump. Almost all these patients will respond to modification of footwear and time.

OTHER CAUSES OF PAIN IN THE HEEL

There are a number of other interesting causes of pain in the heel. A child may traumatise the heel by jumping from a height. Fractures of the os calcis are notoriously difficult to see on X-ray, unless an axial view of the os calcis is taken in addition to the conventional anteroposterior and lateral views (Fig. 29.11).

Infection in the os calcis often runs an unusual subacute course (see Ch. 9) and has been misdiagnosed as a sprain, ligamentous injury or Sever's disease (Antoniou & Connor 1974) (Fig. 29.12).

Generalised bony conditions such as fibrous dysplasia and neurofibromatosis can also present with pain in the heel, as can bone tumours such as bone cysts and osteoid osteomata (Fig. 29.13). The last of these may be very difficult to see, and a bone scan can therefore be very useful in the investigation of obscure pain in the heel region.

FLAT FEET

FLAT FOOT (PES PLANUS)

In the past, there has been great concern among parents and doctors about flat feet. However, a knowledge of the natural history of foot development in the child, and the awareness

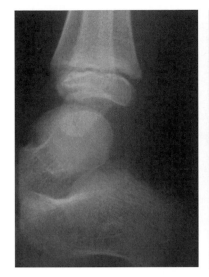
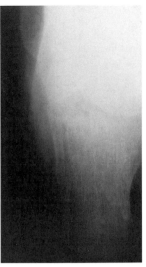

Figure 29.11 Lateral and axial radiographs of a child with a fracture of the os calcis. The longitudinal fracture is seen only with some difficulty in the axial view.

that the ordinary flexible flat foot associated with joint laxity should be considered a normal variant and not a disability, have led to a much more rational attitude to this very common condition.

Natural history

The natural history of foot development in the child is well documented (Staheli et al 1987).

At birth, the most common position for the foot is in slight dorsiflexion and eversion – that is, mild calcaneovalgus. At the end of the first year, when the child begins to stand, the foot nearly always looks flat, particularly because there is a large pad of fat on the medial side of the foot beneath the navicular; this is a normal fat pad, although it can look quite large and sometimes has a considerable vascular element. Between the ages of 1 and 2 years, walking

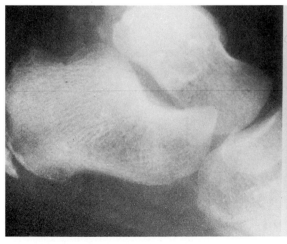

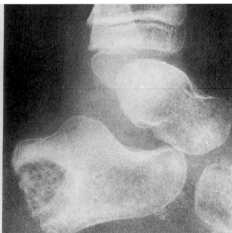

Figure 29.12 Lateral radiographs showing osteomyelitis of the os calcis. The initial radiograph (A) was taken 2 months before the second (B). Note the development of the abcess with time. The patient was initially believed to have a strain of the tendo-Achilles at the time of the first X-ray.

A   B

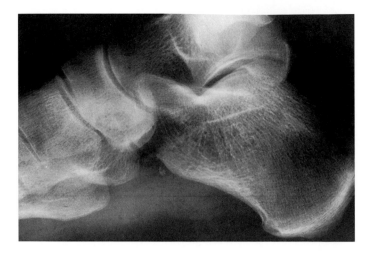

Figure 29.13 Lateral radiograph of a child with pain in the hindfoot region, showing an osteoid osteoma in the tarsal navicular.

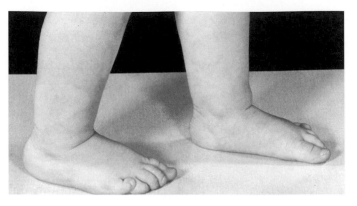

Figure 29.14 Clinical photograph of a child aged 18 months showing the normal weight-bearing appearance of the feet at this age. Note the overlapping 5th toe on the right foot.

becomes established and the child characteristically stands with the feet everted and externally rotated. As a result the feet look very flat, but this should not be considered an abnormality (Fig. 29.14). Between the ages of 2 and 3 years, the medial arch starts to appear. If, at this stage, a child's feet remain significantly flat – with the medial arch resting near or on the ground – it is most important to test for the presence of joint laxity. The majority of these feet will be so-called 'flexible' flat feet, which are asymptomatic and require no treatment. The assessment of joint laxity can be difficult, particularly as it varies considerably between races. Carter & Wilkinson (1964) described five tests for joint laxity in the upper and lower limbs that have become accepted as evidence of familial joint laxity (Fig. 29.15), but these do not take into account considerable racial variations. Cheng et al (1991) have shown that among Chinese children, the tests of Carter & Wilkinson are not sufficiently sensitive for children in Hong Kong because they are generally far more lax than the European children tested by Carter & Wilkinson.

Diagnosis

In the diagnosis of flat foot, the problem is to distinguish the normal variant, usually associated with joint laxity for which no treatment is necessary, from patients who have a significant abnormality causing symptoms for which treatment is necessary and which are often due to some underlying cause not arising in the foot. Morley (1957), in an unselected series of patients attending routine health clinics, showed that 97% of children younger than 18 months have apparent flat feet. By the age of 10 years, only 4% of children had any evidence of flat feet. In this series, there was no evidence that any treatment such as shoe modifications, insoles or exercises made any difference to the natural evolution of the feet. Rose et al (1986) published the results of an important 25-year study designed to distinguish normal anatomical variants from pathological conditions. They stated that tests for flat foot should relate to function and should be dynamic rather than static. They accepted that all except markedly valgus, everted feet in young children were normal, and showed that children progressively developed an arch with time, so that initially broad feet in pre-school children became normal with

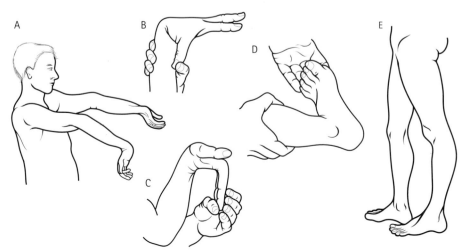

Figure 29.15 Diagrams from Carter & Wilkinson (1964) of the five tests for joint laxity. **A** Hyperextension of elbows: **B** thumb can be placed on the palmar surface of forearm; **C** fingers extend parallel to dorsum of forearm; **D** feet dorsiflex above 30°, and **E** knees hyperextend. (Adapted from Carter C, Wilkinson J 1964 Persistent joint laxity and congenital dislocation of the hip. Journal of Bone and Joint Surgery 46B: 40–45.)

time, irrespective of whether they had any treatment or not.

Rose et al (1986) pointed out that the great-toe extension test is the most useful test for dynamic function of the medial arch. In this test, when the big toe is actively dorsiflexed the medial arch should rise and the tibia externally rotate (Fig. 29.16). The simplest way of testing whether a child has normal flexible flat feet that require no treatment is to get the child to stand on tip-toe. If the arches are restored by this action, the tibia rotates laterally and the heel goes into varus, indicating that the feet are normal. Wenger et al (1989), in a most important prospective study, asked the question 'Can flexible flat feet in children be influenced by treatment?' The conclusion of this study was that flexible flat feet in young children improve with growth. Treatment with corrective shoes, inserts or specially designed insoles does not alter the natural history of the condition. Rao & Joseph (1992), in an interesting study of shod and unshod children, suggested that shoewear in early childhood was detrimental to the development of a normal longitudinal arch, particularly in children with marked joint laxity.

Management

In light of the above, as far as management is concerned, there are two types of flat feet:

a. The common flexible flat foot, which is pain-free, associated with normal muscle power and mobility, and has a normal great-toe extension test. This type of foot should be considered a normal variant. Frequently, it is a familial characteristic and associated with joint laxity. These feet require no treatment and there is no evidence that conservative treatment of any sort alters the natural history of the condition.

b. The pathological type of flat foot. This is often painful. It may have abnormal muscle power, being either weak or

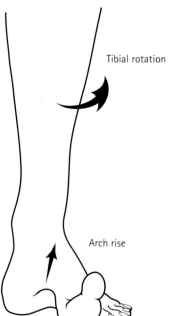

Figure 29.16 Diagram from Rose et al (1986) showing the great-toe extension test. (Adapted from Rose G K, Welton C A, Marshal T 1986 The diagnosis of flat foot in the child. Journal of Bone and Joint Surgery 67B: 71–78.)

Tibial rotation

Arch rise

hypertonic, and may be associated with abnormal mobility, i.e. excessive movement or rigidity. These feet require careful investigation before treatment. Frequently the problem is due to a generalised condition, often neuromuscular in origin, or to some local condition arising in the foot. Treatment with insoles, shoe modifications or exercises may be helpful in this type of foot problem, but it is essential to diagnose the underlying cause if possible.

In the rare severe idiopathic flat foot without any underlying cause, but which is showing symptoms, orthopaedic treatment may be necessary. Supporting the foot with insoles, supportive footwear or orthoses may relieve both symptoms and excessive shoewear. In the older child with severe talo-calcaneal hypermobility, the Grice type of subtalar arthrodesis will stabilise the subtalar joint very satisfactorily, but at the expense of permanent stiffening of the joint and possible later problems in the ankle. Localised naviculo-cuneiform fusion to restore the medial arch has not been successful in the long term (Seymour 1967). The so-called reverse Dillwyn Evans operation, described by Evans in 1975 and recently popularised by Mosca (1995), in which the lateral border of the foot is lengthened by inserting a wedge of bone in the anterior end of the calcaneum, has produced good results. Finally, medial displacement of the os calcis, described by Koutsogiannis (1971) was successful in the short term in some cases.

TARSAL COALITION (PERONEAL SPASTIC FLAT FOOT)

Sir Robert Jones (1897) drew attention to a form of rigid valgus everted foot in which the peroneal muscles were in spasm. This condition became known as 'peroneal spastic flat foot'. The association of this clinical syndrome with tarsal coalition was first described by Slomann in 1921 and Badgely in 1927, who reported the presence of a partial or complete calcaneo-navicular bar in association with peroneal spastic flat foot. In 1948, Harris & Beath described talo-calcaneal coalition, and a wide variety of forms of tarsal coalition have been described since then. The patient, who is usually in the second decade, presents with characteristic clinical signs, often after minor trauma to the foot or ankle, which are initially diagnosed as a simple twist or sprain. However, the symptoms persist. The patient continues to complain of disability, difficulty with walking and running and, if the peroneal spasm is not recognised, may be accused of exaggerating the symptoms and a functional overlay. There are usually clear-cut clinical signs: the foot is held flat and in valgus (Fig. 29.17); the medial arch is not restored when the patient attempts to stand on tip-toe; any attempt to invert the foot at the subtalar joint causes pain, usually over the lateral side of the foot, with spasm of the peroneii. Rarely, spasm of the tibialis posterior may occur with an inversion deformity (Simmons 1965).

Plain anteroposterior and lateral radiographs demonstrate the valgus deformity of the foot. A useful sign of calcaneonavicular coalition, 'the anteater's nose', was reported in

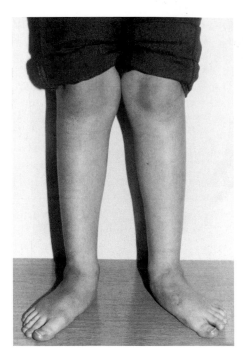

Figure 29.17 Clinical photograph of a patient with bilateral peroneal spastic flat feet.

1987 by Oestreich et al (Fig. 29.18A). A 45° oblique radiograph is very useful when looking for tarsal coalition (Fig. 29.18B), and a 45° axial view of the heel recommended by Harris & Beath (1948) is useful for talo-calcaneal coalition. Computed tomography (CT) is very useful in the diagnosis

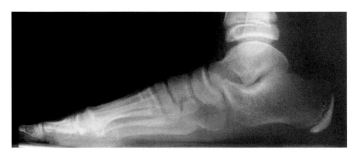

A

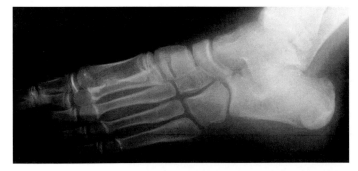

B

Figure 29.18 A Lateral radiograph of the foot, showing a partial calcaneo-navicular bar and the so-called 'anteater's nose' sign. B A 45° oblique radiograph of the same foot, showing the partial calcaneo-navicular bar.

and assessment of all forms of tarsal coalition, and particularly talo-calcaneal bars (Fig. 29.19).

The inheritance of this condition is interesting. Leonard (1974) reported that, among 98 first-degree relatives of 31 patients, 39% had totally asymptomatic tarsal coalition on radiographic examination. The incidence of tarsal coalition in the population is therefore unknown, particularly as it can frequently be entirely asymptomatic. Leonard postulated an autosomal dominant inheritance of almost full penetrance.

Treatment

The management of this condition can be very difficult. If a patient presents with minor symptoms, a medial arch support or medial wedge on the heel may be sufficient to support the medial arch of the foot and relieve the spasm. Frequently, however, the spasm persists. A manipulation under anaesthetic, with or without local injection of hydrocortisone and local anaesthetic into the subtalar region, followed by a below-knee plaster with the foot held in neutral for a period of 6–8 weeks, may be necessary. This often relieves the pain while the patient is in plaster, but it commonly relapses when the plaster is removed. Some surgeons, therefore, recommend prolonged splintage for up to 6 months using a below-knee iron and T-strap or a carefully moulded plastic ankle–foot orthosis. Braddock (1961) published the results of conservative treatment in 56 feet followed up for 21 years. This important review showed that about 50% of the patients had suffered minor symptoms, which did not bother them significantly. Only 10% had had persistent symptoms requiring triple arthrodesis. The prognosis for the foot and the response to treatment bore no relation to the radiological appearances, and symptomatic tarsal arthritis was rare in the long term.

From the surgical point of view, Mitchell & Gibson (1967) recommended excision of the calcaneo-navicular bar in

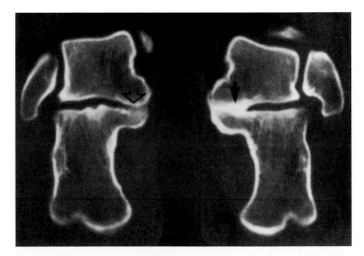

Figure 29.19 A CT scan of the hindfoot, showing a talo-calcaneal bar. (Reproduced with permission from J C Drennan 1992. The child's foot and ankle. Lippincott Williams and Wilkins, Baltimore, p 175.)

patients aged between 10 and 14 years who did not show any secondary changes in the other tarsal joints. Macnicol et al (1986) reviewed 16 feet in 11 patients at an average of 23 years after excision of their calcaneo-navicular bars; 67% had had a good or excellent result. Five feet had poor results that responded well to triple arthrodesis. Beaking of the talus before surgery correlated with a poor result from excision of the calcaneo-navicular bar. Dwyer (1976) suggested os calcis osteotomy to treat the valgus hindfoot. Cain & Hyman (1978) reported the results of a closing medial wedge osteotomy of the os calcis with satisfactory relief of pain and improved movement in the majority of the 40 feet operated upon in their series. CT scanning has made talo-calcaneal bars much easier to diagnose and assess. Olney & Asher (1987) published an early report recommending resection of persistently symptomatic talo-calcaneal middle facet coalition, even in the presence of talar beaking. In 1997, McCormack et al reported a 10-year follow-up of eight of these patients who had operations in nine feet. Eight of the nine feet had done well, and none had required further surgery, although the investigators pointed out that this technique allows the option of a later arthrodesis if the resection does not satisfactorily relieve symptoms.

It is important to remember that a tarsal coalition is not always the cause of a painful peroneal spastic flat foot. It can occur after previous surgery – in particular, overcorrection of the foot in club foot – and in association with juvenile idiopathic arthritis, which frequently affects the subtalar joint in children. It may also be seen in association with infection in the hindfoot and tumours such as an osteoid osteoma. Blockey (1959) drew attention to the fact that peroneal spasm can occur without a tarsal anomaly and that the presence of a tarsal anomaly does not mean that the foot is inevitably stiff. He postulated that a tarsal coalition makes the foot more liable to break down under stress, and that a minor injury may precipitate peroneal spasm. It is important for the orthopaedic surgeon to recognise this condition and treat it energetically, before the spasm becomes established.

THE TOES

CURLY TOES

The majority of babies at birth show significant flexion of the toes, particularly the lateral three toes (Fig. 29.20). This often causes anxiety among parents, even before the child starts to walk, particularly if one of the adults in the family or a close relative has recently had problems from toe deformities. In general, if the toe can be passively straightened and there is no fixed deformity, it is most unlikely to cause any symptoms. However, if there is a fixed deformity this may require treatment once the child is established in walking. Many years ago, Trethowan (1925) recommended over- and under-strapping. Sweetnam (1958) was unable to find any evidence that this type of conservative treatment

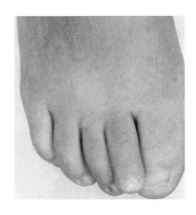

Figure 29.20 Clinical photograph showing typical lateral three curly toes.

influenced the natural history of the disorder. Most parents found it extremely difficult to persist for more than a few months with this treatment. In the majority of patients, the curly toes did not cause any symptoms and should be left alone. In the few cases in which there is persistent deformity causing symptoms, surgical correction by simple tenotomy of the flexor tendon, as reported by Menelaus & Ross (1984), has given good results from a simple procedure that can be performed on a day-case basis and allows the patient to walk within 24 hours of the operation. This is much simpler than formal transfer of the long-toe flexor into the extensor as described by Taylor (1951), which is probably best reserved for patients with severe clawing of the toes associated with neuromuscular imbalance.

OVERRIDING 5TH TOE (CONGENITAL ELEVATION OF THE 5TH TOE)

This is a true congenital deformity of the 5th toe which is hypoplastic, elevated and rotated medially. It overlies the 4th toe (Fig. 29.21). The deformity is fixed, and does not correct spontaneously with time. Treatment is required if problems with shoewear and pressure from the shoes on the toe become troublesome. Conservative measures are rarely successful, and a number of surgical procedures have been described. A simple V–Y plasty, described by Wilson (1953),

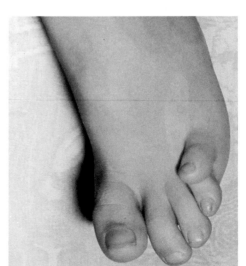

Figure 29.21 Clinical photograph of an overriding 5th toe (congenital elevation of the 5th toe).

releases the dorsal contracture, but often the toe will not remain corrected after this procedure and the deformity recurs. The double V–Y plasty, described by Butler and reported by Cockin (1968) combines a V–Y plasty on the dorsum of the foot and a Y–V plasty on the sole of the foot, connecting the two so that the toe is not only released dorsally, but is also pulled down into the plantigrade position by the Y–V plasty on the sole. This can provide good correction, but must be performed with care to avoid damage to the neurovascular bundles. More radical bony procedures such as proximal phalangectomy or even amputation of the 5th toe should be reserved for patients who have failed previous soft-tissue surgery.

HALLUX VALGUS

Hallux valgus in the young child is rare unless it is associated with other major congenital anomalies affecting the foot, such as Apert's syndrome (acro-cephalo-syndactyly). However, it becomes increasingly common in teenagers. In the past, it was frequently assumed that this condition was caused by poorly fitting shoes, and parents were blamed for their child's hallux valgus. However, the condition is much more likely to be familial rather than acquired. Patients with this type of foot have a characteristically supple, broad forefoot with hallux valgus and a bunion on the medial side and often a bunionette or 5th metatarsal bunion on the lateral side (Fig. 29.22). Ill-fitting shoes do not cause the deformity, but they can certainly cause symptoms by pressure over the medial side of the metatarsal head, leading to development of a bunion and crowding of the toes.

Medial deviation of the first metatarsal (metatarsus primus varus) is common, and may be associated with lateral deviation of the 5th metatarsal and a bunionette. Metatarsus varus is very common in young children and it is tempting to suggest that hallux valgus is the long-term result; however, there is no good evidence for this. Farsetti et al (1994), in their long-term review of metatarsus varus, found only one case of mild hallux valgus in one foot. In 1960, Piggott, in a very useful review, showed that up to 20° of valgus at the first metatarso-phalangeal joint is within normal limits. Between 20° and 25° of valgus, the big toe is deviated but

does not necessarily progress to hallux valgus. Adolescents and young adults with this degree of valgus should be watched. However, once the valgus angle is greater than 25°, progressive deformity is almost inevitable (Fig. 29.23). Similarly, lateral subluxation of the proximal phalanx of the big toe on the first metatarsal head leads to inevitable progression of the deformity and, ultimately, degenerative change. This paper by Piggott (1960) provides a useful rational basis for advising surgical correction: up to 20°, there is no indication for surgery on account of the deformity itself; between 20° and 25°, the situation should be watched; when there is more than 25° of deformity or lateral subluxation of the proximal phalanx on the metatarsal head, it is reasonable to offer surgical correction to prevent further progression and ultimate osteoarthritis in the joint.

Corrective procedures

More than 100 procedures have been described for the correction of hallux valgus. Bony procedures performed before the end of growth in the foot, i.e. before 13–14 years, are likely to fail because of recurrent deformity. Therefore, in the very rare case in which it is necessary to consider surgery before skeletal maturity, McBride's (1928) so-called conservative operation is indicated. If at all possible, the surgeon should try to delay operation until skeletal maturity. Unfortunately, splints, insoles and physiotherapy have little effect on hallux valgus, and the only reasonable conservative treatment is to ensure that adequately fitting shoes are worn that do not press on the toes or the bunion.

Once skeletal maturity is reached, there is a bewildering array of osteotomies. Helal et al (1974) reviewed the results of a number of procedures and came to the conclusion that the oblique or Wilson osteotomy gave the most consistent

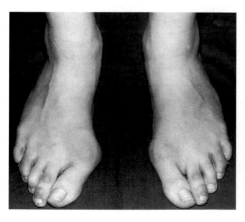

Figure 29.22 Clinical photograph of hallux valgus in a patient aged 12 years. Note the broad forefoot, prominent medial bunion and the tendency to develop a 5th metatarsal bunionette.

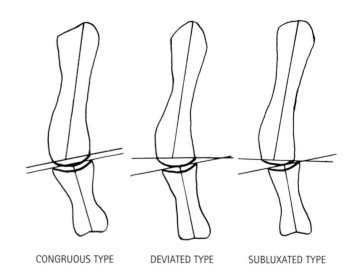

CONGRUOUS TYPE   DEVIATED TYPE   SUBLUXATED TYPE

Figure 29.23 Piggot's (1960) classification of deviation of the hallux in adolescent hallux valgus. (Adapted from Piggott H 1960 The natural history of hallux valgus in adolescents and early adult life. Journal of Bone and Joint Surgery 42B: 749–760.)

results. The problem with this oblique osteotomy is that it can shorten the first metatarsal, and so is unsuitable if the second toe is particularly long. As in all metatarsal osteotomies, it is absolutely essential that the metatarsal head is not allowed to displace dorsally, thus reducing weight bearing on the first metatarsal head and increasing the pressure on the second metatarsal head, leading to metatarsalgia and, occasionally, stress fracture. The Chevron osteotomy, described by Johnson et al in 1979, is aimed at reducing the amount of shortening and holding the metatarsal head more firmly. This operation undoubtedly controls the metatarsal head well, but it is important not to damage the blood supply to the metatarsal head and to avoid avascular necrosis, which leads to pain and joint degeneration. Other popular forms of metatarsal osteotomy are the Hohmann–Thomasen, in which a peg is used to hold the head in position (described by Mygind 1952), and Mitchell et al (1958). Most surgeons will try a variety of these distal osteotomies and then settle on the one which they find works best for them.

In many ways, proximal osteotomy at the base of the metatarsal seems more logical. Clearly, this should be used with great care before skeletal maturity, because the epiphyseal plate is proximal and not distal, and must not be damaged. However, although good results have been reported by Simmonds & Menelaus (1960), it is a more difficult procedure. It is more difficult to correct the metatarsal and obtain long-term satisfactory results. It may be necessary, in severe cases, to combine the McBride procedure with a basal osteotomy to obtain full control of the deformity. Mann et al (1992) reported satisfactory results in 93% of patients in whom the combination of a basal crescentic first metatarsal osteotomy was combined with a modified McBride procedure. However, only seven of 75 patients were younger than 20 years, and the authors made no special mention, in the description of the operative technique, of the care necessary to avoid damage to the epiphyseal plate at the base of the first metatarsal in patients in whom it is still open.

OVERRIDING SECOND TOE

This condition is commonly seen in children's feet, particularly in association with curly 3rd, 4th and 5th toes (Fig. 29.24). The hallux is in mild valgus and the lateral three toes curl medially, so that the 2nd toe is displaced dorsally and lies at a higher level than the 1st metatarsal and other toes. The condition is nearly always passively fully correctable and corrects spontaneously when the child starts to walk. Provided there is no fixed deformity, no treatment is indicated and parents can be reassured that, provided shoes of adequate width are fitted, once the child starts to walk the condition should not cause any further problems. Very occasionally there is a persistent fixed contracture and tenotomy of the extensor tendon is indicated. Fixed flexion deformity of the 2nd toe can also occur. If this does not correct with passive stretching by the mother, then a fixed hammer-toe deformity can develop, causing problems with

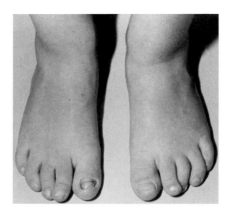

Figure 29.24 Clinical photograph of overriding 2nd toe. Note inward curling of 3rd, 4th and 5th toes.

shoewear and the development of the toenail. Simple flexor tenotomy or, occasionally, flexor-to-extensor transfer may be necessary if the deformity is symptomatic.

HALLUX VARUS

Minor forms of this condition are very common in association with metatarsus varus. Provided the deformity is fully correctable passively, the hallux varus should correct as the forefoot varus corrects, without any specific treatment. It can also occur as an isolated phenomenon in association with a localised fibrous band on the medial side of the foot (Fig. 29.25). If this fails to respond to passive stretching, the contracted fibrous band on the medial side of the great toe, the tight abductor hallucis and shortened medial capsule of the metatarso-phalangeal joint of the big toe can be released. Finally, hallux varus may be associated with localised bony anomalies such as abnormal phalanges, duplication and accessory toes, and congenital short 1st metatarsal, and with generalised conditions such as Apert's syndrome (acro-cephalo-syndactyly) (Fig. 29.26) and diastrophic dwarfism. Quite extensive complex soft-tissue and bony surgery may be necessary to correct hallux varus in these patients. (Mubarak et al 1993, Anderson et al 1999).

HALLUX RIGIDUS

Hallux rigidus occurs in children and adolescents. Unlike the condition in adults, it is more common in girls than in boys. McMaster (1978) has suggested an acute pathogenesis, or that chronic trauma associated with stubbing or stress on the big toe may cause a chondral or

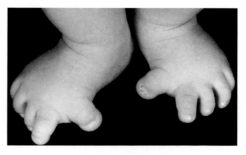

Figure 29.25 Clinical photograph of hallux varus in association with a localised fibrous band.

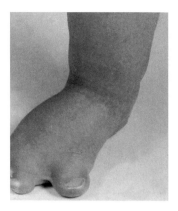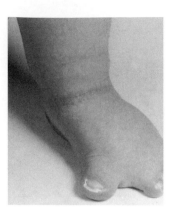

Figure 29.26 Clinical photograph of the feet of a child with hallux varus in Apert's syndrome. Note syndactyly of the other toes.

osteochondral injury to the head of the 1st metatarsal. Radiologically this is often not seen, because it is largely or entirely a chondral lesion. As a result of the injury, the patient develops so-called metatarsus primus elevatus from spasm of the flexor of the big toe, with loss of dorsiflexion of the big toe and tenderness over the dorsum of the metatarso-phalangeal joint. The patient walks awkwardly on the outer side of the foot as a result of loss of the normal 'rock-over' at the 1st metatarso-phalangeal joint. Protection of the joint by a rocker bar may relieve the symptoms, as may a short period of rest in a plaster. If, however, this fails, a dorsal wedge osteotomy of the proximal phalanx of the big toe (as described by Bonney & MacNab 1952) can produce good results, provided the patient has 30° plantarflexion before surgery. Citron & Neil (1987) reported good long-term results at an average follow-up of 22 years in nine of 10 toes treated with dorsal wedge osteotomy of the proximal phalanx. Radiologically, the usual changes of degenerative arthritis are not seen in children, but sometimes a defect similar to that of osteochondritis of the knee may be seen on the metatarsal head, as has been reported by Kessel & Bonney (1958).

METATARSUS PRIMUS ELEVATUS

This condition was believed by Lambrinudi (1938) to be a primary developmental abnormality. Nowadays, most surgeons would consider this to be secondary to plantar flexor spasm of the big toe. This may be seen in association with hallux rigidus and after surgical procedures on the mid- or hindfoot that cause supination of the foot so that the 1st metatarsal is elevated and the big toe has to be held in flexion in order to reach the ground. This is seen after surgery for congenital talipes equinovarus and also in neuromuscular conditions such as poliomyelitis and spina bifida. The patient develops pain over the dorsal bunion and also from the flexion of the big toe. It can be a difficult condition to treat unless muscle balance can be restored. This imbalance is commonly associated with a

strong tibialis anterior, elevating the 1st metatarsal, and weakness of peroneus longus. Lapidus (1940) described transfer of flexor hallucis longus through a tunnel in the 1st metatarsal into the dorsum of the proximal phalanx, with a basal osteotomy of the 1st metatarsal, for this deformity.

INTERPHALANGEAL VALGUS OF THE BIG TOE

Sometimes valgus of the big toe occurs, not at the metatarso-phalangeal joint, but at the interphalangeal joint, usually associated with a congenital anomaly of the distal phalanx. This can cause problems with the distal phalanx pressing on the 2nd toe or even lying underneath it. Radiology may show a malformation of the interphalangeal joint, the epiphysis of the distal phalanx often appearing wedge-shaped, the base of the wedge being on the medial side. If symptoms are sufficient, the deformity can be corrected either by osteotomy of the proximal phalanx, removing a medially based wedge, or after growth has finished by fusion of the interphalangeal joint, provided there is a full range of pain-free movement at the 1st metatarso-phalangeal joint.

DUPLICATION, SYNDACTYLY AND ACCESSORY TOES

Minor anomalies such as duplication, syndactyly and accessory toes are quite common. They may occur on their own or in association with generalised conditions such as chondro-ectodermal dysplasia (Ellis–Van Creveld syndrome) and Apert's syndrome (Fig. 29.26), and also with local abnormalities such as tibial dysplasia. Congenital shortening of the 1st metatarsal is seen in fibrodysplasia (myositis) ossificans progressiva (see Ch. 6) and dysplastic nails in the nail–patella syndrome (onycho-osteodystrophy). It is very important to look at the entire patient in addition to the feet.

Syndactyly frequently needs no treatment. Duplications and accessory toes can sometimes be simply reduced or removed, but occasionally the bony architecture is very complex and careful planning and meticulous surgery are necessary. Parents may frequently ask for the surgery to be performed early, before the child starts to walk, but often it is better to wait until the child has reached at least the age of 1 year, so that the bony architecture of the foot can be more accurately assessed before surgery is decided upon.

CONGENITAL SPLIT OR CLEFT FOOT (LOBSTER-CLAW FOOT)

This is a rare congenital anomaly characterised by failure of development of the central two or three rays of the foot (Fig. 29.27). The 1st metatarsal may be normal or enlarged and the hallux is usually in valgus. There is then a large cleft, and the remainder of the foot is made up of the lateral 4th or

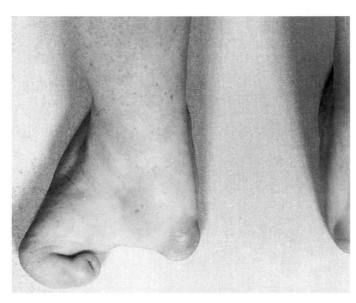

Figure 29.27 Clinical photograph of lobster-claw feet. This is a severe form (Abraham et al 1999).

5th rays, with the phalanges deviating medially. The hindfoot is usually normal. The common form is bilateral and inherited as an autosomal dominant with incomplete penetrance. There is a more rare unilateral form, in which there is usually no family history. The condition can occur on its own or in association with lobster-clawing of the hands. It can also be associated with cleft lip and cleft palate and deafness.

Surgery may be considered to improve footwear and cosmesis. Abraham et al (1999), in a useful review, classified the deformity into three groups according to severity: type I, in which a central partial forefoot cleft is present, can be treated by a soft-tissue syndactylism and correction of the hallux valgus if necessary; type II, with a complete forefoot cleft involving the tarsus, can be treated by a soft-tissue syndactylism with osteotomy of the first ray to aid the soft-tissue closure; in type III, in which there is complete absence of the first to the fourth ray, the patients did not require surgery and managed well in normal shoes with a shoe filler or 'false foot'.

REFERENCES

Abraham E, Waxman B, Shirali S, Durkin M 1999 Congenital cleft foot deformity treatment. Journal of Pediatric Orthopaedics 19: 404–410

Anderson P J, Hall C M, Evans R D, Hayward R B, Jones B M 1999 The feet in Apert's syndrome. Journal of Pediatric Orthopaedics 19: 504–507

Antoniou D, Connor A M 1974 Osteomyelitis of the calcaneus and talus. Journal of Bone and Joint Surgery 56A: 338–345

Badgely C E 1927 Coalition of the calcaneus and the navicular. Archives of Surgery 15: 75–88

Bankart A S B 1921 Metatarsus varus. British Medical Journal 2: 685

Berman A, Gartland J 1971 Metatarsal osteotomy for the correction of adduction of the forepart of the foot in children. Journal of Bone and Joint Surgery 53A: 498–506

Bleck E E 1983 Metatarsus adductus: classification and relationship to outcomes of treatment. Journal of Pediatric Orthopaedics 3: 2–9

Blockey N J 1959 Peroneal spastic flat foot. Journal of Bone and Joint Surgery 37B: 191–202

Bonney G, MacNab I 1952 Hallux valgus and hallux rigidus. A critical survey of operative results. Journal of Bone and Joint Surgery 34B: 366–385

Braddock G T F 1961 A prolonged follow up of peroneal spastic flat foot. Journal of Bone and Joint Surgery 43B: 734–737

Browne R S, Paton D F 1979 Anomalous insertion of the tibialis posterior in congenital metatarsus varus. Journal of Bone and Joint Surgery 61B: 74–76

Cain T J, Hyman S 1978 Peroneal spastic flat foot. Journal of Bone and Joint Surgery 60B: 527–529

Carter C, Wilkinson J 1964 Persistent joint laxity and congenital dislocation of the hip. Journal of Bone and Joint Surgery 46B: 40–45

Cheng J C Y, Chan P S, Hui P W 1991 Joint laxity in children. Journal of Pediatric Orthopaedics 11: 752–756

Citron N, Neil M 1987 Dorsal wedge osteotomy of the proximal phalanx for hallux rigidus. Journal of Bone and Joint Surgery 69B: 835–837

Cockin J 1968 Butler's operation for overriding 5th toe. Journal of Bone and Joint Surgery 60B: 78–81

Cox M J 1958 Kohler's disease. Postgraduate Medical Journal 34: 58–59

Drennan J C 1992 The child's foot and ankle. Lippincott Williams and Wilkins, Baltimore, p 175

Dwyer F C 1976 Causes, significance and treatment of stiffness of the subtaloid joint. Proceedings of the Royal Society of Medicine 69: 97–102

Eastwood D M, Cole W G, Dickens B R B 1996 Idiopathic toe walking: is this a neurological problem 'solved' by surgery? Proceedings of the British Society of Children's Orthopaedic Surgery, Journal of Bone and Joint Surgery 78B: (Suppl 1) p 11

Evans D 1975 Calcaneovalgus deformity. Journal of Bone and Joint Surgery 57B: 270–278

Farsetti P, Weinstein S L, Ponseti I V 1994 The long term functional and radiographic outcomes of untreated and non operatively treated metatarsus adductus. Journal of Bone and Joint Surgery 76A: 257–265

Fowler S B, Banks A L, Parrish T F 1959 The cavovarus foot. Journal of Bone and Joint Surgery 41A: 757

Giannestras J 1973 Foot disorders, medical and surgical management, 2nd edn. Henry Kimpton, London

Hall J E, Salter R B, Bhalla S K 1967 Congenital short tendocalcaneus. Journal of Bone and Joint Surgery 49B: 695–697

Harris N H 1972 Rotational deformities and their secondary effects in the lower extremities in children. Journal of Bone and Joint Surgery 54B: 172

Harris R I, Beath T 1948 Aetiology of peroneal spastic flat foot. Journal of Bone and Joint Surgery 30B: 624–634

Helal B, Gupta S K, Gojaseni P 1974 Surgery for adolescent hallux valgus. Acta Orthopaedica Scandinavica 45: 271–295

Heyman C H, Herndon C H, Strong J M 1985 Mobilisation of the tarso-metatarsal and intermetatarsal joints for the correction of resistant adduction of the forepart of the foot in congenital club foot or congenital metatarsus varus. Journal of Bone and Joint Surgery 40A: 299–310

Johnson K A, Cofield R H, Morrey B F 1979 Chevron osteotomy for hallux valgus. Clinical Orthopaedics and Related Research 142: 44–47

Jones Sir R, 1897 Peroneal spasm and its treatment. Report on a meeting of the Liverpool Medical Institution Journal 17: 442

Katz K, David R, Soudry M 1999 Below knee plaster cast for the treatment of metatarsus adductus. Journal of Pediatric Orthopaedics 19: 49–50

Kessel I, Bonney G 1958 Hallux rigidus in the adolescent. Journal of Bone and Joint Surgery 40B: 668–673

Kite J H 1967 Congenital metatarsus varus. Journal of Bone and Joint Surgery 46A: 388–397

Kohler A 1908 Uber einer haufige bisher anscheinend unbekannte Erkrankung einzelner kindlicher Knocken Munchen. Medizinische Wochenschrift 55: 1923

Koutsogiannis E 1971 Treatment of mobile flat feet by displacement osteotomy of the calcaneus. Journal of Bone and Joint Surgery 53B: 96–100

Lambrinudi C 1938 Metatarsus primus elevatus. Proceedings of the Royal Society of Medicine 31: 1273

Lapidus P W 1940 'Dorsal Bunion' its mechanics and operative correction. Journal of Bone and Joint Surgery 22: 627–637

Leonard M A 1974 The inheritance of tarsal coalition and its relationship to spastic flat foot. Journal of Bone and Joint Surgery 56B: 520–525

Lloyd-Roberts G C, Clark R C 1973 Ball and socket ankle joint in metatarsus adductus varus. Journal of Bone and Joint Surgery 55B: 193–196

Lloyd-Roberts G C, Pilcher M F 1965 Structural idiopathic scoliosis in infancy. Journal of Bone and Joint Surgery 47B: 520–523

McBride E D 1928 A conservative operation for bunions. Journal of Bone and Joint Surgery 10B: 735–739

McCormack T J, Olney B, Asher M 1997 Talocalcaneal coalition resection: a 10-year follow up. Journal of Pediatric Orthopaedics 17: 13–15

McMaster M J 1978 The pathogenesis of hallux rigidus. Journal of Bone and Joint Surgery 60B: 82–87

Macnicol M F, Inglis G, Buxton R A 1986 Symptomatic calcaneonavicular bars. Journal of Bone and Joint Surgery 68B: 128–131

Mann R A, Rudicel S, Grabes S C 1992 Repair of hallux valgus with a distal soft tissue procedure and proximal metatarsal osteotomy. Journal of Bone and Joint Surgery 74A: 124–129

Menelaus M B, Ross E R S 1984 Open flexor tenotomy for hammer toes and curly toes in childhood. Journal of Bone and Joint Surgery 66B: 770–771

Mitchell C L, Fleming J L, Allen R, Glenney C, Sandford G A 1958 Osteotomy bunionectomy for hallux valgus. Journal of Bone and Joint Surgery 40A: 41–59

Mitchell G P, Gibson J M C 1967 Excision of calcaneonavicular bar for painful spasmodic flat foot. Journal of Bone and Joint Surgery 49B: 281–287

Morley A J M 1957 Knock knee in children. British Medical Journal 2: 976–979

Mosca V S 1995 Flexible flat foot and skew foot. Journal of Bone and Joint Surgery 77A: 1937–1945

Mubarak S J, O'Brien T J, Davids J R 1993 Metatarsal epiphyseal bracket: treatment by central physiolysis. Journal of Pediatric Orthopaedics 13: 5–8

Mygind H 1952 Operations for hallux valgus. Report of Danish Orthopaedic Association. Journal of Bone and Joint Surgery 34B: 529

Oestreich A E, Mize W A, Crawford A H, Morgan R C 1987 The 'anteater's nose'. A direct sign of calcaneonavicular coalition on the lateral radiograph. Journal of Pediatric Orthopaedics 7: 709–711

Olney B W, Asher M A 1987 Excision of symptomatic coalition of the middle facet of the talocalcaneal joint. Journal of Bone and Joint Surgery 69A: 539–544

Piggott H 1960 The natural history of hallux valgus in adolescents and early adult life. Journal of Bone and Joint Surgery 42B: 749–760

Ponseti I V, Becker J R 1966 Congenital metatarsus varus. The results of treatment. Journal of Bone and Joint Surgery 48A: 702–711

Rao U B, Joseph B 1992 The influence of footwear on the prevalence of flat foot. Journal of Bone and Joint Surgery 74B: 525–527

Rose G K, Welton C A, Marshal T 1986 The diagnosis of flat foot in the child. Journal of Bone and Joint Surgery 67B: 71–78

Rushforth G F 1978 The natural history of hooked forefoot. Journal of Bone and Joint Surgery 60B: 530–532

Sever J W 1912 Apophysitis of the os calcis. New York Medical Journal 95: 1025–1029

Seymour N 1967 The late results of naviculo-cuneiform fusion. Journal of Bone and Joint Surgery 49B: 558–559

Simmonds F A, Menelaus M B 1960 Hallux valgus in adolescence. Journal of Bone and Joint Surgery 42B: 761–768

Simmons E H 1965 Tibialis spastic varus foot with tarsal coalition. Journal of Bone and Joint Surgery 47B: 533–536

Slomann M C 1921 Coalitio calcaneo navicularis. Journal of Orthopaedic Surgery 3: 586–602

Staheli L T, Chew B E, Corbett M 1987 The longitudinal arch. A survey of 882 feet in normal children. Journal of Bone and Joint Surgery 69A: 426–428

Stark K G, Johanson J E, Winter R B 1987 The Heyman–Herdon tarsometatarsal capsulotomy for metatarsus adductus; results in 48 feet. Journal of Pediatric Orthopaedics 7: 305–310

Stricker S J, Angulo J C 1998 Idiopathic toe-walking: a comparison of treatment methods. Journal of Pediatric Orthopaedics 18: 289–293

Sutherland D M, Olshen R, Cooper L, Woo S L Y 1980 The development of mature gait. Journal of Bone and Joint Surgery 62A: 336–353

Sweetnam D R 1958 Congenital curly toes. An investigation into the value of treatment. Lancet 2: 398–400

Taylor R G 1951 The treatment of claw toes by multiple transfers and flexor to extensor tendons. Journal of Bone and Joint Surgery 35B: 539–542

Trethowan W H 1925 Treatment of hammer toes. Lancet 1: 1257–1258

Waugh W 1958 The ossification and vascularisation of the tarsal navicular and their relation to Kohler's disease. Journal of Bone and Joint Surgery 40B: 765–777

Wenger D R, Mauldin D, Speck G, Morgan D, Lieber R L 1989 Corrective shoes and inserts as treatment for flexible flat foot in infants and children. Journal of Bone and Joint Surgery 71A: 800–810

Wilson J N 1953 V–Y correction for varus deformity of the 5th toe. British Journal of Surgery 41: 133–135

PART 2   Early assessment and management of the club foot

A. Catterall

INTRODUCTION

Despite the interest that has been shown in the condition of club foot over the years, its cause remains unknown and its treatment empirical. New views are beginning to emerge in which the spectrum of the disease is recognised and, with it, a more logical view of treatment.

AETIOLOGY

The incidence of club foot in the UK is approximately 1–3 in 1000 live births; 50% are bilateral, and the male: female ratio is 2.5:1. The incidence varies in different parts of the world, from 0.93/1000 in Sweden to 9.0/1000 in the Polynesian races. The cause remains unclear, but a family history of club foot is present in many cases (Table 29.1).

Table 29.1 Family history in club foot

Normal parents, male patients	2%
Normal parents, female patient	5%
Affected parent and affected child	25%

There are three aspects to the aetiology that should be considered:

1. The effects of intrauterine moulding and environmental factors.
2. Nerve and muscle imbalance.
3. The theory of delayed development.

INTRAUTERINE MOULDING AND ENVIRONMENTAL FACTORS

The temptation to associate foetal position with the club foot deformity is strong (Browne 1934). At the end of pregnancy, foetal moulding may be present, particularly if the amniotic fluid volume is reduced. Postural club foot deformity, calcaneo-valgus of the newborn and plagiocephaly are common in such circumstances. They are, however, self-correcting. Moulding does not explain the calf-wasting present in children with club feet. It would, however, act as an environmental factor, increasing the chances of serious deformity if, for any reason, the foot was unable to move. An interesting environmental factor has recently been identified in relation to amniocentesis. In the Canadian Early and Mid-trimester Amniocentesis Trial (1998), it has been shown that there is a 1.4% incidence of club foot in amniocentesis performed between 11 and 13 weeks of gestation, compared with a 0.1% incidence in the middle trimester. The frequency increases to 15% when the procedure is associated with an amniotic leak. Ultrasound examinations also show that when a club foot is identified there is always evidence of free movement of the feet in the amniotic cavity. This suggests that there is no moulding effect at this stage of development.

NEUROLOGICAL IMBALANCE

The common association between foot deformities, meningomyelocele and spinal dysraphism makes neurological imbalance a probable primary aetiological factor. Relapse or recurrent deformity is commonly associated with a neurological deficit. This may be either muscular or neurological in origin. It would also explain the calf wasting and small feet that characterise the relapsed deformity, particularly when skin changes are also present. However, present techniques of investigation do not always reveal a definable cause in these children (Feldbrin et al 1995, Macnicol & Nadeem 2000).

Handelsman & Badalamente (1981) and Macnicol et al (1992) have identified differences in muscle fibre type, with a high proportion of type I fibres in those with club foot compared with controls. There is also an increased amount of fibrosis and reduced excursion of these muscles. A postural imbalance of muscle tone in the presence of rapid growth is often seen in the progressive deformities associated with poliomyelitis, pes cavus and related conditions. Zimny et al (1985) have also shown an increased number of myofibroblasts in the ligamentous tissue around the medial side of the foot. Such cells are also seen in conditions such as Dupuytren's disease, in which soft-tissue contractures of a progressive nature also occur.

THE THEORY OF DELAYED DEVELOPMENT

There are a number of studies that have demonstrated that the intrauterine foot passes from an initial position of equinovarus to calcaneo-valgus; it has been postulated that an incident occurring *in utero* might prevent this progression. In the experimental animal, exposure to curare, a viral infection, and other agents at approximately the 30-mm stage results in deformities very similar to those of club foot. Associated with this theory of delayed maturation is an observation that the blood supply to the leg and foot is changing from a primordial form to a secondary pattern at about the same time. Hootnick et al (1982) linked this failure of change in the vascular anatomy to a cessation of growth and the production of the club foot deformity. Abnormalities of the dorsalis pedis artery have been described by Sodre et al (1990) and a number of cases are on record in which major vascular catastrophe has occurred in the presence of minimal surgery (Hootnick & Packard 1990). It is postulated that failure of vascular development is the cause of this.

CONCLUSIONS ON AETIOLOGY

This discussion suggests that there is no single cause for club foot. The high familial incidence suggests an inherited anomaly, which could be either neurological or vascular. This results in delayed maturation of the foot, with a subsequent imbalance between the muscles that plantarflex and dorsiflex the foot. The resulting position would tend to be exacerbated by any form of abnormal intrauterine moulding, making the deformity more severe at birth. The environmental factors associated with amniocentesis before 12–13 weeks of gestation would exacerbate this tendency. It would also suggest that there are critical environmental factors operating which, if altered between 10–13 weeks of development, will result in a club foot deformity. The minor resolving or postural club foot deformity could be simply the consequence of environmental moulding, and its quick response to treatment suggests that it has only been of short duration and is not associated with neurological deficit.

DIAGNOSIS BY ULTRASOUND AT MID-TRIMESTER EXAMINATION

The use of ultrasound in the prenatal diagnosis of club foot was first reported by Benacerraf and Frigoletto in 1985. Many cases are now diagnosed at the time of the middle trimester ultrasound examination of the foetus. The families are, therefore, aware that their future baby is abnormal and are seeking counselling from both paediatrian and orthopaedic surgeon. At present there is little data upon which the orthopaedic surgeon can base an opinion. However, review of the recent literature establishes a number of observations. A prospective study by Treadwell et al (1999) has shown that the incidence of identified club foot deformity was 0.43%. Of these, only 30% were an isolated deformity, the remainder being part of multiple abnormalities. In a study by Lochmiller et al (1998) of 285 cases, boys were affected in a ratio of 2:1, and there was a positive family history in 24%. In a study of 4651 pregnancies (Pagnotta et al 1996), 41 club feet were noted in 27 pregnancies; 14 feet in eight patients had isolated deformities, and the remainder had multiple abnormalities of which the club foot was a component part. Woodrow et al (1998) studied 17 patients with positive ultrasound scans and found that six had normal feet at the time of birth. Although these data are not uniform, one may conclude that about 30% of cases have an isolated club foot in the middle trimester, whereas the remainder have a deformity that is part of multiple abnormalities. In approximately 20–25%, there is a family history of club foot. Some cases diagnosed in the middle trimester do not have a serious deformity at birth.

PATHOLOGY

There are four components to the pathology of club foot:

1. Bony abnormalities.
2. Joint deformities and subluxations within the foot.
3. Muscle imbalance.
4. Reduced muscle excursion.

BONY CHANGES

The involved leg in the club foot may be short. This short-ening involves not only the tibia and foot but also the femur, and is more common in girls. Where the condition is unilat-eral, there is an obvious difference in the size of the foot. In the foot itself, many of the bones are of abnormal shape; the most commonly reported is the talus. This has a short neck and greater medial and plantar deviation than that on the normal opposite side. Its ossification centre is situated in the neck and anterior body, and may mislead the inexperienced surgeon in assessing the position of this bone (Howard & Benson 1992, 1993). It must, however, be stressed that the material from which this information has been obtained considered only severe deformity (Irani & Sherman 1972), and it is the author's view that, in the more common milder case, the anatomy of the foot bones may be almost normal at birth. In the long term, after treatment, the dome of the talus may flatten (Hutchins et al 1985). This is almost certainly the consequence of treatment, rather than a primary abnormality.

THE FIXED JOINT DEFORMITIES

These may be considered at a number of individual sites (Fig. 29.28).

The ankle joint

At the ankle, the talus lies in equinus with its head pointing downward and medially out of the mortice. In extreme cases, the degree of forced plantarflexion that occurs results in ante-rior subluxation of the talus in the ankle, such that its great-est vertical height is outside the mortice. This is associated with a posterior movement of the calcaneum on the talus, which exacerbates the problem. The movement of dorsiflexion is

therefore blocked unless a soft-tissue release allows the talus to move backwards in the mortice. The talo-calcaneal joints are in the position of full equinus, with the calcaneum lying directly beneath the talus and not in its normal divergent posi-tion (Carroll et al 1978, Herzenberg et al 1988).

The talo–navicular joint

The navicular lies on the medial side of the head of the talus and is held there by shortening of the tissues forming the medial complex of the ankle joint. Because the head of the talus lies forward of the mortice, the navicular is unable to assume its normal position until either the talus has moved backwards or a soft-tissue release of the navicular allows it to be repositioned on the head of the talus.

The calcaneo–cuboid joint

The cuboid is subluxed medially upon the calcaneum. This is partly the consequence of forced inversion and partly because of inelasticity of the ligaments tethering the cuboid to the navicular. This means that, if the navicular lies in a position of medial subluxation, the cuboid must also be displaced medially in relation to the calcaneum. As a conse-quence, if a soft-tissue release of the forefoot is required to restore the normal divergence of the medial and lateral rays, the Y-shaped ligament between the navicular, cuboid and calcaneum must be released, in addition to the medial capsule of the calcaneo-cuboid joint.

The tarso–metatarsal joints

Shortening of the short and long plantar ligaments together with the plantar fascia will produce a flexion deformity or plantaris of the midfoot, particularly on the medial side. This results in a cavus deformity medially. The plantar fascia is the only structure to bridge the medial and lateral rays of the foot (see below).

THE MUSCLES

In the established condition the calf is always wasted, and this is proportional to the severity of the condition. It also

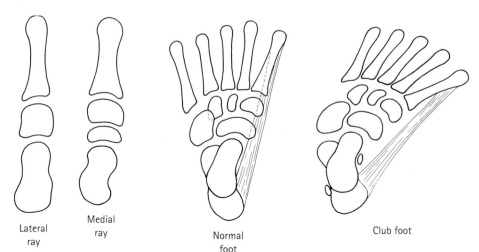

Lateral
ray

Medial
ray

Normal
foot

Club foot

Figure 29.28 Drawings of the rays of the foot, and the link mechanism and changes in the club foot.

correlates with the size of the foot and commonly with its stiffness. The muscles show a variable degree of fibre abnormality. Isaacs et al (1977) and Handelsman & Badalamente (1981, 1982) have shown that in muscle biopsy material there is a preponderance of type 1 fibres, together with an increased amount of fibrosis within the muscle itself. The atrophy of the muscle is due to a decrease in the size of the individual fibres, rather than an overall reduction in their number. This reduction in size is primarily seen in the peronei, whereas the fibrosis is most marked in the triceps surae, tibialis posterior and, to a lesser extent, flexor digitorum communis and flexor hallucis longus. There is therefore a gradient of involvement, with the long toe flexor muscles least involved and the calf and tibialis posterior most involved. This means that in many soft-tissue releases there is no need to lengthen flexor hallucis longus and flexor digitorum communis because they do not have the same reduced excursion as the triceps surae. They may be amenable to conservative treatment once the primary contractures have been released.

The reduced excursion in the tibialis anterior is of interest. This is part of the weaker side of the musculature. Apparent overaction of tibialis anterior due to reduced excursion and tightness is seen in children with residual forefoot varus and supination after primary surgery. On the lateral side of the foot, the peronei are elongated and functionally weak (Porter 1987a,b).

The consequences of these abnormalities is a postural imbalance between the muscles that plantarflex and invert and those that dorsiflex and evert. This imbalance will persist and, if severe, will result in secondary relapse, even if a full soft-tissue release has provided a good correction.

THE IMPACT OF GROWTH ON THE DEFORMITIES

The importance of growth and its relation to persisting deformity are seldom discussed in texts such as this but are, of course, fundamental to the development of the foot. It must be remembered that the foot doubles its size in the first year and if this process is to occur, there must be a simultaneous increase in size of both the osseous and the cartilaginous structures, together with the soft tissues, ligaments, tendons and muscles.

It has already been mentioned that a number of tendons and muscles have reduced excursion and that this prevents correction, particularly in the more severely affected and stiff feet. The success of primary treatment must, in part, involve an improvement in this range of excursion. Acutely, this can be achieved by stretching of the muscle belly, but over-stretching will result in injury and fibrosis, thereby exacerbating the problem. A sustained increase in excursion can only be achieved by growth of the muscle and tendon. This growth occurs at the musculotendinous junction (Ziv et al 1984, Wright & Rang 1990) and requires active contraction and relaxation of the muscle. No growth will occur at the time of tendon lengthening, and release of the muscle in the musculotendinous area may seriously interfere with or even destroy this growth centre.

These observation would go a long way to explaining the lack of overall long-term success of the use of serial corrective plasters. Continuous passive motion, however, by repeatedly stretching and relaxing the muscles, will promote this growth process, at a time when it is occurring at a rate that will not be repeated again in the growing period (Dimeglio et al 1996). A surgical procedure that results in damage to the musculotendinous areas of a muscle may lead to altered growth and recurrent deformity. Damage to muscles that occurs as the result of over-stretching will also be associated with such problems.

A DYNAMIC CONCEPT OF THE FOOT

Although the foot comprises of a large number of bones, from a functional and dynamic aspect it consists of medial and lateral rays together with a tethering link mechanism (Fig. 29.28). The medial ray is formed by the talus, navicular, medial cuneiform and first metatarsal. The lateral ray consists of the calcaneum, cuboid and 5th metatarsal. The two rays lie one above the other posteriorly, but are at the same level anteriorly with the foot in the weight-bearing position. The link mechanism joins the two rays and is formed by the interosseous ligament posteriorly, the remaining tarsal bones in the midfoot and the transverse metatarsal ligament anteriorly. The important Y-shaped ligament joins the navicular to the cuboid and calcaneum. The movements of inversion, eversion, pronation and supination consist of rotatory movements of the medial and lateral rays in which the limitations to full movement are imposed by the elasticity of the link mechanism. These are the joint capsules, the long and short plantar ligaments, and distal attachment of the tibialis anterior.

Dorsiflexion is a composite movement occurring partly at the ankle joint and partly at the subtaloid and midtarsal joints. *Inversion* and *eversion* are a component of subtaloid movement. As dorsiflexion proceeds from the position of full equinus there is a posterior and lateral rotatory movement of the talus in the ankle mortice and the lateral malleolus can be felt to move forward in relation to the heel (Swann et al 1969, Scott et al 1984). At the subtaloid joint there is a rotatory movement of the calcaneum and, hence, of the lateral ray upon the talus and the medial ray. The centre of this rotation is the interosseous ligament, so that the anterior aspect of the calcaneum comes to lie under the head of the talus in plantarflexion and lateral to it in dorsiflexion. There is a corresponding medial displacement of the posterior aspect of the calcaneum. As the foot moves from full equinus and inversion, for every 10° of dorsiflexion there is 10° external rotation of the foot upon the tibia.

Pronation is the downward movement of the medial ray at the naviculo-cuneiform and cuneiform-metatarsal joints. It is often associated with tightness of the plantar fascia. In contrast, *supination* is the elevation of the medial ray in relation to the lateral one. It is commonly associated with inversion at the subtaloid joint. When seen in isolation as a fixed deformity, it is always associated with a tether of the link mechanism, preventing the downward movement of the medial ray upon the lateral ray. There is an associated fixed deformity of the calcaneo-cuboid joint, with the cuboid displaced medially and, to a lesser extent, dorsally upon the calcaneum.

Cavus is a descriptive term for the high arched foot. In practice, there is pronation of the medial ray which, in severe cases, may be associated with plantaris of the lateral ray and the bony link mechanism. There is always a tight plantar fascia.

THE CONCEPT OF TETHERS

The movement of dorsiflexion may be prevented by tethers occurring posterolaterally between the lateral malleolus, talus and calcaneum, medially between the medial malleolus and navicular, and inferiorly and anterolaterally in relation to the link mechanism (Fig. 29.29). The inferior structures that prevent movement are the plantar fascia, the short plantar ligaments and the distal tendon of the tibialis posterior. The anterolateral structures limiting movement are the ligaments between the lateral aspect of the navicular, calcaneum and cuboid. All these tethers need to be released if normal dorsiflexion is to occur.

In the past, the result of surgical release were poor, so that triple arthrodesis at maturity was commonly required. Lloyd-Roberts (1964) referred to this type of management as 'ingenious empiricism'. A review of the literature and, in particular, of the paper by Harrold & Walker (1983) is important. This paper identifies the outcome of treatment related to the severity of the deformity present when first seen by the orthopaedic surgeon shortly after the infant's birth (Table 29.2). In the postural club foot, a small number of children require operation, whereas in the severe deformity, where more than 20% of fixed equinus or varus are present at birth, conservative treatment is almost uniformly unsuccessful. This raises the question whether, for this latter group of patients, primary conservative treatment may possibly do harm.

Table 29.2 Outcome of treatment in relation to severity of deformity at birth

		No.	Success	Operations
Group 1	No fixed deformity	35	31 (89%)	4
Group 2	<20° equinus/varus	28	13 (46%)	15
Group 3	>20° equinus/varus	40	4 (10%)	36

(After Walker & Harrold 1983.)

ASSESSMENT

THE NEED FOR ASSESSMENT

Traditionally, the majority of orthopaedic surgeons treat children with club feet by a standard method. The method of treatment varies from centre to centre. Stretching and strapping or plaster correction is started as soon as possible after birth. If this fails to correct the foot, operation is advised early, or later in the first year, depending upon the philosophy of the surgeon. The type of operation varies, being limited in nature in some centres (Main et al 1977, Main & Crider 1978, Williams et al 1987, Porter & Youle 1993) and radical in others (Turco 1979, Ghali et al 1983). Main et al (1977), Main & Crider (1978) and Green & Lloyd-Roberts (1985) reported that, among children failing primary conservative treatment, 63% can be managed by a simple posterior release; however, other surgeons (Turco 1979, Ghali et al 1983) feel that a radical release is required for satisfactory correction.

An obvious conclusion is that, unless all club feet are the same, there is a spectrum of severity that will require a detailed assessment to identify an 'à la carte' treatment (Bensahel et al 1987). Harrold & Walker (1983) have provided the only report in which the results of conservative treatment are compared with the severity of the deformity presenting to the surgeon shortly after birth (Table 29.2).

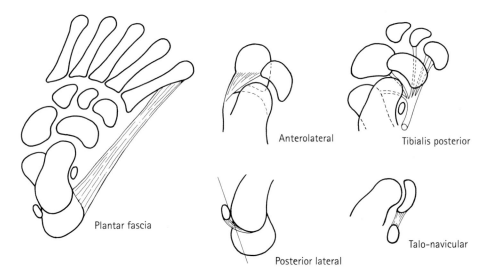

Plantar fascia

Anterolateral

Tibialis posterior

Posterior lateral

Talo-navicular

Figure 29.29 The soft-tissue tethers of the club foot.

This paper raises serious doubts about the value of conservative treatment in group 3 patients in whom, an operation is almost invariably necessary. There is also the worrying observation in the report by Hutchins et al (1985) that, in the long term, flattening of the posterior part of the dome of the talus occurs and might be considered the consequence of conservative treatment.

The need for assessment is essential if the spectrum of disease severity is to be recognised.

Questions that should be asked include:

- Is there a generalised anomaly?
- Is the spine normal?
- Are the hips normal?
- Is there abnormal joint laxity?
- Are there constriction bands?

The *differential diagnoses* are:

- Diastrophic dwarfism
- Larsen's syndrome
- Freeman–Sheldon syndrome
- Spina bifida and spinal dysraphism
- Trisomy 13
- Congenital myopathy.

The indications and contraindications for conservative treatment at birth must be carefully defined. To identify these differences, it is important to be able to describe the foot in terms of its mobility and fixed deformities (Catterall 1991) and to be able to record changes that occur as a result of conservative or surgical treatment.

THE REQUIREMENTS OF ASSESSMENT

If a standard method of assessment is to be developed, the surgeon requires three things:

1. A standard language of terms to allow observations that are observer-independent.

2. The identification of fixed deformities.
3. A knowledge of how the normal foot moves from equinovarus to calcaneo-valgus.

These are important concepts, which need agreement. However, they have been the foundation on which, for instance, scoliosis research has been able to progress over recent years.

The fixed deformities present in the club foot have already been discussed. The use of the term 'varus' is controversial. It is, for the most part, a consequence of forefoot supination and cavus, both of which can be identified. Deformity commonly results from a tendinous or ligamentous tether that restricts the normal movement of the foot, particularly in the area of the link mechanism.

A common language of terms

Catterall (1991) suggested a dictionary of terms with a common method of examination to identify four types of club foot deformity (Table 29.3). The requirements of this method of examination are set out below. Classifications using similar criteria have also been introduced by Dimeglio et al (1995), who identified four patterns of deformity based on the presence of equinus, varus deviation, derotation around the talus, and adduction of the forefoot. His classification defines a soft-soft foot (1–5 points), soft-stiff foot (5–10 points), a stiff-soft foot (10–15 points), and a stiff-stiff foot (15–20 points). Pirani has introduced a method similar to that of Catterall (1991), but has given values to the classification, to make its use in treatment more effective.

THE EXAMINATION

It is important that the child is examined fully before the feet are examined in detail. As the examination proceeds, the examiner must ask specific questions (Table 29.4 and 29.5).

Before proceeding to a radiological examination, a standard method of examination and recording should identify:

Table 29.3 Identifiable types of club foot				
Type	Resolving pattern	Tendon contracture	Joint contracture	False correction
Hind foot				
Lateral malleolus	Mobile	Posterior	Posterior	Posterior
Equinus	No	Yes	Yes	Yes
Creases				
Medial	No	No	Yes	No
Posterior	No	Yes	Yes	Yes
Anterior	Yes	No	No	Yes
Forefoot				
Lateral border	Straight	Straight	Curved	Straight
Mobile	Yes	Yes	No	Yes
Cavus	+/–	+/–	+/–	No
Supination	No	No	Yes	No

Table 29.4 Club foot assessment form 1

Name	Initials	Hospital No.	Research No.	
ADDRESS	Date of birth / /		Consultant	
Position in family	Sex M F	Side R L	Bilateral	
F.H of CTEV Y/N	Other deformities (state)			

PREGNANCY DETAILS

Duration	weeks	Complications Y/N	(state)			
Delivery	Vertex/breech	Caesarean section Y/N	Birth weight	lb		oz or.kg
Neonatal period Normal Y/N if no state why.						

PRIMARY EXAMINATION

Date / /	Facial moulding Y/N	Plageocephaly Y/N				
Upper limbs	Normal/abnormal					
Spine normal Y/N If no state why.						
Hips	Right: Stable Y/N	Abduction-in-flexion	1/4	1/2	3/4	full
	Left: Stable Y/N	Abduction-in-flexion	1/4	1/2	3/4	full
Knees Normal Y/N						

NEUROLOGICAL EXAMINATION Normal Y/N if no state why.

EXAMINATION OF FEET

General appearance	Normal R/L	Long and thin R/L	Short and fat R/L	Trophic changes Y/N

CALF	RIGHT	LEFT
Tibial torsion (degrees)		
Max calf measurement (cm)		

HINDFOOT

Equinus (degrees)
Lateral malleolus
Posterior (Y/N)

FOREFOOT

Lateral border of foot
   Straight/curved (degrees)
   Corrects in equinus
Creases
   Posterior/medial/both
   Anterior
Presence of: Cavus
        Supination
Radiographs taken Y/N   if yes Result
PRIMARY TREATMENT
No treatment
Serial plasters frequency of reapplication/week
Manipulation only number of times per day/week
Manipulation + strapping number of times per day/week
OTHERS (please specify details)

(F.H, family history; CTEV, childhood talipes equinovarus.)

1. The orientation of the tibia and hindfoot.
2. The forefoot in relation to the hindfoot.
3. The dorsiflexion arc.
4. Forefoot supination and cavus.

Orientation of the tibia and hindfoot

The child lies or sits, depending upon age, with the knee flexed. The tibial tubercle and condyles, together with the medial and lateral malleoli, are identified, and from this the

Table 29.5 Club foot assessment form 2

Name	Initials	Hospital No.	Consultant	Date of Birth / /
	Date / /	Date / /	Date / /	Date / /
	Right Left	Right Left	Right Left	Right Left
Length of foot (cm)				
HINDFOOT				
Dorsiflexion/plantarflexion				
Lateral malleolus posterior (Y/N)				
FOREFOOT				
Lateral border of foot				
Straight/curved (degrees)				
Corrects in equinus Y/N				
Creases				
Posterior/anterior/medial				
both				
Presence of: Cavus				
Supination				
RADIOGRAPHS				
Date / / Result				
RESULT OF TREATMENT				
If treatment successful, was position maintained by splints Y/N Type of splint				
Date of stopping conservative treatment / / Duration weeks				
OPERATION				
Date / / Nature (posterior only/posterior and medial)				
Date / / Nature (posterior only/posterior and medial)				
Date / / Nature (posterior only/posterior and medial)				

position of the head of the talus is identified and noted. The relationship with the posterior aspect of the calcaneum identifies any fixed equinus, which is noted and recorded. The length of the foot and the maximum circumference of the calf can be measured in centimetres.

Forefoot/hindfoot alignment and mobility

The forefoot is now viewed and examined from below. A curved lateral border is commonly seen. Attempting to straighten the lateral border by manipulation of the foot in equinus should result in the head of the talus becoming covered by the navicular and a gap developing between the navicular and the medial malleolus. The lateral border of the foot will change from curved to straight. If these three observations are present, the mid-tarsal area or link mechanism is considered mobile and correctable. Stiffness of the mid-tarsus is identified by lack of this movement.

The process of dorsiflexion

As the normal foot dorsiflexes from a position of equinovarus, three things can be noted:

1. The lateral malleolus moves forward in relation to the posterior aspect of the calcaneum.

2. The posterior border of the tibia and heel become straight.

3. The posterior crease becomes obliterated and a crease appears anteriorly over the ankle joint.

The forefoot should externally rotate in relation to the tibia. If this fails to occur, the point at which this happens is noted.

The presence of cavus and supination

Supination is best observed by bringing the heel to the neutral position in relation to the tibia and assessing the position of the heads of the 1st and 5th metatarsals. Cavus is revealed from the medial side by noting tightness of the plantar fascia and whether the line between the medial malleolus and the head of the 1st metatarsal is straight or curved.

Radiological assessment

Plain radiographs will only show the position in which the foot lies. Stress radiographs identify fixed deformity. Two radiographs are of value. A lateral X-ray in maximum dorsiflexion will demonstrate whether the lateral malleolus is opposite the tibia and the forefoot is seen in lateral projection; breeching of the calcaneo-cuboid or cuboid-metatarsal joints suggests false correction with a rocker-bottom foot. A stress antero-posterior radiograph with the foot in eversion shows the alignment of the calcaneo-cuboid joint and whether there is divergence between the talus and calcaneum (Fig. 29.30).

Conclusion of the examination

At the conclusion of the examination, four types of foot can be identified (Table 29.3):

1. *Resolving pattern.* The postural or resolving pattern of foot has no fixed deformity and, if seen at initial examination, may be thought of as a postural club foot. However, when it is present during the course of treatment, it implies that the course of therapy is effective and should be continued.

2. *Tendon contracture* type of foot. Here, there is fixed equinus without serious forefoot deformity, except that a degree of cavus may be present.

3. *False correction.* Here there is persisting equinus of the hindfoot, but a hypermobile forefoot, breeched in the mid-tarsal region at either the calcaneo-cuboid or tarso-metatarsal joints, producing a false correction.

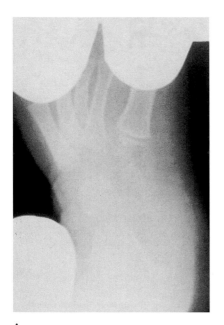
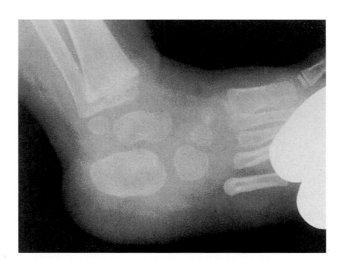

A

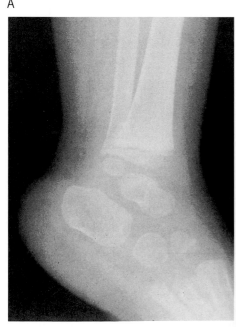
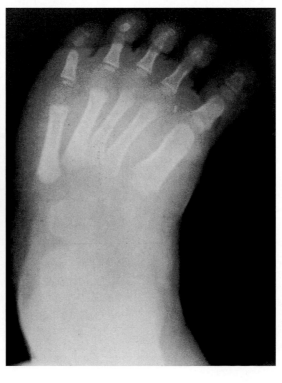

B

Figure 29.30 Stress radiographs used in assessment. **A** Stress anteroposterior radiographs to show the reduction of the calcaneo-cuboid joint. **B** Stress lateral radiographs to show persisting equinus and an early breach at the cuboid-metatarsal joints.

When this is seen during the course of conservative treatment, it is an absolute indication to discontinue conservative treatment and undertake surgery of the posterior release type.

4. *Joint contracture type of foot.* This is a more serious form of club foot, in which both hindfoot and forefoot deformities are present in association with a moderate to marked degree of stiffness. This may be seen either primarily, or after failure of primary treatment.

TREATMENT

Because the cause of this condition is unknown, treatment remains empirical. The objectives should be to convert the tendon or joint contracture types of foot, seen at birth, to the resolving pattern, without injuring the soft cartilaginous structures of the foot. This damage occurs for the most part as a result of excessive pressure exerted via the inelastic soft tissues and ligaments during the course of conservative treatment, particularly if serial plasters are used (Denham 1967). Operations that divide these inelastic structures or tethers may be looked upon as protective, and can thus be considered as an incident in continuing conservative treatment (Lloyd-Roberts 1964).

Movement is never increased after operation, and the foot will have its greatest mobility before the first operative procedure. This means that treatment designed to increase mobility before this first operation may be very important in the long term. In children seen for the first time at the age of 4–5 years who have had no previous treatment the feet remain deformed, but surprisingly supple and mobile in the position of deformity. Soft-tissue correction of these feet is often unexpectedly easy to perform.

THE MANAGEMENT OF THE FAMILY

The realisation that the new baby has a club foot is a dramatic and difficult problem with which parents have to come to terms, particularly when the child is their firstborn. There is the horror of the deformity itself, and anxiety about the potential treatment. Time for discussion must be made available, so that the parents have an understanding, not only of the nature of the club foot deformity, but also of the fact that the foot will always be small, with restricted movement, and the calf thin. Function, however, can be remarkably normal, with athletic activities and games to be expected. These discussions take time, but are necessary for an important bond to be formed between the child, the parents and the doctor. Particularly where a severe deformity of the joint contracture type is present, no rash promises of normality should be given, despite frequent requests from the parents for this reassurance.

CONSERVATIVE TREATMENT

Conservative treatment should be started as soon as possible after delivery of the infant. The questions to be decided are what method should be used and, in particular, what form of splintage? There are three aspects to conservative treatment:

1. Correction of the deformity.
2. Restoration of movement.
3. Maintenance of the correction obtained.

The first two are achieved, in principle, by manipulation and the third by some form of splintage, appliance, strapping or plaster.

Manipulative treatment should concentrate initially on the forefoot, with no attempt being made to correct the hindfoot equinus. The centre of movement is the talo-navicular joint and the mid-tarsal area. The foot should be manipulated by short corrective movements to stretch the supination, cavus and mid-tarsal subluxation. To do this, the thumb is placed over the prominent head of the talus on the superolateral side of the midfoot and the index finger on the medial side of the heel, with the forefoot grasped between the thumb and index finger of the opposite hand. Gentle repeated pressure is applied over the head of the talus to obtain correction. Only when mobility is restored to the mid-tarsal area, with straightening of the lateral border of the foot, can correction of the hindfoot be addressed. In this manipulation, the foot is gently dorsiflexed and externally rotated on the tibia while an attempt is made to move the talus backwards in the mortice. As this movement is performed, care must be taken to ensure that the lateral malleolus remains in the neutral position and that a spurious correction is not being obtained by an elastic external torsion of the tibia. The maintenance of the correction obtained poses problems. Plaster of Paris casts will hold the correction, but will not permit repeated manipulation except when it is removed. Strapping used in the Robert Jones technique is likely to be ineffective until the fixed forefoot deformity is sufficiently corrected for the adhesive strapping between the knee and the outer border of the foot to act satisfactorily as a tension band; Ghali et al (1983) combined a rigid foot plate with strapping to improve its efficiency. More recently, the effect of 'continuous passive motion' has been reported by Dimeglio et al (1996). Using this technique, they have demonstrated remarkable results, with a greatly reduced need for surgery. Even in the most severe stiff–stiff or joint contracture type of foot, they have been able either to correct the foot or to use only limited posterior release surgery.

The author's preferred method

After neonatal examination, the type of foot to be treated is identified. For the resolving pattern, the foot is regularly manipulated and strapped using the Robert Jones technique. For the tendon and joint contracture types, a manipulative stretching programme repeated several times a day by the parents and twice daily by a physiotherapist while the child is an inpatient is commenced. It is appreciated that, although ideal, inpatient treatment is not always possible. If mobility improves to the extent that the lateral border of the foot can be made straight with the foot in equinus, then a modified Robert Jones technique is used. Adjustable velcro strapping is preferred to elastoplast (Fig. 29.31), but is applied in a similar way. This allows the position to be adjusted on a daily basis. The author has no personal experience with the technique of continuous passive motion as described by Dimeglio et al (1996), but it is the logical progression of the Robert Jones method of management.

If, at any stage, the foot becomes swollen, splintage is discontinued but manipulation continued until the swelling resolves. If the forefoot remains uncorrectable, no rigid splint is applied but manipulation by the family continues until operative treatment can be undertaken. A contraindication to conservative treatment is the recognition of false correction with persistent equinus of the hindfoot, breeching of the foot in the mid-tarsal area and the development of an anterior ankle crease. This is an absolute indication for a posterior release, to prevent the false correction becoming worse.

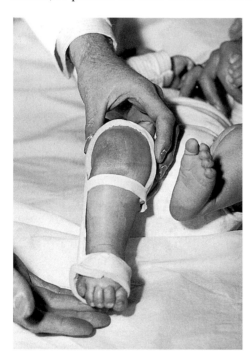

Figure 29.31 Child treated by Robert Jones technique, using velcro rather than elastoplast strapping.

OPERATIVE TREATMENT

In recent years there has been an increasing tendency for operative treatment. In a report from Iowa (Laaveg & Ponseti 1980), in what is often considered to be a very conservative approach, only 13% of the patients did not require some form of operative treatment. The majority of reports suggest that conservative treatment is successful in 30–50% of cases. It must, however, be recognised that the criteria for successful correction are becoming more critical, and that few feet of the tendon and joint contracture types can be managed entirely conservatively. The problem is which operation should be advised and at what stage in the child's development. The results of the conservative method of management, including continuous passive motion advocated by

Dimeglio et al (1996), may improve the results of conservative treatment and reduce both the need for surgery and its severity.

PROCEDURES

In principle, there are three types of procedure. First, there is soft-tissue release, which may be either a simple posterior, posterolateral procedure or an extensive medial, posterior and lateral procedure. Second, there are tendon transfers, which attempt to rebalance the foot; the tibialis anterior transfer is the most common of these. Third, there are more extensive reconstructive procedures in which a soft-tissue release is combined with a bony procedure, usually after the child has reached the age of 5–6 years; these include the Dillwyn Evans procedure (Evans 1961), multiple metatarsal osteotomies and finally, at maturity, triple arthrodesis. The previous discussion has identified that there are a number of fixed deformities present that are partly the consequence of ligamentous and tendinous contracture and partly bony deformity, particularly in the older child. Soft-tissue release will correct the majority of these deformities in the younger child, but the extent of the soft-tissue release will vary. This leads to the concept of a progressive release of tethers, starting with the fixed equinus and proceeding sequentially forward from the hindfoot to the forefoot, releasing the identified contractures established by clinical examination. The indications for these procedures are threefold:

1. Failure of conservative treatment to progress.
2. Recurrent deformity.
3. Persistent cavus that is symptomatic.

THE TIMING OF OPERATION

It must be appreciated that, because of the variable nature of the fixed deformities in club foot, the extent of operation required to correct these deformities will vary from patient to patient. In the foot with the resolving pattern, operation is seldom required and when indicated a posterior release is all that is necessary. For the tendon contracture, examination will have revealed fixed equinus, but no fixed forefoot deformity apart from minimal cavus, and it is possible to correct this by posterior or posterolateral release undertaken at the point when conservative treatment is failing to progress (Attenborough 1966, Hudson & Catterall 1994, Williams et al 1987). This is usually at approximately 6–16 weeks after birth, and should be thought of as an incident in continuing conservative treatment. A similar procedure is also required for false correction and should be advised once the diagnosis of this overcorrection has been established by X-ray.

The more difficult problem is the management of joint contracture. In theory, a more extensive procedure should be undertaken at birth to correct this type of foot. However, the foot is extremely small and the dissection has to be done under the loupe lens or microscope. In these circumstances it is easy to damage the articular surfaces, leading to subsequent stiffness and scarring. Comparison of the results of surgical correction undertaken at birth (Pous & Dimeglio 1978, Ryoppy & Sairanen 1983) and at approximately 1 year (Ghali et al 1983) suggest that similar long-term results are obtained, and hence the need for an early operation is not absolute. In addition, the opportunity for repeated manipulation to mobilise the foot and stretch the skin, particularly on the inner side of the foot, would seem to be important

before surgery. Spontaneous improvement in movement seems to occur in the foot, even though the fixed elements remain unchanged. It is the author's practice, therefore, to advise that the operation is performed when the child is 9–12 months of age, so that once the plaster is removed the child is ready to start walking, which helps to maintain the corrected position.

When an extended soft-tissue release is necessary, two different types of approach may be considered. The

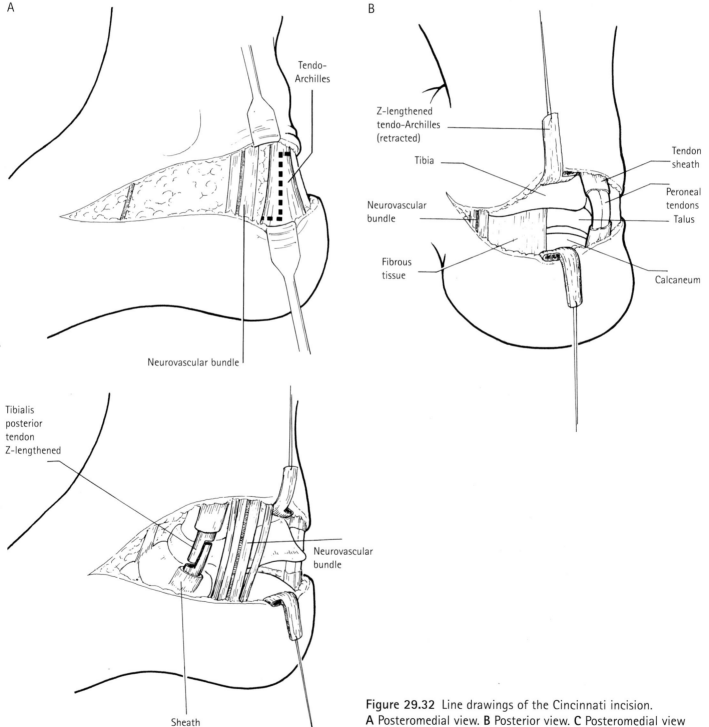

Figure 29.32 Line drawings of the Cincinnati incision.
A Posteromedial view. **B** Posterior view. **C** Posteromedial view showing further dissection.

Cincinnati incision (Crawford et al 1982) (Fig. 29.32) provides the maximum exposure and highlights the three-dimensional complexity of the deformity. The second approach uses two incisions – a posterolateral and a medial incision – from the medial malleolus to the 1st metatarsal. Both incisions allow the surgeon to view the deformity from the medial, posterior and lateral side. The advantage of the two-incision approach is that there is no incision on the medial side of the ankle, and the plantar fascia can be radically released, which is more difficult through the Cincinnati incision. If, as the wound is closed, the stitch tension is too great, the wound should be partially closed and the remainder left open, as in Dupuytren's contracture. The foot is normally corrected to 10–15° less than full correction in the first plaster, which is then changed under anaesthetic at 2 weeks, to obtain the fully corrected position. If Kirschner wires have not been used, the manipulation can be repeated on one or more occasions until a full correction has been obtained. It is important to remember the principle that an operation is an incident in continuing conservative treatment.

THE PLACE OF THE ILIZAROV FRAME AND METHODS IN MANAGEMENT

In recent years a number of reports have been published discussing the use of the Ilizarov frame in the management of deformities of the foot and ankle (Ilizarov et al 1983; Grill & Franke 1987; Wallander et al 1996). These reports are for the most part an audit of the short-term results, and do not give the reader clear indications and precise details of technique.

There is no doubt that after the application of this frame it is possible to correct severe deformity. The early reports (Ilizarov et al 1983, Grill & Franke 1987, Grill 1989, Franke et al 1990, Laville & Collin 1992, Friedman & Levitz 1994) concentrated on the results in feet with severe deformity after previous surgery, which were in addition very stiff. It should not be expected that such feet would have an improved range of movement after such treatment. However, correction using the Ilizarov frame avoids triple arthrodesis, which reduces the size of the foot. The author's experience includes a number of such feet, in the great majority of which triple arthrodesis has been avoided in the short term, and good correction of deformity obtained. Does this method of management have other indications in the management of children with club feet? Joshi has reported the use of a similar type of frame in primary management, and has obtained successful results without the need for surgery. The mobility of these feet in the long term is not known.

Recurrent deformity after surgery would seem to be a good indication for such treatment. Further surgery to such feet will increase the scarring already present within the foot. A frame could have a useful place, provided that correction was achieved in two phases: distraction of the scar tissue in the plane of the deformities, and then correction of the foot sequentially to the plantigrade position.

The author has used these two principles for children over the age of 4 years with persisting or recurrent deformity after surgery and has established one further indication for the treatment. This is the child with persisting deformity who demonstrates a wedge-shaped navicular on plain radiographs or on magnetic resonance imaging. This type of foot seldom improves after further surgical correction and is a good indication for this form of therapy.

The frame should be applied to allow independent correction of the medial and lateral aspects of the foot, together with the equinus. It is important that the first phase of this correction is by downward distraction of the foot on the tibia to create space in the ankle and subtaloid joints to permit correction. Simultaneously with or after this correction, the medial and lateral aspects of the foot are lengthened in the ratio of 2:1. This produces distraction with correction. Only after *this* distraction is the deformity itself corrected. The forefoot and supination are corrected first, followed by the equinus. This normally requires further downward distraction of the heel and an upward movement of the forefoot. In essence, the foot is rotated in distraction into dorsiflexion. Once correction is obtained, the frame is removed and a below-knee plaster of Paris applied, which is changed at 1 week. It is remarkable how supple and mobile these feet are at this stage. The plaster is reapplied for 6 weeks and an ankle–foot orthosis worn for 6 months. To date we have no experience of long-term follow-up of this type of treatment.

CONCLUSION

The cause of club feet is unknown, but in the majority of those affected a degree of muscle imbalance is present from an early stage. The variability of this imbalance suggests a spectrum of severity and implies that a standard method of treatment will not be appropriate for every case. In the long term, the mobility and suppleness of the foot are as important as the correction of the deformity itself (Cooper & Dietz 1995). Conservative treatment that results in stiffness may lead to more radical procedures to correct residual deformity, and the result is a vicious spiral of increasing stiffness. The most important need at the present time is for a language of assessment that is 'observer independent', leading to a standard method of examination and classification before treatment. This identifies the type and severity of deformity, so that specific treatment can be advised. If this can be established, a more scientific approach can be applied to the management of the child with a club foot.

REFERENCES

Attenborough C G 1966 Severe congenital talipes equinovarus. Journal of Bone and Joint Surgery 48B: 31

Benacerraf B R, Frigoletto F D 1985 Prenatal ultrasound diagnosis of club foot. Radiology 155: 211–213

Bensahel H, Csukonyi Z, Desgrippes Y, Chaumien J P 1987 Surgery in residual club foot: one-stage medioposterior release 'à la carte'. Journal of Pediatric Orthopaedics 7: 145–148

Browne D 1934 Talipes equinovarus. Lancet 2: 969

The Canadian Early and Mid-trimester Amniocentesis Trial (CEMAT) Group 1998 Randomised trial to assess safety and fetal outcome of early and midtrimester amniocentesis. [see comments]. Lancet 351: 242–247

Carroll N C, McMurtry R, Leete S F 1978 The pathoanatomy of congenital club foot. Orthopedic Clinics of North America 9: 225–232

Catterall A 1991 A method of assessment of the club foot deformity. Clinical Orthopaedics and Related Research 264: 48–53

Cooper D M, Dietz F R 1995 Treatment of idiopathic club foot A 30 year follow up note. Journal of Bone and Joint Surgery 77A: 1477–1489

Crawford A H, Marxen J L, Osterfeld D L 1982 The Cincinnati incision: a comprehensive approach for surgical procedures of the foot and ankle in childhood. Journal of Bone and Joint Surgery 64A: 1355–1358

Denham R A 1967 Congenital talipes equionvarus. Journal of Bone and Joint Surgery 49B: 583

Dimeglio A, Bensahel H, Souchet P, Mazeau P, Bonnet F 1995 Classification of club foot. Journal of Pediatric Orthopaedics B4: 129–136

Dimeglio A, Bonnet F, Mazeau P, De Rosa V 1996 Orthopaedic treatment and passive motion machine: consequences for the surgical treatment of club foot. Journal of Pediatric Orthopaedics B5: 173–180

Evans D 1961 Relapsed club foot. Journal of Bone and Joint Surgery 43B: 722–733

Feldbrin Z, Gilai A N, Ezra E, Khermosh O, Kramer U, Wiengrab S 1995 Muscle imbalance and the aetiology of idiopathic club foot. An electromyographic study. Journal of Bone and Joint Surgery 77B: 596–601

Franke J, Grill F et al 1990 Correction of club foot relapse using Ilizarov's apparatus in children 8–15 years old. Archives of Orthopaedic and Trauma Surgery 110: 33–37

Friedman H E, Levitz S 1994 A literature review of the Ilizarov technique and some applications for treating foot pathology. Journal of Foot and Ankle Surgery 33: 30–36

Ghali N N, Smith R B, Clayden A D, Silt D D 1983 The results of pantalar reduction in the management of congenital talipes equinovarus. Journal of Bone and Joint Surgery 65B: 1–7

Green A D, Lloyd-Roberts G C 1985 The results of early posterior release in resistant club feet. A long-term review. Journal of Bone and Joint Surgery 67B: 588–593

Grill F 1989 Correction of complicated extremity deformities by external fixation. Clinical Orthopaedics and Related Research 241: 166–176

Grill F, Franke J 1987 The Ilizarov distractor for the correction of relapsed or neglected club foot. Journal of Bone and Joint Surgery 69B: 593–597

Handelsman J E, Badalamente M A 1981 Neuromuscular studies in club foot. Journal of Pediatric Orthopaedics 1: 23–32

Handelsman J E, Badalamente M A 1982 Club foot: a neuromuscular disease. Development Medicine and Child Neurology 24: 3–12

Harrold A J, Walker C J 1983 Treatment and prognosis in congenital club foot. Journal of Bone and Joint Surgery 65B: 8–11

Herzenberg J E, Carroll N C, Christofersen M R, Lee E H, White S, Munroe 1988 Club foot analysis with three-dimensional computer modeling. Journal of Pediatric Orthopaedics 8: 257–262

Hootnick D R, Levinsohn E M, Crider R J, Packard D S Jr 1982 Congenital arterial malformations associated with club foot. A report of two cases. Clinical Orthopaedics 167: 160–163

Hootnick D R, Packard D S Jr, Levinsohn E M 1990 Necrosis leading to amputation following club foot surgery. Foot and Ankle 10: 312–316

Howard C B, Benson M K 1992 The ossific nuclei and the cartilage anlage of the talus and calcaneum. Journal of Bone and Joint Surgery 74B: 620–623

Howard C B, Benson M K 1993 Club foot: its pathological anatomy. Journal of Pediatric Orthopaedics 13: 654–659

Hudson I, Catterall A 1994 Posterolaterol release for resistant clubfoot. Journal of Bone and Joint Surgery 76B: 281–284

Hutchins P M, Foster B K, Paterson D C, Cole E A 1985 Long-term results of early surgical release in club feet. Journal of Bone and Joint Surgery 67B: 791–799

Ilizarov G A, Shevtsov V I et al. 1983 Method of treating talipes equinocavus. Ortopedia Travmatologia Protezirovanie 5: 46–48

Irani R N, Sherman M S 1972 The pathological anatomy of idiopathic club foot. Clinical Orthopaedics 84: 14–20

Isaacs H, Handelsman J E, Badenhorst M, Pickering A 1977 The muscles in club foot – a histological, histochemical and electron microscopic study. Journal of Bone and Joint Surgery 59B: 465–472

Laaveg S J, Ponseti I V 1980 Long-term results of treatment of congenital club foot. Journal of Bone and Joint Surgery 62A: 23–31

Laville J M, Collin J F 1992 Treatment of recurrent or neglected clubfoot by Ilizarov's appliance. Revue de Chirurgie Orthopédique et Réparatrice de l'Appareil Moteur 78: 485–490

Lloyd-Roberts G C 1964 Congenital club foot. Journal of Bone and Joint Surgery 46B: 369

Lochmiller C, Johnston D, Scott A, Risman M, Hecht J T 1998 Genetic epidemiology study of idiopathic talipes equinovarus. American Journal of Medical Genetics 79: 90–96

Macnicol M F, Nadeem R D, Maffulli N, Capasso G et al 1992 Histochemistry of the triceps surae muscle in idiopathic congenital clubfoot. Journal of Foot and Ankle Surgery 13: 80–84

Main B J, Crider R J 1978 An analysis of residual deformity in club feet submitted to early operation. Journal of Bone and Joint Surgery 60B: 536–543

Main B J, Crider R J, Palk M, Lloyd-Roberts G C, Swann M, Kander B A 1977 The results of early operation in talipes equinovarus. A preliminary report. Journal of Bone and Joint Surgery 59B: 337–341

Pagnotta G, Maffulli N, Aureli S, Maggi E, Mariani M, Yip K M 1996 Antenatal sonographic diagnosis of clubfoot: a six-year experience. Journal of Foot and Ankle Surgery 35: 67–71

Porter R W 1987a Congenital talipes equinovarus: I. Resolving and resistant deformities. Journal of Bone and Joint Surgery 69B: 822–825

Porter R W 1987b Congenital talipes equinovarus: II. A staged method of surgical management. Journal of Bone and Joint Surgery 69B: 826–831

Porter R W, Youle K 1993 Factors that affect surgical correction in congenital talipes equinovarus. Journal of Foot and Ankle Surgery 14: 23–27

Pous J G, Dimeglio A 1978 Neonatal surgery in clubfoot. Orthopedic Clinics of North America 9: 233–240

Ryoppy S, Sairanen H 1983 Neonatal operative treatment of club foot. A preliminary report. Journal of Bone and Joint Surgery 65B: 320–325

Scott W A, Hosking S W, Catterall A 1984 Club foot. Observations on the surgical anatomy of dorsiflexion. Journal of Bone and Joint Surgery 66B: 71–76

Sodre H, Bruschini S, Mestriner L A et al 1990 Arterial abnormalities in talipes equinovarus as assessed by angiography and the Doppler technique. Journal of Pediatric Orthopaedics 10: 101–104

Swann M, Lloyd-Roberts G C, Catterall A 1969 The anatomy of uncorrected club feet. A study of rotation deformity. Journal of Bone and Joint Surgery 51B: 263–269

Treadwell M C, Stanitski C L, King M 1999 Prenatal sonographic diagnosis of clubfoot: implications for patient counseling. Journal of Pediatric Orthopaedics 19: 8–10

Turco V J 1979 Resistant congenital club foot – one-stage posteromedial release with internal fixation. A follow-up report of a fifteen-year experience. Journal of Bone and Joint Surgery 61A: 805–814

Walker C J, Harrold A J 1983 Treatment and prognosis in congenital club foot. Journal of Bone and Joint Surgery 65B: 8–11

Wallander H, Hansson G, Tjernstrom B 1996 Correction of persistent clubfoot deformities with the Ilizarov external fixator. Experience in 10 previously operated feet followed for 2–5 years. Acta Orthopaedica Scandinavica 67: 283–287

Williams D H, Grant C E P, Catterall A 1987 Posterolateral release for resistant club foot: early clinical experience. Journal of Bone and Joint Surgery 69B: 155.

Woodrow N, Tran T, Umstad M, Graham H K, Robinson H, de Crespigny L 1998 Mid-trimester ultrasound diagnosis of isolated talipes equinovarus: accuracy and outcome for infants. Australian and New Zealand Journal of Obstetrics and Gynaecology 38: 301–305

Wright J, Rang M 1990 The spastic mouse. And the search for an animal model of spasticity in human beings. Clinical Orthopaedics and Related Research 253: 12–19

Zimny M L, Willig S J, Roberts J M, D'Ambrosia R D 1985 An electron microscopic study of the fascia from the medial and lateral sides of clubfoot. Journal of Pediatric Orthopaedics 5: 577–581

Ziv I, Blackburn N, Rang M, Koreska J 1984 Muscle growth in normal and spastic mice. Developmental Medicine and Child Neurology 26: 94–99

PART 3   Club foot: later problems and relapse
J. A. Fixsen

"The literature on the treatment of club foot is, as a general rule, that of unvarying success. It is often as brilliant as an advertising sheet and yet in practise there is no lack of half cured or relapsed cases, sufficient evidence that methods of cure are not universally understood." This statement by E H Bradford, First Professor of Orthopedic Surgery at Harvard, at a meeting of the American Orthopedic Association in 1889 remains as relevant today as it did more than over 100 years ago. Mr Catterall (see Ch. 29.2) has drawn attention to the importance of classifying this deformity. Almost all the results of treatment as reported in the literature remain flawed, as we have no objective measurement of the severity of the deformity with which the surgeon started. This is perhaps not surprising when one considers that the deformity is three-dimensional, involving 13 joints in the mid- and hindfoot, and that some measure of the stiffness or mobility of the deformity has to be made. Attempts at radiological measurement are at present only two-dimensional. In the young foot, the position of the ossific nucleus not only may be eccentric, as in the talus, but in addition an axis drawn through it may bear little relationship to the axis of the cartilage in which it lies. The elegant three-dimensional computer modelling analysis of club foot published by Herzenberg et al (1988) shows only too clearly the marked deformity already existing in the cartilage models of the bones in a club foot of a neonate. The axis of the talus in the club foot points laterally in the hindpart of the talus and medially in the neck, the talus being much more boomerang-shaped than in the normal foot (Figs 29.33 and 29.34).

The next major problem when surveying the literature is the paucity of maturity reviews or really long-term satisfactory reviews of club feet. There is a great tendency among authors to publish their results with an average follow-up of 4–7 years. When dealing with a condition that is likely to alter throughout growth, it really is not useful to publish long-term results unless the patients surveyed have reached maturity at the time of review. Perhaps the best long-term review in the English literature is that by Laaveg & Ponseti (1980). It is interesting to note that, in this careful study, only 126 of 498 feet with congenital talipes equinovarus obeyed the following criteria:

1. No other congenital abnormality was present.
2. They were all seen and treatment started within 6 months of age.
3. They were all treated by the same orthopaedic team.

Ultimately, only 104 feet were available for follow-up, but the average follow-up was 18.8 years. In this series, only 13 of 104 feet required no surgery whatsoever; 40 required elongation of the tendo-Achilles only and, of the remainder, 49 underwent one relapse at an average age of 3 years and 3 months, 25 underwent a second relapse at an average age

of 4 years and 5 months, 10 feet underwent a third relapse at 5 years and 3 months, and three feet suffered a fourth relapse at 6 years and 5 months. Cooper & Dietz (1995) published a further follow-up of these patients, with a minimum follow-up of 30 years. In a careful and well-planned study in which the investigators used pain and functional limitation as their main outcome criteria, 78% of the patients had good or excellent function, compared with 85% of their control group of patients who did not have any congenital deformity of the foot. They commented that X-ray images could not predict the result, and that studies with short-term follow up relying upon X-ray findings or range of motion may not reflect the factors necessary for good life-long foot function. The type of surgery undertaken in these patients would be considered very conservative nowadays. However, with the publication of these results and the problems we are now seeing from very radical club foot surgery, there has been a resurgence of interest in more conservative methods of treatment, as advocated by Dr Ponsetti.

Posterior release surgery was advocated by Attenborough (1966) for those patients for whom conservative treatment failed. There have been two reasonable long-term reviews of this type of surgery: one by Green & Lloyd-Roberts (1985) with an average follow-up of 15 years (range 10–24 years), and one by Hutchins et al (1985) with a follow up of 15 years and 10 months (range 8–31 years). Green & Lloyd-Roberts

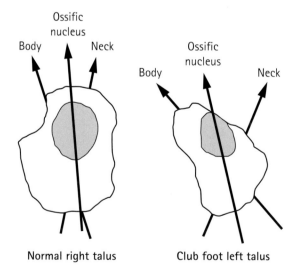

Figure 29.33 Two-dimensional view of the normal and club foot talus, showing that the axes drawn through the talar neck and body do not coincide with an axis drawn through the ossific nucleus. (Reproduced from Herzenberg et al (1988), with permission from the Journal of Pediatric Orthopaedics vol 8, p 258, 1988.)

Clubfoot | Normal
Lateral | Lateral

Anteroposterior | Anteroposterior

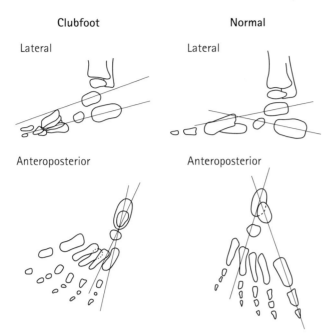

Figure 29.34 Outline drawings from the radiograph of the normal and club foot of a child aged 6 months, showing the talar and calcaneal axes. In the normal foot, these cross in both anteroposterior and lateral views, so that the axes of the so-called 'scissors' are open, whereas in the club foot the axes tend to run parallel to each other or only cross at a very acute angle – i.e. the scissors are closed.

reported a 59% success rate, whereas Hutchins et al reported an 81% success rate, but their criteria were less strict than those of Green & Lloyd-Roberts. The approach described by Porter (1987) in an interesting report used the posterior release described by Attenborough and then, if the foot showed persistent forefoot adduction, a medial release as a second stage in the, 3rd or 4th year of life. Unfortunately, only a small number of feet had been followed to maturity in 1987 when the report was published. Several reports of more extensive surgery have been made, such as those by Turco (1979) and Ghali et al (1983). Both groups claimed 84% good results, but with a much less satisfactory long-term follow-up: an average of 7 years was reported in Turco's paper and 11½ years in that by Ghali's group. This looks satisfactory until one realises that Turco's study included patients with 2-year follow-up and that by Ghali's group included those with 3-year follow-up, which negates the idea of these being long-term reviews.

Whatever the reported long-term results of surgery, it is clear that there are problems of relapse in at least 10–20% of cases, even in the best series. The variability of club foot suggests that there is no one single operation that is correct for all cases, and the 'à la carte' approach as suggested by Bensahel et al (1987) is logical. In the past, relapse has always meant recurrence of deformity, but more recently, particularly in association with the more extensive and radical operations, over-correction has become an increasing problem. Tarraf & Carroll (1992) reported that the most common persistent deformity was residual forefoot adduction and supination; only 3.8% of feet showed over-correction after the first operation. However, this figure increased to 17.5% and 18.2% after the second and third operations.

ASSESSMENT OF RECURRENT DEFORMITY

In the assessment of feet presenting with recurrent deformity, routine X-rays, provided they are taken in a standard fashion, can be helpful in assessing the position of the bones and, to some extent the degree of deformity. It is very important to remember that X-rays do not give a three-dimensional picture. Rotational problems are often hidden in what appears to be a simple angular deformity on the X-ray.

MANAGEMENT OF PERSISTENT DEFORMITY

In the management of patients with persistent deformity, three problems emerge:

1. Recurrence of deformity.
2. Over-correction.
3. Increasing and disabling stiffness of the foot.

This last problem is particularly important, because a mobile foot with some deformity is often more satisfactory to the patient than an anatomically normal foot that is completely stiff. This may explain why the clinical results in several long-term studies do not approximate closely to the anatomical results as measured radiologically because, inevitably, such measurements cannot take any account of the inherent stiffness of the foot.

RECURRENT DEFORMITY

The following should be considered in the assessment of a foot with recurrent deformity:

1. A persistent tendency to inversion.
2. Recurrent equinus.
3. The sagittally breached or 'bean-shaped' foot.
4. Cavo varus foot.

Persistent tendency to inversion

Persistent tendency to inversion is commonly seen after conservative treatment and simple posterior surgery. A child starts to walk, but persistently swings the foot into supination during the swing phase of gait. Provided the foot remains supple and the hindfoot is not in fixed equinus, the tibialis anterior tendon can be used as a dynamic internal splint by transferring it to the lateral side of the foot. Laaveg & Ponseti (1980) noted that the relapse rate among their patients was significantly lower in those who had this transfer. Garceau & Palmer (1967) stated that this procedure should be used in feet showing supination and inversion of the forefoot during the swing phase of gait in the presence of weakness or apparent absence of peroneal muscle function after the hindfoot has been adequately corrected. Contraindications were active eversion of the foot, uncorrected equinus and a rigid foot. Kernohan et al (1985) reported 79% satisfactory results, but there was a 17% over-correction rate in some cases sufficiently severe to require revision.

Initially, over-correction was accepted; however, if progressive planovalgus develops and becomes fixed, it is most important to revise the transfer. Over-correction from whatever cause in club foot can be as much, if not a greater problem as under-correction, for the patient in adult life. An interesting point in the series of Kernohan et al (1985) was that a small number of operations were performed in patients with a rigid deformity, as a means of holding the foot until it was large enough for more extensive bony surgery. Surprisingly, 50% of these patients did not require the expected later surgery, suggesting that, even in a rigid foot, sometimes this tendon transfer can produce sufficient correction to make further surgery unnecessary. More recently, Feldbrin et al (1995) reported good evidence of muscle imbalance, particularly in the more severe and recalcitrant club feet, using electrophysiological studies. Good clinical results in 16 of these patients were reported in a subsequent study from the same unit (Ezra et al 2000).

Recurrent equinus

When considering recurrent equinus, the most important thing is to decide whether it is occurring in the hindfoot, the forefoot, or both. It is also important to consider whether it is true equinus in the sagittal plane, or whether there is some rotational component to the deformity. Repeat posterior soft-tissue surgery becomes increasingly difficult and unrewarding as the surgeon struggles through the previous scar tissue and less and less response is gained from releasing the fibrous tissue and joint capsules. Perhaps the most useful practical point for the surgeon engaged in this difficult and demanding surgery is to resist the temptation to make a new incision, but to use the old scar. If he makes a new incision, the resulting tram-lines down the back of the leg frequently add to his problem and that of any later surgeon. The question of whether to use the Cincinnati incision (Crawford et al 1982), (Fig. 29.32) arises when a previous vertical incision has been used. This is possible, although it will produce a crossover of the two incisions at the junction of the vertical with the horizontal incision.

Lateral X-rays are of considerable value in assessing the state of the bones and joints, the site of the equinus, and whether there is external rotation of the hindfoot giving rise to apparent posterior displacement of the lateral malleolus and the so called 'flat-top' talus. This appearance is commonly caused by external rotation of the hindfoot, so that on the lateral X-ray one sees an oblique view of the hindfoot as it rotates away from the observer and an oblique view of the forefoot as it rotates towards the observer (Fig. 29.35A). In order to assess the hindfoot, the foot should be rotated medially so that a true lateral view of the hindfoot is obtained, which will usually make the apparent flat-top talus disappear and often show that the majority of the deformity is forefoot and midfoot (Fig. 29.35B).

If, in this situation, a repeat posterior operation is performed, the lengthening of the posterior structures will produce a persistent calcaneo-cavus foot. If the X-rays show established bony deformity in the older patient, the surgeon has a variety of choices. He or she may accept a certain amount of equinus, particularly in females, and accommodate for it by a low heel. A classic corrective procedure at or near maturity is the Lambrinudi (1927) type of triple arthrodesis procedure. This will correct the foot, but will add to its inherent stiffness and may lead to problems in the ankle joint in later life. Lower tibial osteotomy can be performed when the growth plate is closed, to bring the foot up to the plantigrade position without risking further stiffening of the foot or ankle (Napiontek & Nazar 1994).

The 'Bean-Shaped' or sagittally breached foot

The bean-shaped foot was well described by Evans (1961) when he reported his collateral operation of medial release and lateral calcaneo-cuboid fusion for this deformity. The basis of this procedure is to release the shortened medial border of the foot and to shorten the lengthened lateral border. It is essential, therefore, to realise that the medial release is a vital part of this operation (Fig. 29.36). Unless the structures are adequately released on the medial side, the calcaneo-cuboid fusion that shortens the convex lateral border of the foot is incapable of correcting the forefoot or the hindfoot. Basically, this is an osteotomy of the midfoot, removing the minimum amount of bone. It is vital that the midfoot is completely released at the site of the operation and that, in addition to correcting the adduction of the forefoot, it can also correct supination. Similarly, it can correct the varus of the hindfoot into valgus so that there is a rotational element at the 'midfoot osteotomy'. Before considering this operation, it is important to ensure that the deformity is at the talo-navicular/calcaneo-cuboid level and not further forwards in the tarsus, and that any hindfoot equinus has been corrected. It is also important that the forefoot is supinated and not pronated, because pronation is produced by the operation. Tayton & Thompson (1979) reported that the results in Evans' own patients were clinically satisfactorily in 85%, provided some degree of stiffening was accepted. Addison et al (1983) reported satisfactory results in 67% of patients using strict criteria, although 90% of their patients were pleased with the clinical result of their operation.

Graham & Dent (1992) have reported a further review of Dillwyn Evans' patients with an average follow-up of 29 years, all of whom were older than 20 years at the time of review. They found that 90% of patients were able to perform all desired activities, and mild residual deformity was compatible with good function. Poor function related to ankle and subtalar stiffness. Another approach to the bean-shaped foot was suggested by McHale & Lenhart in 1991, when they described an opening wedge medial cuneiform osteotomy and a closing cuboid procedure, which they had performed in six patients (seven feet).

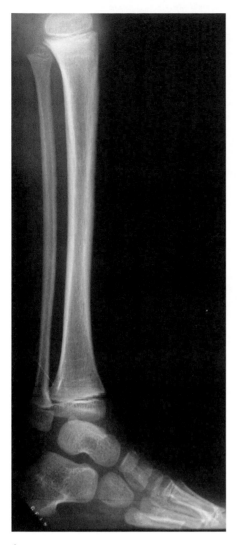

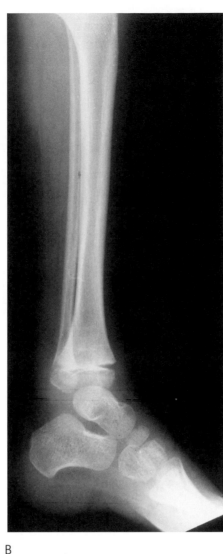

Figure 29.35 **A** Lateral view of the foot and the tibia, showing that the fibula appears posterior because the hindfoot is externally rotated. The talus appears flat-topped because one is looking at an oblique view of the ankle mortice and the forefoot is lying obliquely towards the viewer. **B** Lateral view of the same foot, with the hindfoot properly positioned relative to the X-ray beam so that a true lateral view is taken. The fibula is now in its correct position, so that a true lateral view of the ankle joint is obtained and the talus no longer looks flat-topped. However, now the forefoot shows significant forefoot equinus or plantaris. These two radiographs show how easy it is to be misled by simple two-dimensional radiography when the problem is really a three-dimensional one.

A

B

Cavovarus deformity

Cavovarus deformity may also be seen in the relapsed club foot. Tarraf & Carroll (1992) showed a high statistical significance between residual cavus deformity and failure to release the plantar fascia and short plantar ligaments at the first operation. The classical treatment in the younger patient is the Steindler release (Steindler 1920). Near maturity, a dorsal wedge osteotomy has been advised, but this inevitably stiffens the midfoot. Paulos et al (1980) stressed the importance of assessing the hindfoot mobility, and have pointed out that, if the foot is mobile, the varus of the hindfoot is often dictated by a fixed pronation of the forefoot. The simple 'block' test described by Coleman & Chestnut (1977) (see later Fig. 29.41) is most useful to demonstrate whether there is mobility at the subtalar joint, with fixed pronation of the medial part of the forefoot. If this is the case, the logical way to correct the deformity is by an extended medial soft-tissue release, sometimes including osteotomy of the 1st and 2nd metatarsals to correct the pronation of the medial part of the forefoot. Here again it is important to distinguish the rotational element in the deformity from the varus of the

hindfoot and the adduction of the forefoot. If, however, the foot is stiff, more radical bony procedures such as dorsolateral wedge tarsectomy and triple arthrodesis may be indicated, accepting the stiffness they will inevitably cause.

TALECTOMY

Talectomy remains a radical solution, but still has a place in the management of the really difficult and rigid club foot after previous surgery. This type of foot can either be left in its deformed state until near maturity, when major bony surgery is undertaken, or it can be converted safely and relatively simply into a plantigrade but stiff foot by the removal of the talus. It is important when performing this operation that no remnant of the talus is left behind and that the calcaneum is stabilised on the tibia by a Kirschner wire passed through the heel pad and the calcaneum up into the tibia. If possible, the Kirschner wire should be retained for at least 6–8 weeks. Talectomy is a safe and successful solution to some of the most difficult and scarred recurrent club feet that are too young and too severe to be left until maturity.

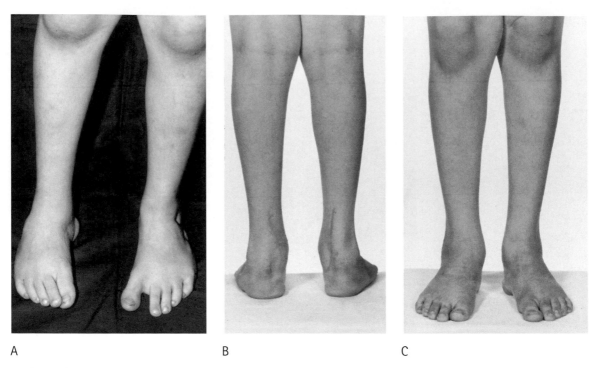

A   B   C

Figure 29.36 A and **B** Bilateral club feet after a previous posterior release. On the right there is forefoot varus and supination with the hindfoot laterally rotated and also in varus. This type of foot is suitable for the Dillwyn Evans collateral release, whereas on the left the forefoot varus is occurring more distally, at the tarso-metatarsal level, and this type of foot would not be suitable for a Dillwyn Evans procedure. **B** and **C** The same feet after Dillwyn Evans procedure on the right and medial release of the abductor hallucis on the left, showing good correction on both sides. The patient was reviewed at the age of 16 years and remained very satisfied with the results in both feet.

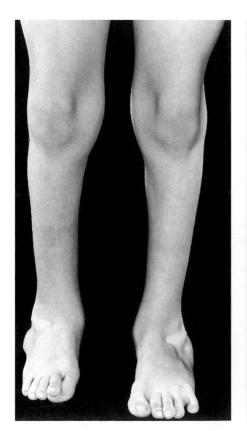
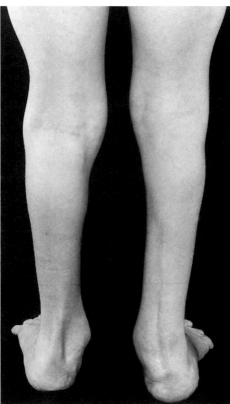

Figure 29.37 Anterior (**A**) and posterior (**B**) views of the feet of a child of 4½ years, after extended posteromedial release at the age of 3 months. The initial result was considered to be excellent, until the child showed signs of over-correction around the age of 4 years.

tends to dev
nerve condu
cavus and s
present to c
and calf wea
sprains, giv
patella, or
form, inheri

Type III F
patients tend
with severe
have a very
other types l
midal signs,
present to th

TREATMEN

Irrespective
demands tha
assessed. It
sible for the
major proble
the 1st and
pronates the
standing the
varus as a re

By carefu
whether or r
documented
on a raise
remainder o
29.41). If the
bility is pres
(1997) descr
foot flexibili
alternative t
held rigidly
'block test' o
are rigid – a
approach.

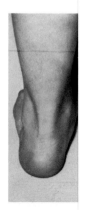

A

THE ILIZAROV METHOD

The Ilizarov method, another useful tool in the correction of recurrent deformity in club foot (Bradish & Noor 2000) and is considered in more detail on page 476.

OVER-CORRECTION

Over-correction (Fig. 29.37) can occur after any form of club foot treatment, surgical or non-surgical. It seems to be increasingly common after the more extensive operations that have been devised to decrease the relapse rate. Unfortunately, it is extremely difficult to correct over-correction once it has occurred. As stated previously, if one remembers the great variability of this condition, it is important not to apply a single surgical solution as an answer to all forms of club feet.

At present there is very little advice about methods of dealing with over-correction. If the heel is grossly valgus, perhaps a medial displacement os calcis osteotomy may be considered. If the forefoot is grossly abducted, some form of midfoot osteotomy may be necessary. However, frequently, the advice is to accept the over-correction and manage it by orthoses or footwear, rather than attempt yet further surgery.

CONCLUSION

The multiplicity of problems in the management of club foot emphasise yet again the importance of Bradford's statement. Despite a plethora of operations and reports of operations, the problem of the relapsed club foot remains relatively common, and until we have an objective measurement of the severity of club foot, progress is unlikely to be made.

REFERENCES

Addison A, Fixsen J A, Lloyd-Roberts G C 1983 A review of the Dillwyn Evans type collateral operation for severe club feet. Journal of Bone and Joint Surgery 65B: 12–14

Attenborough C G 1966 Severe congenital talipes equinovarus. Journal of Bone and Joint Surgery 48B: 31

Bensahel H, Csukonyi Z, Desgrippes Y, Chaumien J P 1987 Surgery in residual club foot; one stage medioposterior release 'à la carte'. Journal of Pediatric Orthopaedics 7: 145–148

Bradish C F, Noor S 2000 The Ilizarov method in the management of relapsed club feet. Journal of Bone and Joint Surgery 82B: 387–391

Coleman S S, Chestnut W J 1977 A simple test for hindfoot flexibility in the cavovarus foot. Clinical Orthopaedics and Related Research 123: 60–62

Cooper D M, Dietz F R 1995 Treatment of idiopathic club foot 30 year follow up. Journal of Bone and Joint Surgery 77A: 1477–1489

Crawford A H, Marxen J L, Osterfeld D L 1982 The Cincinnati incision: a comprehensive approach for surgical procedures for the foot and ankle in childhood. Journal of Bone and Joint Surgery 64A: 1355–1358

Evans D 1961 Relapsed club foot. Journal of Bone and Joint Surgery 43B: 722–733

Ezra E, Hayek S, Gilai A N, Khermosh O, Wientroub S 2000 Tibialis anterior tendon transfer for residual dynamic supination deformity in treated club feet. Journal of Pediatric Orthopaedics B9: 207–211

Feldbrin Z, Gilai A N, Ezra E, Khermosh O, Kramer U, Wiengrob S 1995 Muscle imbalance in the aetiology of idiopathic club foot. An electromyographic study. Journal of Bone and Joint Surgery 77B: 596–601

Garceau G J, Palmer R M 1967 Transfer of the anterior tibial tendon for recurrent club foot. Journal of Bone and Joint Surgery 49A: 207–231

Ghali N N, Smith R B, Clayden A D, Silk F F 1983 Results of pantalar reduction in the management of congenital talipes equinovarus. Journal of Bone and Joint Surgery 65B: 1–7

Graham G P, Dent C M 1992 The Dillwyn Evans operation for relapsed club foot, long term results. Journal of Bone and Joint Surgery 74B: 445–448

Green A D L, Lloyd-Roberts G C 1985 The results of early posterior release in resistant club foot, a long term review. Journal of Bone and Joint Surgery 67B: 588–593

Herzenberg J E, Carroll N C, Christophersen M R, Lee E H, White S, Munroe R 1988 Club foot analysis with 3 dimensional computer modelling. Journal of Pediatric Orthopaedics 8: 257–262

Hutchins P M, Foster B K, Paterson D C, Cole E A 1985 Long term results of early surgical release in club foot. Journal of Bone and Joint Surgery 67B: 791–799

Kernohan J, Kavanagh T G, Fixsen J A, Lloyd-Roberts G C 1985 A long term review of tibialis anterior tendon transfer in congenital club foot. Journal of Bone and Joint Surgery 67B: 490

Laaveg S J, Ponseti I V 1980 Long term results of treatment of congenital club foot. Journal of Bone and Joint Surgery 62A: 23–31

Lambrinudi C 1927 New operation on drop foot. British Journal of Surgery 15: 193

McHale K A, Lenhart M K 1991 Treatment of residual clubfoot deformity – the 'bean-shaped' foot – by opening wedge medial cuneiform osteotomy and closing wedge cuboid osteotomy. Clinical review and cadaver correlations. Journal of Pediatric Orthopaedics 11: 374–381

Napiontek M, Nazar J 1994 Tibial osteotomy as a salvage procedure in the treatment of congenital talipes equinovarus. Journal of Pediatric Orthopaedics 14: 763–767

Paulos L E, Coleman S S, Samuelson K M 1980 Pes cavovarus, review of the surgical approach using soft tissue procedures. Journal of Bone and Joint Surgery 62A: 942–953

Porter R W 1987 Congenital talipes equinovarus; II. A staged method of surgical management. Journal of Bone and Joint Surgery 69B: 826–831

Steindler A 1920 Stripping of the os calcis. Journal of Orthopaedic Surgery 2: 8

Tarraf Y N, Carroll N C 1992 Analysis of the components of a residual deformity in club feet presenting for operation. Journal of Pediatric Orthopaedics 12: 207–216

Tayton K, Thompson T 1979 Relapsing club feet, late results of delayed operation. Journal of Bone and Joint Surgery 61B: 474–480

Turco V J 1979 Resistant congenital club foot. One stage posteromedial release with internal fixation. Journal of Bone and Joint Surgery 61A: 805–814

PART 4   Pes cavus
S. S. Coleman and J. A. Fixsen

INTRODUCTION

Pes cavus, or a high arched foot, is rarely seen at birth or in the first year of life unless it is part of a severe congenital

talipes equinovarus. There is a rare benign form of high arched foot that is called pes arcuatus; this is occasionally seen as an isolated abnormality in the first year of life, and resolves spontaneously. Cavus deformity of the foot

retained for 6–8 weeks and then a decision can be made as to whether tendon transfers are necessary to prevent recurrence of deformity. The degree of correction obtained can be assessed on the lateral weight-bearing X-ray by measuring the angle of Meary (Fig. 29.42).

If both the hindfoot and forefoot are inflexible – i.e. the block test is negative – both components of the deformity must be treated. In young children, this may require a plantar release combined with a medial release. In older children in whom a medial release is not sufficient, the plantar release can be combined with a lateral wedge osteotomy (Dwyer 1959), or simply a valgus displacement osteotomy of the calcaneum. In adolescents and adults, the forefoot correction may require a wedge tarsectomy or even a full triple arthrodesis.

The place of tendon transfers is difficult to assess, particularly if one is dealing with a progressive neurological condition such as HMSN. If there is significant forefoot inversion and overactivity of the tibialis posterior, transfer of this tendon to the dorsum has been advocated at the same time as the medial release. Full transfer of the tibialis anterior should be avoided, but a split transfer, or the procedure described by Fowler et al (1959) in which the tibialis anterior is transferred onto the dorsum of the base of the 1st metatarsal and combined with a wedge osteotomy of the base of the first cuneiform, may be undertaken.

Toe deformities are also a major problem. These patients, because of their disturbance of pain and temperature sensation, are liable to serious soft-tissue lesions, particularly over the pressure areas on the toes. The typical Z deformity of the big toe can be treated by the classical Robert Jones tendon transfer, in which the extensor hallucis longus is transferred to the distal portion of the shaft of the 1st metatarsal, and the interphalangeal joint of the big toe is either fused or

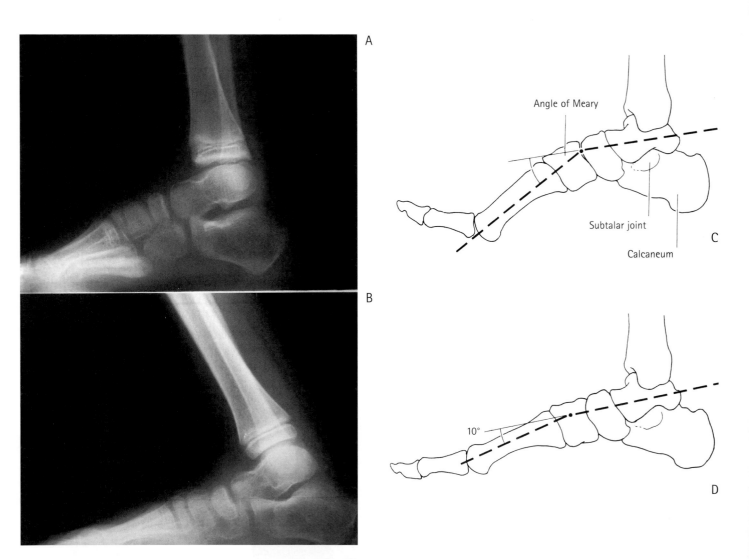

Figure 29.42 A Standing lateral weight-bearing radiograph of a typical cavovarus foot caused by Charcot–Marie–Tooth disease. Note the lack of overlap of the talus on the calcaneum, the clear view through the subtalar joint and the increased angle of Meary (30°). **B** Lateral standing film 1 year later shows almost complete correction of these abnormalities. **C, D** Tracings of the pre- and postoperative radiographs.

tenodesed if the child still has significant growth left in the toe. Clawing of the lesser toes can cause serious problems with the nails and pressure sores. In the past, the so-called Girdlestone toe flexor to extensor transfer was recommended (Taylor 1951). This transfer was described originally for victims of polio, but in the progressive forms of neurological disease the simple flexor tenotomy described by Menelaus & Ross (1984) is simpler and more effective.

PES CALCANEO–CAVUS

This type of foot is characteristic of the paralytic neurological conditions such as poliomyelitis, spinal muscular atrophy and the lower motor neurone type of spina bifida. Characteristically, both the medial and the lateral arches are raised, giving rise to the positive 'coin' sign. The heel is in calcaneus and the subtalar joint stiff, so that the 'block' test is negative and is not appropriate in this type of foot. A lateral X-ray shows the characteristic 'pistol-grip' appearance of the calcaneum (Fig. 29.43).

In younger children, a Steindler (1920) soft-tissue release of the plantar fascia may be helpful. Once bony deformity becomes fixed, a Mitchell (1977) posterior displacement osteotomy of the os calcis combined with a plantar release can be used. In the rigid foot, in adolescents or young adults, the Elmslie triple arthrodesis reported by Chomeley (1953) can be useful. In this procedure, a posterior wedge is excised from the subtalar joint to correct the calcaneus of the heel, and subsequently a wedge tarsectomy is performed to bring

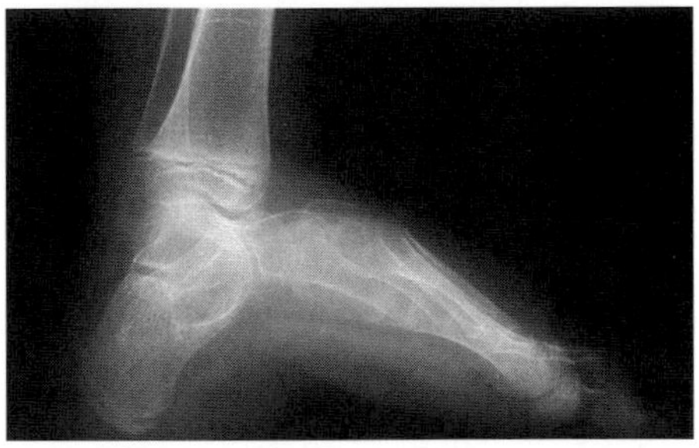

Figure 29.43 Lateral X-ray of a calcaneo-cavus foot, showing the almost vertical position of the calcaneum: the so-called 'pistol grip' appearance of the calcaneum.

the forefoot up on the corrected hindfoot. Attempts to restore power and 'push off' by the so-called Robert Jones transfer, in which the dorsiflexors are transferred into the calf, have never been really successful. Silver et al (1985) pointed out that the calf muscle is approximately six times stronger than the dorsiflexors of the foot as it has to lift the entire body weight, and not just the foot. As a result, it is not surprising that transfers of the dorsiflexors into the calf are unlikely to reproduce good push off. Wilbur Westin et al (1988) described an unusual variant of this procedure. Instead of fixing the tendo-Achilles to the back of the tibia, the tendo-Achilles was transferred into the fibula. This technique was used in a number of patients with calcaneus feet associated with spina bifida, and appears to be useful in preventing progression of calcaneus and valgus in these patients.

REFERENCES AND FURTHER READING

Brewerton D A, Sandifer P H, Sweetnam D R 1963 Idiopathic pes cavus, an investigation into its aetiology. British Medical Journal 2: 659

Chomeley J A 1953 Elmslie's operation for the calcaneus foot. Journal of Bone and Joint Surgery 35B: 46

Coleman S S, Chestnut W J 1977 A simple test for hindfoot flexibility in the cavovarus foot. Clinical Orthopaedics and Related Research 123: 60

Deluca P A, Banta J B 1985 Pes cavovarus as a late consequence of peroneus longus tendon laceration. Journal of Pediatric Orthopaedics 5: 582–583

Dwyer F C 1959 Osteotomy of the calcaneum for pes cavus. Journal of Bone and Joint Surgery 41B: 80

Fowler D, Brooks A L, Parrish T F 1959 The cavovarus foot. Journal of Bone and Joint Surgery 41A: 757

Harding A E, Thomas P K 1980 The clinical features of hereditary motor and sensory neuropathies types I and II. Brain 103: 259

Menelaus M B, Ross E R S 1984 Open flexor tenotomy for hammer toes and curly toes in children. Journal of Bone and Joint Surgery 66B: 770

Mitchell G T 1977 Posterior displacement osteotomy of the calcaneous. Journal of Bone and Joint Surgery 59B: 233

Price A, Maisel R, Drennan J C 1993 Computer tomographic analysis of pes cavus. Journal of Pediatric Orthopaedics 13: 646–653

Price B D, Price C T 1997 A simple demonstration of hindfoot flexibility in the cavovarus foot. Journal of Pediatric Orthopaedics 17: 18–19

Sharrard W J W 1971 Paediatric Orthopaedics and Fractures, 1st edn. Blackwell, Oxford, p 283

Silver R L, De La Garza J, Rang M 1985 The myth of muscle balance. Journal of Bone and Joint Surgery 67B: 432–437

Steindler A 1920 Stripping of the os calcis. Journal of Orthopaedic Surgery 2: 8

Taylor R G 1951 The treatment of claw toes by multiple transfers of flexor into extensor tendons. Journal of Bone and Joint Surgery 35B: 539–542

Westin G W, Dugeman R D, Gausewitz S H 1988 The results of tenodesis of the tendo Achilles to the fibula for paralytic pes calcaneus. Journal of Bone and Joint Surgery 78A: 320–338

PART 5   Congenital vertical talus (congenital convex pes valgus)
S. S. Coleman and J. A. Fixsen

This rare foot deformity has been given many different names, depending upon how various authors view the

pathology and its clinical manifestations. The most common name is 'congenital vertical talus', but perhaps the most accurate has been suggested by Tachdjian (1983) – namely 'teratologic dislocation of the talo-calcaneo-navicular joint'. Irrespective of the term used, it is important to understand that this is a rigid foot deformity. Hamanishi (1984), in a major review of 69 cases, suggested that, from the aetiological point of view, these feet could be grouped according to an association with one of five disorders:

1. Neural defects/spinal anomalies.
2. Neuromuscular disorders.
3. Malformation syndromes.
4. Chromosomal aberrations.
5. Idiopathic.

Coleman (1983), from personal experience of a major series of 40 congenital vertical tali, reported that only two feet in one child were not associated with any other abnormality. It is most important, therefore, that the orthopaedic surgeon presented with a child with a congenital vertical talus examines the child thoroughly for any other problems and considers the treatment of the foot in relation to these other problems.

In infancy, the deformity superficially resembles a severe calcaneo-valgus or plano-valgus foot (Fig. 29.44). It is for this reason that the diagnosis is often delayed. The difference between the two, which is most important from a diagnostic and therapeutic point of view, is that the true congenital vertical talus is rigid and cannot be passively corrected. In older children, it must be distinguished from severe flat foot, paralytic flat foot, flat foot in cerebral palsy and spuriously corrected or rocker-bottomed foot after treatment of club foot (Lloyd-Roberts & Spence 1958). A plantarflexion stress lateral radiograph (the Eyre-Brook view) shows that the rela-

tionships of the bones of the hindfoot do not change and that the navicular remains dorsally dislocated on the talus (Eyre-Brook 1967). It is important to remember that the navicular is the last bone to ossify in the foot, at the age of about 4 years. However, the position of the navicular can be determined in younger children by a line drawn through the longitudinal axis of the 1st metatarsal, which will run through the centre of the navicular (Fig. 29.45).

The pathology of congenital vertical talus includes four basic abnormalities that involve the bones, joints, ligaments and muscles of the foot. Although there is some variability in the degree of severity, certain abnormalities of anatomy are always present. These consist of:

1. A complete irreducible dorsal dislocation of the navicular on a vertically orientated talus.
2. Abnormal displacement of the peroneus longus and posterior tibial tendons so that they function as dorsiflexors rather than plantarflexors.
3. Subluxation of the talo-calcaneal joint.
4. Fixed equinus of the hindfoot as the result of a contracted heel cord and ankle capsule (Fig. 29.46); in some cases there is also a calcaneo-cuboid subluxation or dislocation (Coleman et al 1970).

Once the diagnosis has been established, it is accepted that non-operative treatment will not succeed. Manipulation of the foot into plantarflexion may stretch out the anterior structures, including the skin, but true restoration of the bony relationships rarely, if ever, occurs. Surgical correction is therefore necessary.

Over the years, many methods of surgical treatment have been proposed, but the basic principles remain the same –

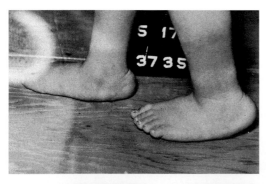
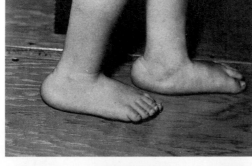
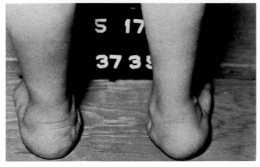
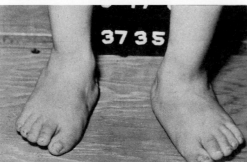

Figure 29.44 Photograph of a patient with congenital vertical talus. Note flattened longitudinal arch and features that simulate a severe plano-valgus or calcaneo-valgus foot.

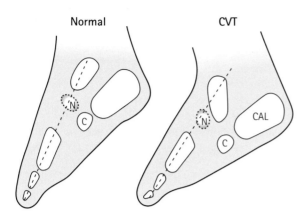

Figure 29.45 Diagrammatic representation of the Eyre-Brook view in the normal and congenital vertical talus (CVT) foot. N, navicular; C, cuboid; CAL, calcaneum.

namely, restoring the bones to their normal relationships and holding them there. Many different techniques have been described but the essential steps are as follows:

1. The talo-navicular dislocation must be reduced and stabilised.
2. The hindfoot equinus must be corrected and the normal talo-calcaneal relationships restored.
3. The forefoot, which is in calcaneus and frequently everted, must be reduced and stablised on the corrected hindfoot.

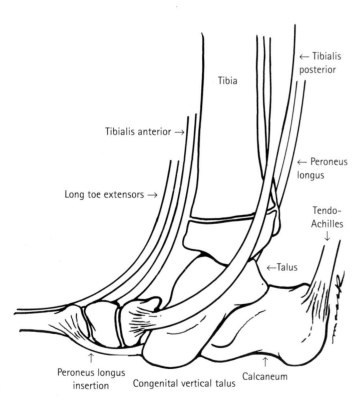

Figure 29.46 Diagrammatic illustration of the basic pathological anatomy of the congenital vertical talus foot as described in the text.

These steps comprise, in essence, an open reduction of the three major deformities present in the foot (Fig. 29.47).

In the past, two-stage reduction was commonly advocated (Stone & Lloyd-Roberts 1963): the forefoot was reduced on the hindfoot at the first stage, and at the second stage the hindfoot was corrected. Stone & Lloyd-Roberts also advised removing the navicular, to shorten the medial column of the foot. This procedure was also reported by Clark et al (1977). More recently, the importance of a full release of the contracted peroneal tendons and reduction of the calcaneo-cuboid subluxation that lengthens the lateral column of the foot has made excision of the navicular and shortening of the medial column unnecessary. Finally, Stone & Lloyd-Roberts (1963) advised transfer of the tibialis anterior into the neck of the talus, to help support the talus in its corrected position.

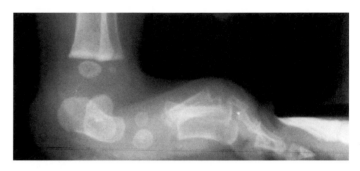

A

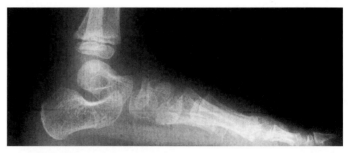

B

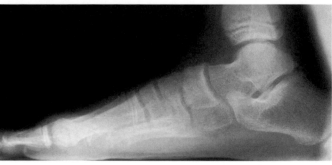

C

Figure 29.47 A Example of the foot of a patient 6 months old with a typical congenital vertical talus. **B** 4 years later, surgery has produced a near-normal foot, clinically and radiographically. **C** 19 years later, the foot has maintained its near-normal radiographic appearance, except for some minor asymptomatic alterations in the talo-navicular joint.

Nowadays, the majority of surgeons prefer a single one-stage complete reduction of the triple deformity without any tendon transfers (Kodros & Dias 1999). It is probably best to perform this operation when the child is between the ages of 6 months and 2 years; many of these children have multiple other problems and it is reasonable to delay surgery until the child's development has been assessed and other problems dealt with. The deformity, although it is unsightly, is unlikely to severely hinder the establishment of walking. Complete reduction of the deformity requires medial surgery to reduce the talo-navicular dislocation, which is normally stabilised with a K wire passed along the first ray and fixing the navicular in its corrected position on the reduced talus. A posterior release is important to correct the heel equinus, and a lateral release to reduce the calcaneo-cuboid displacement and elongate the peroneii. In order to allow satisfactory correction of the forefoot on the hindfoot, the tibialis anterior and the dorsiflexors of the foot, which are always tight, require lengthening. In patients older than 3–4 years it may be difficult to stabilise the talus satisfactorily on the calcaneum, because of the deformation of the subtalar joint. In this situation, Coleman (1983) advises a subtalar arthrodesis to stabilise the unstable talo-calcaneal joint.

Congenital vertical talus is a rare but fascinating condition. It is important to establish the diagnosis clearly and not confuse it with other conditions and milder forms of 'rocker-bottom' feet. The majority of these children will have other major problems and it is very important that the treatment of the foot deformity is seen in relation to these and not in isolation. Inevitably with such a rare condition, most reports are small and anecdotal. Dodge et al (1987) published a useful long-term retrospective review of 36 feet followed up for an average of 14 years. A number of surgical techniques had been used and none produced significantly better results than others. They confirmed the high incidence of other problems in these children, and found that the majority did well after surgery. Kodros & Dias (1999) reviewed 32 patients (42 feet) in whom a one-stage complete reduction was performed using the Cincinnati incision (Fig 29.32). They reported no wound complications and no incidence of avascular necrosis in the talus. They found that the Cincinnati incision provided excellent exposure for this complex procedure, but that 10 feet had required further procedures with time. They pointed out that the overall functional result in many of their patients was determined as much by the underlying condition from which they suffered as by the quality of the result of their foot operation.

REFERENCES

Clark M W, D'Ambrosia R D, Ferguson Q B Jr 1977 Congenital vertical talus. Treatment by open reduction and navicular excision. Journal of Bone and Joint Surgery 59A: 816

Coleman S S 1983 Complex foot deformities in children. Lea & Febiger, Philadelphia

Coleman S S, Stelling F H, Jarrett J 1970 Pathomechanics and treatment of congenital vertical talus. Clinical Orthopaedics and Related Research 70: 62

Dodge L D, Ashley R K, Gilbert R J 1987 Treatment of the congenital vertical talus: a retrospective view of 36 feet with long term follow up. Foot and Ankle 7: 326

Eyre-Brook L 1967 Congenital vertical talus. Journal of Bone and Joint Surgery 49B: 618–627

Hamanishi C 1984 Congenital vertical talus. Classification with 69 cases and new measurement system. Journal of Pediatric Orthopaedics 4: 318

Kodros S A, Dias L S 1999 Single stage correction of congenital vertical talus. Journal of Pediatric Orthopaedics 19: 42–28

Lloyd-Roberts G C, Spence A J 1958 Congenital vertical talus. Journal of Bone and Joint Surgery 40B: 33

Stone K H, Lloyd-Roberts G C 1963 Congenital vertical talus. A new operation. Proceedings of the Royal Society of Medicine 56: 12

Tachdjian M O 1983 Pediatric orthopedics. Congenital convex pes valgus. W B Saunders, Philadelphia, pp 2557–2576

Chapter 30

Congenital disorders of the cervical spine

R. N. Hensinger

Radiological interpretation of the infant's spine may be difficult, and a clear understanding of its appearances at different ages is essential if deformity and malalignment are to be recognised.

In 1912, Klippel & Feil published the first complete description of various congenital disorders of the cervical spine. The 'Klippel–Feil syndrome' in its present usage refers to all patients with congenital fusion of the cervical vertebrae, whether it involves two segments, congenital block vertebrae, or the entire cervical spine. As radiographic techniques improved, it became apparent that certain anomalies of the occipito-cervical junction, atlanto-occipital fusion, basilar impression, and abnormalities of the odontoid should be considered separately from the original syndrome. Although they occur commonly in conjunction with fusion of the lower cervical vertebrae, their significance depends upon their influence on the atlanto-axial joint. Their prognostic and therapeutic implications are distinctly different, and they occur with sufficient frequency to warrant individual analysis.

BASILAR IMPRESSION

Basilar impression (or basilar invagination) is a deformity of the bones of the base of the skull at the margin of the foramen magnum. The floor of the skull appears to be indented by the upper cervical spine. The tip of the odontoid is more cephalad, sometimes protruding into the opening of the foramen magnum, and it may encroach upon the brain-stem. This increases the risk of neurological damage from injury, circulatory embarrassment, or impairment of cerebrospinal fluid flow. There are two types:

1. *Primary basilar impression.* A congenital abnormality often associated with other vertebral defects such as atlanto-occipital fusion, hypoplasia of the atlas, bifid posterior arch of the atlas, odontoid abnormalities, and Klippel–Feil syndrome.
2. *Secondary basilar impression.* A developmental condition attributed to softening of the osseous structures at the base of the skull, with deformity developing later in life. This occurs in conditions such as osteomalacia, rickets, Paget's disease, osteogenesis imperfecta, renal osteodystrophy, rheumatoid arthritis, neurofibromatosis, and ankylosing spondylitis.

RADIOGRAPHIC FINDINGS

Basilar impression is difficult to assess radiographically, and many measurement schemes have been proposed. The most commonly used are those described by Chamberlain (1939), McGregor (1948) and McRae (1960). McRae's line (1960) defines the opening of the foramen magnum and is derived from his observation that 'if the tip of the odontoid lies below the opening of the foramen magnum, the patient will probably be asymptomatic'. McRae's line is a helpful guide in the clinical assessment of patients with basilar impression (Fig. 30.1).

With the development of computed tomography (CT) reconstructions, and more recently magnetic resonance imaging (MRI), it is now possible to view the relationship at the occipital-cervical junction in much greater detail. Clinically, the lateral reference lines (McGregor 1948, McRae 1960) are still important for screening. CT reconstruction and MRI are generally reserved for the patient whose routine examination or clinical findings may suggest the presence of an occipito-cervical anomaly. Rouvreau et al (1998) found occipital and C1 abnormalities were often associated with neurological risk. MRI with lateral flexion/extension views seems to be the best method for detecting impingement of

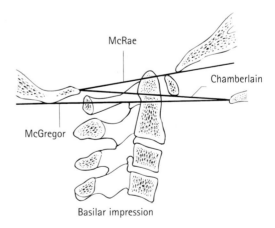

Figure 30.1 Lateral craniometry. The drawing indicates the three lines used to determine basilar impressions. Chamberlain's line (1939) is drawn from the posterior lip of the foramen magnum (opisthion) to the dorsal margin of the hard palate. McGregor's line (1948) is drawn from the upper surface of the posterior edge of the hard palate to the most caudal point of the occipital magnum. McGregor's line is the best method for screening, because the bony landmarks can be clearly defined at all ages on a routine lateral radiograph.

the spine on the spinal cord, especially in patients with odontoid dysplasia and basilar impression.

CLINICAL FINDINGS

Patients with basilar impression frequently have a deformity of the skull or neck; however, these physical findings are also often found in patients without basilar impression (Klippel–Feil syndrome, occipitalisation), and are not considered pathognomonic.

Basilar impression is frequently associated with conditions such as the Arnold–Chiari malformation and syringomyelia, which can cloud the clinical picture. Symptoms are generally caused by crowding of the neural structures (particularly the medulla oblongata) at the level of the foramen magnum. The dominant complaints of symptomatic patients are weakness and paraesthesia of the limbs. In contrast, those who are symptomatic with pure Arnold–Chiari malformation are more likely to have cerebellar and vestibular disturbances (unsteadiness of gait, dizziness and nystagmus). In both conditions, there may be impingement of the lower cranial nerves as they emerge from the medulla oblongata. The trigeminal (V), glossopharangeal (IX), vagus (X) and hypoglossal (XII) nerves may be affected. Headache and pain in the nape of the neck in the distribution of the greater occipital nerve is a common finding. Posterior encroachment may cause blockage of the aqueduct of Silvius, and the presenting symptoms may be caused by increased intracranial pressure (McRae 1960).

There is an increased incidence of vertebral artery anomalies in basilar impression, atlanto-occipital fusion and absence of the C1 facet. In addition, the vertebral arteries may be compressed as they pass through the crowded foramen magnum, causing symptoms suggestive of vertebral arterial insufficiency, such as dizziness, seizures, mental deterioration and syncope. These symptoms may occur alone or in combination with those of spinal cord compression. Erbengi & Oge (1994) have noted that the preoperative evaluation of these patients needs special care, as many have unrecognised low vital capacity and chronic alveolar hypoventilation as a result of chronic slow progressive neurological injury to the brain-stem. Gag and cough reflexes are often depressed.

Although this condition is congenital, many patients do not develop symptoms until the 2nd or 3rd decade of life. This may be due to a gradually increasing instability from ligamentous laxity due to ageing. Patients with this malformation have been mistakenly diagnosed as having multiple sclerosis, posterior fossa tumours, amyotrophic lateral sclerosis, or traumatic injury. It is therefore important to survey this area whenever such a diagnosis is considered and whenever this malformation is in any way suspected.

OCCIPITO–CERVICAL FUSION

Occipito-cervical fusion, which may be partial or complete, is a congenital union between the atlas and the base of the occiput. Synonyms include assimilation of the atlas, occipito-cervical synostosis and occipitalisation of the atlas. The condition ranges from total incorporation of the atlas into the occipital bone, to a bony or even fibrous band uniting one small area of the atlas to the occiput. Basilar impression is commonly associated with occipito-cervical synostosis; other associated anomalies include Klippel–Feil syndrome, occipital vertebrae and condylar hypoplasia.

RADIOGRAPHIC FINDINGS

Standard radiographs of this area can be difficult to interpret. Tomograms and CT reconstruction may be necessary to clarify the pathology. Most commonly, the anterior arch of the atlas is assimilated into the occiput, usually in association with a hypoplastic posterior arch. There is varying loss of height of the atlas, allowing the odontoid to project upward into the foramen magnum and creating a primary basilar impression (Fig. 30.2). There is a high association (up to 70%) with congenital fusion between C2 and C3, which can put an added strain on the C1–C2 articulation, and associated atlanto-axial instability has been reported to develop eventually in 50% of patients with this anatomic configuration.

CLINICAL FINDINGS

Most patients have an appearance similar to the Klippel–Feil syndrome, with a short broad neck, low hairline, torti-

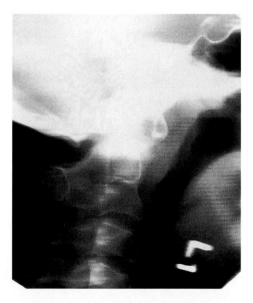

Figure 30.2 A 23-year-old male with the Klippel–Feil syndrome, ataxic gait, hyper-reflexia, and a history of several episodes of unconsciousness. The lateral laminographic view of the cervical spine and base of the skull demonstrates a C2–C3 fusion and fusion of the ring of C1 to the opening of the foramen magnum (occipitalisation). The odontoid is hypermobile. Patients with this pattern of fusion are at great risk. With ageing, the odontoid may become hypermobile, and the space available for the spinal cord may be compromised. (Reproduced with permission from Rothman & Simone (1982).)

collis, high scapula and restricted neck movements. Kyphosis and scoliosis are frequent. Other associated anomalies that are occasionally seen include dwarfism, funnel chest, pes cavus, syndactylies, jaw anomalies, cleft palate, congenital ear deformities, hypospadias and genitourinary tract defects.

Neurological symptoms do not usually occur until midlife, but they can present during childhood. They progress in a slow, unrelenting manner and may be initiated by traumatic or inflammatory processes. McRae (1960) suggested that the odontoid is the key to the development of a neurological lesion and that its position indicates the degree of actual or relative basilar impression. If the odontoid lies below the foramen magnum, the patient is usually asymptomatic. However, with decreased vertical height of the atlas, the odontoid may project well into the foramen magnum and produce brain-stem pressure. Those with instability should be considered for fusion when there are signs of impingement on the spinal cord, nerve roots or cranial nerves.

Anterior compression of the brain-stem from the posteriorly unstable odontoid is the most common problem. This produces a variety of findings, depending on the location and degree of pressure. Pyramidal tract signs and symptoms (spasticity, hyper-reflexia, muscle weakness and wasting, and gait disturbances) are most common; cranial nerve involvement (diplopia, tinnitus, dysphagia and auditory disturbances) is less common. Compression from the posterior lip of the foramen magnum or a constricting band of dura may disturb the posterior columns, resulting in loss of proprioception, vibration and tactile discrimination. Nystagmus, a common occurrence, is probably due to posterior cerebellar compression. Vascular disturbances from vertebral artery involvement may occasionally result in syncope, seizure, vertigo and unsteady gait, amongst other signs and symptoms of brain stem ischaemia.

ANOMALIES OF THE RING OF C1

In 1986, Dubousset called attention to a previously unrecognised problem with the ring of C1, the hemiatlas. Although there had been an occasional case report, he presented the first large study to review the problem in depth. The absence of one facet of C1 leads to a severe and progressive torticollis in the young child. Initially, the deformity is flexible and can be passively corrected. As the child ages, the torticollis becomes more severe and eventually fixed. Radiographic diagnosis using tomograms or CT has been helpful in identifying this deformity (Fig. 30.3). This can also accompany the Klippel–Feil syndrome, with anomalies of the lower cervical spine. Dubousset found these children to have an increased incidence of anomalies of the vertebral vessels, and suggested arteriographic evaluation before traction or surgical intervention, which could further compromise a precarious blood supply to the midbrain and spinal cord.

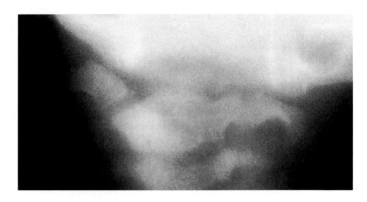

Figure 30.3 Absent facet of C1: anteroposterior tomogram in a 7-year-old with a hemiatlas that has led to a progressive torticollis. The deformity is initially flexible and passively correctible. (Reproduced by permission of L C Fisher III, Jackson, Mississippi.)

LAXITY OF THE TRANSVERSE ATLANTAL LIGAMENT

This is a diagnosis of exclusion suggested by the clinical occurrence of chronic atlanto-axial dislocation without a predisposing cause. There is no history of trauma, congenital anomaly, infection or rheumatoid arthritis to account for the radiological finding. The majority of patients discovered (excluding those with Down's syndrome) have the typical symptoms of atlanto-axial instability, and require surgical stabilisation.

Laxity of the transverse atlantal ligament is common in patients with Down's syndrome, with a reported incidence of 15% (Burke et al 1985) (Fig. 30.4). The lesion may be found in all age groups, without a preponderance at any age (Burke et al 1985). These patients rupture or attenuate the transverse atlantal ligament, with encroachment of the 'safe zone of Steel', but at least initially are protected by the 'check-rein' action of the alar ligaments from spinal cord compression. In other words, many have excessive motion, but relatively few are symptomatic and the majority are discovered only by radiological survey. If radiographs of the upper cervical spine indicate an atlantal–dens interval of more than 4.5 mm, instability is considered to be present. Usually, if symptoms are present, instability of greater than 7 mm or even 10 mm is found. Recent reports suggest an increased incidence of occiput–C1 instability also.

We still know very little about the natural history of atlanto-axial instability in Down's syndrome, despite the radiographic examination of hundreds of children. The findings of some studies have suggested that some children become progressively looser with time; others with small degrees of instability can, on occasion, become stable (Burke et al 1985). Currently, radiographic examination on a routine basis is recommended for children with Down's syndrome only if they plan to compete in athletics. Any child with Down's syndrome who has a musculoskeletal

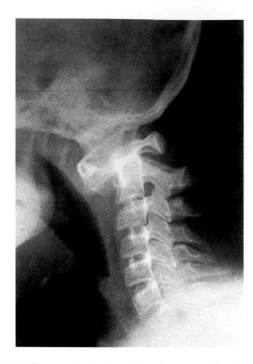

Figure 30.4 The cervical spine of an 11-year-old with Down's syndrome and gross atlanto-axial instability. The gait was clumsy and physical examination revealed poor co-ordination of the extremities. There was no other evidence of motor or sensory impairment or of pathological reflexes. The patient has no symptoms referable to the cervical spine 2 years after surgical stabilisation.

complaint such as subluxating patella, dislocating hips or a wide-based ataxic gait should be investigated. Similarly, if a child with Down's syndrome requires a general anaesthetic, the stability of the cervical spine should be evaluated, because positioning of the head and neck during the procedure could lead to neurological injury. With our present knowledge, prophylactic stabilisation does not appear to be indicated; however, more clinical information is required. Those who have minor degrees of hypermobility or instability should be followed with flexion–extension X-rays on a regular basis. They should not engage in contact sports, somersaults, trampoline exercises or similar activities that favour neck flexion and the potential risks should be discussed with the parents. Any child who has neck symptoms caused by instability or a history of neurological problems should have the lesion surgically stabilised (Burke et al 1985).

ODONTOID ANOMALIES

Various anomalies of the odontoid exist, ranging from aplasia and hypoplasia to os odontoideum. A congenital or developmental aetiology has always been assumed. Hypoplasia and os odontoideum can be acquired secondary to trauma or, rarely, infection (Fielding et al 1980). Several cases of 'os odontoideum' that developed some years after

trauma in a patient in whom a normal odontoid was initially present have been reported (Fielding et al 1980). This has led to the suggestion that some cases of os odontoideum or hypoplasia are due to an unrecognised fracture of the base or damage to the epiphyseal plate of the odontoid during the first few years of life (Fielding et al 1980). This insult could compromise the blood supply to the developing dens, resulting in partial failure, complete absorption, or an os odontoideum. It is probable that both congenital or developmental and post-traumatic forms of hypoplasia and os odontoideum do exist.

CLINICAL FINDINGS

Odontoid hypoplasia and os odontoideum present with similar clinical findings secondary to instability and displacement of the atlas on the axis. The usual age at diagnosis is from 19 to 30 years (Fielding et al 1980). Problems are rarely diagnosed in infancy, although we have seen cases in children younger than 3 years.

Congenital anomalies of the odontoid may be incidental findings in patients who have radiographs taken after trauma to the neck. This trauma may initiate atlanto-axial instability or precipitate symptoms in an already compromised, previously asymptomatic atlanto-axial joint. Patients may present clinically with no symptoms (incidental diagnosis), local neck symptoms (neck pain, torticollis, headache), transitory episodes of paresis after trauma, or myelopathies (cord compression). Neurological manifestations are recognised with increasing frequency. Although accurate statistics are not available, it is believed that a significant percentage, probably more than 50% of patients, either have or will develop neurological problems. Neurological signs and symptoms are varied. Weakness and loss of balance are common complaints. Upper motor neurone signs, proprioceptive and sphincter disturbances are relatively common. Children with odontoid aplasia who may have altered vertebral circulation and develop a stroke in childhood have been reported (Phillips et al 1988).

RADIOLOGICAL FINDINGS

Odontoid aplasia is an extremely rare anomaly. It is best seen in the open-mouth view. The diagnostic feature is the absence of the basilar portion of the odontoid, which normally dips down into and contributes to the body of the axis. The most common form of hypoplasia presents with a short, stubby peg of odontoid projecting just above the lateral facet articulations. Matsui et al (1997) found that the 'round type' which appears to be a very flat C2, has a great deal more instability and a greater risk of severe myelopathy. Often, this causes a Brown–Sequard lesion, which probably represents a more lateral instability in comparison with the ones with the blunt stubby or 'cone-shaped' os odontoideum. Watanabe et al (1996) developed an instability index to help evaluate children who have an os odontoideum. It is defined as the percentage change in the space available for the cord from flexion to extension. Watanabe noted that children with a sagittal plane rotation angle of more than 20° or an instability index of more than 40% are likely to have spinal cord signs. However, the instability associated with os odontoideum is often multidirectional and the more that C1 moves in a side-to-side direction, the more likely is a neurological problem (Matsui et al 1997).

Os odontoideum may be overlooked if tomograms are not taken (Fig. 30.5). It appears as a radiolucent oval or round ossicle with a smooth, dense border of bone. It may be of variable size, located usually in the position of the normal odontoid tip or near the basioccipital bone in the area of the foramen magnum, where it may fuse with the clivus. The base of the dens is almost invariably hypoplastic.

It may be difficult to differentiate an os odontoideum from non-union after an odontoid fracture. With an odontoid non-union, there is a narrow line of separation at the base of the odontoid, which may have either irregular or smooth edges of variable cortical thickness. The preservation of the normal shape and size of the dens on the antero-posterior view is an important distinguishing feature. With os odontoideum, the gap between the os and the hypoplastic dens is wide. It usually lies well above the level of the superior articular facets of the axis. The os generally does not preserve the normal shape or size of the odontoid, usually being half the size, rounded or oval, and having a smooth uniform cortex. If the os is in the area of the foramen magnum, there is little diagnostic problem.

The free ossicle of the os odontoideum usually appears fixed to the anterior arch of the atlas and moves with it in flexion and extension. The C1–C2 articulation is usually most unstable in flexion, less often so in extension, and occasionally unstable in all directions (Fielding et al 1980). In one series of patients, the average displacement in those undergoing surgical stabilisation was 1.1 cm (Fielding et al 1980).

TREATMENT

Patients with congenital anomalies of the odontoid lead a precarious existence. A trivial insult superimposed on an already weakened and compromised structure may be catastrophic.

Patients with local symptoms or transient myelopathies may expect recovery, at least temporarily. Surgical stabilisation is indicated for:

1. Neurological involvement (even if transient).
2. Instability of 10 mm or greater in flexion and extension.
3. Progressive instability.
4. Persistent neck complaints associated with instability.

Controversy exists as to the role of prophylactic stabilisation in asymptomatic patients with instability (Fielding et al 1980). The possible complications of surgery must be weighed against the dangers of instability with secondary spinal cord pressure. In the paediatric age group, it may be difficult or impossible to curtail activity, even in the presence of marked instability (Fielding et al 1980). When fusion is undertaken, regardless of the indication, preoperative halo traction is often required to achieve reduction, which may have to be continued during surgery and postoperatively until transfer to a suitable immobilisation device (Fielding et al 1980).

Generally, a posterior approach is sufficient with atlanto-axial arthrodesis, by the Gallie technique (Fig. 30.6) (Stabler et al 1985). When there are associated bony anomalies at the occipito-cervical junction, the fusion may have to be extended up to the occiput. Koop et al (1984) have reported excellent results with stabilisation, using a technique of flapping the occiput periosteum to the ring of C1, and external stabilisation.

KLIPPEL–FEIL SYNDROME

Congenital cervical fusion is the result of failure of the normal segmentation of the cervical somites during the 3rd to 8th weeks of life. With the exception of a few patients in whom this condition is inherited, the aetiology is as yet

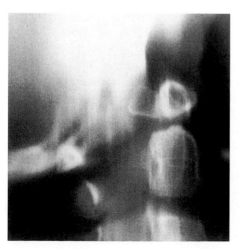

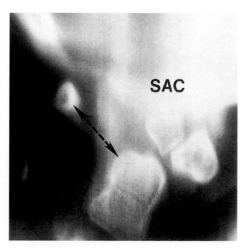

SAC

Figure 30.5 Lateral flexion–extension radiograph of an os odontoideum: **A** extension; **B** flexion. The odontoid ossicle is fixed to the anterior ring of the atlas and moves with it in flexion and extension and lateral slide. The space available for the spinal cord (SAC) decreases with flexion and the ossicle moves into the spinal canal with extension. (Reproduced with permission from Rothman & Simone (1982).)

A   B

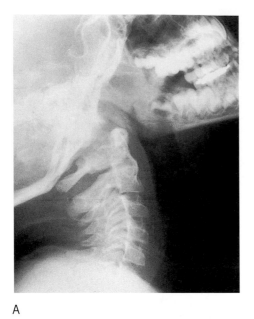

A

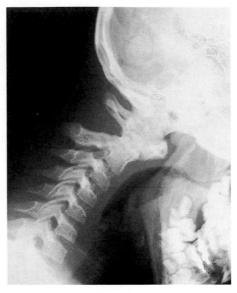

B

Fig. 30.6 This 7-year-old had a 1-year history of peculiar posturing and stiffness of the neck. Flexion (**A**) and extension (**B**) radiographs demonstrated an os odontoideum, and subluxation of C1–C2. **C** Extension and (**D**) flexion radiographs after posterior stabilisation. Reduction must be accomplished before surgery, and if wire stabilisation is selected, care must be take to avoid further flexion of the neck during passage of the wire under C1.

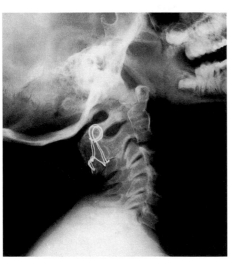

C

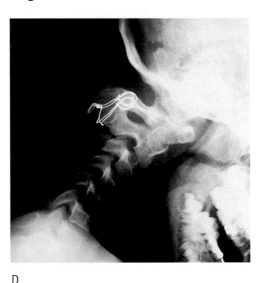

D

undetermined. It is important to note that the effect of this embryological abnormality is not limited to the cervical spine. Patients with the Klippel–Feil syndrome, even those with minor cervical lesions, may have defects in the genitourinary, nervous and cardiopulmonary systems, and even hearing impairment (Hensinger et al 1974). Many of these 'hidden' abnormalities may be more detrimental to the patient's general wellbeing than the obvious deformity in the neck. In the review by Hensinger et al (1974), a high incidence of related congenital anomalies was reported, emphasising that all patients with the Klippel–Feil syndrome should be thoroughly investigated.

CLINICAL APPEARANCE

The classical clinical description of the syndrome is a triad of low posterior hairline, short neck and limitation of neck motion (Fig. 30.7, A and B), but fewer than 50% of the patients have all three signs. Clinically, the most consistent finding is limitation of neck motion.

Shortening of the neck, unless extreme, is a subtle finding. Similarly, the low posterior hairline is not constant. Fewer than 20% of patients with the Klippel–Feil syndrome have obvious facial asymmetry, torticollis or webbing of the neck.

Sprengel's deformity (see Ch. 20.2) occurs in up to 33% of patients. Other clinical features are occasionally found: ptosis of the eye, Duane's contracture (contracture of the lateral rectus muscle), lateral rectus palsy, facial nerve palsy and a cleft or high arched palate. Abnormalities of the upper extremities include syndactyly, hypoplastic thumb, supernumerary digits and hypoplasia of the upper extremity. Abnormalities of the lower extremities are infrequent (Hensinger et al 1974).

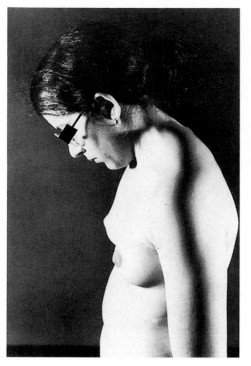

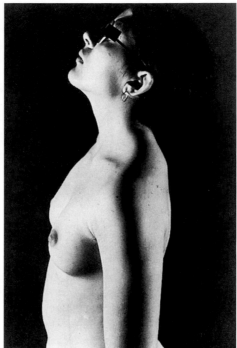

A   B

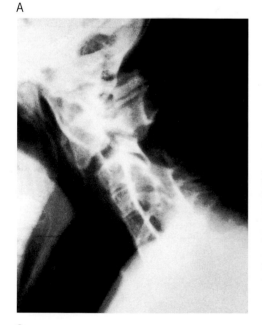

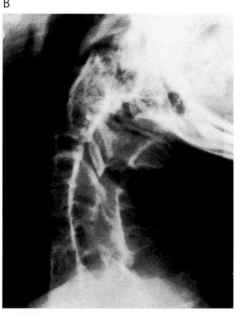

C   D

Figure 30.7 An 18-year-old female with the Klippel–Feil syndrome demonstrating flexion–extension of the cervical spine, both clinically (**A** and **B**) and radiologically (**C** and **D**). The majority of the neck motion is occurring at the C3–C4 disc space. Clinically, the patient is able to maintain adequate range (90°) of flexion–extension. At the time of these examinations, she was asymptomatic, but with ageing this hypermobile articulation may become unstable. (Reproduced with permission from Rothman & Simone (1982).)

RADIOGRAPHIC FEATURES

In the severely affected child, adequate radiographic evaluation can be difficult. Fixed bony deformities frequently prevent proper positioning, and overlapping shadows from the mandible, occiput or foramen magnum may obscure the upper vertebrae. CT scanning coupled with flexion–extension radiographs of the cervical spine (Fig. 30.7, C and D) can delineate more precisely the presence or absence of spinal cord compression. MRI is also useful.

Apart from vertebral fusion, flattening and widening of the involved vertebral bodies and absent disc spaces are the most common findings (Figs 30.8 and 30.9).

Narrowing of the spinal canal, if it occurs, usually manifests in adult life and is due to degenerative changes (osteoarthritic spurs) or hypermobility. Enlargement of the cervical canal is uncommon and, if found, may indicate the presence of conditions such as a syringomyelia, hydromyelia or the Arnold–Chiari malformation.

All these defects may extend into the upper thoracic spine, particularly in the severely affected patient. A disturbance of the upper thoracic spine on a routine chest radiograph may

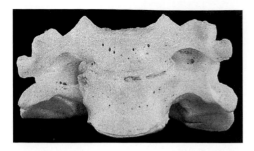

Figure 30.8 Anterior view of a postmortem specimen of a congenital block vertebra of C3–C4. The specimen demonstrates complete fusion, but remnants of the cartilaginous vertebral endplates can still be seen.

be the first clue to an unrecognised cervical synostosis. When a high thoracic congenital scoliosis is being assessed, the radiographic evaluation should routinely include lateral views of the cervical spine.

ASSOCIATED CONDITIONS

Scoliosis/kyphosis

Scoliosis is the most frequent anomaly found in association with the syndrome (Hensinger et al 1974), 60% of these patients having a significant curve.

Renal abnormalities

In the Klippel–Feil syndrome, more than 33% of the children can be expected to have a significant urinary tract anomaly, which is often asymptomatic in the young.

Cardiovascular abnormalities

Up to 14% of patients may have congenital heart disease.

Deafness

The otology literature has reported hearing impairment and deafness in more than 30% of patients with Klippel–Feil syndrome. Other defects include absence of the auditory canal and microtia. There is no characteristic audiological anomaly, and all types of hearing loss have been described.

Mirror motions (synkinesia)

Synkinesia consists of involuntary paired movements of the hands and, occasionally, the arms. It was first described by Bauman (1932), who found it to be present in four of six patients with the Klippel–Feil syndrome. Approximately 20% demonstrate mirror motions clinically (Hensinger et al 1974).

SYMPTOMS

With the exception of the anomalies that involve the atlanto-axial joint, there are no symptoms that can be directly attributed to the fused cervical vertebrae. All symptoms commonly associated with Klippel–Feil syndrome originate at the open segments, where the remaining free articulations may show compensatory hypermobility. Symptoms may then arise from two sources:

1. Mechanical symptoms caused by irritation of the joint.
2. Neurological symptoms caused by root irritation or spinal cord compression.

The majority of patients who develop symptoms are in the 2nd or 3rd decade of life, suggesting that the instability is in part a function of time, with increasing ligament laxity.

TREATMENT

The minimally affected patient with the Klippel–Feil syndrome can be expected to lead a normal active life, with

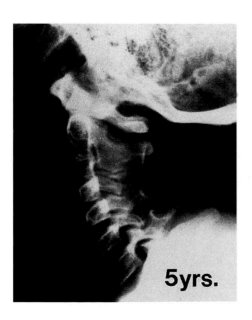

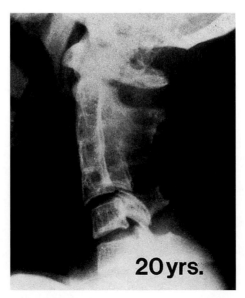

Figure 30.9 A Radiographs of a 5-year-old, demonstrating posterior fusion of the laminae and spinous process, but incomplete fusion of the vertebral bodies anteriorly. B Same patient at age 20 years, now demonstrating complete fusion of the vertebral bodies C2–C5. In children, narrowing of the cervical disc spaces cannot always be appreciated, as ossification of vertebral bodies is not completed until adolescence. The unossified cartilage endplates can give a false impression of a normal disc space.

A   B

no or only minor restrictions or symptoms. Many of the severely affected patients will enjoy the same good prognosis if early and appropriate treatment is instituted when needed. This is particularly applicable in the area of associated scoliosis and renal abnormalities. Prevention of further deformity or complications can be of great benefit to the patient.

Those patients with major areas of cervical synostosis or high-risk patterns of cervical spine motion should be strongly advised to avoid activities that place stress on the cervical spine. Theiss et al (1997) found that 22% of the patients with Klippel–Feil syndrome and congenital scoliosis developed cervical symptoms on long-term follow-up. The patterns of the fusion put them at particular risk. There was greater likelihood of cervical symptoms with fusion at the cervico-thoracic junction and congenital cervical stenosis. Pizzutillo et al (1994) reported on long-term follow-up that individuals with Klippel–Feil syndrome who had hypermobility of the upper cervical segments were at risk of neurological sequelae. Those with alteration in motion in the lower cervical segment were more likely to develop degenerative disease.

Sudden neurological compromise or death after minor trauma has been reported in the Klippel–Feil syndrome and is usually the result of disruption at the hypermobile articulation. The role of prophylactic surgical stabilisation in the asymptomatic patient has not yet been defined.

DIFFERENTIAL DIAGNOSIS OF TORTICOLLIS

Torticollis, or wry-neck, is a common childhood complaint. The aetiology is diverse and identifying the cause can pose a difficult diagnostic problem.

Congenital muscular torticollis is the most common cause of wry-neck posture in the infant and young child, but there are other problems that lead to this unusual posture. Head tilt and rotatory deformity of the head and neck (torticollis) usually indicate a problem at C1–C2, whereas head tilt alone indicates a more generalised problem in the cervical spine. If the posturing of the head and neck is noted at or shortly after birth, congenital anomalies of the cervical spine, particularly those that involve C1–C2, typically present as a rigid deformity, and the sternocleidomastoid muscle is not contracted or in spasm.

Approximately 20% of patients with the Klippel–Feil syndrome have associated torticollis (Hensinger et al 1974, Fielding & Hawkins 1977). With asymmetric development of the occipital condyles or the facets of C1, the head tilt may result in a torticollis unless compensated for by a tilt of the lower cervical spine such as occurs in the milder forms (Dubousset 1986).

Inflammatory conditions can include local irritation from cervical lymphadenitis, which may lead to the appearance of a wry-neck or tilt of the head. Another less frequent cause is a retropharyngeal abscess after inflammation of the posterior pharynx or tonsillitis. Children with polyarticular juvenile idiopathic arthritis frequently develop involvement of the cervical joints; torticollis and limitation of cervical motion may be the only clinical signs. Spontaneous atlanto-axial rotatory subluxation may follow acute pharyngitis (Fielding & Hawkins 1977). A rare inflammatory cause is acute calcification of a cervical disc, which can be visualised on routine radiographic study of the neck.

Traumatic cases should always be considered and carefully excluded early in the evaluation. If unrecognised, they may have serious neurological consequences. In general, torticollis most commonly follows injury to the C1–C2 articulation. Minor trauma can lead to spontaneous C1–C2 subluxation. Fractures or dislocation of the odontoid may not be apparent in the initial radiographic views and, consequently, a high index of suspicion and careful follow-up are required.

Children with bone dysplasia, Morquio's syndrome, spondyloepiphyseal dysplasia and Down's syndrome have a high incidence of C1–C2 instability and should be evaluated routinely.

Intermittent torticollis can occur in the young child. A seizure-like disorder called benign paroxysmal torticollis of infancy is due to many neurological causes, including drug intoxication. Similarly, Sandifer's syndrome, involving gastro-oesophageal reflux with sudden posturing of the trunk and torticollis, is being recognised more often, particularly in the child neurologically handicapped by, for example, cerebral palsy (Sutcliff 1969).

Neurological disorders, particularly space-occupying lesions of the central nervous system, such as tumours of the posterior fossa or spinal column, chordoma and syringomyelia, are often accompanied by torticollis. Generally, there will be additional neurological findings such as long-tract signs and weakness in the upper extremities. Uncommon neurological causes include dystonia musculorum deformans and problems of hearing and vision that can result in head tilt. Although uncommon, hysterical and psychogenic causes exist, but these should be diagnosed only after other causes have been carefully excluded.

RADIOGRAPHIC FEATURES

All children with torticollis should be evaluated with radiographs, to exclude a bony abnormality or fracture. Radiographic interpretation of congenital torticollis may be difficult, because of the fixed abnormal head position and restricted motion. In those with a painful wry-neck, it may be impossible to position the child appropriately for a standard view of the occipito-cervical junction. A helpful guide is that the atlas moves with the occiput, so that if the X-ray beam is directed 90° to the lateral skull, a satisfactory view of the occipito-cervical junction will usually result (Fig. 30.10). Flexion–extension stress films, laminograms or cine-radiography may be necessary to confirm the atlanto-axial instability.

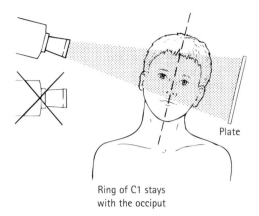

Ring of C1 stays
with the occiput

Figure 30.10 Obtaining a satisfactory radiograph may be hampered by the patient's limited ability to co-operate, fixed bony deformity, and overlapping shadows from the mandible, occiput and foramen magnum. A helpful guide is that the atlas moves with the occiput, and if the X-ray beam is directed 90° to the lateral of the skull, a satisfactory view of the occipito-cervical junction usually results.

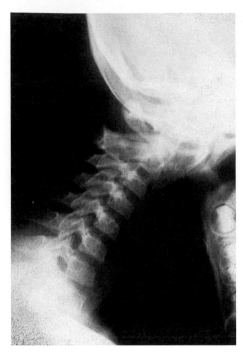

Figure 30.11 Marked anterior displacement of C1 on C2 found in a patient with atlanto-axial rotatory fixation of 2 months' duration.

ATLANTO-AXIAL ROTARY DISPLACEMENT

The onset of the problem may be spontaneous, associated with trivial trauma, or may follow an upper respiratory tract infection. Typically, the child awakes with a 'crick' in the neck and, with little or no treatment, this resolves within 1 week. Rarely, these deformities persist and the child presents with a resistant, unresolving torticollis, best described as atlanto-axial rotary fixation or fixed atlanto-axial displacement.

This problem can occur within the normal range of motion or with anterior shift of the atlas on the axis as a result of fractures of C1 and C2 or ligamentous deficiency, leading to atlanto-axial instability. Neurological deficits may rarely be associated with rotary displacements, particularly with associated anterior displacement.

The aetiology of this type of displacement remains theoretical, because sufficient anatomical and postmortem evidence are unavailable. The obstruction is probably capsular and synovial interposition, which produces pain in the initial stages, with resultant muscle spasms. The condition is complicated by muscle spasm, which holds the neck in flexion and may aggravate the forward displacement of C1 on C2 (Fig. 30.11).

CLINICAL FINDINGS

The torticollis position is likened to a robin listening for a worm or the 'cocked robin' position (Fig. 30.12). The head is tilted to one side and rotated to the opposite side, with slight flexion. When the condition is acute, the child resists attempts to move the head, complaining of marked pain with any passive attempts to do so. Associated muscle spasm, unlike muscular torticollis, is predominantly on the side of the 'long' sternocleidomastoid, because this muscle is

attempting to correct the deformity. If the deformity becomes fixed, the pain will subside but the torticollis will persist, associated with a diminished range of neck motion. In long-standing cases, particularly in younger children, facial flattening may develop on the side of the tilt.

RADIOGRAPHIC FINDINGS

In the acute stages, the diagnosis is primarily dependent on history and clinical evidence, because the radiographic findings on plain films are not diagnostic and can be found in torticollis from other causes.

In the open-mouth anteroposterior and lateral projections,

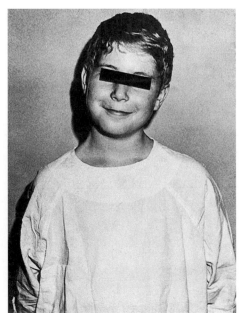

Figure 30.12 Typical torticollis position of atlanto-axial rotatory displacement ('cocked robin'), with head rotated in one direction and tilted to the opposite side, with slight flexion.

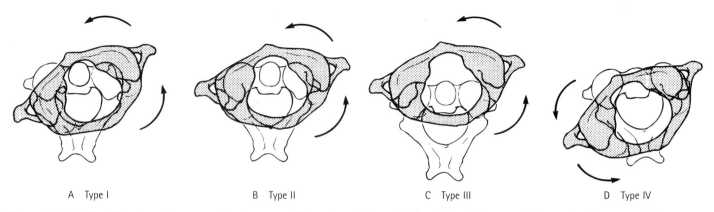

| A Type I | B Type II | C Type III | D Type IV |

Figure 30.13 Classification of rotatory displacement. (Reproduced from Fielding & Hawkins 1977 © Journal of Bone and Joint Surgery.)

the lateral mass of C1 that has rotated forward appears wider and closer to the midline (medial offset), whereas the opposite lateral mass is narrower and away from the midline (lateral offset). One of the facet joints may be obscured because of apparent overlapping.

On the lateral projection, the wedge-shaped lateral mass of the atlas lies anteriorly, where the oval arch of the atlas normally lies. The posterior arches of the atlas fail to superimpose because of head tilt. This may suggest assimilation of the atlas to the occiput because, with head tilt, the skull may obscure C1. Flexion–extension stress films are suggested, to rule out the possible anterior displacement of the atlas on the axis that is occasionally seen with rotary displacement.

Type I rotary displacement is by far the most common form seen in the paediatric age group (Fig. 30.13). It is a much more benign lesion and may be approached with an expectant attitude. The *type II* deformity is potentially more dangerous and must be carefully managed. *Types III and IV* deformities are rare, but because of the problem of neurological involvement or even instant death, they must be very carefully managed.

CT has largely replaced cine-radiology as the radiological technique of choice for this condition (Fig. 30.14).

TREATMENT

Many cases of atlanto-axial rotary displacement probably do not reach medical attention. A stiff neck and a slightly twisted head often resolve over a few days. If the complaints are mild and have been present for less than 1 week, we suggest a simple soft collar and analgesics. If there is no spontaneous improvement or the symptoms have been present for more than 1 week, more aggressive treatment should be instituted. In the more advanced cases that do not respond to simple measures, we suggest bed rest, head halter traction, muscle relaxants and analgesics.

If the atlas is displaced anteriorly on the axis, then gradual reduction should be obtained, followed by immobilisation in the corrected position in a Minerva cast for 6 weeks, to allow ligamentous healing to occur. Careful follow-up is necessary in these patients, because of the potential for continued atlanto-axial instability.

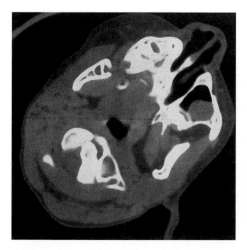

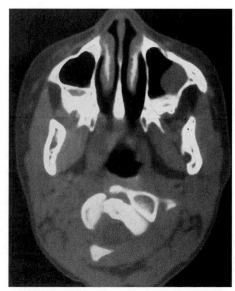

A

B

Figure 30.14 Dynamic CT scan of the upper cervical spine in atlanto-axial rotatory subluxation. **A** The head is rotated approximately 45° to one side, with the contralateral lateral mass of C1 moving forward on the facet of C2. **B** The head cannot be rotated past the midline, and the relationship of C1 to C2 is unchanged. (Reproduced from Phillips & Hensinger 1989 © Journal of Bone and Joint Surgery.)

If the condition has been present for 1–3 months, halo traction is often necessary to achieve reduction. However, the C1–C2 articulation may not stabilise after immobilisation and may require surgical correction and fusion.

If the condition has been present for more than 3 months, the deformity typically is fixed. In those whose spinal canal is compromised by anterior C1 displacement, a further insult could be catastrophic. C1–C2 fusion is indicated to achieve stability and to maintain correction.

CONGENITAL MUSCULAR TORTICOLLIS (CONGENITAL WRY-NECK)

This is a common condition usually discovered in the first 6–8 weeks of life. The deformity is caused by contracture of the sternocleidomastoid muscle, with the head tilted toward the involved side and the chin rotated toward the contralateral shoulder (Fig. 30.15). If the infant is examined within the first 4 weeks of life, a mass or 'tumour' is usually palpable in the neck (Fig. 30.16). It is generally a non-tender, soft enlargement that is mobile beneath the skin and attached to or located within the body of the sternocleidomastoid muscle. The mass attains maximum size within the first 1 month of life and then gradually regresses. If the child is examined after 4–6 months of age, the mass is usually absent, and the contracture of the sternocleidomastoid muscle and the torticollis posture are the only clinical findings (Fig. 30.15).

If the condition is progressive, deformities of the face and skull can result, and they are usually apparent within the first year. Flattening of the face on the side of the contracted sternocleidomastoid muscle may be particularly impressive (Fig. 30.15).

If the condition remains untreated during the growth years, the level of the eyes and ears becomes distorted and may result in considerable cosmetic deformity.

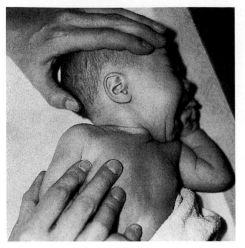

Figure 30.16 Six-week-old infant with swelling in the region of the sternocleidomastoid muscle. The mass is usually soft, non-tender, and mobile beneath the skin, but is attached to the muscle.

AETIOLOGY

Birth records of affected children demonstrate a preponderance of breech or difficult deliveries or primiparous births (MacDonald 1969). However, the deformity has occurred after otherwise normal deliveries, and has been reported in infants born by caesarean section (MacDonald 1969). Microscopic examination of resected surgical specimens and experimental work suggest that the lesion is caused by occlusion of the venous outflow of the sternocleidomastoid muscle. This results in oedema, degeneration of muscle fibres and, eventually, fibrosis. There is some evidence to suggest the problem may be caused by uterine crowding or 'packing syndrome' because in 75% of children in one study the lesion was recorded as being on the right side (MacDonald 1969). In addition, 20% of children with congenital muscular torticollis have congenital dysplasia of the hip, a problem believed to be the result of restriction of infant movement in the tight maternal space. Radiographs of the cervical spine should be obtained, to exclude congenital anomaly of the cervical spine.

TREATMENT

Conservative measures

Excellent results can be obtained in the majority of patients by means of conservative measures (MacDonald 1969, Canale et al 1982). Stretches are performed by the parent with guidance from the physical therapist and physician. Additional treatment measures include positioning of the crib and toys so that the neck will be stretched when the infant is trying to reach and grasp. The use of a 'sleeping helmet' has been suggested to reduce the deformity and hasten face and skull remodelling (Clarren et al 1979), but this is rarely necessary.

Surgery

If the condition persists beyond 1 year of age, non-operative measures are rarely successful (Canale et al 1982). Similarly, established facial asymmetry and limitation of normal

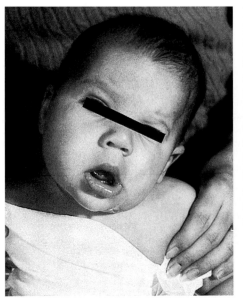

Figure 30.15 A 6-month-old infant with left-sided congenital muscular torticollis. Note the rotation of the skull and asymmetry and flattening of the face on the side of the contracted sternocleidomastoid.

motion of more than 30° usually preclude a good result, and surgical intervention will be required to prevent further facial flattening and poor cosmesis (Canale et al 1982). However, a good (but not perfect) cosmetic result can be obtained as late as 12 years of age. Asymmetry of the skull and face will improve as long as adequate growth potential remains after the deforming pull of the sternocleidomastoid is removed.

Surgery consists of complete section of the sternocleidomastoid muscle, usually at its distal insertion. In the older child, an accessory incision may be required to section the muscle at its origin on the mastoid process. The entire muscle should not be excised, because this may lead to reverse torticollis (MacDonald 1969) or additional deformity. The postoperative regimen includes passive stretching exercises in the same manner as those performed preoperatively. They should begin as soon as the patient can tolerate manipulation of the neck. Bracing or cast correction may be necessary if the deformity is long-standing or if the habit is well established. The results of surgery have been uniformly good, with a low incidence of complications or recurrence and almost all patients are pleased with the results (MacDonald 1969, Canale et al 1982). If the patient is young, the facial asymmetry can be expected to resolve completely, unless there is persistence of the torticollis, particularly from residual fascial bands (MacDonald 1969).

REFERENCES

Bauman G I 1932 Absence of the cervical spine: Klippel–Feil syndrome. Journal of the American Medical Association 98: 129–132

Burke S W, French H G, Roberts J M, Johnston C E, Whitecloud T S, Edmunds J O 1985 Chronic atlanto-axial instability in Down syndrome. Journal of Bone and Joint Surgery 67A: 1356–1360

Canale S T, Griffin D W, Hubbard C N 1982 Congenital muscular torticollis. Long term follow up. Journal of Bone and Joint Surgery 64A: 810–816

Chamberlain W E 1939 Basilar impression (platybasia): bizarre developmental anatomy of occipital bone and upper cervical spine with striking and misleading neurologic manifestation. Yale Journal of Biological Medicine 11: 487–496

Clarren S K, Smith D W, Hampton J W 1979 Helmet treatment for plagiocephaly in congenital muscular torticollis. Journal of Pediatrics 94: 43–46

Dubousset J 1986 Torticollis in children caused by congenital anomalies of the atlas. Journal of Bone and Joint Surgery 68A: 178–188

Erbengi A and Oge H K 1994 Congenital malformations of the craniovertebral junction: classification and surgical treatment. Acta Neurochirurgica (Wien) 127: 180–185

Fielding J W, Hawkins R J 1977 Atlanto-axial rotatory fixation. Journal of Bone and Joint Surgery 59A: 37–44

Fielding J W, Hensinger R N, Hawkins R J 1980 Os odontoideum. Journal of Bone and Joint Surgery 62A: 376–383

Hensinger R N, Lang J R, MacEwen G D 1974 The Klippel–Feil syndrome: a constellation of related anomalies. Journal of Bone and Joint Surgery 56A: 1246–1253

Klippel M, Feil A 1912 Un cas d'absence des vertebras cervicales avec cage thoracique remontant jusqu'à la base du crane. Nouvelle Iconographie de la Salpetrière 25: 223–250

Koop S E, Winter R B, Lonstein J E 1984 The surgical treatment of instability of the upper part of the cervical spine in children and adolescents. Journal of Bone and Joint Surgery, 66A: 403–411

MacDonald C 1969 Sternomastoid tumour and muscular torticollis. Journal of Bone and Joint Surgery 51B: 432–443

McGregor M 1948 The significance of certain measurements of the skull in the diagnosis of basilar impression. British Journal of Radiology 21: 171–181

McRae D L 1960 The significance of abnormalities of the cervical spine. American Journal of Roentgenology 84: 3–25

Matsui H, Imada K, Tsuji H 1997 Radiographic classification of os odontoideum and its clinical significance. Spine 22: 1706–1709

Phillips P C, Lorentsen K J, Shropshire L C, Ahn H S 1988 Congenital odontoid aplasia and posterior circulation stroke in childhood. Annals of Neurology 23: 410–413

Phillips W A, Hensinger R N 1989 The management of rotatory atlanto-axial subluxation in children. Journal of Bone and Joint Surgery 71A: 664–668

Pizzutillo P D, Woods M, Nicholson L, MacEwen G D 1994 Risk factors in Kilppel–Feil syndrome. Spine 19: 2110–2116

Rothman R H, Simone F A (eds) 1982 The spine, 2nd edn. Saunders, Philadelphia

Rouvreau P, Glorion C, Langlais J, Noury H, Pouliquen J C 1998 Assessment and neurologic involvement of patients with cervical spine congenital synostosis as in Klippel–Feil syndrome: study of 19 cases. Journal of Pediatric Orthopaedics 7B: 179–185

Stabler C L, Eismont F J, Brown M D, Green B A, Malinin T I 1985 Failure of posterior cervical fusions using cadaveric bone graft in children. Journal of Bone and Joint Surgery 67A: 370–375

Sutcliff J 1969 Torsion spasms and abnormal postures in children with hiatus hernia: Sandifer's syndrome. Progress in Pediatric Radiology 2: 190–197

Theiss S M, Smith M D, Winter R B 1997 The long-term follow-up of patients with Klippel–Feil syndrome and congenital scoliosis. Spine 22: 1219–1222

Watanabe M, Toyama Y, Fujimura Y 1996 Atlantoaxial instability in os odontoideum with myelopathy. Spine 21: 1435–1439

Chapter 31

Thoraco-lumbar spine

PART 1 Back pain in children
M. A. Edgar

INTRODUCTION

Back pain in childhood, whilst uncommon, is often associated with serious underlying pathology (King 1999). In the author's own series of 210 cases (Burgoyne & Edgar 1998), infection or neoplasia proved to be the underlying cause in 42% of patients younger than 12 years. After this age, there is a relative increase in non-specific causes of backache. Adolescent back pain is associated with decreased mobility of the lumbar spine (Salminen 1984) and stiffness of the hip and knee joints (Fairbank et al 1984). Back pain in this adolescent age group is more common in girls (Salminen et al 1992) and also exhibits a familial pattern (Balagué et al 1999). During later adolescence, trauma, mechanical and early degenerative disorders are more frequent causes of back pain, and serious pathology affects only a small proportion.

In young children, back pain tends to be vague and poorly localised. Consequently spinal or paraspinal pathology in the young may be easily missed or misdiagnosed, with adverse effects on subsequent treatment and outcome. Careful clinical evaluation, appropriate investigation and a grasp of the likely causes for each age group minimise the likelihood of that unsatisfactory state of affairs

ASSESSMENT OF THE CHILD

Localised physical signs may be difficult to elicit in the younger child or infant, and they are often better examined on the mother's lap. With the child prone, palpate for tenderness, swelling, abnormal alignment or muscle spasm. A step deformity in the lower lumbar region indicates spondylolisthesis. Turn the child supine, assess straight leg raising and palpate the abdomen (including the groin for tracking psoas abscess) – discitis can present with deep abdominal tenderness or psoas spasm.

With the child standing, assess overall posture and observe the contour of the back for any asymmetry or deformity. Ask the child to bend forward, distinguishing between flexion at the hip and spine: a kyphotic deformity or the asymmetric rib hump of a structural scoliosis are more clearly seen in this position. Marked stiffness on forward flexion may occur in spondylolisthesis, infection, adolescent disc herniation, rheumatological disease or a neoplastic lesion. Joint stiffness elsewhere may suggest a systemic arthropathy such as ankylosing spondylitis. The spine is then assessed in extension, lateral flexion and rotation.

Finally, examine the gait (see Ch. 23). Leg length discrepancy or neurological causes may be responsible for a limp, yet are rarely painful, whereas discitis is.

Assessment of motor function in the infant is best done by looking for wasting and observing functional activities such as heel walking, tip-toeing and rising from a squat. Sensory testing can be very difficult, but should be performed if the child is able to co-operate. Assessment of all reflexes, including the Babinski response and clonus, are important objective tests and should always be performed. Asymmetric abdominal reflexes may indicate a cervical syrinx in juvenile idiopathic scoliosis, although this is usually painless (Zadeh et al 1995).

CONGENITAL MALFORMATIONS OF THE SPINE

Be wary of attributing troublesome back symptoms to a congenital malformation: it may be a coincidental finding. The various types of congenital scoliosis and kyphosis, even when associated with spinal dysraphism, rarely cause pain unless producing secondary mechanical effects (e.g. congenital asymmetric absence of a lumbar pedicle (Polly & Mason 1991)). Children who have 'idiopathic' scoliosis associated with syringomyelia of the cervico-thoracic cord and a Chiari I malformation (Fig. 31.1) only occasionally suffer backache (Evans et al 1996). Congenital or developmental spinal stenosis in childhood similarly rarely causes pain. Beware the child with an 'idiopathic' scoliosis who complains of pain and stiffness, especially if it is worse at night: an underlying neoplasm (such as an osteoid osteoma or intradural tumour), or severe spondylolisthesis is likely (Taylor 1986). Similarly, an 'idiopathic' left thoracic scoliosis is also unusual and should be thoroughly investigated to exclude other causes such as syringomyelia, tumour or neuromuscular disorder (Conrad et al 1985, Schwend et al 1995, Ramirez et al 1997).

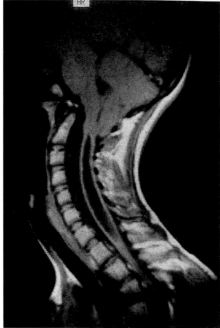
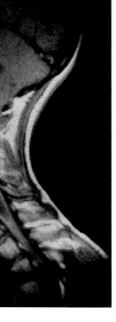
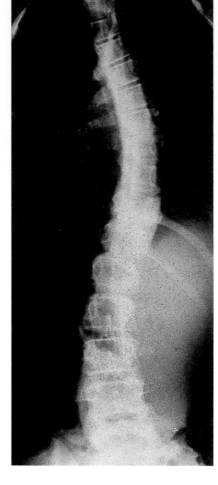
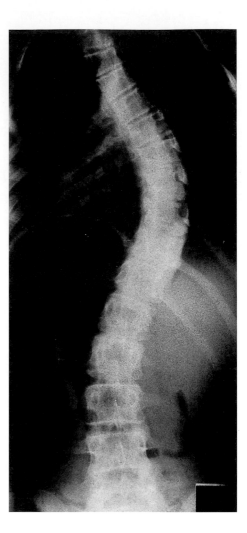

Figure 31.1 Syrinx of the cervicodorsal spine (Chiari I malformation) presenting as a coincidental finding in a child aged 13 years with a slowly progressive juvenile idiopathic scoliosis. She had no neck or back pain.

TRAUMATIC BACK PAIN

In general, children's spines are remarkably resilient to injury. Even when trauma is severe enough to produce a fracture or fracture-dislocation, the incidence of neurological damage is much lower than that in adults. Paradoxically, sporadic cases of trauma with neurological deficit but without fracture (often referred to as spinal cord injury without radiological abnormality, or 'SCIWORA'), have been reported in and are unique to children. The cervical cord is most commonly injured, and younger children tend to suffer a greater neurological loss (Hadley et al 1988). The exact aetiology is unknown, but a combination of traction injury and a vascular insult to the cord have been implicated (Linssen et al 1990).

In infancy, back trauma should raise the possibility of non-accidental injury. Cullen (1975) demonstrated that vertebral collapse, particularly in the thoraco-lumbar region, can be part of the battered baby syndrome. Therefore bruising or tenderness of the back demands an X-ray.

The most potent cause of back pain after trauma is the post-traumatic kyphosis of adolescence following a vertebral burst fracture (Figs 31.2 and 31.3). Pain usually accompanies

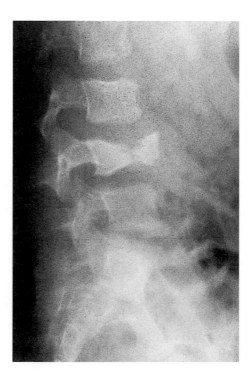

Figure 31.2 Burst fracture of L4 in a 5-year-old boy who fell 12 m from the fourth floor. This was associated with a fractured calcaneum, but the boy was normal neurologically. Fracture healed and remodelled.

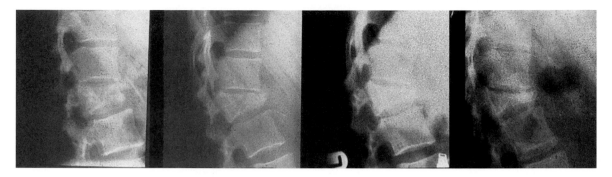

Figure 31.3 Post-traumatic kyphosis. Series of four lateral views of 16-year-old girl's lumbar spine extending over a 2-year period after a road traffic accident. The progressive painful kyphosis is demonstrated.

increasing kyphosis. Fortunately, the kyphotic deformity stabilises by 18 months, but the pain can persist for longer because of mechanical instability. Continued pain and cosmetic deformity may be an indication for corrective anterior and posterior fusion with instrumentation.

Akin to this is the iatrogenic kyphosis that may follow wide decompression, usually of the cervico-thoracic spine for neoplasia or infection. This can be rapidly progressive, particularly during the adolescent growth phase. Again, as with post-traumatic kyphosis, these painful deformities may need correction and stabilisation. Some neurosurgeons use a linear division through the lateral part of the lamina on each side over several levels in children, so that a posterior lid can be taken off the canal and then replaced (laminoplasty).

SPINAL INFECTION

Although the incidence of spinal infection, in parallel with bone and joint infection, has reduced considerably in the past few decades, it still presents sporadically as a cause of back pain in children. There is evidence that the neonatal period may be the time when the child is at greatest risk (Eismont et al 1982). It is also the time when the diagnosis is most difficult to make. On presentation, the neonate is ill, febrile and failing to thrive. Septicaemia is usually the first diagnosis made and the spinal lesion may not be detected for several weeks. Tuberculosis of the spine must be considered if the child is from a part of the world where the disease remains endogenous (Asian and African immigrants are an 'at risk' population). A technetium-99m (^{99m}Tc) bone scan and magnetic resonance imaging (MRI) scan should localise the lesion early, well ahead of X-ray changes.

The problem of diagnosing juvenile spinal infection was recognised in a useful study of six children by Pritchard & Thompson (1960). In one case, psoas spasm misdirected the clinician's attention from the lumbar spine to the hip, and in others the initial clinical diagnosis was a perinephric abscess and low-grade meningitis.

Just as spinal infection has become much less common in children, so the type of infection has changed. Fortunately the classic Potts' tuberculous kyphos, seen earlier this century and still tragically evident in some developing countries, is now almost unheard of in the Western world, although the increase of human immunodeficiency virus infection may herald a reversal of this.

Juvenile discitis (Fig. 31.4) presumably arises by erosion of an initial endplate infection into the disc substance, with further spread being prevented by the body's defence mechanisms. Despite earlier controversy over juvenile discitis, its infective nature was confirmed by Wenger et al (1978) in 41 children ranging in age from 11 months to 16 years. Pre-existing upper respiratory tract or ear infection was common. The diagnosis was delayed in a significant proportion, despite back pain and abnormal back posture. Again, misdiagnosis of a hip or lower limb condition, or even a visceral abnormality was common. Generally, MRI is a more accurate means of diagnosis than a ^{99m}Tc bone scan. Needle biopsy produces positive cultures in only 50% of cases, but the histology usually confirms the diagnosis of pyogenic infection. In Wenger's series, conservative management with rest and antibiotics proved successful in all but two patients, who subsequently required surgical discectomy and fusion.

Yu et al (1989) from Boston demonstrated atypical X-ray changes in children with multifocal osteomyelitis – a condition in which the vertebral infection may present as a vertebra plana without intervening disc collapse. Histiocytosis X (Langerhans' cell histiocytosis) in the form of an eosinophilic granuloma, the classic form of vertebra plana (Fig. 31.5), may be confused with spinal osteomyelitis. Finally, mention needs to be made of the intervertebral disc calcification syndrome, mainly seen in the cervical spine, which was once believed to represent the endstage of infective discitis. However, there is now good evidence that this is of metabolic or traumatic origin (Sonnabend et al 1982).

Therefore, in summary, where there is the slightest suspicion of a possible spinal infection, a ^{99m}Tc bone scan and MRI should be carried out immediately. Where indicated, needle biopsy under CT guidance should then be undertaken. The specimen should be sent, not only for histology and pyogenic culture, but also for tuberculous culture. Most cases diagnosed early respond well to adequate antibiotics and rest. However, in those patients in whom there is recurrent infection or in

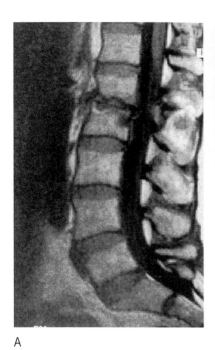

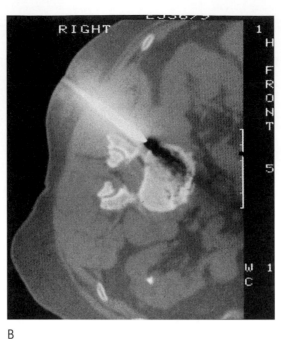

Figure 31.4 A MRI of infective discitis L1–L2. **B** CT-guided needle biopsy.

A

B

whom vertebral collapse produces an unstable or progressive kyphosis, surgical intervention may be necessary.

KYPHOSIS OF ADOLESCENCE AND THE OSTEOCHONDRITIDES

It must not be forgotten that the painful rigid spine (with a developing kyphosis) in adolescence may herald the onset of ankylosing spondylitis or juvenile idiopathic arthritis. In both conditions, the erythrocyte sedimentation rate will be significantly increased and in ankylosing spondylitis there will be evidence of sacro-iliitis.

The main differential diagnosis of a painful adolescent kyphosis is, of course, the more common Scheuermann's osteochondritis or adolescent round back. Note the difference in lateral profile between the two conditions (Fig. 31.6).

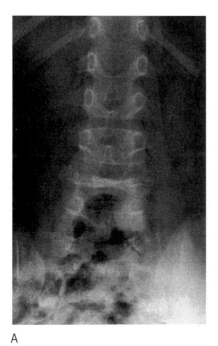

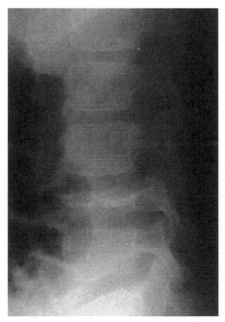

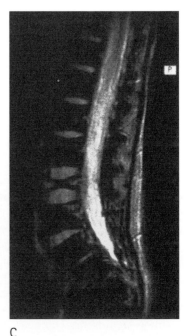

A

B

C

Fig. 31.5 Eosinophilic granuloma of L4, which presented as acute back pain in 7-year-old boy. **A** Anteroposterior X-ray. **B** Lateral X-ray. **C** MRI of lumbar spine.

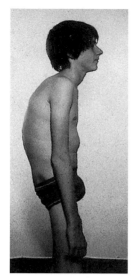
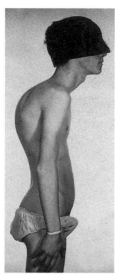

Figure 31.6 Comparison of lateral spinal profile in adolescents with ankylosing spondylitis (left) and Scheuermann's thoracic kyphosis (right).

Scheuermann's disease has a familial pattern and occurs slightly more often in girls. Only 50% of patients complain of backache. Such patients are best followed up in a spinal deformity clinic to monitor progression. Contact sports and activities involving heavy lifting are best avoided.

A painful scoliosis, particularly if the curve is stiff or associated with muscle spasm, should always be taken seriously. In a group of 34 adolescents with painful scoliosis (Burgoyne & Edgar 1998), four had a spinal neoplasm and a fifth had juvenile idiopathic arthritis. Back pain in so-called adolescent idiopathic scoliosis therefore should always be investigated thoroughly with X-rays and a blood count; MRI and ^{99m}Tc scans should be considered. Although mechanical back pain can occur with severe idiopathic deformity, muscle spasm and stiffness are not characteristic.

Osteochondritis can also affect the upper and middle lumbar spine. Undoubtedly, this can be associated with transient stiffness and muscle spasm, sometimes after a strain at sport, to produce the so-called irritable lumbar spine of adolescence. This condition never leads to severe structural kyphosis and should not be called Scheuermann's disease.

MECHANICAL AND DEGENERATIVE DISORDERS

These conditions are generally confined to the adolescent when recreational and sporting demands are greater and, as has been clearly shown from MRI studies, disc degeneration in the low lumbar spine is already beginning to take place. In a consecutive series of 160 adolescents who complained of back pain, 43% fell into this category (Burgoyne & Edgar 1998). Of these, 35 had musculoligamentous strains, 24 had a spondylolysis or spondylolisthesis, six had adolescent disc herniations, and four had fractures after trauma.

Interestingly, Fairbank et al (1984) found that adolescent back pain arising from so-called soft-tissue strains and spontaneous-onset backache were more common in those who tended to avoid sport and showed a stiff range of lower limb joint movement. It may be, therefore, that back strains due to sporting injuries are different and have a better prognosis.

Spondylolysis and spondylolisthesis are probably the next most common causes of low back pain in adolescence. Of 24 consecutive patients in our series, in all but one instance the lumbo-sacral junction was involved. Thirteen were found to have pars fractures without displacement (spondylolysis), and in the remaining 11 a slip had occurred (spondylolisthesis).

Spondylolysis and spondylolisthesis may be coincidental findings, with other pathology the cause of backache. In a remarkable survey in the USA, 500 schoolchildren in the first year of primary education were examined, underwent X-ray, and were followed through to maturity (Fredrickson et al 1984). The incidence of spondylolysis at the age of 6 years was 4.4% and this increased to 6% at maturity; the equivalent figures for spondylolisthesis were 2.6% and 4%, respectively. As expected, the incidence of spondylolisthesis was greater in those keen on sport – particularly gymnastics, which was associated with an incidence of 8–10%. Only one of their cases of spondylolysis healed. The odd finding was that, of the 30 patients who had reached adult life with either a spondylolysis or type II spondylolisthesis, none had back pain. It seems that a longitudinal study involving several thousand children would be necessary to evaluate the prevalence of pain in this condition.

Spondylolysis has not been recorded in children younger than 14 months. It occurs after walking commences and is believed to be a stress phenomenon rather than a failure of bony development, as was confirmed experimentally by Cryon & Hutton (1978). More recent support for this has come from Hardcastle et al (1992) in a study from Australia, in which, in a group of fast bowlers aged 16–18 years, the incidence of spondylolysis was found to be 54% and – even more worrying – the incidence of lower lumbar disc degeneration was 63%.

The other caveat over spondylolysis is that it may be unilateral (Porter & Park 1982). This usually occurs at L3 or L4. Buttressing of the opposite pedicle and lamina may occur, and the X-ray appearance may mimic an osteoid osteoma.

Adolescent disc herniation is now being recognised more frequently, with the advent of MRI. There is general agreement that disc protrusion in the young is different from that seen in the adult (Kamel & Rosman 1984). Stiffness is a more common symptom than back pain. Straight leg raising is markedly reduced, often being less than 30°, with considerable tightness of the hamstrings. Sciatic list is nearly always present, compared with an incidence of only 25% in adult cases. At operation, the bulging disc is usually found to be very soft and the nuclear contents very gelatinous. The nerve root often appears inflamed. The results of operation are far less predictable than in the adult. Therefore it is wise to manage adolescent patients with disc problems conservatively for an extended period. The great majority do settle. However, it is important that investigations are undertaken early to exclude other more serious lesions. There seems to be growing evidence that, if there is a large sequestrated fragment or if the disc material is degenerate and desiccated, the results of disc excision are more reliable.

SPINAL NEOPLASIA

Spinal neoplasms may be grouped into those that occur in the bony vertebrae, those from neurological tissue, and paravertebral tumours.

BONE TUMOURS

Reviewing their series of 1917 primary bony tumours, Delamarter et al (1990) found that only 0.4% occurred in the thoraco-lumbar spine in children and adolescents. Their study also clearly demonstrated that, whereas most primary bone tumours in children are benign (88%), in adults the majority are malignant (81%). The most common benign neoplasms, which usually occur in the adolescent period, are osteoid osteomas, osteoblastomas, aneurysmal bone cysts and giant-cell tumours.

Osteoid osteoma or osteoblastoma

This is the most common benign tumour of the spine and also the most common cause of a painful, stiff scoliosis. The condition has been well reviewed by Ransford et al (1984) in a series of 15 patients presenting between the age of 8 and 19 years. The lumbar spine is by far the most common region, with the lesion usually located in the pedicle or lamina. The scoliosis is typically rigid, with pain often troublesome at night. The ^{99m}Tc bone scan produces a very well localised and characteristic 'hot spot'. The lesion may or may not be seen on plain X-rays: pedicle enlargement with sclerotic bone surrounding a small nidus. More often, the appearance is equivocal and even a CT scan may require careful interpretation. The new technique of tomographic scintillography using ^{99m}Tc is probably the most reliable way of localising the exact position of the lesion in the posterior arch.

Excision of the lesion relieves the pain dramatically and the spine becomes mobile again. In Ransford's series, all but one of the scoliotic curves completely or partially resolved. There has been concern about the stability of the spine after excision of osteoid osteoma or osteoblastoma. Kirwan et al (1984) recommend a posterolateral approach, excising the transverse process and entering the pedicle from the lateral side, to excise the nidus without sacrificing the integrity of the articular facets. Although this can be achieved, in some cases the concern is that the lesion may be incompletely removed or may recur, and it may be better to sacrifice the entire pedicle and associated articular facet on one side, rather than risk recurrence.

Aneurysmal bone cyst of the spine

Ten percent of aneurysmal bone cysts occur in the axial skeleton, mainly in the thoracic and lumbar spine, most commonly in the 2nd and early 3rd decades of life. They predominate in the posterior arch, but can expand anteriorly into the vertebral body (Fig. 31.7). Spinal aneurysmal bone cysts may develop insidiously. They tend to be very vascular: operation can be haemorrhagic, and often entails anterior and posterior approaches. Preoperative embolisation may be helpful in such a situation (Papagelopoulos et al 1998), but because these cysts respond so well to radio-

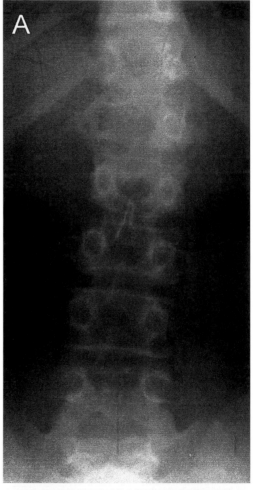

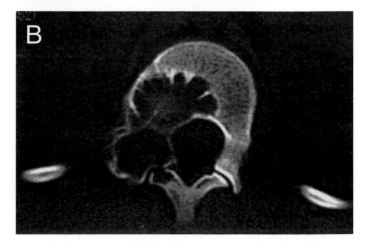

Figure 31.7 Aneurysmal bone cyst in a 14-year-old girl. A Anteroposterior X-ray; note the absent right pedicle of L1. B CT scan of the same vertebra.

therapy, with a low recurrence rate, this form of treatment may be preferable to a difficult surgical excision.

Giant-cell tumour of the spine is rare, being about 2–3% of all reported spinal tumours. The ballooned egg shell appearance of the vertebral body may appear very similar to an aneurysmal bone cyst. However, the peak incidence is usually during the twenties. A recent case report by Biagnini et al (1990) described successful management using arterial embolisation of feeder branches from the spinal arteries, followed by radiotherapy and subsequent spinal fusion.

Of the malignant primary tumours, osteogenic sarcoma and chordoma have both been described in adolescence, but are extremely rare.

Spinal cord and cauda equina tumours

Painful scoliosis is now well established as a presenting symptom for an underlying spinal cord or cauda equina tumour. In the series described by Citron et al (1984), 11 of the 12 patients presented between the ages of 2 and 18 years. Most were initially believed to have idiopathic scoliosis. This study underlines the importance of taking painful spinal deformities seriously and investigating them early.

Benign and malignant tumours of the cauda equina may mimic the back and sciatic pain pattern of lumbar disc herniation. In their review of 32 patients with cauda equina tumours, presenting with a presumptive diagnosis of lumbar disc herniation, Ker & Jones (1985) included a patient aged 8 years. Again, there was considerable delay in making the correct diagnosis. Fortunately, the vast majority of patients had benign conditions, with neurofibroma and ependymoma predominating.

Paraspinal tumours

In infancy, back pain or swelling arising from paravertebral tumours gives rise to serious concern. The likely tumours are nephroblastoma or Wilms's tumour, neuroblastoma and teratoma. Neuroblastoma and teratoma tend to invade vertebral bodies locally and also undergo metastatic spread to bone. Neuroblastoma can be diagnosed early, if suspected, by the detection of vanillylmandelic acid in urine. With adequate excision and radiotherapy, nephroblastoma now carries a good prognosis. Interestingly, these patients tend to present in the juvenile and adolescent period with a postirradiation scoliosis concave to the side of the lesion, with the tell-tale nephrectomy scar and postirradiation skin changes.

SUMMARY

It is clear that the significance of back pain in children tends to be underestimated and that serious conditions are misdiagnosed, with consequent delay in appropriate treatment. Back pain associated with any of the following symptoms or signs demands careful evaluation and appropriate investigation:

- age less than 12 years
- night pain
- pain lasting more than 1 month
- an acutely rigid spine
- a painful scoliosis
- associated systemic symptoms, e.g. weight loss
- associated conditions or syndromes, e.g. neurofibromatosis
- progressive neurological symptoms, including alteration in bowel or bladder function.

Infections, tumour or inflammatory arthropathies may be implicated in such cases.

REFERENCES

Balagué F, Troussier B, Salminen J J 1999 Non specific low back pain in children and adolescents: risk factors. European Spine Journal 8: 429–438

Biagnini R, De Cristofaro R, Ruggieri P, Boriano S 1990 Giant cell tumour of the spine. Journal of Bone and Joint Surgery 72A: 1102–1107

Burgoyne W, Edgar M 1998 The assessment of back pain in children. Current Paediatrics 8: 173–179

Citron N, Edgar M A, Sheehy J P, Thomas D G T 1984 Intramedullary spinal cord tumours present with scoliosis. Journal of Bone and Joint Surgery 66B: 513–517

Conrad R W, Richardson W J, Oakes W J 1985 Left thoracic curves can be different. Orthopaedic Transactions, 9: 126–127

Cryon B M, Hutton W C 1978 The fatigue strength of the lumbar neural arch in spondylysis. Journal of Bone and Joint Surgery 60B: 234–238

Cullen J V 1975 Spinal lesions in battered babies. Journal of Bone and Joint Surgery 57B: 364–366

Delamarter R B, Sachs B L, Thompson G H, Bohlman H H, Makley J T, Carter J R 1990 Primary neoplasms of the thoracic and lumbar spine. An analysis of 29 consecutive cases. Clinical Orthopaedics and Related Research 256: 87–100

Eismont F J, Bohlman H H, Soni P L, Goldberg V M, Freehafer A A 1982 Vertebral osteomyelitis in infants. Journal of Bone and Joint Surgery 64B: 32–35

Evans S C, Edgar M A, Hall-Craggs M A et al 1996 MRI of 'idiopathic' juvenile scoliosis. Journal of Bone and Joint Surgery 78B: 314–317

Fairbank J C T, Pynsent P B, Poortvleit J A Y, Phillips H 1984 Influence of anthropometric factors and joint laxity in the incidence of adolescent back pain. Spine 9: 461–464

Fredrickson B E, Baker D, McHolick W J, Uyan H A, Lubicky J P 1984 The natural history of spondylolysis and spondylolisthesis. Journal of Bone and Joint Surgery 66A: 699–707

Hadley M N, Zabramski J M, Bronner C M, Rekate H, Sonntag V K 1988 Pediatric spinal trauma. Review of 122 cases of spinal cord and vertebral column injuries. Journal of Neurosurgery 68: 18–24

Hardcastle P, Annear P, Foster D H et al 1992 Spinal abnormalities in young fast bowlers. Journal of Bone and Joint Surgery 74B: 421–425

Kamel M, Rosman M 1984 Disc protrusion in the growing child. Clinical Orthopaedics and Related Research 185: 46–52

Ker N B, Jones C B 1985 Tumours of the cauda equina – the problems of differential diagnosis. Journal of Bone and Joint Surgery 67B: 358–362

King H A 1999 Back pain in children. Orthopedic Clinics of North America 30: 467–474

Kirwan E O'G, Hutton P A N, Pozo J L, Ransford A O 1984 Osteoid osteoma and benign osteoblastoma of the spine. Journal of Bone and Joint Surgery 66B: 21–26

Linssen W H J, Praamstra P, Gabreels F J M, Rotteveel J J 1990 Vascular insufficiency of the cervical cord due to hyperextension of the spine. Paediatric Neurology 6: 123–125

Papagelopoulos P J, Currier B L, Shaughnessy W J et al 1998 Aneurysmal bone cyst of the spine. Management and outcome. Spine 23: 621–628

Polly D W Jr, Mason D E 1991 Congenital absence of a lumbar pedicle presenting as back pain in children. Journal of Pediatric Orthopaedics 11: 214–219

Porter R W, Park W 1982 Unilateral spondylolysis. Journal of Bone and Joint Surgery 64B: 344–348

Pritchard A E, Thompson W A L 1960 Acute pyogenic infections of the spine of children. Journal of Bone and Joint Surgery 42B: 86–89

Ramirez N, Johnston C E, Browne R H 1997 The prevalence of back pain in children who have idiopathic scoliosis. Journal of Bone and Joint Surgery 79A: 364–368

Ransford A O, Pozo J L, Hutton P A N, Kirwan E O'G 1984 The behaviour pattern of the scoliosis associated with osteoid osteoma or osteoblastoma of the spine. Journal of Bone and Joint Surgery 66B: 16–20

Salminen J J 1984 The adolescent back. A field survey of 370 Finnish school children. Acta Paediatrica Scandinavica Supplementum 315: 8–122

Salminen J J, Pentti J, Terho P 1992 Low back pain and disability in 14-year-old schoolchildren. Acta Paediatrica 81: 1035–1039

Schwend R M, Hennrikus W, Hall J E, Emans J B 1995 Childhood scoliosis: clinical indications for magnetic resonance imaging. Journal of Bone and Joint Surgery 77A: 46–53

Sonnabend D H, Taylor T K F, Chapman G K 1982 Intervertebral disc calcification syndromes in children and adolescents. Spine 6: 535–537

Taylor L J 1986 Painful scoliosis: a need for further investigation. British Medical Journal 292: 120–122

Wenger D R, Bobechko W P, Gilday D L 1978 Spectrum of intervertebral disc space infection in children. Journal of Bone and Joint Surgery 60A: 100–108

Yu L, Kasser J R, O'Rourke E, Kozakewich H 1989 Chronic recurrent multifocal osteomyelitis association with vertebra plana. Journal of Bone and Joint Surgery 71A: 105–112

Zaden H G, Sakka S A, Powell M P, Mehta M H 1995 Absent superficial abdominal reflexes in children with scoliosis. An early indicator of syringomyelia. Journal of Bone and Joint Surgery 77A: 762–767

PART 2   Spinal deformities

R. A. Dickson

BASIC PRINCIPLES

DEFINITIONS AND TERMINOLOGY

The spine is normally straight in the frontal (coronal) plane. If it is not, a lateral curvature or scoliosis is present. Scolioses are subdivided into structural and non-structural, according to whether the spine is additionally twisted (Leatherman & Dickson 1988). Thus structural scoliosis is defined as a lateral curvature with rotation. As with many orthopaedic descriptions, these terms are accurate neither semantically nor descriptively. The really important attribute of a structural scoliosis is that the problem is intrinsic to the spine, and has the ability to progress with growth to produce a serious deformity that may threaten both good health and quality of life. By contrast, non-structural curves are secondary to some other factor such as leg length inequality or muscle spasm from a painful focus (e.g. disc prolapse, infection, tumour). Significant progression is seen only occasionally in some curves associated with spinal cord tumour. The remainder of these non-structural curves tend to resolve when the underlying problem is dealt with.

In the sagittal plane, it is normal to have lordotic spinal curvatures (curves convex anteriorly) in the cervical and lumbar regions and an intervening kyphosis (a curve convex posteriorly) in the thoracic region. Only if these natural curves are exaggerated or abnormally reduced do they assume pathological significance. For instance, the thoracic kyphosis is increased in Scheuermann's disease, otherwise termed idiopathic hyperkyphosis. The lumbar lordosis is characteristically increased in paralytic conditions such as muscular dystrophy or cerebral palsy.

The distinction between structural and non-structural scolioses is not always easily made, at least on initial inspection. Most non-structural curves occur lower down in the spine, where the lateral profile is naturally lordotic. If a lateral curvature is imposed in this region, for example secondary to a pelvic tilt produced by leg length inequality, then the presence of a spinal curvature in two planes (lordosis plus lateral curvature) will impose a deformity in the third plane, with resultant spinal rotation. It is for this reason that non-structural lumbar scolioses, secondary to a leg length inequality, are found in such large numbers during school screening programmes that focus upon minor alterations in spinal shape.

It is conventional to describe scolioses according to their site and direction and the number of curves present. The site of a curve is determined by the position of the apical vertebra or vertebrae, and thus curves can be, for example, thoracic or lumbar. If the apex occurs at the T12 or L1 levels, it is referred to as thoraco-lumbar; similarly, it is called cervico-thoracic if the apex is at C7 or T1. The direction to which the convexity of the curve points determines the side of the curve, and thus right thoracic or left lumbar curve patterns are common. Multiple curves are more common than single ones. The combined right thoracic and left lumbar pattern is particularly prevalent.

STRUCTURAL AND NON-STRUCTURAL SCOLIOSIS

When Adams in 1865 described his 'forward bending test', he realised that the rotational component of the three-dimensional deformity was increased with spinal flexion (Fig. 31.8). This is why this position is a favoured one for inspecting patients in scoliosis clinics and for screening for scoliosis in the community. Because the deformity is less evident in the erect position, some form of mechanical event must be taking place when the spine is flexed that enhances rotation. This provides an important clue as to the nature of the underlying deformity of structural scoliosis.

When a posteroanterior (PA) radiograph of a structural scoliosis is inspected, the lateral curvature is obvious, but the vertebrae within the curve are also rotated, and this direction of rotation is constant: the posterior elements turn into the concavity and the vertebral bodies into the convexity, irrespective of the type or spinal level of the scoliosis. If the spinous processes and the centres of the vertebral bodies are marked on this PA radiograph, it can be seen that

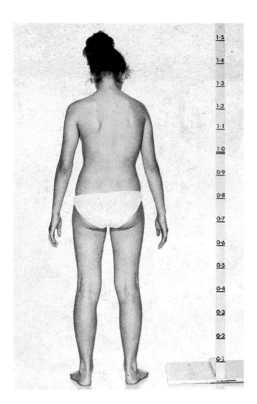

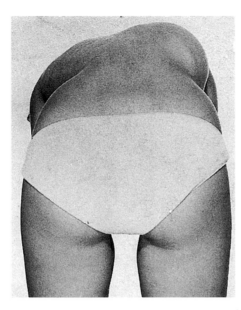

Figure 31.8 Erect and forward-bending views, showing that the rotational prominence is increased on forward bending.

the line joining the spinous processes is shorter than the line joining the vertebral bodies, and thus the back of the spine is shorter than the front (Fig. 31.9). If the back of the spine is shorter than the front in every case of structural scoliosis,

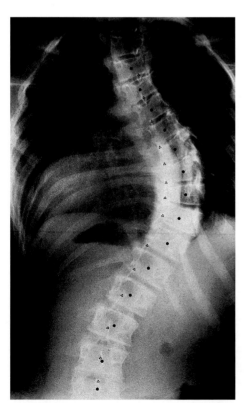

Figure 31.9 PA radiograph of an idiopathic thoracic curve, with the tips of the spinous processes marked with hollow triangles and the centre of the vertebral bodies with black circles. It can be readily seen that the line joining the spinous processes is shorter than the line joining the more anterior vertebral bodies, and thus the back of the spine is shorter than the front.

then all these deformities are lordotic and, reciprocally, there is no such deformity as kyphoscoliosis. This fundamental point was obvious to Adams even before X-rays were discovered, and his careful cadaver dissections demonstrated the essential lordosis beautifully. A significant abnormality in these spines is therefore that the front of the spine is relatively too long and readily buckles to the side on flexion, to produce a positive Adams' forward-bending test. It is the three-dimensional nature of this deformity, with particular reference to the abnormal lateral profile, that holds the key to an understanding of the clinical features, behaviour and treatment.

'Structural' scolioses resulting from solitary congenital hemivertebrae tend to exist in the coronal plane only, tend to exhibit no rotation when the PA radiograph is inspected, and produce no rotational prominence on forward bending. This is because the sagittal profile is not affected. Similarly, a true lordoscoliosis is produced by leg length inequality, by the combination of coronal and sagittal plane curvatures, but the sagittal profile is not abnormal and progressive buckling does not ensue.

THE SIZE OF THE DEFORMITY

Because the deformity encompasses lordosis, rotation and lateral curvature, it exists in three dimensions, with each vertebra occupying a different position in space relative to its neighbours. Planes are two-dimensional, and there is therefore no one plane that adequately describes the deformity. By contrast, if the spine is straight in the coronal plane, a lateral radiograph can be used to measure the amount of cervical or lumbar lordosis and the amount of thoracic kyphosis. Angles are planar measurements, and if there is no one plane that can assess structural scoliosis, the deformity cannot be described by an angular measurement (Dickson 1987). Cobb was aware of this, but in an effort to assess his patients and their response to treatment he devised the angle that bears his name (Cobb 1948). If a PA radiograph of a structural scoliosis in inspected and the vertebrae that are maximally tilted at the top and bottom of the deformity are selected, lines can be drawn along their upper and lower borders, respectively. These lines subtend an angle referred to as the Cobb angle, and it is standard practice to measure the deformity of structural scoliosis in this way (Fig. 31.10).

If the deformity is in only two planes, e.g. a solitary hemivertebra, then this angle accurately reflects the shape of the spine, but the more the spine has twisted the less satisfactory is this measure. It is this undue reliance on the appearance of the spine on PA and lateral views of the patient that has obscured the true nature of the three-dimensional deformity. Because the vertebrae within the structural scoliosis are rotated, the PA projection of the patient must necessarily be an oblique view of the deformity, with each vertebra being portrayed in a different degree of obliquity (Fig. 31.11). Of course, the direction of rotation of the posterior elements indicates that the deformity is unquestionably lordotic, but it does not say by how much. Meanwhile, the lateral view of the patient is another oblique view of the same deformity, this time providing the spurious appearance of kyphosis, which is nothing more than the scoliosis seen in another plane. In simple terms, therefore, it is possible for the three-dimensional deformity to vary greatly in size and perceived shape, merely by altering the plane of projection.

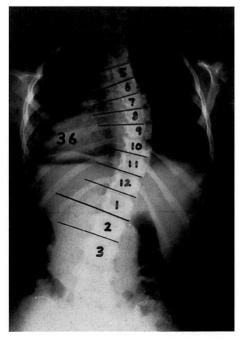

Figure 31.10
Measuring the Cobb angle on a PA radiograph.

This can be simply verified by inspecting, say, a coat-hanger. If the long side (hypotenuse) is vertical, and the hook points due east or west, the angle subtended will be maximal (if we look in a north–south direction), whereas if the hook points north or south the appearance is that of a straight line – i.e. there is no deformity present. As the hook is moved from either due east or west round to north or south, the angle subtended becomes less and less. Stagnara was aware of this and devised an X-ray to be taken truly PA to the apical vertebra (du Peloux et al 1965). If, for example, the apical vertebra was rotated 30° about a vertical axis from neutral, then the X-ray beam was rotated 30° to ensure that this vertebra appeared truly PA. This they termed the 'plan d'élection', which is the plane of projection providing the biggest deformity; 90° round from this would be a true lateral of the curve apex, which unmasks the essential lordosis. Any views in between, such as PA and lateral of the patient, merely show the deformity obliquely (Fig. 31.11). Using Stagnara's principle, it is possible only to obtain true AP and lateral projections of one vertebra at a time, and it would require an excessive dose of radiation to the growing child to build up a radiographic picture of the deformity incrementally.

In order to avoid too many X-rays, and still find out more about true spinal shape, the PA and lateral views of the patient can be taken in biplanar fashion and known landmarks (e.g. pedicles, corners of bodies) can be digitised for computer analysis and graphic display (Fig. 31.12). The deformity can thus be rotated by the computer so that it can be seen in any desired projection without taking further radiographs (Howell & Dickson 1989). This is obviously difficult and time-consuming, and does not produce one single meaningful figure to register the size of the deformity. A curve with a Cobb angle of 60° is more than twice as large as a curve of 30°. It is thus confusing to present data in the form of mean Cobb angles and mean percentage changes.

There is much that can be learnt qualitatively, but not quantitatively, from the PA projection of the patient. In the coronal plane, it can be seen that, above and below the structural curve, there are compensatory curves that straighten the spine. These are convex the opposite way to the structural curve and are referred to as 'compensatory scolioses'. If we consider the direction of rotation of the structural scoliosis and its two compensatory curves, it will be seen that for a single curve – e.g. a right thoracic curve – the spinous processes are rotated towards the left in the region of the structural curve in addition to the first segment or two of the compensatory curves above and below (Fig. 31.9). Bearing in mind that posterior element rotation into the curve concavity implies lordosis, and the reverse kyphosis, the direction of rotation in the compensatory curves is now the opposite of the structural curve – i.e. the compensatory curves are convex left and the posterior elements are rotated to the left. Thus these so-called compensatory scolioses are kyphoses. This is not surprising, because the structural curve is a lordoscoliosis and ought to

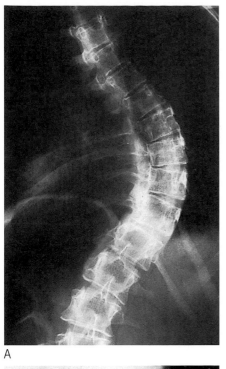

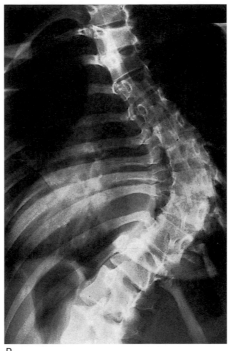

A

B

Figure 31.11 Four X-ray views of the same deformity. A PA of patient. B True PA of the apical vertebra (plan d'élection), showing the deformity to be substantially greater than the PA view of the patient. C Lateral view of the patient, showing the spurious impression of kyphosis. D True lateral of the apical vertebra, unmasking the essential lordosis.

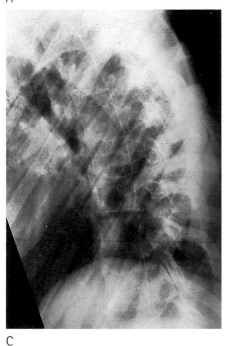

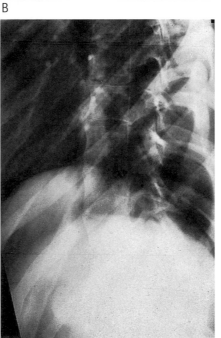

C

D

be balanced in three dimensions above and below by asymmetric kyphoses.

If a PA radiograph of a double structural right thoracic and left lumbar curve is inspected, it will be seen that there is no intervening kyphosis between the two structural curves, but there are kyphoses above the upper one and below the lower one. Triple- or multiple-curve patterns also commonly exist, and on inspection of their PA radiographic appearance the entire spine is lordotic from top to bottom. Thus much about the three-dimensional shape of the spine

in structural scoliosis can be inferred from a PA view of the patient.

CLASSIFICATION OF SPINAL DEFORMITIES

The following is a brief classification, based upon the recommendations of the Scoliosis Research Society:

1. Idiopathic.
2. Congenital.
3. Neuromuscular.

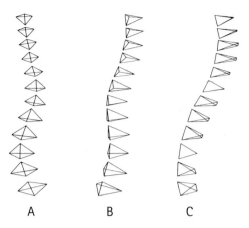

Figure 31.12 Computer graphic representation of a spinal deformity. **A** PA view of patient. **B** True lateral view of the apical region, showing the lordosis. **C** Lateral view, showing the impression of kyphosis.

4. Neurofibromatosis.
5. Mesenchymal disorders.
6. Trauma.
7. Infection.
8. Tumours.
9. Miscellaneous.

Idiopathic spinal deformities are divided into two broad categories: scoliosis and kyphosis. Idiopathic scoliosis is further subdivided into two types according to the patient's age at disease onset – early onset (before the age of 5 years) and late onset (after the age of 5 years). This age of onset distinction is important, because it is only with early onset deformities that health can be jeopardized (Branthwaite 1986). Late-onset scoliosis is a question of appearance and deformity, although there are social and psychological disadvantages therefrom.

Idiopathic kyphosis is Scheuermann's disease, and there are two types according to site. Type I Scheuermann's disease is typical mid-lower thoracic hyperkyphosis apical about T8–T9, whereas Type II Scheuermann's disease is in the thoraco-lumbar or upper lumbar spine and is referred to as 'apprentice's spine', as it can be associated with a more vigorous lifestyle.

Congenital spinal deformities are broadly divisible into two groups: congenital bone deformities and congenital spinal cord deformities. Congenital bone deformities are produced by congenital bony anomalies – either failures of formation (hemivertebrae or wedged vertebrae) or failures of segmentation (congenital fusions or bars across disc spaces). There is a particularly nasty prognosis with a hemivertebra on one side and a unilateral bar on the other, because growth will inexorably lead to severe progression.

Congenital spinal cord deformities include the spina bifida and myelodysplasia syndromes. The underlying anomaly is present before birth, but the prognosis for deformity is much more dependent on the degree of paralysis.

Thus the congenital kyphosis of myelomeningocele is always associated with complete paralysis from the waist down, whereas the time of onset and ultimate severity of the more usual paralytic-type lordoscoliosis with pelvic obliquity is proportional to the degree and level of paralysis.

These congenital spine deformities are often associated with spinal dysraphism (e.g. diastematomyelia, tethered filum, spino-cutaneous fistula), whereby the function of the spinal cord can be further jeopardised (see Ch. 16).

Neuromuscular spinal deformities include conditions such as a cerebral palsy, poliomyelitis, Friedreich's ataxia and the muscular dystrophies. The typical paralytic lordoscoliosis with pelvic obliquity occurs in proportion to the severity of the neurological problem.

Neurofibromatosis deformities are either scoliosis or kyphosis and can be of early onset and very progressive.

Mesenchymal disorders refer to those heritable disorders of connective tissue (e.g. brittle bone disease and Marfan's syndrome), mucopolysaccharidoses, skeletal dysplasias and metabolic bone diseases in which spinal deformities occur.

Traumatic spinal deformities can be produced by trauma to the spine itself (fracture/fracture-dislocation of the spine or paralysis therefrom), or can result from extraspinal trauma such as damage to the chest or abdominal wall from surgery, burns, or retroperitoneal fibrosis.

Infection, which may be pyogenic or tuberculous, typically produces kyphotic deformities.

Deformities associated with tumours can be produced by the presence of the tumour or by its treatment. Non-structural deformities are produced by associated muscle spasm, whereas idiopathic-type scolioses are produced by intradural tumours, probably by a neuropathological mechanism. The widespread laminectomy used to excise the neoplasm produces progressive kyphosis in the growing spine.

A number of other conditions, such as congenital anomalies of the upper extremity, juvenile idiopathic arthritis and congenital heart disease, are also associated with a higher prevalence of spinal deformities.

THE PATHOGENESIS OF STRUCTURAL SPINAL DEFORMITIES

As with all musculoskeletal deformities, the development of structural scoliosis from the straight to the declared deformity is a combination of biological and biomechanical factors (Deacon et al 1987). Innumerable scoliosis screening programmes have shown, and indeed anatomists centuries ago had already described, that a degree or two of lateral spinal curvature can hardly be considered abnormal. Epidemiological surveys have demonstrated that 10% of normal teenagers have a scoliosis measuring 5° or more. Forty percent of these are due to a leg length inequality, but that still leaves a substantial majority (6% of all normal children) with a structural scoliosis somewhere in their spine. However, with increasing curve size the prevalence rate becomes exponentially smaller, with 2% having curves

can be acc
This accou
age of 25 y

Meanwhi
being in fr
inbuilt prot
ling. The b
and lumbar
such that t
before the
pay-out of
that fails,
lordoscolios
lumbar lor
column and
precisely w
Scheuermai

There ai
(Euler's law
critical load
beam lengt
example, bi
ence have s
likely to pro
This has no
chanical, in
likely it is
column, the
to note tha
cantly tall
matched co
are more sl

The ques
refers to an
the spine i
simple term
buckle more
the remainc
conditions s
bone is ch
brittle bone
Recklinghai
dystrophica
foraminae,
therefore ir
both these c
mity and a
produced is
pathic cases

Euler's la
Marfan's a
promotes th
idiopathic t
neuromuscu
quate, and
spinal defor

of 10° or more and 1 in 200 normal children having a curve of 20° or more (Dickson 1984). Clearly, something has to be added to 'schooliosis' in order to make it scoliosis, and not surprisingly this problem exists in the sagittal plane. What is perhaps surprising is that the importance of the lateral profile has been largely ignored, despite the pioneering work of Adams (1865) and Somerville (1952).

Twenty years ago in Leeds an epidemiological survey was commenced, with particular reference to the lateral profile of the spine, involving 16 000 schoolchildren. Every year uring this 5-year longitudinal survey, measurements such as standing height and bone age were recorded and AP and lateral radiographs of the spine were taken. A number of children developed idiopathic scoliosis during the course of the study, but had straight spines when the study was commenced. When their initial lateral profiles were analysed, it was seen that the lordotic abnormality in the sagittal plane preceded the development of the lateral spinal curvature, demonstrating its crucial, aetiological significance.

When a true lateral radiograph of the apex of an idiopathic thoracic scoliosis is compared with a lateral view of the apical region of a patient with type I Scheuermann's hyperkyphosis, the deformities in the sagittal plane would appear to be exactly the opposite (Fig. 31.13). In idiopathic scoliosis, the anterior vertebral height is greater than the posterior and any endplate irregularity or Schmorl node formation is situated more posteriorly, whereas in

Scheuermann's disease anterior vertebral height is reduced in comparison with posterior height and Schmorl node formation is situated anteriorly in the growth plate. The conditions of idiopathic scoliosis and Scheuermann's disease have therefore considerable similarities, and it should be borne in mind that they exist in otherwise normal, entirely healthy children with a similar community prevalence rate and familial trend (Sorenson 1964).

The amount of thoracic kyphosis varies during late childhood and adolescence: in the prepubertal phase it reduces appreciably, only to be regained in the year or two before maturity. It is while the kyphosis is reducing in the prepubertal phase that girls are going through their peak adolescent growth period and are particularly prone to develop idiopathic scoliosis. Boys, with their constant growth velocity during this age period, are relatively protected; however, when the thoracic kyphosis increases just before maturity, boys are then going through their peak adolescent growth period. This may explain why boys have an increased prevalence of the opposite deformity, Scheuermann's disease. Clinically, Scheuermann's disease presents a year or two before maturity, whereas idiopathic scoliosis presents much earlier, during adolescence or even childhood.

Interestingly, 67% of all patients with type I thoracic Scheuermann's disease also have co-existent idiopathic scoliosis, but several segments lower down, in the region of the compensatory lumbar hyperlordosis (Fig. 31.14). As the

A

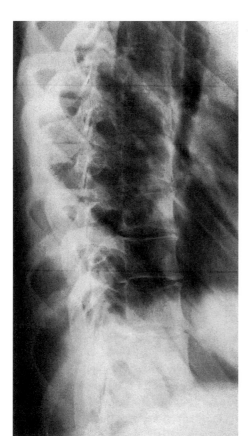

B

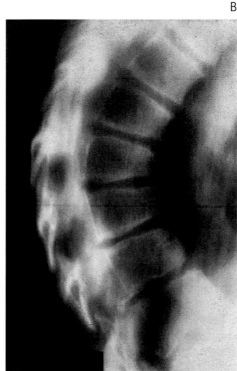

Figure 31.13 **A** True lateral radiograph of the apex of an idiopathic thoracic curve. **B** Lateral radiograph of a patient with Scheuermann's thoracic hyperkyphosis.

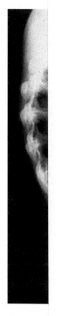

A

thoracic
lumbar
side to
mities,
existing
dren, a
'patholo
scoliosi
ends o
'normal

Acco
the trar
be cons
(Fig. 31
lordose
verse p
cervica
and sho
thoracic
back th
point at
bral co
with th
lumbar
prismat
buckles
base.

It sh
growing
average
discern
althoug
vertical
tenden

subsequent heart and lung problems. Clinically, therefore, it is better to consider only two types of idiopathic scoliosis: early onset (before the age of 5 years) and late onset (after the age of 5 years) (Leatherman & Dickson 1988).

LATE-ONSET IDIOPATHIC SCOLIOSIS (AFTER 5 YEARS OF AGE)

This condition is largely a question of deformity and appearance, as there are few accompanying organic health consequences, and idiopathic scoliosis is not associated with an increased prevalence or severity of back pain, although when the scoliotic back does become painful, symptoms are more recalcitrant than with a straight back. The condition, however, should not be relegated to the realms of pure cosmesis, as the deformity itself can have a very major impact on the quality of life (Bengtsson et al 1974). It is particularly distressing when an adolescent presents with a severe deformity such that, even with optimal treatment, a significant residual deformity will remain for life. Although nowadays there would appear to be fewer such cases attending scoliosis clinics for the first time, curve size at presentation remains a concern and continues to fuel the debate concerning the merits and demerits of routine school screening.

When screening was introduced, decades ago, curve size was the dominant consideration and the importance of age of onset had not been established. Screening implies the systematic examination of a population at regular intervals to harvest those with both the declared and latent forms; subsequent re-examinations separate those with the latent from those with the clinical condition. It has been used for a variety of medical conditions, from which much has been learnt and guidelines and criteria laid down (Whitby 1974). Clearly, an important prerequisite before routine screening is established is that the natural history of the condition should be adequately understood. For instance, if the group affected were a particularly vulnerable subset of the population, the majority of effort could be addressed to this relatively small number, the population 'at risk'. In addition, knowing the natural history allows time intervals between screening episodes to be defined and big curves at presentation to be eliminated.

Screening for scoliosis has major financial implications. Whereas breast cancer kills, late-onset idiopathic scoliosis does not. Moreover, there is no point in acquiring thousands of minor cases if there is no adequate treatment to prevent progression. In addition, there should be a simple test that can be applied to a population: the test should identify that condition and no other, and should not produce too many false positives or false negatives. This is where the validity, sensitivity, and specificity of a screening test are crucial and whereas, for example, the value of screening and early treatment for cervical cancer in women is clearly established, no such certainty exists in scoliosis screening. In particular, recent years have shown a progressive loss of confidence in

any form of conservative treatment, with many studies struggling to differentiate the effects of treatment from the natural history.

Some countries do still insist upon regular routine school screening for scoliosis using some quick measure of rotational asymmetry of the torso on forward bending, such as the scoliometer, but there is a move away from compulsory screening until such time as the natural history of the condition is better understood. However, early detection, as opposed to routine screening, is clearly important, and national orthopaedic associations and scoliosis societies have an important responsibility to increase local community awareness, amongst both lay and medical colleagues, of the need for recognition and prompt referral.

An important by-product from these school-scoliosis-screening programmes has been a body of knowledge concerning normality and abnormality, incidence and prevalence rates, curve patterns, familial trends, and so on (Mardia et al 1999). Interestingly, there is evidence of the condition pursuing a more benign course, with recent prevalence rates being lower and with less obvious progression potential (Stirling et al 1996). If there is evidence of a change in natural history, this reinforces the need for repeated investigations, particularly as regards the efficacy of treatment in relationship to contemporaneous controls.

Clinical features

Patients with late-onset idiopathic scoliosis present as a result of truncal asymmetry, and it is usually the rotational component of the deformity that is the most obvious. Thus thoracic deformities present as a result of the rib hump (Fig. 31.8), and thoraco-lumbar or lumbar deformities present with a loin hump. With these lower curves, there is also asymmetry of the waist, an increased flank recession on the concave side, and a flattening of the waist on the convex side. As a result, the hip on the concave side appears unduly prominent and this can be as cosmetically obvious as a rib hump (Fig. 31.16).

The great majority of patients referred to scoliosis clinics are adolescent females. There is a fairly even sex ratio for very small curves detected by screening, but a steep rise in the female:male ratio with increasing curve magnitude. Patients and parents are frequently alarmed by a Cobb angle of 30° or 40°, and many feel a sense of guilt that they did not recognise the problem earlier. There are two principal reasons for this. First, adolescence is an emotional time and, whereas parents are used to seeing their infants or young children nearly naked, they seldom so see their adolescent children. Adolescent girls, although they cannot see their backs, can notice a problem of a twisting torso with the appearance of a more prominent developing breast on the side opposite the curve convexity. Second, curve size may be appreciable radiographically at presentation because it is the asymmetry of the surface of the body which provokes presentation. The spinal column has to undergo a certain amount of buckling before this adversely affects the shape of

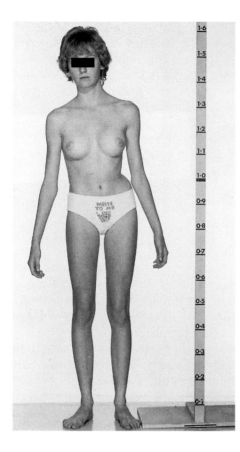

Figure 31.16 Waist asymmetry in a girl with a lumbar curve.

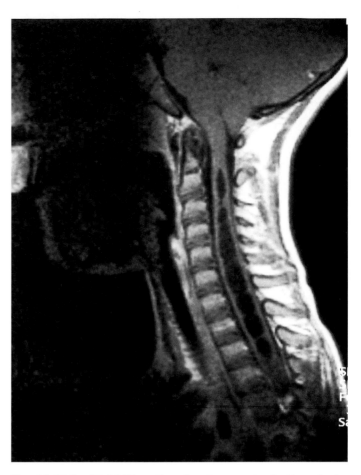

Fig. 31.17 Sagittal MRI section showing a syrinx in the spinal cord.

the outer surface of the body. Although this may be a disadvantage in terms of delayed presentation, it is a positive advantage as regards surgical treatment. If the deformity does not really impinge significantly on surface shape until it has a Cobb angle of say 30°, then the surgeon doesn't have to reduce the deformity to much less than 30° to bring it back into the realms of acceptability.

Pain is not a feature of idiopathic scoliosis, although some fatigue discomfort over the rotational prominence is by no means exceptional. Any suspicion of pain being more significant demands further investigation, particularly if there is any suggestion of night pain, when neoplasm or a syrinx must be excluded. In addition, thought must always be given to the progressive idiopathic deformity in a male: it is wise to submit all males with progressive deformities to MRI, because a syrinx is much more common than generally believed (Fig. 31.17). The usual curve patterns of single right thoracic, single left thoraco-lumbar or lumbar, or double right thoracic and left thoraco-lumbar/lumbar are those we generally see, and any unusual curve pattern, such as a progressive left thoracic curve in a teenager, should arouse suspicion of a possible underlying lesion. MRI scanning should be insisted upon before the diagnosis of a purely idiopathic condition is established. This is particularly important if surgery is considered, because appreciable alteration of spinal shape in the presence of an intradural tumour or syrinx is a recipe for neurological disaster, with a very high paraplegia rate.

In idiopathic scoliosis, the neurological examination should be normal. In the presence of a congenital scoliosis, there may be additional spinal dysraphism and the overlying skin in the midline may be the site of a dimple, sinus, naevus, haemangioma, or hairy patch. Similarly, the presence of spinal dysraphism may result in a short and attenuated lower extremity on one side. Thus a careful assessment of the entire patient, in addition to the neurological system, is important.

At the conclusion of the history and physical examination, it is useful if a permanent record of surface shape can be obtained (Fig. 31.18), as it is surface shape rather than spinal shape that is the most important factor. The deformity buckles further on forward bending, and thus patients should be assessed in this position in addition to the erect position.

Radiographic assessment

Undoubtedly, far too many X-rays are taken of patients with idiopathic scoliosis. At presentation, the patient should have one full set of spine films, which should include AP and lateral views of the spine from C1 to S1 inclusive. The principal purpose of these films is to exclude a congenital spine deformity or other relevant feature. As patients present with problems of surface shape, the only certain way of excluding

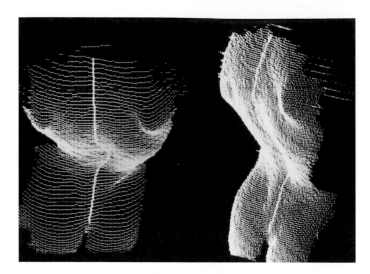

Fig. 31.18 Computerised measurement of surface shape – helpful in reducing the number of X-rays.

a congenital scoliosis is radiographically. In addition, patients with an intradural tumour or syrinx may present with an apparent idiopathic deformity and thus the whole spine should be imaged adequately, to exclude widening of the interpedicular distance or flattening of the internal pedicular surface. Because syringes tend to be cervical in location, the spine should be imaged from C1 down. Although much emphasis is placed upon isotope scanning for painful scoliosis to exclude osteoid osteoma or benign osteoblastoma, these lesions are usually visible on plain X-rays as an expansion of bone, often with a central lucency, at the junction of pedicle and transverse process on the concave side of the curve apex. A PA view of the left hand and wrist should be obtained in the immature patient, in order to assess bone age.

Measurement of the deformity by X-ray is controversial, although most scoliosis surgeons continue to favour measurement of the Cobb angle (Cobb 1948) (Fig. 31.10). There is some merit in taking a de-rotated AP view of the curve apex (the plan d'élection of Stagnara) and a similar true lateral view of the curve apex (du Peloux et al 1965). The plan d'élection and de-rotated lateral views are obtained by inspecting the original AP view of the patient and measuring the amount of rotation of the vertebra at the curve apex, using the method of Perdriolle (1979). If this shows that the apical vertebra is rotated 30° from the straight, either the patient or the incident beam is turned through 30° in order to achieve the plan d'élection, and then 90° from this in order to achieve the de-rotated lateral view. Perhaps the most useful single measure on an AP view of the patient is the amount of apical rotation at the curve apex. This is a much more accurate index of the patient's chief problem (the rotational component of the deformity). Perdriolle's technique was to use a transparent template over the apical vertebra, with particular reference to the pedicle on the concave side, which is sited more and more towards the concave side, with more and more apical rotation. The amount of rotation is read off in degrees from the template. This measurement of rotation can then be repeated with clinical progression or after surgical intervention. Any differences accurately reflect real change compared with alteration in the Cobb angle (Dickson 1987). Unless obscured by metalwork, the convex pedicle is still just as easily seen after a spinal fusion as it was before.

Should the patient undergo surgery and should there be any suspicion of an underlying cord problem, an MRI scan should be performed to exclude a dysraphic anomaly that could endanger the spinal cord if spinal shape was suddenly altered.

X-ray dosage should be kept to a minimum and low-dose techniques are readily available. Thus, although good quality normal-dose films are required at presentation for diagnostic purposes, any subsequent films need only be of the low-dose variety, as they produce quality good enough for measurement. Wherever possible, measurement of surface shape should be used in place of X-rays (Fig. 31.18); although there are sophisticated techniques available, they are still incapable of providing one overall figure that would state how much deformity the patient has.

A useful measurement technique is to take AP and lateral biplanar X-rays and digitise known landmarks, so that spinal shape can be reconstructed by computer graphics (Fig. 31.12).

Treatment

As late-onset idiopathic scoliosis is principally a question of deformity and appearance, it is very much more up to the patient and family than the surgeon as to whether the deformity is acceptable or not. Patients' perceptions change as they go through adolescence to maturity, and they may thus have differing views about acceptability at different times. What 'acceptability' really means is that, if the deformity were not to change appreciably, at that moment the patient and family would be happy enough with it, and the wise counselling of the scoliosis surgeon is crucial to this decision-making process. Although the surgeon cannot, and should not, state whether someone else's deformity is acceptable, he nevertheless has a key role in presenting information about the condition to the patient and family (Dickson 1999).

The only way in which spinal shape can be appreciably improved is by major spinal surgery, which may require both anterior and posterior stages. Risks are being reduced by improved anaesthetic techniques, the routine use of intensive care, careful preoperative history taking, examination and where necessary imaging, electrophysiological monitoring of the spinal cord during surgery, and the routine 'wake-up' test, but there are still definite risks of damage to the spinal cord. Thus acceptability is part of a balance of risks and rewards: the rewards are a much-improved spinal shape, whereas the risks include catastrophic neurological deficit. Acceptability therefore varies very considerably from deformity to deformity and from family, to family, as the balance of risks and rewards is interpreted differently. Thus a deformity with a Cobb angle of 40° may be so upsetting to one patient and family that they would go through thick and thin to have it improved, whereas a deformity with a Cobb angle of 70° might be entirely acceptable to another with concern at one or two very major operations and the possibility of paralysis overriding any thought of undergoing treatment. Although our knowledge of natural history is incomplete, it should be explained that bigger deformities tend to progress more than smaller ones, and more immature patients have a greater progression potential than those approaching maturity. As the spine does not stop growing until the middle of the 3rd decade on average, it is unwise to consider that progression potential is exhausted when the bones of the hand and wrist reach maturity. Under the responsible guidance of the surgeon and with repeat consultations, often over many years, it is usually possible for the patient, family and surgeon to reach the correct therapeutic decision unanimously.

Once acceptability has been decided upon, the management strategy for late-onset idiopathic scoliosis is relatively straightforward. If the deformity is acceptable, then preservation of acceptability throughout the remainder of spinal growth is the objective. This is the place for conservative management. If the deformity is unacceptable, restoration of acceptability and maintenance of that situation throughout the remainder of growth is the objective. This is the place for surgical treatment.

Conservative treatment

Ever since the time of Hippocrates, various orthotic devices have been worn in the belief that progression of an idiopathic scoliotic deformity could be attenuated by so doing. The first popularly prescribed orthosis was the Milwaukee brace, a cervico-thoraco-lumbo-sacral orthosis devised by Blount (Blount & Moe 1973). This was conceived as a postoperative adjunct for poliomyelitic curves. The Milwaukee brace was believed to work by three-point fixation – above, below, and over the apex of the deformity. Thus there was a pelvic mould below, with vertical metal uprights going initially to a ring, which exerted upward pressure on the mandible in front and occipital condyles behind. Problems with dentition and malocclusion led to the use of a simple cervical choker in the later models. Then, slung between the uprights, was a pad held just below the apex of the curve posteriorly, to complete the three-point fixation. An important feature was that, for thoracic curves, the lumbar lordosis should be obliterated in the brace and consequently some 'correction' could be seen when X-rays were taken without and then with the brace on.

However, it would appear that the brace was designed without any clear understanding of the three-dimensional nature of the deformity. Nevertheless, it rapidly became the accepted method of treatment and in its hey-day it would have been almost heretical to suggest a controlled trial of the

efficiency of the brace, let alone not to have prescribed it. It was also empirical for the brace to be worn for 23 hours a day, from diagnosis until after the vertebral ring apophyses had fused. However, the vertebral ring apophyses have nothing to do with spinal growth, nor does their fusion bear any relationship to cessation of spinal growth. General skeletal maturity, as determined by maturation of the carpal bones and fusion of the hand epiphyses, occurs on average during the 15th year in girls and the 17th year in boys, but the cartilaginous vertebral endplates do not fuse until after 20 years of age. Not surprisingly, substantial growth of the spine beyond general skeletal maturity has been demonstrated (Howell et al 1992). As expected, curve progression has been demonstrated well into the twenties and thus, in order for a sustained effect to be achieved, the brace would have to have been worn until the age of 25 years, which does challenge even the most compliant! Interestingly, although it was assumed that children wore their braces assiduously, Houghton et al (1987) showed, by the use of compliance meters, that they only wore them for a small fraction of the prescribed time, to the disappointment of the protagonists of conservative treatment.

So it was that the thresholds for treatment of idiopathic scoliosis evolved: those with a Cobb angle less than 20° were observed; those with an angle between 30° and 50° were braced; those with an angle greater than 50–60° were operated upon. That the results of brace-wearing could merely reflect the natural history of the underlying condition was never challenged until recently, when a limited trial showed that no significant benefit was conferred on brace wearers (Miller et al 1984). The same 'corrective effect' had been previously achieved with plaster casts, and flattening of the lumbar lordosis in the cast was considered a very important point. When the need for superstructure was challenged and the Boston underarm thoraco-lumbo-sacral orthosis was introduced, the point of flattening the lumbar lordosis to induce thoracic hyperextension was reinforced, as there was now only two-point fixation rather than the previous three-point fixation (Watts et al 1977). There is, however, no doubt that a temporary correction during brace-wearing can be achieved by flattening the lumbar lordosis.

Electrospinal stimulation was introduced in the 1970s, in an attempt to treat idiopathic scoliosis conservatively. This concept, rather like orthotic treatment, was principally addressed to the coronal plane, with stimulation of the convex paraspinal muscles; not surprisingly, no evidence could be produced that electrospinal stimulation was effective.

To determine whether bracing alters the natural history of late-onset idiopathic scoliosis, a prospective randomised controlled trial (RCT) was deemed necessary. RCTs are, of course, the highest quality studies in the Cochrane hierarchy, but unfortunately an RCT could not be carried out, for a number of logistical reasons – principally because bracing proponents would not stop bracing, and those who had abandoned bracing would not resume it. Randomisation was therefore impossible, but centres in America and Europe

biomechanical buckling. If anterior and posterior prophylactic fusion is carried out and does not prevent progression, subsequent corrective surgery is difficult or even impossible to perform, because of pleural adhesions from previous surgery.

Moreover, the natural history of congenital scoliosis is not as predictable as we would like, and by no means all potentially serious growth asymmetries go on to produce unacceptable deformities at a young age. These cases may seem a formidable undertaking, particularly in the very young, when much of the growing spine is cartilaginous, but if the prophylactic opportunity is missed, the deformity can rapidly deteriorate and cause irreversible chest problems. With this exception, it is wise to observe the natural history of congenital scoliosis because not all anomalies, particularly single failures of formation, produce unacceptable deformities (McMaster & Ohtsuka 1982).

Once unacceptability has been reached, these rigid deformities are not amenable to the same surgical treatment as their idiopathic counterparts, and the only safe way of significantly altering spinal shape is by two-stage wedge resection at the curve apex, so that correction is not accompanied by tension lengthening of the spinal cord. While Roaf's concept of anteroconvex hemiepiphysiodesis was very sound biologically, it is only reliable for the solitary hemivertebra, which seldom progresses to unacceptability (Roaf 1963). For failures of segmentation it is an ineffective technique, because by the time the biological effect of epiphysiodesis can occur with growth, the lordotic sagittal plane has driven the deformity into further deterioration (Andrew & Piggott 1985). Leatherman & Dickson (1988) concluded that, on balance, it is better to wait for the deformity to declare itself, and to carry out a two-stage closing wedge resection once serious progression has been observed. Removing the apical keystone vertebra in closing wedge fashion is neither difficult nor dangerous, and does not add a great amount of time to a prophylactic anterior fusion of the levels above and below. It is a very much more certain way of controlling asymmetric spinal growth at a young age than is prophylactic fusion with all its uncertainties. Isolated removal of a hemivertebra is usually only indicated for the lumbo-sacral hemivertebra, producing progressive imbalance and torso list. Prophylactic posterior fusion at an earlier age is preferable to excision of the hemivertebra in order to reduce the risk of cord dysfunction.

The principal indication for dealing surgically with congenital kyphosis is the development of unfavourable neurological signs in the lower extremities. Anterior dural decompression by excision of the dorsal hemivertebra plus interbody strut grafting and posterior instrumental support are required. These are better done earlier than later, to prevent the development of atrophic cord changes.

CONGENITAL SPINAL CORD DEFORMITIES

This refers to the spina bifida syndrome. The more significant the myelodysplasia, the more obvious the ensuing spinal deformity. Thus patients with a meningomyelocele and total neurological loss in the lower extremities are most likely to develop the most severe deformities. The majority of these are typical, long C-shaped paralytic lordoscolioses with pelvic obliquity below (Fig. 31.35). Progressive torso imbalance imperils walking and sitting, and undue pressure on the lower buttock may produce recurrent pressure ulceration, the septic effects of which can threaten life itself. However, these are difficult deformities to manage: the

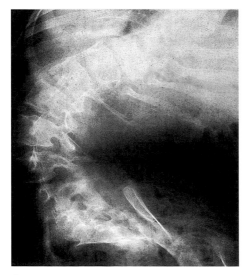

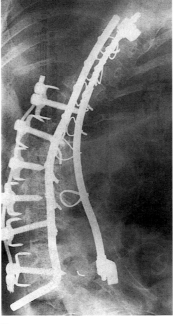

Figure 31.35 A PA radiograph of a collapsing paralytic lordoscoliosis with pelvic obliquity in association with spina bifida. **B** PA radiograph after anterior and posterior instrumentation and fusion.

A   B

extensive anterior and posterior surgery has a high complication rate. Surgical treatment should not be rushed into.

For those who still have sufficient lower limb function to
enable them to walk, spinal surgery is contraindicated because
a rigid lumbar spine can send them off their feet and make them
permanent wheelchair-sitters. Some patients who are wheelchair-sitters with no lower limb function can be adequately
managed by the provision of a total contact Derby seat in the
back of the wheelchair. However, for the patient with progressive torso list, who has to use his upper extremities for support
in the wheelchair, surgical correction and fusion is indicated.

The objective is to try to provide a square pelvis with a
balanced spine above, and this requires anterior and posterior instrumentation and fusion down to the sacrum.
Anterior segmental instrumentation is favoured in the first
stage, and posterior instrumentation in the second stage, has
to be varied in accordance with the local anatomy. Thus
areas of wide posterior element deficiency are fixed by the
transpedicular route, but the spine above can be dealt with
by hooks or segmental wires.

These spines should be carefully assessed before surgery
because as many as 40% of patients with paralytic lordoscolioses also have a significant congenital bony anomaly
(hemivertebra or bar in the thoraco-lumbar region above the
area of spina bifida) and it is this congenital bony anomaly
that can produce the torso imbalance.

Some of the children most severely affected with spina
bifida also have congenital deficiency of the anterior spinal
column in the lumbar region, and they develop severe and
progressive lumbar kyphoses. They are eventually drawn so
far forward that the anterior chest wall can come to rest on
the anterior thighs. All the anterior structures, even as far
forwards as the anterior abdominal wall, contract secon-
darily and need to be surgically released if the deformity is
to be effectively straightened.

Congenital spinal deformity syndromes

Congenital spinal deformities are encountered in a number
of generalised conditions such as Goldenhar's syndrome
(hemifacial dysplasia), Treacher–Collins syndrome
(mandibulo-facial dysostosis), Crouzon's syndrome (cranio-
facial dysostosis), Apert's syndrome (cranio-facial dysostosis
plus syndactyly) and Larsen's syndrome (multiple congenital
dislocations with a characteristic facial abnormality).
Although progressive deformities are not unusual, in these
children there are more often other major clinical considerations that override the spinal deformity.

When congenital anomalies in the cervico-thoracic region
are combined with a short neck, low hairline and restricted
cervical movement, the term Klippel–Feil syndrome is applicable (Fig. 31.36) (see Ch. 30). Progressive deformity, wry-neck,
facial asymmetry, and Sprengel's shoulder can produce a very
unfavourable appearance, but corrective surgery in the cervico-thoracic region is difficult, dangerous and not recommended (see Ch. 30). As congenital intervertebral fusion
reduces the number of motion segments, instability can be a

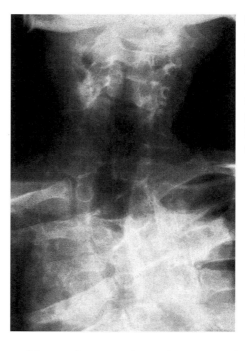

Figure 31.36 PA radiograph of the cervico-thoracic region, showing multiple congenital anomalies of the Klippel–Feil syndrome.

problem and may produce adverse neurological features. This
is particularly so in the upper cervical spine, but may occur
anywhere in the neck where mobility is preserved. Simple
fusion therefore has an important role.

In the lumbo-sacral region, the bony skeleton may
completely or partially fail to form: this is lumbo-sacral
agenesis. With complete lumbar absence, the appearance is
that of a sitting Buddha; however, more often, the lesions are
partial. Many of these patients have significant urogenital or
alimentary tract problems, which override the spine in
priority, but for those with spino-pelvic instability, fusion
may be necessary.

OTHER SPINAL DEFORMITIES

NEUROMUSCULAR DEFORMITIES

The true neuromuscular diseases of childhood refer to those
conditions that affect the spinal cord, peripheral nerves,
neuromuscular junctions and muscles. These include spinal
muscular atrophy, the peripheral neuropathies, Friedreich's
ataxia, arthrogryposis, and the muscular dystrophies. It is
convenient also to include in this section cerebral palsy and
poliomyelitis.

The common denominator here is that spinal column
buckling is favoured by inadequate neuromuscular control.
Therefore, not surprisingly, the most severe neuromuscular
problems tend to cause the most severely progressive spinal
deformities. Thus, in cerebral palsy, those at the milder end
of the spectrum, with minimal brain dysfunction only, may
develop no spinal deformity at all, whereas those with
spastic quadriplegia invariably develop a significant scoliosis. In general there are two types of scoliosis encountered:

1. An idiopathic-type deformity above a square and stable
   pelvis.

Reports of patients with Von Recklinghausen's scoliosis frequently and erroneously refer to the deformity as kyphoscoliosis. There is no doubt that these short, sharp, angular dystrophic curves can look kyphotic, with a posterior chest wall prominence on the convex side, but it is the apical vertebral bodies that are to be found immediately under the convex ribs. It is thus the front of the spine that is pointing backwards, rather than the back – or, in more simple terms, the lordosis has buckled all the way round, so that it now effectively points posteriorly.

As with idiopathic and congenital scolioses, the earlier the onset and the greater the progression potential, the more difficult it is to obtain a lasting correction. In this respect the Von Recklinghausen's curve is notorious, as bone graft material often is rapidly resorbed rather than consolidated. A golden rule is that the dystrophic curve always requires anterior and posterior fusion with excision of the anterior growth plates. If the curve is acceptable, then early anterior and posterior fusion is required. If the deformity is unacceptable, less severe curves can be dealt with by anterior multiple discectomies, followed by posterior instrumentation and fusion (Fig. 31.38). The most severe curves require the Leatherman two-stage wedge resection.

At the mild end of the spectrum, these deformities can be managed like their idiopathic counterparts, but if the patient is young or there are any features suggesting dystrophic change, an anterior stage should be performed.

Pure kyphoses, akin to early-onset severe angular Scheuermann's kyphosis, are much less common than scolioses, but can produce progressive lower-limb paralysis. They should be treated by anterior decompression and strut grafting.

Cervical spine deformities are not uncommon in Von Recklinghausen's disease and can be extremely complex, with an area of lordoscoliosis at one level and angular kyphosis at another. Again, anterior and posterior fusion are necessary, although access can be problematical.

HERITABLE DISORDERS OF CONNECTIVE TISSUE, MUCOPOLYSACCHARIDOSES, AND SKELETAL DYSPLASIAS

Brittle bone disease (see Ch. 6) is caused by defective synthesis of type I collagen, which obviously affects the skeleton, because bone contains type I collagen only. About 70% of patients with osteogenesis imperfecta can be shown to have a scoliosis (Fig. 31.39); even in those that do not, the spine is still abnormal, with changes of juvenile osteoporosis (multiple compression fractures with biconcave vertebrae). Patients presenting with spinal deformity are nearly always those with the severe disease. Again, rather like Von

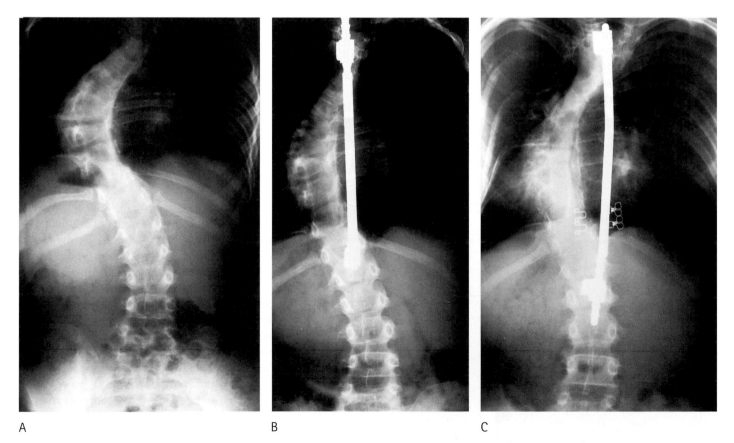

A   B   C

Figure 31.38 **A** AP views showing a progressive curve in Von Recklinghausen's disease. **B** After anterior discectomy and growth arrest and the first growing rod. **C** The last rod ten years later.

growth c
spine, pro
rior deco
establishe
rior fusio

Much h
the tuber
recomme
discecton
strut and
segmenta

DEFORM

There are
spinal de
syringom
tumours i
all impor

Glioma
immature
mental ha
nant and

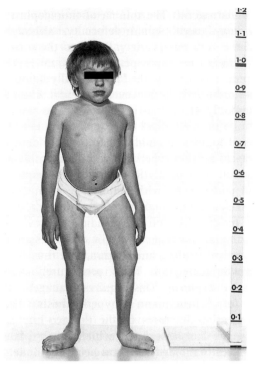

A

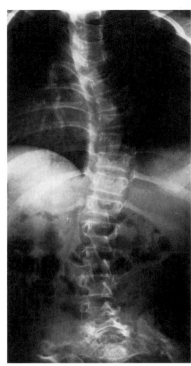

B

Figure 31.39 A Severe osteogenesis imperfecta showing the characteristic leg deformities. **B** All such individuals have a scoliosis.

Recklinghausen's disease, the more the spinal column is disadvantaged by bone weakness, the earlier the onset and the more progressive the ensuing deformity. Because of the problems of quality and strength of bone in relationship to instrumentation, it has been rightly said that progressive curves require stabilisation or nothing at all. In order to spread load, segmental instrumentation is to be preferred. The addition of methyl methacrylate cement to hook sites merely moves the weakness problem to another interface.

Marfan's syndrome, homocystinuria, congenital contractural arachnodactyly, Ehlers–Danlos syndrome, and their various formes frustes, are all associated with a greater prevalence rate of the idiopathic type of scoliosis, as the spinal column is disadvantaged at soft-tissue level in these heritable ligament laxity disorders. The ensuing deformities should be dealt with like their idiopathic counterparts but, where possible, both anterior and posterior spinal fusion should be undertaken because of the inherent soft-tissue weakness of the spinal column. The Marfan's patient may have significant heart valve and aortic disease, but this seldom presents a problem in adolescent scoliosis surgery. With homocystinuria, however, vascular damage may lead to thrombosis and it is important to avoid unnecessary surgery in these patients. Similarly, it is important to differentiate the different types of Ehlers–Danlos syndrome, in order to avoid surgery in those with vascular fragility, in whom excessive bleeding is a serious problem.

Of the mucopolysaccharidoses, MPS4 (Morquio's syndrome) is the most important to the spinal surgeon, because of the two common and major spinal problems: thoraco-lumbar kyphosis and atlanto-axial instability (Fig. 31.40). The thoraco-lumbar kyphosis is associated with local platyspondyly and the apical, anteriorly beaked vertebra may gradually produce cord compression. There is some evidence that an extension trunk brace can be preventive, but once neurological signs develop, anterior decompression and strut grafting become necessary.

Atlanto-axial instability results from a deficient odontoid, and this is a significant source of both mortality and neurological morbidity (Kopits et al 1972). Untreated, most of these patients develop myelopathy. Thus C1–C2 fusion is generally recommended in all cases prophylactically, by the age of 10 years. This can be performed posteriorly, with a supportive halo-vest.

Achondroplasia

There are two important spinal problems that occur in these patients: thoraco-lumbar kyphosis and spinal stenosis (Nelson 1970). Spinal stenosis, which tends to be more marked lower down the spine, is a problem of late adolescence and early adulthood. There is a typical story of leg claudication and weakness related to exercise, and gradually increasing neurological abnormalities in the legs, usually of the lower motor neurone variety. Myelography confirms the diagnosis and decompressive laminectomy is required in order to prevent progressive paralysis and to aid recovery. It is important to note that, if this is performed on the immature spine, a concomitant fusion is required to prevent progressive kyphosis.

Thoraco-lumbar kyphosis is a constant feature of achondroplasia, with a bullet-shaped apical vertebra. Seventy-five percent of these kyphoses resolve with growth, and therefore decompression of the syrinx or excision of the tumour is generally accompanied by resolution of the idiopathic-type lordoscoliosis.

Extradural tumours such as aneurysmal bone cysts, giant-cell tumours and eosinophilic granulomas tend not to produce a spinal deformity, or only a very mild kyphosis. However, osteoblastoma or its smaller equivalent, the osteoid osteoma, are generally associated with an idiopathic-type lordoscoliosis, with the lesion sitting at the junction of the pedicle and transverse process on the concave side of the curve apex, where there is characteristically cystic enlargement on plain films. Bone-seeking isotopes show a typical 'hot spot'. Tomography may, on occasion, be required to define the precise site of the lesion (Fig. 31.42). Excision of the neoplasm nearly always produces resolution of the deformity, although the posterior tethering effect of surgical scarring can induce further progression in some patients.

Wilms' tumour and neuroblastoma constitute the paravertebral tumours in childhood; although they are paravertebral in site, the necessary radiation therapy can induce vertebral changes, particularly in the form of platyspondyly and a thoraco-lumbar kyphosis with a bullet-shaped vertebra. A true structural lordoscoliosis is, however, uncommon. Should progressive kyphosis require surgical treatment, previous spinal irradiation can cause greater rates of pseudarthrosis after autogenous iliac crest grafting.

REFERENCES AND FURTHER READING

Adams W 1865 Lectures on the pathology and treatment of lateral and other forms of curvature of the spine. Churchill, London

American Orthopedic Association Research Committee 1941 End result study of the treatment of idiopathic scoliosis. Journal of Bone and Joint Surgery 23: 963–977

Andrew T A, Piggott H 1985 Growth arrest for progressive scoliosis. Journal of Bone and Joint Surgery 67B: 193–197

Archer I A, Dickson R A 1985 Stature and idiopathic scoliosis. A prospective study. Journal of Bone and Joint Surgery 67B: 185–188

Archer I A, Deacon P, Dickson R A 1986 Idiopathic scoliosis in Leeds – a management philosophy. Journal of Bone and Joint Surgery 68B: 670

Bengtsson G, Fallstrom K, Jansson B, Nachemson A 1974 A psychological and psychiatric investigation of the adjustment of female scoliosis patients. Acta Psychiatrica Scandinavica 50: 50–59

Blount W P, Moe J H 1973 The Milwaukee brace. Williams & Wilkins, Baltimore

Branthwaite M A 1986 Cardiorespiratory consequences of unfused idiopathic scoliosis. British Journal of Diseases of the Chest 80: 360–369

Cobb J R 1948 Outline for the study of scoliosis. American Academy of Orthopedic Surgeons Instructional Course Lectures 5: 261

Deacon P, Archer I A, Dickson R A 1987 The anatomy of spinal deformity: a biomechanical analysis. Orthopedics 10: 897–903

Dickson R A 1984 Screening for scoliosis. British Medical Journal 289: 269–270

Dickson R A 1987 Scoliosis: how big are you? Orthopedics 10: 881–887

Dickson R A, Archer I A 1987 Surgical treatment of late-onset idiopathic thoracic scoliosis. The Leeds procedure. Journal of Bone and Joint Surgery 69B: 709–714

Dickson R A 1999 Spinal deformity – adolescent idiopathic scoliosis: nonoperative treatment. Spine 24: 2601–2606

Dickson R A, Weinstein S L 1999 Bracing (and screening) – yes or no? Review Article. Journal of Bone and Joint Surgery 81B: 193–198

Dubousset J, Graf H, Miladi L, Cotrel Y 1986 Spinal and thoracic derotation with CD instrumentation. Orthopedic Transactions 10: 36

Dwyer A F, Newton N C, Sherwood A A 1969 An anterior approach to scoliosis: a preliminary report. Clinical Orthopaedics and Related Research 62: 192–202

Griss P, Harms J, Zielke K 1984 Ventral derotation spondylodesis (VDS). In: Dickson R A, Bradford D S (eds) Management of spinal deformities. Butterworths International Medical Reviews, London, pp 193–236

Harrenstein R J 1930 Die Skoliose bei Saueglingen und ihre Behandlung. Z Orthop Chir 52: 1–40

Harrington P R 1960 Surgical instrumentation for management of scoliosis. Journal of Bone and Joint Surgery 42A: 1448

Hibbs R A 1911 An operation for progressive spinal deformities. New York Medical Journal 93: 1013–1016

Hodgson A R 1973 Correction of kyphotic spinal deformities. Journal of Bone and Joint Surgery 55B: 211–212

Houghton G R, McInerney A, Tew A 1987 Brace compliance in adolescent idiopathic scoliosis. Journal of Bone and Joint Surgery 69B: 852

Howell F R, Dickson R A 1989 The deformity of idiopathic scoliosis made visible by computer graphics. Journal of Bone and Joint Surgery 71B: 399–403

Howell F R, Mahood J, Dickson R A 1992 Growth beyond skeletal maturity. Spine 17: 437–440

James J I P 1954 Idiopathic scoliosis: the prognosis, diagnosis, and operative indications related to curve patterns and the age at onset. Journal of Bone and Joint Surgery 36B: 36–49

Kopits S E, Perovic M N, McKusick V, Robinson R A 1972 Congenital atlanto-axial dislocations in various forms of dwarfism. Journal of Bone and Joint Surgery 54A: 1349–1350

Leatherman K D, Dickson R A 1979 Two-stage corrective surgery for congenital deformities of the spine. Journal of Bone and Joint Surgery 61B: 324–328

Leatherman K D, Dickson R A 1988 Management of spinal deformities. John Wright, Bristol

Lloyd-Roberts G C, Pilcher M F 1965 Structural idiopathic scoliosis in infancy. Journal of Bone and Joint Surgery 47B: 520–523

Luque E R 1982 The anatomic basis and development of segmental spinal instrumentation. Spine 7: 256–259

Mardia K V, Walder A N, Berry E, Sharples D, Millner P A, Dickson R A 1999 Assessing spinal shape. Journal of Applied Statistics 6: 735–745

Mau H 1968 Does infantile scoliosis require treatment? Journal of Bone and Joint Surgery 50B: 881

McMaster M J, Macnicol M F 1979 The management of progressive infantile idiopathic scoliosis. Journal of Bone and Joint Surgery 61B: 36–42

McMaster M J, Ohtsuka K 1982 The natural history of congenital scoliosis. A study of 251 patients. Journal of Bone and Joint Surgery 64A: 1128–1147

Mehta M H 1972 The rib vertebra angle in the early diagnosis between resolving and progressive infantile scoliosis. Journal of Bone and Joint Surgery 54B: 230–243

Mehta M H, Morel G 1979 The non-operative treatment of infantile idiopathic scoliosis. In: Zorab P A, Siegler D (eds) Scoliosis. Proceedings of the Sixth Symposium Academic London, pp 71–84

Miller J A, Nachemson A L, Schultz A B 1984 Effectiveness of braces in mild idiopathic scoliosis. Spine 9: 632–635

Millner P A, Dickson R A 1996 Idiopathic scoliosis: biomechanics and biology. Review Article. European Spine Journal 5: 362–373

Moe J H 1958 A critical analysis of methods of fusion for scoliosis. Journal of Bone and Joint Surgery 40A: 529–554

Moe J H, Kharrat K, Winter R, Cummine J L 1984 Harrington instrumentation without fusion plus external orthotic support for the treatment of difficult curvature problems in young children. Clinical Orthopaedics 185: 35–45

Nachemson A L 1968 A long term follow up study of non-treated scoliosis. Acta Orthopaedica Scandinavica 39: 466–476

Nachemson A L, Peterson L-E 1995 Effectiveness of treatment with a brace in girls who have adolescent idiopathic scoliosis. Journal of Bone and Joint Surgery 77A: 815–822

Nelson M A 1970 Orthopaedic aspects of the chondrodystrophies. The dwarf and his orthopaedic problems. Annals of the Royal College of Surgeons of England 47: 185–210

du Peloux J, Fauchet R, Faucon B, Stagnara P 1965 Le plan d'élection pour l'examen radiologique des cypho-scolioses. Revue de Chirurgie et Orthopédie 51: 517–524

Perdriolle R 1979 La scoliose – son étude tridimensionnelle. Maloine, Paris

Peterson L-E, Nachemson A L 1995 Prediction of progression of the curve in girls who have adolescent idiopathic scoliosis of moderate severity. Journal of Bone and Joint Surgery 77A: 823–827

Roaf R 1963 The treatment of progressive scoliosis by unilateral growth arrest. Journal of Bone and Joint Surgery 45B: 637–651

Scott J C, Morgan T H 1955 The natural history and prognosis of infantile idiopathic scoliosis. Journal of Bone and Joint Surgery 37B: 400–413

Somerville E W 1952 Rotational lordosis: the development of the single curve. Journal of Bone and Joint Surgery 34B: 421–427

Sorenson K H 1964 Scheuermann's juvenile kyphosis. Munksgaard, Copenhagen

Stirling A J, Howel D, Millner P A, Sadiq S, Sharples D, Dickson M A 1996 Late-onset idiopathic scoliosis in children six to fourteen years old. Journal of Bone and Joint Surgery 78A: 1330–1336

Verbout A J 1985 The development of the vertebral column. Springer, Berlin

Watts H G, Hall J E, Stanish W 1977 The Boston brace system for the treatment of low thoracic and lumbar

scoliosis by the use of a girdle without superstructure. Clinical Orthopaedics 126: 87–92

Whitby L G 1974 Screening for disease. Definitions and criteria. Lancet ii: 819–821

Wynne-Davies R 1975 Infantile idiopathic scoliosis. Journal of Bone and Joint Surgery 57B: 138–141

PART 3 Spondylolisthesis
R. A. Dickson

INTRODUCTION

Spondylolisthesis is the slipping forward of one vertebra and the spine above upon the vertebra immediately below. When the condition first received orthopaedic attention in the latter half of the 20th century, it was believed to be of congenital origin, but now it is recognised that several varieties exist, with most being acquired.

The International Society for Study of the Lumbar Spine proposed a classification (Wiltse et al 1976) that is now generally accepted. Five types are recognised:

- dysplastic
- isthmic
- degenerative
- traumatic
- pathological.

Degenerative spondylolisthesis affects the over-50-year-old age group and is attributable to instability of arthritic posterior facet joints. It is much more common in women, particularly at the L4–L5 level and, because the back of the spine is not left behind, it can lead to spinal stenosis.

Traumatic spondylolisthesis refers to forward subluxation of one vertebra upon another as the result of a fracture in a region other than the pars interarticularis, such as the pedicle; Taillard (1976) questioned whether this should be called spondylolisthesis, rather than simple traumatic vertebral subluxation.

Pathological spondylolisthesis may complicate a number of underlying conditions such as tuberculosis, giant-cell tumour, Paget's disease, rheumatoid disease, Albers-Schönberg disease, arthrogryposis, syphilis, and metastases.

In childhood, the dysplastic and isthmic varieties are encountered. Both forms are strongly familial, with almost one-third of first-degree relations having the same lesion (Wynne-Davies & Scott 1979).

ISTHMIC SPONDYLOLISTHESIS

The isthmus or pars interarticularis is the posterolateral bony element between the upper and lower articular processes. There are theoretically three subtypes of isthmic spondylolisthesis:

- lytic
- attenuation of the pars
- acute pars fracture.

However, there is little convincing evidence that acute pars fractures ever occur, and attenuation and elongation of the pars are seen only with dysplastic spondylolisthesis (Scott 1990). Therefore, for practical purposes 'isthmic spondylolisthesis' and 'lytic spondylolisthesis' are interchangeable terms.

The slippage in lytic spondylolisthesis is caused by a defect in the pars interarticularis (Fig. 31.43) (referred to as a spondylolysis). The development of this defect was originally believed to be congenital, but lyses are now considered to be fatigue or stress fractures in what has been shown biomechanically to be the weakest part of the neural arch (Shah et al 1978). Although lyses have been noted in children younger than 2 years, these lesions do not generally develop until after the age of 5 years, with an increasing prevalence rate from 1–2% at this young end of the age

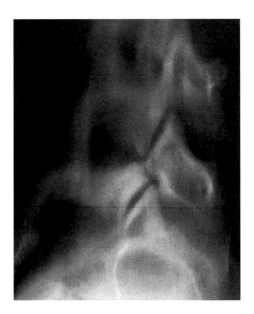

Figure 31.43 Obligue tomogram of the lower lumbar spine, showing a lysis in the L5 pars interarticularis. Oblique plain films are much less reliable; if there is any doubt about the integrity of the pars, oblique tomograms or CT should be taken.

spectrum to a constant 6–7% in the adult population, except in Alaskans who have a prevalence rate in excess of 50%. Slippage (spondylolisthesis) probably only occurs in 10–20% of those with lyses. These fatigue fractures are much more common in those who pursue a particularly active life. Among gymnasts, lyses occur in more than 10% and spondylolisthesis in 6% (Jackson et al 1976). Of course, these prevalence rates are derived from anteroposterior (AP) and lateral plain films of the spine and thus if, for example, oblique tomograms or three-dimensional computed tomography (CT) reconstructions were carried out, these rates could probably be comfortably doubled, if not more. In contrast, the condition does not occur in those who, because of physical handicap, have never walked.

During childhood, the lysis is filled with cartilage in which there are zones of endochondral ossification. Thus there is considerable potential for healing. Despite this, there is an increasing prevalence rate throughout growth. Once adulthood is reached, the nature of the spondylolysis changes towards that of a fracture non-union with hypertrophic callus (Fig. 31.44), with little or no spontaneous healing potential. This explains the constant prevalence rate at maturity. In the adult, the appearance of the lytic defect should not therefore be misinterpreted as a gap, but rather as a mass lesion that may irritate the local nerve root. Radicular symptoms from lyses are not uncommon in the adult, but are rare in the immature.

In the lumbar spine, forces are concentrated at the pars, particularly at the L5–S1 level, which is by far the most common site for spondylolisthesis (Shah et al 1978). Should L5, however, be relatively low-slung below the level of the iliac crests and with broad, strong transverse processes, it is protected and the level above is relatively unprotected, producing an L4–L5 lytic spondylolisthesis. Individuals with type II Scheuermann's disease (thoraco-lumbar kyphosis or 'apprentice's spine') have a much greater incidence of lower lumbar lyses, and these may be multiple.

When slippage occurs, the vertebral body in front of the lyses moves forwards and leaves the back of the spinal arch behind. The spinal canal is therefore locally more capacious, quite unlike degenerative spondylolisthesis, and the step that is visible or palpable is at the junction of the slipped vertebra with the one above. Because the canal is large and the lyses cartilaginous, neurological symptoms and signs are clinically very unusual.

As lytic spondylolisthesis is an acquired condition, both L5 and S1 are reasonably well formed and the slippage tends to be forwards in the sagittal plane, without much in the way of local angular kyphosis (Fig. 31.45).

DYSPLASTIC SPONDYLOLISTHESIS

Originally termed 'congenital', dysplastic spondylolisthesis is caused by hypoplasia or aplasia of the L5–S1 facet joints. The back of the spine is not left behind, so that the AP canal diameter is proportionately reduced. Interestingly, however, only a modest degree of slippage occurs (not usually more than 25% of the sagittal width of the top of the sacrum) before a secondary spondylolysis develops in the pars of L5 which, although allowing further slippage to take place, does not further jeopardise the size of the spinal canal. Therefore, as with lytic spondylolisthesis, neurological symptoms and signs are unusual. It is only when secondary spondylolysis complicates dysplastic spondylolisthesis that attenuation of the pars can be seen before a frank spondylolysis develops (Scott 1990).

Because the condition is congenital and develops at an earlier age than lytic spondylolisthesis, the body of L5 and the upper sacrum may be considerably deformed. L5 becomes increasingly wedge-shaped and the upper sacrum rounds off. Furthermore, in dysplastic spondylolisthesis there is always a spina bifida occulta of L5 or S1 and the sacrum appears more open than normal. It is these X-ray features on both AP and lateral projections that clearly

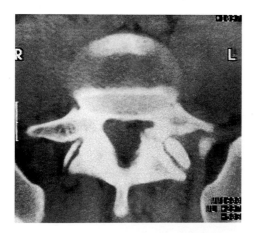

Figure 31.44 CT scan through the pars interarticularis of L5 in a professional cricketer with left L5 radicular pain. There is a lysis on the left side, which appears as a fracture non-union with hypertrophic callus irritating the L5 root.

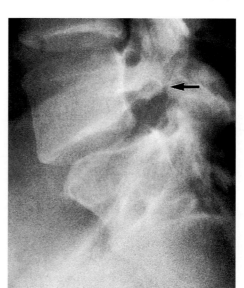

Figure 31.45 Lateral radiograph of the lower lumbar spine, showing a mild L5–S1 slip caused by bilateral lyses (arrowed).

differentiate the dysplastic from the lytic variety (Fig. 31.46). Because the L5 and S1 vertebrae are reciprocally misshapen, the slippage in dysplastic spondylolisthesis is very much more in the nature of a progressive kyphosis than a simple slip forwards in the sagittal plane.

MEASUREMENT

It has become the accepted standard to measure the degree of spondylolisthesis on a standing lateral radiograph (Wiltse & Winter 1983). Although a variety of measurements have been described, two are of particular value:

1. The extent of anterior displacement or slip.
2. The angle of sagittal rotation, also know as the sagittal roll, slip angle, or lumbo-sacral kyphosis (Fig. 31.47).

The *extent of anterior displacement* is the distance between the posterior cortex of L5 and the posterior cortex of S1, expressed as a percentage of the anteroposterior diameter of S1.

A more important clinical correlation is the *angle of sagittal rotation*, which is the relationship between L5 and S1 as subtended by lines drawn parallel to the anterior cortex of L5 and the posterior cortex of S1. The important clinical deformity in spondylolisthesis is lumbo-sacral kyphosis, and the angle of sagittal rotation more accurately defines the clinical problem, as a very considerable lytic spondylolisthesis with, say, a 75% slip purely in the sagittal plane may produce no clinical deformity whatever.

CLINICAL FEATURES

Patients present as a result of pain, deformity, neurological symptoms, hamstring tightness and gait abnormality. The low back pain is mechanical, being worse during activity and hyperextension and relieved by rest. The pain is often referred to the buttock and thigh, but rarely with radicular distribution into the leg. Hamstring spasm or contracture is commonly associated with the more severe degrees of spondylolisthesis, particularly of the dysplastic variety, in which progressive lumbo-sacral kyphosis leads to relative flexion of the hip and knee; in severe degrees of slippage, there is frank hamstring contracture over and above any spasm induced by local discomfort. As the lumbo-sacral kyphosis progresses and the hips and knees take up a Z-deformity, posture becomes increasingly more distressing. Occasionally, with spondyloptosis, the L5 body finishes anterior to the first sacral segment, allowing the upper posterior corner of S1 to indent the canal, producing symptoms of spinal claudication and leg fatigue (Fig. 31.48). Otherwise, the only other neurological symptom encountered is occasional radicular pain in the same nerve root as the slipping vertebra (i.e. L5 for an L5–S1 slip and L4 for an L4–L5 slip).

Above the lumbo-sacral kyphosis, a compensatory thoraco-lumbar hyperlordosis may develop, with an anterior skin crease at umbilical level (Fig. 31.49). Thus from the top of the spine down to the feet a gradually increasing Z-deformity can occur. Neurological examination is usually normal, but attention should be directed to the relevant nerve root. During adolescence, these children may suffer a spondylolisthetic 'crisis' (Scott 1990), with profound muscle spasm such that patients can be deformed in the frontal plane in addition to their lateral profile (Fig. 31.50). Lesions at the L4–L5 level tend to have a worse prognosis than those at the L5–S1 level, in terms of both irritability and progression.

TREATMENT

As with most orthopaedic conditions, there is a considerable divergence of opinion as to how patients should be treated.

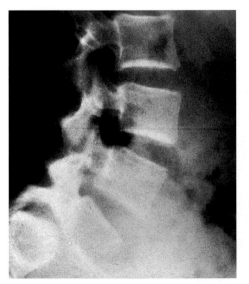

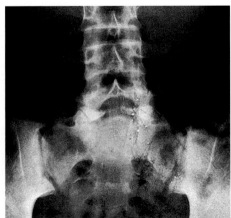

Figure 31.46 Lateral (**A**) and AP (**B**) radiographs of the lower lumbar spine, showing the typical appearances of dysplastic spondylolisthesis of L5 and S1. Note the lumbo-sacral kyphosis and the spina bifida occulta of L5.

A   B

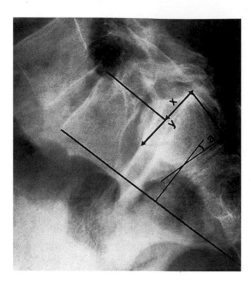

Figure 31.47 Lateral radiograph of the lower lumbar spine, showing the two most useful measures of the degree of displacement: Taillard's percentage slippage (x/y) and the slip angle (angle 'a').

Recent years have seen an exponential increase in the use of operative surgery, particularly in the nature of attempted reduction with transpedicular instrumentation in addition to biological fusion. In many countries, such techniques are currently accepted as 'standard', but there is no convincing evidence that patients fare better.

There is a place for both conservative and operative

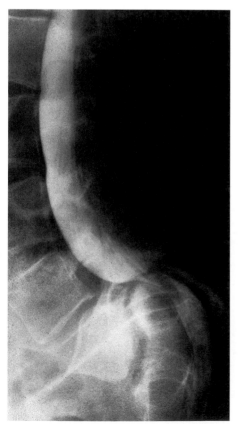

Figure 31.48 Lateral myelogram in a case of spondyloptosis, showing thecal impingement by the upper back corner of S1.

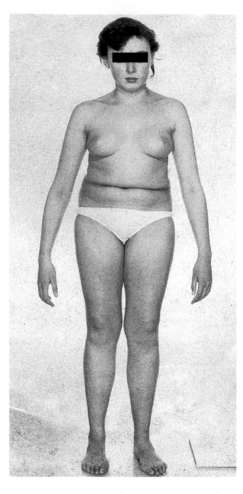

Figure 31.49 The anterior umbilical skin crease typical of severe lumbosacral kyphosis.

management. For the immature with a spondylolysis and considerable potential for healing, an expectant policy should be pursued. The child presenting with mechanical low back pain whose plain X-rays indicate no obvious abnormality and in whom there is no suspicion of any underlying bone destructive lesion (e.g. absence of night pain) should have oblique films taken of the lumbar spine and oblique tomograms, if necessary, to confirm the diagnosis. CT scanning with the gantry angle appropriate for the pars (Fig. 31.44) rather than the intervertebral disc is useful for demonstrating spondylolyses by three-dimensional reconstruction. Spondylolyses with active cartilaginous endochondral ossification zones can be detected with isotope bone scanning.

Many patients with mechanical low back pain do not have a satisfactory diagnosis even after exhaustive investigation, and it is important to bear in mind the possibility of a spondylolysis. As patients approach maturity, they are also vulnerable to intervertebral disc derangements and the two can frequently coexist. Therefore in the older adolescent it is important to take a careful history, with particular reference to nerve root compression. Exuberant tissue around the spondylolysis may compress the local nerve root (L5 for the L5–S1 level) – the same root that will be affected by an L4–L5 disc prolapse; it is therefore quite wrong to rush in to surgical treatment at the level of the

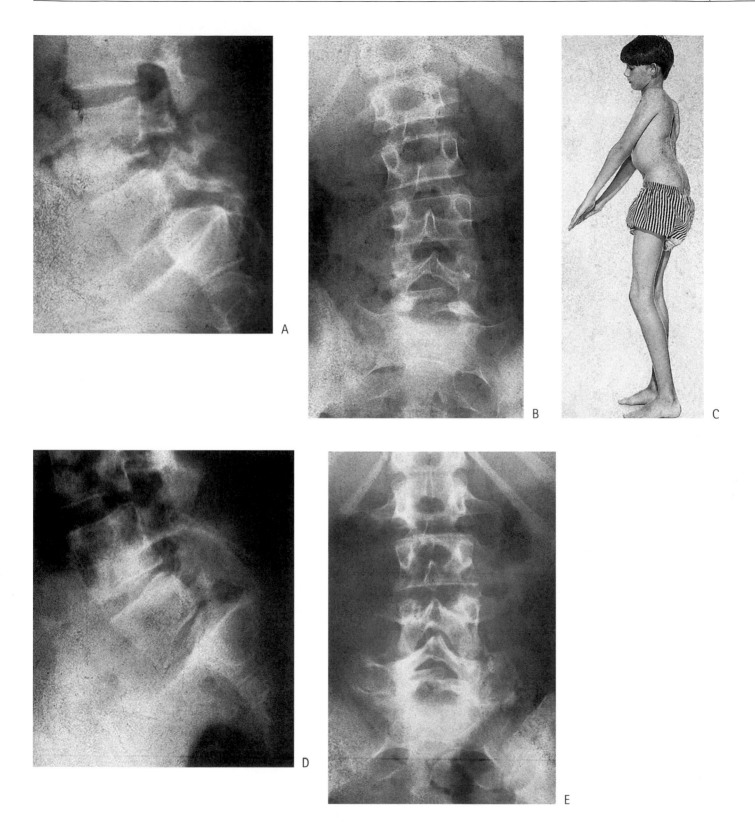

Figure 31.50 A and **B** Lateral and AP radiographs of a boy with moderately severe dysplastic spondylolisthesis with an obvious scoliosis caused by asymmetric muscle spasm. **C** Clinical photograph showing the asymmetric hyperlordotic spasm above the lumbo-sacral kyphosis (the adolescent crisis). **D** and **E** Lateral and AP radiographs after Scaglietti closed-cast treatment and bilateral alar-transverse fusion. There is a solid fusion, and the muscle spasm has been completely abolished.

spondylolisthesis without careful imaging of the adjacent motion segments.

As the majority of spondylolyses heal, or at least become asymptomatic with the passage of time, the condition should be treated symptomatically. Wiltse has a very considerable experience of spondylolysis and spondylolisthesis and advises that treatment of a spondylolysis or a spondylolisthesis of less than 25% should be confined to a period of rest for the acute exacerbation (Wiltse & Jackson 1976). If the degree of slip is less than 50%, sporting activities are not restricted. A concern to many is the risk of further slippage if surgical treatment is not carried out, but long-term studies have shown that progressive slippage occurs only during the first few years (Wiltse & Jackson 1976). If the degree of slippage is 30% or less at presentation, then further slipping is unusual.

If a child has a slip of more than 50% or intractable local symptoms, spinal fusion is indicated. Wiltse & Jackson (1976) advise bilateral intertransverse fusion *in situ* without instrumentation, and have reported excellent results in 90% of cases. Bilateral intertransverse fusion is preferred to either anterior or posterior fusion, for both biomechanical and clinical reasons (Lee & Langrana 1984). The fusion rate is greater and further slippage after surgery is unusual. For those with neurological symptoms, nerve root decompression and removal of the loose, 'rattle' fragment can be performed, but Wiltse & Jackson state that these symptoms always resolve with a solid fusion. Interbody fusion should be reserved for the occasional patient in whom bilateral intertransverse fusion has failed; although usually performed anteriorly, this procedure can also be performed posteriorly (Cloward 1963).

Wiltse & Jackson (1976) also demonstrated clearly that lumbar and hamstring muscle spasm resolve with solid fusion, and body shape improves without the need for reduction. The more severe the slip, and the more severe the clinical disability, the more tempting is the desire to correct the condition surgically. However, with lytic spondylolisthesis the deformity is seldom significant, and what muscle spasm exists in the erector spinae or hamstrings settles with a sound fusion. As lumbo-sacral kyphosis is more important than percentage slip, reduction is particularly attractive in significant dysplastic spondylolisthesis. In 1932, Capener first attempted open reduction of a spondylolisthesis, and since then various open and closed techniques have been advanced. In 1969, Harrington used his scoliosis instrumentation in an effort to reduce spondylolisthesis, and designed and implanted transpedicular screws attached to his rods in an unsuccessful attempt to correct the position of the displaced vertebrae (Harrington & Tullos 1971). Segmental wiring techniques became popular and were followed by staged anterior and posterior multiple procedures, some of which corrected the slippage at the expense of the L5 nerve root (Bradford 1979).

It would seem logical to try closed reduction first and, if that fails and reduction is still considered important, to proceed to operative reduction. The Scaglietti closed-cast system can be very effective, although it is time consuming for the patient (Scaglietti et al 1976). A localiser cast similar to that used for scoliosis is applied under traction on a Risser–Cotrel table, with the spine extended at the lumbo-sacral region as much as can be tolerated. The addition of a spica round one thigh maintains the spine–pelvis relation-

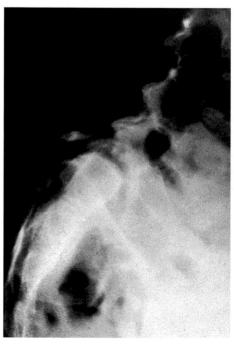 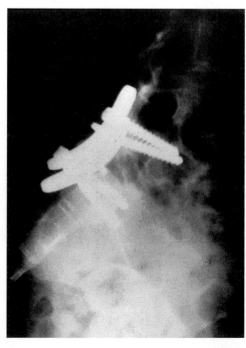

Figure 31.51 A Preoperative lateral lower lumbar radiograph showing a severe L5–S1 dysplastic spondylolisthesis, verging on spondyloptosis. **B** Lateral radiograph after partial reduction and fusion using transpedicular instrumentation.

A   B

ship. Lateral X-rays taken before and after casting demonstrate whether a reduction is being achieved. Further casts are applied over the ensuing weeks until no further correction is obtained, then bilateral intertransverse fusion is performed in the cast, which is retained until the fusion consolidates (Fig. 31.50).

Should this technique be unsuccessful, operative reduction can be achieved, but it is necessary to visualise clearly the L5 nerve roots during the procedure. In fact, the instability produced locally by thorough visualisation of the L5 roots from cauda equina to foramen allows a degree of reduction to occur spontaneously on the operating table, and the subsequent application of metalwork maintains the reduced position rather than achieving it. Transpedicular instrumentation is the best way of securing the reduced position (Fig. 31.51).

The end-point of surgical treatment for spondylolisthesis has to be a sound spinal fusion, and the addition of rigid internal fixation may enhance the fusion rate. While there are distinct advantages in rigidly fixing the spine internally, from the point of view of earlier mobility without a cumbersome cast, it has to be asked that, if a Wiltse-type fusion *in situ* without metalwork produces a fusion in over 90% of cases, can the addition of metalwork be regarded as either justified or advantageous?

REFERENCES

Bradford D S 1979 Treatment of severe spondylolisthesis. A combined approach for reduction and stabilisation. Spine 4: 423–429

Capener N 1932 Spondylolisthesis. British Journal of Surgery 19: 374–386

Cloward R B 1963 Lesions of the intervertebral disks and their treatment by interbody fusion methods. Clinical Orthopaedics and Related Research 27: 51–77

Harrington P R, Tullos H S 1971 Spondylolisthesis in children. Observations and surgical treatment. Clinical Orthopaedics and Related Research 79: 75–84

Jackson D W, Wiltse L L, Cirincione R J 1976 Spondylolysis in the female gymnast. Clinical Orthopaedics 117: 68–73

Lee C K, Langrana N A 1984 Lumbosacral spinal fusion. A biomechanical study. Spine 9: 574–581

Scaglietti O, Frontino C, Bartolozzi P 1976 Technique of anatomical reduction of lumbar spondylolisthesis and its surgical stabilisation. Clinical Orthopaedics and Related Research 117: 164–175

Scott J H S 1990 Spondylolisthesis. In: Dickson R A (ed) Spinal surgery: science and practice. Butterworths, London, ch 22, pp 353–367

Shah J S, Hampson W G J, Jayson M I V 1978 The distribution of surface strain in the cadaveric lumbar spine. Journal of Bone and Joint Surgery 60B: 246–251

Taillard W F 1976 Etiology of spondylolisthesis. Clinical Orthopaedics and Related Research 117: 30–39

Wiltse L L, Jackson D W 1976 Treatment of spondylolisthesis and spondylolysis in children. Clinical Orthopaedics and Related Research 117: 92–100

Wiltse L L, Winter R B 1983 Terminology and measurement of spondylolisthesis. Journal of Bone and Joint Surgery 65A: 768–772

Wiltse L L, Newman P H, Macnab I 1976 Classification of spondylolysis and spondylolisthesis. Clinical Orthopaedics and Related Research 117: 23–29

Wynne-Davies R, Scott J H S 1979 Inheritance and spondylolisthesis. A radiographic family survey. Journal of Bone Joint Surgery 61B: 301–305

Chapter 32

Principles of fracture care

M. F. Macnicol

INTRODUCTION

In childhood, bone has certain characteristics that are quantitatively different from those of the adult. First, the modulus of elasticity is relatively high, and the thick periosteal sleeve adds further resistance to complete fracturing. Hence buckle (torus) and greenstick fractures are relatively common, although they may be more extensive than plain radiographs suggest. Second, it should be appreciated that bone tends to give way before ligament in the prepubertal child: apophyses and other bony points of soft-tissue attachment avulse before the tendon ruptures or the ligament tears.

The aetiology of paediatric fractures is discussed by Lennart Landin (see Ch. 33); to some extent, it is culturally determined. The incidence of skeletal injury varies geographically and between urban and rural communities. In temperate countries, seasonal variations and alteration in the hours of daylight also affect fracture patterns. Epidemiological studies are important, as they identify trends and hazards in relation to our increasingly congested roads, to playgrounds where safety precautions are often lacking, and to sporting and social activities such as the 'craze' for skateboarding. In the first year of life, the frequency of fracturing is equivalent in the two sexes, but boys are twice as likely to fracture during late childhood and adolescence, just as they are more than twice as likely to die from severe injury. Pathological changes in the skeleton may predispose to fracture and are dealt with later in this chapter.

CHARACTERISTICS OF FRACTURES

The sites of bone injury in the child differ from those in the adult, and the most important difference relates to the fact that the bones of a child are actively growing. A paediatric fracture possesses greater potential to unite quickly and to remodel deformity. Whereas approximately 1 in 6 fractures are initially angulated more than 20° after reduction and splintage, 5 years after the injury this figure reduces to approximately 1 in 40. This capacity to realign depends principally upon the reorientation of the epiphysis and growth plate as the bone elongates.

In addition to the tropic change in physeal growth (Fig. 32.1), which accounts for the majority of the correction, differential periosteal activity produces remodelling of the shaft, but does not supplement the growth plate realignment (Friberg 1979).

Correction of malalignment is more likely:

- in the younger child
- the nearer the fracture is to the epiphyseal plate
- if the deformity is angulated in the plane of joint movement.

The history of growth and correction of malalignment is of interest. The monographs of Poland (1898), König (1908), Aitken (1935) and Blount (1954) recorded the pathophysiology of epiphyseal injury and the subsequent physeal response. The speed of correction is exponential rather than linear, and appears to be the result of the redistribution of loading through the growth plate. Little correction occurs if the primary angulation is less than 5°; in contrast, malalignment of more than 20° will usually not correct completely (Fig. 32.2). The correction rate is about 1° per month, but the precise mechanism of this tropic change is unknown. Pauwels (1975) considered that increased pressure on the growth plate results in a stimulus to growth. This may explain the correction of genu varum in the toddler and the eventual lessening of valgus after a proximal tibial metaphyseal fracture. However, it is also known that longitudinal tension across the plate will decrease its growth rate, and Crilly (1972) suggested that the periosteal sleeve may control axial growth by 'reining in' the physis. Whatever the mechanism, the epiphysis tends to reorientate until it lies at 90° to the axial forces passing up the limb.

MANAGEMENT

Although paediatric fractures unite rapidly and are rarely associated with major complications, several management problems may be encountered. The young child, in particular, may be fretful and difficult to examine fully. Worried parents and a crying child pose problems for even the most experienced clinician.

Many fractures are difficult to see, and therefore imaging must be of good quality. In addition to standard anteroposterior and lateral views of the injured site, oblique views and special projections should be requested in cases of uncertainty, particularly at the elbow and the ankle. Radiographs of the opposite, uninjured limb and discussion with the radiologist will improve accuracy. It should be appreciated that fractures missed in the Accident & Emergency department constitute a major source of complaints and possible litigation.

Osteochondral fractures may be seen adequately only by tomography or digital radiography, and it may be ecessary to request arthrography, computed tomography,

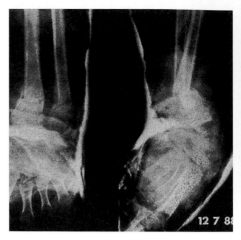
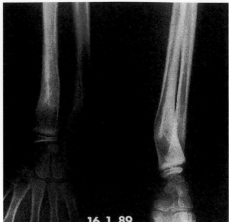
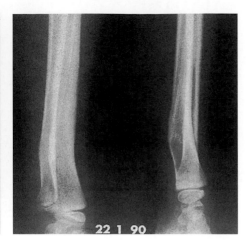

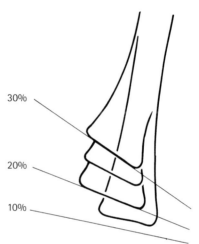

Figure 32.1 The growth plate gradually realigns the epiphysis if anatomical reduction is not achieved. This process will not correct the deformity fully if angulation is excessive.

three-dimensional reconstruction or magnetic resonance imaging. More sophisticated investigation is hampered by the need to sedate or anaesthetise the child.

Once a fracture has been identified, its site and degree of displacement determine whether reduction, and possibly internal fixation, are required. No firm prescription can be given in terms of angulation and malposition. However, as a

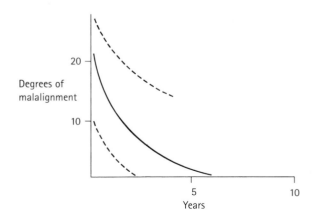

Figure 32.2 Growth plate correction of malalignment is maximal in the first year, proceeding at a rate of approximately 1° per month.

general rule, angulation of more than 10° is unacceptable, particularly in the diaphysis and in the older child. Rotational malalignment should be corrected fully, but the overgrowth that follows long-bone fracture makes an overlap at the fracture site of 1.0–2.0 cm acceptable. When dealing with femoral shaft fractures, an overgrowth of 0.5–1.0 cm can be expected. No more than 10° of varus and 15° of valgus should be accepted, and this presupposes at least 3 years of further skeletal growth in the femur or tibia.

The 'three Rs' of management are:

1. Realign the fracture.
2. Respect the soft tissue.
3. Remember the patient.

These apply to children as much as to adults, although the alignment of long-bone fractures can be slightly less precise and still allow good function eventually.

Disruptions of the growth plate (physis) account for 15–20% of all paediatric fractures. This proportion is an underestimate, because metaphyseal cracks may propagate into the growth plate (Peterson 1994), but may be missed on the X-ray. Growth plate injury is very common in the phalanges or at the distal radius, so that approximately 70% of all these fractures occur in the upper limb. The distal tibia accounts for just under 10% of the total, and the distal femur 1–2%.

A fracture through the growth plate occurs at the zone of hypertrophy: shear produces varying degrees of displacement at the weakest site in the physis, where the matrix is minimal and the cells largest (Haas 1945). The resistance to shearing or angulation is enhanced by the surrounding tissues, principally the periosteum and the musculoligamentous cuff. Of greater importance is the intrinsic structure of the growth plate, including the mammillary or small, cone-shaped projections that interdigitate with the metaphysis, and the overlapping edge (lappet) of the peripheral physis, which fits like a cap upon the ossified metaphysis. Surrounding the physis is the groove of Ranvier, which consists of undifferentiated cells capable of increasing the circumference of the growth plate and of anchoring the plate to the perichondrial sheath. A further fibrous band, the perichondrial ring of Lacroix, attaches to the groove of Ranvier (Rang 1969) and acts as a protective sleeve; this weakens as the skeleton matures. The combination of the Salter–Harris classification and the identification of mechanisms of injury, such as the Lauge-Hanson classification for ankle fractures, allows greater appreciation of the three-dimensional displacement and the best technique for closed reduction (Dias & Giergerich 1983).

As a rule immediate reduction of the fracture is the ideal, and unnecessary delay in treatment of supracondylar humeral fractures, for example, should be avoided. General anaesthesia is required if manipulation of the fracture is necessary and the child and parent should be warned that a further manipulation may be required later in the first week. It is important to recognise the presence of a periosteal hinge, which allows the fracture to be thumbed back into position after increasing the initial angulatory deformity. Gross swelling may make it advisable to apply skin traction and elevate the limb initially. This technique may gradually produce a satisfactory reduction or pave the way for a later closed or open reduction. The positioning of the injured limb is important in order to hasten the return of function, as is the choice of external splints and the timing of their removal.

Circulatory compromise is relatively common, particularly when dealing with supracondylar humeral fractures, with forearm fractures and with fractures involving the femur and tibia. The development of a compartment syndrome must be recognised early: wick catheter studies suggest that pressures of 30 mm of mercury for more than 8 hours (Rorabeck & Clarke 1978) regularly produce nerve and, later, muscle injury. Sensory loss, pain on passive movement and discomfort despite splitting the plaster should encourage early fasciotomy. Distal pallor and an absent pulse are indicative of major arterial injury, but a compartment syndrome can occur in the presence of apparently satisfactory distal circulation.

After fracture reduction and the application of a suitable splint, the position should be monitored carefully with further radiographs. Displacement usually occurs during the first week and hence clinic review must be ensured during this period. Any change of plaster should be accompanied by check X-rays. It is important to encourage weight bearing as soon as possible after lower limb fracture; there is no proof that this increases the likelihood of angulation. Algodystrophy and psychological difficulties occasionally complicate limb fractures in children, and satisfactory function is by no means assured where there has been extensive soft-tissue injury and vascular impairment.

The injured child rarely succumbs to the effects of multiple fractures alone: associated trauma to the brain and spinal cord, the viscera or uncontrolled haemorrhage are usually responsible (see Ch. 34). Post-traumatic sepsis, pulmonary insufficiency or renal failure are relatively rare in children. Nevertheless, polytrauma does occur and the same rules of resuscitation apply as with the adult. Ventilatory difficulties or cardiovascular collapse can occur with alarming rapidity, and the ABC rule of 'airway protection, breathing and circulatory support' must be observed. Assisted ventilation may be required initially after multiple trauma, but must be carefully monitored, as must colloid replacement.

The wound demands the same careful management as in the adult. Wound toilet includes excision of devitalised skin, fat, fascia and muscle, the removal of fragments of avascular bone, thorough irrigation, and the avoidance of skin tension when closing the tissues. Delayed primary closure should be mandatory for any contaminated wound associated with a fracture.

The following grading scale (Matter & Rittman 1978) reflects injury severity:

- type 1: a spike of bone piercing the skin from within outwards, causing a circumscribed soft-tissue wound.
- type 2: an appreciable wound in association with a fracture, including contusion of the surrounding skin and muscle. The extent of comminution and soft-tissue damage is difficult to quantitate.
- type 3: vitality of the limb is threatened by vessel and nerve damage, with significant contamination, skin loss and functional deficit.

Gustilo et al (1984) have recommended a further division of the type 3 open fracture into three subgroups, which are also applicable to the child:

- type 3a: the fracture site still covered with soft tissue, although skin may be extensively lacerated
- type 3b: bone is exposed as a result of extensive soft-tissue loss and periosteal stripping, usually in association with significant contamination
- type 3c: an open fracture is associated with an arterial injury that requires repair and threatens limb salvage.

Compartment syndrome influences recovery and is probably more common in the open fracture than when there is no wound. External fixation is appropriate for the severely compound fracture, particularly in the presence of bone loss. Buckley et al (1990) reported a series of children managed with external fixation and noted that tibial overgrowth may be a concern.

Overgrowth after a long-bone fracture is a well-known

problem, particularly in the lower limb. Reynolds (1981) considered that this was due to increased vascularity at the time of healing, and that the compensatory mechanism thereafter was minimal. The stimulus occurs principally in the first 18 months after trauma, although a further 25% of overgrowth may occur in the subsequent 18 months. Shapiro (1981) found that there was a continual, slight overgrowth until maturity, or certainly for the first 4 years after the fracture. There is no clear influence from the dominant limb, and anatomical reduction with internal fixation does not appear to increase the overgrowth. Boys appear to produce a greater degree of overgrowth than girls, although this is an inconstant feature. It is best to allow a 1 cm overlap at the time of fracture splintage or traction, to accommodate overgrowth of around 1–2 cm. A certain amount of increased growth will also occur in the ipsilateral uninjured bone of the leg, whether tibia or femur.

Throughout the convalescent period, the parents and child should be kept fully informed of any developments, particularly the concern that further manipulation or even internal fixation may be required. Epiphyseal plate injuries should be reviewed carefully for subsequent growth arrest, which may be either temporary or permanent. The Salter–Harris (Salter & Harris 1963) type V, and sometimes type II, fracture may appear innocent initially, but the effects of growth arrest become increasingly obvious with time.

The problem of growth arrest is dealt with in Chapter 35. Type III and IV fractures should be treated by open reduction, as late as 5 or 7 days after the fracture if necessary. Transepiphyseal fixation is safe and it is advisable to excise the periosteum in order to prevent peripheral bridging. When growth arrest occurs from a bridging bar of bone, the periphery is involved in approximately 60% of cases (type I), whereas the central (type II) tether occurs in approximately 20% of cases. A combination of patterns (type III) occur in a further 20%.

Surgical procedures to excise the bar must be carried out with precision after preliminary imaging, particularly computed tomography. At least 50% of the growth plate should be normal, although radiographic projections of the affected area may exaggerate the bulk of the bar (Fig. 32.3). If this surgery is to be effective, it should be carried out with at least 2 years of potential growth available. Langenskiöld & Österman (1983) pointed out that bone shortening may be treated by a lengthening procedure or contralateral epiphysiodesis, and that angular deformity can be realigned by osteotomy or frame distraction. However, these procedures do not prevent the deformation of the joint, which always follows partial closure of a growth plate if the malalignment is allowed to progress (Fig. 32.4).

Baeza Giner & Oliete Sanz (1980) studied the use of interposition materials after the excision of an osseous bar. They considered that fat was more effective than the silastic sheet promoted by Bright (1974) and also stated that methyl methacrylate cement (Mallet 1975) caused growth disturbance in its own right. More recently, interest has centred

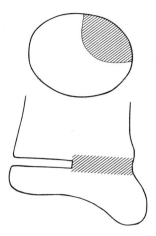

Figure 32.3 Radiographic projections of a growth tether (osseous bar) will tend to exaggerate the size of the bone bridge. Computed tomography affords a more accurate portrayal of the tether.

upon the use of transphyseal fixation using biodegradable pins made of a self-reinforced polyglycolide (Bostman et al 1989). These pins have a diameter of 1.5 mm and can be inserted across the physis because the surface is 1.8 mm² and therefore within the experimentally observed safe limit of 3% of the growth plate area (Mäkelä et al 1987).

Finally, osteoarticular fractures are now being treated more effectively. The structure of juvenile articular cartilage is better defined, and it is appreciated that this tissue has a capacity for healing by gradual creeping substitution. Fibrous tissue is produced initially, to be replaced by fibrocartilage. The inflammatory response from the local haematoma produces granulation tissue, which is gradually organised. After internal fixation (see later in this chapter), the implant should be removed at some stage: in childhood this is advised after 6–12 months, although in the older child the implant may be left *in situ* for longer. The removal of metal from the skeleton is not without hazard, particularly if it becomes buried within the substance of bone or requires extensive dissection. Its removal, therefore, is sometimes unwise, particularly in the forearm or around the knee.

INDICATIONS FOR INTERNAL FIXATION

Many aspects of fracture management in children are discussed in other chapters of this book. The indications for operating upon a fracture in this age group are limited and remain a source of debate. However, it is instructive to focus upon those injuries that cause difficulties if managed conservatively, and the problems of nursing care, delayed mobility, residual deformity and, occasionally, of joint stiffness. For a more extensive discussion about the conservative versus the operative management of children's fractures, recommended reading should include the textbooks by Ogden (1982), Rang (1983) and Rockwood et al (1996).

Three fundamental criteria determine whether a fracture should be dealt with surgically:

- the condition of the child
- the age of the child
- the nature of the fracture.

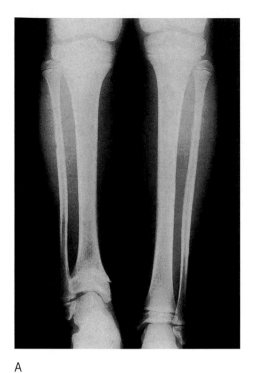

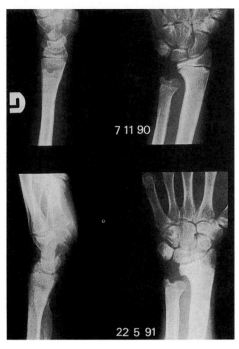

Figure 32.4 A The alignment of a joint surface is significantly affected by growth plate arrest, in addition to the inevitable shortening.
B Disproportionate growth of the forearm bones after physeal injury (7 11 90) may be checked by distal radial epiphysiodesis (22 5 91), but a later ulnar lengthening is the only means of improving the radio-ulnar relationship.

A

B

CONDITION OF THE CHILD

The clinical condition influences the decision about internal fixation, either because the injuries pose problems in effective nursing and rehabilitation (e.g. in polytrauma (Loder 1987) or severe head injury with behavioural disturbance) or because a pre-existing disorder makes conservative management difficult. Some children with skeletal dysplasias, including osteogenesis imperfecta and fibrous dysplasia, cerebral palsy associated with gross muscle spasm, and mental retardation with uncontrollable behaviour, are better managed if the fracture is securely reduced and internally fixed at the outset. Pathological fractures of any sort should be considered for operative treatment; this subject is considered later in this chapter. Occasionally, obesity or the social circumstances of a child will determine in part whether surgical treatment is appropriate.

AGE OF THE CHILD

Internal fixation is indicated more often in the adolescent, particularly if the growth plates are closing. In practice, this means that girls older than 12 years old and boys older than 14 years old may be considered as adults, particularly when dealing with difficult long-bone fractures. Primary or delayed internal fixation should therefore be considered for the following reasons:

1. Impractical or failed manipulative reduction.
2. Redisplacement of the fracture, whether early or late.
3. Multiple injuries, particularly ipsilateral femoral and tibial fractures ('the floating knee').

4. Significant arterial or neurological damage where a stable limb is essential for repair.
5. Rare instances of delayed union, such as the femoral neck and the lateral condyle of the humerus.

These criteria also apply to the younger child, but less frequently. The surgical decision is influenced by the inclinations of the surgeon, the facilities available, and sometimes by the opinion of the parents, as well as by the fracture itself. If safe anaesthesia, surgical skill, fixation devices and blood products are found wanting, conservative management may be safer.

NATURE OF THE FRACTURE

The clinical characteristics of a fracture are determined by:

- its site in the bone
- its behaviour.

Before a discussion of the specific anatomical sites at which fixation is often advisable, factors affecting fracture behaviour should be considered. Oblique, comminuted or pathological fractures are usually unstable, and their control may be achieved only by internal fixation. If there is additional bone loss or type III compounding (see Ch. 34), external fixation may be required, at least initially. Fracture reduction may be obstructed by the surrounding soft tissues as a result of:

1. Buttonholing through muscle or fascia (lower femoral shaft, clavicle, proximal humerus).
2. Periosteal entrapment (proximal tibia).
3. Joint incarceration (medial humeral epicondyle, talus).

Nerve entrapment in the fracture site should also be suspected, particularly in the upper limb at the mid-humeral level, around the elbow, and in the mid-forearm where nerve trunks in relatively anchored sites are close to bare areas of bone between muscle attachments (Macnicol 1978). Muscle contraction may displace fractures, producing an unacceptable gap (olecranon and other avulsion injuries) or malalignment (single or double forearm fractures, subtrochanteric femoral fractures).

INTERNAL FIXATION

The sites at which fractures may need internal fixation will be considered briefly. Further details are presented in later chapters.

UPPER LIMB

Shoulder girdle

The clavicle may be fractured at birth and must be differentiated from congenital pseudarthrosis and cleidocranial dysostosis. Brachial plexus injuries (see Ch. 21) may be sustained in association with the fracture, but fixation is never indicated. In the older child, fixation may be required for the relatively rare outer one-third fracture (Fig. 32.5), lateral to the conoid and trapezoid ligaments, if there is buttonholing and no apposition of bone ends. Severe (type III) displacement of the acromio-clavicular joint with disruption of the clavicular periosteal tube (Ogden 1982) may also merit control with axial K wire fixation. The distal end of the clavicle should never be excised during these operative procedures. The danger of neurovascular injury at the root of the neck must be appreciated: this is of particular concern if medial (sternal head) epiphyseal separation of the clavicle is considered for operative treatment.

Scapular fractures are uncommon in childhood and indications for fixation are very unusual. Displaced glenoid intra-articular fractures and wide avulsions of the coracoid process and acromion merit compression screw fixation in

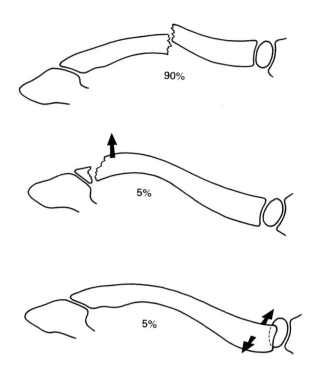

Figure 32.5 The incidence of clavicular fractures at three sites: 90% of fractures occur in the central one third and 5% in each of the end thirds. The lateral third may remain unacceptably displaced owing to the surrounding soft tissues; both it and the medial epiphyseal disruption merit temporary fixation.

the older child. Laceration of the subclavian vessels in a child with multiple injuries may also make it appropriate to stabilise the clavicle or segments of the scapula.

Humerus

Proximal epiphyseal fractures of the humerus are usually Salter–Harris type I or II injuries. The former occur in the neonate after a difficult obstetrical delivery, resulting in an initial 'pseudoparalysis' of the limb. They are occasionally encountered up to the age of 4 years. From 5 to 11 years, a

Figure 32.6 The contesting pull of the pectoral and abductor muscle groups maintains displacement of the unstable type II proximal epiphyseal fracture of the humerus.

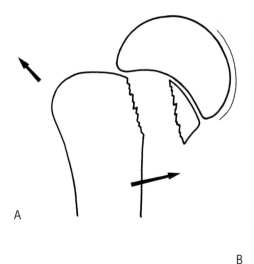

A

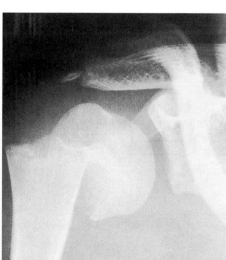

B

metaphyseal torus or transverse fracture is more common, and at the end of childhood (before closure of the growth plate) the type II epiphysial fracture is produced. Soft-tissue buttonholing, residual malalignment (especially humerus varus) and growth impairment are recognised complications. Reduction may prove impossible owing to anatomical factors (Fig. 32.6), and the use of a shoulder spica in the 'salute position' (Fig. 32.7) is both ineffectual and uncomfortable. Fixation with smooth K wires is advisable in awkward cases, followed by removal of the implants 1 month before movement is permitted.

Humeral shaft fractures complicated by complete radial nerve palsy or secondary to a pathological lesion may be stabilised with a plate and screws, or by an intramedullary device in the adolescent. Open fractures provide a rare indication for external fixation: great care should be taken with the placement of the transfixion pins.

As with the supracondylar humeral fracture (see Ch. 37), displaced condylar fractures of the distal humerus should be anatomically reduced and internally fixed, so that irregularities of the trochlear and capitellar surfaces are avoided. The Milch type II (Fig. 32.8) (Milch 1964) and comminuted condylar fractures are particularly unstable. Avulsed medial epicondylar fractures are usually best dealt with by fixation, particularly if they are rotated or trapped within the joint as a result of elbow dislocation. Pinning or lag screw fixation allows early movement after 2 weeks of back-shell support.

Radius and ulna

Avulsed olecranon fractures should be reduced and fixed with tension band wiring or an oblique compression screw. If the radiographs reveal radial or proximal ulnar fractures, or both, or features to suggest a fracture-dislocation of the

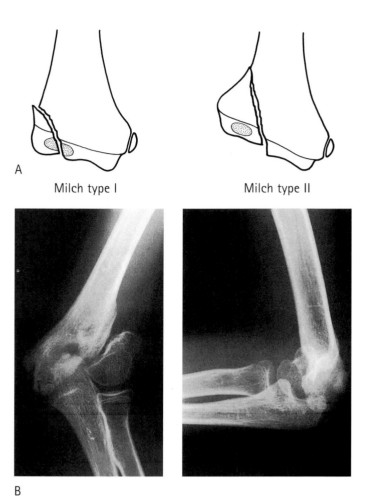

Milch type I   Milch type II

A

B

Figure 32.8 Milch type I and II fractures of the lateral (and rarely the medial) humeral condyle (A) should be accurately fixed with K wires or a small fragment cancellous screw, because the type II fracture (Salter–Harris grade II) is particularly unstable (B).

elbow, internal fixation is indicated (Macnicol 1987). This also applies to Monteggia fracture variants in the older child (Fig. 32.9) and displaced Galeazzi fractures; these injuries, together with poorly reducible mid-forearm fractures, should be treated as displaced articular fractures, because the resumption of normal forearm rotation depends upon their accurate reduction. Intramedullary flexible nails are

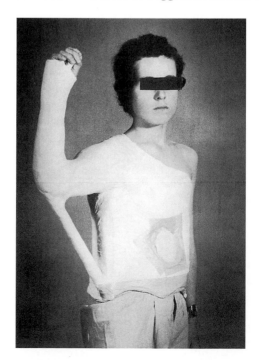

Figure 32.7 A shoulder spica in the salute position is poorly tolerated, so K wire fixation is usually preferred after closed reduction.

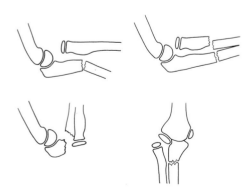

Figure 32.9 Monteggia fracture variants should be reduced accurately in order to ensure reduction of the radial head and the restitution of normal radio-ulnar relationships.

very effective and usually avoid the need to expose the fractures. Plating of the radius and ulna in the adolescent should be performed through separate incisions, generally over the volar surface for the radius and the subcutaneous, dorsal border for the ulna. Radial head fractures can usually be pieced together and held with small-fragment or Herbert-screw fixation. Lesser fragments, representing osteochondral shear injuries, may be reparable with fibrin glue, polyglycolic pegs or K wires, as with comparable patello-femoral and talar lesions.

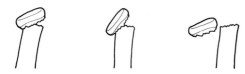

Figure 32.10 Radial neck fractures should be reduced if they are significantly tilted.

Radial neck fractures (Fig. 32.10) with significant tilting of the radial head (>60°) can generally be manipulated back into alignment, utilising a percutaneous wire as a temporary lever if necessary. If the reduction appears to be unstable, placement of an oblique Kirschner wire or screw across the fracture line will give acceptable fixation (Fig. 32.11), the wire being removed at 1 month. A transcondylar (capitellar) pin fixation along the line of the radial neck is not advised, because the elbow joint is penetrated unnecessarily and the wire may break while the fracture is uniting. Dissection of soft tissue around the radial head must be cautious, as the proximal radius may be devascularised.

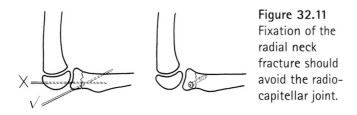

Figure 32.11 Fixation of the radial neck fracture should avoid the radio-capitellar joint.

Distal radial fractures can usually be manipulated satisfactorily, although the unstable metaphyseal injury should be stabilised with an oblique Kirschner wire inserted at the radial styloid (Fig. 32.12). Muscle interposition may prevent closed reduction, and exploration is sometimes warranted if neurological loss is present. When segmental radial fractures are present, distal fixation achieves satisfactory stability when combined with a long arm plaster (Campbell 1990). In comminuted fractures, particularly if compound, external fixation is of value, inserting transverse pins through the radius proximal to the fracture, and the metacarpals distally. The very rare distal radial type III and IV epiphyseal fractures are effectively managed with transverse, intraepiphyseal lag screw fixation. Trans-scapho-perilunate dislocations are also best dealt with operatively in the adolescent.

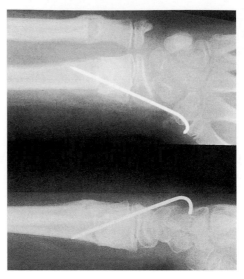

Figure 32.12 Irreducible or unstable distal radial fractures warrant open reduction and K wire fixation until union has occurred. The wire is withdrawn at 4 weeks.

Hand

Fixation of carpo-metacarpal fracture-dislocations and certain metacarpal fractures may be advisable in the child older than 10 years. Mid-shaft metacarpal fractures with more than 45° of angulation, and multiple unstable fractures, merit either longitudinal or transverse wire fixation after reduction by manipulation. Shear fractures of the metacarpal head, although prone to avascular necrosis and often compound, should be fixed with fine Kirschner wires for 3–4 weeks, with the metacarpo-phalangeal joint held flexed in a boxing-glove bandage or plaster slab. Open reduction and internal fixation are also advisable if a metacarpo-phalangeal joint proves to be irreducible or if rotational malalignment persists.

Fractures of the shafts of the phalanges can usually be manipulated and held with a volar slab or rigid finger splints, maintaining the interphalangeal joints in extension. Internal fixation is indicated if a type III or IV basal epiphyseal fracture separation is present, or if volar angulation of a proximal shaft fracture persists. Fractures of the neck and distal condyles prove difficult to control conservatively, but K wire fixation and immobilisation often fail to reduce the fragment completely and regularly lead to stiffness of the affected interphalangeal joint. The difficulties associated with the management of these intra- or juxta-articular fractures are often exacerbated by their late presentation after inadequate conservative treatment (Fig. 32.13).

Parallel or crossed Kirschner wires are preferred to small fragment screws or wire loops; longitudinal wires should be used only in rare instances when an irreducible interphalangeal dislocation has been operated upon to reduce the volar plate, or when a mallet fracture (type I, II or III epiphysial separations) of the distal phalanx cannot be splinted adequately by the repositioned finger and external strapping (Figs 32.14 and 32.15). A type III splitting fracture of the basal epiphysis of the terminal phalanx occurs in adolescence, but rarely requires fixation unless separation is more than 2 mm. Buddy taping (garter strapping) between the injured finger

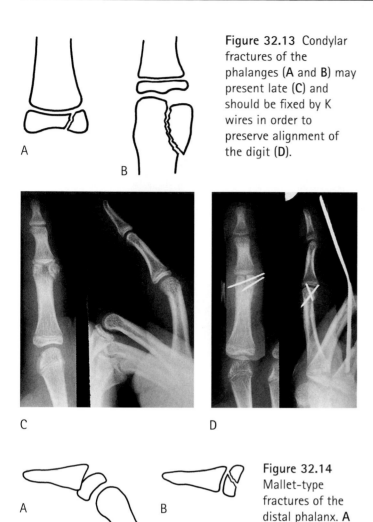

Figure 32.13 Condylar fractures of the phalanges (**A** and **B**) may present late (**C**) and should be fixed by K wires in order to preserve alignment of the digit (**D**).

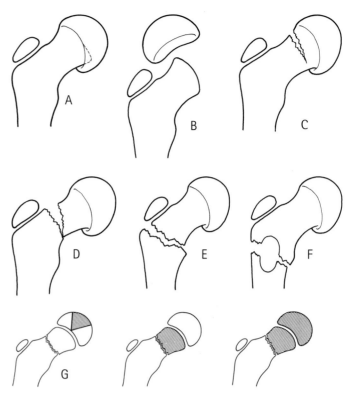

Figure 32.16 Proximal femoral fractures are classified as transepiphyseal (minimally displaced) (**A**), significantly displaced (**B**), transcervical (**C**), cervico-trochanteric (basal) (**D**), trochanteric (**E**) and subtrochanteric (pathological) (**F**). The patterns of avascular necrosis (**G**) relate largely to the degree of fragment separation and the level of the fracture.

Figure 32.14 Mallet-type fractures of the distal phalanx. **A** Type I. **B** Type III.

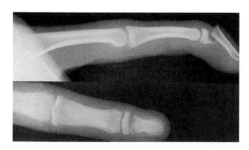

Figure 32.15 The type II epiphyseal fracture of the distal phalanx is stable and requires reduction and fixation only if significantly displaced through the nail bed.

and its neighbouring digit offers an excellent, dynamic form of splintage for the more stable phalangeal fractures, or later in the convalescence after an unstable fracture.

LOWER LIMB

Hip

The principles of femoral neck fracture management include early release of the haemarthrosis in order to reduce the risk of tamponade, perfect reduction by open operation if neces-sary, and sound internal fixation, preferably with compres-sion screws. The implants are normally removed within 1 year of the fracture. Complications are related to the level of the fracture (Fig. 32.16) and the fixation achieved: avas-cular necrosis, growth plate arrest, deformities and non-union remain significant problems. Necrosis largely reflects the ischaemia produced by the initial displacement of the fracture, although the prognosis is demonstrably improved by better surgical care and fixation (Canale 1990).

Pelvis

Fractures of the pelvis (see Ch. 38) are usually stable and require no fixation. In severe, crushing injuries the larger fragments can be secured with lag screws rather than flex-ible plates, although adolescent fractures of the acetabulum may require reinforcing buttress plates for the anterior or posterior columns. External fixation is indicated for pubic diastasis and certain unstable pelvic ring fractures.

Distal femur

Distal femoral epiphyseal fractures comprise approximately 1% of all growth plate injuries. Type I fractures occur in young children, and occasionally as a result of birth injury; internal fixation is not usually required unless vascular injury is present. Type II fractures are seen in early adolescence and merit fixation by pins (Fig. 32.17), screw re-attachment of the metaphyseal fragment if it is large enough, or plate stabilisation at the cessation of skeletal growth (Fig. 32.18). Growth arrest is seen in a considerable proportion of the type II fractures, because the mechanism of injury is usually violent. Type III and IV fractures are rare; they should be carefully reduced and secured with lag screws, avoiding the growth plate.

Patella

Patellar fractures are usually produced by repeated stress (Sindig–Larsen-Johansson syndrome) or patellar lateral dislocation. The latter produces marginal or osteochondral fractures (see Ch. 38.3). It is rarely necessary to re-attach these fragments, and arthroscopy allows the surgeon to decide whether to remove or replace intra-articular fragments. Fibrin glue (Tussacol) could eventually offer an alternative to wire transfixion, although the strength of the adhesive is at present inadequate to resist the shearing forces transmitted through the patello-femoral joint. Absorbable pins may also prove to have a role in the management of these fractures. Transverse and sleeve fractures of the patella should be accurately reduced and held with tension band wiring or lag screws. Early knee movement can then be allowed, provided that weight bearing is restricted.

Proximal tibia

Fractures of the proximal tibia include epiphyseal displacements (Burkhart & Paterson 1979, Shelton & Canale 1979)

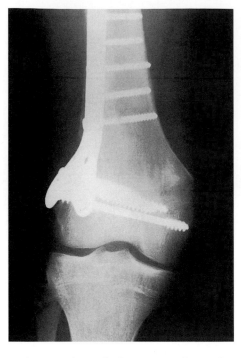

Figure 32.18 A rare instance of distal femoral plating, using a T-plate in preference to a blade plate.

and metaphyseal fractures of varying severity, with or without fibular fracture. The epiphysis is protected by the collateral ligaments that extend distal to the physis, but, conversely, this makes the reduction and stabilisation more uncertain with conservative methods than with the distal femoral epiphysis. Steinmann pins or Kirschner wires can be used, crossed from either side of the knee at angles that keep the pins apart as they transverse the growth plate into the

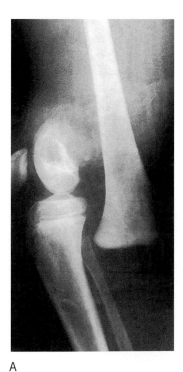
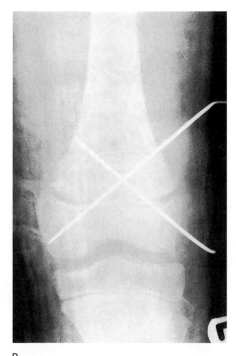
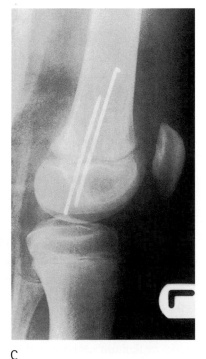

A   B   C

Figure 32.17 A severely displaced distal femoral epiphyseal fracture (A) internally fixed by Kirschner wires (B and C).

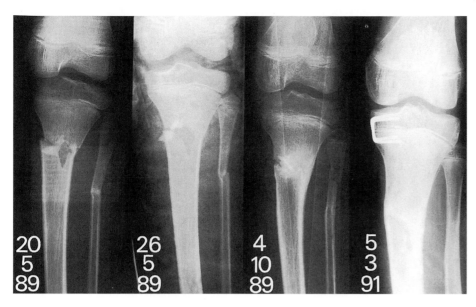

Figure 32.19 Valgus deformity persisted in spite of closed reduction, and an eventual corrective medial tibial stapling was deemed necessary. In most cases, the valgus angulation corrects gradually after the first year after fracture.

tibial metaphysis. The proximal ends of the pins should be bent to prevent inward migration, as with all pin or wire fixation. Implants can be removed at 4–6 weeks, depending upon the age of the child. Plaster splint support should be retained for a further 2 weeks before knee movements are commenced.

Open reduction of the proximal tibial epiphysis may be necessary if the periosteal sleeve and collateral structures fold into the fracture gap (Fig. 32.19) or when the hyperextension forces have been sufficiently violent to injure the popliteal vessels. The very rare type III and IV fractures should also be operated upon, with insertion of a transverse lag screw, and early movement using a continuous passive motion machine. Displaced tibial tuberosity fractures merit open reduction and fixation (Fig. 32.20). Chow et al (1990) recommended the combination of a cancellous screw and tension band wiring, thus allowing the early return of knee flexion. As this fracture occurs as the growth plate is closing, recurvatum and overgrowth do not pose the same problems as injury to the proximal tibial growth plate in childhood (Fig. 32.21). However, the skin overlying the tibial tuberosity may heal poorly if the incision is placed over it, and residual prominence and tenderness persist, together with the usual risk of some flexion loss, particularly if the re-attachment is too distal (producing patella baja).

Hyperextension injury of the knee may also avulse the intercondylar eminence as a result of the pull of the cruciate ligaments, which partially tear but do not rupture. Meyers & McKeever (1959) graded the displacement of this fragment, which is always bigger than it appears radiographically (Fig. 32.22). Splintage of the knee using a plaster cylinder in full extension will prove sufficient for type I fractures and the type II fracture, provided that it reduces completely when compressed by the femoral condyles. However, malreduction leaves the child with a possibly permanent block to knee extension, and the medial and lateral cartilaginous wings of the eminence often overly the anterior meniscal horn(s) at exploration. Therefore open reduction, either arthroscopically aided or by conventional arthrotomy, is recommended, together with the insertion of a small fragment, intraepi-

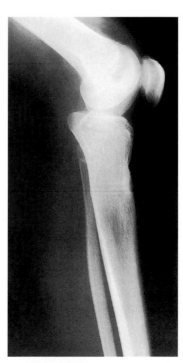

Figure 32.21 Recurvatum and an oblique tibial articular surface result from partial growth arrest of the proximal growth plate.

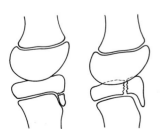
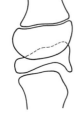

Figure 32.20 The types of tibial tuberosity fracture.

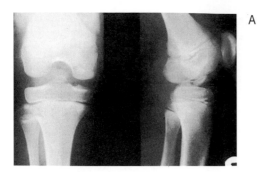

A

B

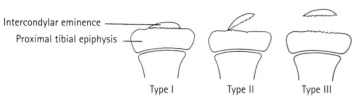

Intercondylar eminence
Proximal tibial epiphysis

Type I   Type II   Type III

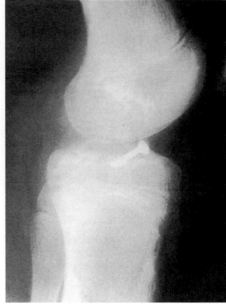

C

Figure 32.22 A The radiographic appearances of a significantly displaced fracture of the tibial intercondylar eminence. **B** Meyers & McKeever (1959) graded the separation into three groups. **(C).** Fixation of the fracture shown in **A**, by means of a small fragment cancellous screw.

physial lag screw (Fig. 32.22) or a wire loop through the epiphysis, brought out over the tibial tuberosity anteriorly. Anterior cruciate laxity may persist (Smith 1984), although this lessens if the child still has some years of growth ahead.

Ankle

Ankle fractures are dealt with in Chapter 38.4. These injuries are common in children, those of the distal tibial epiphysis being second in frequency to those of the distal radius. Surgical reduction and fixation are indicated when closed reduction proves impossible or inadequate, particularly when the articular surfaces are involved in type III and IV epiphysial separations of the distal tibia (Fig. 32.23), triplane fractures and the juvenile Tillaux fracture (Fig. 32.24) (Kling et al 1984). Small intraepiphysial compression screws (Fig.

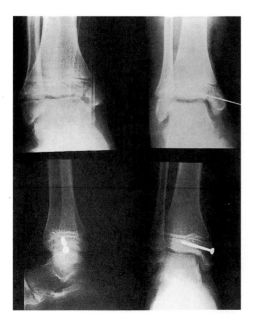

Figure 32.23 Accurate fixation of ankle fractures is readily achieved with lag screws.

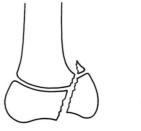

Figure 32.24 The Tillaux fracture represents an avulsion injury (see Ch. 38.4).

32.25) are preferred to wire or pin fixation, although the Tillaux fracture occurs at the cessation of skeletal growth, and hence the implant can be directed across the closing growth plate. The fibular epiphyseal fracture usually does not require fixation because a below-knee cast will stabilise it adequately, in conjunction with the distal tibial fixation. However, tension band wiring is sometimes indicated, and plate fixation of the distal fibular shaft is required when there is significant shortening and external rotation.

Foot

Crushing injuries of the foot may cause splitting injuries of the tarsal bones. Calcaneal, talar, navicular and cuboid

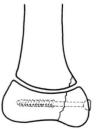

Figure 32.25 Intraepiphyseal screw fixation allows accurate reduction and fixation of both the metaphyseal and epiphyseal components of the fracture.

fractures should be reduced and fixed with a small fragment cancellous screw if comminution permits. Early movement of the subtalar joint, with protected weight bearing, should be encouraged as stiffness is common, even in childhood. Midfoot fracture-dislocations and metatarsal fractures should be manipulated and secured with percutaneous Kirschner wires because the morbidity from malunion is considerable. Cast fixation is inadequate if displacement or malalignment persist. Late correction of deformity is seldom satisfactory.

PATHOLOGICAL FRACTURES

Pathological fractures in childhood may occur at any site in the long bones, vertebrae or pelvis, although they are extremely rare in flat bones. Relatively minor injuries produce the fracture. Characteristically there is no history of convincing trauma, or the incident may be relatively trivial. The child complains of pain, which is usually persistent and sufficient to limit walking if the lower limb is involved. Although the periosteal tube usually prevents significant displacement, the effects of the fracture cannot be ignored.

Internal fixation (see above) will be indicated only in specific cases, particularly femoral and tibial shaft fractures secondary to osteogenesis imperfecta, and certain other skeletal dysplasias in which treatment of the primary condition is as yet impossible. External support in the form of plaster casts or orthoses is the mainstay of orthopaedic treatment, because the child should remain as active as possible throughout the convalescence.

Skeletal alterations leading to pathological fracture may be considered as follows:

- generalised
- localised to one limb
- localised to the lesion.

The skeletal changes may be either congenital or acquired; the biochemical and biomechanical changes vary, affecting both the composition and the architecture of the bone.

GENERALISED CONDITIONS

Generalised conditions may be present at birth. Osteogenesis imperfecta type II (Sillence et al 1979) is an autosomal recessive disease that results in multiple fractures and death at the time of delivery. Birth fractures will be described in Chapter 36 and may be caused by other congenital conditions such as hypophosphatasia and the Silverman syndrome. The child with arthrogryposis who has stiff joints (see Ch. 19) may also present with a long bone fracture (Fig. 32.26). Proximal femoral pseudarthrosis associated with congenital short femur and pseudarthrosis of the clavicle may prove confusing.

In later childhood, pathological fractures occur in osteogenesis imperfecta (Figs 32.27 and 32.28), whether it is autosomal recessive (type III) or dominant (types I and IV). Certain of the other skeletal dysplasias such as polyostotic

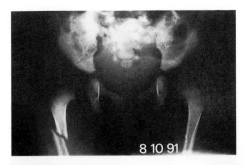

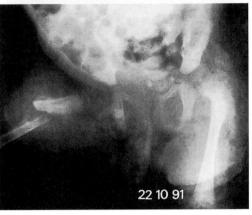

Figure 32.26 Oblique fracture of the right femoral shaft after the difficult delivery of an arthrogrypotic child. Abundant callus formed a fortnight later.

fibrous dysplasia, pycnodysostosis and osteopetrosis (Fig. 32.29) predispose to pathological or stress fractures, as does idiopathic osteoporosis of adolescence or the rare juvenile form (Fig. 32.30). The metabolic bone disease associated

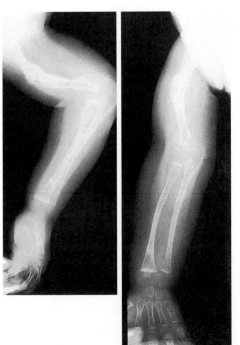

Figure 32.27 Typical upper limb deformities after multiple fracture in osteogenesis imperfecta

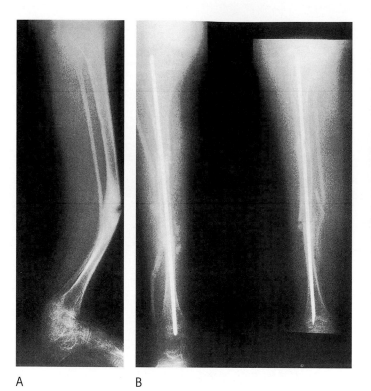

A   B

Figure 32.28 Tibial fracture in osteogenesis imperfecta before (A) and after (B) intramedullary rodding.

with endstage renal or hepatic failure is also associated with an increased incidence of fracture, particularly in the convalescent phase after organ transplantation, when steroid

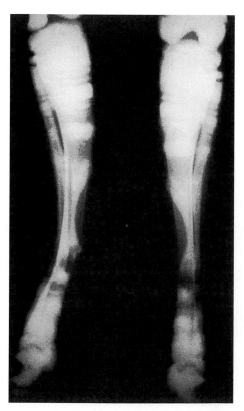

Figure 32.29 Pathological tibial fractures in a child with osteopetrosis.

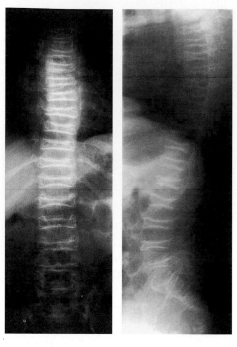

Figure 32.30 Compression fractures of the vertebrae in idiopathic osteoporosis.

therapy and immunosuppression are required. Unusual metabolic conditions such as Bartter's syndrome (Gill 1985) may be encountered (Fig. 32.31).

Acquired diseases that affect the entire skeleton include the leukaemias, renal osteodystrophy, hyperparathyroidism, pituitary dysfunction and infiltrative disorders such as histiocytosis X. Malnutrition leads to rickets, scurvy and the wasting diseases (kwashiorkor and marasmus), with concomitant weakening of the skeleton and a predisposition to fracture. These children with their acquired systemic disease are unwell, and the diagnosis must be established if the underlying condition is to be treated effectively. Multiple fractures should also arouse suspicion that the injuries are non-accidental (see Ch. 36).

SINGLE-LIMB INVOLVEMENT

Fractures localised to one limb may be secondary to congenital conditions affecting one or more bones in the limb, such as fibrous dysplasia (Fig. 32.32) or Ollier's disease. More commonly, the pathological fracture occurs when disuse osteoporosis results from congenital or acquired conditions. Immobilisation and paralytic conditions cause significant bone loss, and rehabilitation must always be graduated and carefully supervised. Myelodysplasia, poliomyelitis, severe cerebral palsy and arthrogryposis are associated with an increased incidence of fractures, as are chronic osteomyelitis, tuberculosis, septic arthritis, juvenile idiopathic arthritis, post-irradiation osteoporosis and chemotherapy.

Fractures occur in up to 30% of children with spina bifida (Menelaus 1980) and may involve the diaphysis, metaphysis or growth plate (Korhonen 1971). The diagnosis is often delayed, as the child may not feel pain. Local warmth, erythema, swelling and progressive deformity should alert the surgeon to the likelihood of pathological fracture. It is

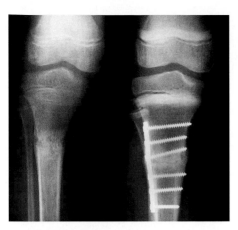

Figure 32.31
Stabilisation of
stress fractures of
the tibia (**A**) and
femoral neck (**B**) in
Bartter's syndrome.

A

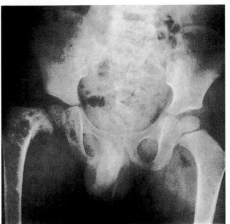

Figure 32.32
Fibrous dysplasia
of the femora,
with a
pathological
fracture and varus
deformity on the
right side.

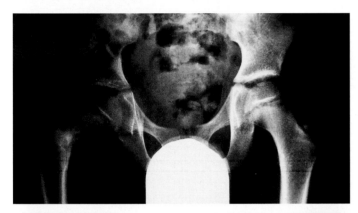

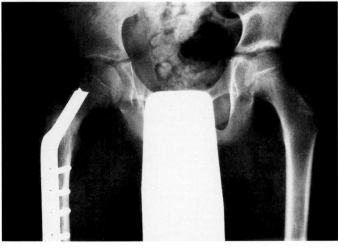

B

stress may promote further pathological fracture and a hypertrophic callus response may lead to thickening and deformity around the knee and ankle, together with altered growth (see Ch. 35). Epiphysiolysis typically produces an initial widening of the growth plate before major slipping occurs. If stress is minimal, the displacement will not progress and the type I epiphyseal fracture (Salter & Harris 1963) will heal slowly.

MONOSTOTIC LESIONS

Benign cystic conditions of bone are the most common cause of single pathological fracture, which occurs most often in the upper humerus (Fig. 32.33). Although the fracture itself may cause the underlying lesion to heal, needle decompression and injection with steroid or the insertion of bone marrow, or cancellous bone graft (Fig. 32.34) may be

easy to confuse the finding with infection. The radiographic appearances may be quite alarming and mimic chronic osteomyelitis (Townsend et al 1979) or tumour. Congenital insensitivity to pain (Kuo & Macnicol 1996) and post-traumatic neurological loss may also lead to repeated fractures of the weight-bearing bones and to osteolysis. However, blood tests are usually normal and the temptation to take a biopsy of the lesion should be resisted.

The healing of these fractures may be delayed (Wenger et al 1980), but orthotic support and graduated weight bearing will usually ensure a satisfactory outcome. However, recurrent

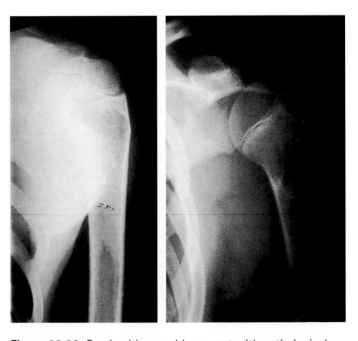

Figure 32.33 Proximal humeral bone cyst with pathological fracture of the lateral cortex (left) leading to later healing (right).

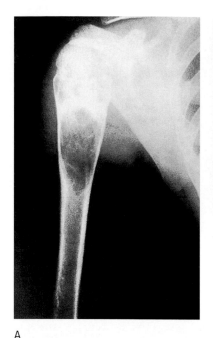
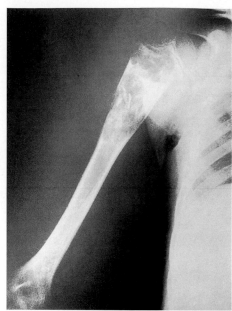

A   B

Figure 32.34 A larger humeral bone cyst (**A**), treated by cortico-cancellous bone grafting (**B**). Multiple puncture aspiration and steroid instillation is less invasive but may require repeated interventions.

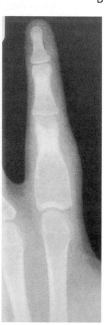
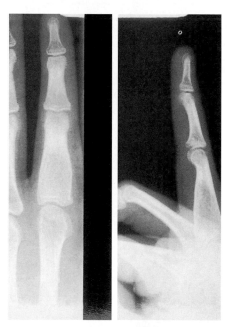

Figure 32.35 A minor pathological fracture of a proximal phalangeal cyst (left) was treated by strapping to the adjacent digit. The cyst healed subsequently (right).

required before the condition resolves. Splintage may be sufficient in some patients (Fig. 32.35), but unicameral bone cyst or fibrous dysplasia involving the proximal femur (Fig. 32.32) should be internally fixed in order to prevent varus deformity.

Benign and malignant neoplasms (see Ch. 13) and infection (see Ch. 9) may cause pathological fracture if cortical destruction exceeds 50% of the normal bone strength. A metastatic deposit from nephroblastoma or neuroblastoma (Figs 32.36 and 32.37) should be included in any differential diagnosis. Fracture may also occur where the bone has been weakened by the insertion or removal of a screw, pin or plate, or if blood supply has been impaired by previous trauma, with resultant scarring of the surrounding soft tissues.

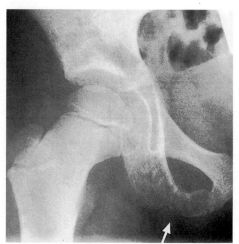

Figure 32.36 A neuroblastoma metastasised to the pelvis, producing a pathological fracture of the inferior ramus (arrow).

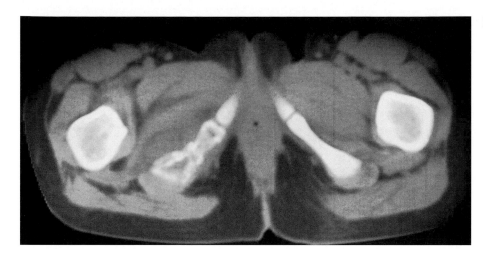

Figure 32.37 CT scan of the pelvic lesion.

The typical radiographic appearances include a transverse fracture with little comminution, and a relatively indistinct fracture line. Displacement is usually minimal and significant soft-tissue wounding is rare. The fracture is usually missed because radiographs are not obtained, although it may be difficult to discern at certain sites, particularly in the spine and ribs. Perthes' disease (see Ch. 25) and other examples of osteonecrosis, such as osteochondritis of the femoral condyles, also produce a form of pathological fracture when the ischaemic trabeculae are revascularised during the healing process. Finally, congenital pseudarthrosis may sometimes mimic the localised form of pathological fracture, particularly in the absence of cutaneous neurofibromatosis.

STRESS FRACTURES

Stress fractures, while not in themselves 'pathological', may also be confusing if a history of repetitive, relatively minor trauma is not sought. In the adolescent, stress fracture of the femoral neck (Figs 32.38 and 32.39) may occur transversely across the inferior or superior aspects of the neck (Devas 1963). The inferior, compression fracture is less likely to displace, but varus deformity resulting from delayed union and persisting symptoms are indications to fix the lesion internally. Stress fractures of the tibia (Fig. 32.40), fibula (Griffiths 1952), patella, ulna and metatarsal have also been described. Spondylolysis secondary to pathological changes in the pars interarticularis and spondylolisthesis are discussed in Chapter 31.3, and chronic stress lesions of the neck, humerus and ulna are also recognised as rare pathological conditions in childhood.

The tibia usually develops a linear shadow in the proximal metaphysis, and the posteromedial or posterolateral border eventually shows a resorptive fracture line. The mid-shaft may also thicken anteriorly, similarly to the shin splint fracture in the adult. As the fracture line is difficult to see by conventional radiography in the early stages, technetium-99m isotope scanning or tomography are valuable investigations. CT is less applicable, but demonstrates the cortical response well. MR scanning is less specific.

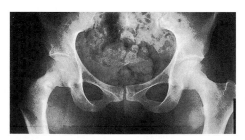

Figure 32.38 Inferior stress fractures of the femoral neck.

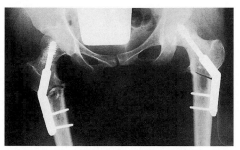

Figure 32.39 Internal fixation after valgus osteomoties, to produce healing.

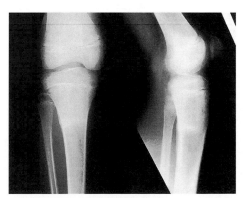

Figure 32.40 Stress fracture of the proximal tibial shaft in an athletic boy.

REFERENCES

Aitken A P 1935 The end results of the fractured distal radial epiphysis. Journal of Bone and Joint Surgery 17: 302–308

Baeza Giner V, Oliete Sanz V 1980 Profilaxis de los puentes osseos del cartilago de crecimiento. Estudio experimental. Revisa de Orthopedia y Traumatologica 24: 305–320

Blount W P 1954 Fractures in children. Williams & Wilkins, Baltimore

Bostman O, Mäkelä E A, Tormala P, Rokkanen P 1989 Transphyseal fracture fixation using biodegradable pins. Journal of Bone and Joint Surgery 71B: 706–707

Bright R W 1974 Operative correction of partial epiphyseal plate closure by osseous-bridge resection and silicone rubber implant. Journal of Bone and Joint Surgery 56A: 655–664

Buckley S L, Smith G, Sponseller P D, Thompson J D, Griffin P P 1990 Open fractures of the tibia in children. Journal of Bone and Joint Surgery 72A: 1462–1469

Burkhart S S, Peterson H A 1979 Fractures of the proximal tibial apophysis. Journal of Bone and Joint Surgery 61A: 996–1002

Campbell R M 1990 Fractures and dislocations of the hand and wrist region. Orthopedic Clinics of North America 21: 217–344

Canale S T 1990 Fractures of the hip in children and adolescents. Orthopedic Clinics of North America 21: 341–352

Chow S P, Lam J J, Leong J C Y 1990 Fracture of the tibial tubercle in the adolescent. Journal of Bone and Joint Surgery 72B: 231–234

Crilly R G 1972 Longitudinal overgrowth of chicken radius. Journal of Anatomy 112: 11–18

Devas M B 1963 Stress fractures in children. Journal of Bone and Joint Surgery 45B: 528–541

Dias L S, Giergerich C R 1983 Fractures of the distal tibial epiphysis in adolescence. Journal of Bone and Joint Surgery 65A: 438–444

Friberg S 1979 Remodelling after distal forearm fractures in children: correction of residual angulation in fractures of the radius. Acta Orthopaedica Scandinavica 50: 731–739

Gill J R 1985 Bartter's syndrome. In: Gonick H C, Buckalen V M eds. Renal tubular disorders: pathophysiology, diagnosis and management. Marcel Dekker, New York

Griffiths A L 1952 Fatigue fracture of the fibula in childhood. Archive of Diseases in Childhood 27: 552–557

Gustilo R B, Mendoza R M, William D N 1984 Problems in the management of type III (severe) open fractures: a new classification. Journal of Trauma 24: 742–746

Haas S L 1945 Retardation of bone growth by a wire loop. Journal of Bone and Joint Surgery 27: 25–36

Kling T F Jr, Bright A W, Hensinger R N 1984 Distal tibial physeal fractures in children that may require open reduction. Journal of Bone and Joint Surgery 66A: 647–657

König F 1908 Die späteren Schicksale deform-geheiter Knochenbruche, besonders bei Kindern. Archiv für Klinische Chirurgie 85: 187–211

Korhonen B J 1971 Fractures in myelodysplasia. Clinical Orthopaedics and Related Research 79: 145–150

Kuo R, Macnicol M F 1996 Congenital insensitivity to pain: orthopaedic implications. Journal of Pediatric Orthopaedics B5: 292–295

Langenskiöld A, Österman K 1983 Surgical elimination of post-traumatic partial fusion of the growth plate. In: Houghton G R, Thompson G H (eds) Problematic musculoskeletal injuries in children. Butterworth, London, pp 14–31

Loder R 1987 Polytrauma in children. Orthopaedic Trauma 1: 48–54

Macnicol M F 1978 Roentgenographic evidence of median nerve entrapment in a greenstick fracture. Journal of Bone and Joint Surgery 60A: 998–1000

Macnicol M F 1987 Elbow injuries in children. Current Orthopaedics 1: 412–419

Mäkelä E A, Vainionpia S, Vihtonen K 1987 The effect of a penetrating biodegradable implant on the epiphyseal plate: an experimental study on growing rabbits with special regard to polyglactin. Journal of Pediatric Orthopaedics 7: 415–420

Mallet J 1975 Les epiphysiodèses partielles traumatiques de l'extremité inférieure du tibia chez l'enfant. Revue de Chirurgie Orthopédique 61: 5–16

Matter P, Rittman W W 1978 The open fracture. Huber, Bern

Menelaus M B 1980 The orthopaedic management of spina bifida cystica, 2nd edn. E & S Livingstone, Edinburgh, pp 63–65

Meyers M H, McKeever F M 1959 Fracture of the intercondylar eminence of the tibia. Journal of Bone and Joint Surgery 41A: 209–222

Milch H 1964 Fractures and fracture-dislocations of humeral condyles. Journal of Trauma 4: 592–607

Ogden J A 1982 Skeletal imaging in the child. Lea & Febiger, Philadelphia

Pauwels F 1975 Eine Klinische Beobachtung als Beispiel und Beweis fur funktionelle anpassung des Knochens durch Langenwachstum. Zeitschrift für Orthopadie 113: 1–5

Peterson H A 1994 Physeal fractures: Part 2. Two previously unclassified types. Journal of Pediatric Orthopaedics 14: 431–438

Poland J 1898 Traumatic separation of the epiphysis. Smith Elder, London

Rang M C 1969 The growth plate and its disorders. Churchill Livingstone, Edinburgh

Rang M C 1983 Children's fractures, 2nd edn. J B Lippincott, Philadelphia

Reynolds D A 1981 Growth changes in fractured long bones: a study of 126 children. Journal of Bone and Joint Surgery 63B: 83–88

Rockwood C A Jr, Wilkins K E, Beaty J H 1996 Fractures in children, 4th edn Lippincott-Raven, Philadelphia, New York

Rorabeck C H, Clarke K M 1978 The pathophysiology of the anterior tibial compartment syndrome: an experimental investigation. Journal of Trauma 18: 299–304

Salter R B, Harris R W 1963 Injuries involving the epiphyseal plate. Journal of Bone and Joint Surgery 45A: 587–622

Shapiro F, 1981 Fractures of the femoral shaft in children: the overgrowth phenomenon. Acta Orthopaedica Scandinavica 52: 649–655

Shelton W R, Canale S T 1979 Fractures of the tibia through the proximal tibial epiphyseal cartilage. Journal of Bone and Joint Surgery 61A: 167–173

Sillence D O, Senn A, Danks D M 1979 Genetic heterogeneity in osteogenesis imperfecta. Journal of Medical Genetics 16: 101–116

Smith J B 1984 Knee instability after fractures of the intercondylar eminence of the tibia. Journal of Pediatric Orthopaedics 4: 462–464

Townsend P F, Cowell H R, Steg N L 1979 Lower extremity fractures simulating infection in myelomeningocele. Clinical Orthopaedics and Related Research 144: 256–259

Wenger D R, Jeffcoat B T, Herring J A 1980 The guarded prognosis of physeal injuries in paraplegic children. Journal of Bone and Joint Surgery 62A: 241–246

Chapter 33

Fracture epidemiology

L. A. Landin

The purpose of fracture epidemiology, as of epidemiology in general, is to identify and describe the aetiology of disease in a population, with the ultimate goal of finding methods of prevention. By tradition and out of necessity, the interest of orthopaedic surgeons has focused on diagnosis and therapy, but it is also our duty to participate in preventive programmes to reduce accidents and to recognise any new hazards, that may affect the children in our society. Therefore it is important to have some knowledge of what, why, when and how fractures occur in children.

In surveys of paediatric trauma, fractures are found to contribute 10–25% of all injuries in childhood and adolescence (Sibert et al 1981, Nathorst Westfelt 1982). In a series of 23 915 patients seen at four major hospitals for injury-related symptoms, 17.8% had fractures; thus close to 20% of patients who present to hospitals with injuries have a fracture (Wilkins 1996).

DEFINITIONS

1. *Incidence.* The number of new cases occurring in a defined population during a certain time interval. Thus the age-specific annual incidence is the risk, for an individual or a group of individuals of a certain age, of catching a disease or incurring an accident during 1 year.
2. *Prevalence.* The total number of persons with a disease or a condition at a certain time in a defined population.
3. *Frequency or rate.* The percentage of a specific disease or fracture in relation to the total number of cases in a series.

The incidence is dependent upon the accuracy of the sampling procedure and a knowledge of the size of the population at risk: minor fractures can escape diagnosis, and severe fractures might be referred to other centres and thus not be recorded. These sources of error should be estimated and non-residents in the population excluded in order to arrive at as precise an incidence as possible. The ultimate goal is to produce reliable data, allowing comparison with other populations, and to detect secular changes. The term incidence is unfortunately often confused with frequency, but they are two different entities.

INCIDENCE

The risk of sustaining a fracture, or the incidence, is closely related to age (Worlock & Stower 1986a) The incidence of childhood fractures has been calculated in studies from Malmö, Sweden (Landin 1983, Tiderius et al 1999), covering 8682 fractures between 1950 and 1979, and 1673 fractures between 1993 and 1994. The risk of fracture increased in children of both sexes up to the age of 11–12 years and then decreased in girls, but further increased in boys to the age of 13–14 years (Fig. 33.1). Boys are more common in all age groups, accounting for 62% of all fractures. From the incidence figures in the Malmö studies, it can be calculated that the cumulative risk of having at least one fracture from birth to the age of 16 years is 42% for boys and 26% for girls, which means that nearly every second boy and every fourth girl will sustain a fracture during the period from birth to the age of 16 years.

The overall annual incidence of fractures was 193 per 10 000, which means that approximately 2% of the children in the population sustain a fracture each year.

FREQUENCY

The unique mechanical properties of the growing skeleton, characterised by increased mineralisation with age, the function of the periosteum, the presence of physes, physical activity, and psychomotor development, make the fracture pattern in children different from that seen in adults, or in

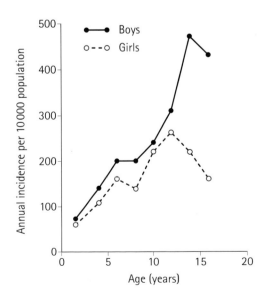

Figure 33.1 Age- and sex-specific incidence of fractures among children in Malmö, Sweden. (From Landin 1983, with permission.)

the elderly, in whom the loss of bone mass causes the typical pattern of fragility fractures.

In addition, the frequency of the different fracture types, and the incidence of fractures, will be influenced by factors such as age, cultural and environmental factors, and the climate.

The frequencies of the different fracture types in a series of fractures in an urban population of Malmö, Sweden, are shown in Table 33.1. The most common skeletal injury in children is fracture of the distal end of the forearm, which contributes 25% of all fractures, followed by fractures of the hand phalanges and of the carpal and metacarpal regions. Overall, the hand is the most common location of skeletal injury, although many fractures are minor avulsions of little consequence (Worlock & Stower 1986b). Paediatric fracture patterns are similar in different parts of the world, with some exceptions: in Austria, for example, the tibia is most commonly affected, contributing 13% (Jonasch & Bertel 1981), the cause being falls during down-hill skiing.

When the different fracture types are related to age, some patterns can be discerned (Fig. 33.2). The *late peak pattern* is mostly sport- and equipment-related. The *bimodal pattern* includes an early increase in incidence as a result of low-energy trauma, followed by a late incidence peak attributable to high- or moderate-energy trauma, again from sport or road accidents. The *decreasing pattern* is typical of skull fractures only. The *rising pattern* is closely related to sports, skateboarding, cycling and similar activities, which increase with age, particularly in boys. Finally, the *early peak pattern* of the supracondylar fracture of the humerus, mostly caused by falling from a height, and the *irregular pattern* of the tibial shaft are unique for those particular fractures.

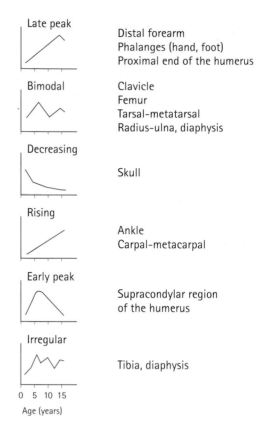

Figure 33.2 Patterns of fracture frequency. (From Landin 1983, with permission.)

AETIOLOGY

ENVIRONMENTAL FACTORS

Fracture aetiology reflects levels of activity during growth. Falls are the predominant cause in small children, whereas playground equipment and sports-related accidents are more common in the older age groups. Traffic accidents account for approximately 12% of cases; 50% of these were bicycle accidents in the Malmö study. Sports-related accidents contribute about 21% of cases.

ENDOGENOUS FACTORS

There has been much debate about whether the aetiology of accidents among children reflects not only environmental hazards, but also personality traits and social factors. In some investigations, injured children have been found to be impulsive, overactive, impatient and energetic (Mechem Fuller 1948, Bijur et al 1986), whereas other studies have shown no personality differences between accident-prone children and a control group – "all children are accident-prone sometimes" (Gustafsson 1977).

Children aged 3–6 years and 13–14 years who have sustained one fracture have an increased risk of an additional fracture compared with the overall incidence (Landin 1983). Boys are more likely than girls to be 'fracture

Table 33.1 The frequency of various fracture types	
Type	**Frequency (%)**
Distal forearm	22.7
Hand (phalanges)	18.9
Carpus or metacarpal (scaphoid excluded)	8.3
Clavicle	8.1
Ankle	5.5
Tibial shaft	5.0
Tarsus or metatarsal (talus, os calcis excluded)	4.5
Foot (phalanges)	3.4
Forearm shafts	3.4
Supracondylar region of the humerus	3.3
Proximal end of the humerus	2.2
Facial skeleton	2.1
Skull	1.8
Femoral shaft	1.6
Radial neck	1.2
Vertebrae	1.2

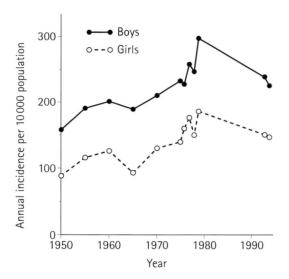

Figure 33.3 Changes in the incidence of fractures in boys and girls in Malmö, Sweden, from 1950 to 1979, and in the early 1990s.

repeaters', which supports the theory that psychological factors have an aetiological role.

Children with an evidently fragile skeleton as a result of osteogenesis imperfecta, neurological disorders (such as cerebral palsy, epilepsy and myelomeningocele), juvenile idiopathic arthritis and renal osteodystrophy sustain fractures more often than expected from the overall incidence, but the scarcity of these conditions makes their contribution to the total number of fractures small. This is in contrast to fractures in the elderly, among whom the majority of patients are osteoporotic or present with associated conditions such as metabolic bone disease, neurological disorders with impaired balance, or rheumatoid arthritis.

Gammaphotoabsorptiometry has been used to compare the bone mineral content of children sustaining fractures with that in a control group without a fracture. The bone mineral content was reduced in the 8% of children who sustained fractures from low-energy trauma, whereas there was no difference in children who sustained their fractures from moderate- or high-energy trauma. So, although there is no distinct pattern of bone fragility, the quality of the skeleton or degree of mineralisation probably is of importance, even in paediatric fractures (Landin & Nilsson 1983, Bailey et al 1989).

PRESENT TRENDS

From 1950 to 1979, the incidence of fractures in children in Malmö, Sweden, almost doubled. The increase was due to a greater number of fractures caused by slight trauma, such as sports-related accidents, whereas high-energy trauma, such as traffic accidents, decreased over the period. The recorded increase over the years was not explained by improved medical care and access, as the rate of minor avulsions compared with diaphysial fractures remained constant over the years (Landin 1983). A fracture incidence similar to that in Malmö for 1975–1979 was found in Nottingham children in 1981 (Worlock & Stower 1986a).

To investigate any further changes in the epidemiology of children's fractures in Malmö, a study covering the years 1993–1994 was performed (Tiderius et al 1999). The data collection procedure and organisation of the medical facilities were the same as for the study in 1950–1979, allowing for the analysis, over half a century, of paediatric fracture epidemiology in an urban population of western Europe. An overall reduction of 9% in the incidence since 1979 was recorded (Fig. 33.3). It could not be attributed to any single type of skeletal injury or group of fractures. Since the late 1970s, participation in organised sports has increased, whereas unsupervised play has decreased (Engström 1996). By 1992, not many more than 50% of 15-year-old Swedish youths engaged in jogging or a corresponding physical effort at least once a week. Although these observations do not constitute direct proof, they can be regarded as circumstantial evidence of the effects of a more sedentary life-style upon the risk of fracture. Another explanation could be the effect of safety programmes and an increasing awareness of safety among the public in western Europe, exemplified by the use of protective equipment in sports, and safety-belts in the back seats of cars. The latter, together with the extensive use of specially designed children's seats in cars have resulted in a threefold reduction in the number of children killed in traffic accidents annually, comparing the periods 1975–1979 and 1993–1994 (Swedish National Road Administration 1998).

FUTURE DEVELOPMENTS

New sports and activities, such as the introduction of skateboards and roller skates, invariably cause new hazards; virtual epidemics of injuries were reported by Allum in 1977 and Bunker in 1983. The incidence of fractures in children thus seems to mirror the affluence of our society with sporting 'crazes' increasing the risk of injury, against a background life-style that is more protective and sedentary governed by videogames and computers.

REFERENCES

Allum R L 1977 Skateboard injuries, a new epidemic. Injury 10: 152–153

Bailey D A, Wedge J H, McCulloch R G, Martin A D, Bernhardson S C 1989 Epidemiology of fractures of the distal end of the radius in children as associated with growth. Journal of Bone and Joint Surgery 71A: 1225–1230

Bijur P E, Stewart-Brown S, Bather N 1986 Child behaviour and accidental injury in 11 966 preschool children. American Journal of Diseases of Children 140: 487–492

Bunker T D 1983 The 1982 epidemic – roller skating injuries. British Journal of Sports Medicine 17: 205–208

Engström L-M 1996 Sweden. In: De Knop P, Engström L-M, Skirstad B, Weiss M R (eds) Worldwide trends in youth sport Human kinetics, ch 20. Champaign, Illinois pp. 231–243

Gustafsson L H 1977 Childhood accidents. Three epidemiological studies on the etiology. Scandinavian Journal of Social Medicine, 5–13

Jonasch E, Bertel E, 1981 Injuries in children up to 14 years of age. Medico-statistical study of over 263,166 injured children [article in German]. Hefte Unfallheilkund 150: 1–146

Landin L A 1983 Fracture patterns in children. Analysis of 8682 fractures with special reference to incidence, etiology and secular changes in a Swedish urban population 1950–1979. Acta Orthopaedica Scandinavica Supplementum 202: 1–109

Landin L A, Nilsson B E 1983 Bone mineral content in children with fractures. Clinical Orthopaedics and Related Research 178: 292–296

Mechem Fuller E 1948 Injury prone children. American Journal of Orthopsychiatry 18: 708–723

Nathorst Westfelt J A R 1982 Environmental factors in childhood accidents. A prospective study in Göteborg, Sweden. Acta Paediatrica Scandinavica Supplementum 53: 291

Sibert J R, Maddocks G B, Brown B M 1981 Childhood accidents – an endemic of epidemic proportions. Archives of Disease in Childhood 56: 225–234

Swedish National Road Administration 1998 Annual statistics. Vägverket Trafikantavdelningen, Borlänge, Sweden

Tiderius C J, Landin L A, Düppe H 1999 Decreasing incidence in fractures in children. An epidemiological analysis of 1673 fractures in Malmö, Sweden 1993–1994. Acta Orthopaedica Scandinavica 70: 622–626

Wilkins K E 1996 The incidence of fractures in children. In: Rockwood C A, Wilkins K E, Beaty J H (eds) Fractures in children. Lippincott-Raven, Philadelphia, New York, pp 3–17

Worlock P, Stower M 1986a Fracture patterns in Nottingham children. Journal of Pediatric Orthopaedics 6: 656–660

Worlock P, Stower M 1986b The incidence and pattern of hand fractures in children. The Journal of Hand Surgery 11B: 198–200

Chapter 34

Polytrauma in children

M. J. Bell

INTRODUCTION

Trauma is the most common cause of death in childhood. The multiply injured child presents specific problems in management because of anatomical and physiological differences from the adult. Children are not just small adults. The clinicians involved in the management of the multiply injured child must be aware of the significant differences.

A child with multiple injuries should be managed according to the principles of advanced paediatric trauma life support (APLS/ATLS) laid down by the Royal Colleges of Surgeons (Advanced Life Support Group 2000) and the American College of Surgeons (1997). All children with multiple system injury should be transferred to a centre with paediatric intensive care facilities, full paediatric support and, of course, an appropriate orthopaedic surgeon who can deal with their musculoskeletal injuries. In the multiply injured child, it is the other injuries that are the more pressing and life threatening than the orthopaedic injuries.

The most common cause of these injuries are road traffic accidents, either inside the car or as a pedestrian. The other significant cause is falling from a height.

The clinician treating children must always be aware that multiple injuries may result from child abuse.

SPECIFIC DIFFERENCES

HEAD

A child has a large head in relationship to its body size. The large head, which raises the fulcrum of neck motion, may explain why children have a significant increase in injuries of the upper cervical spine.

With the child lying in the supine position, the prominent occiput produces a relative flexion of the cervical spine so that a pseudosubluxation at the level of C2–C3 is a common finding. This should not be interpreted as a cervical spine injury (see Ch. 39.1).

AIRWAY

Infants are obligate nasal breathers. Children between the age of 3 and 8 years have the significant problem of adenotonsillar hypertrophy. The larynx of a child is in a more anterior cranial position and, as a result, intubation techniques are modified and different equipment is required. The epiglottis has to be lifted forwards to expose the cords. The child's airway is narrow compared with that of an adult and a relatively small reduction of the airway can significantly affect flow. Mucosal secretions and mucosal hypertrophy can significantly affect the airway in a child.

BLOOD VOLUME

The blood volume of a child varies according to age (Table 34.1). In the neonate, the volume is approximately 100 ml per kilogram of body weight. This changes to 70 ml/kg in the adolescent. Given the relatively small blood volume in a young child, a femoral fracture or even a scalp laceration may produce sufficient blood loss to lead to cardiovascular decompensation.

CARDIAC FUNCTION

At rest, infants and children have a pulse rate much higher than that of adults, and this may well be increased by fear and anxiety. They also have a much lower blood pressure. Awareness of these factors when trying to assess blood loss in the child is important, because the child compensates very satisfactorily in the early stages of haemorrhage, but once

Table 34.1 Vital signs: approximate range of normal				
Age (years)	Ventilatory rate (breaths/min)	Systolic BP (mmHg)	Heart rate (beats/min)	Blood volume (ml/kg)
<1	30–40	70–90	110–160	100
2–5	25–30	80–100	95–140	90
5–12	20–25	90–110	80–120	80
>12	15–20	100–120	60–100	70

BP, blood pressure.

The cervical spine should be immobilised and radiographically screened by anteroposterior, lateral and oblique views. Multiple levels of injury and pseudo-subluxation at the C2 and C3 levels may catch out the unwary.

Another important injury which appears to be unique in children is 'SCIWORA' – spinal cord injury without obvious radiological abnormality. These children have a neurological problem, but X-rays fail to identify a problem within the cervical spine. A rare but fatal injury is separation of the occiput from C1.

Pelvic fractures

The greater plasticity of bone and increased flexibility and elasticity of the sacro-iliac joint and the symphysis pubis in the child mean that more trauma is required to fracture the paediatric pelvis. This also results in the energy of the accident being transmitted to underlying structures, as with the thorax, and therefore the fracture of a child's pelvis seen on an initial X-ray should be an indication that associated life-threatening soft-tissue injuries may be present. Of course, these take a priority over the management of the fracture.

Quimby (1966) and Rang (1983) divided pelvic fractures in children into three categories:

- uncomplicated fractures
- fractures with missile injuries requiring surgical exploration
- fractures associated with massive haemorrhage.

Most pelvic fractures unite with a favourable result after minimal treatment. However, it is the complications of pelvic fractures that require treatment, as they can be life-threatening.

Physical signs

There are three signs that describe a significant pelvic injury, making a pelvic X-ray mandatory:

1. *Destot's sign*. Large haematoma formation superficially beneath the inguinal ligament or in the scrotum.
2. *Roux's sign*. A decreased distance from the greater trochanter to the pubic spine on the affected side in lateral compression fractures.
3. *Earle's sign*. A bony prominence or large haematoma as well as tenderness on rectal examination indicating a significant pelvic fracture.

Neurological examination

Because of concomitant injuries to the lumbo-sacral plexus and sciatic, femoral and obturator nerves, a thorough neurological examination of the lower limbs is essential after pelvic injury. The presence of a nerve injury should be identified before treatment is commenced.

Blood loss

Pelvic injuries are associated with significant blood loss. There is a place for the early stabilisation of pelvic fractures using external fixators. If blood loss continues, then consultation with a vascular surgeon and interventional radiologist is essential, to consider other methods of controlling the haemorrhage.

Concomitant injuries

Concomitant injuries associated with pelvic fractures are divided into two distinct groups:

1. *Remote injuries* include skull fractures, subdural haematoma, cervical fractures, facial injuries, long bone fractures, lung contusions, haemothorax, ruptured diaphragm and abdominal injuries, including splenic, renal and liver lacerations.
2. *Related injuries* include tears of major blood vessels in the pelvis, retroperitoneal bleeding, rectal tears and rupture or lacerations of the urethra and bladder.

It is paramount that, if a pelvic fracture is identified, these injuries are considered.

Spinal injuries

The phenomenon of SCIWORA appears to be unique to children. Predisposing factors include ligamentous laxity, cervical spine hypermobility and immature vascular supply to the cord. Reported incidences vary from 7% to 66% of patients with cervical spine injury, usually in children younger than 8 years of age (see Ch. 39.1). Younger patients appear to be more prone to upper cervical trauma, (occiput to C3) and to suffer greater neurological injury than the older child. Approximately 50% of young children with SCIWORA suffer a complete spinal cord injury, whereas older children usually have incomplete neurological deficits and injuries that involve the sub-axial cervical spine. This condition creates significant problems in the management of the cervical spine in the multiply injured patient, especially if the child is unconscious, or paralysed and ventilated. Careful radiological evaluation is essential but, in the absence of fracture, subluxation or obvious soft-tissue injury, the cervical spine should still be protected until careful dynamic flexion/extension radiographic studies can be performed to evaluate pathological ligamentous laxity at any suspected level. This can only be done in the awake and co-operative child.

ORTHOPAEDIC INJURIES IN THE MULTIPLY INJURED CHILD

Long bone fractures should be stabilised as soon as possible. The need for intensive care is an indication for surgical stabilisation of long bone fractures in both adults and children. Surgical stabilisation aids nursing care within the intensive care unit and facilitates rehabilitation. The method chosen depends upon the experience of the surgical team. Surgical stabilisation with external fixation (Fig. 34.2), intramedullary elastic nails, or open reduction with plate and screw fixation have their respective indications and advantages.

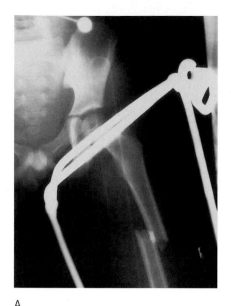

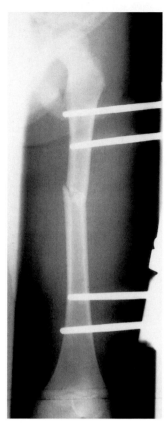

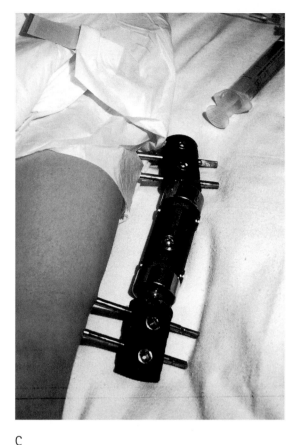

A

B   C

Figure 34.2 A Radiograph of a femoral fracture in a Thomas splint. **B** Same fracture with unilateral external fixator. **C** Clinical photograph of the external fixator *in situ*.

In the assessment of long bone injuries, it is essential to evaluate the limb and then the fracture. A distal neurovascular examination is important, as the deformity that must have taken place at the time of injury makes concomitant neurological or vascular injury likely. It is accepted that, in the unconscious patient, neurological examination may be difficult, but at least the circulation should be thoroughly assessed; in this respect, Doppler studies have been shown to be useful. If significant swelling of the limb has taken place in the unconscious patient, compartmental monitoring should be undertaken, as the unconscious patient will not complain of pain.

After long bone fractures in children, overgrowth of both the femur and tibia has been reported (see Ch. 38). This depends upon age, and may well relate to release of the periosteal tether or increased vascularity. Clinicians must be aware that this is a complication that may occur following treatment, especially after external or internal fixation.

Compound fractures

Most open fractures in children are caused by high-velocity trauma from road traffic accidents, but they can occur from low-energy trauma such as falls and football injuries. The presence of an open fracture suggests significant trauma, and a large number of these children have additional injuries. The presence of an open fracture should alert the clinician to the possibility of more serious injuries elsewhere.

Compound injuries are best classified according to Gustilo & Anderson (1976); modified in 1984 by Gustilo et al (see Ch. 32). This system describes the size of the wound, the extent of the soft tissue injury, the degree of contamination and the presence or absence of associated vascular injury (Table 34.3).

Table 34.3 Classification of open fractures	
Type I	An open fracture with a wound <1 cm long and clean
Type II	An open fracture with a laceration >1 cm long without excessive soft tissue damage, flaps or avulsions
Type III	Massive soft tissue damage, compromised vascularity, severe wound contamination, marked fracture instability
Type III A	Adequate soft tissue coverage of a fractured bone despite extensive soft tissue laceration or flaps or high-energy trauma irrespective of the size of the wound
Type III B	Extensive soft tissue injury loss with periosteal stripping and bone exposure; usually associated with massive contamination
Type III C	Open fracture associated with arterial injury requiring repair

Type I

Type I usually results in a spike of bone puncturing the skin from within outwards. In these cases, stabilisation can be with the use of plates, intramedullary nails or external fixation. The wound should be treated with copious irrigation (limited excision and antibiotics are satisfactory).

Type II

It may be possible to treat Type II fractures in a manner similar to that used for Type I, with excision of the wound edges, inspection of the depths of the wound, removal of all devitalised tissue and stabilisation of the fracture. Antibiotics should be given. With these wounds, it is often appropriate that a second look should be carried out at 48 hours, to ensure that no necrotic tissue has been left behind. At this stage it may be possible to close the wound. If not, the wound could be closed by skin grafting or other reported techniques for slowly bringing skin edges together.

Type III

Type III fractures present different problems for the orthopaedic surgeon. The problems are the extensive soft tissue injury, comminution of the fracture, bone loss and vascular injury.

The principles of management of Type III fractures are the same in children as in adults. The fracture should be stabilised, the best form being that of external fixation. This can be carried out with either unilateral fixation or a circular frame. The unilateral device is probably the best in the emergency situation. The fracture can be stabilised and length maintained. However, definitive treatment may be achieved more effectively with a circular frame, because of its greater versatility in the management of the comminuted fracture, especially with bone loss (Fig. 34.3). If a vascular injury is present, the fracture should be stabilised by external fixation before the vascular repair is carried out.

With these extensive wounds, advice should be obtained from a plastic surgeon as, after extensive debridement, there may be major soft tissue defects. If large areas of bone are exposed, soft tissue cover should be obtained by mobilising a local flap. Occasionally, free flaps are required and the timing of plastic surgical intervention depends on the extent and severity of the soft tissue injury.

Bone loss

In the rare situation in which a child with a compound fracture presents with bone loss, limb reconstruction should be planned at an early stage. Initial management of the fracture should maintain its length, and this is best achieved with an external fixator (Hull et al 1997). The opportunities that are available are:

1. Bone grafting of the defect.
2. Bone transport.
3. Acute limb shortening followed by proximal limb lengthening.

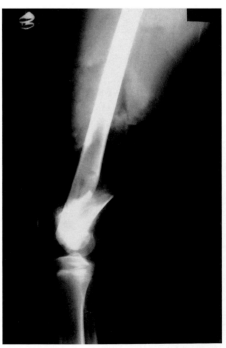
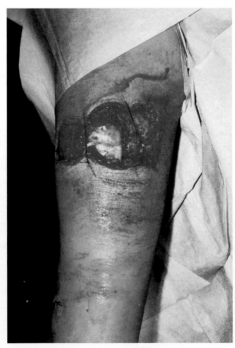
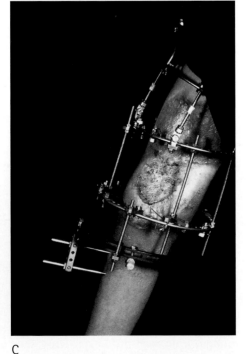

A B C

Figure 34.3 A Compound femoral fracture with bone loss. **B** The wound after debridement. **C** The grafted wound with circular frame *in situ*.

Bone transport or acute shortening with subsequent proximal lengthening should not be carried out anywhere other than in a unit with expertise in this form of treatment. There are significant pitfalls, irreversible complications must be avoided, and professional support from ancillary staff is essential, especially from physiotherapists, orthotists and occupational therapists (see Ch. 28).

OUTCOMES OF POLYTRAUMA

Improved care of the multiply injured child, from field contact to rehabilitation, has decreased both mortality and morbidity. Van der Sluis et al (1997) analysed patients younger than 15 years with an Injury Severity Score of 16 or greater. Eighty percent of the patients survived. One year after injury, 22% were disabled, mainly by brain injury. Nine years after injury, 42% showed cognitive impairment, but only 12% had significant physical disability. Seventy-six percent were in employment or attended school.

Even though treatment is improving, every attempt must continue to be made to reduce the number of major injuries. Car safety, traffic control, suitable play areas for children, crash helmets for cyclists, and adequate policing are some of the measures by which this reduction may be achieved.

REFERENCES AND FURTHER READING

Advanced Life Support Group 2000 Advanced Paediatric Life Support. The Practical Approach, 3rd Edn. BMJ Books, London

American College of Surgeons 1997 Advanced trauma life support program for doctors. Chicago, American College of Surgeons

Cramer K E 1995 The pediatric polytrauma patient. Clinical Orthopaedics and Related Research 318: 125–135

Gustilo R B, Anderson J T 1976 Prevention of infection in the treatment of 1025 open fractures of long bones. Retrospective and respective analysis. Journal of Bone and Joint Surgery 58A: 453–458

Gustilo R B, Mendoza R M, Williams D M 1984 Problems in the management of Type III (severe) open fractures. A new classification of Type III open fractures. Journal of Trauma 24: 742–746

Hull J B, Sanderson P L, Rickman M, Bell M J, Saleh M 1997 External fixation of children's fractures: use of the Orthofix Dynamic Axial Fixation. Journal of Pediatric Orthopaedics B6: 203–206

Jennett B, Teasdale J B, Galbraith S et al 1977 Severe head injuries in three countries. Journal of Neurosurgery and Psychiatry 40: 291–298

Milch H, Milch R A 1959 Fractures of the pelvic girdle In: Milch H, Milch R A (eds) Fracture surgery. Paul B Hoeber, New York

Quimby W C Jr 1966 Fractures of the pelvis and associated injuries in children. Journal of Pediatric Surgery 1: 353–364

Rang M 1983 Children's fractures, 2nd Edn. JB Lippincott, Philadelphia

Rockwood C A, Wilkins K E, Beatey J H 1996 Fractures in children, 4th Edn. Lippincott Raven, Philadelphia

Tolo V T 1983 External fixation in children's fractures. Journal of Pediatric Orthopaedics 3: 435–442

Van der Sluis C K, Kingma J, Fisma W H, Fen Duis H J 1997 Pediatric polytrauma: short-term and long-term outcomes. Journal of Trauma 43: 501–506

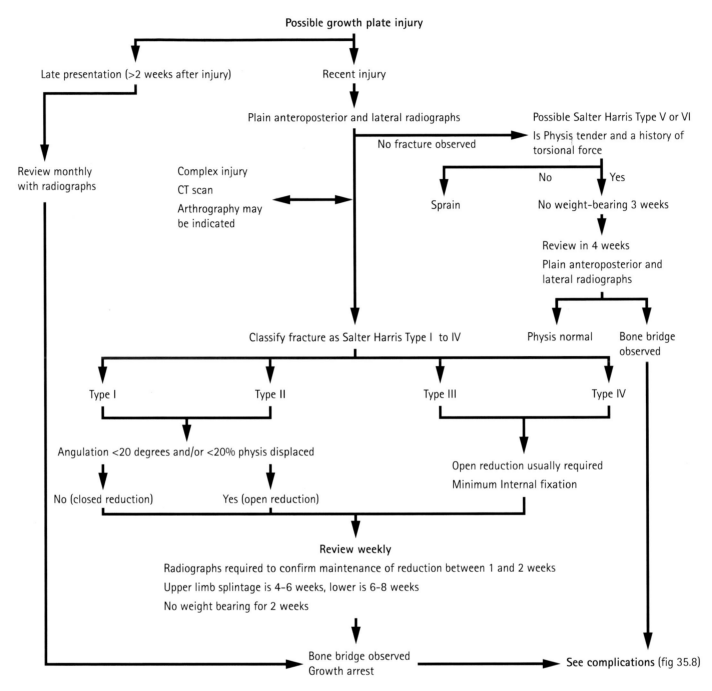

Figure 35.5 The flow diagram covers the basics of the clinical management of physeal fractures.

An illustrative case of a 6-year-old boy with a Gustillo compound grade 3 comminuted fracture of the right tibia and fibula is presented (Fig. 35.7A). He sustained this in a motor vehicle accident. The wound extended to the medial aspect of the ankle joint which was open. The growth plate of the distal medial tibia was abraded to the bone for 1 cm (Fig. 35.7A: distal arrow) as in a type VI Rang and Kessel physeal injury. Initially the wound was debrided and the fracture stabilised with an external fixator (Fig. 35.7B). An acute Langenskiöld procedure was performed for the distal tibial growth plate injury. This included debridement of the

exposed peripheral physis with a dental burr and fat interposition. Additionally a rectus abdominis free flap was carried out to cover the bone lesion, with split thickness skin graft to the exposed muscles. The ruptured tibialis anterior tendon was repaired. The patient has been followed up regularly and at 3 years 6 months after injury this representative X-ray confirms ongoing physeal growth (Fig. 35.7C, D). A CT scan at 4 years and 6 months showed peripheral growth plate repair (Fig. 35.7E) and at final follow up 5.5 years later there was no angular deformity of the leg. The distal tibial growth plate was open and the

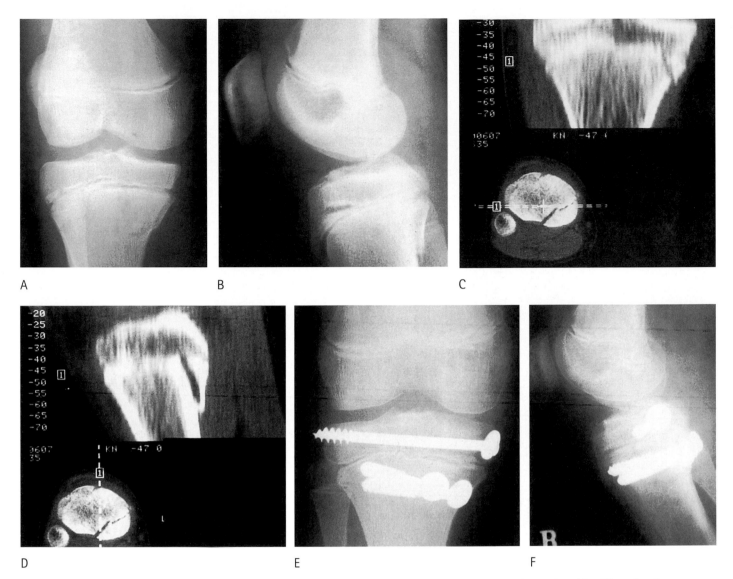

Figure 35.6 Open reduction of a type IV triplane fracture of proximal tibia. Preoperative planning assisted by CT evaluation. Interfragment screw fixation provides intra-epiphyseal and metaphyseal stable fixation.

affected limb was 1.5 cm longer than the normal side (Foster et al 2000).

Intermediate presentation

The displaced growth plate fracture seen 2 weeks after injury always poses a management dilemma. Late closed manipulation may further injure the growth plate and it may be prudent to defer treatment and perform a realignment osteotomy later. However, if an open procedure is undertaken, a circumferential metaphyseal–periosteal release may allow gentle repositioning of the grossly displaced epiphysis.

Late presentation

This is considered under 'Salvage procedures' below.

COMPLICATIONS

Early removal of Kirschner wires after open reduction and internal fixation should prevent pin track infection. For example, following lateral condylar fractures the wires are removed after 2–3 weeks. Biodegradable implants made of synthetic polymers may obviate the need to remove implants but may still prove problematical because of local inflammation or their mechanical characteristics. Nevertheless, biodegradable wires have been proved useful in animals and humans (Bostman et al 1987, 1989, 1992a,b, Makela et al 1992, Partio et al 1992a,b, Hara et al 1994).

With fractures of the distal femoral and proximal tibial physes the risk of associated vascular injury needs to be emphasised. Similarly, compression of the median nerve

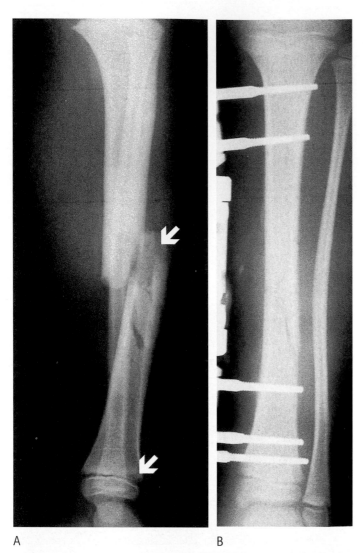

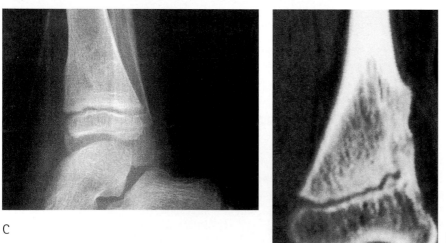

Figure 35.7 An illustrative case of a 6-year-old boy who presented with a Gustillo compound grade 3 comminuted fracture of the right tibia and fibula. He underwent an anticipatory Langenskiöld procedure. **A** Comminuted compound fracture with abraded physis (Rang type VI injury). **B** External fixator in position. **C** Growth normal after 3½ years. **D** CT peripheral growth plate repair at 4½ years.

may occur with markedly displaced distal radial injuries. The site of the growth plate injury is important prognostically. The distal femoral physis, for instance, is most at risk of bone bridge formation and significant premature arrest.

SALVAGE PROCEDURES

Once it has been established that bone growth has become compromised, techniques used to correct the problem depend upon the physis involved and the age of the patient.

Peterson has reviewed the treatment in detail (Peterson 1984, 1996, 1998). A clinical flow diagram of the complications is presented in Figure 35.8.

Possible treatment regimens are described below.

Conservative

If the physeal arrest has occurred at or near the end of skeletal growth, or in a physis whose contribution to the total length of the limb is minor, the need to repair the bone bridge is small. Limb-length discrepancy in the upper limbs is very well tolerated and up to 2.5 cm is acceptable in the lower limbs (Peterson 1984).

Orthoses

Small variations in lower limb length may be corrected with orthotic support.

Epiphysiodesis (injured physis)

Angular deformity in a limb that is almost at the end of skeletal growth may be reduced by destruction of the undamaged portion of the injured physis. This can be performed by placing a staple or screw across the physis. If the limb already has considerable deformity, a corrective wedge osteotomy should be performed (see below).

Epiphysiodesis (contralateral physis)

Limb-length discrepancy can be reduced be premature closure of the corresponding physis on the adjacent leg. This can be achieved by the placement of staples that span the physis on both the lateral and medial side (Zuege et al 1979). Percutaneous drill epiphysiodesis is now the favoured procedure in our centre. Screw fixation techniques are sometimes advocated.

Physiolysis

When the bone bridge will lead to unacceptable deformity, the bone bridge itself can be surgically removed. Angular deformity and shortening as a consequence of bone bridge formation can be substantially reduced by timely surgical intervention (Mizuta et al 1987).

The management of growth arrest involves the assessment of angular deformity as well as the extent of the bone bridge. Langenskiöld (1981) recommends that, if angulation is greater than 25° at the time of the interpositional physiolysis, a concomitant osteotomy to correct the axis should be undertaken. Interpositional physiolysis may be undertaken within 12 months of normal growth plate closure with an anticipation of correction of length and angulation.

In experimental peripheral growth arrest studies a bridge lesion of up to 17.2% of total physeal area can be treated successfully (Foster 1989) (Table 35.3). With central lesions as much as 50% of the growth plate area may be resected and still allow continued longitudinal growth (Langenskiöld 1981, Klassen & Peterson 1982). Growth arrest is reversed by creating a physiological non-union at the site of the tether so that the remaining physis continues to grow. This is satisfactory if the critical area of physeal resection is not exceeded and the bone bridge does not reform.

Evaluation of the growth plate lesion is an essential part of the preoperative planning and is best undertaken by CT scans, although this may be replaced in the future with MRI.

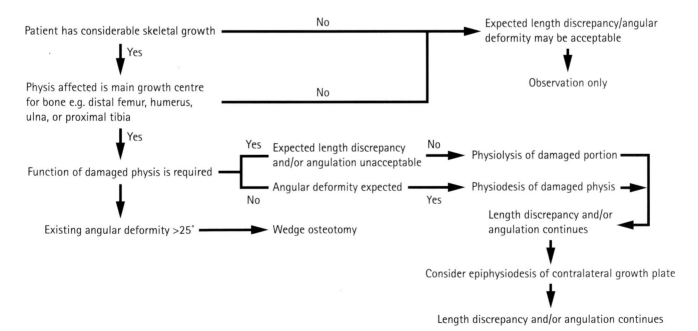

Figure 35.8 The flow diagram covers the basics of clinical management of the complications that may be expected following physeal trauma.

Ilizarov G A, Soybelman L M 1969 Some clinical and experimental data concerning bloodless lengthening of the lower extremities. Eksperimental'naya Khirurgiya i Anesteziologiya 14: 27–32

Johnson J T H, Southwick W O 1960 Growth following transepiphyseal bone grafts. An experimental study to explain continued growth following certain fusion operations. Journal of Bone and Joint Surgery 42A: 1381–1395

Johnstone E W, Leane P B, Kolesik P, Byers S, Foster B K 2000 Spatial arrangement of physeal cartilage chondrocytes and the structure of the primary. Journal of Orthopedic Sciences 5: 302–306

Kamegaya M, Shinohara Y, Kurokawa M, Ogata S 1999 Assessment of stability in children's minimally displaced lateral humeral condyle fracture by magnetic resonance imaging. Journal of Pediatric Orthopaedics 19: 570–572

Kaufmann H 1984 Appearance of secondary ossification centers. In: Lentner C (ed.) Geigy Scientific Tables, physical chemistry, composition of blood, hematology, somatometric data. Ciba-Geigy, Basle, pp 316–318

Klassen R A, Peterson H A 1982 Excision of physeal bars: The Mayo Clinic experience 1968–1978. Orthopaedic Transactions 6: 65

Kronenberg H M, Lanske B, Kovacs C S et al 1998 Functional analysis of the PTH/PTHrP network of ligands and receptors. Recent Progress in Hormone Research 53: 283–301; discussion 301–3

Langenskiöld A 1975 An operation for partial closure of an epiphysial plate in children, and its experimental basis. Journal of Bone and Joint Surgery 57B: 325–330

Langenskiöld A 1981 Surgical treatment of partial closure of the growth plate. Journal of Pediatric Orthopaedics 1: 3–11

Lee E H, Chen F, Chan J, Bose K 1998 Treatment of growth arrest by transfer of cultured chondrocytes into physeal defects. Journal of Pediatric Orthopaedics 18: 155–160

Macnicol M F, Anagnostopoulos 2000 Arrest of the growth plate after arterial cannulation in infancy. Journal of Bone and Joint Surgery 82B: 172–175

Makela E A, Bostman O, Kekomaki M et al 1992 Biodegradable fixation of distal humeral physeal fractures. Clinical Orthopaedics and Related Research 283: 237–243

Mizuta T, Benson W M, Foster B K, Paterson D E, Morris L L 1987 Statistical analysis of the incidence of physeal injuries. Journal of Pediatric Orthopaedics 7: 518–523

Monticelli G, Spinelli R 1981 Distraction epiphysiolysis as a method of limb lengthening. III. Clinical applications. Clinical Orthopaedics and Related Research 154: 274–285

Ogden J A 1982 Skeletal growth mechanism injury patterns. Journal of Pediatric Orthopaedics 2: 371–377

Partio E K, Hirvensalo E, Bostman O et al (1992a) Absorbable rods and screws: a new method of fixation for fractures of the olecranon. Int Orthop 16: 250–254

Partio E K, Hirvensalo E, Partio E et al (1992b) Talocrural arthrodesis with absorbable screws, 12 cases followed for 1 year. Acta Orthopaedica Scandinavica 63: 170–172

Peterson H A 1984 Partial growth plate arrest and its treatment. Journal of Pediatric Orthopaedics 4: 246–258

Peterson H 1996 Physeal and apophyseal injuries. In: Rockwood C, Wilkins K, Beaty J (eds) Fractures in children. Lippincott-Raven, Philadelphia, pp 103–165

Peterson H 1998 Treatment of physeal bony bridges by means of bridge resection and interposition of cranioplast. In: de Pablos J (ed.) Surgery of the growth plate. S.A. Ediciones Ergon, Madrid, pp 299–307

Phemister D B 1933 Operative arrestment of longitudinal growth of bones in the treatment of deformities. Journal of Bone and Joint Surgery 15: 1–15

Poland J 1898 Separation of the epiphysis. Smith Elder, London

Rang M 1969 The growth plate and its disorders. Churchill Livingstone, Edinburgh

Rubin P 1964 Dynamic classification of bone dysplasias. Year Book Medical Publishers, Chicago

Salter R B 1970 Textbook of disorders and injuries of the musculoskeletal system. Williams & Wilkins, Baltimore

Salter R B, Harris W R 1963 Injuries involving the epiphyseal plate. Journal of Bone and Joint Surgery 45A: 587–622

Sims C D, Butler P E, Casanova R, Lee B T et al 1996 Injectable cartilage using polyethylene oxide polymer substrates. Plast Reconstr Surg 98: 843–850

Smith B G, Rand F, Jaramillo D, Shapiro F 1994 Early M R imaging of lower-extremity physeal fracture-separations: a preliminary report. Journal of Pediatric Orthopaedics 14: 526–533

Trueta J, Amato V P 1960 The vascular contribution to osteogenesis III. Changes in the growth cartilage caused by experimentally induced ischaemia. Journal of Bone and Joint Surgery 42B: 571–587

Trueta J, Morgan J D 1960 The vascular contribution to osteogenesis I. Studies by the injection method. Journal of Bone and Joint Surgery 42B: 97–109

Vortkamp A, Lee K, Lanske B, Segre G V, Kronenberg H M, Tabin C J 1996 Regulation of rate of cartilage differentiation by Indian hedgehog and PTH-related protein [see comments]. Science 273: 613–622

White P G, Mah J Y, Friedman L 1994 Magnetic resonance imaging in acute physeal injuries. Skeletal Radiol 23: 627–631

Zuege R C, Kempken T G, Blount W P 1979 Epiphyseal stapling for angular deformity at the knee. Journal of Bone and Joint Surgery 61A: 320–329

Chapter 36

Birth injuries and non-accidental injuries

P. J. Witherow

GENERAL CONSIDERATIONS

INTRODUCTION

Fracture patterns in early childhood differ from those in later childhood and adult life (Ogden et al 1996). An appreciation of the anatomy of growing bones helps one to understand the reasons for these different modes of failure, particularly in the context of the low-velocity, low-energy skeletal injuries seen in birth trauma and child abuse.

ANATOMY

The physis or growth plate tends to be weakest in zones three and four, the hypertrophic and calcifying zones, except in infancy when the plane of greatest weakness is through the ossifying calcified cartilage columns in the metaphysis, rather than through the deeper layers of the physis, so that fracture separations tend to take off a thin shell of juxtaphyseal bone. Peripherally there is a small indentation around the resting and proliferating parts of the growth plate called the groove of Ranvier (Shapiro et al 1977) containing a zone of increased cellularity. This is associated with bone deposition at the interface between the perichondrium and the physis, producing a thin cuff of bone described by Lacroix as the perichondrial bone bark which extends a few millimetres beyond the physis–metaphysis junction, reinforcing it. There is then a zone of bone resorption concerned with maintaining tubulation of the metaphysis prior to the start of the deposition of laminar bone at the metaphyseal–diaphyseal junction. This zone of resorption is associated with a honeycomb-like surface which, particularly in the younger infant, represents a point of weakness (Marks 1998).

The shafts of the long bones in the neonate are composed largely of woven bone as Haversian systems are relatively under-developed at the time of birth.

The child's periosteum is thick. It is continuous with the perichondrium of the chondro-epiphysis and at this level is densely adherent. In the area of metaphyseal remodelling where the bone is widely fenestrated the periosteum is also quite adherent to the fibrovascular tissue of the intertrabecular marrow spaces (Ogden et al 1996). This stabilises those metaphyseal fractures which follow the plane of weakness adjacent to the shaft side of the physis so that they tend to heal with minimal subperiosteal new bone. Once the periosteal–bone bond at the level of the metaphysis is broken, however, the diaphyseal periosteum, which is loosely applied, can be widely stripped and extensive subperiosteal new bone follows (Fig. 36.1).

BIOMECHANICS

The bone of the neonate and infant is more flexible than that of the older child or adult, although it is not as strong. The load–deformation curve has a long plastic deformation region prior to failure, a characteristic that slows the rate of crack propagation (Curry & Butler 1975). In the metaphysis and also in the diaphysis of young children there is relatively little dense lamellar bone and the surface of the propagating crack tends to be irregular rather than relatively smooth. Greater energy is required to drive the fracture line and this restricts the extent of the fracture.

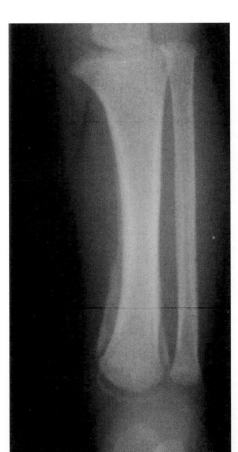

Figure 36.1 Fracture-separation of the distal tibial epiphysis. The hoop-like appearance is probably a combination of subperiosteal new bone and the metaphyseal rim fracture.

FRACTURE PATTERNS

Transverse and spiral fractures of the shafts of the long bones occur as in adults and the majority of these are complete fractures. Incomplete spiral fractures can occur in toddlers, particularly in the tibia, but also sometimes in the femur.

Separation of the chondro-epiphyses (only the distal femur regularly has an ossific nucleus at the time of birth) occurs through a plane which can vary between zones three and four of the physis and the metaphyseal zone in which the cartilage columns are becoming ossified. After the neonatal period, a peripheral fragment which is backed up by the perichondrial bone ring of Lacroix frequently remains, with the epiphysis forming a chip or bucket handle appearance on X-ray (Fig. 36.2).

Greenstick fractures occur with low-velocity, low-energy injuries when there is failure in tension on one side with plastic deformation or buckling on the other. The woven bone of the young child can also fail largely in compression, which gives rise to metaphyseal torus or buckle fractures usually occurring at the junction between metaphysis and diaphysis where the transition between the flexible

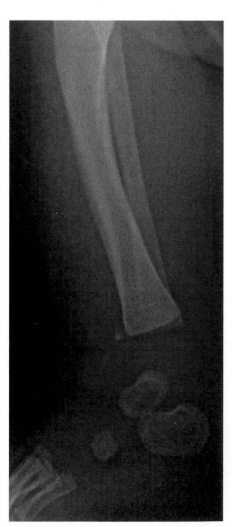

Figure 36.2 Metaphyseal chip fracture of classic type.

fenestrated and the stiffer cortical bone produces a stress concentration.

HEALING

The rate of growth of long bones in the first year of life, although decaying, will not be approached again until puberty. Compared with the adult the young child's bones are more vascular and more porous with increased endosteal and periosteal osteogenic potential.

In the neonate, diaphyseal fractures are frequently sticky at a week and stable at three: a toddler may take twice as long to reach the same end points. Remodelling occurs probably by a combination of periosteal appositional growth and resorptive remodelling together with differential epiphyseal growth. Remodelling potential is greatest in the first year of life. Misalignment in the plane of the adjacent joint tends to be best corrected and rotational misalignment worst.

The metaphysis is well vascularised, being a region of intense bone deposition and remodelling activity. Metaphyseal fractures usually heal rapidly.

BIRTH INJURIES

INTRODUCTION

Advances in obstetric practice, particularly the more widespread use of caesarean section to deliver babies presenting by the breech, and the better assessment of fetal maturity, have led to a decrease in both the number and severity of birth injuries. Most of these are now either fractures of the clavicle or mild brachial plexus palsies, but a few serious injuries remain and can pose difficult problems of diagnosis and treatment.

INCIDENCE

The combined incidence of fractures and brachial plexus injuries has fallen steadily: 20 per thousand in the 1930s, seven per thousand in the 1950s and a current level of approximately two to three per thousand (Thorndike & Pierce 1936, Rubin 1964, Wickstrom et al 1988). The clavicle is most commonly injured followed by the brachial plexus, the humerus and the femur.

Cervical cord injuries are often present in fatal cases (Gresham 1975), but unidentified fractures of the cervical spine associated with more limited cord or root damage occur more frequently than is appreciated.

The risk of birth injury is increased if manipulation is needed at delivery, if the baby's weight is over 4.5 kg (Wickstrom et al 1988) and following breech delivery.

AETIOLOGY

In vertex presentations cervical cord injuries can occur during instrumental rotation of the head from occipitoposterior to anterior in mid-cavity. They can also result if strong head traction is used to deliver arrested shoulders or, in breech presentations, if heavy traction is used to deliver the after-coming head.

Forceful groin traction during delivery of the extended breech can result in femoral shaft fractures. Humeral fractures may be caused in breech babies when bringing down the arms, particularly when there is shoulder dystocia or the arms are in the nuchal position. Fractures can even occur during caesarean section delivery (Nadas et al 1993).

SPECIFIC INJURIES

Clavicle

Clavicular fractures account for 40–50% of all birth injuries. The fracture usually occurs in the mid-third of the bone and is commonly greenstick, although it may be complete and either transverse or oblique. Both shoulder dystocia and large birth weight are risk factors (Oppenheim et al 1990). The majority of clavicular fractures follow vertex deliveries. Complete fractures of the clavicle are recognised by pseudoparalysis of the ipsilateral arm and pain on handling, but greenstick fractures may not become apparent until 2 weeks or more from the time of delivery when the fracture callus mass becomes obvious.

It is important to exclude an associated brachial plexus palsy because 5% of clavicular fractures are associated with plexus damage (Oppenheim et al 1990) and 13% of infants with brachial plexus palsy have a fractured clavicle (Greenwald et al 1984). It may be difficult to rule out neural injury in the first few days after birth as pain may produce pseudoparalysis or an asymmetrical Moro reflex. The diagnosis normally becomes clear by the end of the first week as the clavicular fracture firms up. Other conditions to be considered in the differential diagnosis of pain around the shoulder are upper humeral osteomyelitis and separation of the proximal humeral epiphysis. Both of these can be differentiated on the basis of a careful clinical examination.

Congenital pseudarthrosis of the clavicle, although rare, should not be forgotten (Owen 1970). The abnormality may be noted shortly after birth or, more significantly, after discharge home when questions of undiagnosed birth trauma and of possible child abuse may be raised. The pseudarthrosis, unless bilateral, is on the opposite side to the heart, the bone ends are smooth on X-ray without callus formation and there is no local tenderness.

Most fractured clavicles need no treatment apart from careful handling. If the fracture is displaced and the baby is in pain, a simple sling made from a crêpe bandage is all that is required.

Shoulder and proximal humerus

In the neonate and young infant the junction between the metaphysis and physis is a point of weakness, particularly when rotational loads are applied. The joint capsule and ligaments fail very infrequently so that dislocations are rare. Therefore most apparent dislocations of the shoulder are, in fact, fracture separations between the cartilaginous head of

the humerus and the metaphysis. This injury produces pain with pseudoparalysis, local swelling and tenderness around the shoulder (Lemperg & Liliequist 1970). Crepitus can be felt on examination.

The radiographic appearances mimic a dislocation because the chondro-epiphysis often lacks an ossific centre in the neonate. If there is any uncertainty ultrasonography (Broker & Burbach 1990) or arthrography will help to confirm the location of the humeral head in the glenoid.

Treatment is by immobilising the arm in internal rotation with a sling and swathe. Periosteal new bone will appear between the sixth and tenth days and immobilisation should be continued for 2–3 weeks.

Distal humerus and elbow

Again, dislocation is extremely uncommon although medial dislocation of the radial head due to presumed forced pronation has been reported (Bayne & Rang 1984). Apparent posterior dislocation of the elbow represents a fracture separation of the distal chondro-epiphysis (Downs & Wirth 1982, Barrett et al 1984) (Fig. 36.3).

Local swelling, tenderness and possibly crepitus are evident despite the normal relationship between the epicondyles and the tip of the olecranon. The X-ray appearances suggest a posteromedial dislocation but the proximal ends of the radius and ulna will be too close to the lower end of the humerus due to the lack of the spacer effect of the chondro-epiphysis. Arthrography will confirm the diagnosis.

Treatment should be by re-alignment with splintage of the elbow in a sling and swathe or a posterior slab for 2–3 weeks. The reported results are satisfactory with a full or virtually full recovery in most cases.

Humeral and femoral shaft fractures

Most fractures are mid-third, transverse and complete. For the humerus, immobilisation with the forearm across the chest will be needed for 2–3 weeks. For the femur, properly applied and supervised Bryant's traction can be used until

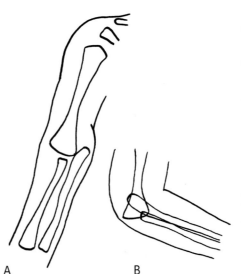

Figure 36.3
Separation of the distal epiphysis of the right humerus in a neonate simulating dislocation. The ossific centre of the capitellum is not present at birth. **A** Anteroposterior view. **B** Lateral view.

A   B

the fracture is reasonably firm at about 1 week, followed by a further week or two in a plaster spica. If the fracture has occurred in a baby who has been in the extended breech position *in utero*, the proximal fragment will tend to flex strongly and a marked degree of angular malunion can follow if this is not appreciated (Fig. 36.4). Although angular malunions of up to 40° will normally correct quite rapidly with growth, this problem can be avoided by immobilising the baby in the squat position in a spica cast after 5–7 days of traction.

Overlap and angulatory malunion normally correct quite quickly and full functional recovery is the rule. However, rotational malalignment should be corrected whenever possible to prevent long-term abnormality (Hagglund et al 1988).

Proximal femur

Fracture separation of the upper femoral epiphysis is uncommon but can be confused with developmental dysplasia. The leg lies flexed, abducted and externally rotated at the hip. There is local swelling and pain on gentle examination. The X-ray appearances (Fig. 36.5) suggest congenital dislocation or proximal femoral dysplasia. However, the acetabular appearance is normal (acetabular angle less than 30°). The metaphysis tends to buttonhole anteriorly and laterally through the torn periosteum, leaving an intact posterior hinge (Ogden et al 1984). Ultrasound will confirm that the femoral head is in the acetabulum and an arthrogram can be carried out if doubt persists. The displacement can usually be reduced by putting the leg in abduction, internal rotation and slight flexion. Immobilisation in a spica in this position, or treatment on overhead traction in abduction, will minimise the risk of late femoral neck retroversion and coxa vara.

Distal femur

Separation of the distal chondro-epiphysis can occur, particularly after breech delivery. This is usually incomplete and

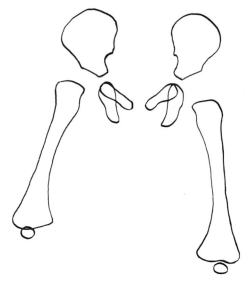

Figure 36.5 Separation of the proximal epiphysis of the femur simulating congenital dislocation of the hip. The metaphysis of the right femur is displaced proximally and laterally.

produces a picture similar to that seen in child abuse with varying degrees of periosteal stripping. Assessment of the degree of displacement is easier at the knee than it is at the elbow because the epiphyseal ossific centre is present in most term infants (Hensinger 1986).

Cervical spine

Cervical cord and cervical vertebral injuries are most likely to happen during breech delivery when there is difficulty with the after-coming head or in vertex deliveries when there is a shoulder dystocia.

The historical experiments of Duncan (Byers 1975) indicate that the cervical spine tends to fail when sustained loads of the order of 100 lb (45 kg) are applied. In traction the meninges and cord usually fail before the vertebrae (Lanska et al 1990). Cervical cord injury has been implicated in up to 10% of those infant deaths which occur at the time of delivery. Cervical spine injuries are normally associated with marked dystocia and sometimes the obstetrician feels a snap or 'give' during traction to deliver the after-coming head in breech deliveries or the shoulder in vertex presentation.

Vertebral injuries do occur (Stanley et al 1985) and may be associated with respiratory distress or brachial plexus palsy. The mode of vertebral failure is usually a fracture-separation between the body and the physis of the vertebral end-plate. Because the facet joints are relatively horizontal in infancy, cervical fractures are both unstable and easily reduced in extension.

The normal failure mode is through the upper vertebral end-plate with forward displacement of the more cephalad vertebrae at this level. Rarely, the displacement may be posterior with a vertical separation at the body-arch synchondroses.

Because of the relative prominence of the occiput in the infant, babies with cervical spine injuries should be nursed supine on a sponge support with a hollow for the back of the

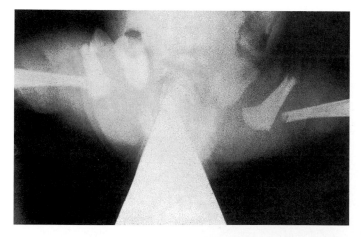

Figure 36.4 Bilateral femoral fractures which occurred during breech extraction. The proximal fragments will remain flexed and the distal fragments need to be aligned with them.

head. If they are nursed on a flat surface the cervical spine will be brought into flexion and displacement at the fracture site increased.

DIFFERENTIAL DIAGNOSIS OF NEONATAL INJURY

The neonate tends to adopt a flexed posture and when awake normal limb mobility is evident. Abnormal immobility of arm or leg is due either to true weakness from brachial plexus or spinal cord injury or to pseudoparalysis which occurs when the limb is painful. In the first few days of life the diagnosis is between plexus injury and clavicular fracture or epiphyseal fracture-separation, bearing in mind that both conditions can co-exist. After the first few days, osteomyelitis needs to be considered. Infantile osteomyelitis has a propensity to cause physeal damage with partial growth arrest so that prompt treatment is highly desirable. Complete cervical spinal cord damage produces tetraplegia and the diagnosis is obvious. Incomplete cord damage may be mistaken for spinal muscular atrophy, myotonia congenita or hypoxic-ischaemic brain damage; it should be appreciated that X-rays are usually normal.

NON-ACCIDENTAL INJURY

INTRODUCTION

Children who have been the victims of physical abuse are often brought to accident and emergency departments some days after they sustain their injuries. It is not always appreciated that although there are fracture patterns which are suggestive of child abuse (Akbarnia et al 1974), the most common presentation is with a single fracture rather than with multiple fractures and with a fracture which is diaphyseal rather than metaphyseal.

If a non-accidental injury is not recognised as such, there is a real risk of further injury which may result in permanent neurological damage (Morse et al 1970). The risk of subsequent injury may be as high as 20%, and of death 5%. Against this background it is important that all doctors dealing with injured children should consider the possibility of non-accidental injury carefully and involve a paediatrician at an early stage if in doubt.

The decision as to whether the child has suffered an accidental or a non-accidental injury has to be based on an assessment of probabilities because the history will often be misleading. It is helpful to consider the appropriateness of the history, the presence or absence of any risk factors, and the injury itself, before coming to a final decision.

Because of the importance of not missing the diagnosis on the one hand and not wrongfully accusing carers on the other, everyone treating injured children should be familiar with the local child protection policies and act on them if there is any suspicion of child abuse. Most errors are caused by either not sharing information or not revising an assessment when new information becomes available (Munro 1999).

AETIOLOGY

Very little is known about the mechanisms of injury in child abuse, although there is reasonable certainty about the effects of shaking, impact and of asphyxial injury from chest compression or airway obstruction. Deductions can be made about the mechanism of limb fractures by extrapolating from accidental falls in the toddler age group (Caffey 1972), but it is necessary to be very careful when extrapolating from injuries in older children whose bones have a more compact structure and different modes of failure.

DIAGNOSIS

The history

The history may be inappropriate and may change if the initial explanation is rejected or more injuries come to light. The perpetrators virtually never make a frank admission as to the cause of the injury, although they may make partial admissions such as "I may have picked him up rather roughly".

Babies do not fracture their limbs by catching them between the bars of the cot and hospital studies of children who have fallen from a bed or cot show that the injuries which result are usually minor (Nimityongskul & Anderson 1987). The explanation 'he bruises easily' is only acceptable if the bruises are at appropriate sites. All bruises in infants under 9 months should be regarded with some suspicion, especially if the bruising is on the trunk and face. The age of the child may be a helpful pointer since 80% of physical child abuse occurs under the age of 2 years.

Schemes for the estimation of the age of bruises based on colour changes from red through blue, purple, yellow and brown have been suggested but in practice there is wide variation in the rate of colour change. In one report yellow colouration was seen between day two and day thirteen (Stephenson & Bialas 1996).

It is important to appreciate that most fractures in child abuse represent transmitted rather than direct trauma to the bone and bruising at the fracture site should not be expected (Eastwood 1998).

Delay in taking the child to a doctor is not unreasonable in the case of a minor skull fracture or a minor greenstick limb fracture, but becomes highly suspicious when there is a complete fracture of a long bone. The attitude of the parents can also provide useful clues. The parents of a baby who has been injured accidentally are usually upset and frequently angry, whereas the parents of abused children may have an inappropriately flat emotional response.

Risk factors

Risk factors can be assessed with regard to the child, the carers and the home environment. Prematurity or serious neonatal illness can lead to a failure of bonding. A proportion of normal children cry more than average and are difficult to console. The parents or carers may be young, immature or unrealistic. Drug abuse and social deprivation increase the likelihood of non-accidental injury.

The parents themselves may well have been abused in childhood and lack parental skills, particularly the ability to cope with a crying baby. It is helpful if those dealing with families in which there has been child abuse adopt a sympathetic and non-judgemental attitude.

The injury

The injury itself may give a strong indication that child abuse has occurred. Certain fracture patterns are much more common in child abuse than in accidental injury. Those with a high specificity for child abuse include metaphyseal corner or bucket handle, rib, scapular, outer clavicle, complex skull and bilateral fractures. There may be characteristic cutaneous injuries. The fractures may be of an inappropriate age and undisclosed fractures may show up on a skeletal survey. It must be emphasised, however, that most cases presenting with skeletal injuries have an isolated fracture rather than multiple or typical non-accidental injury fractures.

CUTANEOUS INJURIES

These are present in a high proportion of physically abused children, possibly over 70%. The head and neck should be examined for fingertip bruises, usually about a centimetre across, and for the crescentic abrasions or drag marks produced by fingernails. The eyes should be examined for both subconjunctival and retinal haemorrhages: these may be associated with injury from asphyxia or shaking. Inside the mouth there may be tears of the labial frenulum from airway obstruction or forcible bottle feeding.

Examination of the mouth and fundi is not always easy but should be carried out unless it is planned to involve a paediatrician. When a toddler permits inspection of the mouth without protest this in itself can indicate an abnormally passive attitude.

The trunk and limbs should be inspected as part of a general check for joint range and skeletal tenderness. Fingertip bruising may be present on the back and patterned bruises from a belt or other object may be found on the trunk or legs.

The crescentic bruises of human bites may be seen, usually on either the hands, feet or buttocks. If suspected, the skin should be swabbed with a saline-soaked piece of absorbent paper which, with appropriate controls (of the saline and the paper), can be sent for forensic examination. Bite marks can be associated with the more serious forms of child abuse.

SKELETAL INJURIES

Periosteal elevation

Periosteal elevation with subperiosteal new bone formation may be seen in child abuse (Kleinman 1998a) either as an isolated finding along the shafts of long bones, where it is probably a response to forcible handling, or in association with epiphyseal fracture-separations. Care has to be exercised, however, in the case of babies, because after the age of 1 month up to 40% of normal infants show some degree of periosteal elevation. This is normally mid-shaft and symmetrical, affecting mainly the humeri, femora and tibiae (Schopfner 1966). Recent periosteal new bone may be seen between 1 and 3 months of age. A double cortex appearance may persist into the second year of life.

Metaphyseal fractures

These fall into two groups: a spectrum of metaphyseal change, representing degrees of fracture-separation of the epiphysis on the one hand (Kleinman et al 1986) and torus compression and transverse greenstick fractures of the metaphysis on the other (Fig. 36.6).

Reference has been made to the way the anatomy of the physis and the perichondrial ring influences the track of the fracture plane in partial or complete separations of the chondro-epiphysis. The bone collar of Lacroix supports the peripheral part of the juxta-physeal metaphysis which tends to remain with the physis. Appearances can vary from a linear translucency paralleling the physis, to a rim or corner fracture. If the X-ray plane is oblique to the bone, the peripheral fragment has a bucket handle or hoop configuration.

The rim fragment unites rapidly. Within a month there may be no X-ray evidence of a previous injury. Periosteal stripping is usually minimal with undisplaced metaphyseal fractures, but displaced fracture-separations are associated with extensive subperiosteal new bone during healing.

Transverse metaphyseal supracondylar fractures and torus, or greenstick buckle fractures, occur in child abuse but these fractures can be, and often are, accidental.

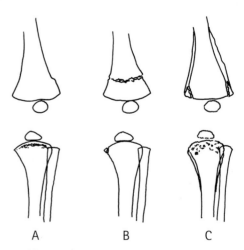

Figure 36.6 Metaphyseal fracture patterns. Femur: **A** buckle or torus fracture; **B** transverse metaphyseal fracture; **C** epiphyseal separation. Tibia: **A** linear metaphyseal lucency; **B** corner fracture; **C** diffuse metaphyseal irregularity. Tibia: **A** and **B** with femur **C** represent progression along the spectrum of fracture separations of the physis.

Diaphyseal fractures

These are the most common fractures found in child abuse and transverse fractures are more common than spiral ones (King et al 1988). The younger the child the greater the chance of the fracture being non-accidental (Rex & Kay 2000). Spiral fractures of the humerus (Worlock et al 1986) are more likely to be non-accidental than accidental but it is still necessary to pay attention to the appropriateness of the history, to any delay in bringing the child to hospital, to the age of the fracture and to the presence or absence of other injuries.

Rib fractures

These are significant indicators of non-accidental injury and probably result from the infant's chest being compressed in an attempt to stop it crying. The fractures are commonly at the rib head–neck junction (Kleinman 1998b) or the rib–costal cartilage junctions (Fig. 36.7). They may also be posterolateral. The ribs most frequently fractured are the sixth to eleventh with an average of four fractures per patient (Feldman & Brewer 1984). Ribs are not commonly fractured in children during cardiopulmonary resuscitation.

Skull and cerebral injury

Between 5% and 10% of victims of non-accidental injury have skull fractures (Hobbs 1984). Accidental fractures are likely to be parietal, linear, not depressed and less than 1 mm in width. In non-accidental injury simple linear fractures often occur but the pattern may be complex, and involve more than a single cranial bone. Growing fractures (diastatic fractures) are more frequent following child abuse than they are after accidental injury.

Cerebral injury is an important cause of mortality and morbidity in child abuse (Hobbs 1984). Shaking and impact can produce diffuse brain damage, particularly of the occipital lobes, or may result in subdural haematomas (Tzioumi &

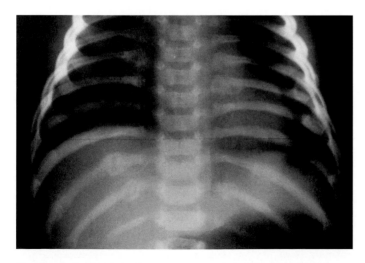

Figure 36.7 Multiple healing rib fractures. Posterolateral fractures of ribs 10 and 11, and rib head–neck fractures (e.g. ribs 6 and 7 left).

Oates 1998). Skull fractures may also be associated with subdural bleeding.

The outcome following cerebral whiplash injury includes paresis, visual loss and mental handicap (Dykes 1986).

INVESTIGATION

The definitive history and examination is best carried out by an experienced doctor. Detailed notes should be made with sketches and measurements. Any cutaneous injuries should be photographed.

The question of whether to carry out a skeletal survey is difficult. The total body X-ray dose is not inconsiderable but at first presentation, particularly in children less than 2 years old, a single skeletal survey is justified in most cases where there is a reasonable suspicion of child abuse. Repeat skeletal surveys should not normally be necessary unless there is a strong likelihood of further occult fractures.

Good-quality X-rays in two planes should be taken of all skeletal injuries. Compromise exposures of the whole limb are satisfactory for the location of fractures but not for the assessment of fracture age nor for giving an opinion on the possible mechanism of injury. Radiographs should be repeated wherever practicable, if possible 5 days after admission and at two intervals a week apart thereafter if the age of the fractures is likely to be of importance.

The isotope bone scan is more sensitive than plain X-rays in picking up recent undisplaced fractures and rib fractures, but the concentration of isotope adjacent to the growth plate results in quite large local radiation doses and metaphyseal fractures may be obscured.

Further investigations should include coagulation studies and a full blood count if there are bruises or petechiae, and a serum copper estimation if copper deficiency is postulated.

FRACTURE AGEING

Although a complete fracture will remain painful for a week, incomplete fractures in infants can become relatively painless within a few days and may be missed if the clinical examination is not sufficiently methodical (Fig. 36.8).

In assessing the age of a fracture from X-rays (Chapman 1992, O'Connor & Cohen 1998) it is helpful to look at the degree of soft-tissue swelling, loss of definition of the fracture line, the time at which the very earliest calcification appears, and the density and homogeneity of both the subperiosteal new bone and the fracture callus.

DIFFERENTIAL DIAGNOSIS

In general the skeletal injuries of child abuse are not likely to be confused with pathological fractures. However, patients with undiagnosed haemophilia and osteogenesis imperfecta have been the subject of child-care proceedings. Nevertheless, both of these conditions and child abuse can coexist (Johnson & Coury 1988).

With bruising and petechiae, mild haemophilia, purpura

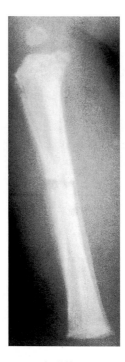
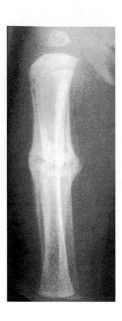

A

B

Figure 36.8 A diffuse metaphyseal irregularity and a transverse tibial fracture not obvious clinically on admission with gastroenteritis. Two days later when this X-ray was taken the callus is past the 6–10-day stage. **B** Twelve days later the callus is at the 3-week plus stage and the metaphyseal changes have almost resolved.

and leukaemia have to be considered and ruled out. A family history should always be taken.

Metaphyseal spurs and osteoporotic fractures occur in the rare condition of copper deficiency seen in malnourished and often premature infants. It is normally associated with characteristic motor delay, anaemia, leukopenia and X-ray changes (Shaw 1988).

Osteogenesis imperfecta poses particularly difficult problems (Smith 1995). Osteopenia may not be present at the time of the first fracture The injury may occur with minimal violence so that the carers' story may appear unconvincing.

The common type I disease with blue sclerae is autosomal dominant so there will usually (but not always) be a family history. In the first year of life infants tend to have a thinner and hence bluish sclerae — another reason for taking care. Type II and type III osteogenesis are unlikely to be confused since intrauterine and birth fractures occur, type II is usually lethal and the diagnosis in both types is obvious at birth. A particular problem arises with the less well delineated type IV osteogenesis imperfecta in which inheritance is also autosomal dominant and the sclerae are white. However, the statistical probability of osteogenesis in the presence of a normal facial shape, white sclerae, no family history, normal bone density and no excess of wormian bones in the skull is low.

Other conditions to be considered include fractures in neuropathic limbs, particularly in patients with spina bifida, the fractures which occur in small premature babies with osteopenia, and congenital pseudarthrosis of the tibia and clavicle. Periosteal reaction may be seen in normal infants, Caffey's disease, congenital syphilis and in association with the bone changes of leukaemia.

REFERENCES

Akbarnia B, Torg J S, Kirkpatrick J, Sussman S 1974 Manifestations of the battered-child syndrome. Journal of Bone and Joint Surgery 56A: 1159–1166

Barrett W P, Almquist E A, Staheli L T 1984 Fracture separation of the distal humeral physis in the newborn. Journal of Pediatric Orthopaedics 4: 617–619

Bayne O, Rang M 1984 Medial dislocation of the radial head following breech delivery: a case report and review of the literature. Journal of Pediatric Orthopaedics 4: 485–487

Broker F H, Burbach T 1990 Ultrasonic diagnosis of separation of the proximal humeral epiphysis in the newborn. Journal of Bone and Joint Surgery 72A: 187–191

Byers R K 1975 Spinal-cord injuries during birth. Developmental Medicine & Child Neurology 17: 103–110

Caffey J 1972 The parent–infant traumatic stress syndrome; (Caffey–Kempe syndrome), (battered babe syndrome). American Journal of Roentgenology, Radium Therapy and Nuclear Medicine 114: 218–229

Chapman S 1992 The radiological dating of injuries. Archives of Disease in Childhood 67: 1063–1065

Curry J D, Butler G 1975 The mechanical properties of bone tissue in children. Journal of Bone and Joint Surgery 57A: 810–814

Downs D M, Wirth C R 1982 Fracture of the distal humeral chondroepiphysis in the neonate. Clinical Orthopaedics and Related Research 169: 155–158

Dykes L J 1986 The whiplash shaken infant syndrome: what has been learned? Child Abuse and Neglect 10: 211–221

Eastwood D 1998 Breaks without bruises are common and can't be said to rule out non-accidental injury. British Medical Journal 317: 1095–1096

Feldman K W, Brewer D K 1984 Child abuse, cardiopulmonary resuscitation, and rib fractures. Pediatrics 73: 339–342

Greenwald A G, Schute P C, Shiveley J L 1984 Brachial plexus palsy. A 10 year report on the incidence and prognosis. Journal of Pediatric Orthopaedics 4: 689–692

Gresham E L 1975 Birth Trauma. Pediatric Clinics of North America 22: 317–328

Hagglund G, Hansson L I, Wiberg G 1988 Correction of deformity after femoral birth fracture 16-year follow-up. Acta Orthopaedica Scandinavica 59: 333–335

Hensinger R N 1986 Standards in pediatric orthopedics. Raven Press, New York, p 284

Hobbs C J 1984 Skull fracture and the diagnosis of abuse. Archives of Disease in Childhood 59: 246–252

Johnson C F, Coury D L 1988 Bruising or hemophilia: accident or child abuse? Child Abuse and Neglect 12: 409–415

King J, Diefendorf D, Apthorp J, Negrete V F, Carlson M 1988 Analysis of 429 fractures in 189 battered children. Journal of Pediatric Orthopaedics 8: 585–589

Kleinman P K (1998a) Skeletal trauma: general considerations. In: Kleinman P K (ed) Diagnostic imaging of child abuse, 2nd edn. Mosby, St Louis, pp 8–25

Kleinman P K (1998b) Bony thoracic trauma. In: Kleinman P K (ed) Diagnostic imaging of child abuse, 2nd edn. Mosby, St Louis, pp 110–148

Kleinman P K, Marks S C, Blackbourne B 1986 The metaphyseal lesion in abused infants: a radiologic–histologic study. American Journal of Roentgenology 14: 895–905

Lanska M J, Roessmann U, Wiznitzer M 1990 Magnetic resonance imaging in cervical cord birth injury. Pediatrics 85: 760–764

Lemperg R, Liliequist B 1970 Dislocation of the proximal epiphysis of the humerus in newborns: report of two cases and discussion of diagnostic criteria. Acta Paediatrica Scandinavica 59: 377–380

Marks S C Jr 1998 The structural and developmental contexts of skeletal injury. In: Kleinman P K (ed) Diagnostic imaging of child abuse, 2nd edn. Mosby, St Louis, pp 2–7

Morse C W, Sahler O J Z, Friedman S B 1970 A three-year follow up study of abused and neglected children. American Journal of Diseases of Children 120: 439–446

Munro E 1999 Common errors of reasoning in child protection work. Child Abuse and Neglect 23: 745–758

Nadas S, Gudinchet F, Capasso P, Reinberg O 1993 Predisposing factors in obstetrical fractures. Skeletal Radiology 22: 195–198

Nimityongskul P, Anderson L D 1987 The likelihood of injuries when children fall out of bed. Journal of Pediatric Orthopaedics 7: 184–186

O'Connor J F, Cohen J 1998 Dating fractures. In: Kleinman P K (ed) Diagnostic imaging of child abuse, 2nd edn. Mosby, St Louis, pp 168–177

Ogden J A, Ganey T M, Ogden D A 1996 The biological aspects of children's fractures. In: Rockwood C A, Wilkins D E, Beaty J H (eds) Fractures in children, 4th edn. Lippincott-Raven, Philadelphia, pp 19–52

Ogden J A, Lee K E, Rudicel S A, Pelker R R 1984 Proximal femoral epiphysiolysis in the neonate. Journal of Pediatric Orthopaedics 4: 282–292

Oppenheim W L, Davis A, Growdon W A, Dorey F J, Davlin L B 1990 Clavicle fractures in the newborn. Clinical Orthopaedics and Related Research 250: 176–180

Owen R 1970 Congenital pseudarthrosis of the clavicle. Journal of Bone and Joint Surgery 52B: 644–652

Rex C, Kay P R 2000 Features of femoral fractures in non-accidental injury. Journal of Pediatric Orthopaedics 20: 411–413

Rubin A 1964 Birth injuries: incidence, mechanisms and end results. Obstetrics and Gynecology 23: 218–221

Schopfner C E 1966 Periosteal bone growth in normal infants. American Journal of Roentgenology, Radium Therapy and Nuclear Medicine 97: 154–163

Shapiro F, Holtrop M E, Glimcher M J 1977 Organisation and cellular biology of the perichondrial ossification groove of Ranvier. A morphological study in rabbits. Journal of Bone and Joint Surgery 59A: 703–723

Shaw J C L 1988 Copper deficiency and non-accidental injury. Archives of Disease in Childhood 63: 448–455

Smith R 1995 Osteogenesis imperfecta, non-accidental injury, and temporary brittle bone disease. Archives of Disease in Childhood 72: 169–176

Stanley P, Duncan A W, Isaacson J, Isaacson A S 1985 Radiology of fracture-dislocation of the cervical spine during delivery. American Journal of Radiology 145: 621–625

Stephenson T, Bialas Y 1996 Estimation of the age of bruising. Archives of Disease in Childhood 74: 53–55

Thorndike A, Pierce F R 1936 Fractures in the newborn. A plea for adequate treatment. New England Journal of Medicine 215: 1013–1018

Tzioumi D, Oates R K 1998 Subdural haematomas in children under 2 years. Accidental or inflicted? A 10 year experience. Child Abuse and Neglect 22: 1105–1112

Wickstrom I, Axelsson O, Bergstrom R, Meirik O 1988 Traumatic injury in large-for-dates infants. Acta Obstetrica et Gynecologica Scandinavica 67: 259–264

Worlock P, Stower M, Barbor P 1986 Patterns of fractures in accidental and non-accidental injury in children: a comparative study. British Medical Journal 293: 100–102

Chapter 37

Fractures of the shoulder, upper limb and hand

J. de Pablos and A. Tejero

INTRODUCTION

Fractures of the upper limb in children, especially distal fractures (forearm, wrist and hand), are up to three times more frequent than those of the lower limb (de Pablos & Gonzalez 1999). Published series have shown that 7 out of 10 fractures in children involve the upper limb and that 50% of children's fractures affect the forearm and the hand (Landin 1983, 1997). This fact, together with the serious sequelae that may follow late diagnosis or inadequate treatment (or even correct treatment), makes it especially important to consider fractures in this area with particular care. Most occur in children over 6 years old and are the result of injuries suffered at sport, open-air games at school or traffic accidents (Cheng & Shen 1993). In younger children, household accidents are obviously the most frequent cause of these fractures. As with almost all fractures in children, those that involve the upper limb heal rapidly and non-union and delayed union are rare. Very active remodelling may occur in malunited fractures, especially in young children and in areas close to the growth cartilages. Few fractures remodel as swiftly and completely as those at the proximal end of the humerus (Gasco & de Pablos 1997). The overgrowth phenomenon after healing of long bone fractures in children is much less important in the upper limb than in the lower, and is practically non-existent in fractures of the forearm (de Pablos et al 1994). Joint stiffness is very unusual and is mostly associated with severe fractures at the elbow, or with aggressive surgical treatment of some fractures into or adjacent to the joint. Growth cartilage fractures may lead to premature physeal closure and its consequences (shortening and/or angular deformities). In general, however, and with exceptions such as the premature closure of the distal ulnar growth cartilage, the functional repercussions are not so severe as those in the lower limb, especially those at the knee.

These factors, above all the rapid healing and remodelling ability, allow for conservative treatment of most fractures of the upper extremities in children. However, there are some cases where reduction and surgical fixation of the fracture, percutaneously or by means of conventional open surgery, is necessary. The most common fixation methods involve the insertion of Kirschner wires (K-wires) for epiphyseal-metaphyseal fractures, and intramedullary nailing of diaphyseal fractures using flexible rods. Some specific injuries need external fixation or osteosynthesis plates (DCP type), particularly for the fixation of diaphyseal fractures.

Whatever method is used, special care should be taken to avoid potential iatrogenic injuries, especially physeal injuries and pin track infections. The rest of this chapter is devoted to analysing the main features of fractures of the shoulder girdle and upper limb in children, in topographical order.

SHOULDER AND HUMERAL SHAFT

CLAVICULAR FRACTURES

Clavicular fractures in children account for 10–15% of all fractures in children (Landin 1997). About half occur in children over 10 years of age. The mechanism of injury is usually indirect. In 75% the fracture is caused by a fall on the lateral side of the shoulder: the majority occur in the mid third of the clavicle. Fractures of the outer end of the clavicle usually result from forces transmitted through the humerus. Fractures caused by direct trauma are rare.

The clavicle can fracture in three main sites: diaphyseal, medial and lateral.

Diaphyseal fractures

Diaphyseal fractures are usually located in the middle third and are by far the most frequent (over 90% of all clavicular fractures). They may be complete, but it is more common to find a 'greenstick' fracture, associated with a greater or lesser degree of angulation. When the fracture is complete, the proximal fragment is normally displaced upwards by the action of the sternocleidomastoid muscle, while the distal fragment moves downwards as a result of the contraction of the pectoralis major and deltoid muscles. Contraction of the subclavius muscle tends to cause overlapping of the fragments.

Treatment should always be conservative since healing is almost invariable and, although there may be some malunion, excellent remodelling usually occurs (Fig. 37.1). Hence open reduction, with or without internal fixation, should always be avoided. The most frequently recommended conservative treatment is a simple sling or a 'figure-of-8' bandage for 3–4 weeks (Curtis et al 1991a). The aim of such bandaging is more to immobilise the fracture than to reduce it, and this must be clearly explained to parents. They should be aware that although the fracture fragments may overlap, it is almost certain adequate healing and remodelling will occur within 12–18 months, especially in children under 6–8 years of age.

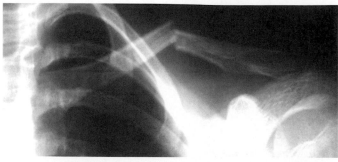

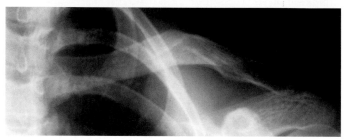

Figure 37.1 Complete fracture of the clavicular shaft in a 12-year-old boy (**A**). Note the remodelling that takes place by 9 months (**B**) after the fracture.

In order to place the 'figure-of-8' bandage, which is normally applied without anaesthesia, or with local anaesthesia instilled into the fracture site, the physician stands behind the child, who should be sitting with arms raised (in the position of surrender) or akimbo. When placing the bandage, backward pressure is applied on both shoulders, in an effort to distract the fracture site. The figure-of-8 bandage must be adjusted periodically (this may be done easily by the patient's relatives), in order to improve immobilisation and thus reduce the level of pain. Care should be taken with such adjustments, since excessive tightening of the bandage can cause skin lesions and/or neurovascular problems due to excessive axillary compression.

The figure-of-8 bandage remains the most popular form of treatment for fractures of the mid third of the clavicle, but other types of support, such as a simple sling, can be used for incomplete (greenstick) fractures, or complete fractures with only slight displacement. These simpler forms of treatment are often more comfortable and produce similar results to those of the figure-of-8 bandage. As healing occurs in 3–4 weeks, the sling or bandage should be kept on for this time. Recovery of shoulder movement usually takes place spontaneously without the need for physiotherapy.

Fracture of the medial end

This is the rarest location for fractures of the clavicle (about 2% of all clavicular fractures). In this rare group, sternoclavicular dislocation is the most common type of injury in adults, while in patients of up to 20 or 25 years of age (due to the extremely slow fusion of the medial growth plate (Post

1989)) proximal clavicular displacements are usually epiphyseal detachments (Salter–Harris types I and II). Clinical suspicion helps to establish the diagnosis, as the pain is localised and aggravated by palpation of the sternoclavicular junction. More importantly, there is protrusion when the displacement is anterior, or depression when it is posterior. With posterior displacement there may be dyspnoea and/or dysphagia due to compression of the trachea and/or the oesophagus. It is currently popular to confirm the diagnosis by transverse imaging techniques (CT), but conventional radiology using Rockwood views (45° tube inclination) is simpler and nearly always adequate.

Conservative or surgical treatment of fractures with anterior displacement is controversial: it is difficult to achieve reduction by conservative means and open reduction with internal fixation by K-wires or simple sutures is gaining popularity.

When the displacement is posterior, closed reduction is almost impossible and treatment, especially in the presence of tracheo-oesophageal compression, is surgical. If K-wires are used for fixation, it is wise to bend the free end of the wire to avoid potential migration (Lemire & Rosman 1984, Lyons & Rockwood 1990). Nonetheless, especially in anterior displacement fractures it may be reasonable to leave the arm in a sling, for 3–4 weeks (Curtis 1990), as healing and remodelling may avoid the need for surgery.

Fractures and dislocations of the outer end

These are also rare in children, although less so than those of the medial end. Most are fractures (particularly type I and II epiphysiolysis) without dislocation, since a small epiphyseal fragment of the distal clavicle usually remains attached to the acromio-clavicular joint. Such fragments are often difficult to detect and it is easy to confuse such fractures with acromio-clavicular dislocations. As with proximal fractures, conservative reduction is difficult to achieve, and the deformity may dictate the need for surgical reduction and fixation with K-wires. Precautions should again be taken to avoid potential wire migration (Lemire & Rosman 1984, Lyons & Rockwood 1990). The K-wires should be removed 4 weeks following the fracture. In fractures with minor displacement treatment is always conservative (a sling or Velpeau bandage for 3–4 weeks).

During fracture healing, if reduction was not anatomical, a 'double distal clavicle' may develop temporarily, but will undergo spontaneous remodelling over time. This is due to ossification of the periosteal cuff that remains in place when the clavicle is displaced proximally.

Among the complications of clavicular fractures are:

1. *Neurovascular injury*. The most common cause is acute compression of the subclavian vessels, the brachial plexus or the carotid artery by the displaced fracture fragments. Very rarely the callus that develops after these fractures causes neurovascular compression (Curtis et al 1991a).

2. *Tracheo-oesophageal compression.* This is most common in proximal fractures with posterior displacement. It normally responds well to open reduction with or without fixation of the fracture fragments.
3. *Non-union.* Non-unions are rare, and must be differentiated from congenital pseudoarthrosis of the clavicle (either isolated or syndrome related, such as in cleidocranial dysostosis). Treatment, especially in older children, generally only requires refreshing of the bone ends and stabilisation with a DCP plate and screws, and may not even necessitate bone graft.
4. *Malunion.* This is rare in children, as although most fractures heal with some overlap or angulation, remodelling allows cosmetic and functional improvement in a few months.
5. *Pain.* This is very unusual but may occur particularly after unreduced fractures of the lateral end.

FRACTURES OF THE SCAPULA

These fractures are rare and often occur in association with multiple trauma. They hardly ever need surgical treatment and usually respond well to conservative treatment immobilising the affected upper limb in a sling for 3–4 weeks.

TRAUMATIC DISLOCATION OF THE SHOULDER

This is another rare injury in the skeletally immature. An apparent dislocation in the newborn is usually a Salter–Harris type I epiphysiolysis, rather than a dislocation of the glenohumeral joint. Although shoulder dislocations may occur in other directions, anterior dislocations are by far the most frequent (Marans et al 1992). Clinical ('epaulette' shoulder and functional incapacity) and radiological diagnosis, especially if the cephalic nucleus is ossified, is not difficult.

As in the adult, treatment should be attempted by closed reduction, if necessary under general anaesthesia, in the emergency room. Following reduction, it is important to apply secure immobilisation using a Velpeau or Gilchrist (Gilchrist 1967) type bandage for 3–4 weeks. This may reduce the likelihood of future chronic instability (recurrent dislocation), which is very high in immature patients (up to 50% of cases) (Marans et al 1992, Hovelius et al 1996).

It is important to distinguish between traumatic dislocation (and potential subsequent chronic instability) and voluntary dislocation of the shoulder. The latter is not caused by trauma and the patients, who normally suffer from joint hyperlaxity, should be informed and discouraged from repeating the manoeuvre that led to dislocation. The problem may then resolve with growth.

FRACTURES OF THE PROXIMAL HUMERUS

These fractures account for less than 1% of all fractures in children. They occur through the growth plate or more distally in the metaphysis.

Fractures of the proximal humeral physis

These physeal fractures are either Salter–Harris type I (typically in neonates and in children under 8–10 years of age) or more commonly type II (in children over 10 and adolescents). Types III, IV and V are exceptional in the proximal humerus (Gregg-Smith & White 1992): they are usually caused by falling on the hyperextended hand with the shoulder also in hyperextension or, less frequently, by direct trauma to the posterolateral shoulder.

Clinically (pain, potential deformity and functional impairment) and radiologically, they are not difficult to diagnose. The distal fragment tends to displace anterolaterally while the proximal fragment remains normally located. When the distal fragment displaces laterally, it may protrude below the deltoid muscle, as Moore described over a century ago (Moore 1874).

Neer & Horowitz classified these fractures by grades, depending on the degree of displacement (Neer & Horowitz 1965):

- Grade I: less than 5 mm
- Grade II: up to one-third of the diaphysis
- Grade III: up to two-third of the diaphysis
- Grade IV: more than two-third of the diaphysis, or complete displacement.

These fractures have an extraordinary ability to heal and remodel, and are therefore usually treated conservatively, (Baxter & Wiley 1986, Larsen et al 1990).

Slightly displaced type I and II fractures do not require reduction and may be treated using immobilisation, whereas in more displaced fractures the most appropriate treatment is reduction under anaesthesia and immobilisation. If closed reduction proves impossible, open reduction should be used; this does not need to be anatomical, thanks to the high remodelling capacity. Such remodelling potential is inversely proportional to the age of the patient, allowing greater residual displacement in small children than in adolescents. Curtis et al (1991b) suggest certain acceptable values for residual angulation/displacement based on age; these may help the surgeon decide upon the therapeutic options. Specifically, acceptable values of angulation and displacement in children 1–5 years of age would be 70° and 100% respectively. Between 5 and 12 years of age up to 50° of angulation and 50% of displacement may be considered reversible. Children over 12 years old have less predictable remodelling potential and less displacement is allowable. In this group of patients no more than 30% of displacement (Neer–Horowitz type II) should be accepted.

The most commonly used methods of immobilisation are slings or a Velpeau type bandage for 3–4 weeks, after which progressive mobilisation should be encouraged. Other non-operative treatments include: bed rest with the arm in abduction for very unstable fractures; skin traction for 2 weeks, followed by the use of a sling – the efficiency of this method is doubtful – and plaster casts of the 'Statue of

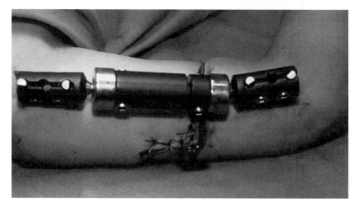

A

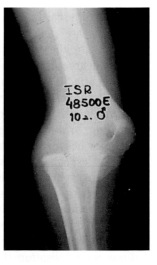

B

Figure 37.5 Compound fracture of the humeral shaft in a 9-year-old boy. The radial nerve (arrow) is observed adjacent to the bone crossing the fracture site, which explains its vulnerability (**A**). Debridement and external fixation were carried out (**B**).

6 years. The incomplete and complex ossification patterns of the distal humerus make identification of the fracture fragments hard. Secondly, treatment difficulties arise: reduction and maintenance of the fracture fragments is often problemmatical, and can be hazardous. The percentage of neurovascular complications of these fractures – both before and after treatment – is high. Elbow fractures and dislocations may be complicated also by malunion, non-union and functional limitation.

ELBOW DISLOCATION

Elbow dislocations occur mainly in adolescents (13–14 years of age), and are rare in children under 8 years. These lesions account for approximately 5% of all elbow injuries in the skeletally immature.

The most widely accepted classification is based on the integrity of the radio-ulnar joint and the direction of displacement of the segments. It is similar to that used in adults.

Type I. Intact proximal radio-ulnar joint:

  A. Posterior
    1. Posteromedial
    2. Posterolateral
  B. Anterior
  C. Medial
  D. Lateral.

Type II. Dislocated proximal radio-ulnar joint:

  A. Divergent
    1. Anteroposterior, with the radius displaced anteriorly and the ulna displaced posteriorly
    2. Transverse, with the ulna displaced medially and the radius displaced laterally
  B. Radio-ulnar translocation (radius displaced medially and ulna laterally)
  C. Isolated dislocation of the radial head.

The vast majority (over 90%) of elbow dislocations are posterior (Fig. 37.6) (Carlioz & Abols 1984). The mechanism of injury in posterior dislocations is a fall on the outstretched hand with the arm in supination and the elbow in extension or partial flexion. Anterior dislocations may be caused by a direct blow to, or fall upon, the olecranon. Medial or lateral displacements result from direct trauma, violent rotation of the forearm or a fall on the hand.

The clinical and radiological diagnosis is not usually difficult; however, care may be required to distinguish a supracondylar fracture. Compared with the latter, an elbow dislocation exhibits less swelling, a shortened forearm, no crepitation, and a loss of the normal triangular relationship between the epicondyles and the vertex of the olecranon. In posterolateral dislocations the radial head may be palpated. The radiograph should be carefully examined to evaluate the fractures which are commonly associated with elbow dislocation; i.e., fractures of the radial head or neck, coronoid

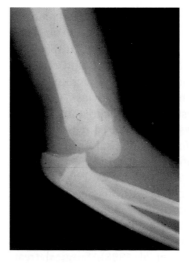

Figure 37.6 Posterolateral dislocation of the elbow in a 10-year-old boy.

process and medial epicondyle (Carlioz & Abols 1984). Before commencing treatment, it is crucial to have evaluated, as far as possible, the integrity of the neurovascular structures, which are frequently damaged in these dislocations. This is most important since neurovascular injuries can be produced, not only by the fracture itself, but also by the reduction. Information about the neurovascular situation prior to treatment allows correct assessment *before* reduction and guides decision-making in treatment.

The treatment recommended involves closed reduction under general anaesthesia and immobilisation with a plaster cast for 2–3 weeks. Reduction should be carefully planned. In posterior dislocations, two kinds of forces must be applied: the first is along the humeral axis, applying humeroulnar distraction, and the second follows the axis of the forearm, drawing it anteriorly with respect to the humeral condyles (Hankin 1984). In posterolateral dislocations, the forearm is placed in supination, and lateral displacement is first reduced, followed by reduction of the posterior displacement.

When associated fractures are present, once reduction of the dislocation is complete, the adequacy of their reduction must be assessed. Special attention should be paid to potential displacement of an associated fracture of the medial epicondyle. It is sometimes possible to see an epitrochlear fragment incarcerated in the humero-ulnar joint. If necessary, reduction and internal fixation of the fracture or fractures should be undertaken after reduction of the dislocation. Early diagnosis and treatment of associated fractures is critical, since treatment becomes increasingly difficult and hazardous if delayed.

Complications are rare but must not be overlooked. Perhaps the most frequent and severe (together with vascular problems) are the neurological injuries that may occur before, during or after treatment. The most commonly damaged nerve is the ulnar nerve. The median nerve may also be damaged by entrapment, either intra-articularly or at the fracture site itself (Ayala et al 1983). Ulnar lesions, usually neuropraxias, occur in about 10% of elbow dislocations in children and usually resolve spontaneously. Due to their anatomical features, lesions of the median nerve may lead to permanent sequelae requiring surgical repair. Vascular lesions are generally related to serious trauma with compound fractures. Stiffness, usually an extension deficit of 10° to 20°, is relatively frequent.

Other complications, such as chronic elbow instability, myositis ossificans and radio-ulnar synostosis, are more infrequent.

PULLED ELBOW OR NURSEMAID'S ELBOW

This is the most common elbow injury in children and, at the same time, one of the most trivial. It is practically a daily occurrence for frightened parents to bring children to the emergency room of orthopaedic departments, thinking that their child is suffering from painful paralysis of the upper limb.

The medical history and clinical signs are remarkably consistent. The upper limb has usually been subjected to sudden violent traction from the hand (hence the term 'pulled elbow') and the child, usually about 3 years old, suffers acute pain in the forearm, associated with an almost complete functional loss of the elbow, forearm and hand, that may be taken for paralysis. The limb, which in most cases is completely immobile, adopts a characteristic posture, with the elbow in 90° of flexion, the forearm in pronation, and the hand in a 'drooping' position. In addition, the child cries bitterly upon any attempt at passive mobilisation of the limb.

Anatomical investigations undertaken by Salter and Zaltz (1971) led them to conclude that the condition is caused by a reversible interposition of the annular ligament between the radial head and the capitellum, following sudden violent traction of the hand (Fig. 37.7).

Diagnosis is usually simple and is based exclusively on the clinical signs described above, since there are no specific radiological signs.

Treatment is also quite simple, but requires the surgeon to be familiar with the problem, and to diagnose it correctly. The reduction manoeuvre involves extension of the elbow while simultaneously placing the forearm in supination. When complete extension and supination are achieved, a 'click' can be heard, and this is felt more clearly by placing a thumb at the level of the radial head. Within minutes of this manoeuvre, the child begins to use the injured arm spontaneously, showing the problem has been solved. No plaster or bandaging is required after reduction; at most, a sling might be used for 2 or 3 days.

Complications are rare, but may include a recurrence of the problem, especially if the parents jerk the child's arm again. If this occurs treatment again involves closed reduction and advice to the parents not to repeat the traction. However, exceptional cases of irreducible 'pulled elbow', requiring open reduction, have been described (Salter & Zaltz 1971).

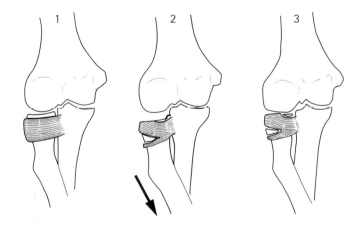

Figure 37.7 The pathoanatomical mechanism of production of pulled elbow in children according to Salter & Zaltz (1971). (Reproduced from Rang 1983.)

Graves S C, Canale S T 1993 Fractures of the olecranon in children: long-term follow-up. Journal of Pediatric Orthopaedics 13: 239–241

Greene M H, Hadied A M, Lamont R L 1984 Scaphoid fractures in children. Journal of Hand Surgery (Am) 9: 536–541

Greene W B, Anderson W J 1982 Simultaneous fracture of the scaphoid and radius in children. Journal of Pediatric Orthopaedics 2: 191–194

Gregg-Smith S J, White S H 1992 Salter–Harris III fracture dislocation of the proximal humeral epiphysis. Injury 23: 199–200

Hankin F M 1984 Posterior dislocation of the elbow. A simplified method of closed reduction. Clinical Orthopaedics and Related Research 190: 254–256

Hove L M, Engesaeter L B 1997 Corrective osteotomies after injuries of the distal radial physis in children. Journal of Hand Surgery (Br) 22: 699–704

Hovelius L, Agustini B G, Fredin H, Johansson O, Norlin R, Thorling J 1996 Primary anterior dislocation of the shoulder in young patients. A ten-year prospective study. Journal of Bone and Joint Surgery 78A: 1677–1684

Jakob R, Fowles J V 1975 Observations concerning fractures of the lateral humeral condyle in children. Journal of Bone and Joint Surgery 57A: 430–436

Jeffery C C 1950 Fractures of the head of the radius in children. Journal of Bone and Joint Surgery 32B: 314–324

Josefsson P O, Danielsson L G 1986 Epicondylar elbow fracture in children: 35-year follow-up of 56 unreduced cases. Acta Orthopaedica Scandinavica 57: 313–315

Kaempffe F A 1999 Biplane osteotomy and epiphisiodesis of the distal radius for correction of wrist deformity due to distal ulnar growth arrest. Orthopedics 22: 84–86

Kasser J R 1993 Forearm fractures. In: MacEwen G D, Kasser J R, Heinrich S D (eds) Pediatric fractures. A practical approach to assessment and treatment. Williams & Wilkins, Baltimore, pp 165–190

Kay S, Smith C, Oppenheim W L 1986 Both bone midshaft forearm fractures in children. Journal of Pediatric Orthopaedics 6: 143–146

Kjaer-Petersen K, Junk A C, Petersen L K 1992 Intrarticular fractures at the base of the fifth metacarpal. A clinical and radiographical study of 64 cases. Journal of Hand Surgery (Br) 17B: 144–147

Landfried M J, Stenclik M, Susi J G 1991 Variant of Galeazzi fracture–dislocation in children. Journal of Pediatric Orthopaedics 11: 332–335

Landin L A 1983 Fracture patterns in children: analysis of 8682 fractures with especial reference to incidence, etiology and secular changes in Swedish urban populations. Acta Orthopaedica Scandinavica 84(suppl 202): 1–100

Landin L A 1997 Epidemiology of children's fractures. Journal of Pediatric Orthopaedics 6B: 79–83

Larsen C F, Kiaer T, Lindquist S 1990 Fractures of the proximal humerus in children. Nine year follow-up of 64 unoperated on cases. Acta Orthopaedica Scandinavica 61: 255–257

Larson B, Light T R, Ogden J A 1987 Fracture and ischemic necrosis of the immature scaphoid. Journal of Hand Surgery (Am) 12: 122–127

Lascombes P, Prévot J, Ligiér J N, Metaizeau J P, Poncelet T 1990 Elastic stable intramedullary nailing. Journal of Pediatric Orthopaedics 10: 167–171

Lee B S, Esterhain J L, Das M 1984 Fracture of the distal radial epiphysis. Clinical Orthopaedics and Related Research 185: 90–96

Lemire L, Rosman M 1984 Sternoclavicular epiphyseal separation with adjacent clavicular fracture. Journal of Pediatric Orthopaedics 4: 118–120

Lesko P D, Georgis T, Slabaugh P 1987 Irreducible Salter–Harris type II fracture of the distal radial epiphysis. Journal of Pediatric Orthopaedics 7: 719–721

Ligiér J N, Metaizeau J P, Prévot J, Lascombes P 1988 Elastic stable intramedullary nailing in children. Journal of Bone and Joint Surgery 70B: 74–77

Luhmann S J, Gordon J E, Shoenecker P L 1998 Intramedullary fixation of unstable both-bone forearm fractures in children. Journal of Pediatric Orthopaedics 18: 451–456

Lyons F A, Rockwood C A 1990 Migration of pins used in operations on the shoulder. Journal of Bone and Joint Surgery 72A: 1262–1267

Mann D C, Rajmaira S 1990 Distribution of physeal and non-physeal fractures in 2650 long-bone fractures in children aged 0–16 years. Journal of Pediatric Orthopaedics 10: 713–716

Mansat M, Mansat Ch, Martinez Ch 1983 L'articulation radio-cubitale inférieur. Pathologie traumatique. In: Razemon J P, Fisk G R (eds) Le poignet. Paris: Expansion Scientifique Francaise, Paris, pp 187–195

Marans H J, Angel K R, Schemitsch E H, Wedge J H 1992 The fate of traumatic anterior dislocation of the shoulder in children. Journal of Bone and Joint Surgery 74A: 1242–1244

Marzo J M, d'Amato C, Strong M 1990 Usefulness and accuracy of arthrography in management of lateral humeral condyle fractures in children. Journal of Pediatric Orthopaedics 10: 317–321

Metaizeau J P, Prévot J, Schmitt M 1980 Reduction et fixation des fractures et dÈcollement Èpiphysaires de la tête radial par broche centromedullaire. Revue de Chirurgie Orthopedique et Reparatrice de l'Appareil Locomoteur 66: 47–49

Mintzer C M, Waters P M, Brown D J 1994 Percutaneous pinning in the treatment of displaced lateral condyle fractures. Journal of Pediatric Orthopaedics 14: 462–465

Monteggia G 1814 Insituzione Chirugiche 5: 130

Moore E M 1874 Epiphyseal fracture of the superior extremity of the humerus. Transactions of the American Medical Association 25: 296–300

Nafie S A 1987 Fractures of the carpal bones in children. Injury 18: 117–119

Neer C S, Horowitz B S 1965 Fractures of the proximal humeral epiphyseal plate. Clinical Orthopaedics and Related Research 41: 24–31

Ogden J A 1991 The uniqueness of the growing bones. In: Rockwood C A, Wilkins K E, King R E (eds) Fractures in children. Lippincott, Philadephia, pp 1–86

Post M 1989 Current concepts in the treatment of fractures of the clavicle. Clinical Orthopaedics and Related Research 245: 89–101

Price C T, Scott D S, Kurzner M E, Flynn J C 1990 Malunited forearm fractures in children. Journal of Pediatric Orthopaedics 10: 705–712

Rang M 1983 Children's fractures. J B Lippincott, Philadelphia pp 139–142

Richter D, Ostermann P A W, Ekkernkamp A, Murh G, Hahn M P 1998 Elastic intramedullary nailing: a minimally invasive concept on the treatment of unstable forearm fractures in children. Journal of Pediatric Orthopaedics 18: 457–461

Roy D R 1989 Completely displaced distal radius fractures with intact ulna in children. Orthopedics 12: 1089–1092

Royce R O, Dutkowsky J P, Kasser J R, Rand F R 1991 Neurologic complications after K-wire fixation of supracondylar humerus fractures in children. Journal of Pediatric Orthopaedics 11: 191–194

Salter R B, Harris W R 1963 Injuries involving the epiphyseal plate. Journal of Bone and Joint Surgery 45A: 587–622

Salter R B, Zaltz C 1971 Anatomic investigation on the mechanism of injury and pathologic anatomy of 'pulled elbow' in young children. Clinical Orthopaedics and Related Research 77: 134–143

Sanders R A, Frederick H A 1991 Metacarpal and phalangeal osteotomy with miniplate fixation. Orthop Rev 20: 449–456

Shaw B A, Kasser J R, Emans J B 1990 Management of vascular injuries in displaced supracondylar humerus fractures without arteriography. Journal of Orthopedic Trauma 4: 25–29

Sponseller P D 1996 Injuries of the humerus and elbow. In: Richards B S (ed) Orthopaedic knowledge update, Pediatrics. American Academy of Orthopaedic Surgeons, Rosemont, pp 239–250

Vahvanen V, Westerlungd M 1980 Fracture of the carpal scaphoid in children. A clinical and roentgenological study of 108 cases. Acta Orthopaedica Scandinavica 51: 909–913

Van der Reis W L, Otsuka N Y, Moroz P, Mah J 1998 Intramedullary nailing versus plate fixation for unstable forearm fractures in children. Journal of Pediatric Orthopaedics 18: 9–13

Vandenberk P, De Smet L, Fabry G 1996 Finger fractures in children treated with absorbable pins. Journal of Pediatric Orthopaedics 5B: 27–30

Walsh H P J, McLaren C A N, Owen R 1987 Galeazzi fractures in children. Journal of Bone and Joint Surgery 69B: 730–733

Wiley J J, Galey J P 1985 Monteggia injuries in children. Journal of Bone and Joint Surgery 67B: 728–736

Wilkins K E 1991a Fractures of the distal humerus. In: Rockwood C H, Wilkins, K E, King R E (eds) Fractures in children. Lippincott, Philadelphia, pp 526–728

Wilkins K E 1991b Fractures of the proximal radius and ulna. In: Rockwood C H, Wilkins K E, King R E (eds) Fractures in children. Lippincott, Philadelphia, pp 728–779

Wilkins K E 1998 Operative management of children's fractures. Is it a sign of impetuousness or do the children really benefit? Journal of Pediatric Orthopaedics 18: 1–3

Williamson D M, Coates C J, Miller R K 1992 Normal characteristics of the Baumann (humerocapitellar) angle: an aid in assessment of supracondylar fractures. Journal of Pediatric Orthopaedics 12: 636–639

Zionts L E, McKellop H A, Hathaway R 1994 Torsional strength of pin configurations used to fix supracondylar fractures of the humerus in children. Journal of Bone and Joint Surgery 76A: 253–256

Chapter 38

Fractures of the pelvis, femoral neck, lower limb and foot

PART 1   Fractures of the pelvis

P. Engelhardt

FREQUENCY AND MECHANISM OF INJURY

Pelvic fractures are uncommon in children (Canale & King 1991). The infrequency is due to the greater volume of cartilage which provides a buffer for energy absorption. Also the bones are less brittle than in the adult. Usually fractures of the pelvis are seen in polytraumatised children who have been struck by a motor vehicle. Isolated fractures include all kinds of avulsion-type fractures of the apophyses of the pelvis. These avulsions can occur in children playing football and result from sudden contraction of the muscle which inserts into the apophysis. Fractures of the acetabulum are rare.

CLASSIFICATION

This follows the same principle as adults and can be divided according to the AO Classification system into ABC groups: A = stable, B = rotational instability, C = additional vertical instability. The classification of Torode & Zieg (1985) is simple and follows a logical progression of injury status from mild to severe (Fig. 38.1). For practical purposes fractures of the acetabulum need special attention due to the potential for severe growth disturbances (Ogden 1990).

TYPE I

Avulsion of parts of the anterior iliac apophysis, the ischial tuberosity or the anterior inferior iliac spine as a chondro-osseous injury, especially in the adolescent athlete (Fig. 38.2).

TYPE II

Iliac wing fractures. Occur as a result of direct force against the pelvis.

TYPE III

Simple pelvic ring fracture, usually involving the pubic rami or disruption of the pubic symphysis.

TYPE IV

Instability of the pelvis is the result of a fracture or joint disruption creating instability (Group C in the AO classification). Included here are bilateral pubic rami fractures, fractures involving either the right or left pubic ramus or the symphysis, and additional fracture-dislocation of the posterior elements of the pelvis.

ASSESSMENT

Fractures of the pelvis need a multidisciplinary approach. Additional injuries of the genitourinary system, the abdomen and CNS must be ruled out and properly treated. There is no place for routine X-ray examination by the alar, obturator or inlet and outlet projections due to radiation exposure. A CT scan should be arranged when there is suspicion of posterior element disruption particularly around the sacro-iliac joint (Type IV).

TREATMENT

It is generally accepted that children have greater potential for healing and remodelling their bony injuries. As is reflected by most authors, conservative treatment of fractures of the pelvis is the rule (Torode & Zieg 1985, Garvin et al 1990). A careful work up of associated injuries in the emergency room is mandatory for the appropriate treatment.

AVULSION FRACTURES OF THE ISCHIAL TUBEROSITY (TYPE I)

Bed rest for 2–3 weeks. In rare cases of non-union surgery is necessary. Therapy can be managed on an outpatient basis.

AVULSION FRACTURES OF THE ANTERIOR SUPERIOR AND ANTERIOR INFERIOR ILIAC SPINES (TYPE I)

In cases of no or slight displacement bed rest with the hip joint flexed is sufficient (Fig. 38.2). Near the end of growth

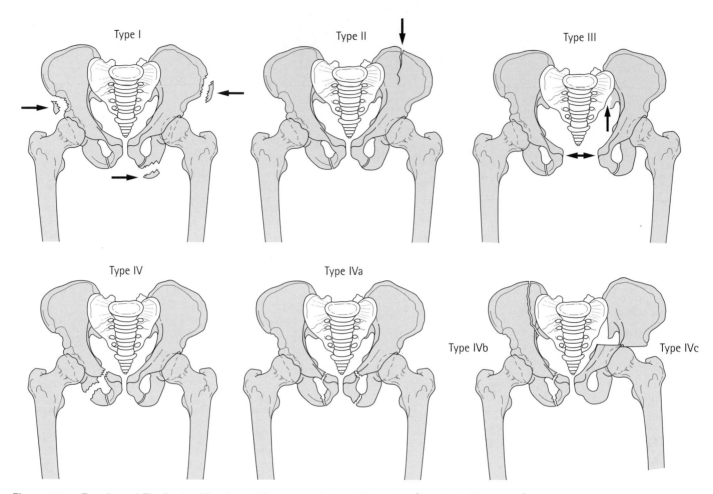

Figure 38.1 Torode and Zieg's classification of fractures of the childs pelvis (Torode & Zieg 1985).

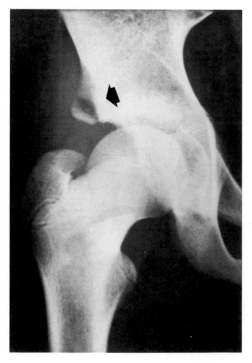

Figure 38.2 Radiograph of a 14-year-old boy showing avulsion of the inferior iliac spine.

termination a severely displaced apophysis may be openly reduced and fixed with sutures.

MARGINAL FRACTURES OF THE PELVIC RING (TYPE II)

The strength and rigidity of the pelvis is not affected. Cracks in the iliac wing heal without sequelae. Bed rest until the pain subsides is sufficient.

ANTERIOR AND POSTERIOR FRACTURES OF THE PELVIC RING, MALGAIGNE FRACTURES (TYPE III/IV)

Rotational and vertical instability have to be analysed by X-rays or under fluoroscopy. Anterior disruption of the ring heals conservatively. Additional posterior lesions need to be carefully checked by CT scan. Occasionally, open reduction and the application of an anterior external fixation frame is indicated. Always have a high suspicion of intra-abdominal trauma or bladder and urethral disruption! Beware of misinterpreting a widened symphysis or sacro-iliac joint: due to the larger cartilage layers (growth cartilage) of these bones, the interval is proportionally wider than in adults. Disruption through the sacro-iliac joint can result in severe growth disturbance of the whole pelvis (Engelhardt 1992).

FRACTURES OF THE ACETABULUM

These fractures are best seen on CT scan. The potential hazard of premature closure of the triradiate cartilage must be kept in mind, but may not be prevented by open reduction. In Salter–Harris type V lesions fusion may occur with progressive subluxation of the hip. It is doubtful if the adult approach to fractures of the acetabulum can be applied to children. Secondary reconstructive procedures, such as a shelf operation, or Chiari and intertrochanteric osteotomies, may be necessary to contain the femoral head (Heeg et al 1990).

OUTCOME

Type I, II and III fractures usually heal without sequelae. Initially they need close observation in the presence of additional soft-tissue injury. Disruption of the symphysis pubis heals even in the presence of diastasis because the lesion is separate from the bone cartilage on either side rather than disrupting the fibrous joint, as in the adult (Fig. 38.3).

Depending upon the severity of the bony lesion together with vertical instability, permanent disability may result. Injury of the growth cartilage may lead to permanent deformity of the pelvis, with leg-length discrepancy and pelvic obliquity as well as fusion of the sacro-iliac joint (Schwarz et al 1998). In the case of triradiate cartilage damage a shallow acetabulum can be expected, with the need for secondary reconstructive procedures.

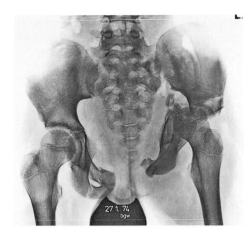

A

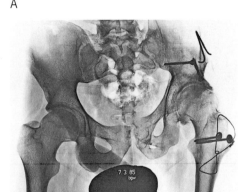

B

Figure 38.3 A A 15-year-old boy with Malgaigne and acetabular fractures. **B** After 10 years severe asymmetry of the pelvis with femoral head subluxation can be seen.

REFERENCES

Canale S, King R 1991 Pelvic and hip fractures. In: Rockwood C Jr, Wilkins K, King R (eds) Fractures in children, 4th edn. Lippincott, Philadelphia, 991–1046

Engelhardt P 1992 Die Malgaigne-Beckenringverletzung im Kindesalter. Orthopäde 21: 422–426

Garvin K, McCarthy R, Barnes C, Dodge B 1990 Pediatric pelvic ring fractures. Journal of Pediatric Orthopaedics 10: 577–582

Heeg M, Klasen H, Visser J 1990 Acetabular fractures in children and adolescents. In: Heeg M (ed) Fractures of the acetabulum. Van Denderen BV, Groningen, Netherlands, pp 63–70

Ogden J 1990 Skeletal injury in the child. Saunders, Philadelphia

Schwarz N, Posch E, Mayer J, Fischmeister F M, Schwarz A F, Ohner T 1998 Long term result of unstable pelvic ring fractures in children. Injury 29: 431–433

Torode I, Zieg D 1985 Pelvic fractures in children. Journal of Pediatric Orthopaedics 5: 76–84

PART 2 Femoral neck fractures
P. Engelhardt

FREQUENCY AND MECHANISM OF INJURY

Hip fractures are uncommon in children and result from violent force. They can occur in children of all ages, but the highest incidence is in 11- and 12-year-olds, with 60–75% occurring in boys. Age-related differences in the mechanical property of bone account for the greater frequency of hip fractures among adults than among children. The ratio of adult to childhood fracture is, according to Ratliff (1962), 130:1.

A fracture of the femoral neck may be caused by a force that acts directly over the greater trochanter, producing valgus angulation, or is directed along the shaft of the femur, causing varus deformity. A fracture caused by relatively slight trauma may complicate pathological conditions such as a cyst, disuse osteopenia or neurological disorders. Large series of femoral neck fractures have been published by Ratliff (1970) (132 cases), Boitzy (1971) (40 cases, 22 with complications), Canale & Bourland (1977) (61 cases, 26 with avascular necrosis) and a recent comparative series by Canale (1990) in which improvements in management and fixation significantly reduced the complication rate.

A stress fracture of the femoral neck in a patient with an open epiphysis is rare (Canale & King 1991). The youngest reported is by Wolfgang (1977) in a child of 10 years. Figure 38.4 shows a stress fracture with the typical 'internal callus' of a compressive fracture as classified by Devas (1965).

CLASSIFICATION

Hip fractures in children were classified morphologically by Delbet, as cited by Colonna (1929), at four levels (Fig. 38.5: Table 38.1):

Intracapsular

1. *Transepiphyseal.* Acute traumatic separation of a previously normal epiphysis (Fig. 38.6)
2. *Transcervical.* Mid–femoral neck (Fig. 38.7)
3. *Cervicotrochanteric.* Base of the femoral neck (Fig. 38.8)

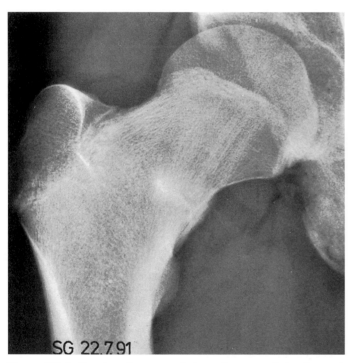

Figure 38.4 Compression type of stress fracture of the femoral neck in a 13-year-old boy who was an active football player. (X-ray taken 9 weeks after onset of right hip pain.)

Extracapsular

4. *Intertrochanteric.* Between both trochanters.

Subtrochanteric fractures (below the lesser trochanter) are classified as femoral shaft fractures and are not considered here. They are usually pathological.

ASSESSMENT

When the fracture is complete the leg is externally rotated. The child is fearful of any passive limb motion and unable to move actively. The diagnosis is confirmed by anteroposterior and lateral radiographs. Computed tomography may be used to assess the degree of displacement and intracapsular haematoma (Fig. 38.9). With an undisplaced fracture of the femoral neck, the X-ray may not be diagnostic initially. A bone scan at 3 months is helpful in detecting femoral head necrosis, the most common complication. Magnetic resonance imaging scan detects avascularity even earlier.

TREATMENT

The principles of management include:

- restriction of vascular complications by careful technique
- avoidance of injury to the physeal plate
- anatomically precise reduction of the fragments
- stabilisation with pins or screws allowing early protected weight bearing.

Urgent operative treatment is advisable in practically all cases, according to Ratliff (1970), Boitz (1980) and Canale (1990), in order to evacuate the intracapsular haematoma and establish normal skeletal anatomy. Care must be taken to prevent movement between the fragments.

The fracture site is exposed using Watson–Jones' anterolateral incision. An anterior capsulotomy exposes the fragments and their orientation. A Kirschner wire (K wire) is inserted laterally below the greatest trochanter and advanced to the fracture site using an image intensifier. After carefully checking the reduction in all planes the K wire is driven across the fracture. Two lag screws are inserted parallel to the K wire, securing firm fixation of

Table 38.1 Classification of proximal femoral fractures				
Classification	Type I	Type II	Type III	Type IV
Avascular necrosis risk	Very high	High	High	Low
Urgency of treatment	Emergency	Emergency	Emergency	Delay possible
Treatment undisplaced	eventually conservative	eventually conservative	eventually conservative	Conservative
Treatment displaced	Operative	Operative	Operative	Operative
Conservative treatment (aspiration of haemarthrosis)	Hip spica	Hip spica	Hip spica	Hip spica
Operative treatment	K wires, cannulated screws	K wires, cannulated screws	K wires under 3 years, or cannulated screws	K wires, or Blade plate

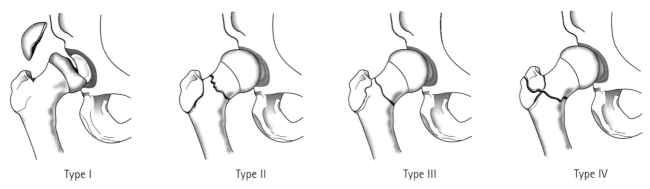

Type I   Type II   Type III   Type IV

Figure 38.5 Classification of proximal femoral fractures.

the fragments without crossing the growth plate (Fig. 38.10). Cannulated screws may also be used inserted over the K wires.

The use of several small pins seems to be sufficient in most cases, as suggested by Miller (1973) and Canale & Bourland (1977), but can lead to pin distraction of the fragments. The large Smith-Petersen nail is not recommended for hip fractures in children because it may fail to penetrate the hard bone of the proximal fragment, causing wide separation or comminution at the fracture site. Closure of the joint capsule is not necessary. The child is kept in bed for 2 weeks in a single hip spica cast to control rotation if there is any concern about the fixation. Movement of the hip is encouraged when the symptoms allow.

COMPLICATIONS

The following complications may arise:

- avascular necrosis (AVN)
- growth arrest
- coxa vara
- non-union
- osteoarthritis.

Avascular necrosis

This is the most feared complication because it leads to a very unfavourable result (Fig. 38.7). First described by Johansson (1927), the aetiology of AVN is presumed to

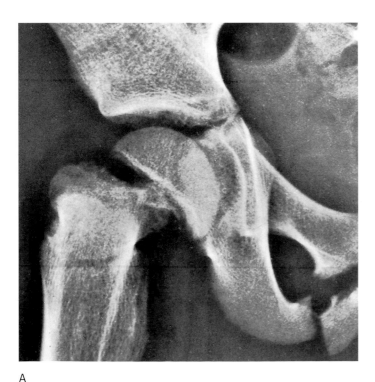

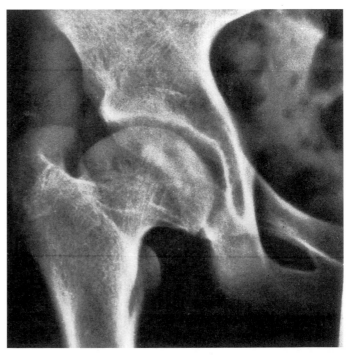

A   B

Figure 38.6 Transepiphyseal femoral neck fracture in a 10-year-old boy. **A** The traumatic nature of the injury was confirmed by the persence of an ipsilateral fracture of the ischium. A closed reduction was carried out, and 6 years after injury there is shortening of the femoral neck and coxa vara due to growth disturbance of the proximal femoral epiphysis with trochanteric overgrowth (**B**).

Immediate spica cast application as a low-risk treatment is used in some centres, at least in the age group up to 10 years (Ferguson & Nicol 2000). Between 6 and 8 weeks after injury the cast is removed; the results are good. There may be compliance problems for some children and parents, especially if they hear about the alternatives of early mobilisation with other protocols (Hughes et al 1995).

External fixators of different design (AO, Orthofix and others) have become popular around the world during the past 15 years (Tolo 1983, Krettek et al 1989, Aronson & Tursky 1992, Blasier et al 1997, Hull & Bell 1997, Weinberg et al 2000). Stable fixation of the fracture allows early weight bearing and early return to school activities (Fig. 38.15) There are some compliance problems in connection with screws and pins but pin tract infections are not common. In transverse fractures the fixator must stay in place for 3 months, while spiral fractures are stable after 2 months or less. Re-fracture after fixator removal may

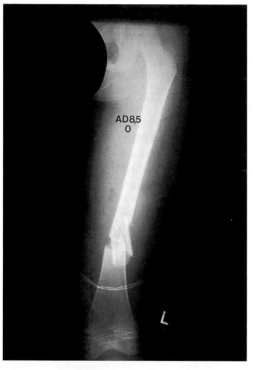

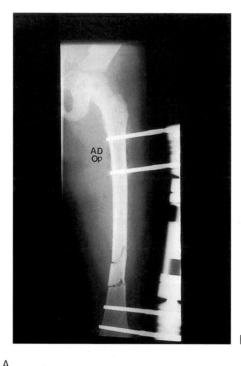

A

B

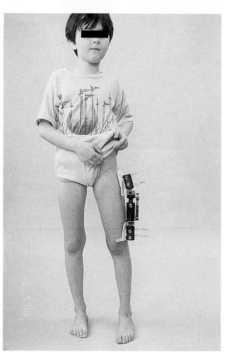

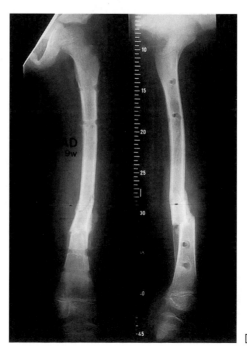

C

D

Figure 38.15 A Complex segmental fracture in a 9-year-old boy. **B** Alignment of the fracture with external fixator. **C** The boy bears weight after 2 weeks. **D** After 10 weeks and fixator removal, good alignment of the fracture in both planes.

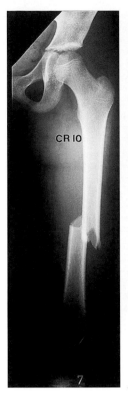
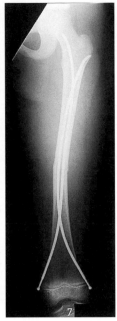
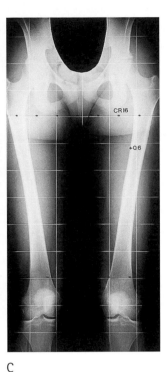

A

B

C

Figure 38.16 **A** Midshaft transverse fracture in a 10-year-old boy. **B** Intramedullary fixation by two elastic nails introduced from the distal metaphysis. **C** Fully functioning femur at 16 years showing minor overgrowth of 0.6 cm.

occur in up to 10% of cases causing a second period of morbidity.

The indications for external fixation are second and third degree open fractures of the femur, comminuted fractures or with an open tibial fracture necessitating an 'exfix' in combination with a closed femoral fracture.

Elastic intramedullary titanium nails have become the treatment of choice for the standard femoral shaft fracture of the school child up to the age of 15 in some centres. The French school of paediatric orthopaedics in Nancy and Metz have shown that mid-shaft and proximal femoral fractures can be stabilised by introducing two titanium nails from the metaphysis past the fracture into the femoral neck and greater trochanter. This 'Eiffel tower system' offers axial and rotatory stability and allows early mobilisation and weight bearing (Ligier et al 1988, Metaizeau 1988, Dietz et al 1997, Parsch 1997) (Fig. 38.16). Distal fractures are fixed by using the titanium rods in antegrade fashion, descending from below the greater trochanter, past the fracture ending in the distal femur, short of the growth plate. The complication rate is low and the infection rate less then 1%. Soft tissue irritation and bursitis around the knee area disappeared with the introduction of an olive-ended nail. The nails are removed after 4–6 months depending on the age of the child. Overgrowth of the fractured femur is common and averages 0.6 cm. The highest rate of overgrowth is seen in mid-shaft transverse fractures in the younger age group around 7 years. The lowest is encountered in long spiral fractures.

Flexible Ender nails introduced from below the greater trochanter into the distal metaphysis, or in the retrograde approach, ascending from the medial and lateral metaphysis into the femoral neck and greater trochanter, also have their proponents (Mann et al 1986, Heinrich et al 1994).

Intramedullary stable nails with an interlocking mechanism have been introduced in the treatment of femoral shaft fractures in adolescents in the USA. They can be compared to the Küntscher nails used in the 1950s and 1960s, but offer an antirotatory locking mechanism with additional screws set in the trochanter and the distal femur (Beaty et al 1994, Canale & Tolo 1995). Interlocking nails allow early weight bearing; nail removal is undertaken an average of 14 months post injury. The risk of partial or segmental avascular necrosis (AVN) of the femoral head has been mentioned by several authors. This is caused by injury to the posterior superior ascending branch of the medial circumflex artery (O'Malley et al 1995).

REFERENCES

Aronson D D, Singer R M, Higgins R F 1987 Skeletal traction for fractures of the femoral shaft in children. Journal of Bone and Joint Surgery 69A: 1435–1439

Aronson J, Tursky E A 1992 External fixation of femur fractures in children. Journal of Pediatric Orthopaedics 12: 157–163

Beals R K, Tufts E 1983 Fractured femur in infancy: the role of child abuse. Journal of Pediatric Orthopaedics 3: 583–586

Beaty J H, Austin S M, Warner W C, Canale S T, Nichols L 1994 Interlocking intramedullary nailing of femoral shaft fractures in adolescents: preliminary results and complications. Journal of Pediatric Orthopaedics 14: 178–183

Blasier R D, Aronson J, Tursky E A 1997 External fixation of pediatric femur fractures. Journal of Pediatric Orthopaedics 17: 342–346

Canale S T, Tolo V T 1995 Fractures of the femur in children. Journal of Bone and Joint Surgery 77A: 294–315

Daly K E, Calvert P T 1991 Accidental femoral fractures in infants. Injury 22: 337–338

Dietz H G, Schmittenbecher P P, Illing P 1997 Intramedulläre Osteosynthese im Wachstumsalter. Urban & Schwarzenberg, München

Ferguson J, Nicol R O 2000 Early spica treatment of pediatric femoral shaft fractures. Journal of Pediatric Orthopaedics 20: 189–192

Gross R H, Stranger M 1983 Causative factors responsible for femoral fractures in infants and young children. Journal of Pediatric Orthopaedics 3: 341–343

Hedlund R, Lindgren U 1986 The incidence of femoral shaft fractures in children and adolescents. Journal of Pediatric Orthopaedics 6: 47–50

Heinrich S D, Drvaric D M, Darr K, MacEwen G D 1994 The operative stabilization of pediatric diaphyseal femur fractures with flexible intramedullary nails: a prospective analysis. Journal of Pediatric Orthopaedics 14: 501–507

Henderson O L, Morrissy R T, Gerdes M H, McCarthy R E 1984 Early casting of femoral shaft fractures in children. Journal of Pediatric Orthopaedics 4: 16–21

Hughes B F, Sponseller P D, Thompson J D 1995 Pediatric femur fractures: effects of spica cast treatment on family and community. Journal of Pediatric Orthopaedics 15: 457–460

Hull J B, Bell M J 1997 Modern trends for external fixation of fractures in children: a critical review. Journal of Pediatric Orthopaedics B6: 103–109

Irani R N, Nicholson J Z, Chung S M K 1976 Long-term results in the treatment of femoral-shaft fractures in young children by immediate spica immobilization. Journal of Bone and Joint Surgery 58A: 945–951

Kasser J R 1996 Femoral shaft fractures In: Rockwood C A, Wilkins K E, Beaty J H (eds) Fractures in children, 4th edn. Lippincott-Raven, Philadelphia, pp 1195–1229

King J, Diefendorf D, Apthorp J, Negrete V F, Carlson M 1988 Analysis of 429 fractures in 189 battered children. Journal of Pediatric Orthopaedics 8: 585–589

Krettek C, Haas N, Tscherne H 1989 Versorgung der Femurschaftfraktur im Wachstumsalter mit dem Fixateur externe. Acta Traumatologica 19: 255–261

Landin L A 1983 Fracture patterns in children. Analysis of 8682 fractures with special reference to incidence, etiology and secular changes in Swedish urban population 1950–1979. Acta Orthopaedica Scandinavica Supplement 202: 1–109

Ligier J N, Metaizeau J P, Prévot J, Lascombe P 1988 Elastic stable intramedullary nailing of femoral shaft fractures in children. Journal of Bone and Joint Surgery 70B: 74–77

Mann D C, Weddington J, Davenport K 1986 Closed Ender nailing of femoral shaft fractures in adolescents. Journal of Pediatric Orthopaedics 6: 651–655

Metaizeau J P 1988 L'ostéosynthèse chez l'enfant. Embrochage centromédullaire élastique stable. Sauramps, Montpellier

Mueller M E, Nazzarin S, Koch P 1987 Classification AO des fractures. 1: Les OS Longs. Springer, Berlin.

O'Malley D E, Mazur J M, Cummings R J 1995 Femoral head necrosis associated with intramedullary nailing in an adolescent. Journal of Pediatric Orthopaedics 15: 21–23

Newton P O, Mubarak S J 1994 Financial aspects of femoral shaft fracture treatment in children and adolescents. Journal of Pediatric Orthopaedics 14: 505–512

Nicholson J T, Foster R M, Heath R D 1955 Bryant's traction. A provocative cause of circulatory complications. Journal of the American Medical Association 157: 415–418

Nork S E, Hoffinger S A 1998 Skeletal traction versus external fixation for pediatric femoral shaft fractures: a comparison of hospital costs and charges. Journal of Orthopedic Trauma 12: 563–568

Parsch K 1997 Modern trends in internal fixation of femoral shaft fractures in children. A critical review. Journal of Pediatric Orthopaedics B6: 117–125

Saxer U 1978 Femurschaftfrakturen. In: Weber BG, Brunner Ch, Freuler F (eds) Die Frakturenbehandlung bei Kindern und Jugendlichen. Springer, Berlin

Staheli L T, Sheridan G W 1977 Early spica cast management of femoral shaft fractures in young children. Clinical Orthopaedics and Related Research 126: 162–166

Sullivan J A, Gregory P, Herndon W A, Yngve D A, Goradia V K 1994 Management of femoral shaft fractures in children ages 5 to 13 by traction and spica cast. Orthopedics 2: 567–571

Tolo V T 1983 External skeletal fixation in children's fractures. Journal of Pediatric Orthopaedics 3: 435–442

Ward W T, Levy J, Kaye A 1992 Compression plating for child and adolescent femur fractures. Journal of Pediatric Orthopaedics 12: 626–632

Weinberg A M, Hasler C C, Leitner A, Lampert C 2000 External fixation of pediatric femoral shaft fractures. European Journal of Trauma 1: 25–32

PART 4   Fractures of the knee and tibia
C. Hasler

INTRA-ARTICULAR INJURIES OF THE KNEE

ACUTE PATELLAR DISLOCATION

Epidemiology and mechanism of injury

The first episode of patello-femoral dislocation occurs most often in adolescence with a peak incidence at 15 years of age. It affects about one in 1000 children annually between the ages of 9 and 15 years (Nietosvaara et al 1994). Typically, external rotation and valgus stress on the flexed knee causes the dislocation. In children patellar dislocation accounts for almost half of all acute traumatic haemarthroses and is the most common injury responsible for osteo-chondral fragments in the knee. Although medial and superior dislocations have been described, lateral dislocation is by far the most common.

There are three main goals of treatment:

- relocation of the patella
- recognition, repair or removal of osteo-chondral lesions
- prevention of re-dislocation.

Clinical findings

Most patients present after the patella has spontaneously relocated. They are often unaware of what happened, and indeed sometimes believe something displaced medially when they notice the prominent medial femoral condyle. If one encounters a patella which is still displaced, it is relocated by gradual passive extension of the knee with the hip flexed to relax the quadriceps muscles. When the patella has relocated, diagnosis is confirmed by finding a haemarthrosis and tenderness over the medial patellar retinaculum. Fat globules in the aspirated fluid do not necessarily mean the presence of an associated osteochondral fracture.

Radiological findings

Radiographic evaluation after acute dislocation should include an axial (skyline) film of the patella with the knee flexed 20° to detect associated osteochondral lesions. They may be found at the medial border of the patella as an extra-articular avulsion of the medial retinaculum, at the lateral femoral condyle (intra-articular) and as loose bodies anywhere in the joint.

Children with an acute patellar dislocation often show predisposing osseous and ligamentous anatomical factors which need to be thoroughly assessed. Most have some radiological and ultrasonographic signs of patello-femoral dysplasia such as a shallow cartilaginous sulcus (Nietosvaara 1994) associated with maltracking in early flexion. In addition, general ligamentous laxity is associated with hereditary conditions (Downs, Ehlers–Danlos, Larsen's syndrome, or osteogenesis imperfecta); muscular imbalance and dysplastic femoral condyles may be evident. Genu valgum, genu recurvatum and increased external torsion of the tibia also contribute to patello-femoral instability. Most patients have a combination of these factors so that precise clinical assessment, aided by CT, is a prerequisite for patients in whom a realignment procedure is contemplated.

Associated injuries

There is a 40% risk of an associated osteochondral lesion. Half are intra-articular, and half are extra-articular. In a prospective study intra-articular fragments were found after spontaneous relocation only when the medial patellar facet impacted against the lateral femoral condyle on its way back into the sulcus (Nietosvaara et al 1994). Arthroscopy is indicated if there are signs of loose bodies. Very few are big enough for re-attachment and most simply need removal. Rarely, a large soft-tissue gap proximal and medial to the patella indicates avulsion of the vastus medialis muscle and warrants open suture.

Prognosis

Primary surgical repair of the torn medial retinacular structures yields results no better than conservative treatment, often leaves cosmetically ugly scars, or puts the infrapatellar nerve at risk. In both groups the rate of recurrent instability is reported to be 46% in a randomised controlled treatment trial (Nietosvaara 1996).

Treatment of acute dislocation of the patella

When there is a tense haemarthrosis aspiration quickly relieves pain. Acute arthroscopy is indicated only if there is radiological or clinical evidence of an osteochondral fragment. Immobilisation in a cylinder cast for 3 weeks, with full weight bearing permitted, allows healing of the torn medial patellar retinaculum. After cast removal, strengthening exercises for the quadriceps muscles, and range of motion exercises, should be started. A careful re-evaluation of the knee joint should rule out associated injuries of the cruciate and medial collateral ligaments.

OSTEOCHONDRAL FRACTURES OF THE KNEE

Mechanism of injury

Most osteochondral fractures of the knee complicate acute dislocations of the patella and have their origin either from the medial margin of the patella or from the lateral femoral condyle. Occasionally a direct fall upon the knee or a flexion-rotation injury with shearing forces damage the surface of the medial or lateral femoral condyle.

Clinical and radiological findings

Depending upon the severity of the trauma, the size and origin of the fragment, as well as delay in presentation, the symptoms and clinical signs will differ. If standard AP, lateral and skyline radiographs of the patella are not conclusive, a tunnel view should be ordered to demonstrate clearly the intercondylar area. Radiographs may fail to detect small fragments or those consisting mainly of cartilage. The differential diagnosis includes acute osteochondral fractures, chondral flaps and separations, and osteochondritis dissecans.

Late presentation

In some patients the initial clinical and radiological examination may not have revealed a fragment, or the the fragment was overlooked. A history of intermittent swelling and locking of the knee suggests either a meniscal tear or a loose body following osteochondral fracture. Large fragments are often palpable, even by the patient, and visible on an X-ray. If the diagnosis is not clear and the X-ray is negative, an MRI scan, possibly with gadolinium enhancement, is recommended.

Treatment

Arthroscopic examination and clinical assessment of ligament integrity under anaesthesia give precise information about the size, composition and origin of the fragment and associated injuries. In a fresh injury large fragments (>2 cm) separated from a weight-bearing area should be reattached. Stable fixation, with the implant buried beneath the articular cartilage, can be performed with a Herbert screw, an AO mini fragment screw or biodegradable pins inserted through a lateral or medial mini-arthrotomy. Smaller fragments should be removed. Longstanding fragments lose their original size and and shape and their margins become rounded so that refixation is difficult or impossible. Removal of the fragment should prevent further locking and effusions of the knee and, if there is a large crater in a weight-bearing area, a procedure to reconstruct the cartilaginous surface should be considered as the crater will otherwise be symptomatic.

FRACTURES OF THE PATELLA

Mechanism of injury

Fractures of the patella are rare in children and are due either to a direct blow or to a forceful contraction of the quadriceps muscle (avulsion fractures).

Fracture types

The most frequent type is an osteochondral avulsion fracture of the medial border after patellar dislocation. Longitudinal fractures are usually undisplaced and visible only on an axial view (Fig. 38.17). Transverse fractures and sleeve

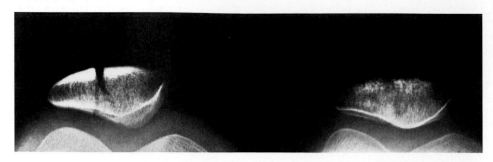

Figure 38.17 **A** Longitudinal fracture of the patella without intra-articular displacement; **B** consolidation after 6 weeks.

fractures of the inferior pole show varying amounts of displacement due to the tension of the extensor muscles. The latter should be regarded as an avulsion injury which has to be differentiated from the Sinding–Larsen–Johansson syndrome. The avulsed fragment, if small, may not be radiologically apparent until the cartilage ossifies. Avulsion may also occur from the superior and medial margins. Transverse stress fractures occur exceptionally in cerebral palsy and spina bifida patients or in athletes (Brunner & Döderlein 1996). A bipartite patella with an accessory ossicle in the superolateral quadrant should not be confused with a fracture. Radiological differentiation is possible because of the typical localisation of the ossicle and its rounded margin.

Treatment

When a tense haemarthrosis is present, aspiration relieves pain. For undisplaced fractures 4–5 weeks in a cylinder cast, with weight bearing as tolerated, is recommended. For displaced fractures the articular surface and the extensor tendon should be reconstructed and fixed by tension band wiring as in the adult (Maguire & Canale 1993). Early passive motion is allowed but weight bearing is restricted for 5 weeks. For avulsion fractures, treatment depends upon the extent of separation of the fragments.

INTRA-ARTICULAR FRACTURES OF THE DISTAL FEMUR

Fracture types

Salter–Harris types III, IV and transitional fractures of the distal femur are rare. Type III fractures consist of a vertical fracture line extending from the physis into the joint, most commonly through the intercondylar notch. The type IV fracture starts from the metaphyseal cortex, crosses the physis and extends into the joint. As the fracture may reduce spontaneously, it can be overlooked or mistaken for a ligamentous injury. Transitional fractures occur during adolescence when the physis has already partially closed. Due to the asymmetry of this process the non-fused part of the epiphysis may break off with a sagittal epiphyseal and a horizontal physeal fracture line (two-plane fracture). There may be an additional frontal metaphyseal plane (three-plane fracture). Careful inspection of the lateral radiographic view helps to differentiate a transitional fracture from a Salter–Harris type I epiphysiolysis.

Treatment

When intra-articular displacement of more than 2 mm occurs, open anatomical reduction and stable internal fixation with lag screws should be performed to prevent displacement and later osteoarthritis. Although the risk of growth disturbance is significantly diminished by an anatomical 'waterproof' osteosynthesis, partial growth arrest with subsequent malalignment may occur. In a transitional fracture the indication for open reduction and internal fixation is the same as for all intra-articular fractures. For a two-plane fracture epiphyseal lag screw fixation is adequate; in a triplane fracture the metaphyseal part of the fragment should be fixed with an additional lag screw. Growth disturbances are unlikely since the physis closes within a year of fracture.

FRACTURES OF THE TIBIAL SPINE

Mechanism of injury

Fractures of the anterior tibial spine in childhood are the most common intra-articular fracture of the proximal tibia in children. Biomechanically they correspond to a rupture of the anterior cruciate ligament (ACL) in adults. In children the tibial spine is less resistant to tensile stress than the ACL. However, prior to avulsion of the tibial spine, the ACL stretches due to sequential failure of its fibres (Noyes et al 1974, particularly in low-velocity injuries. A fall from a bicycle causing a direct blow on the distal femur with the knee flexed is most frequently reported as the mechanism of injury, followed by trauma sustained during such athletic activities as skiing and soccer.

Clinical and radiological findings

Patients usually present with a painful haemarthrosis and inability to weight bear. Clinically they show pathological Lachman and anterior drawer tests. According to Meyers & McKeever (1959), fractures of the intercondylar eminence can be radiologically classified on a standard lateral view as type I (undisplaced), type II (partially displaced, posteriorly hinged) or type III (fully displaced). Zaricznyj (1977) suggested an additional type IV comminuted fracture. Reviews suggest that 12% are type I, 41% type II and 47% type III (Grönkvist et al 1984). When the physis is still open the whole eminence is avulsed, while in the closed physis only one of the tubercles may be avulsed. As the fracture often runs through the subchondral plate, the size of the fragment is underestimated on the X-ray. Associated injuries to the medial collateral ligament and the menisci (lateral more frequent than medial) occur, mainly with type III fractures. However, there seems to be a high potential for spontaneous healing since only rarely is subsequent treatment necessary for those treated conservatively without arthroscopy (Molander et al 1981).

Treatment

A painful haemarthrosis should be aspirated under sterile conditions, followed by:

1. *Type I.* Immobilisation in a cylinder cast for 4 weeks.
2. *Type II.* Closed reduction by extension of the knee followed by a cylinder cast (Fig. 38.18). Arthroscopic or open reduction is recommended when a large fragment is irreducible due to interposition of the anterior horn of a meniscus.
3. *Type III.* Arthroscopic or open reduction is achieved and the fragment fixed with a wire, wire suture, non-metallic osteosuture or small-calibre lag screw, according to surgical preference. The fragment should be anatomically reduced, or even countersunk (Grönkvist et al 1984), to compensate for ACL elongation.

Prognosis

A transepiphyseal screw may cause a partial growth arrest of the proximal tibial physis (Mylle et al 1993), but this may be complicated if the fracture is entirely within the physis.

Chronic anterior instability and loss of full extension, despite union of the fracture in an anatomical position, are the most frequently reported long-term problems. In 38–70% of the patients who have sustained a type II or III injury, there is objective evidence (Lachman test, KT 1000 arthrometer) of anterior cruciate laxity. However, few have subjective complaints if the secondary restraints remain intact. It is possible that post-traumatic overgrowth of the tibial spine may prevent pivoting and the ACL may remain elongated with further growth. An anatomical reduction of the fracture does not therefore prevent cruciate laxity and the results of open and closed methods are similar, provided that the fragment unites in an anatomical position.

RUPTURES OF THE ANTERIOR CRUCIATE LIGAMENT

Ruptures of the anterior cruciate ligament in skeletally immature patients are rare but have become more frequently recognised and reported. The gold standard technique of ACL reconstruction in adults, using the central one third bone–patellar–bone graft, may be applied to adolescents with little growth left (McCarroll et al 1994). In patients with an open physis harvesting the graft and drilling holes may injure the tibial and femoral physes with a real risk of growth disturbance. Conservative treatment, direct repair and extra-articular reconstructions give poor results. Thus, an intra-articular reconstruction has to be considered for instability-related symptoms if rehabilitation is not achieved after a period of conservative treatment, or if there are

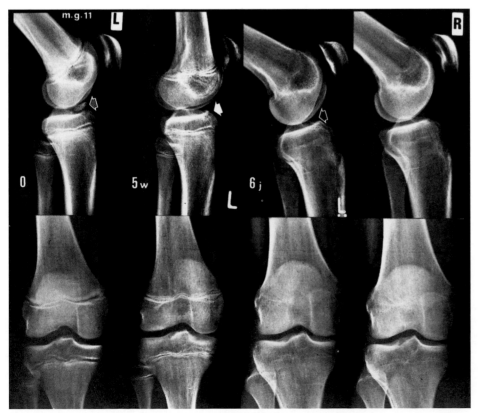

Figure 38.18 Meyers and McKeevers type II fracture of the tibial spine: closed reduction on extension of the knee. From left to right: at injury, after 5 weeks, at 6 years follow up.

associated meniscal injuries. Technically, intra-articular reconstruction without risk of a growth disturbance is possible if the physes are not breached or if reconstruction with a soft-tissue graft (semtendinosus or gracilis tendon) is performed through a small-diameter tibial drill hole in combination with a femoral 'over the top' graft insertion. However long-term results of knee stability and the prevention of osteoarthritis have not been reported.

INTRA-ARTICULAR PHYSEAL FRACTURES OF THE PROXIMAL TIBIA

Salter–Harris type III, IV and transitional fractures are even more rare than at the distal femur and are mostly encountered in late adolescence. Fracture patterns and treatment are basically the same as for distal intra-articular femoral fractures. Special attention should be paid to concomitant ligamentous injury to prevent later instability.

METAPHYSEAL FRACTURES OF THE PROXIMAL TIBIA

AVULSION OF THE TIBIAL TUBEROSITY

Mechanism of injury
This fracture occurs mainly in adolescents either after acute violent contraction of the quadriceps muscle or after acute flexion of the knee against the contracted quadriceps such as in landing after a jump. Growth disturbances are rare, but in younger patients a genu recurvatum may develop (Christie & Dvonch 1981).

Clinical and radiological findings
Patients present with marked pain, a local haematoma over the tuberosity and inability to perform a straight-leg raise, or to weight bear. The patella is displaced proximally and anterior tibial pain may result from a compartment syndrome following displaced intra-articular fractures. A lateral radiograph confirms the diagnosis and shows the size and displacement of the fragment, which may be much larger than is visible on the X-ray.

There are extra- and intra-articular (Salter–Harris type III) avulsion fractures of the tibial tuberosity (Fig. 38.19). The former are called displaced if there is an elevation of the tuberosity of more than 5 mm, the latter if there is a step-off of greater than 2 mm as with all intra-articular fractures.

Treatment

Undisplaced fracture
Conservative treatment comprises a cylinder cast for 5–6 weeks.

Displaced fractures
Open reduction and internal fixation with lag screws through a midline vertical incision lateral or medial to the tuberosity. Interposition of a periosteal flap under the avulsed fragment should be relieved before anatomical reduction and fixation of the fragment with the knee extended. The isolated osseous lesion is not splinted and partial weight bearing is recommended for 6 weeks. If the avulsion is mainly of the soft tissues (periosteum, patellar ligament), a cylinder cast is applied for 6 weeks. After 6 weeks union is confirmed radiographically and full weight bearing permitted. The patient should be followed until skeletal maturity.

EPIPHYSIOLYSIS

Mechanism of injury
Separation of the proximal tibial epiphysis (Salter–Harris types I and II fractures) is rare. The tibial tuberosity is part of the proximal tibial epiphysis and displaces with the epiphysis. The mechanism of injury is most often an indirect, valgus force. Forceful hyperextension with severe anterior displacement of the epiphysis can put the popliteal vessels at risk.

Clinical and radiological findings
Signs of circulatory or neurological impairment (particularly the peroneal nerve) should be looked for carefully. Undisplaced fractures, usually a Salter–Harris type I, may be overlooked if indirect clinical and radiological signs are not considered such as pain and swelling over the proximal tibia, an associated fracture of the proximal fibula, and callus formation at the proximal tibia after 4–6 weeks. On the initial X-ray, the angle between the epiphysis and the diaphysis of the tibia should be measured to avoid missing any varus or valgus angulation as remodelling is poor.

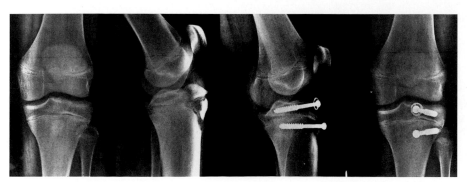

Figure 38.19 Displaced avulsion fracture of the tibial tuberosity with extension into the joint. Anatomical open reduction and internal fixation.

Treatment

Undisplaced fractures are treated by a long-leg plaster.

Displaced fractures are reduced under anaesthesia. The primary goal is to correct malrotation and angulation in the frontal plane. Reduction is only necessary when there is interposition of soft tissues, e.g. pes anserinus or periosteum. Closed or open reduction is secured by percutaneous, crossed Kirschner wires and the leg splinted in a long-leg plaster.

Radiological review after 8–10 days is recommended. Any secondary displacement may be corrected by simple wedging of the plaster. Total plaster time is 4–5 weeks with a final cast-free X-ray. Clinical follow-up for 2 years is necessary with 6-month assessments of leg length and axial alignment.

Growth disturbances

Transient stimulation of the proximal tibial physis, with slight overgrowth of the tibia, is of minor clinical significance. Total or partial growth arrest is rare but may follow Salter–Harris type I or II fractures (Burkhart & Peterson 1979). It is usually caused by the primary trauma and is therefore not preventable. A wise surgeon informs the parents of this risk prior to treatment.

TORUS FRACTURES

These compression fractures do not show any displacement or angulation and are treated by immobilisation in a long-leg plaster for 4–5 weeks. They are stable and there is no risk of secondary angulation. After plaster removal union is confirmed by the absence of tenderness over the fracture site and the ability to weight bear on the leg. Further follow-up is unnecessary as growth disturbances do not occur (Von Laer et al 1982).

BENDING FRACTURES

Mechanism of injury and complications

Forces acting upon the lateral aspect of the proximal tibia may either result in a complete metaphyseal fracture of the tibia and fibula, or in a partial (greenstick) fracture of the medial cortex of the proximal tibia with or without a fibular fracture.

Clinically, a progressive valgus deformity may develop and even minor angulations may worsen. Long-term follow-up may reveal later correction of the valgus (Fig. 38.20). There are two theories to explain this complication:

1. *Mechanical reasons.* Entrapment of soft tissues in the fracture gap (periosteum, medial collateral ligament, pes anserinus) by loss of medial tethering caused by avulsion of the pes anserinus in combination with normal lateral tethering by the intact fibula.
2. *Asymmetrical growth.* Lack of compression on the fractured medial cortex independent of any interposition leading to delayed union, a well-known phenomenon in greenstick fractures. The associated (long-lasting) hyperaemia produces an asymmetrical stimulation of the adjacent proximal growth plate of the tibia, demonstrated by bone scans (Zionts et al 1977).

Treatment

There are two important and easy steps to prevent post-traumatic valgus deformity:

1. Recognition of even minor valgus deformities since a fracture gap on the medial side in combination with intact lateral cortex indicates a valgus deformity. It can be quantified by measuring the angle between the physis and the long axis of the tibia.

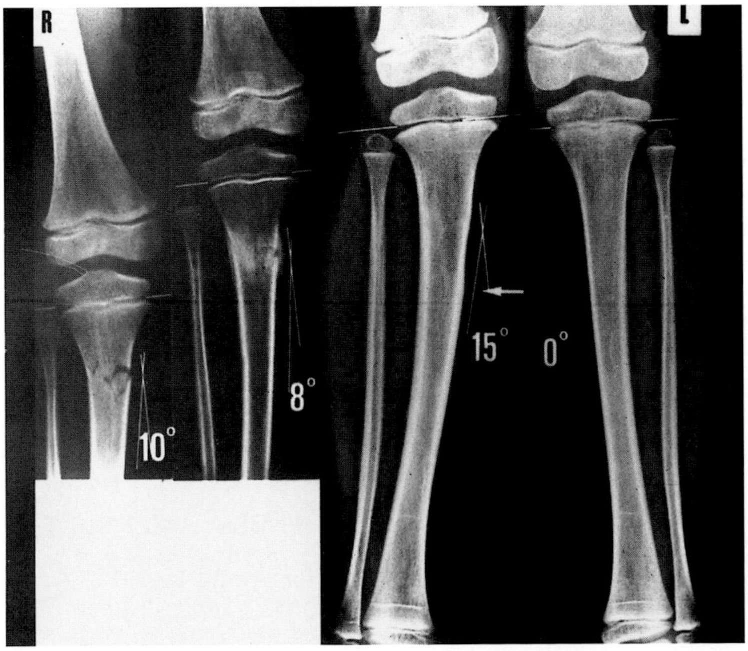

Figure 38.20 Bending fracture of the proximal tibia: primary valgus deformity with subsequent enhanced medial growth and increase of the deformity.

2. Compression of the fracture at the medial tibial cortex:

- Primary angulation of less than 10°: apply an above-knee cast with the knee extended and apply varus stress. After 8 days, the cast is wedged by cutting transversely at the fracture site laterally and opening with a cast spreader. A wooden spacer is placed into the gap, compressing the medially fractured cortex. Closed reduction under anaesthesia is advisable if the subsequent X-ray shows a persisting gap. When the fracture is resistant to manipulation and plastering, compression by external fixation or open reduction is recommended. If external fixation is used, care must be taken to avoid the growth plate of the apophysis to prevent growth disturbance.
- Primary angulation of more than 10° or fully displaced fractures: initial closed reduction with subsequent radiological follow-up after 8 days. Minor residual angulation can be corrected by wedging and the plaster cast is retained for 4 weeks.

Follow up 6 monthly for the first 2 years after injury to monitor any valgus malalignment.

DIAPHYSEAL FRACTURES OF THE TIBIA

The treatment and prognosis of tibial diaphyseal fractures tibia depends considerably upon the fracture pattern. It is important to distinguish between fractures with an intact fibula and those where the fibula is also fractured, the former being twice as common. Isolated fractures of the fibula are rare and always due to direct trauma.

Clinical and radiological findings

Pain and swelling at the fracture site make clinical diagnosis straightforward, and severe deformity should be reduced by manipulation. Although disruption of the posterior tibial artery is rare in children with closed fractures, the pulses of the dorsalis pedis and posterior tibialis arteries should be checked clinically and, if absent, by a Doppler examination. Unremitting pain, particularly on passive movement of the toes, may be the first sign of a compartment syndrome.

ISOLATED TIBIAL FRACTURES

Mechanism of injury, fracture pattern and prognosis

Isolated tibial fractures are the most frequent fractures of the lower extremity. They are usually the result of indirect rotational forces and present as long, oblique or spiral fractures at the junction between the middle and distal thirds. The fracture line spirals from the anteromedial cortex and up to the posterolateral cortex. They generally occur in children below the age of 10 years.

Incomplete fractures: present as torus or greenstick fractures and account for only about 10% of all tibial fractures. As they are stable they can always be treated conservatively by a wedging plaster to correct minor angular deformity.

Complete tibial fractures: with an intact fibula do not shorten. The initial angulation of the tibia rarely exceeds 10°. However, the more medially concentrated forces of the calf muscles lead to progressive varus of the tibia in about 50% of the patients. Subsequent remodelling is age dependent so that varus deformities of 10–15° will reliably correct in children under 10 years; in older children remodelling is unpredictable. Spontaneous remodelling of up to 20° of recurvatum can be expected in patients under 10 years. Antecurvatum of the tibia is rare. Rotational deformities (usually external rotation) will persist (Shannak 1988) but they are compensated for at the hip. Internal rotation deformity is the one to prevent. Stimulation of the tibial physis may cause tibial overgrowth of 0.5–1 cm in a child under the age of 10 years (Von Laer et al 1989). In older children, by contrast, premature closure of the physis may result in slight shortening. In summary, most initial deformities in the sagittal and coronal planes will remodel with time.

Treatment

Children with isolated tibial fractures should be treated conservatively by cast immobilisation even if closed reduction with anaesthesia is necessary. Rotational deformity should be assessed by comparing it with the bimalleolar axis of the uninjured leg. One should strive for angular and/or rotational deformity of less than 10° at union regardless of the age group. In all cases the alignment of the fracture should be monitored closely after 1 week. Wedging of the cast to correct primary or secondary angular deformities of up to 20° is best performed after 8–10 days when the patient is pain free, swelling has reduced and early callus has begun to form (Fig. 38.21). Technically an *open* wedging technique is easier as it avoids pinching the skin and has less risk of provoking an increase in compartment pressure. The cast is cut at right angles to the long axis of the tibia in the concavity of the angulation at the level of the fracture, leaving about one-quarter to one-half of the circumference of the cast intact. The cast is then opened with a cast spreader and a wooden or plastic block of appropriate size placed into the gap.

In older children or adolescents with undisplaced fractures, a patellar tendon bearing cast (Sarmiento cast) may be an alternative. The plaster is removed after 4–5 weeks. If tenderness persists at the fracture site, a below-knee cast is applied for a further 2–3 weeks.

Completely displaced, unstable transverse fractures, open fractures, and patients at risk of a compartment syndrome can be effectively treated by external fixation (Von Laer et al 1989) or by intramedullary elastic stable nails (Ligier et al 1988). When there is an associated femoral fracture ('floating knee') either or both the femur and tibia need stabilisation using external or intramedullary fixation.

DIAPHYSEAL FRACTURES OF THE TIBIA AND FIBULA

Mechanism of injury and prognosis

These are usually the result of direct trauma in road traffic accidents and, in contrast to isolated tibial fractures, the

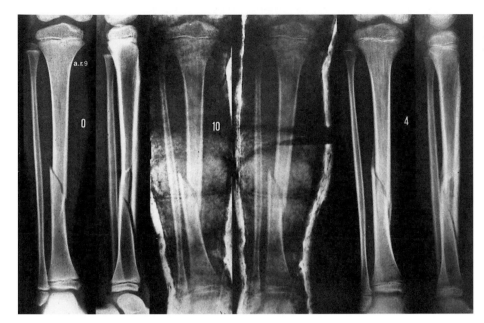

Figure 38.21 Isolated diaphyseal fracture of the tibia: correction of a secondary varus deformity by wedging of the plaster.

muscles of the anterior compartment act to cause a valgus deformity. Spontaneous remodelling may be expected after mild varus deformities following isolated tibial fractures but *not* for valgus deformities. Both rotational and valgus deformities should be prevented by proper radiological monitoring and treatment (Fig. 38.22). Pseudarthrosis after paediatric shaft fractures of the tibia is extremely rare but may be encountered after high-energy trauma with or without subsequent osteomyelitis, following open reduction and unstable fixation, or if there has been segmental bone loss. In open fractures union is usually delayed in younger children whereas non-union may occur in patients older than 11 years.

METAPHYSEAL FRACTURES OF THE DISTAL TIBIA

TORUS AND GREENSTICK FRACTURES

Simple torus fractures may bow posteriorly, but are not angulated in the frontal plane. True greenstick fractures with impaction of the anterior border and complete fracture of the posterior cortex result in a mild recurvatum. The latter may increase if the deformity is not controlled initially by applying a below-knee plaster with the foot slightly plantarflexed.

BENDING FRACTURES

Distal bending fractures pose the same problems as the proximal tibia, although distally the subtalar joint may compensate for mild deformities in the frontal plane. In patients older than 10 years, varus or valgus angulation should be corrected or asymmetrical stimulation of growth will lead to a progressive and then persistent deformity. In younger patients spontaneous correction of up to 20° of valgus, varus and recurvatum may be expected. Anterior bowing rarely develops.

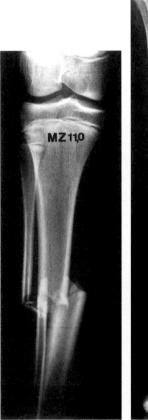
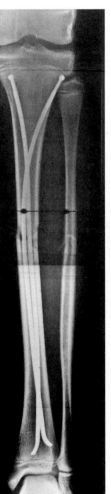
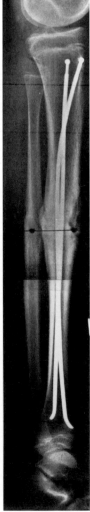

A   B

Figure 38.22 A Fully displaced diaphyseal fracture of the tibia and fibula in an 11-year-old boy. **B** Intramedullary flexible nailing (Prévot nailing).

REFERENCES

Brunner R, Doederlein L 1996 Pathological fractures in patients with cerebral palsy. Journal of Pediatric Orthopaedics 5: 232–238

Burkhart S S, Peterson H A 1979 Fractures of the proximal tibial epiphysis. Journal of Bone and Joint Surgery 61A: 996–1002

Christie M J, Dvonch V M 1981 Tibial tuberosity avulsion fracture in adolescents. Journal of Pediatric Orthopaedics 1: 391–394

Grönkvist H, Hirsch G, Johansson L 1984 Fracture of the anterior tibial spine in children. Journal of Pediatric Orthopaedics 4: 465–468

Ligier J N, Metaizeau J P, Prevot J, Lascombes P 1988 Elastic stable intramedullary nailing of femoral shaft fractures in children. Journal of Bone and Joint Surgery 70B: 74–77

McCarroll J R, Shelbourne K D, Porter D A, Rettig A C, Murray S 1994 Patellar tendon graft reconstruction for midsubstance anterior cruciate ligament rupture in junior high school athletes. American Journal of Sports Medicine 22: 478–484

Maguire J K, Canale S T 1993 Fractures of the patella in children and adolescents. Journal of Pediatric Orthopaedics 13: 567–571

Meyers M H, McKeever F M 1959 Fracture of the intercondylar eminence of the tibia. Journal of Bone and Joint Surgery 41A: 209–220

Molander M L, Wallin G, Wikstad I 1981 Fracture of the intercondylar eminence of the tibia. Journal of Bone and Joint Surgery 63B: 89–91

Mylle J, Reynders P, Broos P 1993 Transepiphyseal fixation of anterior cruciate avulsion in a child. Report of a complication and review of the literature. Archives of Orthopedic and Trauma Surgery 112: 101–103

Nietosvaara Y 1994 The femoral sulcus in children. An ultrasonographic study. Journal of Bone and Joint Surgery 76B: 807–809

Nietosvaara Y 1996 Acute patellar dislocation in children and adolescents. Academic Dissertation, Aurora Hospital and Department of Orthopaedics and Traumatology, Helsinki University

Nietosvaara Y, Aalto K, Kallio P E 1994 Acute patellar dislocation in children: incidence and associated osteochondral fractures. Journal of Pediatric Orthopaedics 14: 513–515

Noyes F R, Delucas J L, Torvik P J 1974 Biomechanics of anterior cruciate ligament failure: an analysis of strain-rate sensitivity and mechanisms of failure in primates. Journal of Bone and Joint Surgery 56A: 236–253

Shannak A O 1988 Tibial fractures in children: a follow-up study. Journal of Pediatric Orthopaedics 8: 306–310

Von Laer L, Jani L, Cuny T, Jenny P 1982 Die proximale Unterschenkelfraktur im Wachstumsalter. Unfallheilkunde 85: 215–225

Von Laer L, Kaelin L, Girard T 1989 Late results following shaft fractures of the lower extremities in the growth period. Zeitschrift für Unfallchirurgie und Versicherungsmedizin 82: 209–215

Zaricznyj B 1977 Avulsion fracture of the tibial eminence: treatment by open reduction and pinning. Journal of Bone and Joint Surgery 59A: 1111–1114

Zionts L E, Harcke H A T, Brooks K M, MacEwen G D 1977 Post-traumatic tibia valga: a case demonstrating asymmetric activity at the proximal growth plate on technetium bone scan. Journal of Pediatric Orthopaedics 7: 458–462

PART 5   Fractures of the foot
P. Engelhardt

TALUS

FREQUENCY AND MECHANISM OF INJURY

Fractures of the talus in children are infrequent, with only 0.08% of all injuries seen in childhood. They are almost always the result of an accidental fall from great heights such as from a balcony or window. They are usually associated with other injuries (Fig. 38.23).

CLASSIFICATION

As in adults the classification of fractures of the talus in children is divided into two groups:

1. Fractures of the periphery, such as the posterior process of talus, osteochondral lesions and shearing fractures of the head of talus.
2. Central fractures involving the body or the neck of the talus.

The fracture pattern at termination of growth resembles that of the adult foot. In the older child the fracture classification by Hawkins is most commonly used for talar neck fractures; it is based on the amount of disruption of the blood supply to the talus (Canale & Beaty 1991):

Type I—Fractures through the neck with minimal displacement.

Type II—The same with subluxation of the subtalar joint.
Type III—The body of talus is dislocated out of the ankle mortise.
Type IV—The same with additional dislocation of the head of the talus.

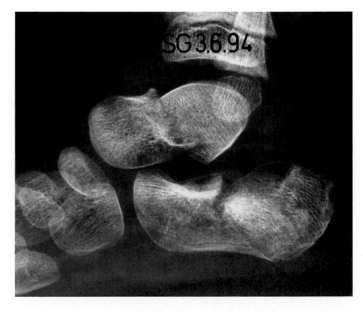

Figure 38.23 Calcaneal and talar neck fractures, sustained by a 5-year-old boy.

ASSESSMENT

Swelling of the hindfoot is severe in central fractures of the talus. Osteochondral lesions of the talus can be easily overlooked. An X-ray, or better a CT scan, is helpful in determining the amount of displacement. Late sequelae such as avascular necrosis of the talus can be evaluated by bone scan or MRI.

TREATMENT

Minor fractures of the periphery can be treated with early mobilisation and limited weight bearing. A major fracture of the posterior process of the talus is best exposed surgically and fixed with resorbable implants (Ethipin). Osteochondral fractures of the talus are not an emergency and can be treated later if problems arise. The stability of the ankle mortice should be assessed at the same time because of potential ligamentous laxity.

All fractures with dislocation of the central part of the talus need the same open reduction and internal fixation. Anatomical reduction (Fig 38.24) is mandatory in order to obtain perfect joint congruity and to reduce the risk of avascular necrosis (AVN). Recently, fixation by counter sunk Herbert screws has seemed promising.

COMPLICATIONS

Several factors are associated with the risk of developing ischaemic necrosis. Displaced fractures of the neck, crush injuries and dislocations carry the highest risk of subsequent ischaemic necrosis (Letts & Gibeault 1980). When considering the remodelling potential of the child's talus, less harm will be done by accepting minor displacement (Ogden 1990). In cases of AVN the talus has a higher bone density on X-ray than the surrounding bones. When there is severe

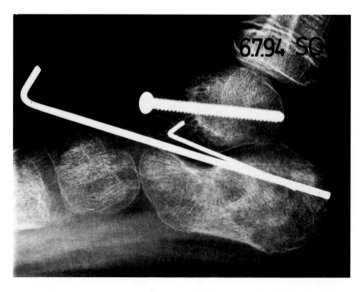

Figure 38.24 Fractures of the calcaneum and talus operatively reduced with internal fixation. Bony union is seen after 4 weeks.

malalignment or AVN, fusion of the subtalar joint is an alternative to wearing orthopaedic orthoses (Marti 1980).

CALCANEUM

FREQUENCY AND MECHANISM OF INJURY

Fractures of the os calcis are infrequently seen in childhood, in contrast to adults. The largely cartilaginous nature of the child's calcaneum, combined with the greater elasticity of the child's bone, probably distributes the applied forces throughout the foot without concentrating it on the calcaneum. A fall striking the heel is the most common mechanism of injury. Bilateral calcaneal fractures are rare (Van Frank et al 1998).

ASSESSMENT

Diagnosis of calcaneal fractures in children on plain X-rays is sometimes difficult. The joint involvement is often subtle and the fracture is easily overlooked. CT gives valuable information regarding the size and location of the fracture fragments (Pablot et al 1985).

CLASSIFICATION

The classification of Schmidt & Weiner which divides fractures into those with subtalar involvement and those without continues to be most used, especially in the adolescent foot (Schmidt & Weiner 1982). For practical purpose it seems sufficient to identify those fractures involving the subtalar joint and to separate them from peripheral fractures (Schantz & Rasmussen 1987).

TREATMENT

Conservative treatment is recommended even for severe depression type fractures (Brunet 2000). The prognosis is invariably favourable and the results are satisfactory, regardless of the extent of comminution (Wiley & Profitt 1984, Schantz & Rasmussen 1988). Children under 10 years of age have adequate remodelling potential at the damaged articular surface of the calcaneum. This is in marked contrast to adult cases. In the rare case of multiple fractures in the same foot, open reduction can be considered. In the very young child the 'Cincinnati approach' gives a very good exposure of the hindfoot (Van Frank et al 1998).

TARSAL, METATARSAL AND PHALANGEAL FRACTURES

FREQUENCY AND MECHANISM OF INJURY

Fractures and dislocations of the midfoot and forefoot are usually the result of direct trauma often with concomitant damage to the soft tissue with severe swelling. Fractures of the phalangeal bones are common because children often play barefoot and injure their toes quite easily. Stress fractures of the metatarsal shaft or neck may occur in children, particularly in those involved in sports that demand chronic, repetitive, stressful activity (Canale & Beaty 1991). Fractures of the base of the fifth metatarsal are caused by sudden contraction of the peroneus brevis muscle. In older adolescents Jones fractures are also the result of repetitive stress (Canale & Beaty 1991).

CLASSIFICATION

A classification system is not very helpful. Treatment is most often conservative even without reduction. Greenstick and buckle fractures are common.

ASSESSMENT

In situations where it is questionable whether a fracture is present or not (e.g. confusion with epiphyseal lines), an X-ray of the other foot is helpful in detecting fractures or dislocations. In cases of severe crush injury care must be taken to avoid a foot compartment syndrome.

TREATMENT

Greenstick fractures of the metatarsal and phalangeal bones do not need reduction. Cold compresses until the swelling subsides, crutches and 2–3 weeks non-weight bearing are sufficient. In severe displacement closed reduction should be undertaken immediately in order to avoid skin necrosis. Kirschner wire transfixation for 3 weeks followed by plaster immobilisation for 2–3 weeks is usually sufficient for uneventful healing (Cehner 1980). The prognosis in terms of ray shortening can be problematic in cases of epiphyseal separation. Open reduction of a severely dislocated metatarsal epiphysis can thus be necessary.

REFERENCES

Brunet J 2000 Calcaneal fractures in children. Journal of Bone and Joint Surgery 82B: 211–216

Canale S, Beaty J 1991 Operative pediatric orthopaedics. Mosby, St Louis

Cehner J 1980 Fractures of the tarsal bones, metatarsals, and toes. In: Weber B G, Brunner Ch, Freuler F (eds) Treatment of fractures in children and adolescents. Springer, Berlin, pp 385–399

Letts R, Gibeault D 1980 Fractures of the neck of the talus in children. Foot and Ankle 1: 74–78

Marti R 1980 Fractures of the talus and calcaneus. In: Weber B G, Brunner Ch, Freuler F (eds) Treatment of fractures in children and adolescents. Springer, Berlin, pp 373–384

Ogden J 1990 Skeletal injury in the child. Saunders, Philadelphia

Pablot S, Daneman A, Stringer D, Carroll N 1985 The value of computed tomography in the early assessment of comminuted fractures of the calcaneus: a review of three patients. Journal of Pediatric Orthopaedics 5: 435–438

Schantz K, Rasmussen F 1987 Calcaneus fracture in the child. Acta Orthopaedica Scandinavica 58: 507–509

Schantz K, Rasmussen F 1988 Good prognosis after calcaneal fracture in childhood. Acta Orthopaedica Scandinavica 59: 560–563

Schmidt T, Weiner D 1982 Calcaneal fractures in children. Clinical Orthopaedics and Related Research 171: 150–156

Wiley J, Profitt A 1984 Fractures of the os calcis in children. Clinical Orthopaedics and Related Research 188: 131–138

Van Frank E, Ward J, Engelhardt P 1998 Bilateral calcaneal fracture in childhood. Archives of Orthopaedic and Trauma Surgery 118: 111–112

Chapter 39

Spinal fractures

PART 1 Traumatic disorders of the cervical spine
R. N. Hensinger

INTRODUCTION

The child's cervical spine often presents a diagnostic dilemma. The presence of cervical growth plates, lack of complete ossification, unique developmental aspects and hypermobility are causes of confusion in the interpretation of cervical radiographs in children with neck pain or stiffness (Cattell & Filtzer 1965). Cervical spine radiographs in children are notoriously difficult to interpret. Lack of familiarity with normal growth and development and poorly positioned films makes diagnosis difficult and can lead to problems in management.

NORMAL DEVELOPMENT AND VARIATIONS

A knowledge of normal physeal development is essential when interpreting a child's radiograph. Physeal plates are generally smooth, regular, in predicted locations and have subchondral sclerotic lines. Fractures are irregular, without sclerosis and usually in unpredictable locations. The upper two cervical vertebrae are unique in their development (Figs 39.1, 39.2); the remaining five develop essentially uniformly.

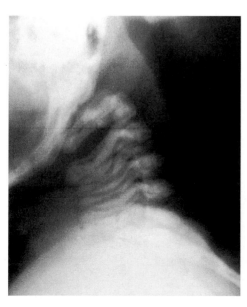

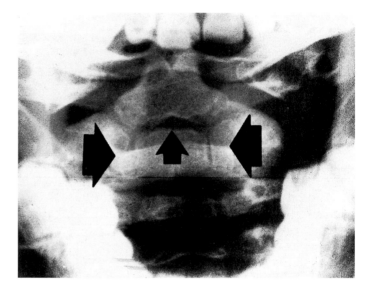

Figure 39.2 The epiphysis at the base of the odontoid process is shown (small arrow). This is well below the level of the superior articular facet of the axis. The synchondroses between the body of the axis and the neural arches are illustrated (large arrows). Just above this are the synchondroses between the odontoid process and the neural arches. The odontoid process, therefore, surmounts the body of the axis and is sandwiched between the neural arches. The epiphyseal line and synchondroses combine to form the letter H. (From Fielding 1973.)

Figure 39.1 An extension radiograph of a 6-week-old child; the anterior arch of the atlas may slide upward to protrude beyond the ossified part of the dens, giving a mistaken impression of odontoid hypoplasia. Note that the anterior portion of the ring of C1 is not yet ossified.

UPPER CERVICAL VERTEBRAE (C1 AND C2)

At birth the atlas is composed of three ossification centres – one for the body (anterior ring) and one for each of the two neural arches. The anterior ring is occasionally bifid and is not usually present at birth, appearing during the first year of life (Fig. 39.1). On rare occasions it is absent and may close by fusion of the neural arches anteriorly. The posterior arch of the first cervical vertebra usually closes by the third year. Occasionally its development is incomplete or remains completely absent throughout life. The neurocentral synchondroses link the neural arches to the body of the atlas and are best seen in the open-mouth view (Fig. 39.2). They close by the seventh year of life and should not be mistaken for fractures.

The developing axis has four ossification centres at birth; one for each neural arch, one (occasionally two) for the body and a fourth for the dens. In the anteroposterior open-mouth view of a young child, the dens (odontoid process) is 'sandwiched' between the neural arches (Fig. 39.2). It surmounts the body of the axis and is separated from it by a synchondrosis, or vestigial disc space of the odontoid. Below this are the synchondroses between the body and the neural arches which together combine to form the letter 'H' (Fig. 39.2).

The epiphysis or synchondrosis of the odontoid runs well below the level of the articular processes of the axis. In the adult, a persistent epiphyseal line is not seen at the base of the odontoid process where fractures often occur, but within the body of the axis well below the level of the articular facets. Cattell & Filtzer (1965) found that this basilar epiphysis of the odontoid may persist up to 11 years of age as a narrow, sclerotic line and can resemble a non-displaced fracture.

The odontoid fuses with the neural arches and the body of the axis between 3 and 6 years of age, essentially the same time that the remainder of the vertebral body joins the neural arches. Therefore, no epiphysis or synchondrosis should be present in the axis in the open-mouth view of a child over 6 years of age. The normal synchondrosis between the dens and the arch of C2 is not seen on the lateral view of the cervical spine, but is easily visible on the oblique view and should not be mistaken for a fracture (Swischuck et al 1979). The ossification centre of the inferior vertebral ring (ring apophysis) of the second cervical vertebra should cause little confusion. It ossifies during the late years of childhood and fuses with the body at approximately 25 years of age.

The tip of the odontoid is not ossified at birth and it has a V-shaped appearance (Fig. 39.2). A mistaken impression of odontoid hypoplasia may be given by a lateral extension X-ray in a very young child because the anterior arch of the atlas slides upward and protrudes beyond the ossified portion of the dens to lie against the unossified tip (Fig. 39.1) (Cattell & Filtzer 1965). A small ossification centre, known as the summit ossification centre, appears at its tip at age 3–6 years and fuses with the main portion of the odontoid by age 12 years. Its persistence is referred to as an ossiculum terminale and should not be confused with an os odontoideum (Fielding et al 1980).

LOWER CERVICAL VERTEBRAE (C3–C7)

The third to seventh cervical vertebrae ossify from three centres: one from the body and one from each neural arch. The neural arches close at the second or third year, and the neurocentral synchondroses between the neural arches and the vertebral body fuse from the third to sixth years. In the lateral radiograph, the ossified portion of the vertebral body in the young child is wedge shaped until it becomes squared off at about 7 years of age (Cattell & Filtzer 1965). The bodies, neural arches and pedicles enlarge radially by periosteal apposition, similar to the periosteal growth seen in long bones.

At birth, the vertebral bodies possess superior and inferior cartilage plates firmly bonded to the disc (Sherk et al 1976). The interface between vertebral body and endplate is similar to the physis of a long bone. The vertebral body is analogous to the metaphysis and the clear space between both it and the endplate represents the physeal plate where longitudinal growth occurs (Caffey 1974). Clinically as well as experimentally stress applied to the vertebral bodies results in splitting of the cartilage endplate at the growth zone in the area of columnar and calcified cartilage rather than at the stronger junction between it and the vertebral disc.

The apophyseal rings on the upper and lower surfaces of the vertebral body begin to ossify late in childhood and fuse to the vertebral body by the age of 25. Apophyseal fractures in the cervical spine have been reported. The inferior endplates are believed to be more susceptible to fracture than the superior because of the mechanical protection afforded by the developing uncinate processes (Lawson et al 1987).

MOBILITY

The cervical region is normally the most flexible area of the spine, especially in children. It may be difficult to determine normal from abnormal mobility in a young child's neck. The most mobile articulation in the cervical spine is between the atlas and axis. Half of all cervical rotation occurs here. Some side-to-side bending is also present, but hyperextension is limited by the dens. In 3–10-year-old children, subluxation is present if there is more than 10° of forward flexion at C1–C2 or if the distance between the posterior spines of C1 and C2 is greater than 10 mm in the neutral radiograph. The atlanto-occipital joint allows some flexion and extension but very little rotation. The C2–C3 joint is slightly mobile in flexion and extension, but not in rotation. Thus, the relatively mobile C1–C2 joint is located between two relatively stiff joints. This concentrates forces at the atlanto-axial joint, and partly explains the high percentage of cervical injuries at this level.

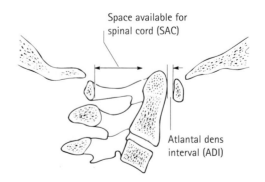

Figure 39.3 Sagittal views of the atlanto-axial joint demonstrating the atlanto–dens interval (ADI). The space available for the cord (SAC) is the distance between the posterior aspect of the odontoid and the posterior ring of C1. (Redrawn from Hensinger & Fielding 1990.)

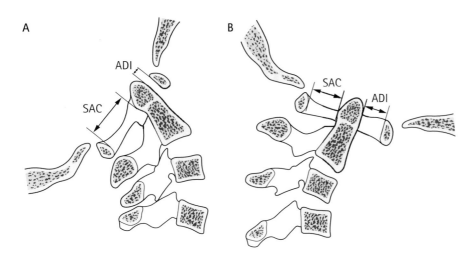

The crit
been de
but may
In child
diagnos
the inte
distance
Increase
processe
space ar
injuries

RETROF

The spac
region c
in adult
evidenc
dislocat
for the
base of
15 years
ryngeal
space is

In ins
while in
logical'
sue shac
the laryn

Figure 39.4 Atlanto-axial instability with intact odontoid. **A** Flexion – forward sliding of the atlas with an increased ADI and decreased SAC. **B** Extension – the ADI and SAC return to normal as the intact odontoid provides a bony block to subluxation in hyperextension. (Redrawn from Hensinger & Fielding 1990.)

The anterior arch of the atlas is firmly held against the odontoid process by the transverse atlantal ligament (Fielding et al 1974). This space is called the atlanto-dens interval (ADI) and on the lateral radiograph is measured from the anterior edge of the dens to the posterior edge of the anterior arch of the atlas (Fig 39.3). Further stability is provided by accessory ligaments such as the alar ligaments that connect the tip of the odontoid process with the medial aspect of the occipital condyles and the capsular ligaments. In the adult anterior displacement of the ring of C1 up to 3 mm from the odontoid is within the range of normal (Fielding et al 1974). When the distance between the odontoid process and the anterior arch of C1 is 4.5 mm or greater the transverse ligament is ruptured and when the distance is 10–12 mm all ligaments have failed (Fielding et al 1974).

Radiographic surveys of children suggest that an ADI of up to 4 mm may be normal (Pennecot et al 1984). (If the space between the dens and anterior arch of C1 is not symmetrical on the flexion view, the atlanto-dens interval should be measured at the mid-portion of the dens.) The

larger normal limit in children is probably due to greater ligamentous laxity and incomplete ossification. A slight increase in the neutral ADI may indicate an injury of the transverse atlantal ligament. This can be a useful sign of acute injury, where flexion-extension views are potentially hazardous.

The ADI is not helpful in chronic atlanto-axial instability due to congenital anomalies, rheumatoid arthritis or Down's syndrome. In these conditions, the odontoid is frequently found to be hypermobile with a widened ADI, particularly in flexion (Burke et al 1985) (Fig. 39.4). Here attention should be directed to the amount of space available for the spinal cord (SAC) by measuring the distance from the posterior aspect of the odontoid or axis to the nearest posterior structure (foramen magnum or posterior ring of the atlas) (Fig. 39.3). This measurement is particularly helpful in non-union of the odontoid or os ondontoideum, because in both the ADI may be normal, yet in flexion or extension there is considerable reduction in the space available for the spinal cord (Fig. 39.5). McRae (1960) measured the distance from

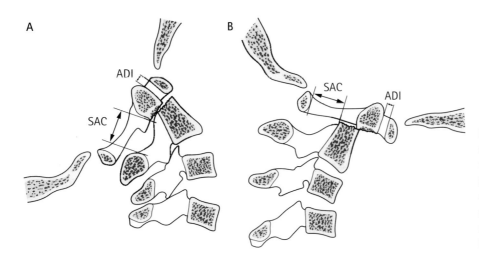

Figure 3
widening
Medical I
Science N
New York
UK.)

Figure 39.5 Atlanto-axial instability with os odontoideum, absent odontoid or traumatic non-union. **A** Flexion – forward sliding of the atlas with reduction of the SAC, but no change in ADI. **B** Extension – posterior subluxation with reduction in SAC and no change in the ADI. (Redrawn from Hensinger & Fielding 1990.)

C

A

the
arch
whi
ical
It sh
drar

P:
ated
at r
spir
the

S
alar
afte
39.€
role
defi
vert
into
'spa
safe
logi
vers
chrc
whe
area
secc
ther

PSE

One
diat
flex
mor
39.7
betv
to 7
ion,
mal
tenc
in f

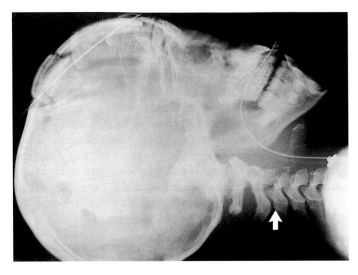

Figure 39.9 Supine lateral radiography of a 6-year-old child struck by an automobile. There is an unstable tear-drop fracture of the body of C3, with kyphosis at the fracture site (arrow). Cervical injuries in children are often associated with head or facial trauma as seen in this case of a massive depressed skull fracture. (From Herzenberg & Hensinger 1989.)

have been used to assess the extent of the bony injury but have been largely replaced by computed tomography (CT). CT should not be used as a screening tool but rather as a method to further elucidate suspicious areas found on plain films (Berne et al 1999). CT may identify occult fractures in the posterior elements that are not clearly seen or appreciated on X-rays. As there is such a high incidence of cervical spine injuries in patients with severe, blunt multiple injury, CT scan can be helpful particularly in the intensive care unit. Woodring noted that while CT scans are particularly helpful

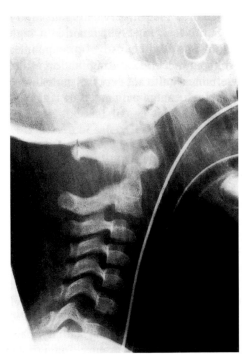

Figure 39.10 Cervical injury in a 3 year old. Initial lateral radiograph in traction demonstrating multiple injuries of the cervical spine. Note the distraction at occiput–C1, C1–C2, and C6–C7.

for C1–C2 problems plain films were better at detecting fractures of the vertebral body, dens and spinous processes, and subluxation and dislocation (Woodring & Lee 1992). However, plain films may show a vertebral body fracture where CT would show an additional fracture through the posterior elements of the same vertebra. CT is recommended for all fractures of C1, C7–T1 when plain films are not helpful (Tan et al 1999) and for surgical planning.

Interestingly, tomograms, particularly with flexion and extension views, continue to be very good in demonstrating atlanto-occipital dislocation, subluxation of the vertebral bodies, and fractures of the lateral masses and processes.

SPINAL CORD INJURY WITHOUT OBSERVABLE RADIOGRAPHIC ABNORMALITIES (SCIWORA)

It is well recognised that children may have partial or complete paralysis without radiographic evidence of spine fracture or dislocation. Pang & Wilberger (1982) coined the phrase 'spinal cord injury without observable radiographic abnormalities' (SCIWORA). Yngve et al (1988) reported the SCIWORA phenomenon in 16 of 17 spinal cord injured children and noted that they tended to be younger than those with osseous fracture.

Magnetic resonance imaging (MRI) demonstrates parenchymal spinal cord injuries (Fig. 39.11) and disc herniation better than CT. Katzberg et al (1999) noted that MRI imaging is more accurate than radiography in the detection of a wide spectrum of neck injuries. It is superior for haemorrhage, oedema, anterior/posterior longitudinal ligament injury, traumatic disc herniation, cord oedema and cord compression. CT remains preferable for the classification of bony injuries.

NEONATAL TRAUMA

The normal infant is unable to support the head adequately until about 3 months of age. Infants, therefore, are incapable of protecting the cervical spine and spinal cord against excessive torsional and traction forces that may occur during delivery and the months following birth. Bony injury usually involves the upper cervical spine, but lower cervical injuries have been reported. These forces may exceed the stretch capability of the neck. According to Stern & Rand (1959), the lax ligaments of a child's neck may not be able to protect the less elastic spinal cord, possibly explaining the occurrence of severe cord injuries without skeletal injury. Spinal cords removed from newborns dying from obstetric trauma show changes over long segments suggesting that longitudinal traction was a major factor.

Skeletal injury due to obstetric trauma is probably underreported because the infantile spine, with its large percentage of cartilage, is difficult to evaluate radiologically, especially if the lesion occurs through cartilage or at the cartilage–bone interface. If routine radiographs are normal, then flexion-extension views are necessary. MRI is better than CT in the diagnosis of upper cervical spinal cord

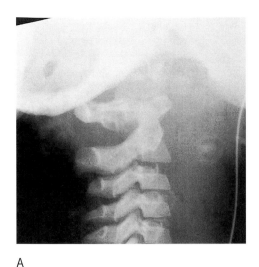

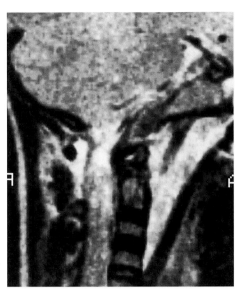

A

B

Figure 39.11 An 8 year old who sustained an occiput–C1 dislocation in a motor vehicle accident. The patient had a complete respiratory arrest and was resuscitated at the accident scene. **A** Lateral radiograph demonstrating vertical displacement between the occiput and the ring of C1. **B** MRI demonstrating the spinal cord lesion at the cervicomedullary junction. The child has no neurological function below C1 and is ventilator dependent.

compression. A cervical spine lesion should be considered in the differential diagnosis of infants who are found to be floppy at birth, particularly if the delivery was a difficult one. Complete flaccid paralysis with areflexia are usually followed by the typical pattern of hyperreflexia once spinal cord shock is over. Brachial plexus birth palsies also warrant a cervical spine radiograph.

Caffey (1974) and Swischuck (1969) described a form of child abuse called the 'whiplash shaken infant syndrome'. The weak infantile neck musculature cannot support the head when it is subjected to whiplash stresses. Intracranial and intraocular haemorrhages resulting in death, or latent cerebral injury, retardation and permanent visual or hearing defects have been reported, together with fractures of the spine and spinal cord injuries.

OCCIPUT–C1 LESIONS

Atlanto-occipital injuries may occur during traumatic deliveries or major blunt trauma and imply an injury to the tectorial membrane and the alar ligaments (Fig. 39.11). Occiput–C1 lesions are infrequently reported in surviving patients as they often result in lethal cervicomedullary cord damage. Many occiput–C1 dislocations may spontaneously reduce and are initially unrecognised. These injuries are probably a result of sudden deceleration. The head is carried forward with a sudden cranio-vertebral dislocation and immediate spontaneous reduction and, hence, normal X-ray findings. Autopsy findings include disruption of the craniovertebral joints, spinal cord and vertebral arteries.

For the rare individual who survives this injury, gentle reduction by positioning and minimal traction is recommended. Great care must be taken not to overdistract the injury site (Fig. 39.10). Halo fixation followed by posterior occipital cervical fusion is the definitive treatment. Chronic or late instability of occiput–C1 can be difficult to diagnose. Carefully controlled flexion-extension lateral views or reconstructed CT which allows calculation of the Powers ratio is helpful (Powers et al 1979). Fracture of an occipital condyle was infrequently reported and very difficult to diagnose (Cottalord et al 1996).

FRACTURES OF THE ATLAS

Fracture of the ring of C1, the so called 'Jefferson fracture', is not a common paediatric cervical fracture. The aetiology is an axial compression load applied to the head, transmitted through the lateral occipital condyles to the lateral masses of C1. The ring of C1 is usually broken in more than one spot (Fig. 39.12). In children isolated single fractures have been described, probably hinging on the synchondroses. Fractures have been reported through the synchondroses. As the lateral masses separate, the transverse atlantal ligament may rupture, or be avulsed (Fig. 39.13), and result in C1–C2 instability.

While plain radiography may show the fracture in certain cases, CT is far superior in visualising the arch of C1 both acutely and in the follow-up period to assess healing (Fig. 39.12). Treatment should consist of a Minerva cast or halo immobilisation. Surgery is rarely necessary to stabilise these fractures.

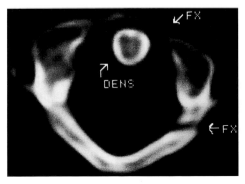

Figure 39.12 A 4 year old who sustained a skull fracture and associated Jefferson fracture in a motor vehicle accident. CT of C1 shows the ring broken in two locations (FX).

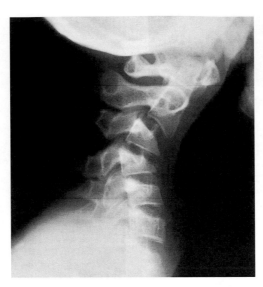

A   B

Figure 39.17 A Lateral radiogram of a 14-year-old male who sustained a ligamentous injury of the cervical spine while playing football. **B** Four weeks later; note the marked cervical kyphosis at C3–C4.

divided into rigid types made out of plastic and soft types made out of foam (Fig. 39.19) (Millington et al 1987). While the rigid types perform better than soft foam in mechanical testing, even the best device allows 17° flexion, 19° extension, 4° rotation and 6° lateral motion. To gain more control following an acute injury, Huerta et al (1987) recommended that these devices be supplemented with tape, bean-bags and other supports.

The child with a cervical injury is at particular risk of further displacement during resuscitation. In a study in four patients with unstable cervical injuries who failed resuscitation in the emergency room, it was found that longitudinal axial traction during emergency intubation actually increased the deformity (Bivins et al 1988). The authors recommended that intubation of trauma patients with suspected unstable cervical injuries prior to radiographic evaluation should be attempted first by the nasotracheal

route rather than with axial traction and a standard laryngoscope. Cricothyroidotomy is another option.

While adults may be positioned safely supine on a flat backboard to immobilise the cervical spine, small children are different. Young children have disproportionately larger heads and are at risk of developing kyphosis and anterior translation of the upper cervical segment in an unstable fracture pattern (Fig. 39.20A,B). Curran et al (1995) showed on lateral views of the cervical spine that 60% of the children were immobilised in over 5° of kyphosis and 37% had 10° or more. One must be more cognisant of how we are transferring these children in a neutral position. We recommend positioning and transporting children less than 6 years of age using a split mattress technique to elevate the thorax 2–4 cm and lower the occiput (Fig. 39.20 C, D). However, this immobilisation protocol does tend to reduce displaced fractures and make their

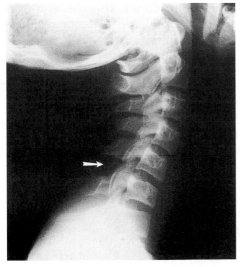

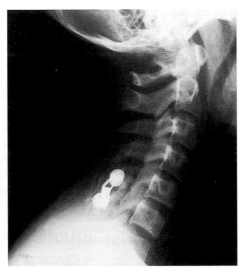

A   B

Figure 39.18 A Unstable ligamentous flexion injury in a teenage boy who fell backward while weight-lifting, striking the back of his head on a table. Note the kyphosis at C5–C6 and the small fleck of bone avulsed from the C5–C6 posterior facet joint (arrow). This injury would not heal adequately with immobilisation alone. **B** The same patient after surgical stabilisation by posterior C5–C6 fusion. (From Herzenberg & Hensinger 1989).

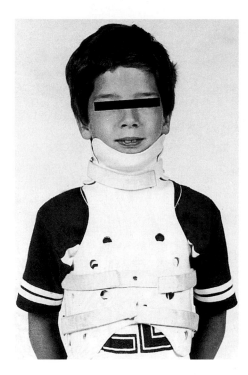

Figure 39.19 A child immobilised in a SOMI brace.

recognition and diagnosis more difficult (Herzenberg & Hensinger 1989).

A plaster Minerva jacket is an excellent means of immobilising the paediatric cervical spine-injured patient (Fig. 39.21). Thermoplastic bracing may be of value in the older child (Millington et al 1987).

Skull tongs and halo devices can be used in the young child (Letts et al 1988). However, excessive pressure by halo pins or Crutchfield tongs can lead to perforation of the skull and brain abscess. The biomechanics and anatomy of halo pin placement in children have been studied and, in general, the pins should be placed anterolaterally, posterolaterally and perpendicular to the skull (Fig. 39.22). In the small child, CT of the skull should be obtained to ensure there is sufficient bone for pin placement. A modified low-torque multiple pin technique of halo application will permit the use of the halo in children down to the age of 7 months.

The halo body cast represents the most rigid form of external immobilisation for cervical spine injuries in children. A halo vest does not limit motion sufficiently (Letts et al 1988).

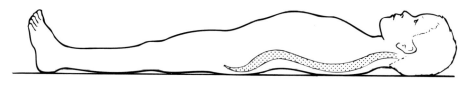

A

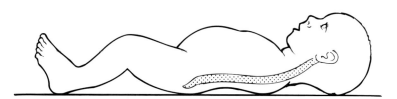

B

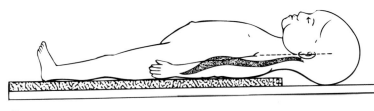

C

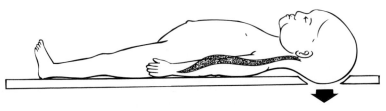

D

Figure 39.20 A Adult immobilised on a standard backboard. **B** Young child on a standard backboard. The relatively large head forces the neck into a kyphotic position. **C** Young child on a modified backboard that has a double-mattress pad to raise the chest, obtaining safe supine cervical positioning. **D** Young child on a modified backboard that has a cut-out to recess the occiput, obtaining safe supine cervical positioning. (From Herzenberg et al 1989 © The Journal of Bone and Joint Surgery.)

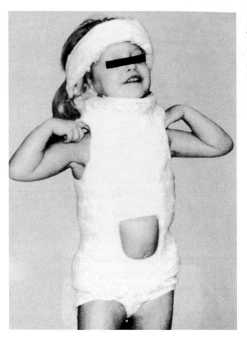

Figure 39.21 A 3 year old with a fracture of the odontoid following 6 weeks of immobilisation in a Minerva cast.

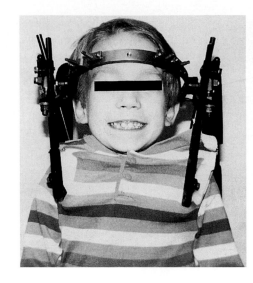

Figure 39.22 Child immobilised in a halo cast following surgical stabilisation of C1–C2 for instability secondary to Morquio's syndrome. Eight halo pins, four anteriorly and four posteriorly, help to distribute the forces on the skull over a larger area.

SURGICAL STABILISATION

Surgery in the child's spine differs little from that in the adult but fusion occurs much more rapidly. Children's spines fuse easily and it is prudent to expose only the relevant area (Stabler et al 1985). Extension of the dissection above or below the area will frequently result in an unwanted creeping fusion to the closely approximated lamina above and below. Homologous bone grafting is not recommended. Stabler et al (1985) reported six of seven children, aged 6–15 years, with pseudarthrosis following posterior wiring and fusion with cadaveric bone graft. Anterior cervical fusion in young children is not recommended for trauma.

Atlanto-axial arthrodesis in children is performed using the same techniques as that used in the adult, the only difference being in the use of smaller gauge wire. The vertebral arteries are locked in a groove on the upper surface of the posterior arch of C1 approximately 2 cm from the midline in the young child, leaving a narrower margin of safety. Halo immobilisation may be indicated to increase the rate of successful fusion. Many children who undergo posterior spine fusion for cervical fractures will experience long-term mild chronic neck pain. McGrory & Klassen (1994) reported on a large series of children who underwent surgical stabilisation of the spine for fractures and dislocations: 76% had excellent results. Complications included spontaneous extension of the fusion mass, continued pain at the iliac crest donor site, and superficial infection of the bone graft. Several authors have reported using internal fixation, including the Halifax interlaminar clamp, transarticular screws, transpedicular screws and a transodontoid anterior screw with excellent results (Abumi et al 1994, Lowry et al 1997, Mizuno & Nakagawa 1999).

REFERENCES

Abumi K, Itoh H, Taneichi H, Kaneda K 1994 Transpedicular screw fixation for traumatic lesions of the middle and lower cervical spine: description of the techniques and preliminary report. Journal of Spinal Disorders 7: 19–28

Berne J D, Velmahos G C, El-Tawil Q et al 1999 Value of complete cervical helical computed tomographic scanning in identifying cervical spine injury in the unevaluable blunt trauma patient with multiple injuries: a prospective study. Journal of Trauma 47: 896–902 discussion 902–903

Bivins H G, Bezmalinovic Z, Price H M, Williams J L 1988 The effect of axial traction during orotracheal intubation of the trauma victim with an unstable cervical spine. Annals of Emergency Medicine 17: 25–29

Burke S W, French H G, Roberts J M, Johnston C E, Whitecloud T S, Edmunds J O 1985 Chronic atlanto-axial instability in Down syndrome. Journal of Bone and Joint Surgery 67A: 1356–1360

Caffey J 1974 The whiplash shaken infant syndrome. Pediatrics 54: 396–403

Cattell H S, Filtzer D L 1965 Pseudosubluxation and other normal variations in the cervical spine in children. Journal of Bone and Joint Surgery 47A: 1295–1309

Connolly B, Emery D, Armstrong D 1995 The odontoid synchondrotic slip: an injury unique to young children. Pediatric Radiology 25(Suppl 1): S129–133

Cottalord J, Allard D, Dutour N 1996 Fracture of the occipital condyle. Journal of Pediatric Orthopaedics 5: 61–63

Curran C, Dietrich A M, Bowman M J, Ginn-Pease M E, King D R, Kosnik E 1995 Pediatric cervical-spine immobilization: achieving neutral position? Journal of Trauma 39: 729–732

Eleraky M A, Theodore N, Adams M, Rekate H L, Sonntag V K 2000 Pediatric cervical spine injuries: report of 102 cases and preview of the literature. Journal of Neurosurgery 92(1 Suppl): 12–17

Fielding J W 1973 Selective observations on the cervical spine in the child. In: Ahstrom J P Jr (ed) Current practice in orthopaedic surgery, vol 5. C V Mosby, St Louis, pp 31–35

Fielding J W, Cochran G V B, Lawsing J F III, Hohl M 1974 Tears of the transverse ligament of the atlas: a clinical and biomechanical study. Journal of Bone and Joint Surgery 56A: 1683–1691

Fielding J W, Hensinger R N, Hawkins R J 1980 Os odontoideum. Journal of Bone and Joint Surgery 62A: 376–383

Furnival R A, Street K A, Schunk J E 1999 Too many pediatric trampoline injuries. Pediatrics 103: e57

Gonzalez R P, Fried P O, Bukhalo M, Holevar M R, Falimirski M E 1999 Role of clinical examination in screening for blunt cervical spine injury. Journal of the American College of Surgeons 189: 152–157

Griffiths S C 1972 Fracture of the odontoid process in children. Journal of Pediatric Surgery 7: 680–683

Hause M, Hoshino R, Omata S, Kuramochi E, Furnikawa K, Nakamura T 1977 Cervical spine injuries in children. Clinical Orthopaedics and Related Research 129: 172–176

Hensinger R N, Fielding J W 1990 The cervical spine. In: Morrisey R T (ed) Lovell and Winter's pediatric orthopaedics, 3rd edn. J B Lippincott, Philadelphia, ch 19

Herzenberg J E, Hensinger R N 1989 Pediatric cervical spine injuries. Trauma Quarterly 5: 73–81

Herzenberg J E, Hensinger R N, Dedrick D K, Phillips W A 1989 Emergency transport and positioning of young children who have an injury of the cervical spine. The standard backboard may be hazardous. Journal of Bone and Joint Surgery 71A: 15–22

Huerta C, Griffin R, Joyce S M 1987 Cervical spine stabilization in pediatric patients: evaluation of current techniques. Annals of Emergency Medicine 16: 1121–1126

Katzberg R W, Benedetti P F, Drake C M et al 1999 Acute cervical spine injuries: prospective MR imaging assessment at a level 1 trauma center. Radiology 213: 203–212

Kleinman P K, Shelton Y A 1997 Hangman's fracture in an abused infant: imaging features. Pediatric Radiology 27: 776–777

Lawson J P, Ogden J A, Bucholz R W, Hughes S A 1987 Physeal injuries of the cervical spine. Journal of Pediatric Orthopaedics 7: 428–435

Letts M, Kaylor K, Goruw G 1988 A biomechanical analysis of halo fixation in children. Journal of Bone and Joint Surgery 70B: 277–279

Lowry D W, Pollack I F, Clyde B, Albright A L, Adelson P D 1997 Upper cervical spine fusion in the pediatric population. Journal of Neurosurgery 87: 671–676

McGrory B J, Klassen R A 1994 Arthrodesis of the cervical spine for fractures and dislocations in children and adolescents. A long-term follow-up study. Journal of Bone and Joint Surgery 76A: 1606–1616

McRae D L 1960 The significance of abnormalities of the cervical spine. American Journal of Roentgenology 84: 3–25

Millington P J, Ellingsen J M, Hauswirth B E, Fabian P J 1987 Thermoplastic minerva body jacket – a practical alternative to current methods of cervical spine stabilization. Physical Therapy 67: 223–225

Mizuno J, Nakagawa H 1999 Spinal instrumentation for unstable C1–2 injury. Neurologia Medico-Chirurgica (Tokyo) 39: 434–439, discussion 439–441

Morandi X, Hanna A, Hamla A, Brassier G 1999 Anterior screw fixation of odontoid fractures. Surgical Neurology 51: 236–240

Nachemson A 1960 Fracture of the odontoid process of the axis. A clinical study based on 26 cases. Acta Orthopaedica Scandinavica 29: 185–217

Odent T, Langlais J, Glorion C, Kassis B, Bataille J, Pouliquen L C 1999 Fractures of the odontoid process: a report of 15 cases in children younger than 6 years. Journal of Pediatric Orthopaedics 19: 51–54

Pang D, Wilberger J E 1982 Spinal cord injury without radiologic abnormalities in children. Journal of Neurosurgery 57: 114–129

Pennecot G F, Gouraud D, Hardy J R, Pouliquen J C 1984 Roentgenographical study of the stability of the cervical spine in children. Journal of Pediatric Orthopaedics 4: 346–352

Powers B, Milla M D, Kramer R S, Martinez S, Gehweiler J A Jr 1979 Traumatic anterior atlanto-occipital dislocation. Neurosurgery 4: 12–17

Rachesky I, Boyce W T, Duncan B, Bjelland J, Sibley B 1987 Clinical prediction of cervical spine injuries in children. Radiographic abnormalities. American Journal of Disease in Children 141: 199–201

Schwarz N, Genelin F, Schwarz A F 1994 Post-traumatic cervical kyphosis in children cannot be prevented by non-operative methods. Injury 25: 173–175

Sherk H H, Nicholson J T, Chung S M K 1978 Fractures of the odontoid process in young children. Journal of Bone and Joint Surgery 60A: 921–924

Sherk H H, Schut L, Lane J 1976 Fractures and dislocations of the cervical spine in children. Orthopedic Clinics of North American 7: 593–604

Stabler C L, Eismont F J, Brown M D, Green B A, Malinin T I 1985 Failure of posterior cervical fusions using cadaveric bone graft in children. Journal of Bone and Joint Surgery 67A: 370–375

Steel H H 1968 Anatomical and mechanical consideration of the atlanto-axial articulation. In: Proceedings of the American Orthopedic Association. Journal of Bone and Joint Surgery 50A: 1481–1482

Stern W E, Rand R W 1959 Birth injuries to the spinal cord. Report of 2 cases and review of the literature. American Journal of Obstetrics and Gynecology 78: 498–512

Swischuck L E 1969 Spine and spinal cord trauma in the battered child syndrome. Radiology 92: 733–738

Swischuck L E 1977 Anterior displacement of C2 in children: physiologic or pathologic? A helpful differentiating line. Radiology 122: 759–763

Swischuck L E, Hayden C K Jr, Sarwar M 1979 The densarch synchondrosis versus the hangman's fracture. Pediatric Radiology 8: 100–102

Tan E, Schweitzer M E, Vaccaro L, Spetell A C 1999 Is computed tomography of nonvisualized C7–T1 cost-effective? Journal of Spinal Disorders 12: 472–476

White A A, Johnson R M, Penjabi M M 1975 Biomechanical analysis of clinical stability in the cervical spine. Clinical Orthopaedics and Related Research 100: 85–96

Wholey M H, Bruwer A J, Baher H L Jr 1958 The lateral roentgenogram of the neck; with comments on the atlanto-odontoid-basion relationship. Radiology 71: 350–356

Woodring J H, Lee C 1992 The role and limitations of computed tomographic scanning in the evaluation of cervical trauma. Journal of Trauma 33: 698–708

Yngve D A, Harris W P, Herndon W A, Sullivan J A, Gross R H 1988 Spinal cord injury without osseous spine fracture. Journal of Pediatric Orthopaedics 8: 153–159

PART 2   Fractures of the thoracic and lumbar spine
R. N. Hensinger and C. L. Craig

GENERAL AND BASIC PRINCIPLES

Injuries of the thoracic and lumbar spine in children are rare. The potential for continued growth, the presence of healthy disc tissue, elasticity of the soft tissue and well-mineralised bone distinguish these injuries from comparable injuries in the adult. The immature spine has the capacity to remodel the vertebral body, but not the posterior elements. Restoration of height of a compressed vertebra is in part due to the hypervascularity of the reparative response and stimulation of the apophysis. This probably accounts for the infrequent occurrence of kyphosis in children with multiple compression fractures.

ANATOMY

The development of the thoraco-lumbar spine in children is more straightforward than that of the cervical spine. One should be aware of the following: (i) an increased cartilage to bone ratio; (ii) the presence of the ring apophysis, and (iii) hyperelasticity. In the newborn and in early childhood the vertebrae are largely cartilaginous, and radiographically the intervertebral spaces appear widened in relation to the vertebral bodies (Fig. 39.23). With ageing the ossification centres enlarge and this cartilage–vertebral ratio gradually reverses. The vertebral apophyses are secondary centres of ossification that develop in the cartilaginous endplates located at the superior and inferior surfaces of the vertebral bodies. They are thicker at their periphery than the centre, and thus appear as a ring with early ossification. These are seen initially between the eighth and twelfth years and normally fuse with the vertebral bodies by the twenty-first year. They may be confused with an avulsion fracture. The vertebral apophysis is equivalent to the epiphysis of a long bone and is separated from the vertebral body (the metaphysis) by a narrow cartilaginous

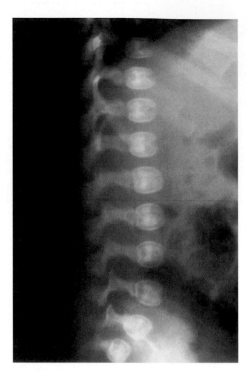

Figure 39.23 X-ray of a normal spine in a 10-week-old infant. The superior and inferior vertebral endplates, vertebral apophysis, are cartilaginous. Thus, the apparent widening of the intervertebral spaces is relative to the ossific portion of the vertebrae. The anterior and posterior notching of the walls of the vertebral body are due to the normal vascular channels and may be confused with fracture.

physis. Vertical growth of the vertebrae occurs equally at the top and the bottom.

In the infant, on the lateral X-ray there appear horizontal conical shadows of lessened density extending inward from the anterior and posterior walls of the vertebral bodies, which may be confused with fracture (Fig. 39.23) (Wagoner & Pendergrass 1939). The posterior notch results from an actual indentation in the posterior vertebra wall at the point of entrance and emergence of the posterior arteries and veins. This indentation is present in all vertebrae, and at all ages (Wagoner & Pendergrass 1939). In the infant, the anterior conical shadow is usually more obvious than the posterior, and results from the presence in this area of a large sinusoidal space within the vertebra (Wagoner & Pendergrass 1939). This anterior notch is not permanent, and disappears with ossification of the anterior and lateral walls of the vertebral body, usually in the first year of life.

Leventhal demonstrated that in the infant and young child the cervical vertebral bodies were simply a series of elastic cartilages and can be stretched up to 2 inches (5 cm) without disruption, while the less elastic cervical spinal cord tolerates only a quarter of an inch (6 mm) (Leventhal 1960). This elasticity probably accounts for the frequent occurrence in the young child of spinal cord damage without radiological evidence of bony injury, both in the

cervical and thoraco-lumbar spines (Melzak 1969, Glasauer & Cares 1972, Babcock 1975, Scher 1976, Banniza von Bazan & Paeslack 1977–78, Kewalramani & Tod 1980, Yngve et al 1988). Magnetic resonance imaging has been helpful in confirming the spinal cord lesion in children with traumatic paraplegia from stretching, blunt injury following dislocation and spontaneous reduction, or vascular compromise (Choi et al 1986, Yngve et al 1988).

By 8–10 years of age, the bony thoraco-lumbar spine has approached the biomechanical properties of the adult, and the fracture patterns are very similar, with the exception of the late development of progressive spinal deformity. Paralytic scoliosis occurs in essentially all children who sustain a complete spinal cord injury prior to the adolescent growth spurt age (less than 11 years in girls and 13 years in boys) (Mayfield et al 1981). Possible causes include injury to the growth plate of the vertebral body as well as resultant muscle imbalance, spasticity and the influence of gravity (Lancourt et al 1981, McPhee 1981, Mayfield et al 1981). As with the cervical spine, laminectomy in the thoracic region increases the likelihood of a progressive kyphotic deformity (36%) (Yasuoka et al 1982). Disc space narrowing and spontaneous interbody fusion following injury is uncommon in children, as the healthy intervertebral discs typically transmit the force to the vertebral bodies (McPhee 1981). Thus, there is a stronger case for initial conservative management of the spine in children than in adults, since the majority (two-thirds) have a stable spine.

INCIDENCE

Fractures of the spine in children are uncommon, with a reported incidence of 2–5% of all spinal injuries (Aufdermaur 1974, Babcock 1975, Hachen 1977–78, Kewalramani & Tod 1980, Hadley et al 1988). Most occur in the cervical spine; however, significant and disabling injuries do take place in the thoracic and lumbar regions. The mechanism of injury varies with the age of the patient. Neonates are more prone to cervical than to dorsal or lumbar spine injury (Leventhal 1960, Koch & Eng 1979). Occasionally, infant spinal injuries are due to child abuse and battering (Swischuk 1969). The young child in the first decade is more often involved in pedestrian/motor vehicle injuries, as a passenger in a car, or in falls from heights (Begg 1954, Glasauer & Cares 1972, Horal et al 1972, Hegenbarth & Ebel 1976, Scher 1976, Abel 1989). In the second decade spinal injuries are often (44%) the result of sports and recreational activities, such as tobogganing, cycling, motorcycling (Odom et al 1976; Banniza von Bazan & Paeslack 1977–78; Herkowitz & Samberg 1978; Shrosbree 1978) and motor vehicle accidents (37%) (Kewalramani & Tod 1980). It is believed that as many as 50% of children who have mild vertebral injuries are never admitted to the hospital, and thus the reported statistics are skewed towards the more severely injured (Anderson & Schutt 1980, Kewalramani & Tod 1980). One should be particularly

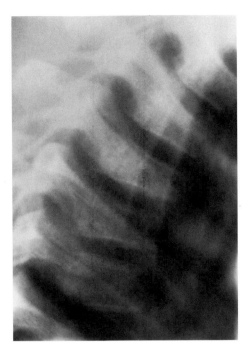

Figure 39.24 X-ray of a 5-year-old girl who sustained compression fractures of three vertebrae from a sledding accident. Note reversal of the normally convex endplate, beaking and wedging of the vertebral bodies. Overlapping of the spongiosum may appear as increased density. The child was asymptomatic within 6 weeks, and complete restitution of the vertebral height can be expected.

suspicious in the multiply injured child, as it is quite possible to overlook a significant vertebral fracture. Children are relatively more elastic than adults and the force is transmitted over many segments with multiple vertebral fractures the rule (Hubbard 1974, Hegenbarth & Ebel 1976, McPhee 1981, Hadley et al 1988) (Fig. 39.24). Similarly, innocuous appearing fractures of the lumbar or thoracic transverse processes are often associated with serious abdominal injury (20%) particularly to the spleen and liver (35%), the pelvis and urinary tract with haematuria (59%) or chest injury (Sturm & Perry 1984, Sclafani et al 1987).

MECHANISMS OF INJURY

The three-column system described by Denis (1983, 1984) permits vertebral injuries to be divided into four major types (Fig. 39.25):

1. Compression fracture: failure of the anterior column with an intact middle column.
2. Burst fracture: failure under compression (usually axial) of both the anterior and middle columns.
3. Seatbelt fracture: compression injury of the anterior column with distraction of the middle and posterior columns through either bony or ligamentous elements.
4. Fracture-dislocation: all three columns fail in compression with rotation and shear of the anterior

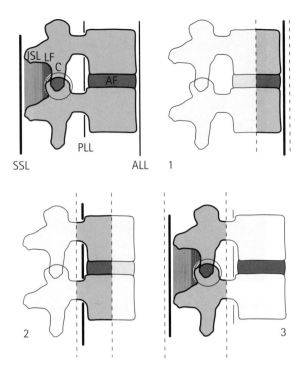

Figure 39.25 Illustration of the anterior middle and posterior columns after Denis (1983). Supraspinous ligament (SSL), the posterior longitudinal ligament (PLL) and anterior longitudinal ligament (ALL), and annulus fibrosus (AF). (1) The anterior column includes the anterior longitudinal ligament, the anterior portion of the annulus fibrosis and the anterior portion of the vertebral body. (2) The middle column is formed by the posterior longitudinal ligament, the posterior annulus fibrosis and posterior wall of the vertebral body. (3) The posterior column includes the posterior bony complex, the posterior arch and the posterior ligamentous complex (supraspinous ligament, infraspinous ligament [ISL], capsule [C]) and ligamentum flavum (LF). (Reproduced by permission from Denis 1983.)

column, distraction and shear of the middle column, and distraction with rotation and shear of the posterior column (Fig. 39.26).

COMPRESSION

Compression injuries due to hyperflexion are more common than distraction, shear or subluxation/dislocation injuries (Horal et al 1972, Ruckstuhl et al 1976). In the immature spine, the intact disc is more resistant to vertical compression than the vertebral body. Roaf experimentally loaded the vertebrae vertically with a slow increase in pressure and demonstrated that the major distortion was a bulge in the vertebral endplate, with only a slight change of the annulus, and no alteration in the shape of the nucleus pulposus (Roaf 1960). He observed that the bulging of the endplate caused the blood to be squeezed out of the cancellous bone, and this led him to suggest that the blood in the spongiosa was a major shock-absorbing mechanism. With further increase of

surgical stabilisation will prevent late deformity (McPhee 1981). In the older child, Lancourt has suggested extending the fusion to include the sacrum, as a guard against the late onset of scoliosis (Lancourt et al 1981). Early reduction of the deformity and surgical stabilisation will prevent the problems of progressive kyphosis or late neurological injury (Westerbarn & Olsson 1953, Jackson 1975).

Laminectomy is seldom helpful, particularly in the child without bony injury (Burke 1974, Jackson 1975, Flesch et al 1977, Mayfield et al 1981, McPhee 1981, Bradford & McBride 1987, Hadley et al 1988). The indications for immediate surgical decompression are the same as those in the adult: (i) an open wound, (ii) progressive neurological deficit in an incomplete injury, and (iii) reduction of an unstable fracture-dislocation (Campbell & Bonnett 1975; Hadley et al 1988). Removal of the posterior elements frequently accentuates the already unstable condition and may lead to progressive deformity (Yasuoka et al 1982). Laminectomy is not a significant factor leading to the development of scoliosis. However, many children develop significant kyphosis following the procedure, which is difficult to manage (Burke 1974, Flesch et al 1977, Herkowitz & Samberg 1978, Lancourt et al 1981, Yasuoka et al 1982). It would seem advisable, if a laminectomy is deemed necessary, that it be accompanied by a short segment fusion.

NEUROLOGICAL INJURY

The most devastating problem for the child with a thoracolumbar spine injury is paraplegia. The spinal cord-injured child can be expected to have all the problems found in the adult: increased susceptibility to long bone fractures, hip dislocation, pressure sores, joint contractures and genitourinary complications (Audic & Maury 1969, Campbell & Bonnett 1975, Banniza von Bazan & Paeslack 1977–1978). In addition, the child can be expected to develop progressive spinal deformity (scoliosis, kyphosis and lordosis) that will significantly complicate management (Burke 1974, Campbell & Bennett 1975, Bedbrook 1977–78, Mayfield et al 1981). For many, the original injury is often overshadowed by the severity of these late spinal deformities (Banniza von Bazan & Paeslack 1977–78). Scoliosis seriously erodes the child's ability to sit easily, and in the young child the pelvic obliquity leads to subluxation of the hip and ischial pressure sores (Kilfoyle et al 1965, Lancourt et al 1981). Kilfoyle et al noted in 1965 that "Surgical intervention is now considered an expression of conservatism". Inexplicably, this recommendation continues to be rediscovered with each subsequent article on the problem of progressive scoliosis in the immature paraplegic and quadriplegic.

In immature children, usually girls under 12 years of age, and boys less than 14 years, the incidence of progressive spine deformity following traumatic paraplegia is 86–100% (Fig. 39.34) (Audic & Maury 1969, Melzak 1969, Banniza von Bazan & Paeslack 1977–78, Lancourt et al 1981, Mayfield et al 1981). The onset of curvature has been reported as early as 3 years of age (Aufdermaur 1974). The fracture seldom determines the direction of the spinal curvature, rather the majority develop a long paralytic thoracolumbar curve believed to be due to the influence of gravity and uneven forces of spasticity (Kilfoyle et al 1965, Lancourt et al 1981). Similarly, on lateral X-rays the predominant

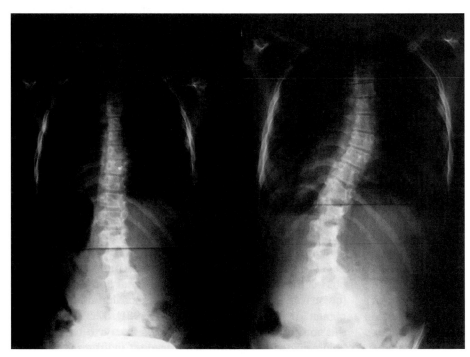

A   B

Figure 39.34 X-ray of a 9-year-old girl who sustained multiple trauma in a motor vehicle accident. There was no vertebral fracture identified but she had a complete transverse myelitis at T10, believed to be due to vascular injury. **A** Anteroposterior view at 11 years demonstrates a mild collapsing type curvature. **B** At 14 years the curve has increased to 50° despite vigorous management with an underarm orthosis and excellent compliance by the patient. Surgical stabilisation and correction of the spine are required to prevent further deformity. (Reproduced by permission from Rockwood C A, Wilkin K E, Beaty J H 1996 Fractures in Children, Volume 3, Fourth Edition. Lippincott-Raven, Philadelphia.)

finding (57%) is a reversal of the normal lumbar lordosis with the development of a long thoraco-lumbar kyphosis, with its apex at the dorsolumbar junction (Lancourt et al 1981, Mayfield et al 1981). Progressive lumbar lordosis is less common (18%) and usually associated with hip flexion contractures, particularly in the ambulatory patient (Kilfoyle et al 1965, McSweeney 1969, Mayfield et al 1981). Progression of the spinal curvature is directly related to the age of the child, spasticity and the level of the lesion (Lancourt et al 1981, Mayfield et al 1981). Children with more proximal injuries are more likely to have a progressive deformity than those injured at or below the level of the conus medullaris (McSweeney 1969, Campbell & Bonnett 1975, Banniza von Bazan & Paeslack 1977–78).

In adolescents, who are nearly skeletally mature at the time of injury, spinal deformity is more often due to a fracture-dislocation (Mayfield et al 1981). Progressive kyphosis and pain at the fracture site is common (42%), particularly in those who underwent laminectomy (Kilfoyle et al 1965, Burke 1974, Bedbroock 1977–78, Mayfield et al 1981).

If the kyphotic deformity is progressive, long-term neurological sequelae may develop with further loss of function from tenting of the spinal cord over the kyphus. Thus, early surgical stabilisation should be considered (Mayfield et al 1981).

Treatment of scoliosis should be initiated soon after the injury, prior to developing a severe curve. The Milwaukee brace has not been effective in controlling a collapsing paralytic curve; however, a total contact underarm plastic orthosis (TLSO) has been helpful (Campbell & Bennett 1975). Treatment recommendations are similar to those developed for idiopathic scoliosis. Curves under 40–45° may be controlled by bracing, or at least surgery can be delayed until the child is of optimum age (Koch & Eng 1979, Lancourt et al 1981, Bedbrook 1977–78). Once the curve exceeds 45–50 degrees, surgical stabilisation should proceed promptly (Campbell & Bonnett 1975, Bedbrook 1977–78, Mayfield et al 1981). In Mayfield's series, 68% required surgical correction (Mayfield et al 1981). It is helpful if the sacrum is not included in the fusion, as this significantly increases the incidence of pseudarthrosis.

POST-TRAUMATIC SYRINX

With the more frequent use of MRI, the relatively rare problem of post-traumatic syringomyelia is being discovered with greater frequency (Betz et al 1987). Symptoms can develop many years after injury (average 4.5 years), even as late as 17 years (William et al 1981, Lyons et al 1987). Pain is the initial symptom in over half followed by progressive neurological deterioration, sweating below the original lesion, loss of motor function and deep tendon reflexes are indications of a progressive syrinx (Williams et al 1981). MRI is excellent for identifying the lesion and Betz advocates an initial baseline MRI in these children to facilitate later detection (Betz et al 1987, Lyons et al 1987).

DIFFERENTIAL DIAGNOSIS

CHILD ABUSE

Vertebral injuries due to child abuse are less common than those of the extremities (Swischuk 1969, Aufdermaur 1974). The injuries are usually due to hyperflexion, and may be simple compression of the vertebral bodies, avulsion of the secondary centre of ossification of the spinous process, less frequently herniation of the nucleus pulposus into the vertebral body, and rarely a fracture-dislocation and kyphosis due to a severe disruption (Swischuk 1969, Kogutt et al 1974, Cullen 1975, Dickson & Leatherman 1978, Kleinman & Ziko 1984) (Fig. 39.35). A striking example is the report of subluxation of T12 on L1 with complete paraplegia from spanking (Renard et al 1978–79). There are no radiological vertebral changes specific for battering. Similarly, the classic epiphyseal and metaphyseal fractures of the long bones associated with battering are present in only 15% of all abused children (Kogutt et al 1974). Clinically, a high index of suspicion is more helpful than a specific radiographic finding. The children may exhibit other signs of neglect, such as poor nutrition and poor hygiene.

Carrion et al (1996) noted that certain dorsolumbar junction injuries in the young child may be from spanking, representing child abuse and is analogous to Salter–Harris type I fracture in the long bone. The fracture is usually through the vertebral body at T12 along the neural central synchondrosis across the inferior endplate and intervertebral disc, exiting anteriorly in the superior (or inferior) endplate of L11 (Carrion et al 1996).

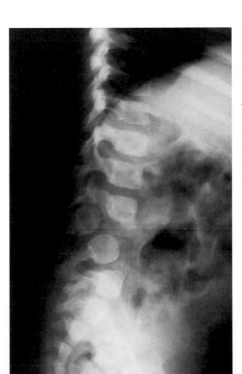

Figure 39.35 Fracture-dislocation of the dorsal lumbar junction (T12–L1), secondary to child abuse. This injury is believed to be secondary to spanking with resultant partial paraplegia.

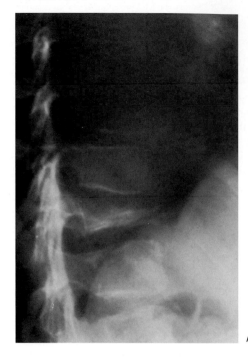

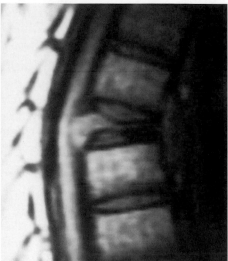

A

B

Figure 39.36 **A** An 8 year old with spontaneous onset of vertebral plana in the thoracic spine. The diagnosis was not confirmed by biopsy, as the clinical presentation was typical of vertebral eosinophilic granuloma. She was treated symptomatically in a TLSO with complete recovery and about 40% reconstitution. No further signs of histocytosis X were found. (Reproduced by permission from Rockwood C A, Wilkin K E, Beaty J H 1996 Fractures in Children, Volume 3, Fourth Edition. Lippincott-Raven, Philadelphia.) **B** A 7-year-old child demonstrating a herniation of the eosinophilic granuloma into the thoracic spinal column. The child presented with clonus and hyperreflexia. Anterior excision confirmed the eosinophilic granuloma. The lesion was bone grafted and healed without incident.

SYSTEMIC DISEASES

Spontaneous collapse of a single vertebra should alert one to the possibility of *eosinophilic granuloma* of the spine. Most of the children are between 2 and 6 years old (Maccartee et al 1972). Usually there is a complete collapse of the body (vertebra plane), and seldom does one see the lytic appearance that is typical of skeletal involvement in other areas (Fig. 39.36). The intervertebral disc is not affected and its thickness is retained. An adjacent soft-tissue mass is uncommon, and if present, suggests an infectious process such as tuberculosis. Several vertebral bodies may be involved, and as many as 11 have been reported (Nesbit et al 1969). The prognosis is excellent with some growth in height of the vertebral body and little residual deformity. However, complete restitution seldom occurs. We have seen Ewing's sarcoma present as vertebra plana, usually with a soft-tissue mass.

Multiple vertebral collapse is commonly seen in *Gaucher's disease* the *mucopolysaccharidoses*, *lymphoma*, (Fig. 39.37) and *neuroblastoma* (Amstutz & Carey 1966, Ribeiro et al 1988). The abnormal cells displace normal bone, the vertebra becomes structurally weak and collapses with minor trauma. Usually the children have visceral as well as skeletal involvement at other sites. A bone scan and survey should be obtained to identify other sites. Typical symptoms are persistent back pain localised to the region of the collapse. Neurological complications seldom occur.

In *Gaucher's disease* (Amstutz & Carey 1966) the bone-forming elements are replaced by an infiltrate of carosen-containing reticulum cells. This can usually be confirmed by aspiration of the marrow and finding the atypical cells (Amstutz & Carey 1966). One or more vertebrae may collapse, but a gibbus is rare (Fig. 39.38) (Amstutz & Carey 1966). Schmorl's node formation may occur.

The mucopolysaccharidoses, chondrodystrophies and lipidoses are similar to Gaucher's, with cellular storage of an abnormal metabolite and structural weakness. Vertebral changes are typically first noted at the dorsolumbar junction, with anterior herniation of the nucleus pulposus, and radiologically appears as a 'beaking' of the vertebral body (Fig. 39.39). Depending on the severity of the disease, the process may involve the entire spine (Begg 1954).

Compression fractures are common in *osteogenesis*

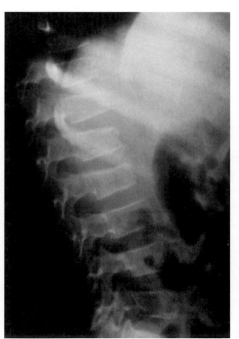

Figure 39.37 A 6 year old with acute leukaemia who presented with back pain and multiple compression fractures of the lumbar spine. This was a spontaneous onset with no history of trauma. This was initially believed to represent child abuse until leukaemia was diagnosed.

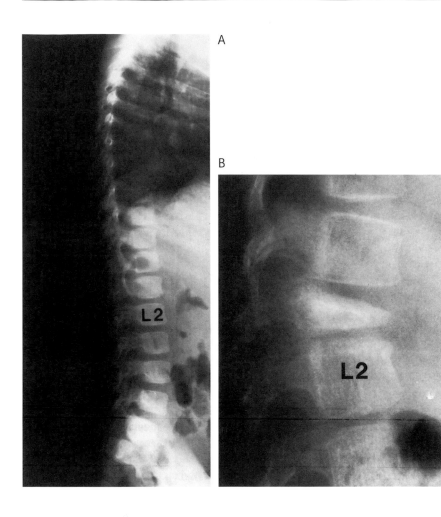

A

B

imperfecta (Fig. 39.40) and may develop serially, similar to the storage diseases. However, the children can be expected to have the typical stigmata, blue sclerae, fragility of the long bones and deformity of the extremities. Progressive spinal deformity, scoliosis and kyphosis, is common in the severely involved children. Certain conditions are associated with systemic osteoporosis and can lead to compression fractures with kyphosis such as cystic fibrosis or as a consequence of treatment, such as steroid-induced osteoporosis in children who have severe juvenile idiopathic arthritis (Ross et al 1987, Varonos et al 1987).

Compression fractures occur with *idiopathic juvenile osteoporosis*, an unusual acquired systemic condition characterised by profound osteoporosis in an otherwise normal prepubertal child, typically between age 8 and 15 years (Jones & Hensinger 1981). The condition may be confused with osteogenesis imperfecta, however it is of limited duration, usually 1–4 years, and is followed by near normal restoration of the skeleton. Osteoporosis is evident radiologically, and fractures occur with minimal trauma. There is no family history, and they do not have the blue sclerae, or poor teeth characteristic of osteogenesis imperfecta, nor do they have the wormian bone skull changes (Jones & Hensinger 1981). Initial complaints are usually related to the spine, and if the condition is recognised, early treatment with a spine brace will improve appearance, and reduce the degree of kyphosis and residual deformity (Jones & Hensinger 1981).

LUMBAR AND DORSOLUMBAR SCHEUERMANN'S DISEASE

Scheuermann's disease is a common cause of thoracic kyphosis. The condition is seldom painful, and typically children present with concerns related to the appearance of the deformity. The children are subsequently found to have the characteristic vertebral changes. Sorenson's radiographic criteria have been generally accepted to confirm the diagnosis, and include three or more adjacent vertebrae wedged greater than 50% (Sorensen 1964, Lippitt 1976, Tribus 1998). Endplate irregularity, Schmorl's node formation, and narrowing of the disc space are common accompaniments, but are not in themselves diagnostic (Bradford et al 1974). Lumbar or dorsolumbar osteochondritis is less common, but more often accompanied by pain (Greene et al 1985, Blumental et al 1987). Several authors, including Scheuermann, suggest that the lumbar vertebral changes are the result of trauma (Scheuermann 1921, Greene et al 1985, Blumental et al 1987). By contrast, the typical thoracic Scheuermann's disease is limited to the thoracic vertebrae, spontaneous in onset, and due to hereditary influences

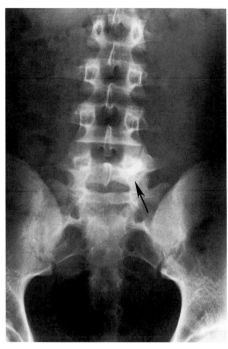

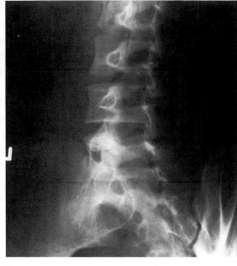

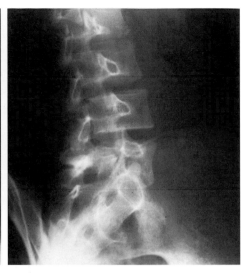

B   C

Figure 39.49 X-rays of a 15-year-old boy with low back pain. **A** Anterior and posterior and oblique views demonstrate reactive sclerosis and hypertrophy of one pedicle and lamina (arrow), and a contralateral spondylolysis of the same vertebral segment. **B** Oblique view demonstrating the reactive sclerosis. Radiologically this may be confused with an osteoid osteoma.

A

those in whom healing is still progressing and may benefit from immobilisation (Letts et al 1986, Van Den Oever et al 1987). The bone scan is not recommended in those whose symptoms are more than 1 year's duration or for those who do not have symptoms (Van Den Oever et al 1987). The bone scan is particularly helpful to those caring for the young athlete whose activities are highly associated with spondylolysis, such as gymnastics (Jackson et al 1976). Early detection of the stress reaction may lead to appropriate treatment measures and, as a consequence, shorten the recovery period. Similarly, the bone scan can be used to assess recovery and performed prior to the athlete returning to competitions (Jackson et al 1976). The bone scan is not indicated once the lesion has become established, unless one suspects bone tumour such as osteoid osteoma, infection or malignancy.

Treatment

Several authors have reported children and young adults who have been able to heal the spondylolytic defect with a cast or brace (TLSO) (Micheli 1979, Van Den Oever et al 1987). Typically, the children have an acute onset of symptoms and the episode of injury can be clearly documented. Unfortunately, not all heal with immobilisation. However, immobilisation should be considered if the injury can be documented to be of recent origin. A bone scan may be helpful to indicate a continuing process versus one of long duration (Letts et al 1986).

Although healing is unlikely, in children and teenagers in whom the spondylolysis is of long duration they can be

expected to respond clinically to simple conservative measures (Hensinger et al 1986). Restriction of vigorous activities and back and abdominal strengthening exercises are usually successful in controlling those with mild backache and hamstring tightness (Hensinger 1983). Patients with more severe or persistent complaints may require bed rest, immobilisation in a cast or brace, and non-narcotic analgesics. Hamstring tightness is an excellent clinical guide to the success or failure of the treatment programme. The majority of affected children can be expected to have excellent relief of symptoms or only minimal discomfort on long-term follow-up (Turner & Bianco 1971).

Any child or adolescent with symptoms due to spondylolysis, especially those under 10 years of age, should be followed closely for progression to spondylolisthesis (Hensinger 1983). We do not advise those with asymptomatic spondylolysis or those with minimal symptoms to restrict their activities; 7.2% of asymptomatic young men, age 18–30 years, have the pars defect, and relatively few have persistent symptoms. Thus, limitation of activity in a growing child would not seem justified (Micheli 1979, Hensinger 1983).

It must be emphasized that it is quite uncommon for spondylolysis to be symptomatic in adolescence, and one should be particularly wary of the child whose symptoms do not respond to bed rest or who has objective neurological findings. In this situation, myelographic and electromyographic evaluations should be considered.

A small percentage of young people with spondylolysis do not respond to conservative measures or are unwilling to curtail their activities, and may require surgical stabilisation. If surgery for spondylolysis is found necessary, a lateral column fusion from L5 to S1 and employing iliac bone is usually sufficient. In those who, in addition, have a spondylolisthesis of grade III or greater, the fusion is usually extended to L4 (Hensinger 1983). Nachemson (1976) reported solid healing of the defect using a bone graft coupled with an intertransverse process fusion. In those patients in whom the defect is small (6–7 mm) and the degree of spondylolisthesis is slight, a variety of techniques have been described to reduce the defect directly. These include widening of the transverse process or screw placement across the pars, coupled with bone graft (Buck 1970, Bradford & Iza 1985, Nicol & Scott 1986, Pedersen & Hagen 1988). These procedures are usually recommended for the older teenager and young adult less than 30 years of age with a minimal degree of displacement and degenerative change (Nicol & Scott 1986). The best candidates are those with defects between L1 and L4 or in situations of multiple levels of spondylosis (Buck 1970, Bradford & Iza 1985, Nicol & Scott 1986, Pedersen & Hagen 1988). This is an attractive alternative to the traditional transverse process fusion because it repairs the defect at one vertebral level rather than involving a second non-affected vertebrae (Bradford & 1985, Pedersen & Hagen 1988). In properly selected patients, 80–90% obtain a solid fusion with 80% good–excellent results (Bradford & Iza 1985, Pedersen & Hagen 1988). The Gill procedure or laminectomy is never indicated without an associated fusion in children (Sherman et al 1979). Removal of the posterior elements may in fact be harmful, leading to increased instability and spondylolisthesis in the postoperative period.

REFERENCES

Abel M S 1989 Transverse posterior element fractures associated with torsion. Skeletal Radiology 17: 556–560

Agran P, Dunkle D, Winn D 1987 Injuries to a sample of seatbelted children evaluated and treated in a hospital emergency room. Journal of Trauma 27: 58–64

Akbarnia B A 1999 Pediatric spine fractures. Orthopedic Clinics of North America 30: 521–535

Alexander C J 1977 Scheuermann's disease; a traumatic spondylodystrophy. Skeletal Radiology 1: 209–221

Amstutz H C, Carey, E J 1966 Skeletal manifestations and treatment of Gaucher's disease. Journal of Bone and Joint Surgery 48A: 670–701

Anderson J M, Schutt A H 1980 Spinal injury in children. A review of 156 cases seen from 1950 through 1978. Mayo Clinic Proceedings 55: 499–504

Audic B, Maury M 1969 Secondary vertebral deformities in childhood and adolescence. Paraplegia 7: 11–16

Aufdermaur M 1974 Spinal injuries in juveniles. Necropsy findings in twelve cases. Journal of Bone and Joint Surgery 56B: 513–519

Babcock J L 1975 Spinal injuries in children. Pediatric Clinics of North America 22: 487–500

Baker D R, McHollick W 1956 Spondyloschisis and spondylolisthesis in children. Journal of Bone and Joint Surgery 38A: 933–934

Banniza von Bazan U K, Paeslack V 1977–78 Scoliotic growth in children with acquired paraplegia. Paraplegia 15: 65–73

Bedbrook G M 1977–78 Correction of scoliosis due to paraplegia sustained in paediatric age-group. Paraplegia 15: 90–96

Begg A C 1954 Nuclear herniations of the intervertebral disc. Journal of Bone and Joint Surgery 36B: 180–193

Betz R R, Gelman A J, DeFilipp G J, Mesgarzadeh M, Clancy M, Steel H H 1987 Magnetic Resonance imaging (MRI) in the evaluation of spinal cord injured children and adolescents. Paraplegia 25: 92–99

Blasier R D, LaMont R L 1985 Chance fracture in a child: a case Report with nonoperative treatment. Journal of Pediatric Orthopaedics 5: 92–93

Blumental S L, Roach J, Herring J A 1987 Lumbar Scheuermann's: a clinical series and classification. Spine 12: 929–932

Boechat M I 1987 Spinal deformities and pseudofractures. American Journal of Roentgenology 148: 97–98

Bradford D S, Iza J 1985 Repair of the defect in spondylolysis or minimal degrees of spondylolisthesis by segmental wire fixation and bone grafting. Spine 10: 673–679

Bradford D S, McBride G G: 1987 Surgical management of thoracolumbar spine fractures with incomplete neurologic deficits. Clinical Orthopaedics and Related Research 218: 201–216

Bradford D S, Moe J H, Montalvo F J, Winter R B 1974 Scheuermann's kyphosis and roundback deformity. Journal of Bone and Joint Surgery 56A: 740–758

Bryant C E, Sullivan J A 1983 Management of thoracic and lumbar spine fractures with Harrington distraction rods supplemented with segmental wiring. Spine 8: 532–537

Buck J E 1970 Direct repair of the defect in spondylolisthesis. Journal of Bone and Joint Surgery 52B: 432–437

Bulos S 1973 Herniated intervertebral lumbar disc in the teenager. Journal of Bone and Joint Surgery 55B: 273–278

Burke D C 1971 Spinal cord trauma in children. Paraplegia 9: 1–14

Burke D C 1974 Traumatic spinal paralysis in children. Paraplegia 11: 268–276

Callahan D J, Pack L L, Bream R C, Hensinger R N 1986 Intervertebral disc impingement syndrome in a child; report of a case and suggested pathology. Spine 11: 402–404

Campbell J, Bonnett C 1975 Spinal cord injury in children. Clinical Orthopaedics and Related Research 112: 114–123

Carrion W V, Dormans J P, Drummond D S, Christofersen M R 1996 Circumferential growth plate fracture of the thoracolumbar spine from child abuse. Journal of Pediatric Orthopaedics 16: 210–214

Choi J U, Hoffman H J, Hendrick E B, Humphreys R P, Keith W S 1986 Traumatic infarction of the spinal cord in children. Journal of Neurosurgery 65: 608–610

Cullen J C 1975 Spinal lesions in battered babies. Journal of Bone and Joint Surgery 57B: 364–366

Denis F 1983 The three column spine and its significance in the classification of acute thoracolumbar spinal injuries. Spine 9: 817–831

Denis F 1984 Spinal instability as defined by the three column spine concept in acute spinal trauma. Clinical Orthopaedics and Related Research 189: 65–76

Dickson R A, Leatherman K D 1978 Spinal injuries in child abuse: case report. Journal of Trauma 18: 811–812

Dietemann J L, Runge M, Badoz A et al 1988 Radiology of posterior lumbar apophyseal disc fractures: report of 13 cases. Neuroradiology 30: 337–344

Fernandez L, Usabiaga J, Curto J M, Alonso A, Martin F 1989 Atypical multivertebral fracture due to hyperextension in an adolescent girl. Spine 14: 645–646

Flesch J R, Leider L L, Erickson D L, Chou S N, Bradford D S 1977 Harrington instrumentation and spine fusion for unstable fractures and fracture-dislocations of the thoracic and lumbar spine. Journal of Bone and Joint Surgery 59A: 143–153

Fredrickson B E, Baker D, McHolick W J, Yuan H A, Lubicky J P 1984 The natural history of spondylolysis and spondylolisthesis. Journal of Bone and Joint Surgery 66A: 699–707

Gellad F E, Levine A M, Joslyn J N, Edwards C C, Bosse M 1986 Pure thoracolumbar facet dislocation: clinical features and CT appearance. Radiology 161: 505–508

Gheiman B, Freiberger R H 1976 The lumbus vertebra: an anterior disc herniation demonstrated by discography. American Journal of Roentgenology 127: 854–855

Glasauer F E, Cares H L 1972 Traumatic Paraplegia in Infancy. Journal of the American Medical Association 219: 3841

Glasauer F E, Caves H C 1973 Biomechanical fractures of traumatic paraplegia in infancy. Journal of Trauma 13: 166–170

Greene T L, Hensinger R N, Hunter L Y 1985 Back pain and vertebral changes simulating Scheuermann's disease. Journal of Pediatric Orthopaedics 5: 1–7

Gumley G, Taylor T K F, Ryan M D 1982 Distraction fractures of the lumbar spine. Journal of Bone and Joint Surgery 64B: 520–525

Hachen H J 1977–78 Spinal cord injury in children and adolescents: diagnostic pitfalls and therapeutic considerations in the acute stage. Paraplegia 15: 5564

Hadley M N, Zabramski J M, Browner C M, Rekate H, Sonntag V H 1988 Pediatric spinal trauma: review of 122 cases of spinal cord and vertebral column injuries. Journal of Neurosurgery 68: 18–24

Hafner R H V 1952 Localized osteochondritis (Scheuermann's disease). Journal of Bone and Joint Surgery 34B: 38–40

Handel S F, Twiford F W, Reigel D H L, Kaufman H H 1979 Posterior lumbar apophyseal fractures. Radiology 130: 629–633

Hegenbarth R, Ebel K D 1976 Roentgen findings in fractures of the vertebral column in childhood. Examination of 35 patients and its results. Pediatric Radiology 5: 34–39

Hensinger R N 1983 Spondylolysis and spondylolisthesis in children. Inst. Course Lecture Series 32: 132–150

Hensinger R N, Lang J R, MacEwen G D 1976 Surgical management of spondylolisthesis in children and adolescents. Spine 1: 207–216

Herkowitz H N, Samberg C 1978 Vertebral column injuries associated with tobogganing. Journal of Trauma 18: 806–810

Hitchcock H H 1940 Spondylolisthesis. Observations on its development, progression, and genesis. Journal of Bone and Joint Surgery 22: 1–16

Horal J, Nachemson A, Schaller S 1972 Clinical and radiological long term follow-up of vertebral fractures in children. Acta Orthopaedica Scandinavica 43: 491–503

Hubbard D D 1974 Injuries of the spine in children and adolescents. Clinical Orthopaedics and Related Research 100: 56–65

Hubbard D D 1976 Fractures of the dorsal and lumbar spine. Orthopedic Clinics of North America Am, 7: 605–614

Jackson D W, Wiltse L L, Cirincione R J 1976 Spondylolysis in female gymnasts. Clinical Orthopaedics and Related Research 117: 68–73

Jackson R W 1975 Surgical stabilization of the spine. Paraplegia, 13: 71–74

Jayson M I V, Herbert C M, Barks J S 1973 Intervertebral discs: nuclear morphology and bursting pressures. Annals of the Rheumatic Diseases 32: 308–315

Johnson D, Falci S 1990 The diagnosis and treatment of pediatric lumbar spine Injuries caused by rear seat lap belts. Neurosurgery 26: 434–441

Jones E T, Hensinger R N 1981 Spinal deformity in idiopathic juvenile osteoporosis. Spine 6: 1–4

Keller R H: 1974 Traumatic displacement of the cartilaginous vertebral rim: a sign of interverterbral disc prolapse. Radiology 110: 21–24

Kewalramani L S, Tod J A 1980 Spinal cord trauma in children: neurologic patterns, radiologic features, and pathomechanics of injury. Spine 5: 11–18

Kilfoyle R M, Foley J J, Norton P L 1965 Spine and pelvic deformity in childhood and adolescent paraplegia. A study of 104 cases. Journal of Bone and Joint Surgery 47A: 659–682

Kleinman P K, Zito J L 1984 Avulsion of the spinous processes caused by infant abuse. Radiology 151: 389–391

Koch B M, Eng G M 1979 Neonatal spinal cord injury. Archives of Physical Medicine and Rehabilitation 60: 378–381

Kogutt M S, Swischuk L E, Fagan G J 1974 Patterns of injury and significance of uncommon fractures in the battered child syndrome. American Journal of Roentgenology Radium Therapy. Nuclear Medicine 121: 143–149

Kolowich P, Phillips W 1986 Seat belt lumbar fractures in children. Orthopaedic Transactions 10: 566

Lancourt J E, Dickson J H, Carter R E 1981 Paralytic spinal deformity following traumatic spinal-cord injury in children and adolescents. Journal of Bone and Joint Surgical 63A: 47–53

Letts M, Smallman T, Afanasiev R, Gouw G 1986 Fracture of the pars interarticularis in adolescent athletes: a clinical-biomechanical analysis. Journal of Pediatric Orthopaedics 6: 40–46

Leventhal H R 1960 Birth injuries of the spinal cord. Journal of Pediatrics 56: 447–453

Libson E, Bloom R A, Shapiro Y 1984 Scoliosis in young men with spondylolysis or spondylolisthesis. Spine 9: 445–447

Libson E, Bloom R A, Dinari G, Robin G C 1984 Oblique lumbar spine radiographs: importance in young patients. Radiology 151: 89–90

Lippitt A B 1976 Fracture of a vertebral body end plate and disk protrusion causing subarachnoid block in an adolescent. Clinical Orthopaedics and Related Research 116: 112–115

Lowrey J J 1973 Dislocated lumbar vertebral epiphysis in adolescent children. Report of three cases. Journal of Neurosurgery 38: 232–234

Lyons B M, Brown D J, Calvert J M, Woodward J M, Wdedt C H R 1987 The diagnosis and management of post traumatic syringomyelia. Paraplegia 25: 340–350

McArdle C B, Crofford M J, Mirfakhraee M, Amparo E G, Calhoun J S 1986 Surface coil MR of spinal trauma: preliminary experience. American Journal of Nuclear Radiology 7: 885–893

McCall I W, Park W M, O'Brien J P, Seal V 1985 Acute traumatic intraosseous disc herniation. Spine 10: 134–137

Maccartee C C Jr, Grifin P O, Byrd E B 1972 Ruptured calcified thoracic disc in a child. Journal of Bone and Joint Surgery 54A: 1272–1274

McPhee I B 1981 Spinal fractures and dislocations in children and adolescents. Spine 6: 533–537

McSweeney T 1969 Spinal deformity after spinal cord injury. Paraplegia 6: 212–221

Mayfield J K, Erkkila J C, Winter R B 1981 Spine deformity subsequent to acquired childhood spinal cord injury. Journal of Bone and Joint Surgery, 63A: 1401–1411

Melzak J 1969 Paraplegia among children. Lancet, ii: 45–48

Micheli L J 1979 Low back pain in the adolescent: differential diagnosis. American Journal of Sports Medicine 7: 362–364

Nachemson A 1976 Repair of the spondylolisthesis defect and intertransverse fusion for young patients. Clinical Orthopaedics and Related Research 117: 101–105

Nicol R O, Scott J H S 1986 Lytic spondylolysis: repair by wiring. Spine 11: 1027–1030

Nesbit M E, Kieffer S, D'Angio G J 1969 Reconstitution of vertebral height in histiocytosis X: a long-term follow-up. Journal of Bone and Joint Surgery 121: 1360–1368

Odom J A, Brown C W, Messner D G 1976 Tubing injuries. Journal of Bone and Joint Surgery 58A: 733

Ogilvie J W, Sherman J 1987 Spondylolysis in Scheuermann's disease. Spine 12: 251–253

Papanicolaou N, Wilkinson R H, Emans J B, Treves S, Mitchell L J 1985 Bone scintigraphy and radiography in young athletes with low back pain. American Journal of Roentgenology 145: 1039–1044

Peck F C 1957 A calcified thoracic intervertebral disk with herniation and spinal cord compression in a child. Journal of Neurosurgery 14: 105–109

Pedersen A K, Hagen R 1988 Spondylolysis and spondylolisthesis. Treatment by internal fixation and bone grafting the defect. Journal of Bone and Joint Surgery 70A: 1524

Povaz F 1969 Behandlungsergebnisse und Prognose von wirbelbruchen bei kindern. Chirurg 40: 30–33

Renard M, Tridon P, Kuhnast M, Renauld J M, Dolifus P 1978–79 Three unusual cases of spinal cord injury in childhood. Paraplegia 16: 130–134

Resnick D, Niwayama G 1978 Intravertebral disk herniations: cartilaginous (Schmorl's) nodes. Radiology 126: 57–65

Ribeiro R C, Pui C H, Schell M J 1988 Vertebral compression fracture as a presenting feature of acute lymphoblastic leukemia in children. Cancer 61: 589–592

Roaf R 1960 A study of the mechanics of spinal injuries. Journal of Bone and Joint Surgery 42B: 810–823

Ross J, Gamble J, Schultz A, Lewiston N 1987 Back pain and spinal deformity in cystic fibrosis. American Journal of Diseases of Children 141: 1313–1316

Rothman S L G 1986 Computed tomography of the spine in older children and teenagers. Clinics in Sports Medicine 2: 247–270

Rowe G G, Roche M B 1953 The etiology of separate neural arch. Journal of Bone and Joint Surgery 35A: 102–110

Ruckstuhl J, Morscher E, Jani L 1976 Behandlung und Prognose von Wirbelfrakturen im Kindes-und Jugendlichen. Chirurg 47: 458–467

Scheuermann H W 1921 The classic, kyphosis dorsalis juvenilis. Z Orthop Chir, 41: 305–317

Scher A T 1976 Trauma of the spinal cord in children. South African Medical Journal 50: 2023–2025

Sclafani S J A, Florence L O, Phillips T F et al 1987 Lumbar arterial injury: radiologic diagnosis and management. Radiology 165: 709–714

Sherman F C, Rosenthal R K, Hall J C 1979 Spine fusion for spondylolysis and spondylolisthesis in children. Spine 4: 59–67

Sherman F C, Wilkinson R H, Hall J E 1977 Reactive sclerosis of a pedicle and spondylolysis in the lumbar spine. Journal of Bone and Joint Surgery 59A: 49–54

Shrosbree R D 1978 Spinal cord injuries as a result of motorcycle accidents. Paraplegia 16: 102–112

Smith W S, Kaufer H 1969 Patterns and mechanisms of lumbar injuries associated with lap seat belts. Journal of Bone and Joint Surgery 51A: 239–254

Sorensen K H 1964 Scheuermann's juvenile kyphosis: clinical appearances. radiography, aetiology and prognosis. Copenhagen, Munksgaard

Sovio O M, Bell H M, Beauchamp R D, Tredwell S J 1985 Fracture of the lumbar vertebral apophysis. Journal of Pediatric Orthopaedics 5: 550–552

Sturm J T, Perry J F 1984 Injuries associated with fractures of the transverse processes of the thoracic and lumbar vertebrae. Journal of Trauma 24: 597–599

Swischuk L E 1969 Spine and spinal cord trauma in the battered child syndrome. Radiology 92: 733–738

Tarr R W, Drolshagen L F, Kerner T C et al 1987 MR Imaging of recent spinal trauma. Journal of Computer Assisted Tomography 11: 412–417

Taylor G A, Eggli K D 1988 Lap-belt injuries of the lumbar spine in children. A pitfall in CT diagnosis. American Journal of Roentgenology 150: 1355–1358

Techakapuch S 1981 Rupture of the lumbar cartilage plate into the spinal canal in an adolescent. A case report. Journal of Bone and Joint Surgery 63A: 481–482

Tribus C B 1998 Scheuermann's kyphosis in adolescents and adults: diagnosis and management. Journal of the American Academy of Orthopedic Surgery 6: 36–43

Turner R H, Bianco A J Jr 1971 Spondylolysis and spondylolisthesis in children and teenagers. Journal of Bone and Joint Surgery 53A: 1298–1306

Van Den Oever M, Merrick M V, Scoff J H S 1987 Bone scintigraphy in symptomatic spondylolysis. Journal of Bone and Joint Surgery 69B: 453–456

Varonos S, Ansell B M, Reeve J 1987 Vertebral collapse in juvenile chronic arthritis: its relationship with glucocorticoid therapy. Calcified Tissue International 41: 75–78

Wagoner G, Pendergrass E P 1939 The anterior and posterior 'notch' shadows seen in lateral roentgenograms of the vertebrae of infants: an anatomic explanation. American Journal of Roentgenology 42: 663–670

Wertzberger K L, Peterson H A 1980 Acquired spondylolysis and spondylolisthesis in the young child. Spine 5: 422–437

Westerborn A, Olsson O 1953 Mechanics, treatment and prognosis of fractures of the dorso-lumbar spine. Acta Chirurgica Scandinavica 102: 59–83

Williams B, Terry A F, Jones H W F, McSweeney T 1981 Syringomyelia as a sequel to traumatic paraplegia. Paraplegia 19: 67–80

Wiltse L L, Newman P H, MacNab I 1976 Classification of spondylolysis and spondylolisthesis. Clinical Orthopaedics and Related Research 117: 23–29

Wynne-Davies R, Scott J H S 1979 Inheritance and spondylolisthesis. A radiographic family survey. Journal of Bone and Joint Surgery 61B: 301–305

Yasuoka S, Peterson H A, MacCarty C S 1982 Incidence of spinal column deformity after multilevel laminectomy in children and adults. Journal of Neurosurgery 57: 441–445

Yngve D A, Harris W P, Herndon W A, Sullivan J A, Gross R H 1988 Spinal cord injury without osseous spine fracture. Journal of Pediatric Orthopaedics 8: 153–159

Section VI
Appendix

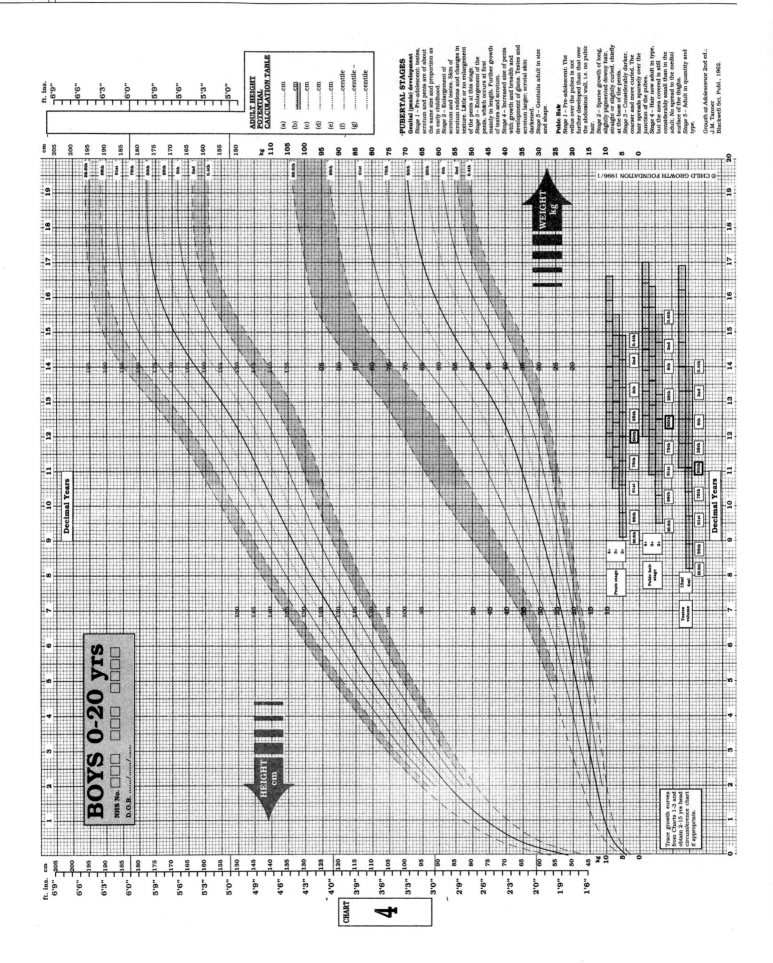

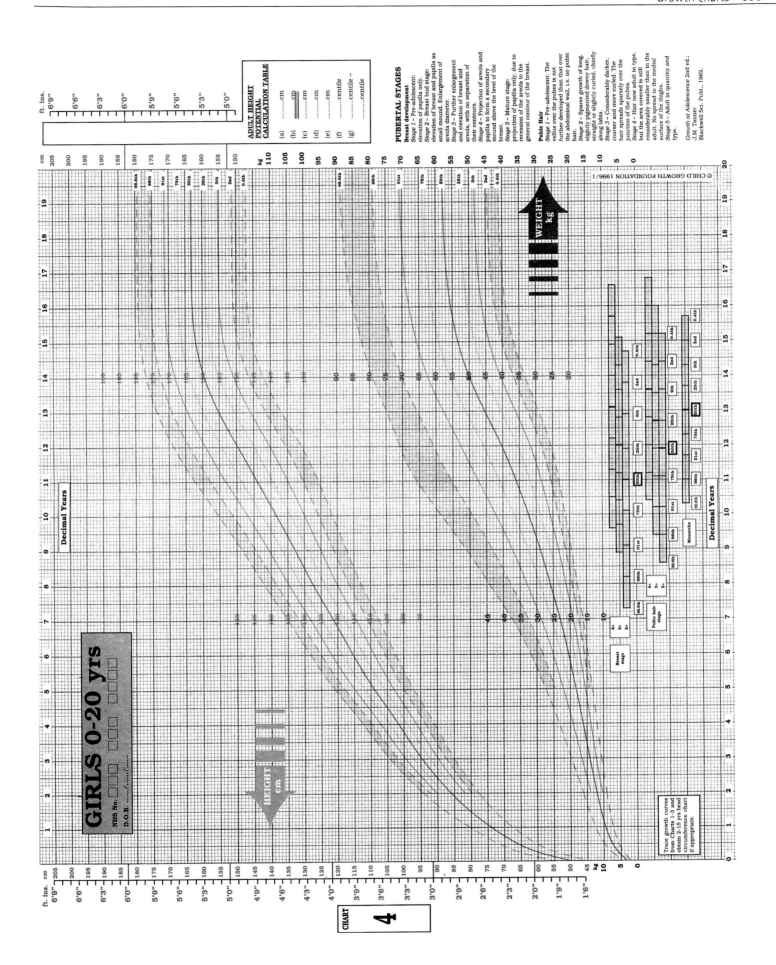

GIRLS 0-20 yrs

NHS No.
D.O.B. ....../....../......

CHART 4

ADULT HEIGHT POTENTIAL CALCULATION TABLE

(a)	.........cm
(b)	.........cm
(c)	.........cm
(d)	.........cm
(e)	.........cm
(f)	.........centile
(g)	.........centile – ....centile

PUBERTAL STAGES

Breast development
Stage 1 – Pre-adolescent: elevation of papilla only.
Stage 2 – Breast bud stage: elevation of breast and papilla as small mound. Enlargement of areola diameter.
Stage 3 – Further enlargement and elevation of breast and areola, with no separation of their contours.
Stage 4 – Projection of areola and papilla to form a secondary mound above the level of the breast.
Stage 5 – Mature stage: projection of papilla only, due to recession of the areola to the general contour of the breast.

Pubic Hair
Stage 1 – Pre-adolescent: The vellus over the pubes is not further developed than that over the abdominal wall, i.e. no pubic hair.
Stage 2 – Sparse growth of long, slightly pigmented downy hair, straight or slightly curled, chiefly along labia.
Stage 3 – Considerably darker, coarser and more curled. The hair spreads sparsely over the junction of the pubes.
Stage 4 – Hair now adult in type, but the area covered is still considerably smaller than in the adult. No spread to the medial surface of the thighs.
Stage 5 – Adult in quantity and type.

Growth at Adolescence 2nd ed.; J.M. Tanner. Blackwell Sci. Publ. 1962.

© CHILD GROWTH FOUNDATION 1996/1

Trace growth curves from Charts 1-3 and obtain 2-15 yrs head circumference chart if appropriate.

Decimal Years

Index

Note: page numbers in *italics* refer to figures or tables

abduction osteotomy 337, 395, 436
abortion, attempted 165
abscesses 119, 120, 150
  Brodie's 59
  cold 149, 155, 168
  detection of 59, 123–9
  in osteomyelitis 121, 137, 166
  in tuberculosis 149, 152, 155, 168
  paraspinal 155, 168
  retropharyngeal 499
  soft-tissue 127, 167
  subperiosteal 59, 166
acetabular deformity, salvage procedure
    378–9
acetabular dysplasia
  in Perthes' disease 393
  in spina bifida 254–5
  ultrasound in assessment 55, *56*
acetabular index, radiography in 365–6
acetabuloplasty, Pemberton's procedure
    254, *255*, 377–8
acetabulum
  fractures of 565, 633, 635
  imaging 363, *364*, 365–6
  in congenital short femur 337, 338
  intrauterine development 359–60
  surgical remodelling 376–8
Achilles tendon *see* tendo-Achilles
achondrogenesis 79
achondroplasia 67, 69, 73–6
  body proportions 68
  bow legs 413
  joint laxity 73, 76
  limb lengthening 76, 440
  neurological abnormalities 543
  radiographic features 74–5
  spinal deformities 74, 543–4
acid maltase deficiency 235
acidosis
  in sickle-cell disease 115–16
  tourniquet use and 42
acquired immunodeficiency syndrome
    (AIDS) 116–17, 231
acro-cephaly-syndactyly *see* Apert's
    syndrome
acromelic dysplasias 68
acromio-clavicular dislocation 610
acrosyndactyly 306, 312
actinomycosis, fungal infection 170
adamantinoma, bone tumour 211
Adams' 'forward bending test' 512–13

adenosine triphosphate (ATP) 13
adolescence
  back pain in 505, 508–9
  fractures, internal fixation of 561
  growth spurt 11
    spondylolysis in 684, 686
  knee meniscal lesions 421
  normal spinal curves in 515–18
  SCFE in 397
  see also sport; trauma
advanced paediatric life support
    (APLS/ATLS) 579, 580–1
Aerobacter spp. 141
age
  age-specific conditions, limp in 347,
    355–6
  assessment of 52
  fracture incidence 575
  gait and 348
  growth plate injuries 591, *592*, 594–5
  idiopathic scoliosis and 519–20
  osteomyelitis features 121
  Perthes' disease prognosis 387, 388
AIDS (acquired immunodeficiency
    syndrome) 116–17, 231
  see also HIV (human immunodeficiency
    virus)
air, in synovitis 422
airway, and polytrauma 579, 580
alar ligaments 659–60, 663
Albers-Schönberg disease (osteopetrosis)
    103–4, 547
Albright's syndrome *see* fibrous dysplasia
alkaline phosphatase 94, 96, 97, 102–3
allograft reconstruction, limb salvage 209
alopecia 100
α-fetoprotein concentration 246
'alphabet soup' histology 201
aluminium bone disease 100, 107
aluminium monostearate therapy 169
amethocaine, topical cutaneous anaesthesia
    44
amniocentesis
  club foot incidence and 464–5
  neural tube defects, diagnosis 246
amniotic band syndrome *see* constriction
    band syndrome
ampicillin 116, 123, 134
amputation
  in the tropics 175–6
  intrauterine 164–5, *166*

landmine injuries 174–5
lower limb anomalies 336, 341–3, 344,
    431–2
tumour surgery 197, 209
amyoplasia congenita *see* arthrogryposis
    multiplex congenita
anaesthesia 41–2
  fear of 8
  in juvenile idiopathic arthritis 178, 181,
    182, 188
  in myasthenia gravis 238
  MRI and 54, 218
  subarachnoid anaesthesia 46
analgesia
  central neuraxial blockade 45–6
  continuous infusion 47
  epidural 45–6
  infiltration analgesia 44
  muscle biopsy 227
  nerve blocks 44–6
  opioid drugs 43, 46–7, *48*
  patient-controlled 47
  postoperative 42–4
  topical cutaneous 44, 181
anencephaly *see* neural tube defects
aneurysmal bone cysts 193, *199*, *200*, *204*,
    206–7
  differential diagnosis 157, 199, 204, 206
  spinal tumours 170, 510–11
angiography 54, 194
angle of sagittal rotation 549
angular deformities 19–26, 87, 432, 595
ankle
  avulsion injuries 568
  ball and socket 452
  deformities
    after pathological fracture 571
    in cerebral palsy 286, 287–9
    in club foot 467
    in neuromuscular disorders 231, 269–70
    in poliomyelitis 268–70
    in spina bifida 252
  disorders, limp in 356
  flexion
    dorsiflexion 270, 275
    plantar flexion 16, 270
  fractures of 559, 568
  in epiphyseal dysplasias 78, 86
  in haemophilia 111–12
  instability 85–6, 89
  kinematics in gait 16, 277

explosives, injuries caused by 162, *163*, 174, 175-6
external oblique transfer 266
extra-articular subtalar arthrodesis 270
eyes
    blue sclerae 70, 103
    cataracts 102, 237
    chronic anterior uveitis 172
    corneal clouding 82
    cystine crystals in 99
    haemorrhages, in non-accidental injury 604
    iridocyclitis (chronic) 178
    lens subluxation 88
    myopia 88
    optic atrophy 220
    retinal detachment 79, 80, 88
    retinoblastoma 192
    vitreous humor disorders 79

facial deformity
    fibrous dysplasia 201
    torticollis 500, 502
facial injuries, explosives as cause *163*, 174
facies
    achondroplasia 73
    acrodysplasia 85
    Beal's syndrome 88
    congenital short femur and 337
    cretinism 102
    idiopathic hypercalcemia 105
    Klippel-Feil syndrome 496, 539
    Marfan's syndrome 88
    Menkes' syndrome 107
    myotonic dystrophy 237
    osteogenesis imperfecta 71
    spondyloepiphyseal dysplasia congenita 79
    Stickler syndrome 81
    thalassaemias 114
    see also cranio-facial anomalies
facio-scapulo-humeral muscular dystrophy 219, 234
factor VIII/IX, plasma coagulation factors 109, 112, 113, 114
faecal incontinence 38
Fairbanks' triangle 336
family stress
    disability in 29-30
    polytrauma in 580
Fanconi syndrome 99, 303
fascia iliaca compartment block 45
fasciculation, in neuromuscular disorders 216, 226
fat, interpositional material 436, 560, 591, 592, 596
feeding, in cerebral palsy 31-2
femoral condyle, osteochondritis dissicans 420-1
femoral epiphyses
    achondroplasia 74-5

dysplasias 78-9, 81
    fractures 565-6, 590
    slipped capital (SCFE) 57, 356, 403-6
femoral head
    blood supply 360
    intrauterine development 359-60
    ossific nucleus and 366, 368
femoral head deformities 391-2
    hip dislocation and 361, *362*, 363, *364*
        cerebral palsy 285
        surgery 376-8
    in Perthes' disease 383-6, 387, 389
    ischaemic necrosis 111
    ossification absent 80
    pistol grip 403, *405*
    salvage procedure 378-80
    'shepherd's crook' *71*, 91, 107
        with coxa vara 201, 336, *337*
femoral nerve block 45
femoral osteotomy
    femoral neck 403-6
    in hip dislocation 375-6
    in Ollier's disease 87-8
    in Perthes' disease *390*, 394, 395
    in pseudoachondroplasia 77-8
    intertrochanteric 80, 402, 405, 406
femur
    anteversion 275
    cysts 199-200
    fibrous dysplasia 91, *199*, 201
    fractures 565-6
        circulatory compromise 559
        femoral neck 565, 573, 635-40
        intra-articular 648
        neonatal 601-2
        overgrowth in 558
    lengthening *see* leg lengthening
    proximal focal deficiency (PFFD) 335, 336-9, 432
    shaft, fractures 640-5
    short 337-9, 467
        congenital 335, 337-8
    shortening 374, 375, 434-5
    torsion 21, 24-6
fetal ultrasonography 219-20, 246
fever, with limp 353, 354, 355, 356
fibre-type disproportion myopathy 236
fibrocartilage periferal structure, of growth plate 14
fibrodysplasia (myositis) ossificans progressiva 104-5, *106*, 462
fibronectin abnormality (Ehlers-Danlos syndrome type X) 90
fibrous cortical defect, bone dysplasia *199*, 200-1, 202
fibrous disorders 88-92
fibrous dysplasia 91
    benign latent lesion 193, *201*
    differential diagnosis 199, 203, 344, 352
    fractures 91, 561, 570, *571*
    heel pain 455

knee tumour 423
    polyostotic 107-8, 569
    see also skeletal dysplasias
fibula
    anomalies 74, 335, 337, 339-45
    fractures 351, 566
fibular hemimelia with equinus deformity 442, *443*, 444
'figure-of-8' bandage 609-10
finger-sucking deformities 314, *315*
fingers
    flexion deformities 297-8, 326
        clawed 167, 265, 290
        windblown hand 307
    fractures 564-5, 630, 631
    hyperaemia 237
    hypoplasia 303-4
    lumps 84-5, 86, 87
    short 78, 115
    tremor 216
    see also arachnodactyly; camptodactyly; clinodactyly; digits
fishing, injuries from explosives *163*, 174
'fishtail' humeral deformity 621
fixation
    bone fragment 421
    external 582, *583*, 609, 643-4
    halo 663
    internal 560-2
        biodegradable pins 560
        intramedullary 72-3, 609
        K-wire problems 622, 631
        nails, elastic intramedullary 643, 645
        pin 564, 566-7
        transepiphyseal/transphyseal 560
flat foot (pes planus) 17-18, 455-9, 488
    peroneal spastic *187*, 457-9
flexorplasty *see* Steindler flexorplasty
floppy infant syndrome *see* hypotonia
flucloxacillin 134, 142-3, 423
fluoroquinolone therapy 154
fluorosis 107
focal myotonia 416
'folded wing' arm position 224
folic acid 242, 245, 246
foot 6, 16-18, *466*, 467
    bone erosion 172-3
    calcaneo-valgus 452-3
    cavus deformity 483-7
    cleft foot 306, 462-3
    contractures 88, 231
    drop foot 167, 235, 281, 287
    flexibility 485
    fractures of 568-9, 654-6
    function, tethers in 468
    fungal bone infections 170
    Ilizarov frame for deformities 444-5
    in arthrogryphosis multiplex congenita *293*, 295
    in cerebral palsy 281, 283, 286, 287-9
    in juvenile idiopathic arthritis 17, 186-7

in poliomyelitis 268–70
in spina bifida 250–2
in spinal dysraphism 219–20, 245, 257–9
in tibial dysplasia 339, 340–3, 345
invertor insufficiency 269
limp in deformities of 350, 356
medial ray *466, 467*
medial release surgery 480, *482*, 486
osteopathia striata 104
sagitally breached 480
serpentine *450*, 451–2
shoes and 18
valgus deformity 250, 252, *253*, 457
varus deformity 250
Z-foot *450*, 451–2
see also club foot; equinus deformity;
    flat foot; heel; hindfoot; pes
foot-progression angle, in torsional profile 22
forearm
    contractures 264–5
    fractures
        circulatory compromise 559
        distal forearm 626–9
        K-wire fixation 627
        nerve entrapment 562
        proximal and middle forearm 624–6
        rotational deformity 626
    length discrepancy 313, *314*
    obstetrical palsy 326
    proximal forearm absence 301, 302
    pseudoarthrosis 314, *315*
foreign bodies, and knee pain 416, 422
'forward bending test' 505, 512–13
fracture-dislocation, thoraco-lumbar spine
    671, *672*, 676, 677
fractures 557–60, 575–7, 599
    ageing of 62, *63*, 605
    bending 651–2
    bilateral 603
    buckle 518–19, 557, 600, 656
        see also fractures, torus
    burst 671, 677
    Chance 675–6
    compound
        external fixation 559, 584
        in polytrauma 583–4
    compression 671–3, 676–7
    fatigue 547–8
    healing 600
    imaging in 53, 61–2
    internal fixation
        indications for 560–2
        lower limb 565–9
        upper limb 562–5
    Jefferson fracture 663
    limp and 351–2
    non-accidental 174, 352, 603, 604–5
    open fractures 559, 583
    pathological 561, 569–73
        in acute haematogenous osteomyelitis
            134

in congenital syphilis 170
in haemophilia 112
in juvenile idiopathic arthritis 187
in thalassaemias 114
motor neurone lesions 245
organ transfer patients 570
solitary bone cysts 199
patterns of 600, 603, 604
personality traits and 576
rotational malalignment 558, 626, 631, 652
spiral 612–13, 630, 642, 644–5
    non-accidental injury 352, 605
stress 352, 573
    femoral neck 635–6
technetium, isotope scanning, in fracture
    590–1
torus 604, 626, 627, 651, 652
    see also fractures, buckle
traditional bone-setters 162–4, 173
    see also greenstick fractures; stress
        fractures
Freeman-Sheldon (whistling face) syndrome
    294, 307, 469
Freiberg's disease (osteochondrosis of the
    head of the 2nd metatarsal) 356
frequency, definition 575
Friedreich's ataxia
    differential diagnosis 218, 219, 220
    spinal deformities 539, 540–1
frog position 296, *297*
frostbite 310, 590
Fukuyama congenital muscular dystrophy
    235
fungal infection 151, 157, 170

gadolinium-enhanced MRI 60, 127, 133, 218
Gage's sign, 'head at risk', in Perthes'
    disease 386
gait 15–16, 275–6
    analysis 248–9, 347–9
        in cerebral palsy 277, *278–9*
    antalgic (anti-pain) gait 348
    ataxia 217, 273
    in cerebral palsy 277, 280–1, 349
    in club foot, recurrent 479–80
    in dislocated hip 373
    in neuromuscular disorders 223–4, 349,
        541
    in-toed gait 21, 23, 25, 449–51
    leg length discrepancy 349
    short-leg gait 373
    tip-toe walking 16, 218, 232, 453
    Trendelenburg 349, 373
    waddling 79, 83, 103
    see also limp
Galeazzi fractures 563, 624
Gallie technique 495
Gardner's syndrome 192
gastric effects, of NSAIDs 48–9
Gaucher's disease 680, *681*
genes, skeletal dysplasias, web site 67

genetic counselling 69, 245–6
genetic factors
    in limb anomalies 301, 302, 335
    in neural tube defects 242
    in osteogenesis imperfecta 70
    in SCFE 397, 398
    in skeletal dysplasias 67
genitourinary system *see* renal system;
    urinary
gentamicin 123, 134, 142–3
gentamicin-impregnated PMMA beads *124,
    125*, 131, 132, 134, 137
genu, *see also* knee
genu recurvatum 267–8, 409–11, 442
genu valgum 20, *21*, 412
    'flat feet' and 17
    Marfan's syndrome and 89
    spina bifida and 253
genu varum 19–20, 412, 413
    achondroplasia and 73, 76
    familial 19, 20
    Ilizarov frame in correction of *443*
    metaphyseal chondrodysplasia and 83, *84*
    vitamin-D-deficiency rickets and 97, *98*
geographic bone destruction
    benign active lesion 194, *200, 204, 206*
    benign aggressive lesion 194, *203*
    benign latent lesion 194, *200, 207*
germinal or reserve zone, of growth plate
    13
giant cells 203–4, 206
giant-cell tumours
    benign aggressive lesion 193, *200, 204,
        206*
    calcified osteoid in *199*, 211
    differential diagnosis 201, 204, 206, 207,
        209
    spinal 511, 547
'giving way' ankle or knee 419, 420, 484
gliomas 545
global health initiatives 162
glucocorticoid therapy 103, 104
gluteal paralysis, treatment 266
gonad protection, during imaging 51
Gower's sign 6, *7*, 224
Graf's classification of hip dysplasia 363,
    364
graphic display, in spinal shape 513–15
grasp function, forearm anomalies 302–3
great-toe extension test 457
greater trochanteric osteotomy, for SCFE
    403, *406*
greenstick fractures 557, 600
    clavicle 601, 609, 610
    femur 641
    foot 656
    forearm 624–5, 626
    humerus 612, 613
    non-accidental injury 604
    tibia 651, 652
Grice subtalar arthrodesis 270, 457

groove of Ranvier 559
'ground glass' bone lesions 91, 105, *199*, 201
ground reaction force, in gait 277
growing pains 15
growth 11–15
  impact on deformities 467
  oncogenesis and 192
growth charts 694–5
growth disturbance
  acute haematogenous osteomyelitis and
    134
  arrest 590
  delay 78, 95, 100, 102
  juvenile idiopathic arthritis and 179, *180*
  Perthes' disease and 383, 384, 391
  tibial fractures 649, 651, 652–3
growth hormone 14, 93, 94
  physeal function and 587, 597
  SCFE and 397, 398, 403
growth plate 12–15, 587–8, 599
  realignment after fracture 557–8
  shear resistance 397, 559, 588
growth plate anomalies
  Blount's disease and 413
  epiphyseal dysplasias and 79, 83
  Perthes' disease and 384, 386
  tuberculosis and 150
growth plate arrest
  premature 627, 628
  reversal 436, 595
  surgical 20, 432–4, 533
growth plate injuries 427, 560, 580, 587–97
  femur 638
  fractures 71, 558–9
    classification of 588, *589*
    humerus 611–12
    lower limb 565–6, 567
    pelvis 635
  genu recurvatum and 410–11
  treatment 591–7
    complications 593–4
    Langenskiöld procedure 587, 592, *594*
    reduction 588, 590, 591
    salvage procedures 594–7
    splints 591
Gruca procedure 340, 432
Guillain-Barré polyneuritis 216, 262
Gustillo compound fracture 592, *594*

haemangiomas 86, 202–3, 521
  differential diagnosis 157, 177, 312
haemarthrosis 109–14
  traumatic 646, 647, 648, 649
haematogenous osteoarticular disease 119,
    121, 147
haematoma 61, 355, 582
  intracapsular, hip fracture 636
haemoglobin C disease (HbSC) 115
haemoglobinopathies 115–16
haemolytic (sickling) crisis 115
haemophilia 109–14

differential diagnosis 141, 605
  HIV infection and 117
  surgery and 113, 114, 117
haemophilia centres 114
haemophilic pseudotumours 172–3
Haemophilus influenzae
  osteomyelitis 123, 166
  septic arthritis 123, 141, 143
haemorrhage
  aneurysmal bone cyst 206–7
  chondroblastoma 203–4
  haemophilia 109–14
  juvenile idiopathic arthritis 181
  retropharyngeal 661
haemorrhagic cysts 57
Haglund's (Sever's) disease (calcaneal
    apophysitis) 352, 454
hair, steely 107
'hair-on-end' skull radiograph 114
hairline low
  Klippel-Feil syndrome 496, 539
  occipito-cervical fusion and 492
hairy patch, on lumbar spine 219, 242,
    257–9, 349, 521
hallux rigidus 461–2
hallux valgus 289, 460–1
hallux varus 461, *462*
hamstring tightness
  cerebral palsy 275, 281, 287, *288*, 290
  Scheuermann's disease type I 534
  spondylolisthesis 549
  spondylolysis 686, 688
hand 52
  bony erosion 172–3
  fractures
    epiphyseal 629
    fixation 564–5
  fungal bone infections 170
  juvenile idiopathic arthritis 182, 188
  obstetrical palsy 326
  osteopathia striata 104
  short 78, 102
  tuberculosis 148
  see also digits; fingers
hand deformities 313–15
  arthrogryphosis multiplex congenita
    297–8
  cleft hand 301, 303, 306
  endochondroma 202–3
  syndactyly 306–7
  ulnar dysplasia and 305–6
  windblown 307
  see also digits; fingers
hand injury 626–31
  explosives as cause *163*, 174, *175*
  workplace accidents *163*, 174
Hand-Schüller-Christian disease 208
handedness, development of 215
handicap, imparting bad news 9–10
handouts/booklets for parents 7, 9
Handy 1 robotic aid to eating 32

hangman's fracture 664, *665*
Harrington instrumentation 271, 524–6, 552
Hawkins classification, talar neck fractures
    654
head, in trauma 579, 580, 581
head lag
  car accidents 676
  hypotonia 225
head tilt 218, 499, 500
hearing impairment 70, 74, 81, 498
heel
  foot fractures and 655
  painful 453–5, *456*
  'pistol grip' deformity 251–2, 269, 487
  see also hindfoot
heel lift (shoe) 454, 458
helical computed tomography 53
hemiatlas anomalies 493
hemiplegia
  cerebral palsy 31, 215, 277, *280*
  limb growth velocity 216–17
  spastic 224
hemivertebrae 536
hepatic disease 112–13, 114, 570
hepatitis C transmission 112, 114
hereditary motor and sensory neuropathies
    (HMSN) 218, 220–1, 484–5
  see also Charcot-Marie-Tooth disease
hereditary multiple exostoses (diaphyseal
    aclasis) *14*, 84–6, 192, 313, *314*
hereditary sensorimotor neuropathy *see*
    hereditary motor and sensory
    neuropathies (HMSN)
heredopathia atactica polyneuritiformis
    (Refsum's disease) 220
Herring classification, in Perthes' disease
    388–9
hidden agenda, in consultation 5
hindfoot
  club foot 470–1, 474
  equinus 437–8, 488, 489, 490
  flexibility 484, *485*
  juvenile idiopathic arthritis 187
  see also heel
hip 359–60
  abductors 14, 21, 171, 254–5
  anomalies
    gait in 348, 349, 350
    limb length discrepancy 429, *430*
    spina bifida 253
  assymetry, in scoliosis 520, *521*
  ball and socket joint 385
  containable hip 392, 394–5
  contractures 231, 265–7
  developmental dysplasia *see* hip
    dislocation, congenital
  epiphyseal dysplasias 78, 81
  flail hips 253, 254, 267
  flexion deformities 110, 265–6
    cerebral palsy 274–5, 283, 285
    fixed 253, 296, *297*

pseudo 155
fracture 565, 635–40
haemophilia and 110, 111
infection, outcome 143–4
instability 452
irritable hip 56–7, 141, 390, 400
    see also synovitis
joint effusions, septic arthritis 56–7, 127, 167
juvenile idiopathic arthritis 179, 182, 183
overuse syndromes 352
pain 57, 79, *351*, 352–4
Perthes' disease 385, 392, *394*, 395
postnatal growth 360
roller bearing hip joint 385, 386
rotation 22, 25
rotational deformity 287
subluxation 361, *362*, 370–1, 384–5
    management 255, 376–7, 379–80
surgery
    cerebral palsy 285–6, 287
    joint replacement 185–6
    salvage 406
tuberculosis 148, *149*, 168
uncontainable hip 392, 395
see also coxa vara
hip capsule, normal 370, *371*
hip dislocation 361–6, 380–1
    assessment of 55–6, 363–6, 370
    associated anomalies 361, 362, 410, 452
    congenital
        arthrogryphosis multiplex congenita 296
        differential diagnosis 336, 391
        examination for 362–3
        familial 361
        fibrous disorders 88, 89, 90
        imaging in 55–6
        in the tropics 164
    irreducable, in infancy 370
    leg length discrepancy 368, 376–7
    limp in 355–6
    neuromuscular disorders 231, 253–5, *255*, 285–6
    paralytic poliomyelitis 266–7
    septic arthritis 126
    traumatic 640
    treatment
        childhood 374–8
        closed reduction 371–2
        infant 368–73
        neonatal 366–7
        open reduction 372–8
        osteotomy 375–8
        outcomes 380–1
        salvage procedures 378–80
        spica plaster 371, 373
        splints 55, 366–7, *368*
        toddler 373–4
hip dysplasia *see* hip dislocation
hip guidance orthosis (HGO) 37, *38*, 249

hip-knee-ankle-foot orthoses (HKAFO) 249
histiocytosis-X (Langerhan's cell histiocytosis LCH) 357, 507, *508*, 680
histology
    bone infection 129
    neuromuscular disorders *232, 233, 235, 236, 237, 238*
history taking
    in clinic 5
    neurological abnormality 215–16
HIV (human immunodeficiency virus) 116–17
    haemophilia and 113, 114, 117
    tuberculosis and 168
    see also AIDS (acquired immunodeficiency syndrome)
HMSN *see* hereditary motor and sensory neuropathies
Hoffa's syndrome 416
Holt-Oram syndrome 301, 303
homocystinuria 69, 88, 543
hormones, skeleton and 14, 93, *95*, 102, 403
Horner's sign 321, 322, 323
host defence mechanisms, joint infection and 119–20
host-tumour interaction 193
human immunodeficiency virus *see* HIV (human immunodeficiency virus)
humeral epiphyseal detachment, neonatal 619–20
humerus
    benign cystic conditions 571–2
    birth injury 601–2
    distal, injuries 616–21
    epiphyseal detachment 619–20
    fractures
        condyle 562, 619, 620–1
        epicondyle 621
        external fixation for 562
        internal fixation 562–3
        spiral, non-accidental 605
        supracondyle 616–19
    lateral rotation osteotomy, operation discredited 331–2
    proximal, injuries 611–13
    shaft, injuries 609–11
    solitary bone cysts, dysplasias of bone 199
    valgus deformity 621
Hunter's syndrome 83
Hurler's syndrome 82–3, *682*
hydrocephalus
    in achondroplasia 73, 74
    neural tube defects and 36, 219, 241, 256
hydrosyringomyelia 256
hypercalcaemia 101, 102–3, 105
hyperlordosis, in cerebral palsy 285
hyperparathyroidism 94, 101
    pathological fractures 570
    primary 94
    vascular calcification in 104
    vitamin-D-deficiency rickets 96, 97
hyperphosphataemia 99, 104

hyperplastic callus 211
hypertonus 217
hypertrophic interstitial neuropathy (Dejerine-Sottas disease) 220–1, 485
hypocalcaemia 97, *98*, 101
hypoparathyroidism 101–2, 104
hypophosphataemia 94, 98, 104, 105, 107
hypophosphatasia 94, 102–3, 569
hypothyroidism 102, 391, 397, 398
hypotonia 216, 225, *226*
    in cartilage disorders 73, 79, 81
    in congenital myotonic dystrophy 237
    in Marfan's syndrome 88
    neonatal 235, 532
hypoxia, in sickle-cell disease 115–16

ibuprofen, NSAID *48*, 49
idiopathic coxa vara *see* coxa vara
idiopathic hyperkyphosis *see* Scheuermann's disease
ifosfamide chemotherapy 211
iliac apophysitis 352
iliac osteotomy 379
iliac spines, fractures 633, *634*
ilio-psoas haematoma 111, 112
ilio-psoas transfer 266
Ilivarov, Gavril Abramovich, external fixation frame of 440–1
Ilizarov technique 440–1
    deformity management 250, *251*
        arthrogryphosis multiplex congenita 295, 296
        club foot 476, 483
        knee flexion deformity 411–12
    hinged frame 441, 442
    limb lengthening 340, 438, 440–5
imaging 51–63
    cervical spine injuries 661–2
    club foot 471–2
    femoral neck fractures 636
    femoral torsion 24–5
    fracture management 557–9
    growth plate injuries 590–1
    infection site 123–9
    inflammatory conditions 218
    juvenile idiopathic arthritis 181
    Klippel-Feil syndrome 497–8
    limp assessment 350
    osteochondritis dessicans 421
    osteomyelitis 135–6
    Perthes' disease 390–1
    septic arthritis 140
    stress films 471–2, 499, 502
    tarsal coalition 458
    thoraco-lumbar spine injuries 676–7, 679, 686–8
    torticollis 499, 500–1
    tumours 193–4, 204–6, 208
    see also computed tomography (CT); magnetic resonance imaging (MRI) ; radiographs; X-rays

immigrant or foreign families, in clinic 5, 7–8
immobilisation
  bone loss in 570
  upper limb injuries 609–10, 611–12, 613
immune deficiency states 116–17, 151, 154, 423
immunological factors 177, 178, 193, 398
immunomodulation therapy 154
in-toed gait 21, 23, 25, 449–51
incidence, definition 575
Indian Hedgehog protein 587
infantile coxa vara see coxa vara
infection
  aspiration and biopsy 129–30
  causative agents 122–3
  definition 119
  diagnosis, tests 129
  differention 197, 336, 414, 454, 571
  growth plate damage 427, 428, 590, 597
  imaging 61, 123–9
  inflammatory process 120
  multifocal 138
  post-operative 182
  treatment 129–32
  tropical 162
  see also bacterial infection; bone infection; joint infections
injections
  fibrosis caused by 171, 220
  intra-articular steroid therapy 164, 181, 182, 187, 422
innominate osteotomy 376–7, 378, 394–5
instability index 494–5
interpositional materials 436, 560, 591, 592, 596
interpositional physiolysis 587, 592, 594
intervertebral disc see disc
intra-articular fracture line 587, 589–90
intra-articular injection 164, 181, 182, 187, 422
intracranial injuries 62, 174, 218
intracranial pressure 492
intramedullary fixation see fixation
intraosseous access 42
intrauterine crowding 244, 293, 452, 464–5, 502, 530
intrauterine diagnosis 54, 69, 246
  see also ultrasound, fetal
invasiveness, definition 119
iridocyclitis, chronic 178
iron chelation therapy 115
irradiation, deformities caused by 398, 546, 590
irritable hip see hip, irritable
ischaemic necrosis see avascular necrosis
ischial tuberosity, fractures 633, 634
isoniazid therapy 152–3

joint infections 119–22
  antibiotic therapy 130–1

aspiration 349–50, 355
diagnostic tests 122–3, 129
differentiatial diagnosis 129, 245, 262
imaging 123–9
management 129–32
mechanism 121–2
see also osteomyelitis; septic arthritis; synovitis
joints
  contractures 314–15, 473
    management 442, 474–5
    soft-tissue-release 183–4
  granulomatous lesions in 151
  haemarthrosis 109–12
  laxity 361, 456
  normal fluid characteristics 122
  replacement 185–6
  rigid 293
  see also synovial; synovitis
juvenile chronic arthritis (Europe) see juvenile idiopathic arthritis
juvenile idiopathic arthritis 177–88, 354
  deformities, toes 186–7
  differentiation 141, 353, 355
  feet 17, 186–7, 459
  fractures 187–8
  imaging in 59–60
  in the tropics 172
  knee flexion deformity 411
  limb length discrepancy 182, 183, 188
  management 178–82
  manipulation under anaesthesia 180, 182
  motivation and rehabilitation 181
  osteoporosis in 179, 180, 181, 186, 681
  pain in 179, 180, 182, 185–6
  pauci-articular 177–8, 179, 182, 183
  physiotherapy 180, 181, 182, 183
  soft tissue problems 182
  spinal 188, 508, 509, 516
  stiffness and deformity 179–83
  surgery
    foot 186–7
    joint replacement 185–6
    osteoporosis, risks in 181, 186
    osteotomy 184–5
    soft-tissue release 183–4
    spine 188
    synovectomy 182, 183
  synovitis in 60, 179, 180, 422
  systemic illness 177–8
juvenile rheumatoid arthritis (USA) see juvenile idiopathic arthritis
juxta-articular osteotomy 154

kanamycin therapy 153
Kirner deformity 302, 310
Klebsiella 162, 166–7
Klein's sign, in SCFE 399
Klippel-Feil syndrome 492–3, 495–9, 539
knee 409–25
  angular deformities 18–26, 86

contractures 88, 231, 267–8, 287
deformities 409–12
  arthrogryphosis multiplex congenita 293, 295–6
  cerebral palsy 275, 280, 283, 287
  extension 287, 295–6
  flexion 110, 111, 411–12, 418
  poliomyelitis 267–8
  spina bifida 252–3
flail knee 253, 268
fractures 424, 424, 425, 646–53
  intercondylar eminence 567, 568
hyperextension 280, 567
infrapatellar fat pad, enlarged 416
intra-articular steroids 182
joint laxity 76, 77
joint replacement 186
knock knee and bow leg 412–14
leg length discrepancy and 429, 430, 442
ligament problems 423–4
limp 352, 356
meniscal lesions 418, 421–2
osteochondritis dissecans 350, 420–1
pain 398–9, 407, 414–17
  psychosomatic 424
popliteal cysts 423
reduction anomalies and 337, 340
septic arthritis 167, 423
snapping 410
stiffness
  after femoral lengthening 438, 439
  post-injection muscle fibrosis 171
surgery
  cerebral palsy 286
  contractures 267–8
  juvenile idiopathic arthritis 182–5, 186
synovial pathology 415, 422–3
tuberculosis in 149, 168
tumours 209–10, 416, 423
see also genu
Kniest dysplasia 79
knock knees see genu valgum
Köhler's disease (osteochondritis of the navicular) 356, 453–4
Kugelberg-Welander spinal muscular atrophy 232
Küntscher's intramedullary femoral shortening 434–5
kyphoscoliosis 71, 73, 79, 80, 83
kyphosis
  adolescent (traumatic) 506–7
  cerebral palsy 285
  cervical spine 665, 666
  congenital 535, 538
  iatrogenic 507, 516, 545–6
  painful 155, 508–9
  postural 73, 75–6
  progressive, infection 544–5
  spina bifida 256
  spinal tuberculosis 160
  surgery 527

see also Scheuermann's disease; thoracic
 kyphosis

labrum, hip 374, 376, 378
lachrymocutaneous reflex 6
Lacroix, perichondrial bone bark ring 14,
 397, 559, 599
laminectomy 516, 543, *544*, 678, 679
laminoplasty 507
landmine injuries 174–5
Langenskiöld procedure 436, 587, 592, *594*
Langerhans' cell histiocytosis LCH
 (histiocytosis-X) 357, 507, *508*, 680
Langerhans' giant cells 149
Larsen's syndrome 409, *410*, 452, 539
laryngeal mask airway 41
lateral shelf acetabuloplasty 395
lead poisoning 107
Leatherman two-stage wedge resection 530,
 542
leg
 bowed *see* genu varum
 examination 6
 growth calculations 14–15
leg length discrepancy 427–45
 after femoral neck osteotomy for SCFE 404
 assessment 349, 428–31
 gait 349
 prediction 430–1
leg lengthening 435–6
 bone division 436–8
 deformity and 442–5
 distraction apparatus 441–2
 soft tissues in 438–40
leg shortening 432–5
Legg-Calvé-Perthes' disease *see* Perthes'
 disease
leprosy 168–9
Leri-Weill disease (dyschondrosteosis) 85, 313
Letterer-Siwe disease 208
leukaemia 211, 356–7, 680
 differential diagnosis 100–1, 129, 166, 606
levamisol therapy 154
ligaments
 calcification of 105, 107
 cervical spine 665, *666*
 discoid meniscus attachments 422
 laxity 216, 493–4, 543, 646, 649
  see also fibrous disorders
 thoraco-lumbar spine *671*, 677, 678
 see also individual ligaments
ligamentum teres 361, *362*
limb
 development 301
 exsanguination, acidosis risk 42
 growth velocity and length 11–15
 intrauterine amputation 164–5, *166*
 malalignment correction 69
 reduction defects 54, 301–15
 salvage surgery 191, 197, 209–10
limb length discrepancy 12, 428, 429

equalisation 432–6
limb lengthening
 acute pain in 440
 bifocal 438, 442, *443*
 Ilizarov technique 440–5
 imaging in 57
 physiology of 435–6
 principles of 436–40
limb shortening 432–5, 584, 585
limb-girdle muscular dystrophies 234–5, 540
limbus, in hip dislocation 361, *362*, 373
limp
 age-related conditions 355–6
 causes of 351–7
 diagnostic investigations 349–51
 gait analysis 347–9
 history in 347
 infection and 348, 354–5
 inflammation in *351*, 352–4
 physical examination 349
'lobster claw hand', discontinued term *see*
 hand deformities, cleft
local anaesthesia *see* anaesthesia; analgesia
Lodwick system, bone tumour growth rate
 193–4
Looser's zones 97
lordoscoliosis
 collapsing 519, 544
 early-onset 533
 tumours and 545, 546
lordosis 11, 512
lower limb blocks, analgesia 45
lower limbs
 contractures 265–71
 fractures 565–9
 reduction anomalies 335–45
lower motor neurone disease 226, *226*
lumbar spine *see* thoraco-lumbar spine
lumbo-sacral agenesis 539
lumbo-sacral kyphosis, in spondylolisthesis
 549, *550*, 552
lumbosacral lipoma 257
'Luque trolley', instrumentation 39, 533
Lyme disease 355
lymph node enlargement, in tuberculosis
 148, 150
lytic spondylolisthesis 547–8

macrodactyly 302, 312
Madelung's deformity 85, 302, 313, 597
maduramycosis, fungal infection of bone 170
Maffucci's syndrome 86, 88, 202–3
magnesium deficiency 102
magnetic resonance imaging (MRI) 53–4
 bone bridges 590, *591*
 gadolinium-enhanced 60, 127, 133, 218
 neurological disorders 218
 non-accidental injury 62
 osteomyelitis 59, *60*, 127–9, 136
 Perthes' disease 392, *393*
 scoliosis evaluation 58–9

spinal dysraphism 258, *259*
spinal tuberculosis 155–6
STIR sequences 127, 133
tumour evaluation 61, 194, *198*
malabsorption, rickets in 98
Malgaigne fractures 634, *635*
malignant hyperthermia 236, 237
malignant tumours 192–3
 bone 193, *198*
 criteria of 194, *198*
 decision-making in management 195, *196*
 in the tropics 162
 nature of 191
 pathological fracture and 109, 572
 types of 208–11
 see also Ewing's sarcoma; osteosarcoma
mallet fracture, phalangeal 564, *565*, 631
Mallet's system, shoulder function
 assessment 329–30, *333*
Malmo splint, for hip dysplasia 367
malnutrition 107, 154, 570, 606
mandibular osteomyelitis 104
Mantoux test, for tuberculosis 151
marble bone disease (osteopetrosis) 99,
 103–4, 569, *570*
Marfan's syndrome 67, 69, 88–9
 patellar instability 417
 spinal deformities 88, 89, 519, 543
Mayo's excision of the first metatarsal head
 187
McBride's metatarsal osteotomy 460
McCune-Albright syndrome 91, 107
McGregor's/McRae's lines, in basilar
 impression 491
mechanical stress
 patellar dislocation 417, 418
 SCFE 397, 403
medial adductor surgical approach 372
medial release, in foot surgery 480, *482*,
 486
medullary blood supply, in bone division
 436–7
medullary cavity, widening in
 thalassaemias 114
meningocele
 atrophic meningocele 258
 spina bifida cystica 242, *243*
meningocele manqué, spinal dysraphism
 257
meningomyelocele 218, 219, 465
meniscal lesions, knee 418, 421–2
Menkes' syndrome 107
mental impairment
 hypoparathyroidism and 102
 hypotonia and 216, 225
 idiopathic hypercalcemia 105
 mucopolysaccharidoses 82
 neuromuscular disorders 235, 237
mercury poisoning 107
merosin, in congenital muscular dystrophy
 235

mesomelic dysplasias 68
metabolic bone disease 93–5
metacarpals 102, 564, 629, 630
metacarpo-phalangeal dislocation/fracture 564, 631
Metaizeau technique 622, *623*
metaphyseal dysostosis 336, *337*
metaphyseal dysplasia 68
metaphyseal fractures 425, 600, 604
    non-accidental injury 352, 603, 604
metaphyseal lucency (leukaemic lines) 356
metaphyseal spiky protrusions 107
metaphyseal torus 600
metaphysis 13–14
metaplasia, definition 191
metastases, from bone tumours 54, 193, 547
metatarsal fractures 568–9, 655–6
metatarsal osteotomy 460–1, 485
metatarso-pharyngeal joint 461
metatarsus adductus, in in-toe gait 449–50
metatarsus primus elevatus 461–2
metatarsus primus varus 460
metatarsus varus 449–50, 461
methyl methacrylate, interpositional material 560, 596
midfoot inversion, procedure 289
Milwaukee brace, for scoliosis 523
mineralisation 93–5
    ectopic 104–5, *106*
        failure in aluminium excess 107
        growth plates and 587
minerals, and bone anomalies 105–7
minicore myopathy 236
mirror motions (synkinesia) 498
mitochondrial myopathy 236, *237*
mobility *see* orthoses; physiotherapists; wheelchairs
monodactylous symbrachydactyly 303
monostotic lesions 571–3
Monteggia fractures 563, 621, 622, 623–4
Morquio's syndrome 499, 543, 544
mortality
    acute haematogenous osteomyelitis 134
    osteoarticular tuberculosis 150, 151
Moseley's straight line graph 431
Mose's rings 366
moth-eaten bone
    congenital syphilis 170
    tumour 194, *210*, *211*
motor development delayed 73–4, 79, 485
motor function, assessment 505
motor neurone lesions 243–4
motor-impaired children, education programme for 36
motorcycle, road traffic accidents, in the tropics 174
moulded baby syndrome *see* intrauterine crowding
mouth, non-accidental injury 604
mucopolysaccharidoses 82–3
    biochemical diagnosis in 68

intrauterine diagnosis 69
    radiology in diagnostic imaging 218
    spinal deformities in 543, 680
multidisciplinary training, for the disabled child 30
multidrug-resistant tuberculosis 154
multiple epiphyseal dysplasia 78–9, 313, 391
muscle biopsy
    neuromuscular disorders 234, 238
    technique 219, 227
muscle contraction, in gait 276–7, 348
muscle disorders
    diagnostic criteria *228–9*, *230*
    see also dystrophic disorders; muscular dystrophies
muscle fibre type, in club foot 465, 467
muscle imbalance, and deformity 242–4, 261, 409, 466–7
muscle myopathies 235–6
muscle spasm
    atlanto-axial rotary displacement 500
    poliomyelitis 261, 262
    spinal tuberculosis 155
    spondylolisthetic crisis 549, *551*
muscle tension, and bone shape 14, 21, 23
muscles
    atrophy 226
    fasciculations 226
    fatigue (growing pains) 15
    haematomas 109, 112
    hypertrophy 226
    post-injection fibrosis 171, 220
    testing 224–6
    wasting 150, 216–17
    weakness *230*, 234, 279, 348
    see also myositis ossificans
muscular atrophy
    peroneal 453, 484
        see also Charcot-Marie-Tooth disease
muscular dystrophies 232–5
    creatine phosphokinase levels in 226
    differential diagnosis 232, 540
    facio-scapulo-humeral dystrophy 219, 234
    gait *223*, 349, 453
    Gower's sign 6, *7*, 224
    muscle testing 224–6
    risk in anaesthetic 42
    scapulo-humeral *224*, 234
    spinal deformities 539
    see also Duchenne muscular dystrophy; Emery-Dreyfuss muscular dystrophy; Fukuyama congenital muscular dystrophy
muscular torticollis *see* torticollis
musculoskeletal inherited disorders 67–9
musculoskeletal injuries 580
musculoskeletal tumours 170–1, 194–5
Mustard procedure 266
myasthenia, definition 238

myasthenia gravis 226, *228–9*, *230*, 238
mycobacteria 122–3, 150
Mycobacterium bovis 123
Mycobacterium leprae 167
Mycobacterium tuberculosis 123
mycotic infection 151, 157, 170
myelocele, spina bifida cystica 242, *243*
myelodysplasia 258, 516
    see also neurological disorders
myelography
    brachial plexus injuries 322, 323
    scoliosis 59
    tuberculous paraplegia 158–9
    with computed tomography 218, 258, 323
myelomeningocele
    associated abnormalities 241–2
    spina bifida cystica 242, *243*
    ultrasound detection *54*, 55
    see also neural tube defects; spina bifida
myeloschisis, spina bifida cystica 242, *243*
myoblast implantation, in Duchenne muscular dystrophy 233
myopathies 227, *228–9*, *230*
    cardiac function in 219
    central core 216, 235–6
    contractures in 217, 231
    fibre-type disproportion 236
    hypotonia in 225
    nemaline 236
    posture in *224*
    proximal, in vitamin-D-deficiency rickets 97
    scoliosis in 235, 236
    surgical risks 541
    see also muscular dystrophies
myositis ossificans *199*, 211
    progressiva (fibrodysplasia) 104–5, *106*
myotonia, definition 236
myotonias *228–9*, 236–7
    'dive-bomber' noise on electromyography 226, *227*, 237
    myotonia atrophica *see* myotonic dystrophy
    myotonia congenita 226, 237
myotonic dystrophy (myotonia dystrophica) 237
myotonic muscular dystrophy *see* myotonic dystrophy
myotubular myopathy 236

naevus, cutaneous lesion 257–9, 521
nail-bed deformity, in polydactyly 312
nail-patella syndrome (onycho-osteodystrophy) 417, 462
navicular bone 356, 453–4, 488
neck
    limited motion 234, 496
    mass, on sternocleidomastoid muscle 502
    mobility 658–60
    short (brevicollis) 319, 492, 496, 539
    trauma 494, 579, 581–2

see also torticollis
necrosis in bone 149, 629
necrotising fasciitis 167–8
Neisseria meningitidis 123, 141
neonatal bone flexibility 599–600
neonatal feet, postural calcaneo-valgus 452
neonatal hip dislocation, screening 362–5
neonatal hip infection, outcome *143*, 144
neonatal HIV infection 116
neonatal hypoparathyroidism 101–2
neonatal injury
  differential diagnosis 603
  see also birth injuries; brachial plexus
    injuries
neonatal jaundice, tip-toe walking and 453
neonatal necrotising fasciitis 167–8
neonatal septic arthritis *128*, 139–40,
  166–7
neonatal spinal infection 507
neoplasms
  pathological fracture and 572
  see also bone tumours; malignant
    tumours; spinal neoplasms; tumours
nephroblastoma 511, 572
nephrocalcinosis 103, 105
nerve biopsy 219
nerve fibre disorders *228–9*, *230*
nerve grafting 323, 325
nerve root compression 550–2
nerve territory orientated macrodactyly 312
neural arch defects 256
neural involvement
  leprosy 167
  poliomyelitis 261
neural tube, *see also* spinal cord
neural tube defects 219–20, 241
  antenatal diagnosis 54
  maternal factors 242
  see also myelomeningocele; spina bifida;
    spinal dysraphism
neuroblastoma 511, 545, 546, 680
  in the tropics 170
  metastases 572
neurofibromatosis
  congenital pseudoarthrosis and 314, *315*,
    344
  diagnostic imaging 218
  dystrophic bone change 541–2
  heel pain 455
  leg length discrepancy in 427, 428
  macrodactyly and 302, 312
  spinal deformities 516, 519
neurofibromatosis type NF-1 (Von
  Recklinghausen's disease) 541–2
neurological assessment, in polytrauma
  581, 582, 583
neurological damage
  cervical spine injuries 661
  forearm fracture 562, 613, 617, 618, 626,
    627
  growth plate injury 593–4

limb lengthening 440
Monteggia fractures 624
thoraco-lumbar spine injuries 674, 676,
  678–9
neurological disorders
  investigation 218–21
  leg length discrepancy in 427–8
  management 227–31
  orthopaedic surgery 230–1
  pes cavus and 484
  physiotherapy 227–30
  scoliosis in 218, 230–1
  torticollis and 499
  see also myelodysplasia; sacral agenesis;
    spina bifida; spinal dysraphism;
    spinal muscular atrophy
neurology, overview 215–21
neuroma, knee pain and 416
neuromuscular disorders 223–6, 227, *228–9*
  electromyography 226–7
  muscle biopsy 227
  surgery and 42, 230–1
  tip-toe walking 453
neuromuscular spinal deformities 516,
  539–41
neuropraxias 615, 618
neurotisation, in brachial plexus injuries
  324, 325
neurovascular injuries
  clavicular fracture and 562, 610
  elbow injuries and 614, 615
night pain *see* pain, night
Nocardia madurae, maduramycosis 170
nodules, tumour formation 193
non-accidental injuries 62–3, 603–6
  cutaneous injuries 604
  differential diagnosis 72, 105, 109, 170,
    602, 612–13
  fractures
    femur 640–1, 642
    patterns 603, 604–5
  imaging 62–3
  in the tropics 162, 174
  limp and 352
  neonatal humeral epiphyseal detachment
    619–20
  polytrauma 579
  risk factors 603–4
  shaking 663
  spanking 679
  spinal 506, 664, 679
non-Hodgkin lymphomas 117
non-ossifying fibroma 100, *199*, 200–1, 203
'Notta's node' 310
NSAIDs (non-steroidal analgesic drugs) 43,
  48–9, 204, 205
nuclear imaging 54, 135–6, 350
nurse-controlled analgesia 47
nursemaid's elbow 615
nutritional rickets *see* vitamin-D-deficiency
  rickets

obesity
  genu valgum and 17, 20
  muscle wasting and 216
oblique metatarsal osteotomy 460–1
observation hip *see* synovitis, transient
obstetrical brachial plexus injuries *see*
  brachial plexus injuries
obstetrical injuries *see* birth injuries
occipital horn syndrome (Ehlers-Danlos
  syndrome type IX) 90
occipitalisation of the atlas *see* occipito-
  cervical fusion
occipito-cervical fusion 492–3
occipito-cervical junction 491
occipito-cervical stenosis *see* occipito-
  cervical fusion
occiput-C1 lesions 663
occult spina bifida *54*, 55
occupational therapy 30, 230, 295
ocular problems *see* eyes
ocular-scoliotic type (Ehlers-Danlos
  syndrome type VI) 89
odontohypophosphatasia 103
odontoid process 493, 494–5, 499, 657–60,
  664, *665*
oestrogens 93, 94
OI *see* osteogenesis imperfecta
olecranon fractures 563, 621–2
Ollier's disease (enchondromatosis) 86–8,
  202–3, 313
oncogenic rickets 100
onion-skin
  nerve lesions 220–1
  periostial lesions 125, 210, *211*
Online Mendelian Inheritance in Man
  website 67, 303
onycho-osteodystrophy (nail-patella
  syndrome) 417, 462
open muscle biopsy, technique 219, 227
ophthalmalogical examinations, in clinic 69
opioid drugs, analgesia 43, 46–7, 48
opioid-sparing effect, of NSAIDs 48
Orthofix distraction apparatus 438
orthoses
  ankle-foot (AFO) *see* ankle-foot orthoses
    (AFO)
  Boston orthosis 523
  elbow 91
  extension 431
  floor reaction 281
  hip guidance orthosis (HGO) 37, *38*, 249
  hip-knee-ankle-foot (HKAFO) 249
  knee 91
  knee-ankle-foot (KAFO) 20, 230, 249, 281
  parapodium 249
  parawalker 249
  polypropylene external support 72, 666,
    667
  reciprocating gait orthosis (RGO) 37, *38*,
    249, *250*
  rocker sole 280–1

orthoses (contd)
  Scottish Rite 394
  standing 31, 249
  swivel walkers 37, 249
  thoraco-lumbar spinal 230
  underarm 281, 283–4
  see also braces
Ortolani's test, for hip dislocation 363
os calcis
  fractures 655
  heel pain 454, 455
  medial displacement 457
  medial wedge osteotomy 459
os odontoideum 494–5
Osgood-Schlatter's disease 352, 414
ossicum terminale 658
ossific nucleus 367, 368
ossification 12
  cervical vertebrae 657–8
  endochondral 12, 83, 587
  thoraco-lumbar vertebrae 669
ossification centres, and age assessment 52
ossification groove, around growth plate 14
osteitis, chronic 166
osteitis fibrosa cystica 101
osteoarthritis
  epiphyseal dysplasias and 78–9, 80, 81
  hip joint 639–40
  recurrent patella dislocation and 418
osteoblastoma 205–6
  fatal outcome 206
  spinal neoplasm 510, 522, 546
osteoblasts 14, 93, 94
  disordered 105, 107
osteochondral fractures 417, 418, 557–8,
  566, 646, 647
osteochondritis
  back pain in 508–9
  femoral condyles 573
  navicular (Köhler's disease) 356, 453–4
  see also Scheuermann's disease
osteochondritis dissecans 420, 421
  capitellum 314
  knee 415, 420–1
  talar dome 356
osteochondroma 199, 201–2
  dyaphyseal aclasis and 84–6
  epiphyseal (Trevor's disease) 84, 86
  knee 414, 423
osteochondromatosis (hereditary, multiple)
    see diaphyseal aclasis
osteochondrosis, of metatarsals 356
osteoclasts 93, 103, 193
  bone resorption 93, 94
osteocytes 93
osteodystrophy, aluminium excess 107
osteogenesis imperfecta (OI) 67, 69–73
  bone density assessment 54
  differential diagnosis
    from child abuse 352, 605, 606
    from idiopathic coxa vara 336, 337

fractures 71–2
  internal fixation 72–3, 569, 570
  management 561
  stress 351
  hyperplastic callus in 211
  intrauterine diagnosis 69
  lethal perinatal 70–1
  mobility 73
  spinal deformities in 73, 542, 543,
    680–1, 682
osteoid osteoma 199, 204–5, 510
  heel pain 455, 456
  limp and 351, 356, 357
  spinal neoplasm 510, 522, 546
    differential diagnosis 687, 688
osteomalacia 96, 97
osteomyelitis
  acute 131–2, 140–1, 162
  acute haematogenous 121, 127, 133–5,
    165–6
  acute spinal pyogenic osteomyelitis
    (spondylitis) 156–7
  bone destruction in 123–6
  chronic 121, 131, 138, 166
    after acute haematogenous
      osteomyelitis 134
  chronic recurrent multifocal (CRMO) 138
  chronic sclerosing type (Garré's) 135,
    138, 139
  clinical features and age 121
  imaging 54, 59, 60, 123–9
    bone scintigraphy 59, 127, 350
    normal appearance on radiographs 53
    technetium bone scan 133
  in the tropics 165–6, 175–6
  infantile, differential diagnosis 603
  laboratory tests 129
  mandibular 104
  multifocal 138, 507
  os calcis 454, 455
  outcome 134–5, 143
  pelvic, limp in 353, 354–5
  sickle-cell disease and 115, 116
  subacute 121, 135–7
    differential diagnosis 197, 204
  see also Salmonella, osteomyelitis
osteonecrosis 53, 99, 573
osteopathia striata 104
osteopetrosis (marble bone disease) 99,
  103–4, 569, 570
osteoporosis
  bone density scans 54
  fractures 100
    copper deficiency 606
    pathological 570
    stress 351
  genetically determined see osteogenesis
    imperfecta
  idiopathic 100–1, 569, 570
  spinal deformities in 100, 542, 681
osteoporosis pseudoglioma syndrome 100

osteosarcoma 193, 197, 199, 208–10
  in the tropics 170
osteosclerosis see osteopetrosis
osteosynthesis (DCP) plates 609, 621, 625
osteotomy
  distraction opening wedge anterior 411
  juvenile idiopathic arthritis 184–5
  limb lengthening 57, 437
  metatarsal 460–1
  wedge procedures 411, 462, 486
  see also individual names of procedures
Outerbridge classification, chondral damage
  417
overuse syndromes, limp and 351, 352
overweight babies, birth injuries 321
oxygen consumption, growth plate 13

pain
  assessment 42–3, 44
  fatigue discomfort 521, 534
  gait in (antalgic) 348
  muscle cramps 233–4
  night
    growing pains 15
    limb pain 78, 79, 83
    osteoid osteoma 204, 357, 510
    spinal disorders 155, 505, 521
    tuberculosis 150, 155
    see also kyphosis, painful; scoliosis,
      painful
pancytopenia 103, 104
para-amino salicylic acid therapy 153
paracetamol, NSAID 48, 49
Paracolon bacillus 141
paradiscal lesions, imaging 155–6
paralysis
  bone loss in 570
  detection 676
  growth plate and 14
  pes calcaneo-cavus and 487
paralytic convex pes valgus 252
paralytic spinal deformities
  collapsing lordoscoliosis 519, 538–9, 540
  lumbar lordosis 512
  spinal cord damage 544
paraplegia
  spastic 31, 220
  traumatic 670, 676, 678–9
  tuberculous 158–9
parapodium, standing aid 249
paraspinal abscesses 155, 168
paraspinal muscles, ossification 104–5
paraspinal tumours 511
parathyroid disorders 101–2
parathyroid hormone (PTH) 93, 94–5
parathyroid-hormone-related protein
  (PTHrP) 94, 587
paravertebral shadows, imaging 155–6
paravertebral tumours 545, 546
parenteral nutrition, copper deficiency and
  107

parents
  attitude in non-accidental injury 603
  father, in the clinic 4–5
  in clinic 3, 4–8
    expectations 5, 6, 61
  medical 5
  mother
    in the clinic 4–8
      pre-admission fears 8–9
  multidisciplinary training and 30
  post-operative management in cerebral
      palsy and 290–1
  support for 8, 74
    in arthrogryposis multiplex congenita
        293, 294, 298
parosteal sarcoma 193
pars articularis, slippage 547
pars fractures, without displacement *see*
    spondylolysis
pars interarticularis defect *683*, *684*, *686*
patella
  bipartite 414–15, 425
  fractures of 566, 647–8
  instability 356, 417–20
  knee pain 414–15
  lateral subluxation 416–17, 419
  Q angle in alignment 416
  re-alignment surgery 419–20
patella alta 416, 418
patella baja 567
patellar dislocation
  acute 418, 419, 646–7
  congenital 418
  exercise programme 419
  instability and 417–20
  lateral 566
  recurrent 171, 416, 418–19
patellofemoral malalignment 416–17, 418,
    646
patellofemoral pain, overuse syndrome 352
pathogenicity, definition 119
pathological fractures *see* fractures
Pauwel's Y-shaped osteotomy 80
Pavlik harness 367, *368*, 371, 642
pectoralis major transfer 297
pelvic obliquity
  congenital spinal deformity syndromes
      538, 539, 540
  limb length discrepancy 429, *430*
  poliomyelitis 267, 271
pelvic osteomyelitis *353*, 354–5
pelvic osteotomy 376–8
pelvic tilt 171, *183*, 188, 349
pelvis
  bone density 104, 105
  fractures 565, 633–5
    CT imaging 61
    polytrauma 582
Pemberton acetabuloplasty 254, *255*, 377–8
penicillin
  benzyl/phenoxymethyl 134

drug sensitivity 123
procaine 169, 170
percutaneous epiphysiodesis 433
perichondrial bone bark, ring of Lacroix 14,
    397, 559, 599
perinatal lethal hypophosphatasia 102
periodic paralysis 226
periodontitis type (Ehlers-Danlos syndrome
    type VIII) 90
periosteal chondroma 203
periosteal hinge 559
periosteum 599
  bone division and 436
  elevation 604
  remodelling by 612
  stripping injury 602
peripheral nerve blocks 44–5
peripheral neuropathies 539, 540–1
peripheral physeal injury *589*, 590
peroneal muscular atrophy 453, 484
    see also Charcot-Marie-Tooth disease
peroneal spastic flat foot *see* flat foot
peroneal tendons 488, 489
Perthes' disease 383–96
  broomstick plaster 394
  diagnosis 386, 387, 388
  differential diagnosis 57, 78, 141, 353
  epiphyseal infarction 383, 384, 386, *387*
  growth disturbance 391, 590
  healing phase 383, 384
  hip containability 392–5
  imaging
    dynamic arthrogram 392
    MRI 392
    technetium bone scan 391, 392, *393*
  in the tropics 172
  joint congruity 391
  leg length discrepancy 391–2
  limp in 350, 351, 356, 390
  management 390–95
  metaphyseal signs, Catterall classification
      386, *387*
  pain in 390, 391
  pathological fractures 573
  prognostic factors 386–9
  splints in 394–5
  susceptibility 383
pes, *see also* foot
pes arcuatus 483
pes calcaneo-cavus 484, 487
pes cavovarus 484–7
pes cavus 217–19, 483–90, 540–1
pes planus (flat foot) 455–7
pes valgus 289, 487–90
pes varus 289
Peto Institute, conductive education 36
PFFD (proximal femoral focal deficiency)
    335, 336–9, 432
phalanges
  cyst *572*
  dislocations 631

fractures 558–9, *572*, 630, 655–6
  fixation 564, *565*, 631
growth plates 558–9, 629
Kirner deformity 302, 310
phasic spasticity 273
Phemister's epiphysiodesis 433
phophorus 94, 107
phrenic nerve lesions 321, 324
physeal chondrocytes 587
physeal plates, cervical spine 657–8
physiolysis, bone bridge removal 595–7
physiotherapists 5, 30, 31
physis *see* growth plate
Piggot's classification, in hallux valgus 460
pigmented naevus 219, 242
pigmented villo-nodular synovitis 422–3
pin track infection 439
pins, biodegradable 560
'pistol grip' heel 251–2, 269, 487
'pithed frog' posture 231, *232*
plain film *see* X-ray
'plan d'election', Stagnara's principle 514,
    515, 522
plano-valgus deformity 91, 488
plantalar arthrodesis 270
plantar release 485–6
plantar responses 226
plasma cell osteomyelitis 136
plasma coagulation factors, in haemophilia
    109, 112, 113, 114
plaster casts
  broomstick plaster 394
  elongation-de-rotation flexion (EDF)
      532–3
  halo body cast 667, 668
  hip spica 9, 371–2, 642, 643
  in the tropics 163
  insensitive skin and 245, 259
  Minerva 663, 664, 667, *668*
  Risser 271
  shoulder spica in the 'salute position'
      562
  wedging in angular deformities 651, 653
plating *see* fixation
plicae, in the knee 415
PMMA beads (gentamicin-impregnated)
    124, *125*, 131, 132, 134, 137
Poland's syndrome 306
poliomyelitis 261–71
  contractures 263–4
    lower limbs 265–71
      surgical correction 263–71
    upper limbs 264–5
  deformities 261, 262, *263*
    hip 265–7
    knee 267–8, 409
    spinal 271, 539, 540
  foot and ankle deformities 268–71, 444,
      484, 487
    Ilizarov frame in correction of 444
  management 262–3

poliomyelitis (*contd*)
  muscles in 216, *230*
  osteoporotic bone 263
  paralysis in 162, 261–2
  physiotherapy 263
pollicisation, technique 308
polydactyly 54, 301, 311–12
polymyositis-dermatomyositis 226, *228–9*,
  237–8
polyneuritis (Guillain-Barré) 216, 262
polyneuropathy, congenital infantile 225
polyposis coli (multiple) 192
polytrauma 579–85, 666
  fractures 561, 580
    long bones 582–3
    spinal 671, 675–6
  head injury 580
  orthopaedic injuries 582–5
  outcomes 585
  see also trauma
'popcorn' radiographic appearance 71
popliteal angle 275
popliteal cysts 423
popliteal web (pterygium syndrome) 294,
  412
positron emission tomography (PET) 218
posterior release surgery, for club foot
  478–9
posterior surgical approach 372–3
postural calcaneo-valgus, neonatal 452
postural support
  in cerebral palsy 33–5
  see also orthoses; wheelchairs
posture
  cerebral palsy 277–9, *280*
    orthoses and 280–1
  limb length discrepancy 429, *430*
  neonatal, motor neurone lesions and
    244–5
  neuromuscular disease 224
  scoliosis 255, 256
  side-lying child 368, *370*
  spina bifida 247
Potts disease *see* spinal tuberculosis
Pott's paraplegia 159–60
preadmission policy 8–9
pre-operative anxiety 41
premature babies
  fractures in 603, 606
  neurological abnormality 215
pressure sores 46, 245
prevalence, definition 575
primary spongiosum 14
proliferative zone of growth plate 13, 587
pronation, in foot function 467
pronator contracture 264
prone-lying infants 450
prophylaxis, opportunistic infections 117,
  147
prostheses
  forearm 302

limb salvage 209
lower limb 336, 339
proteoglycans 82, 94
Proteus spp. 141, 162, 166–7
prothionamide therapy *153*
proximal femoral focal deficiency (PFFD)
  335, 336–9, 432
pseudarthrosis
  congenital 573
    forearm 314, *315*
    tibia 339, 343–5, 444
  metacarpal fractures 630
  spinal fusion surgery 524
pseudo-hip flexion deformity 155
pseudoachondroplasia 76–8
pseudohypoparathyroidism (PHP) 101, 102
Pseudomonas aeruginosa 123, 137, 166
pseudoparalysis
  birth injuries 562, 601
  bone or joint infection 129, 140
  congenital syphilis 170
pseudosubluxation of cervical spine 660
pseudotumours, haemophilic 112, 172–3
psoas abscesses 155, 355
psychological disturbance
  growing pains in 15
  torticollis in 499
psychological effects
  deformity/disability 23, 29, 519
  long-term splintage 395
  polytrauma 580
psychosomatic symptoms, knee pain 409,
  424, 425
pterygium syndrome (popliteal web) 294,
  412
PTH (parathyroid hormone) 93, 94–5
PTHrP (parathyroid hormone related
  protein) 94, 587
pubic symphasis, fractures of 565, 633,
  634, 635
pulse oximetry 48
puncture injury 35
purpura, differential diagnosis 141, 605–6
pus 120, 122
pyarthrosis *see* septic arthritis
pycnodysostosis, skeletal dysplasia 569
pyramidal tract signs, in occipito-cervical
  fusion 493
pyrazinamide therapy 153, *153*

Q angle, patella dislocation 416, 418
quadriceps apparatus
  paralysis 268
  patella dislocation 416–17, 418, 419, 650
  tibial dysplasia 341, 343

radial distal epiphysiolysis 627–8
radial dysplasia 301, 303–5
  associated conditions 303, 304, 307
radial head dislocation
  congenital 301, 311

obstetrical palsy and 326
  ulnar fracture and 623–4
radial head enlargement 111
radial head fractures 622–3
  fixation 564, 622, *623*
    Metaizeau technique 622, *623*
    Steinmann pins 622
radial neck fractures 564
radial polydactyly 301, 311–12
radiation, in imaging 51–2, 53, 54
radio-ulnar dislocation 614–15, 624, 628–9
radio-ulnar synostosis
  congenital 301, 310–11
  forearm fractures and 623, 625
radiographs
  achondroplasia 74–5
  diaphyseal aclasis 85
  dysplasia epiphysealis hemimelica 86
  fibrous dysplasia 91
  hip dislocation 285–6, 365–6
  humeral supracondylar fracture 616
  idiopathic coxa vara 336
  metaphyseal chondrodysplasia 83
  multiple epiphyseal dysplasia 78–9
  Ollier's disease (endochromatosis) 87
  osteogenesis imperfecta 72
  pseudoachondroplasia 77
  SCFE 399–400
  spondyloepiphyseal dysplasia congenita
    81
  Stickler syndrome 81–2
  vitamin-D-deficiency rickets 97
  see also X-rays
radioisotope imaging 127, 687–8
radiotherapy 210, 211, 510–11
radius
  dislocation 623–4
  distal epiphysiolysis 627–8
  fractures
    associated injuries 624, 626
    fixation 563–4
    growth plate injury 558–9
    head 622–3
    metaphyseal 626–7
  hereditary multiple exostoses 313, *314*
  Madelung's deformity 85, 313
Rang's classification of physeal fracture
  589
Ranvier zone injury *589*, 590
rash
  Lyme disease 355
  polymyositis-dermatomyositis 237
rate, definition 575
reciprocating gait orthosis (RGO) 37, *38*,
  249, *250*
reflex activity 244
reflex sympathy dystrophy 416
reflexes, in neuromuscular disorders 226
Refsum's disease (heredopathia atactica
  polyneuritiformis) 220
Reimer's migration index 285

renal dialysis, aluminium bone disease 100, 107
renal failure
nephrocalcinosis 103, 105
pathological fractures 570
SCFE and 397, 398, 403
renal glomerular rickets (renal glomerular osteodystrophy) 99–100
renal system
anomalies in Klippel-Feil syndrome 496, 498, 499
in calcium homeostasis 94
renal tubular rickets 98–9
reserve zone of growth plate 13, 587
respiratory function
analgesic drugs and 42, 47–8
neurological disorders and 39–40, 230–1
surgery and 42
respiratory tract infection, and bone and joint infections 165–6, 167, 507
reticulo-endothelial system, in tubercular infection 148–9
rhabdomyosarcoma 171
rheumatic fever 141, 177, 354
rhizotomy, selective posterior 283
rib hump, in scoliosis 59, 513, 520
rib-vertebra angle difference (RVAD) 532
ribs
bone density 105, 107
'rickety rosary' 97
'rice bodies', in synovial fluid 148
rickets 83, 96–100, 413–14, 588
rifampicin therapy 153, 167
'rim syndrome', hip pain 378
ring of C1 493, 663, 664
road accidents
fracture incidence 576, 577
in the tropics 174
polytrauma 579, 583
seatbelt injuries 671, 675–6
spinal injury 670, 673–4
see also trauma
Robert Jones strapping 474–5
Robert Jones tendon transfer 486
rocker sequence, in gait 277
rotationplasty 209, 210, 339
'rotting stump' appearance, long bones 99, 100
Roux-Goldthwaite procedure 418, 419, 420
Roux's sign, pelvic injury 582
'rugger jersey' spine 99
Russell-Silver dwarfism 427

sacral agenesis 294
sacrum, in dysplastic spondylolisthesis 548
safety helmets 174
Salmonella spp.
arthritis
reactive 354
septic 123, 141
osteomyelitis 116, 123

acute haematogenous 166
in sickle-cell disease 135, 428
subacute 136
tibial overgrowth 428
Salmonella typhimurium, in osteomyelitis in typhoid fever 167
Salter-Harris classification of growth plate injuries 544, 588–90
Salter's osteotomy 378, 436
Sandifer's syndrome 499
Scaglietti closed-cast system 551, 552–3
scanogram, measurement of limb length discrepancy 429
scaphoid, carpal fracture 629
scapula
congenital elevation see Sprengel's shoulder
fractures 562, 603, 611
winging 85, 224, 234–5
scapulo-humeral muscular dystrophy 224, 234
'scarf sign', shoulder girdle weakness 225, 226
SCFE see slipped capital femoral epiphysis
Scheuermann's disease (idiopathic kyphosis) 508–9, 512, 516, 533–5, 674, 681–3
type I 516, 517, 518, 533–4
type II ('apprentice's spine') 516, 534–5, 548, 682
Schmid metaphyseal chondrodysplasia 83, 84
Schmorl nodes 516, 519, 534, 674, 677, 681–3
school, for the handicapped child 9–10
school leavers, disabled 40
sciatic nerve block 45
scintigraphy 54, 127, 350, 510
SCIWORA (spinal cord injury without obvious radiological abnormality) 506, 582, 662, 676
scoliosis 535–8
assessment 58–9, 513–15
collapsing 541, 679
compensatory 514
curvature in 58–9, 528–30
early signs 224
idiopathic 519–20
early-onset 530–3
in the tropics 172
late-onset idiopathic 520–30
clinical features 520–1
radiographic assessment 521–2
treatment 522–30
conservative 523–4
surgical 524–30
limb length discrepancy and 429
malignant progressive curves 530
non-structural 512–13
painful 204, 205, 206, 508–9
tumours and 510, 511, 545
paralytic 670, 678–9

post-irradiation 511
progressive paralytic 39
rotation 512, 513–15, 522
surgical correction 526–8
screening 512, 516, 517, 520
structural 188, 512–13
surface shape 521, 522
surgery
Duchenne muscular dystrophy 233
electroencephalography during 219
instrumentation systems 271, 524–30, 541
scotty dog of Lachapele 686
screw fixation, in SCFE 400–3
scurvy (vitamin C deficiency) 105, 107, 588
seats/chairs, for cerebral palsy 31, 32, 33–5
sedation
intra-articular steroids and 181
MRI and 54, 218
SEDL gene disorder 80–1
segmental demyelination 219
segmentation, failures of 536, 537
semimembranous bursa, popliteal cyst 423
semitendinous tendon, re-routing 419, 420
sensorimotor neuropathies 220–1
sensory loss 36, 217
sensory neuropathies 217, 220, 257
separation fear 8
septic arthritis 120–2, 138–44, 423
diagnosis
differential 353–4, 355, 590
laboratory signs 122, 140
radiological appearance 126, 128
hip 56–7, 353–4
multifocal 138
neonatal 128, 139–40, 166–7
in the tropics 162, 166–7
outcome 143–4
pathological fractures in 570
sickle-cell disease and 115
systemic illness 423
treatment 141–4
antibiotic therapy 131
irrigation 141
surgery 131–2
Sequoia circular external fixator 443
seronegative polyarthritis 177, 178
serpentine foot 450, 451–2
Serratia marcescens, in septic athritis 141
serum enzymes
in neuromuscular disorders 226
see also creatine phosphokinase
Severin's radiographic classification of hip dysplasia 366
Sever's (Haglund's) disease (calcaneal apophysitis) 352, 454
sex hormone deficiency 397, 398
sexual precocity 91, 107
Shapiro's patterns of discrepancy, in leg length 431

Sharrard procedure 254, 266
shear injury
    fracture 559, 622
    growth plate 588, 590
    spinal 671, 673
'shepherd's crook' deformity
    femur 71, 91, 107
        with coxa vara 201, 336, 337
shock, in polytrauma 581
shoe discomfort 459
shoes
    deformities caused by 18, 454–5
    insoles 457
    raises 336, 431
    wedges 20, 25
short finger symbrachydactyly 303
short stature 83, 91, 103, 398, 407
    disproportionate 383
    see also dwarfism
short time inversion recovery (STIR)
        sequences 127, 133
shoulder
    Benjamin double osteotomy 186
    brachial plexus injuries 326, 331–3, 601
        sequelae
            deformity 328–9, 331, 332–3
            dislocation 327–8, 329, 330
            surgery 331–3
            subluxation 329, 330, 331
            surgery 324–5, 326
    contractures
        abduction 220
        medial rotation 327, 328, 329
            treatment 331, 332
        posterior gleno-humeral 331
        surgical correction 264–5
    damage in haemophilia 111
    developmental anomalies 316–20
    dislocation
        acquired 316
        congenital 316
        joint laxity 316, 611
        neonatal 601
            see also shoulder, brachial plexus
                injuries
        recurrent 316–17
        traumatic 317, 611
    function
        assessment, Mallet's system 329–30,
            333
        recording 329–31, 333
    injuries 601, 609–13
    obstetrical palsy injuries see shoulder,
        brachial plexus injuries
    stiffness, muscle fibrosis 171
    see also Sprengel's shoulder
shoulder arthrodesis 264
shoulder girdle
    diaphyseal aclasis and 84–5
    fractures 562–5
    weakness 225, 226

shoulder spica in the 'salute position' 562
sickle-cell disease 115–16, 123
    limb length discrepancy 428
    osteomyelitis and 135, 166
    septic arthritis and 423
    surgery 115–16
SICWORA (spinal cord injury without
        radiological abnormality) 506, 662,
        670
side-lying child 368–70, 530
silastic, interpositional material 560, 596
Silverskiöld's test 275
simple bone cysts 193, 207, 423
Sinding-Larsen-Johansson disease 352, 414,
        566
single limb stance, and gait 16
single-photon emission CT (SPECT) 218
sinus 152, 155, 257–9
sitting posture 283–4
skeletal age assessment 11–12, 430
skeletal congenital disorders 54, 68
skeletal dysplasias
    fractures 561, 569
    genes, web site 67
    stature in 95
    see also fibrous dysplasia; osteogenesis
        imperfecta
'skew baby', side-lying child 368–70
skew foot 452
skin
    anaesthesia 241, 245
    cholecalciferol synthesis 95
    fragility 89, 90
    infection 165–6
    laxity 89, 90
    necrosis 173
skin lesions 6
    desquamating 170
    marks in child abuse 352
    papillomatous 169
    pigmented 91, 219, 242
    ulceration 256
skull
    bossing 73, 115
    'hair on end' radiograph 114
    hyperkeratosis 169
    in achondroplasia 73
    sutures widened 107
    thickened 107
skull fractures, non-accidental 603, 605
sleeve fracture 414, 415, 425
slip angle 549, 550
slipped capital femoral epiphysis (SCFE)
        397–407
    bilateral 403
    complications 406–7
    differentiation from septic arthritis 355
    endocrine factors in 397–8
    'figure 4' position 399
    fixation
        pin 400–3, 406

    screw 400–3
    immunological factors in 398
    inflammation in 398, 399
    mechanical factors in 397
    periosteal oedema 398
    radiological signs 399–400
    treatment 400–6
slipped upper femoral epiphysis (SUFE) 57,
        356
snake bites 173, 175–6
snapping hip 640
snapping knee 410
soap-bubble appearance 205–6
Social Services Department, and disability
        40
soft-tissue
    buttonholing 562
    contractures 265–6, 374
    interposition in fractures 561, 627, 650,
        651
    limb lengthening and 438–9, 440
    release
        club foot 474, 475–6, 481
            in arthrogryphosis multiplex
                congenita 293, 295
        juvenile idiopathic arthritis 183–4
        pes calcaneo-cavus 487
        seating in cerebral palsy 283
    tethers 468
    trauma damage 583–4, 631
    tumours 171, 423
    upper limb anomalies and 301–2, 306–10
solitary bone cysts 199–200
Southwick biplane/triplane osteotomy 405
space-occupying lesions of central nervous
        system 220
spastic cerebral palsy 273, 279
spastic hemiplegia 224
spastic paraplegia 31, 220
spastic quadriplegia 31, 539–40
spasticity 31, 273, 281–2
    asymmetric 220
    gait 224, 415
    tonic 273
speckled calcification 203–4
speech therapists 30, 31, 32–3
spica see plaster casts
spina bifida 242
    deformities 242–5
        foot 444, 484, 487
        knee 409, 411
        management 250–7
        spinal 255–6, 538–9
        spinal cord 36–8, 516
    family recurrence risk 246
    fractures 570–1, 606
    management
        deformities 250–7
        orthopaedic 247–50
        prenatal 245–6
    neonatal care 247

prevention 245
see also myelomeningocele; neural tube
 defects; neurological disorders
spina bifida cystica 36–8, 242
spina bifida occulta 55, 219, 242, *243*, 450
 dysplastic spondylolisthesis and 548, *550*
 Sprengel's shoulder and 319
spinal anaesthesia 46, 181
spinal cord
 compression 492, 497–8
 congenital cysts 217–19
 congenital deformities 516, 538–9
 decompression surgery 159, 160
 injuries
  birth 600, 602–3
  trauma 544, 582
 poliomyelitis and 261
 space available for the (SAC) *658*, 659–60
 stretch injuries 670, 676
 tethered *54*, 55, *241*, *259*
  filum 258, 537
  scoliosis and 58
 tumours 356, 484, 511
 see also neural tube
spinal cord injury without obvious
  radiological abnormality 506, 582,
  662, 676
spinal dysraphism 219–20, 241, 257–9
 foot deformities 465, 469, 484
 sensory impairment in 217
 tip-toe walking 453
 vertebral deformities and 521, 537
 see also neural tube defects; neurological
  disorders
spinal fusion
 prophylactic 537–8
 scoliosis and 230–1, 524, 533
 spondylolisthesis and *551*, 552, 553
 thoraco-lumbar injuries and 677–8, 689
spinal muscular atrophy 216, 225, 231–2
 diagnostic criteria *226*, *228–9*, *230*
 foot deformities 450, 487
 'jug-handle' arm position *232*
 spinal deformities 230–1, 539, 540
 see also neurological disorders
spinal neoplasms 510–11
 bone-forming 204–6
 diagnosis 157, 218
 in the tropics 170
 painful 505, 510–11
  scoliosis and 509, 521
 'spinal tumour syndrome' 155, 159
spinal tuberculosis 154–60, 507
 diagnosis
  differential 156–7
  imaging 155–6, 507
 in the tropics 168, 507
 incidence of 154
 kyphosis in 160, 507
 neurological complications in 157–60
 'spinal tumour syndrome' 155

treatment 157–8
 vertebrae 152, 154, 155–6, 168
spine
 arthrodesis 284–5
 bone density anomalies 79, 105, 107
 buckle 518–19
 deformities 512, 515–19
  congenital 505, *506*, 516, 535–8, 539
   heritable disorders and 218, 539–41,
    542–4
  irradiation and 546
  tumours and 545–6
 disorders
  diagnosis of 6, 54, 55
  limb length discrepancy 427, *430*
  limp and 348, 350, 355
 infection 516, 544–5
  back pain in 507–8
  imaging in 59, 127
 injuries
  backboard *665*, 666, *667*
  polytrauma 582
 shape
  assessment 513–15
  curves of 512, 532
  normal shape changes 11
 stenosis 73, 76, 543
 Z-deformity 549, *551*
 see also cervical spine; discs; scoliosis;
  thoraco-lumbar spine; vertebrae
spiral CT *see* helical computed tomography
splints
 containment 395
 Denis Browne 24, 26
 intermittent compression 39
 polypropylene 113
 thermoplastic 72
 Von Rosen 367
split hand/foot deformities 301, 303, 306,
 462–3
spondylitis *135*, 156–7, 178
 ankylosing 354, 491, 508, *509*
spondylodiscitis *135*
spondyloepiphyseal dysplasias 67, 68,
 79–82, 544
 congenita 79–80, *81*
 ophthalmalogical examinations in 69
 tarda 80–1, 82
 torticollis in 499
spondylolisthesis 505, 549
 cervical spine 664, *665*
 crisis 549, *551*
 dysplastic 548–9
 isthmic 547–8
 lumbo-sacral kyphosis in 549, *550*, 552
 lytic 547–8
 pain in 509, 549
 thoraco-lumbar 688–9
 treatment of 549–53
spondylolysis 352, 509, 550–2
 traumatic *673*, 684–9

spondyloptosis 549, *550*
sport
 back pain and 509
 cervical spine injuries 661
 foot injuries 656
 fractures 415, 576, 577, 583
 knee problems 414, 421, 423–4, 650
  patellar damage 415, 417, 418
 lytic spondylolisthesis and 548
 orthoses for 91
 overuse syndromes 352
 SCFE and 397, 403
 thoraco-lumbar spine injuries 670–3,
  674, 684–6, 688
 upper limb injuries 609
Sprengel's shoulder 316, 318–20
 Klippel-Feil syndrome and 496, 539
 physiotherapy 319
 spinal anomalies with 218, 319
 surgical technique 319–20
Stagnara's principle, 'plan d'election' 514,
 515, 522
Staheli
 hip extension test 274–5
 torsional profile tool 22
stance phase in gait 276, 348
Staphylococcus albus 141
Staphylococcus aureus
 in osteomyelitis 116, 122–3
  acute haematogenous 133–4, 166
  chronic 138
  subacute 136, 137
 in septic arthritis 122–3, 141, 423
  tropical neonatal 162, 166–7
 in tropical muscle abscess 167
Staphylococcus epidermis 123, 136
Staphylococcus spp. 142–3, *197*
stapling 185, 412, 418, 432
Steindler flexorplasty 297, 326
Steindler release 481
Steinhert disease *see* myotonic dystrophy
step length, and gait 16
sternocleidomastoid muscle 500, 502, 503
steroid therapy
 growth plate and 14
 intra-articular 164, 422
 intrathecal 182
Stickler syndrome (arthro-opthalmopathy)
 69, 81–2, 416
Still's disease 105, 177, 178
STIR (short time inversion recovery
 sequences) 127, 133
Streeter's dysplasia *see* constriction band
 syndrome
Streptococcus agalactiae 123
Streptococcus faecalis 136
Streptococcus β-haemolytic 123, 133–4
Streptococcus pneumoniae 123, 141
Streptococcus pyogenes 123, 141
Streptococcus spp. 142–3, 162, 166–7
streptomycin therapy 153

stress fractures 351–2, 573, 656
  lytic spondylolisthesis and 547–8
  patellar 415, 566, 647
stress phenomenon 509
stress shielding 73
subluxation of the hip *see* hip
subperiosteal haemorrhage 105
subscapularis muscle 326, 328
subscapularis recession, operation
    discredited 331
subtalar arthrodesis of Grice 457
subtalar valgus 252
sunray radiological appearance 208
supination of foot 467, 471
supinator contracture, forearm 264
supracondylar fractures 173–6, 559, 614,
    616–19
surgery
  biopsy margins 197
  infection and 119, 131–2, 325
  myositis following 105
  wound care in EDS 91
swelling, in humeral supracondylar fracture
    616
swing phase, gait cycle 276, 348
symbrachydactyly 302–3
Symes through-ankle disarticulation of the
    foot 432
synchondroses, cervical spine 657–8, 663
syndactyly
  fingers 165, 301, 305, 306–7
  toes 165, 245, 462
synkinesia (mirror motions) 498
synovial chondromatosis 422
synovial fluid 122
synovitis
  acute and transient 422
  pigmented villo-nodular 422–3
  transient 57, 350, *351*, 352–4
synovium, oedematous 398, 399
syphilis 157, 169–70, 547, 606
syringomyelia *54*, 55, 241
  pes cavus and 217–19
  post-traumatic 679
  spinal deformity and 218, 505, *506*, 545
syrinx 220, 521, 522, 545

Taillard's percentage slippage *550*
talectomy 270, *293*, 295, 481
talipes calcaneo-valgus 452–3, 488
talipes equinovarus *see* club foot
tall stature 88
talo-calcaneal joint 457, 488, 489, 490
talo-calcaneo-navicular joint 487–90
talo-navicular joint 467, 489, 490
talus
  club foot and 467, 478, *479*, 480, *481*
  congenital vertical 252, 295, 452,
      487–90
  fractures 654–5
  haemophiliac damage 111–12

plantar flexed 17
  see also ankle
TAR (thrombocytopenia absent radius)
    syndrome 303, 361, 412
'target joint', repeated haemarthroses 111,
    113, 114
tarsal coalition (peroneal spastic flat foot)
    17, 351, 457–9
tarso-metatarsal joints 467
tarsus
  fractures 655–6
  splitting injuries 568–9
  wedge tarsectomy 487
teardrop fractures 616, *617*, 662, 665
technetium-phosphate compounds, in
    radioisotope imaging 127, 510
telangiectatic osteosarcoma 208
tendo-Achilles
  Sever's disease 454
  surgery
    lengthening 31, 289, 290
    shortening 16, 17, 18, 270, 453
    tenotomy 39
    transfer 487
tendon reflexes 217, 220, 226
tendon transfer
  foot deformities 270, 474, 486–7
  hand deformities 307, 309
  shoulder deformity 326
tendons
  anomalies in forearm 303, 304
  contracture type, in foot deformity 472,
      473
  synovial sheaths 187
tenotomy, adductor tenotomy 371, 374
'tension-stress' effect, in bone lengthening
    436, 438, 441
tensor fasciae latae transfer 266
teratogenic agents 301, 302, 335
teratologic dislocation of the talo-calcaneo-
    navicular joint 487–90
teratoma, paraspinal 511
thalassaemias 114–15
thiacetazone therapy *153*
thigh-foot angle 22, 275
Thomas's test 274
Thomsen's myotonia congenita 237
thoracic kyphosis 160, 512, 681–4
thoracic spine *see* thoraco-lumbar spine
thoraco-lumbar hypolordosis 549
thoraco-lumbar kyphosis 88, 543
thoraco-lumbar spine 505–53
  assessment 505
  back pain 505–11
  congenital malformations 505
  deformities 512–46
    congenital bony 535–8
    congenital spinal cord 538–9
    definitions 512–16
    heritable dysplasias 542–4
    infection and 544–5

neuromuscular 539–41
pathology of 516–19
scoliosis, idiopathic 519–35
tumours and 545–6
von Recklinghausen's disease and
    541–2
see also kyphosis; scoliosis
development of 669–70
fractures
  differential diagnosis 679
  imaging 676–7
  incidence 670–1
  mechanisms 671–6
  neurological injury 676, 678–9
  systemic diseases and 680–3
  traumatic spondylolysis 684–9
  treatment 677–9
infection 507–8
kyphosis of adolescence 508–9
mechanical and degenerative disorders
    509–10
neoplasia of 510–11
traumatic back pain 506–7
thoracoplasty/thoracotomy, risk in 544
three-dimensional kinematics and kinetics,
    in gait analysis 248
thrombocytopenia absent radius (TAR)
    syndrome 303, 361, 412
thrombophlebitis, snake bite *173*
thumb
  adduction deformities 290
  complex clasped thumb 307
  congenital clasped 301, 307
  duplication, classification of 311–12
  floating *303*, 307, 308
  hypoplasia 303, 307–9
  supple clasped 307
  'thumb-in-palm' deformity 290, 298
  triphalangeal 301, 302, 303, 312
thymic hyperplasia 238
thyroid hormone 14
thyroid protection, during imaging 51
tibia
  bowing 339–40, 343, *344*, 345
    see also tibia vara
  club foot and 467, 470–1
  congenital dysplasia 335, 339–45
    with intact fibula 341–3
  congenital short
    lengthening 340–1
    with absent fibula 339–41, 431–2
  distal, metaphyseal fractures 653
  epiphysiolysis 650–1
  fractures 559, 566–8, 646–53
    diaphyseal 652–3
    intra-articular physeal 650
    metaphyseal 650–2, 653
    stress 351, 573
    triplane, CT evaluation 590, *593*
  growth rate 431
  leg lengthening 436

osteotomy 24, 83, *84*
pain in osteoporosis 100
physis damage 413, 590
posterior ligaments 422
posteromedial angulation 345
proximal, metaphyseal fractures 650–2
pseudoarthrosis, congenital 343–5, 444
shortening, technique 435
torsion 21, 23–4, 73, 76, 418
  Denis Browne splints 24, 26
tibia recurvatum 345
tibia valga 69, 79, 80, 651, 652
tibia vara
  Blount's disease 19, 20, 412, 413, *443*
  musculoskeletal disorders and 69, 83, *84*
  post-traumatic 651, 652, 653
tibial spines 420–1, 648–9
tibial tubercle 414, 419, 420
tibial tuberosity fractures 567, 650
tibialis anterior tendon transfer 479–80
ticarcillin therapy 123
Tillaux fracture 568
tip-toe walking *see* gait
tissue culture 122
toes
  accessory 462
  big toe anomalies 462
  clawing 187, 269, 270–1
  congenital elevation of the 5th toe
    459–60
  curly 459
  hammer-toe 461
  injuries 655–6
  lumps 86, 87
  monophalangic 104–5, *106*
  over-riding *456*, 459–60, 461
  transfer, in proximal forearm anomalies
    303
  ulcers on 484
  Z deformity 486
  see also digits; hallux
Tom Smith's arthritis *see* septic arthritis
tomography 126, 662
tonic spasticity 273
topical cutaneous analgesia 44, 181
Torode & Zieg classification, pelvic
  avulsion fractures 633, *634*
Torpin's Triad 165
torsion
  birth injuries 662
  lower limb 21–6, 413
  see also femur, torsion; tibia, torsion
torsional profile 22
torso, asymmetry 520–1, 536, 538–9, 544
torticollis 218, 499–500
  benign paroxysmal of infancy 499
  congenital muscular 499–500, 502–3
  intermittent 499
  ring of C1 anomalies 493
tourniquets
  Bier's block and 45

complications in 42, 115–16
toxic synovitis *see* transient synovitis of
  the hip
trabecular fracture 383, 384
tracheo-oesophageal compression 610, 611
traction
  Bryant's traction 601–2
  femoral fractures 601, 602, 642, 643
  gallows traction 370, 374
  halo traction 271, 495, 664, 667
  head traction 501, 502
  in osteoarticular tuberculosis 152
  in soft tissue contractures 374, 439
traditional healers, in the tropics 162–4,
  170
trans-scapho-perilunate dislocations 564
transient synovitis of the hip (coxalgia
  fugax) *see* synovitis, transient
transmalleolar axis 23
transpedicular instrumentation 552, 553
transverse absence, upper limb anomalies
  301, 302–3
transverse atlantal ligament laxity 493–4
transverse atlantal ligaments 659–60
transverse deficiency, lower limb anomalies
  335
trauma
  bone loss 444
  femoral neck fractures 635–40
  femoral shaft fractures 640–5
  haemophilia and 113–14
  imaging in 61–2
  in the tropics 162, 173–6
  joint effusion 141, 590
  jumping, heel pain 455
  pelvic injuries 633–5
  physeal injuries 427, 428, 590
  repetitive, running 352, 397
  spinal 506–7, 516, 544, 547
    cervical spine 493, 499, 500, 666
    kyphosis of adolescence 506–7
  wound size in compound fractures 583–4
  see also fractures; non-accidental
    injuries; polytrauma; road accidents
Trendelenburg gait 349, 373
Treponema pallidum 169–70
Treponema pertenue 169
Trethowan's sign 399, *401*
Trevor's disease (dysplasia epiphysealis
  hemimelica) 84, 86
triamcinalone hexacetonide therapy 182
triceps brachii transfer 264, 297
triceps surae 269, 289
trigger digits 301, 307, 310
triple antigen therapy 154
triple arthrodesis
  for foot deformities 270, 486, 487
    club foot 474, 476, 480
    peroneal spastic flat foot 458, 459
triple therapy *see* antibiotic therapy
trochlea fractures 621

trochlear groove, shallow 418
tropics, orthopaedics in 161–76
tuberculoid leprosy 151
tuberculosis 147–54
  bone 148–9, 162
    healing 153–4
    metaphyseal lesions 148
  diagnosis 122, 150–1
  in the tropics 117, 162, 168
  infection dissemination 147
  joints *149*, 150, *151*, 162
    effusions 152
    movement, in staging *152*
    'position of function' splintage 152,
      154
    sequestrae (kissing lesions) 148, 149,
      151
  management 151–4
    anti-tubercular drugs 152–3
  movement limitation 150, 152, 168
  osteoporosis in 149, 150
  pain in 150, 155
  prophylaxis against 147
  relapse/recurrence 154
  spinal 154–60
    deformity in 160, 544–5
    neonatal 507
    neurological complications 157–60
    spondylolisthesis in 547
  surgery in 154
  synovial lesions 148, *152*, 153–4, 422
  tubercle formation 148–9, 150
  see also spinal tuberculosis
tumours
  hyperparathyroidism 101
  limp and 356
  soft tissue, imaging 60–1
  spinal cord 499, 511
  spinal deformities 516, 545–6
  staging of 194–5
  technetium bone scan 194, *198*
  see also bone tumours; giant-cell
    tumours; malignant tumours;
    osteoid osteoma
typhoid fever 157, 167

ulcers, skin lesions 169, 217, 484
ulna
  distal epiphysiolysis 627, 628
  dysplasia 301, 305–6
  fractures
    fixation 563–4
    greenstick 626
    metaphyseal 626–7
    radial head dislocation and 623–4
  hereditary multiple exostoses 313, *314*
  radial dysplasia and 303
  styloid damage 626, 627
  see also Madelung's deformity
ulnar nerve injury 111, 615, 617, 620
ulnar polydactyly 311

ultrasound 53
  fetal 54
    bone dysplasias 69
    club foot 465
    neural tube defects 219–20, 246
  hip
    dislocation 55–6, 363–5
    irritable 56–7
    transient synovitis 353
  limb lengthening 57–8
  limp, assessment of 350–1
  septic arthritis 127, 128, 140
  slipped upper femoral epiphysis 56–7
  spinal dysraphism 258
  trauma 61–2
upper limbs
  anomalies 301–15
  contractures 264–5, 289–90, 297–8
  fractures 562–5, 609
urinary incontinence 37–8
urinary retention 46
uterine crowding 244, 293, 452, 464–5,
  502, 530

VACTERL, proximal forearm and other
  anomalies 303
Van Nes rotationplasty 209–10, 339, 432
vanillylmandelic acid detection 511
vascular anomalies
  brachial plexus injury surgery 324, 325
  cervical spine 493, 494
  Ehlers-Danlos syndrome 89–91
  elbow fracture 618, 619
  failure theory, in club foot 465
  forearm fracture 627
  growth plate injuries 587–8, 593
  in compound fractures 583–4
  radial dysplasia 303
  tibial fractures 650, 652
vascular perfusion, diagnostic imaging 218
vascular response, to malignant tumour
  192, 193
vasti lateralis muscles 171
vastus medialis advancement 419, 420
venous access 42
ventilatory function disorders 238, 255,
  256, 261
vertebra plana 680
vertebrae
  abnormal density 104, 107
  abscesses 152
  anterior vertebral height, analysis 516
  collapse 100, 156, 168, 188, 680
  compression injuries 671–3
  deformities
    beaked 680, 682
    bullet-shaped 543, 544
    flattened 71
    hemivertebrae 536
    imaging 218

intervertebral fusion 539
  irregular and biconvex 77
  scalloping 541
  segmentation anomalies 256, 536
  wedge-shaped 534, 536
elasticity of 670, 676
injuries, neonatal 602–3
notching 670, 677
posterior height analysis 517
subluxation 677
trauma 506, 544
wedge resection 530, 538
see also cervical spine; discs; spine;
    spondylitis; thoraco-lumbar spine
vincristine chemotherapy 211
viral infection
  discitis 355
  reactive arthritis 354
  synovitis 353, 354, 422
  transmission by factor VIII/IX 114
  see also poliomyelitis
virulence, definition 119
vision see eye
vitamin A excess 105
vitamin C deficiency (scurvy) 105, 107, 588
vitamin D (1,25(OH)U2uD) 94, 95, 101
vitamin D toxicity 105
vitamin-D-deficiency rickets 96, 97–8,
  99–100
vitamin-D-dependent rickets 95, 96, 100
vitamin-D-resistant rickets 98, 100
vitamins, and bone anomalies 105
Volkmann's ischaemic contracture 112
Volkmann's syndrome 616–19, 626, 627
  see also compartment syndrome
Von Recklinghausen's disease
  (neurofibromatosis type NF-1) 519,
  541–2
Von Rosen splint 367

Wagner distraction apparatus 438
walking
  assisted see orthoses
  in clinic 6
  neuromuscular disorders 230–1, 233
  spina bifida 247–9, 250
walking patient, surgery in cerebral palsy
  286–9
walking velocity, and gait 16
'wandering acetabulum' 149
'wandering hip' 371
Wassel classification of thumb duplication
  311–12
wasting 216–17
weakness 216
  cerebral palsy 274
  cervical spine anomalies 492, 494
  gradual 237
website
  Online Mendelian Inheritance in Man

303
  skeletal dysplasias 67
Werdnig-Hoffman disease 216, 225, 231, 232
wheelchairs
  cerebral palsy 33–5
  Duchenne muscular dystrophy 39, 233
  neurological disorders 230–1
  spina bifida 36, 249
whiplash shaken infant syndrome 663
whistling face syndrome (Freeman-Sheldon)
  294, 307, 469
Wiberg centre-edge angle 285
Wiberg III patella 418
Williams' syndrome (idiopathic
  hypercalcemia) 105
Wilms's tumour 511, 546
Wilson oblique metatarsal osteotomy 460–1
Wilson's sign 420–1
windblown hand 301, 307
'windswept' deformity, hip 285
'windswept' legs 31, 34, 35, 77
wire-threaded beads see gentamicin-
  impregnated PMMA beads
work-place injuries, tropical 162, 163, 174
wormian bones 107
Wrisberg meniscus 422
wrist
  arthrodesis 290, 298
  drop 265, 326
  dysplasia epiphysealis hemimelica 86
  flexion deformities 290, 297–8, 315
  injuries 626–31
  radial dysplasia 303–4
  surgery in juvenile idiopathic arthritis 188
wry-neck see torticollis

X-linked (Ehlers-Danlos syndrome type IX)
  90
X-rays 53
  femur 57, 338, 399–400
  limp 350
  Monteggia fractures 624
  non-accidental injury 62, 63
    fracture ageing 62, 63, 605, 606
  parental expectations 6, 61
  phalanges 630
  recurrent equinus 479, 480, 481
  scaphoid fractures 629
  spinal deformity 513–15
    scoliosis 59, 521–2
    spondylolisthesis 548–9
    tuberculosis 155–6
  tibia 339–40, 341, 342
  see also radiographs

Yamshidi needle biopsy 195–7
yaws 169

Zielke's anterior segmental instrumentation
  and fusion 271, 527–8